Oncologic Critical Care

Joseph L. Nates • Kristen J. Price
Editors

Oncologic Critical Care

Volume 1

With 225 Figures and 278 Tables

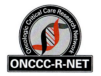

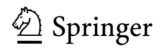

Editors
Joseph L. Nates
Department of Critical Care and
Respiratory Care
The University of Texas MD Anderson
Cancer Center
Houston, TX, USA

Kristen J. Price
Division of Anesthesiology
Critical Care and
Pain Medicine
Department of Critical Care and
Respiratory Care
The University of Texas MD Anderson
Cancer Center
Houston, TX, USA

ISBN 978-3-319-74587-9   ISBN 978-3-319-74588-6 (eBook)
ISBN 978-3-319-74589-3 (print and electronic bundle)
https://doi.org/10.1007/978-3-319-74588-6

This Springer imprint is published by the registered company Springer Nature Switzerland AG.
The registered company address is: Gewerbestrasse 11, 6330 Cham, Switzerland

*We dedicate this book to our families
for their patience and understanding during the long hours of
work away from them
We hope that this pioneering work leads
to improvements in the care of the critically ill cancer patients
around the world*

Preface

The Growing Need for Organized Oncologic Critical Care Services

The world population continues its inexorable growth. Based on the United Nations' latest report on world population, we have reached a population of 7.5 billion people of which 1 billion are over 60 years of age. Currently, there are more than 549 million people over the age of 60 in Asia, practically doubling today's US population. This trend has been named the "silver tsunami" and its social and healthcare impact worldwide is of great concern. As the population rises, so does the number of new cancer cases a year. For the past two decades, cancer has been the second cause of death for all ages in most of the world. In 2012, the World Cancer Research Fund and the American Institute for Cancer Research estimated that there were more than 14 million new cases of cancer and 8.2 million related deaths. In 2018, the age-standardized rate for all cancers was 197.9 per 100,000 habitants. By 2030, the global burden of the disease is expected to reach 21.7 million new cases and 13 million deaths per year.

As the burden of cancer rises, the needs for supportive and critical care healthcare services expand. Unfortunately, multiple factors are at work against a timely and proportionate response from the critical care world. First, the supply and demand for critical care services is growing apart. The timely Committee on Manpower for Pulmonary and Critical Care Societies (COMPACCS) report of the distribution of critical care services in the USA clearly showed clearly this threat. Second, as the currently trained personnel age, they retire and increase the growing deficit. Third, the need for critical care services increases as we get older, ranging from less than 1 specialist per 100,000 habitants at 44 years of age or younger to more than 9 specialists per 100,000 habitants when we reach 84 years of age or older. Fourth, the sharp increase in healthcare costs has overloaded national budgets. The high cost of numerous new technologies, drugs, and the inefficiency of most services are in part to blame. Even the organ-based approach, where among others, all heart, lung, and brain problems are managed by the cardiologist, pulmonologist, and neurologist/neurosurgeon, respectively, contributes to the problem. Unfortunately, there are so many other factors that continue compounding the above challenges that we cannot discuss them all. However, perhaps the greatest of all is that oncologic critical care does not exist as such.

For decades, critically ill onco-hematologic patients have been denied admission to intensive care units around the world with the excuse of poor predicted outcomes. Most critical care organizations have not acknowledged this lack of access, do not have an oncologic section, and allocate minimal space for lectures in their congresses about the specific problems only seen in these populations. Specialty colleges do not recognize this as a subspecialty or dedicate a significant portion of their training to it.

There is an urgent need to develop a robust and organized response from our specialty. This textbook, the first of its class, and our international efforts in education and research are part of this response. As the frontline leaders and pioneers of this new field, namely *Oncologic Critical Care*, I appeal to all of you to join us in the prevention and fight against cancer-related critical illnesses.

Founding President of the   Joseph L. Nates
Oncologic Critical Care Research Network
October 2019

Introduction

Oncologic Critical Care: The Birth of a New Subspecialty

The field of Critical Care has grown rapidly since its beginning in the 1950s. With the increasing proportion of persons above 65 years of age with a 50% overall risk of developing cancer during their lifetimes, cancer rates continue to play a role in the utilization of healthcare services–particularly in the intensive care unit (ICU). This, coupled with a shortage of critical care providers in the next two decades, makes identifying the outcomes of the available oncologic critical care resources imperative.

Currently, no oncologic journals, subspecialty societies in the field, or adequate understanding about the current availability of oncologic/hematologic ICUs exist. Except for our publication in Spanish, no other comprehensive textbooks in oncologic critical care are available. As such, there are major knowledge gaps about outcomes (e.g., ICU utilization, mortality, costs), healthcare disparities (e.g., racial, geographic), and almost all aspects of intensive care delivery to the critically ill cancer patient.

This book, by serving as the first comprehensive source in Oncologic Critical Care, seeks to close these knowledge gaps and serve as a vehicle of education for the current and successive generations of healthcare providers dedicated to the practice of Oncologic Critical Care. The book's target audience encompasses intensivists, medical oncologists, surgical oncologists, general physicians, hospitalists, advance practice providers, nurses, fellows, residents, medical students, and other healthcare providers that take care of cancer patients. This work is a collaborative effort among international experts aimed at specifically focusing on challenges encountered in the diagnosis and management of the critically ill cancer patient population.

This novel resource has 19 parts with over 140 chapters and more than 2,000 pages of care focused on the management of the critically ill cancer patient. It covers all aspects of what we consider a new subspecialty, *Oncologic Critical Care*, that are scarcely covered in standard critical care books. The included chapters explore the following topics in oncologic critical care: organization and management of an oncologic critical care unit, multidisciplinary care and the integration of advance practice providers in this environment, all aspects of clinical pharmacy, and dermatologic complications, and also neurologic, respiratory, cardiovascular, gastrointestinal, genitourinary, renal, and hematological diseases. In addition, we discuss

metabolic/endocrine and vascular complications, transfusion medicine practices, infectious diseases, perioperative care of the critically ill cancer patient,
care of special populations, critical care procedures and their challenges in
coagulopathic patients, ethics, pain management, palliative care, and
outcomes.

Finally, we hope you enjoy and take full advantage of this amazing
resource!

Joseph L. Nates
Kristen J. Price

Acknowledgments

We want to thank Mr. Kian K. Azimpoor and Dr. Andrés F. Laserna for their outstanding and enthusiastic logistical support throughout the planning and execution of this invaluable project.

Contents

Volume 1

Part I Organization and Management of an Oncologic Critical Care Unit **1**

1 **Oncologic Critical Care Department Organization** 3
Kristen J. Price

2 **ICU Utilization** 11
Karen Chen, Susannah K. Wallace, and Joseph L. Nates

3 **Critical Care Admissions and Discharge Criteria in Cancer Patients** 19
Ignacio Pujol Varela and Isidro Prieto del Portillo

4 **ICU Staffing, Models, and Outcomes** 33
Karen Chen and Joseph L. Nates

5 **Multidisciplinary Care of Critically Ill Cancer Patients** 43
Ninotchka Brydges, Brandi McCall, and Tiffany Mundie

6 **Advanced Practice Providers in the Oncologic Intensive Care Unit** 65
Ninotchka Brydges, Tiffany Mundie, and Garry Brydges

7 **Early Warning Systems and Oncological Critical Care Units** 75
Michelle O'Mahony and Tim Wigmore

8 **Rapid Response Team (RRT) in Critical Care** 87
Ninotchka Brydges and Tiffany Mundie

9 **Quality Assurance and Improvement in the Intensive Care Unit** 95
Mary Lou Warren

10 **Patient Risk Prediction Model** 107
Michelle O'Mahony and Tim Wigmore

11 **Outcomes in Critically Ill Oncologic Patients** 121
Silvio A. Ñamendys-Silva

**Part II   Pharmacologic Considerations for the ICU
Cancer Patient** 127

12   **Role of the Clinical Pharmacist in the Oncologic
     Intensive Care Unit** 129
     Brian M. Dee

13   **Stress Ulcer Prophylaxis in the Critically Ill Oncology
     Population** 137
     Reagan D. Collins

14   **Antimicrobial Prophylaxis in High-Risk Oncology
     Patients** 153
     Jeffrey J. Bruno and Frank P. Tverdek

15   **Considerations for Medications Commonly Utilized in
     the Oncology Population in the Intensive Care Unit** 169
     Anne Rain Tanner Brown, Michelle Horng, and Terri Lynn
     Shigle

16   **Complications and Toxicities Associated with Cancer
     Therapies in the Intensive Care Unit** 201
     Melvin J. Rivera, Bryan Do, Jeffrey C. Bryan, Terri Lynn
     Shigle, and Rina Patel

17   **Supportive Care Considerations and Nutrition Support
     for Critically Ill Cancer Patients** 229
     Anne M. Tucker, Jacob W. Hall, Christine A. Mowatt-Larssen,
     and Todd W. Canada

Part III   Dermatologic Complications 247

18   **Graft Versus Host Disease (GHVD) in Critically Ill
     Oncologic Patients** 249
     Ulas Darda Bayraktar

19   **Stevens–Johnson Syndrome (SJS) and Toxic
     Epidermal Necrolysis (TEN)** 267
     Danielle Zimmerman and Nam Hoang Dang

20   **Mycosis Fungoides in Critically Ill Cancer Patients** 281
     Brian H. Ramnaraign and Nam Hoang Dang

Part IV   Neurologic Diseases 297

21   **Delirium and Psychosis in Critically Ill Cancer Patients** ... 299
     Kimberly F. Rengel, Daniel A. Nahrwold, Pratik P.
     Pandharipande, and Christopher G. Hughes

22   **Medication-Induced Neurotoxicity in Critically Ill
     Cancer Patients** 319
     Monica E. Loghin and Anne Kleiman

23 **Seizures and Status Epilepticus in Critically Ill Cancer Patients** 335
Vishank A. Shah and Jose I. Suarez

24 **Posterior Reversible Encephalopathy Syndrome (PRES) in Cancer Patients** 353
Bryan Bonder and Marcos de Lima

25 **Stroke in Critically Ill Cancer Patients** 367
Ritvij Bowry and James C. Grotta

26 **Intracranial Hemorrhage Focused on Cancer and Hemato-oncologic Patients** 381
Yasser Mohamad Khorchid and Marc Malkoff

27 **Increased Intracranial Pressure in Critically Ill Cancer Patients** 395
Abhi Pandhi, Rashi Krishnan, Nitin Goyal, and Marc Malkoff

28 **Leptomeningeal Disease in Solid Cancers** 409
Nazanin K. Majd and Monica E. Loghin

29 **Metastatic Spinal Cord Compression** 429
John W. Crommett

30 **Frequent Central Nervous System (CNS) Infections in the Immunosuppressed Patient** 435
Rafael Araos and Grecia Aldana

Part V   Respiratory Diseases 443

31 **Acute and Chronic Respiratory Failure in Cancer Patients** 445
Steven P. Sears, Gordon Carr, and Christian Bime

32 **Noninvasive Oxygen Therapies in Oncologic Patients** 477
Michael C. Sklar, Bruno L. Ferreyro, and Laveena Munshi

33 **Respiratory Support Strategies and Nonconventional Ventilation Modes in Oncologic Critical Care** 499
Yenny R. Cardenas and Joseph L. Nates

34 **Prone Ventilatory Therapy in Critically Ill Cancer Patients** 509
Alex Pearce and Rebecca E. Sell

35 **Extracorporeal Membrane Oxygenation (ECMO) Critically Ill Cancer Patients** 517
Thomas Staudinger, Peter Schellongowski, and Philipp Wohlfarth

36 **Cancer Treatment-Related Lung Injury** 531
Vickie R. Shannon

**37 Acute Respiratory Distress Syndrome in Cancer
Patients** 557
Alisha Y. Young and Vickie R. Shannon

**38 Diffuse Alveolar Hemorrhage in Critically Ill Cancer
Patients** 583
Brian W. Stephenson, Allen H. Roberts II, and Charles A. Read

**39 Differentiation (Retinoic Acid) Syndrome in Critically Ill
Cancer Patients** 593
Cristina Prata Amendola, Ricardo André Sales Pereira Guedes,
and Luciana Coelho Sanches

40 Pneumonia in the Cancer Patient 607
Ala Eddin S. Sagar and Scott E. Evans

**41 Late Noninfectious Pulmonary Complications in
Hematopoietic Stem Cell Transplantation** 625
Kevin Dsouza, Cameron Pywell, and Victor J. Thannickal

**42 Pleural Disease: Malignant and Benign Pleural
Effusions** 643
María F. Landaeta and Macarena R. Vial

**43 Management of Tracheobronchial Diseases in Critically Ill
Cancer Patients** 653
Donald R. Lazarus and George A. Eapen

44 Tracheostomy 667
Macarena R. Vial and Joseph L. Nates

**45 Pulmonary Hypertension in an Oncologic Intensive
Care Unit** 675
Lilit A. Sargsyan and Saadia A. Faiz

46 Sleep Disorders in Critically Ill Cancer Patients 699
Matthew Scharf, Niki Kasinathan, and Jag Sunderram

Volume 2

Part VI Cardiovascular Diseases **709**

**47 Acute Coronary Syndrome, Thrombocytopenia, and
Antiplatelet Therapy in Critically Ill Cancer Patients** 711
Teodora Donisan, Dinu Valentin Balanescu, Gloria Iliescu,
Konstantinos Marmagkiolis, and Cezar Iliescu

48 Arrhythmias in Cancer Patients 733
Peter Kim, Abdulrazzak Zarifa, Mohammed Salih, and
Kaveh Karimzad

**49 Hemodynamic Evaluation and Echocardiography in the
Oncologic Intensive Care Unit** 753
Raymundo A. Quintana, Nicolas Palaskas, and Jose Banchs

50 Hemodynamic Evaluation and Minimally Invasive Hemodynamic Monitoring in Critically Ill Cancer Patients 775
Phornlert Chatrkaw and Kanya Kumwilaisak

51 Interventional Cardiology in the Cancer Patient 787
Dinu Valentin Balanescu, Teodora Donisan, Konstantinos Marmagkiolis, and Cezar Iliescu

52 Management of Pericardial Effusions/Tamponade in Cancer Patients 807
Sana Shoukat and Syed Wamique Yusuf

53 Chemotherapy-Related Cardiovascular Complications 815
Muzna Hussain and Patrick Collier

54 Outcomes After Cardiopulmonary Resuscitation in the Cancer Patient 837
Cristina Gutierrez

Part VII Gastrointestinal Disease 845

55 Acute Abdomen in Cancer Patients 847
Celia Robinson Ledet and David Santos

56 Gastrointestinal Bleeding in Critically Ill Cancer Patients 857
David M. Richards and William A. Ross

57 Endoscopic and Pharmacologic Management of Upper GI Bleeding 869
David M. Richards, Sajini Thekkel, and William A. Ross

58 Malignant Ascites in Critically Ill Cancer Patients 885
Cristina Prata Amendola, Luís Gustavo Capochin Romagnolo, and Raphael L. C. Araujo

59 Hepatobiliary Diseases in the Cancer Patient Leading to Critical Illness 893
Faisal S. Ali, Hamzah Abu-Sbeih, Emmanuel Coronel, and Yinghong Wang

Part VIII Renal and Genitourinary Disease 919

60 Acute Renal Failure in Critically Ill Cancer Patients 921
Aisha Khattak and Kevin W. Finkel

61 Renal Replacement Therapy in Critically Ill Cancer Patients 937
Kevin W. Finkel and Jaya Kala

62 Hematuria in the Critically Ill Cancer Patients 949
Chukwuma O. Kalu and Ala Abudayyeh

63 **Hemorrhagic Cystitis in the Critically Ill Cancer Patient** ... 959
Chukwuma O. Kalu and Ala Abudayyeh

64 **Obstructive Uropathy in Critically Ill Cancer Patients** 969
Chukwuma O. Kalu and Ala Abudayyeh

Part IX Metabolic/Endocrine Complications **977**

65 **Adrenal Emergencies in Critically Ill Cancer Patients** 979
Ryan P. Richard, Julie A. Grishaw, and Kyle B. Enfield

66 **Carcinoid Crisis in the Intensive Care Unit** 995
Ozge Keskin and Suayib Yalcin

67 **Thyroid Emergencies in Critically Ill Cancer Patients** 1003
Sarimar Agosto and Sonali Thosani

68 **Electrolytic Abnormalities Related to Calcium in
Critically Ill Cancer Patients** 1017
Agamenón Quintero, Jorge Racedo, and Manuel González
Fernández

69 **Electrolytic Abnormalities Related to Phosphate in
Critically Ill Cancer Patients** 1029
Agamenón Quintero, Jorge Racedo, and Roger de Jesús
Durante Flórez

70 **Electrolytic Abnormalities Related to Sodium in
Critically Ill Cancer Patients** 1041
Agamenón Quintero, Jorge Racedo, Carlos Andrés Pérez
Acosta, and Sandra Aruachán

71 **Electrolytic Abnormalities Related to Potassium in
Critically Ill Cancer Patients** 1053
Agamenón Quintero, Jorge Racedo, and Aaron Rafael
Quintero Hernández

72 **Electrolytic Abnormalities Related to Magnesium in
Critically Ill Cancer Patients** 1067
Agamenón Quintero, Jorge Racedo, and Heinznel Negrete

73 **Hypoglycemia and Hyperglycemia in Critically Ill Cancer
Patients** 1079
Seda Hanife Oguz, Ugur Unluturk, Sahin Lacin, Alper Gurlek,
and Suayib Yalcin

Part X Hematologic Diseases **1093**

74 **Benign Hematological Diseases in Cancer Patients** 1095
Kelly N. Casteel and Michael H. Kroll

75 **Thrombotic Thrombocytopenic Purpura and Hemolytic
Uremic Syndrome in Cancer Patients** 1109
Peter J. Miller

76 Tumor Lysis Syndrome in the Cancer Patient 1119
O'Dene Lewis and Stephen M. Pastores

77 Blast Crisis of Chronic Myeloid Leukemia (CML) 1135
Rita Assi and Nicholas Short

78 Hyperleukocytosis in Cancer Patients 1147
Lohith Gowda and Chitra Hosing

**79 Hemophagocytic Lymphohistiocytosis in the Cancer
Patient** 1155
Olakunle Idowu, Jeanneé Campbell, and Naval Daver

Part XI Transfusion Medicine **1163**

80 Statistics in Blood Collection and Transfusion 1165
Fernando Martinez

81 Blood Components 1171
Fernando Martinez and Faysal Fedda

82 Transfusion Reactions 1177
Adriana Maria Knopfelmacher

83 Transfusion-Related Acute Lung Injury (TRALI) 1191
Adriana Maria Knopfelmacher

84 Alternatives to Blood Products 1197
James M. Kelley

**85 Massive Transfusion Protocols (MTPs) in Cancer
Patients** 1205
Adriana Maria Knopfelmacher and Fernando Martinez

86 Guidelines for Blood Transfusion in Patients 1213
Fernando Martinez

Part XII Vascular Complications **1221**

**87 Management of Arterial Bleeding in Critically Ill
Cancer Patients** 1223
T. T. T. Huynh and R. A. Sheth

**88 Prevention and Management of Venous Thromboembolism
in the Cancer Patient** 1243
Sajid A. Haque and Nisha K. Rathi

**89 Superior Vena Cava Syndrome in Critically Ill Cancer
Patients** 1253
Victor J. Matos

**90 Catheter-Related Deep Vein Thrombosis in Critically Ill
Cancer Patients** 1265
Sajid A. Haque and Nisha K. Rathi

Part XIII Infectious Diseases **1273**

91 Infection Prevention in Critical Care Settings 1275
Gabriela Corsi-Vasquez and Luis Ostrosky-Zeichner

**92 Antimicrobial Stewardship in Critically Ill Cancer
Patients** 1287
Kenneth V. I. Rolston and Lior Nesher

93 Neutropenic Fever in the Intensive Care Unit 1297
R. Scott Stephens

94 Sepsis and Septic Shock in Cancer Patients 1313
Imrana Malik and Joseph L. Nates

**95 Management of Multidrug-Resistant
Enterobacteriaceae in Critically Ill Cancer Patients** 1323
Juan David Plata and Ximena Castañeda

96 Fungal Infections in Cancer Patients 1337
Bruno P. Granwehr, Nikolaos V. Sipsas, and Dimitrios P.
Kontoyiannis

97 Viral Infections in Critically Ill Cancer Patients 1361
Gabriela Corsi-Vasquez and Luis Ostrosky-Zeichner

**98 Bacterial and Atypical Infections in Critically Ill
Cancer Patients** 1379
Alejandro De la Hoz and Jorge Alberto Cortés

**99 Catheter- and Device-Related Infections in Critically Ill
Cancer Patients** 1401
Alexandre Malek and Issam Raad

**100 Nosocomial Infections and Ventilator-Associated
Pneumonia in Cancer Patients** 1419
J. V. Divatia, Jacob George Pulinilkunnathil, and Sheila
Nainan Myatra

101 Parasites in Cancer Patients 1441
Juan David Plata and Ximena Castañeda

102 Tropical Diseases in Cancer Patients 1451
Jorge Enrique Sinclair Ávila, Jorge Enrique Sinclair De Frías,
and Felix Liu Wu

**103 Skin and Soft Tissue Infections Among Cancer
Patients** 1465
Ariel D. Szvalb and Kenneth V. I. Rolston

Volume 3

Part XIV   Special Patient Populations 1477

104   Practical Approach to the Critically Ill Obstetric Patient with an Oncological Disease 1479
Sandra Olaya, Paula Velásquez, and Jacobo Bustamante

105   What the Intensivist Needs to Know About Leukemia Patients 1489
Mahesh Swaminathan and Kiran Naqvi

106   What the Intensivists Need to Know About Critically Ill Lymphoma Patients 1499
Ranjit Nair and Krina Patel

107   What the Intensivists Need to Know About Critically Ill Myeloma Patients 1513
Ranjit Nair and Krina Patel

108   What the Intensivist Needs to Know About Hematopoietic Stem Cell Transplantation? 1531
Brion V. Randolph and Stefan O. Ciurea

109   Radiation Therapy Complications Leading to Critical Illness 1547
Shalini Moningi, Geoffrey V. Martin, and Jay P. Reddy

Part XV   Critical Care Procedures 1555

110   Management of Airway in the Cancer Patients 1557
Gang Zheng and Carin A. Hagberg

111   Critical Care Procedures by the Advanced Practice Provider 1571
Ninotchka Brydges, Brandi McCall, and Garry Brydges

112   Point-of-Care Ultrasound for Oncologic Critical Care 1579
Wendell H. Williams, Anna D. Dang, and Dilip R. Thakar

113   Interventional Radiology Procedures in Critically Ill Cancer Patients 1597
Steven M. Yevich

**Part XVI Perioperative Management of the Surgical Cancer
Patient** 1609

114 **Enhanced Recovery After Surgery (ERAS) in the
     Oncologic Patient** 1611
     Joshua Botdorf, Celia Robinson Ledet, Ninotchka Brydges,
     Danilo Lovinaria, and Garry Brydges

115 **Neurosurgery and Post-Surgical Care of the Critically Ill
     Cancer Patients** 1641
     Gilda V. Matute and Thomas M. McHugh

116 **Skull Base and Endoscopic Procedures in Cancer
     Patients** 1653
     Garry Brydges, Ninotchka Brydges, and Charles Cowles

117 **Neurosurgery and Spine Procedures in Cancer Patients** ... 1667
     John Wiemers and Claudio E. Tatsui

118 **Neurosurgery and Pituitary Resection in Cancer
     Patients** 1683
     Nicole Luongo, Peter Slivinski, Adrian M. Smith, and
     Danilo Lovinaria

119 **Anesthesia for Free Flap Reconstruction After Head and
     Neck Surgical Resection** 1693
     Jennifer Jones and Faisal I. Ahmad

120 **Head and Neck Surgery in Oncologic Patients:
     Laryngectomy and Radial Neck Dissection** 1709
     Pamela Amakwe Uzoigwe, Maxie Pollard, and Ursula Uduak
     Williams

121 **Plastic Surgery and Flap Graft Management of Radial
     Forearm, VRAM, and TRAM Flaps in Critically Ill
     Cancer Patients** 1719
     Jason Silva, Amy Jackson, and Justin Broyles

122 **Perioperative Care of the Thoracic Oncologic Patient
     Undergoing EBUS, Thoracotomy, and Pneumonectomy** ... 1727
     Marion W. Bergbauer, Johnny Dang, and George A. Eapen

123 **Thoracic Surgery and Rigid Bronchoscopy** 1741
     Jen Chang and Mona Sarkiss

124 **Thoracic Surgery and Esophagectomy** 1753
     Melissa Morris Puskac and Robert A. Hetz

125 **Tumor Thrombectomy Overview and General Concepts** ... 1765
     Yelena Livshits and Juan E. Marcano

126 **Perioperative Management of the Oncologic Patient
     Undergoing Gastrointestinal Surgery** 1775
     Bobby Bellard, Jasmin Eapen, Suma Joseph, and Maxy
     Mathew

127 Perioperative Management of the Oncologic Patient Undergoing Cytoreductive Surgery with Hyperthermic Intraperitoneal Chemotherapy (HIPEC) 1783
Darline Hurst and Pascal Owusu-Agyemang

128 Care of the Postoperative Patient with Liver Cancer in the Intensive Care Unit 1793
Clint Westaway, Nizy Samuel, and Jean Nicolas Vauthey

129 Pancreatic Surgery in Cancer Patients 1809
Kristine McCarthy, Wei Zhang, Jose Soliz, and Danilo Lovinaria

130 Perioperative Management of the Genitourinary Oncologic Patient Undergoing Partial/Radical Nephrectomy 1825
Clarissa Stapleton, Christina Duffy, and Jonathan Duplisea

131 Total Abdominal Hysterectomy, Bilateral Salpingo-oophorectomy, and Pelvic Lymphadenectomy in Cancer Patients 1837
Ninotchka Brydges, Lesley Boyko, and Javier D. Lasala

132 Orthopedic Surgery and Femoral/Humeral Fracture Repairs 1851
Matthew John Byars and Javier D. Lasala

133 Magnetic Resonance Imaging (MRI) for the Acute Care Oncology Patient 1861
Tamra Kelly and David Ferson

134 Perioperative Management of Breast Cancer Surgery 1869
Ninotchka Brydges, La Sonya D. Malbrough, Danilo Lovinaria, and Joseph R. Ruiz

Part XVII Pain Management 1885

135 Acute Pain in Critical Care Oncologic Patients 1887
Keyuri Popat and Catherine Vu

136 Pathophysiology, Assessment, and Treatment of Chronic Cancer Pain in Critically Ill Patients 1901
Christina Le-Short and Dhanalakshmi Koyyalagunta

137 Substance Withdrawal in ICU Environment 1913
Nuria Martínez and María-Consuelo Pintado

Part XVIII Ethics and Palliative Care 1935

138 Ethical Issues at the End-of-Life in the Cancer Patient 1937
Colleen M. Gallagher, Jessica A. Moore, and Allen H. Roberts II

139 Palliative Care in Critically Ill Cancer Patients 1963
Ali Haider, Ahsan Azhar, and Kevin Madden

Part XIX Pediatric Oncologic Critical Care 1983

140 Oncologic Emergencies in Pediatric Critical Care 1985
José A. Cortes and Rodrigo Mejía

**141 Pain Management of Children with Terminal Cancer
in the Critical Care Unit** 2005
Karen Moody and Veronica Carullo

**142 Delirium in the Pediatric Critical Care Oncologic
Patient** 2021
Sydney Nicole Ariagno and Chani Traube

**143 Chimeric Antigen Receptor (CAR) T-Cell Therapy in
the Pediatric Critical Care** 2035
Sajad Khazal and Kris Mahadeo

Index 2049

About the Editors

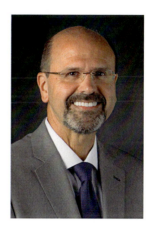

Dr. Joseph L. Nates is a Professor at the University of Texas MD Anderson Cancer Center. He has lived and practiced medicine in several countries. Currently, he is the Deputy Chair of the Department of Critical Care in the Division of Anesthesiology, Critical Care, and Pain Medicine. Dr. Nates is also the Medical Director of the 70-bed Oncologic Surgical and Medical Intensive Care Units and the Founder and President of the Oncologic Critical Care Research Network (ONCCC-R-NET), a global organization dedicated to the advancement of oncologic critical care research and education. Through his organization, Dr. Nates has been leading the pioneering efforts to establish *Oncologic Critical Care* as a new subspecialty and disseminate this knowledge worldwide. As the foundation for this objective, he has led and coauthored the first two comprehensive oncologic critical care textbooks, in both Spanish and English languages. He has also established regional and global collaborative networks and organized several *Oncologic Critical Care* symposiums.

Throughout his career, Dr. Nates has occupied multiple leadership positions and received numerous awards, among them the Presidential Award for "Outstanding Achievement and Leadership for Elimination of Ventilator-Associated Pneumonia" from the Department of Health and Human Services and the four leading Critical Care Societies in the USA in 2012, the "Bill Aston Award for Quality" from the Texas Hospital Association, and Distinguished Service Award in 2015, as well as many other research awards during his career. In 2018, for his contributions to critical care, the American College of

Critical Care Medicine awarded him the title *Master of Critical Care Medicine*. The same year, for his international contributions to the development of *Oncologic Critical Care*, the Chilean Society of Critical Care and Emergency Medicine awarded him the title *International Master of Critical Care Medicine*.

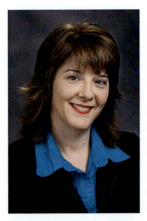

Dr. Kristen J. Price was born and raised in New Orleans, Louisiana. She received her undergraduate degree in Marine Science from the University of Tampa followed by a Doctor of Medicine degree from Louisiana State University Medical Center in New Orleans. She completed an Internal Medicine residency, Chief Medical Residency, and Pulmonary and Critical Care fellowship at the University of Texas Health in Houston. Following training, she joined the faculty at the University of Texas MD Anderson Cancer Center and currently holds the title of Professor and Chair, Department of Critical Care and Respiratory Care. Under her leadership, the number of faculty and advance practice providers has grown substantially. She also oversees the Respiratory Care Department and the Section of Integrated Bioethics in Cancer Care. Dr. Price developed the multifaceted "Intensive Care Unit Organizational Infrastructure" to systematically organize, establish, and sustain evidence-based clinical, educational, and research initiatives in the ICU. Her main focus of research has been in the outcomes of critically ill oncology patients, particularly those with hematologic malignancies and respiratory failure. She is an active member of the Society of Critical Care Medicine and currently serves on the "Academic Leaders in Critical Care Medicine" task force. Dr. Price has four grown children and currently resides in Houston, Texas.

Section Editors

Pharmacologic Considerations for the ICU Cancer Patient
Jeffrey J. Bruno The University of Texas MD Anderson Cancer Center, Houston, TX, USA

Todd W. Canada Critical Care/Nutrition Support, The University of Texas MD Anderson Cancer Center, Houston, TX, USA

Neurologic Diseases
Yenny R. Cardenas Critical Care Department, Universidad del Rosario Hospital Universitario Fundacion Santa Fe de Bogota, Bogota, Colombia

Respiratory Diseases
Yenny R. Cardenas Critical Care Department, Universidad del Rosario Hospital Universitario Fundacion Santa Fe de Bogota, Bogota, Colombia

Critical Care Procedures
Garry Brydges Anesthesiology – CRNA Support, The University of Texas MD Anderson Cancer Center, Houston, TX, USA

Division of Anesthesia, Critical Care and Pain Medicine, Department of Anesthesiology, The University of Texas MD Anderson Cancer Center, Houston, TX, USA

Ninotchka Brydges Department of Critical Care and Respiratory Care, The University of Texas MD Anderson Cancer Center, Houston, TX, USA

Perioperative Management of the Surgical Cancer Patient
Garry Brydges Anesthesiology – CRNA Support, The University of Texas MD Anderson Cancer Center, Houston, TX, USA

Division of Anesthesia, Critical Care and Pain Medicine, Department of Anesthesiology, The University of Texas MD Anderson Cancer Center, Houston, TX, USA

Pediatric Oncologic Critical Care
Rodrigo Mejía MD Anderson Cancer Center, Houston, TX, USA

Contributors

Ala Abudayyeh Division of Internal Medicine, Section of Nephrology, The University of Texas MD Anderson Cancer Center, Houston, TX, USA

Hamzah Abu-Sbeih The Department of Gastroenterology, Hepatology and Nutrition, The University of Texas MD Anderson Cancer Center, Houston, TX, USA

Sarimar Agosto Department of Endocrinology, University Health System and University of Texas Health San Antonio, San Antonio, TX, USA

Faisal I. Ahmad Department of Head and Neck Surgery, The University of Texas MD Anderson Cancer Center, Houston, TX, USA

Grecia Aldana Department of Pulmonary Medicine, The University of Texas MD Anderson Cancer Center, Houston, TX, USA

Faisal S. Ali The Department of Gastroenterology, Hepatology and Nutrition, The University of Texas MD Anderson Cancer Center, Houston, TX, USA

Rafael Araos Genomics and Resistant Microbes (GeRM) Lab, Facultad de Medicina Clínica Alemana Universidad del Desarrollo,Millennium Nucleus for Collaborative Research on Bacterial Resistance (MICROB-R), Santiago, Chile

Raphael L. C. Araujo Fundação Pio XII – Hospital de Câncer de Barretos, Barretos, São Paulo, Brazil

Sydney Nicole Ariagno Weill Cornell Medicine, New York, NY, USA

Sandra Aruachán Department of Clinical Research, Instituto Médico de Alta Tecnología IMAT Oncomedica, Montería, Colombia

Rita Assi Department of Leukemia, The University of Texas MD Anderson Cancer Center, Houston, TX, USA

Lebanese American University Medical Center-Rizk Hospital, Beirut, Lebanon

Ahsan Azhar Department of Palliative Care, Rehabilitation and Integrative Medicine, The University of Texas MD Anderson Cancer Center, Houston, TX, USA

Dinu Valentin Balanescu Department of Cardiology, The University of Texas MD Anderson Cancer Center, Houston, TX, USA

Jose Banchs Department of Cardiology, Division of Internal Medicine, The University of Texas MD Anderson Cancer Center, Houston, TX, USA

Ulas Darda Bayraktar Division of Hematology and Oncology, Aras Medical Center, Ankara, Turkey

Bobby Bellard Department of Anesthesiology and Perioperative Medicine, Division of Anesthesiology and Critical Care, The University of Texas MD Anderson Cancer Center, Houston, TX, USA

Marion W. Bergbauer Department of Anesthesiology and Perioperative Medicine, The University of Texas M.D. Anderson Cancer Center, Houston, TX, USA

Christian Bime University of Arizona School of Medicine and Banner-University Medical Center – Tucson, Tucson, AZ, USA

Bryan Bonder Division of Hematology and Oncology, University Hospitals Cleveland Medical Center, Cleveland, OH, USA

Joshua Botdorf Department of Critical Care and Respiratory Care, Division of Anesthesia, Critical Care and Pain Medicine, The University of Texas MD Anderson Cancer Center, Houston, TX, USA

Ritvij Bowry Department of Neurosurgery, Division of Neurocritical care, McGovern Medical School, University of Texas Health Science Center, Houston, TX, USA

Lesley Boyko Division of Anesthesia, Critical Care and Pain Medicine, The University of Texas MD Anderson Cancer Center, Houston, TX, USA

Anne Rain Tanner Brown Critical Care/Nutrition Support, The University of Texas MD Anderson Cancer Center, Houston, TX, USA

Justin Broyles The University of Texas MD Anderson Cancer Center, Houston, TX, USA

Jeffrey J. Bruno The University of Texas MD Anderson Cancer Center, Houston, TX, USA

Jeffrey C. Bryan Leukemia, The University of Texas MD Anderson Cancer Center, Houston, TX, USA

Ninotchka Brydges Department of Critical Care and Respiratory Care, The University of Texas MD Anderson Cancer Center, Houston, TX, USA

Garry Brydges Anesthesiology – CRNA Support, The University of Texas MD Anderson Cancer Center, Houston, TX, USA

Division of Anesthesia, Critical Care and Pain Medicine, Department of Anesthesiology, The University of Texas MD Anderson Cancer Center, Houston, TX, USA

Ninotchka Brydges Division of Anesthesia, Critical Care and Pain Medicine, Department of Critical Care and Respiratory Care, The University of Texas MD Anderson Cancer Center, Houston, TX, USA

Jacobo Bustamante Universidad Tecnológica de Pereira y Hospital Universitario San Jorge (HUSJ), Pereira, Colombia

Matthew John Byars Department of Anesthesiology, Critical Care and Pain Medicine, UTMD Anderson Cancer Center, Houston, TX, USA

Jeanneé Campbell Department of Critical Care, Division of Anesthesiology and Critical Care, The University of Texas MD Anderson Cancer Center, Houston, TX, USA

Todd W. Canada Critical Care/Nutrition Support, The University of Texas MD Anderson Cancer Center, Houston, TX, USA

Yenny R. Cardenas Critical Care Department, Universidad del Rosario Hospital Universitario Fundacion Santa Fe de Bogota, Bogota, Colombia

Gordon Carr Banner-University Medical Center Tucson, Tucson, AZ, USA

Veronica Carullo Departments of Anesthesiology and Pediatrics, Weill Cornell Medical Center, New York, NY, USA

Ximena Castañeda Los Cobos Medical Center, Bogotá, Colombia

Kelly N. Casteel UT MD Anderson Cancer Center, Houston, TX, USA

Jen Chang Department of Anesthesiology and Perioperative Medicine, The University of Texas MD Anderson Cancer Center, Houston, TX, USA

Phornlert Chatrkaw Department of Anesthesiology, Faculty of Medicine, Chulalongkorn University, Pathumwan, Bangkok, Thailand

Karen Chen Department of Critical Care and Respiratory Care, The University of Texas MD Anderson Cancer Center, Houston, TX, USA

Stefan O. Ciurea The University of Texas MD Anderson Cancer Center, Houston, TX, USA

Patrick Collier Robert and Suzanne Tomsich Department of Cardiovascular Medicine, Sydell and Arnold Miller Family Heart and Vascular Institute, The Cleveland Clinic Foundation, Cleveland, OH, USA

Case Western Reserve University, Lerner College of Medicine, Cleveland, OH, USA

Reagan D. Collins Critical Care/Nutrition Support, Division of Pharmacy, The University of Texas MD Anderson Cancer Center, Houston, TX, USA

Emmanuel Coronel The Department of Gastroenterology, Hepatology and Nutrition, The University of Texas MD Anderson Cancer Center, Houston, TX, USA

Gabriela Corsi-Vasquez McGovern Medical School, University of Texas at Houston, Houston, TX, USA

Jorge Alberto Cortés Department of Internal Medicine, National University of Colombia, Bogota, DC, Colombia

José A. Cortes MD Anderson Cancer Center, Houston, TX, USA

Charles Cowles Division of Anesthesia, Critical Care and Pain Medicine, Department of Anesthesiology, The University of Texas MD Anderson Cancer Center, Houston, TX, USA

John W. Crommett Department of Critical Care Medicine, The University of Texas M.D. Anderson Cancer Center, Houston, TX, USA

Anna D. Dang University of Texas Health Science Center at Houston, Houston, TX, USA

Johnny Dang Department of Anesthesiology and Perioperative Medicine, The University of Texas M.D. Anderson Cancer Center, Houston, TX, USA

Nam Hoang Dang University of Florida Health Cancer Center, Gainesville, FL, USA

Naval Daver Department of Leukemia, Division of Cancer Medicine, The University of Texas MD Anderson Cancer Center, Houston, TX, USA

Alejandro De la Hoz Grupo de Investigación en Enfermedades Infecciosas, Hospital Universitario San Ignacio, Bogotá, Distrito Capital, Colombia
School of Medicine, Pontificia Universidad Javeriana, Bogotá, DC, Colombia

Marcos de Lima Stem Cell Transplant Program, Seidman Cancer Center, University Hospitals Cleveland Medical Center, and Case Western Reserve University, Cleveland, OH, USA

Brian M. Dee The University of Texas MD Anderson Cancer Center, Houston, TX, USA

Isidro Prieto del Portillo Department of Critical Care, Hospital MD Anderson Cancer Center, Madrid, Spain

J. V. Divatia Department of Anaesthesia, Critical Care and Pain, Tata Memorial Hospital, Homi Bhabha National Institute, Mumbai, India

Bryan Do Lymphoma and Myeloma, The University of Texas MD Anderson Cancer Center, Houston, TX, USA

Teodora Donisan Department of Cardiology, The University of Texas MD Anderson Cancer Center, Houston, TX, USA

Kevin Dsouza Division of Pulmonary, Allergy and Critical Care Medicine, Department of Medicine, University of Alabama at Birmingham, Birmingham, AL, USA

Christina Duffy Department of Anesthesiology, Division of Anesthesia, Critical Care and Pain Medicine, The University of Texas MD Anderson Cancer Center, Houston, TX, USA

Jonathan Duplisea Department of Urology, Division of Anesthesia, Critical Care and Pain Medicine, The University of Texas MD Anderson Cancer Center, Houston, TX, USA

Roger de Jesús Durante Flórez Department of Critical Care Medicine, Instituto Médico de Alta Tecnología IMAT Oncomedica, Montería, Colombia

George A. Eapen Department of Pulmonary Medicine, Division of Internal Medicine, The University of Texas MD Anderson Cancer Center, Houston, TX, USA

Jasmin Eapen Department of Anesthesiology and Perioperative Medicine, Division of Anesthesiology and Critical Care, The University of Texas MD Anderson Cancer Center, Houston, TX, USA

Kyle B. Enfield Division of Critical Care and Pulmonary Medicine, Department of Medicine, University of Virginia, Charlottesville, VA, USA

Scott E. Evans Department of Pulmonary Medicine, Division of Internal Medicine, The University of Texas MD Anderson Cancer Center, Houston, TX, USA

Saadia A. Faiz Department of Pulmonary Medicine, Division of Internal Medicine, The University of Texas MD Anderson Cancer Center, Houston, TX, USA

Faysal Fedda Department of Laboratory Medicine, The University of Texas MD Anderson Cancer Center, Houston, TX, USA

Manuel González Fernández Department of Hematology and Oncology, Instituto Médico de Alta Tecnología IMAT Oncomedica, Montería, Colombia

Bruno L. Ferreyro Interdepartmental Division of Critical Care Medicine, Mount Sinai Hospital, Sinai Health System, University of Toronto, Toronto, ON, Canada

David Ferson Department of Anesthesiology and Perioperative Medicine, UT MD Anderson Cancer Center, Houston, TX, USA

Kevin W. Finkel Division of Renal Diseases and Hypertension, University of Texas Health Science Center at Houston, Houston, TX, USA

Department of Medicine, Division of Renal Diseases and Hypertension, UTHealth Science Center at Houston–McGovern Medical School, Houston, TX, USA

Colleen M. Gallagher Section of Integrated Ethics in Cancer Care, The University of Texas MD Anderson Cancer Center, Houston, TX, USA

Lohith Gowda Division of Hematologic Malignancy and Stem Cell Transplant, Yale School of Medicine, New Haven, CT, USA

Nitin Goyal Department of Neurology, University of Tennessee Health Science Center, Memphis, TN, USA

Bruno P. Granwehr Department of Infectious Diseases, Infection Control and Employee Health, The University of Texas MD Anderson Cancer Center, Houston, TX, USA

Julie A. Grishaw University of Virginia, Charlottesville, VA, USA

James C. Grotta Clinical Innovation and Research Institute, Memorial Hermann Hospital, Houston, TX, USA

Ricardo André Sales Pereira Guedes Fundação Pio XII – Hospital de Câncer de Barretos, Barretos, São Paulo, Brazil

Alper Gurlek Department of Internal Medicine, Division of Endocrinology and Metabolism, Hacettepe University School of Medicine, Ankara, Turkey

Luís Gustavo Capochin Romagnolo Fundação Pio XII – Hospital de Câncer de Barretos, Barretos, São Paulo, Brazil

Cristina Gutierrez Division of Anesthesia and Critical Care, Critical Care and Respiratory Care Department, The University of Texas MD Anderson Cancer Center, Houston, TX, USA

Carin A. Hagberg Department of Anesthesiology and Perioperative Medicine, The University of Texas MD Anderson Cancer Center, Houston, TX, USA

Ali Haider Department of Palliative Care, Rehabilitation and Integrative Medicine, The University of Texas MD Anderson Cancer Center, Houston, TX, USA

Jacob W. Hall Critical Care/Nutrition Support, The University of Texas MD Anderson Cancer Center, Houston, TX, USA

Sajid A. Haque Department of Critical Care, The University of Texas MD Anderson Cancer Center, Houston, TX, USA

Robert A. Hetz Department of Thoracic and Cardiovascular Surgery, The University of Texas M.D. Anderson Cancer Center, Houston, TX, USA

Michelle Horng Critical Care/Nutrition Support, The University of Texas MD Anderson Cancer Center, Houston, TX, USA

Chitra Hosing Department of Stem Cell Transplantation and Cellular Therapy, The University of Texas MD Anderson Cancer Center, Houston, TX, USA

Christopher G. Hughes Department of Anesthesiology, Division of Anesthesiology Critical Care Medicine, Vanderbilt University Medical Center, Nashville, TN, USA

Darline Hurst Department of Anesthesiology and Perioperative Medicine, The University of Texas MD Anderson Cancer Center, Houston, TX, USA

Muzna Hussain Robert and Suzanne Tomsich Department of Cardiovascular Medicine, Sydell and Arnold Miller Family Heart and Vascular Institute, The Cleveland Clinic Foundation, Cleveland, OH, USA

T. T. T. Huynh Department of Thoracic and Cardiovascular Surgery, The University of Texas MD Anderson Cancer Center, Houston, TX, USA

Department of Interventional Radiology, The University of Texas MD Anderson Cancer Center, Houston, TX, USA

Olakunle Idowu Department of Critical Care, Division of Anesthesiology and Critical Care, The University of Texas MD Anderson Cancer Center, Houston, TX, USA

Cezar Iliescu Department of Cardiology, The University of Texas MD Anderson Cancer Center, Houston, TX, USA

Gloria Iliescu Department of General Internal Medicine, The University of Texas MD Anderson Cancer Center, Houston, TX, USA

Amy Jackson The University of Texas MD Anderson Cancer Center, Houston, TX, USA

Jennifer Jones Division of Anesthesiology, Critical Care and Pain Medicine, The University of Texas MD Anderson Cancer Center, Houston, TX, USA

Suma Joseph Department of Anesthesiology and Perioperative Medicine, Division of Anesthesiology and Critical Care, The University of Texas MD Anderson Cancer Center, Houston, TX, USA

Jaya Kala Division of Renal Diseases and Hypertension, UTHealth Science Center at Houston, Houston, TX, USA

Chukwuma O. Kalu UTHealth and MD Anderson Cancer Center, Houston, TX, USA

Kaveh Karimzad Department of Cardiology, Division of Internal Medicine, The University of Texas MD Anderson Cancer Center, Houston, TX, USA

Niki Kasinathan Department of Medicine, Division of Pulmonary and Critical Care, Rutgers-Robert Wood Johnson Medical School, New Brunswick, NJ, USA

James M. Kelley Department of Laboratory Medicine, The University of Texas MD Anderson Cancer Center, Houston, TX, USA

Tamra Kelly Department of Anesthesiology and Perioperative Medicine, UT MD Anderson Cancer Center, Houston, TX, USA

Ozge Keskin Department of Medical Oncology, Selçuk University, Konya, Turkey

Aisha Khattak Division of Renal Diseases and Hypertension, University of Texas Health Science Center at Houston, Houston, TX, USA

Sajad Khazal Department of Pediatrics, Pediatric Stem Cell Transplantation and Cellular Therapy, The University of Texas MD Anderson Cancer Center, Houston, TX, USA

Yasser Mohamad Khorchid Department of Neurology, University of Tennessee Health Science Center, Memphis, TN, USA

Peter Kim Department of Cardiology, Division of Internal Medicine, The University of Texas MD Anderson Cancer Center, Houston, TX, USA

Anne Kleiman Department of Neuro-Oncology, The University of Texas MD Anderson Cancer Center, Houston, TX, USA

Adriana Maria Knopfelmacher Department of Laboratory Medicine, The University of Texas MD Anderson Cancer Center, Houston, TX, USA

Dimitrios P. Kontoyiannis Department of Infectious Diseases, Infection Control and Employee Health, The University of Texas MD Anderson Cancer Center, Houston, TX, USA

Dhanalakshmi Koyyalagunta The University of Texas MD Anderson Cancer Center, Houston, TX, USA

Rashi Krishnan Department of Neurology, University of Tennessee Health Science Center, Memphis, TN, USA

Michael H. Kroll UT MD Anderson Cancer Center, Houston, TX, USA

Kanya Kumwilaisak Department of Anesthesiology, Faculty of Medicine, Chulalongkorn University, Pathumwan, Bangkok, Thailand

Sahin Lacin Department of Medical Oncology, Hacettepe University Institute of Cancer, Ankara, Turkey

María F. Landaeta Lincoln Medical and Mental Health Center, New York, NY, USA

Javier D. Lasala Department of Anesthesiology and Perioperative Medicine, The University of Texas MD Anderson Cancer Center, Houston, TX, USA

Department of Anesthesiology, Critical Care and Pain Medicine, UTMD Anderson Cancer Center, Houston, TX, USA

Donald R. Lazarus Baylor College of Medicine, Houston, TX, USA

Celia Robinson Ledet Department of Surgical Oncology, The University of Texas, MD Anderson Cancer Center, Houston, TX, USA

Christina Le-Short Pain Medicine, John Mendelsohn Faculty Center (FC13.3016), Houston, TX, USA

O'Dene Lewis Critical Care Medicine Fellow, Department of Anesthesiology and Critical Care Medicine, Memorial Sloan Kettering Cancer Center, New York, NY, USA

Felix Liu Wu University of Panama, Panama City, Panama

Yelena Livshits Department of Anesthesiology, Critical Care and Pain Medicine, The University of Texas MD Anderson Cancer Center, Houston, TX, USA

Monica E. Loghin Department of Neuro-Oncology, The University of Texas MD Anderson Cancer Center, Houston, TX, USA

Danilo Lovinaria University of Minnesota Nurse Anesthesia Program, Minneapolis, MN, USA

Nicole Luongo Department of Anesthesiology and Perioperative Services, The University of Texas MD Anderson Cancer Center, Houston, TX, USA

Kevin Madden Department of Palliative Care, Rehabilitation and Integrative Medicine, The University of Texas MD Anderson Cancer Center, Houston, TX, USA

Kris Mahadeo Department of Pediatrics, Pediatric Stem Cell Transplantation and Cellular Therapy, The University of Texas MD Anderson Cancer Center, Houston, TX, USA

Nazanin K. Majd Department of Neuro-Oncology, The University of Texas MD Anderson Cancer Center, Houston, TX, USA

La Sonya D. Malbrough Department of Anesthesiology and Perioperative Medicine, The University of Texas M.D. Anderson Cancer Center, Houston, TX, USA

Alexandre Malek Department of Infectious Diseases, Infection Control and Employee Health, The University of Texas MD Anderson Cancer Center, Houston, TX, USA

Imrana Malik Department of Critical Care, The University of Texas MD Anderson Cancer Center, Houston, TX, USA

Marc Malkoff Department of Neurology, University of Tennessee Health Science Center, Memphis, TN, USA

Juan E. Marcano Department of Surgery, Division of Cardiothoracic Surgery, Baylor College of Medicine, Houston, TX, USA

Konstantinos Marmagkiolis Florida Hospital Pepin Heart Institute, Tampa, FL, USA

Nuria Martínez Intensive Care Unit, Hospital MD Anderson Cancer Center, Madrid, Spain

Geoffrey V. Martin Department of Radiation Oncology, UT MD Anderson Cancer Center, Houston, TX, USA

Fernando Martinez Department of Laboratory Medicine, The University of Texas MD Anderson Cancer Center, Houston, TX, USA

Maxy Mathew Department of Anesthesiology and Perioperative Medicine, Division of Anesthesiology and Critical Care, The University of Texas MD Anderson Cancer Center, Houston, TX, USA

Victor J. Matos National Institute of Cancer, Santo Domingo, Dominican Republic

Gilda V. Matute Department of Anesthesiology and Perioperative Services, The University of Texas MD Anderson Cancer Center, Houston, TX, USA

Brandi McCall Department of Critical Care and Respiratory Care, The University of Texas MD Anderson Cancer Center, Houston, TX, USA

Kristine McCarthy The University of Texas MD Anderson Cancer Center, Houston, TX, USA

Thomas M. McHugh Department of Anesthesiology and Perioperative Medicine, Division of Anesthesiology and Critical Care, The University of Texas MD Anderson Cancer Center, Houston, TX, USA

Rodrigo Mejía MD Anderson Cancer Center, Houston, TX, USA

Peter J. Miller Department of Internal Medicine – Section on Pulmonary, Critical Care, Allergy and Immunologic Diseases, Section on Hematology and Oncology, Department of Anesthesiology – Section on Critical Care Medicine, Wake Forest University School of Medicine, Winston-Salem, NC, USA

Shalini Moningi Department of Radiation Oncology, UT MD Anderson Cancer Center, Houston, TX, USA

Karen Moody Department of Pediatrics, The University of Texas M.D. Anderson Cancer Center, Houston, TX, USA

Jessica A. Moore Section of Integrated Ethics in Cancer Care, The University of Texas MD Anderson Cancer Center, Houston, TX, USA

Christine A. Mowatt-Larssen Critical Care/Nutrition Support, The University of Texas MD Anderson Cancer Center, Houston, TX, USA

Tiffany Mundie Department of Critical Care and Respiratory Care, The University of Texas MD Anderson Cancer Center, Houston, TX, USA

Laveena Munshi Interdepartmental Division of Critical Care Medicine, Mount Sinai Hospital, Sinai Health System, University of Toronto, Toronto, ON, Canada

Sheila Nainan Myatra Department of Anaesthesia, Critical Care and Pain, Tata Memorial Hospital, Homi Bhabha National Institute, Mumbai, India

Daniel A. Nahrwold Department of Anesthesiology, Moffitt Cancer Center, Tampa, FL, USA

Department of Oncologic Sciences, University of South Florida, Morsani College of Medicine, Tampa, FL, USA

Ranjit Nair Department of Lymphoma and Myeloma, Division of Cancer Medicine, The University of Texas MD Anderson Cancer Center, Houston, TX, USA

Silvio A. Ñamendys-Silva Department of Critical Care Medicine, Medica Sur Clinic and Foundation, Mexico City, Mexico

Department of Critical Care Medicine, Instituto Nacional de Cancerología, Mexico City, Mexico

Department of Critical Care Medicine, Instituto Nacional de Ciencias Médicas y Nutrición Salvador Zubirán, Mexico City, Mexico

Kiran Naqvi Leukemia, The University of Texas MD Anderson Cancer Center, Houston, TX, USA

Joseph L. Nates Department of Critical Care and Respiratory Care, The University of Texas MD Anderson Cancer Center, Houston, TX, USA

Heinznel Negrete Department of Critical Care Medicine, Instituto Médico de Alta Tecnología IMAT Oncomedica, Montería, Colombia

Lior Nesher Infectious Disease Institute, Soroka Medical Center, Ben-Gurion University of the Negev, Beer-Sheba, Israel

Michelle O'Mahony Department of Anaesthesia, Critical Care and Pain Medicine, Royal Marsden Hospital, London, UK

Seda Hanife Oguz Department of Internal Medicine, Division of Endocrinology and Metabolism, Hacettepe University School of Medicine, Ankara, Turkey

Sandra Olaya Universidad Tecnológica de Pereira y Hospital Universitario San Jorge (HUSJ), Pereira, Colombia

Luis Ostrosky-Zeichner Infectious Diseases, The University of Texas Health Science Center at Houston, Houston, TX, USA

Pascal Owusu-Agyemang Department of Critical Care, The University of Texas MD Anderson Cancer Center, Houston, TX, USA

Nicolas Palaskas Department of Cardiology, Division of Internal Medicine, The University of Texas MD Anderson Cancer Center, Houston, TX, USA

Pratik P. Pandharipande Department of Anesthesiology and Surgery, Division of Anesthesiology Critical Care Medicine, Vanderbilt University Medical Center, Nashville, TN, USA

Abhi Pandhi Department of Neurology, University of Tennessee Health Science Center, Memphis, TN, USA

Stephen M. Pastores Department of Anesthesiology and Critical Care Medicine, Memorial Sloan Kettering Cancer Center, New York, NY, USA
Weill Cornell Medical College, New York, NY, USA

Krina Patel Department of Lymphoma and Myeloma, Division of Cancer Medicine, The University of Texas MD Anderson Cancer Center, Houston, TX, USA

Rina Patel Critical Care / Nutrition Support, The University of Texas MD Anderson Cancer Center, Houston, TX, USA

Alex Pearce Department of Internal Medicine, University of California San Diego, La Jolla, San Diego, CA, USA

Carlos Andrés Pérez Acosta Department of Critical Care Medicine, Instituto Médico de Alta Tecnología IMAT Oncomedica, Montería, Colombia

María-Consuelo Pintado Intensive Care Unit, Hospital MD Anderson Cancer Center, Madrid, Spain

Juan David Plata School of Medicine and Health Sciences, MeDeri University Hospital, Bogotá, Colombia
Rosario University, Bogotá, Colombia

Maxie Pollard UT MD Anderson Cancer Center, Houston, TX, USA

Keyuri Popat The University of Texas MD Anderson Cancer Center, Houston, TX, USA

Cristina Prata Amendola Fundação Pio XII – Hospital de Câncer de Barretos, Barretos, São Paulo, Brazil

Kristen J. Price Division of Anesthesiology, Critical Care and Pain Medicine, Department of Critical Care and Respiratory Care, The University of Texas MD Anderson Cancer Center, Houston, TX, USA

Ignacio Pujol Varela Department of Critical Care, Hospital MD Anderson Cancer Center, Madrid, Spain

Jacob George Pulinilkunnathil Department of Anaesthesia, Critical Care and Pain, Tata Memorial Hospital, Homi Bhabha National Institute, Mumbai, India

Melissa Morris Puskac Department of Anesthesiology and Perioperative Medicine, The University of Texas M.D. Anderson Cancer Center, Houston, TX, USA

Cameron Pywell Department of Medicine, University of Alabama at Birmingham, Birmingham, AL, USA

Raymundo A. Quintana Division of Cardiology, Department of Medicine, Emory University School of Medicine, Atlanta, GA, USA

Agamenón Quintero Department of Critical Care Medicine, Instituto Médico de Alta Tecnología IMAT Oncomedica, Montería, Colombia

Aaron Rafael Quintero Hernández Department of Critical Care Medicine, Instituto Médico de Alta Tecnología IMAT Oncomedica, Montería, Colombia
School of Medicine, Universidad del Sinú, Montería, Colombia

Issam Raad Department of Infectious Diseases, Infection Control and Employee Health, The University of Texas MD Anderson Cancer Center, Houston, TX, USA

Jorge Racedo Department of Critical Care Medicine, Instituto Médico de Alta Tecnología IMAT Oncomedica, Montería, Colombia

Brian H. Ramnaraign University of Florida Health Cancer Center, Gainesville, FL, USA

Brion V. Randolph Hematology/Oncology, Medical University of South Carolina, Charleston, SC, USA

Nisha K. Rathi Department of Critical Care, The University of Texas MD Anderson Cancer Center, Houston, TX, USA

Charles A. Read Division of Pulmonary, Critical Care, and Sleep Medicine, Department of Medicine, MedStar Georgetown University Hospital, Washington, DC, USA

Jay P. Reddy The University of Texas MD Anderson Cancer Center, Houston, TX, USA

Kimberly F. Rengel Department of Anesthesiology, Division of Anesthesiology Critical Care Medicine, Vanderbilt University Medical Center, Nashville, TN, USA

Ryan P. Richard University of Virginia, Charlottesville, VA, USA

David M. Richards Department of Gastroenterology, Hepatology & Nutrition, Division of Internal Medicine, The University of Texas MD Anderson Cancer Center, Houston, TX, USA

Melvin J. Rivera Thoracic / Head and Neck Medicine, The University of Texas MD Anderson Cancer Center, Houston, TX, USA

Allen H. Roberts II Division of Pulmonary, Critical Care, and Sleep Medicine, Department of Medicine, MedStar Georgetown University Hospital, Washington, DC, USA

Kenneth V. I. Rolston Department of Infectious Diseases, Infection Control and Employee Health, The University of Texas MD Anderson Cancer Center, Houston, TX, USA

William A. Ross Department of Gastroenterology, Hepatology & Nutrition, Division of Internal Medicine, The University of Texas MD Anderson Cancer Center, Houston, TX, USA

Joseph R. Ruiz Department of Anesthesiology and Perioperative Medicine, The University of Texas M.D. Anderson Cancer Center, Houston, TX, USA

Ala Eddin S. Sagar Department of Pulmonary Medicine, Division of Internal Medicine, The University of Texas MD Anderson Cancer Center, Houston, TX, USA

Mohammed Salih Department of Cardiology, Division of Internal Medicine, The University of Texas MD Anderson Cancer Center, Houston, TX, USA

Nizy Samuel Department of Anesthesiology, Critical Care and Pain Medicine, The University of Texas MD Anderson Cancer Center, Houston, TX, USA

Luciana Coelho Sanches Fundação Pio XII – Hospital de Câncer de Barretos, Barretos, São Paulo, Brazil

David Santos Department of Surgical Oncology, The University of Texas MD Anderson Cancer Center, Houston, TX, USA

Lilit A. Sargsyan Divisions of Critical Care, Pulmonary, and Sleep Medicine, Department of Internal Medicine, McGovern Medical School at The University of Texas Health Science Center at Houston, Houston, TX, USA

Mona Sarkiss Department of Anesthesiology and Perioperative Medicine, Department of Pulmonary Medicine, The University of Texas MD Anderson Cancer Center, Houston, TX, USA

Matthew Scharf Department of Medicine, Division of Pulmonary and Critical Care, Rutgers-Robert Wood Johnson Medical School, New Brunswick, NJ, USA

Department of Neurology, Rutgers-Robert Wood Johnson Medical School, New Brunswick, NJ, USA

Peter Schellongowski Department of Medicine I, Intensive Care Unit, Medical University of Vienna, Vienna General Hospital, Vienna, Austria

Steven P. Sears Pulmonary and Critical Care Medicine, University of Arizona, Tucson, AZ, USA

Rebecca E. Sell Department of Internal Medicine, University of California San Diego, La Jolla, San Diego, CA, USA

Division of Pulmonary and Critical Care, University of California San Diego, San Diego, CA, USA

Vishank A. Shah Stroke and Neurocritical Care, Department of Neurology, University of Arkansas for Medical Sciences College of Medicine, Little Rock, AR, USA

Vickie R. Shannon Department of Pulmonary Medicine, Division of Internal Medicine, The University of Texas at MD Anderson Cancer Center, Houston, TX, USA

R. A. Sheth Department of Interventional Radiology, The University of Texas MD Anderson Cancer Center, Houston, TX, USA

Terri Lynn Shigle Oncology, The University of Texas MD Anderson Cancer Center, Houston, TX, USA

Stem Cell Transplantation and Cellular Therapy, The University of Texas MD Anderson Cancer Center, Houston, TX, USA

Nicholas Short Department of Leukemia, The University of Texas MD Anderson Cancer Center, Houston, TX, USA

Sana Shoukat Department of Cardiology, The University of Texas MD Anderson Cancer Center, Houston, TX, USA

Jason Silva The University of Texas MD Anderson Cancer Center, Houston, TX, USA

Jorge Enrique Sinclair Ávila University of Panama, Panama City, Panama

Jorge Enrique Sinclair De Frías University of Panama, Panama City, Panama

Nikolaos V. Sipsas Athens Laikon General Hospital and Medical School, National and Kapodistrian University of Athens, Athens, Greece

Michael C. Sklar Interdepartmental Division of Critical Care Medicine, Mount Sinai Hospital, Sinai Health System, University of Toronto, Toronto, ON, Canada

Peter Slivinski Department of Anesthesiology and Perioperative Services, The University of Texas MD Anderson Cancer Center, Houston, TX, USA

Adrian M. Smith Department of Neurosurgery, The University of Michigan MidMichigan Health System, Midland, MI, USA

Jose Soliz The University of Texas MD Anderson Cancer Center, Houston, TX, USA

Clarissa Stapleton Department of Anesthesiology, Division of Anesthesia, Critical Care and Pain Medicine, The University of Texas MD Anderson Cancer Center, Houston, TX, USA

Thomas Staudinger Department of Medicine I, Intensive Care Unit, Medical University of Vienna, Vienna General Hospital, Vienna, Austria

R. Scott Stephens Oncology and Bone Marrow Transplant Critical Care, Division of Pulmonary and Critical Care Medicine, Johns Hopkins University, Baltimore, MD, USA

Brian W. Stephenson Division of Pulmonary, Critical Care, and Sleep Medicine, Department of Medicine, MedStar Georgetown University Hospital, Washington, DC, USA

Jose I. Suarez Division of Neurosciences Critical Care, Departments of Anesthesiology and Critical Care Medicine, Neurology, and Neurosurgery, The Johns Hopkins University School of Medicine, Baltimore, MD, USA

Jag Sunderram Department of Medicine, Division of Pulmonary and Critical Care, Rutgers-Robert Wood Johnson Medical School, New Brunswick, NJ, USA

Mahesh Swaminathan Leukemia, The University of Texas MD Anderson Cancer Center, Houston, TX, USA

Ariel D. Szvalb Department of Infectious Diseases, Infection Control and Employee Health, The University of Texas MD Anderson Cancer Center, Houston, TX, USA

Claudio E. Tatsui MD Anderson Cancer Center, Houston, TX, USA

Dilip R. Thakar Department of Anesthesiology and Perioperative Medicine, The University of Texas MD Anderson Cancer Center, Houston, TX, USA

Victor J. Thannickal Division of Pulmonary, Allergy and Critical Care Medicine, Department of Medicine, University of Alabama at Birmingham, Birmingham, AL, USA

Sajini Thekkel Division of Anesthesiology, Critical Care and Pain Medicine, The University of Texas MD Anderson Cancer Center, Houston, TX, USA

Sonali Thosani Department of Endocrine Neoplasia and Hormonal Disorders, Division of Internal Medicine, The University of Texas MD Anderson Cancer Center, Houston, TX, USA

Chani Traube Department of Pediatrics, Division of Pediatric Critical Care Medicine, Weill Cornell Medicine, New York, NY, USA

Anne M. Tucker Critical Care/Nutrition Support, The University of Texas MD Anderson Cancer Center, Houston, TX, USA

Frank P. Tverdek The University of Texas MD Anderson Cancer Center, Houston, TX, USA

Ugur Unluturk Department of Internal Medicine, Division of Endocrinology and Metabolism, Hacettepe University School of Medicine, Ankara, Turkey

Pamela Amakwe Uzoigwe UT MD Anderson Cancer Center, Houston, TX, USA

Jean Nicolas Vauthey Hepato-Pancreato-Biliary Section, Department of Department of Surgical Oncology, The University of Texas MD Anderson Cancer Center, Houston, TX, USA

Paula Velásquez Universidad Tecnológica de Pereira y Hospital Universitario San Jorge (HUSJ), Pereira, Colombia

Macarena R. Vial Interventional Pulmonology Unit, Clínica Alemana de Santiago-Universidad del Desarrollo, Santiago, Chile

Servicio de Enfermedades Respiratorias, Unidad de Neumologia Intervencional, Clinica Alemana de Santiago, Vitacura, Santiago, Chile

Catherine Vu Department of Anesthesiology, The University of Texas MD Anderson Cancer Center, Houston, TX, USA

Susannah K. Wallace Department of EHR Analytics and Reporting, The University of Texas MD Anderson Cancer Center, Houston, TX, USA

Yinghong Wang The Department of Gastroenterology, Hepatology and Nutrition, The University of Texas MD Anderson Cancer Center, Houston, TX, USA

Mary Lou Warren Department of Critical Care, UT MD Anderson Cancer Center, Houston, TX, USA

Clint Westaway Department of Anesthesiology, Critical Care and Pain Medicine, The University of Texas MD Anderson Cancer Center, Houston, TX, USA

John Wiemers MD Anderson Cancer Center, The University of Texas, Houston, TX, USA

Tim Wigmore Department of Anaesthesia, Critical Care and Pain Medicine, Royal Marsden Hospital, London, UK

Ursula Uduak Williams UT MD Anderson Cancer Center, Houston, TX, USA

Wendell H. Williams The University of Texas MD Anderson Cancer Center, Houston, TX, USA

Philipp Wohlfarth Department of Medicine I, Intensive Care Unit, Medical University of Vienna, Vienna General Hospital, Vienna, Austria

Suayib Yalcin Department of Medical Oncology, Hacettepe University Institute of Cancer, Ankara, Turkey

Steven M. Yevich The University of Texas MD Anderson Cancer Center, Houston, TX, USA

Alisha Y. Young Department of Pulmonary Medicine, University of Texas at McGovern Medical School, Houston, TX, USA

Syed Wamique Yusuf Department of Cardiology, The University of Texas MD Anderson Cancer Center, Houston, TX, USA

Abdulrazzak Zarifa Department of Cardiology, Division of Internal Medicine, The University of Texas MD Anderson Cancer Center, Houston, TX, USA

Wei Zhang The University of Texas MD Anderson Cancer Center, Houston, TX, USA

Gang Zheng Department of Anesthesiology and Perioperative Medicine, The University of Texas MD Anderson Cancer Center, Houston, TX, USA

Danielle Zimmerman University of Florida Health Cancer Center, Gainesville, FL, USA

Part I

Organization and Management of an Oncologic Critical Care Unit

Oncologic Critical Care Department Organization

Kristen J. Price

Contents

Introduction 4

The ICU Best Practice Committee 5
ICU Clinical Operations Committee 6
Quality and Safety Committee 7
Staff Education Committee 7
ICU Clinical Practice/Effectiveness and Evidence-Based Healthcare Committee 7
Clinical Informatics Committee 7
ICU Staff Wellness Committee 8
Patient/Family and Caregiver Engagement Committee 8
Research and Publications Committee: Critical Care 8

Conclusion 9

References 9

Abstract

Intensive care units (ICUs) are highly complex areas with the delivery of care provided by numerous disciplines with different reporting structures. These multidisciplinary care models are being redesigned as a result of increased emphasis on quality and safety, efficiency, and patient/family experience. The structure and governance of Critical Care departments vary widely in academic medical centers across the United States. Historically, ICUs were governed by individual Critical Care departments with significant focus on education, research, and training. In large centers, there can be several ICUs with completely different structure and organization. The push to improve the quality and safety of care in a streamlined and cost-efficient manner has organizations looking at more innovative ways to structure ICU care models such as institutes or centers. These "Critical Care Organizations" are few in number and are continuing to evolve at the present time. This chapter outlines The University of Texas MD Anderson Cancer Center intensive care unit organizational infrastructure which was designed over a decade and a half ago with the vision to systematically organize, establish, and sustain evidence-based clinical and

K. J. Price (✉)
Division of Anesthesiology, Critical Care and Pain Medicine, Department of Critical Care and Respiratory Care, The University of Texas MD Anderson Cancer Center, Houston, TX, USA
e-mail: kjprice@mdanderson.org

© Springer Nature Switzerland AG 2020
J. L. Nates, K. J. Price (eds.), *Oncologic Critical Care*,
https://doi.org/10.1007/978-3-319-74588-6_1

research initiatives in our oncologic intensive care unit. While some changes in the model have occurred over time, the basic structure and function of our intensive care unit organizational infrastructure model has been remarkably stable and highly successful.

Keywords
"Oncologic Critical Care" · Organization · Administration · Committees

Introduction

Academic medical centers (AMC) in the United States have traditionally focused on patient care, education, and research, with divisions and departments within these centers often functioning in silos. This has been true of Critical Care departments whose structure and governance have varied widely. Historically, intensive care units (ICUs) have been governed by individual Critical Care departments, and in large centers, there can be several ICUs with completely different structure and organization. The highly complex nature of an ICU along with care provided by numerous disciplines with different reporting structures has led to inefficiencies and higher costs not necessarily associated with improved outcomes. Thus, multidisciplinary ICU care models are being redesigned as a result of increased emphasis on quality and safety, efficiency, and patient/family experience. This push to improve the quality and safety of care in a streamlined and cost-efficient manner has organizations looking at more innovative ways to structure ICU care models such as institutes or centers. These "Critical Care Organizations" are few in number and are continuing to evolve at the present time [1–3].

Caring for the critically ill cancer patient is particularly challenging as the critical illness must be addressed in the context of the patient's stage and prognosis from the underlying malignancy. MD Anderson Cancer Center (MDACC) is a tertiary center with cutting-edge research sought after from patients all over the world. Patients once deemed untreatable are now seeking target therapies specific to their individual malignancies. This, along with an aging population with increasing comorbidities, significantly contributes to the challenge of oncologic Critical Care. The department of Critical Care at MDACC was established in 1997 and is comprised of highly specialized faculty members who are board-certified intensivists trained in anesthesiology, pulmonary medicine, and internal medicine. In close collaboration with the primary oncology staff, and in partnership with our advanced practice providers (APP), our intensivists lead a large multidisciplinary team to provide evidence-based, state-of-the-art care to critically ill oncologic patients in a 52-bed combined medical and surgical intensive care unit (ICU). The department of Critical Care provides academic support to the Section of Integrated Ethics in Cancer Care which offers consulting services, academics, research, and policy development for all of MD Anderson's components including regional, national, and international affiliates. The Critical Care department is also responsible for providing respiratory care services throughout the entire hospital.

This chapter outlines The University of Texas MD Anderson Cancer Center intensive care unit organizational infrastructure which was designed over a decade and a half ago with the vision to systematically organize, establish, and sustain evidence-based clinical and research initiatives in our oncologic intensive care unit. While some changes in the model have occurred over time, the basic structure and function of our intensive care unit organizational infrastructure model have been remarkably stable and highly successful. When created, the vision of the multifaceted ICU organizational infrastructure model aligned with MDACC's institutional goal to "enhance the excellence, value, safety and efficiency of our patient care." The model centers around the ICU Best Practice Committee which is comprised of key leaders from all of the disciplines represented in ICU. Eight additional committees, described in this chapter, have bidirectional reporting to the ICU Best Practice Committee. Each committee, charged with developing, planning, and implementing processes in their specialty area, is chaired by a member of the Critical Care faculty, co-chaired by a member of nursing or other disciplines' leadership, and is comprised of key multidisciplinary team members. The Best Practice Committee coordinates all activities related to the ICU initiatives to enhance best and safe patient care. ICU staff are encouraged to electronically submit ideas for process improvement projects via our Best Practice form link on the Critical Care website. The projects are vetted and sent to the appropriate committee for action. Once all project requirements are completed, that committee reports back to the Best Practice Committee for final endorsement and implementation. At the beginning of each fiscal year, every committee presents their goals to the ICU Best Practice Committee. At the end of each year, each committee summarizes their goals and accomplishments and presents their year-end summaries to the Best Practice Committee as well. A description of the organizational infrastructure as well as the purpose and goals of each committee follows.

The ICU Best Practice Committee

The ICU Best Practice (BP) Committee, chaired by the department chair of Critical Care and co-chaired by the associate director of ICU nursing, coordinates all clinical evidence-based activities related to the initiatives of the eight committees in the ICU organizational infrastructure (Fig. 1). The members of BP are, for the most part, leaders in the disciplines of ICU nursing, pharmacy, respiratory care, infection control, APP, nutrition, laboratory, social work, patient advocacy, chaplaincy, housekeeping/facilities, and information services. Each has a passion for ensuring that the best and safest care is provided to our critically ill ICU patients. The group is divided into teams of three to four, and each is responsible for performing at least one comprehensive Joint Commission endorsed tracer in the ICU per month. When at all possible, tracer feedback and education take place with the staff in real time.

The data is collected, and the results of the tracers are discussed at each Best Practice meeting. The data is trended, and quarterly reports are generated which are reviewed, posted on our internal website, and reported up to the institution's senior leadership.

Committee membership is critically reviewed on an annual basis to ensure attendance and engagement. There are three standing strategic goals of the BP committee:

1. To enhance best practices in the department of Critical Care, utilizing an evidence-based and a clinical effectiveness approach
2. To enhance quality and safety initiatives in the ICU, utilizing an interdisciplinary approach with collaboration and cooperation among appropriate disciplines at MD Anderson Cancer Center
3. To enhance clinical outcome measurements of the ICU infrastructure and support the implementation of any corresponding action plans

A critical summary is performed by the group at the end of every fiscal year; often, new goals are added and removed as needed.

The BP committee has two meetings per month on the first and third Wednesdays. The core group meets on the first with standing reports from each of the disciplines and a detailed review of the tracer reports. All new projects submitted electronically are reviewed and assigned to the appropriate infrastructure committee for analysis. The second meeting of the month follows the same format; however, the chairs and/or co-chairs of all of the infrastructure committees are present to give updates on all of the activities and projects they are engaged in. Once projects are completed and endorsed by the BP committee, they are funneled through the staff education committee who determine which disciplines need to be educated on that particular project. The need for cyclical education is also determined and carried out under this committee.

The adequate coordination of all committees is pivotal to keep the unit functioning at a high level of organization and productivity.

Intensive Care Unit Organizational Infrastructure

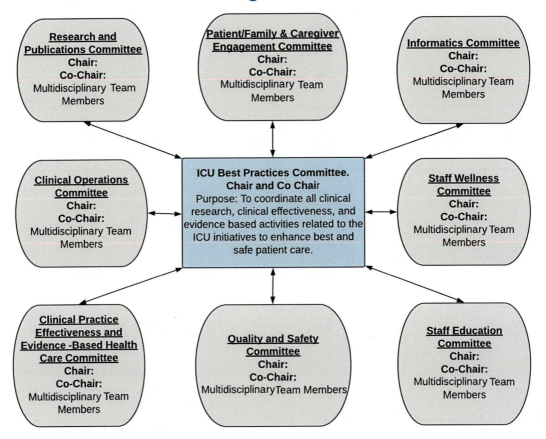

Fig. 1 Intensive care unit organizational infrastructure model

ICU Clinical Operations Committee

Purpose: To continuously review and improve clinical and operational practices in the intensive care unit (ICU)

General Goals

1. Monitor daily clinical activities and develop strategies to correct ineffective practices in the ICU.
2. Generate, support, and implement strategies to deliver excellent patient care.
3. Implement policies recommended by government agencies (e.g., Centers for Disease Control, Agency for Healthcare Research and Quality) to improve safety and prevent and ultimately abolish preventable complications (e.g., ventilator-associated pneumonia, catheter-related blood stream infections, wound infections).
4. Evaluate quality indicators pertaining to operational issues in the ICU.
5. Advise the Best Practice Committee on projects with foreseeable positive impact on administrative, clinical, and economical outcomes (quality improvement and clinical practices projects).
6. To increase patient safety by continuing to work with legal to finalize an institutional policy regarding audio and videotaping in the ICU.
7. To review the implementation of the rounding checklist.

8. To collaborate with Best Practice regarding the possible implementation of an intermediate unit.
9. Continue to sustain the initiatives implemented by the SCCM collaborative workgroup.
10. Implement the massive transfusion protocol for the ICU.

Quality and Safety Committee

Purpose: To identify and address opportunities to continuously improve organizational processes that will positively affect patient outcomes and patient satisfaction as well as lower costs for the ICU

General Goals
1. To continue to monitor current multidisciplinary indicators and add new indicators as appropriate to the quality and safety report
2. To review ICU data on multidisciplinary incident reports, errors, and high-risk clinical activities and develop plans and interventions to reduce risks and improve system and care processes to prevent such events
3. To collaborate with the Best Practice Committee on Joint Commission initiatives and Best Practice projects
4. To consolidate, analyze, and disseminate information via the ICU Best Practice Committee monthly and the institution's Acute and Critical Care Subcommittee meetings as needed
5. Specific committee goals include:
   (a) Report compliance on universal protocol/time-outs on a quarterly basis
   (b) Establish a monthly quality and safety report in collaboration with the epic team
   (c) Continue the device-related infection control ad hoc group to evaluate each CLABSI and add any incidences of CAUTI and PVAP for full review
   (d) Continue early nutrition initiative to evaluate sustainability of FY 18 project with identification of interventions to promote early nutrition in the ICU

Staff Education Committee

Purpose: To promote and coordinate the education of ICU staff, patients and families, faculty, fellows, advanced practice providers, residents, and students

General Goals
1. To provide instruction to the ICU staff, faculty, fellows, advanced practice providers, residents, and students on all new or updated order sets and protocols.
2. To provide instruction to the ICU staff, faculty, fellows, advanced practice providers, residents, and students on the Joint Commission guidelines based on tracer round results.
3. To continue to provide education for fellows, residents, and students with didactic lectures and bedside teaching.
4. To continue to support nursing staff development.
5. To educate the ICU staff on new or updated ICU operations.
6. To continue to implement education for identified low-compliance areas.

ICU Clinical Practice/Effectiveness and Evidence-Based Healthcare Committee

Purpose: To coordinate, evaluate, and recommend practice changes related to ICU operations and patient care

General Goals
1. To facilitate practice changes in clinical care for enhancing patient care experience.
2. Reduce practice variability through the implementation of standardized order sets and/or algorithms.
3. Enhance multidisciplinary planning to ensure safe delivery of patient care.

Clinical Informatics Committee

Purpose: A multidisciplinary group focused on informatics issues in the Critical Care environment to include electronic health record issues and enhancements, IT devices used in our environment, and quality and performance improvement projects with an informatics focus.

General Goals

1. Continue to address incoming concerns with our new electronic health record.
2. Review and prioritize parking lot issues for optimization.
3. Periodic evaluation and revision of documentation for efficiency and compliance.

ICU Staff Wellness Committee

Purpose: Take the lead in exploring ways to provide emotional and social well-being to our staff and to provide programs/activities addressing the needs of staff

General Goals

1. The committee will continue to provide emotional well-being to the ICU staff by providing four quarterly debriefing sessions.
2. The committee will continue to provide emotional well-being stress relief opportunities by hosting a stress busters twice a quarter.
3. The committee will provide a staff survey to determine areas of need for overall wellness (e.g., meditation room; working mothers' room).

Patient/Family and Caregiver Engagement Committee

Purpose: Create a more patient- and family-centered environment and facilitate healing through enhanced communication and empowerment

General Goals

1. Enhance the use of a daily goal board with a multidisciplinary approach.
2. Review current visitation guidelines and amend to include open visitation.
3. Encourage patients and families to be active participants in the healing process.

4. Improve the overall experience for patients and families through enhanced communication, engagement, and empowerment.

Research and Publications Committee: Critical Care

Purpose: To encourage research and publication in the Critical Care department by enhancing collaborations within the department and other departments

1. To maintain a current and updated list of all research projects, case reports, and QI projects that might lead to publications from all Critical Care staff
2. To enhance the involvement of all Critical Care staff in research activities and guide them in the process
3. To encourage department members to present their research findings to other faculty and staff in the department.

General Goals

The following significant changes were made in the past fiscal year:

1. A biyearly newsletter continues to be published updating all Critical Care staff regarding all ongoing projects, published abstracts, and papers.
2. The "Frontiers in Critical Care Multidisciplinary Research Sessions" were a success with presenters from different disciplines presented (MDs, APPs, pharmD).
3. Two vetting process through the committee for all prospective studies in the ICU is in place.
4. We have continued an updated list of all ICU staff projects (includes faculty, nursing, APPs, and pharmacy) which can be found at the research committee website http://inside.mdanderson.org/departments/ccm/icu-research-and-publications-committee.html.
5. We have kept an updated list of all congress relevant to Critical Care, for people to have access to.

New Committee Objectives

1. Will continue to maintain a list of *departmental resources and projects* via the research website.
2. Continue newsletters and quarterly/semester meetings with the committee.
3. The "Frontiers in Critical Care Multidisciplinary Research Sessions" will now invite researchers from other specialties to present their studies that are relevant to Critical Care (i.e., lymphoma and cardiology).
4. We will see if we can record the "Frontiers in Critical Care Multidisciplinary Research Sessions" so that all staff can access it if they were unable to attend to the talk.
5. The committee will guide APPs in the following: creating research ideas and identifying objectives, developing and writing of protocols for IRB or QI approval, understanding of statistical analysis of data, and writing abstracts and manuscripts.

Conclusion

The ICU organizational infrastructure was developed to bring the multidisciplinary team members together for the purpose of establishing and sustaining evidence-based clinical patient safety initiatives. This novel staffing model brings together all disciplines with different reporting structures to focus on efficiency and appropriate resource utilization in our critically ill oncologic patients. While the basic structure of each committee is the same, each chair and co-chair has autonomy in the way they select members, conduct their meetings, complete projects, and accomplish their goals each year. Listing specific accomplishments of each committee is beyond the scope of this chapter; however, quite remarkably, the model has been sustained for over two decades now. Committees have been added and retired under the governance of the multidisciplinary infrastructure, and the results have been truly outstanding. As regulations and reimbursement processes continue to be based on value and outcomes, academic medical centers will face ongoing challenges in the years to come. As Critical Care Organizations continue to evolve, models such as our ICU organizational infrastructure will be instrumental in improving the quality and safety of care in a streamlined efficient manner.

References

1. Leung S, Gregg SR, Coopersmith CM, Layon AJ, Oropello J, Brown DR, Pastores SM, Kvetan V, Academic Leaders in Critical Care Medicine Task Force of the Society of the Critical Care Medicine. Critical care organizations: business of critical care and value/performance building. Crit Care Med. 2018;46(1):1–11.
2. Moore JE, Oropello JM, Stoltzfus D, Masur H, Coopersmith CM, Nates J, Doig C, Christman J, Hite RD, Angus DC, Pastores SM, Kvetan V, Academic Leaders in Critical Care Medicine (ALCCM) Task Force of the Society of the Critical Care Medicine. Critical care organizations: building and integrating academic programs. Crit Care Med. 2018;46(4):e334–41.
3. Pastores SM, Halpern NA, Oropello JM, Kostelecky N, Kvetan V. Critical care organizations in academic medical centers in North America: a descriptive report. Crit Care Med. 2015;43(10):2239–44.

ICU Utilization

2

Current Trends in ICU Beds, Use, Occupancy, and Costs in the United States

Karen Chen, Susannah K. Wallace, and Joseph L. Nates

Contents

Introduction 12

ICU Beds and Utilization 12

ICU and Hospital Mortality 13

Costs 14

Specialty ICUs 14

Best Practices in ICU Optimization 15

Critical Care Organizations 15

Conclusion 16

References 16

Abstract

Oncologic critical care units specialize in the care of patients with critical illness related to their malignancy, treatment, or other conditions. Intensive care unit (ICU) beds, utilization, and costs have continuously increased in general acute care hospitals in the United States over the past three decades. This chapter reviews and summarizes current literature related to ICU beds, utilization, and costs in general and oncologic critical care units as well as recommendations to improve access, quality, and costs of healthcare. The concept of the specialty ICU and its associated outcomes is briefly covered. Evidence-based recommendations of best practices for ICU resource optimization are delineated. In conclusion, effective critical care organizations will develop and align the multiple facets of research, quality improvement, culture of safety, and outcomes to improve the value of critical care units in healthcare delivery.

K. Chen · J. L. Nates (✉)
Department of Critical Care and Respiratory Care, The University of Texas MD Anderson Cancer Center, Houston, TX, USA
e-mail: kachen@mdanderson.org; jlnates@mdanderson.org

S. K. Wallace
Department of EHR Analytics and Reporting, The University of Texas MD Anderson Cancer Center, Houston, TX, USA
e-mail: skishwall@mdanderson.org

© Springer Nature Switzerland AG 2020
J. L. Nates, K. J. Price (eds.), *Oncologic Critical Care*,
https://doi.org/10.1007/978-3-319-74588-6_5

Keywords

ICU beds · Utilization · Optimization ·
Mortality · Costs · Quality · Value ·
Outcomes · Specialty ICU · Critical care
organizations

Introduction

There is significant variation in treatment of the same disease by physicians and hospitals throughout the United States [40]. In addition, there is no systematic classification and organization of intensive care units; some combine MICU and SICU, some have subspecialty ICUs, whereas community hospitals may place less sick patients in the ICU solely for more concentrated nursing care. Furthermore, there is no national database describing ICU utilization with any specific details due to this lack of a standardized definition and reasons for admission to intensive care units.

Unfortunately, this poses a problem as to comparative groups. Based on the literature available, it appears that less than half and in some circumstances as low as 10–20% of the ICU patients require the most intensive treatment described as "fairly continuous physician involvement and various forms of life support" [45, 26]. On the other end of the spectrum, patients who receive monitoring and intensive nursing care make up about 20–30% of patients in general ICUs, with a higher percentage of "monitoring" patients in ICUs which also serve as CCUs.

ICU Beds and Utilization

Between 2000 and 2010, the number of ICU beds in non-federal acute care hospitals in the United States has increased from 88,235 to 103,900 (17.8%). The ratio of ICU to total hospital beds has also increased from 13.5% to 16.2% (a change of 20.4%) [15].

There are significant variations in ICU practices and policies throughout the healthcare system thus highly impacting ICU utilization rates. Many of these factors, such as practitioner discretion, hospital capacity, policies, and procedures of the hospital, are based on subjective and at times arbitrary considerations as opposed to evidence-based decisions. In a study conducted within the US Veterans Affairs Health System, the rate of ICU admission for low-risk hospitalized patients varied from 1.2% to 38.9% [9]. In this same study, the variations in the ICU utilization did not alter outcomes. Thus, many of these patients should have been treated in less acute lower cost settings [9]. In addition, when patients are unnecessarily placed in ICUs or keeping them in the ICU longer than necessary may cause harm in the form of complications such as increased healthcare- associated infections, medication errors, adverse drug events, agitation, and delirium with associated long-lasting sequelae [19, 20, 29].

In a different study, certain conditions such as DKA, GI bleed, PE, CHF which frequently utilize ICU care but which may not always be necessary, institutions that utilized ICUs more frequently performed more invasive procedures and incurred higher costs but had no improvement in hospital mortality. Of note, many of these hospitals with high ICU utilization were small (<99 beds) or teaching hospitals, thus ICU admission provided either specialized nursing or physician skill sets [5]. In this study, hospitals had similar ICU utilization patterns across the conditions [5]. However, lack of clear-cut guidelines for ICU admissions and differences in institutional resources, policies, and culture have resulted in significant variability in utilization among hospitals [1, 8, 43]. Thus, Chang and Shapiro concluded, in order to improve the value of critical care services, factors that lead clinicians to admit to a higher level of care when equivalent care can be delivered in a less costly setting will need to be addressed by the institutions within the confine of their healthcare system [5].

In another study, many patients who required monitoring but no acute ICU intervention may not have needed ICU-level care but benefitted from higher level of care than that available on a regular medical/surgical ward. This suggests that an increased allocation of intermediate care unit beds likely will improve ICU resource utilization [26]. In a single center oncology unit, this theory was once again demonstrated by decreased ICU utilization rate over time with the advent of surgical intermediate units as noted by Wallace [41].

Contrary to popular belief that elderly people may require more intensive care than their proportion of the general population or that the elderly might receive less intensive care than their younger counterparts due to scarcity of ICU beds, analysis of the data does not show this [16]. As opposed to other developed countries, age does not appear to be an important determination for ICU admission in the United States based on MEDPAR data showing about 15–18% of beneficiaries utilizing the ICU or CCU for various age groups ranging from <65 to >85 years [16].

In 2010, the average national ICU occupancy rate based on the midnight bed census was 66% [14]. A 2005–2007 study using Project IMPACT data reported a mean hourly ICU occupancy rate of 68.2% [44]. According to a 2003 SCCM survey [46], occupancy was highest in Surgical ICUs (79%), ICUs in federal hospitals (80%), and ICUs of hospitals with 301–750 beds (77%). Mortality remained stable despite variations in the occupancy rate [18]. Unfortunately, the data sets used in these large national studies did not include specific information regarding oncologic critical care.

Due to early detection and more treatment options for cancer, survival of cancer patients has increased over the last three decades [4]. Unfortunately, many of these therapies cause increased side effects and significant toxicities that require life support and/or life-sustaining measures, which have resulted in ICU referrals and admissions [2].

It is estimated that as high as 20% of patients admitted to ICUs hold a cancer diagnosis [7, 34]. The authors found that the presence of clinical pharmacists in the ICU, presence of ICU protocols, and daily meetings between oncologists and intensivists were associated with lower hospital mortality even after adjustment for hospital case volume [35]. Protocols and daily meetings were also associated with more efficient resource utilization [35].

Wallace et al. [41] described the results of two decades of ICU utilization and hospital outcomes in a comprehensive cancer center in the United States. The ratio of ICU to total hospital beds was 8.2% in 2013 and remained stable throughout the time period. ICU utilization was 12% and decreased over time with the advent of specialty step-down units such as surgical intermediate care units and neuro progressive units. Average ICU and hospital lengths of stay were 3.9 and 7.4 days, respectively, in comparison to patients in general hospitals with average lengths of stay of 4.4 days [41].

The proportion of hospital days spent in the ICU (6.9%) was lower than that in national studies (14.4–21.1%). Patients with cancer are often admitted to the hospital to receive anticancer therapy which may account for the lower percentage [41]. Given the increase in the incidence of cancer and improved survival rates along with more chemotherapeutic and surgical options, cancer patients are requiring advanced life support for cancer-related complications, treatment-related toxicities, and severe infections [22]. Some examples include structural problems such as spinal cord compression, superior vena cava syndrome, and cerebral metastasis with associated edema; metabolic problems such as hypercalcemia, tumor lysis syndrome, hyponatremia related to syndrome of inappropriate antidiuretic hormone; and hematologic problems such as hyperleukocytosis and leukostasis, disseminated intravascular coagulation, and infectious problems due to myelosuppression. Length of stay varies by service line. For example, length of stay for hematopoietic stem cell transplantation recipients increased over time possibly due to the increasing use of cord blood and haploidentical transplants which require a longer time to achieve hematologic recovery [41].

ICU and Hospital Mortality

In a JAMA study published in 2013, a comparison of data between 2009, 2005, and 2000 showed a lower percentage of patients died in an acute care hospital in 2009 as compared to 2005 and 2000 but admission to ICU and the rate of health care transitions increased in the last 30 days of life, despite growth in hospital-based palliative services [39]. This study questions the notion that there is a trend toward less aggressive care at the end-of-life as reported by the CDC based on the fact that more patients aged 65 and older were likely to die at home [39].

Wallace et al. in a 20 year study of ICU utilization and outcomes reported hospital mortality to be 3.6% among patients with cancer: 16.2% among patients with an ICU stay and 1.8% among non-ICU patients [41]. The observed mortality rate was less than the expected mortality rate for almost all services, and the overall standardized mortality ratio was 0.71. The hospital mortality rates were 3.9% for surgical ICU patients and 33.8% for medical ICU patients (42.7% in the hematological patients and 25.2% in the solid tumor patients).

ICU mortality rates vary by type of malignancy and are reported to be 18.3–31.2% among patients with solid tumor malignancies, 36.6–47.8% in patients with leukemia, and 27.8–50.0% in patients with lymphoma [17, 31, 41]. Over the past two decades, there has been a decreasing hospital mortality for hematopoietic stem cell transplantation recipients thought to be due to reduced intensity conditioning regimens and other global changes in pretransplant protocols [10, 41].

Costs

Intensive care unit utilization contributes to a significant portion of health care costs. In 2010, intensive care services accounted for 13.2% of total hospital expenditures, 4.1% of national healthcare expenditures, and 0.72% of the gross domestic product [15]. Annual costs for critical care services increased by 92.2% from $56 to $108 billion dollars between 2000 and 2010, which was double the rate of increase of the GDP during the same time period. The proportion of critical care costs to GDP increased 32.1%. Hospital stays that involved ICU services were two and a half times more costly than other hospital stays. Hospital stays with ICU services accounted for just over one-quarter of all discharges (26.9%) but nearly one-half of aggregate total hospital charges (47.5%) [3].

Intensive care is also expensive. And the Medicare reimbursement rate for intensive care covers only 83% of its costs as compared to 105% in those without an ICU stay [6]. In this chapter, an analysis performed in the year 2000 analyzing costs and reimbursements concluded that hospitals lose money on patients who spend at least 1 day in an ICU versus making money on those patients that do not spend any times in ICUs [6].

Several initiatives have been established to decrease ICU utilization and contain costs such as noninvasive mechanical ventilation, intermediate or low intensity surgical patients, and palliative and end-of-life care outside of the ICU. Other initiatives include patient safety and quality mandates, participating in hospital performance metrics, optimizing ICU design, staffing and coverage mechanisms, maximizing ICU throughput and patient flow, dealing with capacity strain, rationing ICU beds, containing ICU costs, standardizing ICU technologies and alarms, developing and managing rapid response and sepsis teams, and fostering interdisciplinary collaboration and interacting with hospital networks in critical care organizations [24].

Specialty ICUs

Do critically ill patients in ICUs at cancer centers perform better than those in ICUs at general hospitals after adjustment for severity? The findings in ORCHESTRA suggest that admission to an ICU in cancer centers was not associated with lower ICU mortality, hospital mortality, or better resource utilization when compared to ICU admissions in general hospitals [22, 34]. In a more recent study by Romano et al., early palliative care in oncologic patients significantly reduced the utilization of ICU services and in hospital mortality but does not change utilization of chemotherapy or radiation therapy [32]. Although palliative care has not shown an impact on critically ill patients, it has shown improved survival and improved quality of life in ambulatory cancer patients [38]. In a large European study, patients with cancer were more often admitted to the ICU for sepsis and respiratory complications than other ICU patients. Overall, the outcome of patients with solid cancer was similar to that of ICU patients without cancer, whereas patients with hematological cancer had a worse outcome [37].

Although ICU patients with cancer still have a higher mortality than ICU patients without malignancy, published survival rates of critically ill patients with cancer are approaching those of severely ill patients without cancer, and it no longer seems justified to universally deny patients with cancer access to intensive care medicine [33]. Of utmost importance, close collaboration among medical and surgical oncologists with the intensivists will ensure the establishment of clear goals and a multidisciplinary approach to treatment for every patient with cancer who requires ICU admission [11].

Best Practices in ICU Optimization

Although implementing change to optimize ICU utilization is quite a formidable task, significant potential benefits, including but not limited to improved patient outcomes, increased bed capacity and patient throughput, decreased payment penalties, as well as increased patient satisfaction, abound for an organization that succeeds in this realm [24]. Accurate data to drive change cannot be overly emphasized in this challenging but rewarding endeavor.

Here are some common tenets and best practices in ICU resource utilization management [24]. First, establishing and diligently using care bundles. These bundles are usually implemented as a checklist to reduce the complications of ICU care, namely, infections, pain, delirium, immobility, prolonged ventilatory support, etc. [25, 30]. Secondly, establishing end-of-life planning and palliative care treatment plans can improve patient satisfaction, duration of survival while reducing ICU length of stay and ICU admissions thus reducing ICU costs [21, 38]. Thirdly, establishing admission, discharge, and triage criteria as well as operating an intermediate care unit [28, 36]. Fourthly, multidisciplinary teams daily rounding utilizing checklists have shown improved patient outcomes as well as decreased length in ICU stay [42]. Fifthly, ICU staffing that includes a specialty team led by an intensivist, a board-certified physician with advanced training

who provides specialty care to critically ill complex patient [42]. Finally, there needs to be focused ongoing review of operational efficiencies, variations in practice, and outcomes leading to a quality metric scorecard and a performance improvement plan [24].

Critical Care Organizations

Changing healthcare regulations and reimbursement structures provide challenges for hospitals and healthcare systems. The Society of Critical Care Medicine developed a task force of successful leaders of critical care organizations in North America to provide guidelines for adult critical care medicine leaders in academic and non-academic settings [27]. The task force members have expertise in critical care administration, healthcare management, and clinical practice. They describe two phases of care integration within critical care organizations: horizontal – an initial phase that includes regionalization of care, and vertical, which includes continuum of care following acute and intensive care.

After integration of business and operational aspects of critical care, the next step is to integrate critical care organizations within academic medical centers to improve healthcare delivery. The key elements of critical care organizations include patient care and safety, quality improvement, research, education, and professional development [23]. The culture of safety should include reporting, review, and open discussion of adverse events, patient safety education, and checklist development. Seamless interoperability between electronic health records and incident reporting systems is important to improve value for patients. Clinical outcomes, health services research, quality improvement benchmarking, and the use of severity scoring systems (APACHE, MPM, SAPS) are important for describing the population health of critical care organizations. As a result of technological advancements, electronic health records, publicly reported metrics, emphasis on patient safety and experience, in addition to the value of care, critical care organizations will need to effectively and efficiently utilize their resources.

Conclusion

As there is no standardized classification system for intensive care units and reasons for ICU admission, ICU utilization may vary significantly from hospital to hospital. As high as 20% of patients admitted to general ICUs carry a cancer diagnosis [34]. Wallace et al. described the results of two decades of ICU utilization and found hospital mortality reported to be 3.6% among patients with cancer, 16.2% among patients with an ICU stay, and 1.8% among non-ICU patients [41]. The observed mortality rate was less than the expected mortality rate for almost all services, and the overall standardized mortality ratio was 0.71. As ICU utilization contributes to a significant proportion of health care costs and with costs rising, several initiatives have been established to decrease ICU utilization and contain costs such as noninvasive mechanical ventilation, intermediate or low intensity surgical patients, and palliative and end-of-life care outside of the ICU just to name a few. In addition, best practices such as utilizing checklists, multidisciplinary team rounds led by intensivists, establishing admission, discharge and triage criteria, as well as tracking performance metrics in a quality improvement plan will improve ICU utilization optimization. In the future, two phases of care will need to be integrated within critical care organizations. Horizontal integration which includes regionalization of care and a vertical one that incorporates the continuum of medical care following the ICU stay [27].

References

1. Admon AJ, Seymour CW, Gershengorn HB, Wunsch H, Cooke CR. Hospital-level variation in ICU admission and critical care procedures for patients hospitalized for pulmonary embolism. Chest. 2014;146(6):1452–61.
2. Azoulay E, Soares M, Dramon M, Benoit D, Pastores S, Afessa B. Intensive care of the cancer patient: recent achievements and remaining challenges. Ann Intensive Care. 2011;1:5.
3. Barrett, ML, Smith MW, Elixhauser A, Honigman LS, Pines JM. Utilization of Intensive Care Services, 2011. Available at: https://www.hcup-us.ahrq.gov/reports/statbriefs/sb185-Hospital-Intensive-Care-Units-2011.pdf. Accessed 9 Sept 2018.
4. Brenner H. Long-term survival rates of cancer patients achieved by the end of the 20th century: a period analysis. Lancet. 2002;360(9340):1131–5.
5. Chang DW, Shapiro MF. Association between ICU utilization during hospitalization and costs, use of invasive procedures and mortality. JAMA Intern Med. 2016;176(10):1492–9.
6. Cooper L, Line-Zwirble. Medicare intensive care unit use: analysis of incidence, cost, and payment. Crit Care Med. 2004;32(11):2245–53.
7. Encina B, Lagunes L, Morales-Codina M. The immunocompromised oncohematologial critically ill patient: considerations in severe infections. Ann Transl Med. 2016;4(17):327–30.
8. Gershengorn HB, Iwashyna TJ, Cooke CR, Scales DC, Kahn JM, Wunsch H. Variation in use of intensive care for adults with diabetic ketoacidosis. Crit Care Med. 2012;40(7):2009–15.
9. Gooch RA, Kahn JM. ICU bed supply, utilization, and health care spending: an example of demand elasticity. JAMA. 2014;311(6):567–8.
10. Gooley TA, Chien JW, Pergam SA, et al. Reduced mortality after allogeneic hematopoietic-cell transplantation. N Engl J Med. 2010;363(22):2091–101.
11. Gutierrez C, Pastores S. When should ICU patients get an ICU bed? Available at: http://learnicu.org/Lists/Web%20Contents/Attachments/7824/When%20Should%20the%20Cancer%20Patient%20Get%20an%20ICU%20Bed.pdf. Accessed 29 Aug 2018.
12. Halpern NA, Pastores SM, Greenstein RJ. Critical care medicine in the United States 1985–2000: an analysis of bed numbers, use, and costs. Crit Care Med. 2004;32(6):1254–9.
13. Halpern NA, Pastores SM. Critical care medicine in the United States 2000–2005: an analysis of bed numbers, occupancy rates, payer mix, and costs. Crit Care Med. 2010;38(1):65–71.
14. Halpern NA, Pastores SM. Critical care medicine beds, use, occupancy and costs in the United States: a methodological review. Crit Care Med. 2015;43(11):2452–9.
15. Halpern NA, Goldman DA, Tan KS, Pastores SM. Trends in critical care beds and use among population groups and Medicare and Medicaid beneficiaries in the United States: 2000–2010. Crit Care Med. 2016;44(8):1490–9.
16. Helbing C, Supervisory Statistician, office of Research, Division of Beneficiary Studies, health Care financing administration, US Dept of Health and Human services, June 6, 1983, data from MedPar File.
17. Horster S, Stemmler HJ, Mandel PC, et al. Mortality of patients with hematological malignancy after admission to the intensive care unit. Onkologie. 2012;35(10):556–61.
18. Iwashyna TJ, Kramer AA, Kahn JM. Intensive care unit occupancy and patient outcomes. Crit Care Med. 2009;37(5):1545–57.
19. Jain M, Miller L, Belt D, King D, Berwick DM. Decline in icu adverse events, nosocomial infections and cost through a quality improvement initiative

focusing on teamwork and culture change. BMJ Qual Saf. 2006;15(4):235–9.

20. Kane-Gill SL, Dasta JF, Buckley MS, Devabhakthuni S, Liu M, Cohen H, et al. Clinical practice guideline: safe medication use in the ICU. Crit Care Med. 2017;45(9):e877–915.

21. Khandelwal N, Curtis JR. Economic implications of end-of-life care in the icu. Curr Opin Crit Care. 2014;20(6):656–61.

22. Koch A, Checkley W. Do hospitals need oncological critical care units? J Thor Dis. 2017;9(3):E304–9.

23. Leung S, Gregg SR, Coopersmith CM, Layon AJ, Oropello J, Brown DR, et al. Critical care organizations: business of critical care and value/performance building. Crit Care Med. 2018;46(1):1–11.

24. Margin of Excellence: Intensive Care Unit (ICU) Utilization. Available at: https://www.premierinc.com/downloads/icu-utilization-whitepaper.pdf. Accessed 20 Aug 2018.

25. Marra A, Ely EW, Pandharipande PP, Patel MB. The ABCDEF bundle in critical care. Crit Care Clin. 2017;33(2):225–43.

26. Matthews K, Jenq G, Siner J, Long E, Pisani M. ICU utilization by "subacute" patients reasons for admission and opportunities for improvement. Crit Care Med. 2012;40(12):1–328.

27. Moore JE, Oropello JM, Stoltzfus D, Masur H, Coopersmith CM, Nates J, et al. Critical care organizations: building and integrating academic programs. Crit Care Med. 2018;46(4):e334–41.

28. Nates JL, Nunnally M, Kleinpell R, Blosser S, Goldner J, Birriel B, Fowler CS, Byrum D, Miles WS, Bailey H, Sprung CL. ICU admission, discharge, and triage guidelines: a framework to enhance clinical operations, development of institutional policies, and further research. Crit Care Med. 2016;44(8):1553–602.

29. Nordon-Craft A, Moss M, Quan D, Schenkman M. Intensive Care unit- acquired weakness: implications for physical therapist management. Phys Ther. 2012;92(12):1494–506.

30. Optimizing critical care with the ABCDEF Bundle. Available at: http://www.sccm.org/ICULiberation/News/Optimizing-Critical-Care-with-the-ABCDEF-Bundle. Accessed 16 Oct 2018.

31. Puxty K, McLoone P, Quasim T, Kinsella J, Morrison D. Survival in solid cancer patients following intensive care unit admission. Intensive Care Med. 2014;40(10):1409–28.

32. Romano AM, Gade KE, Nielsen G, Havard R, Harrison JH Jr, Barclay J, et al. Early palliative care reduces end-of life Intensive Care (ICU) use but not ICU course in patients with advanced cancer. Oncologist. 2017;22(3):318–23.

33. Shimabukuro-Vornhagen A, Boll B, Kochanek M, Azoulay E, von Bergwelt-Baildon MS. Critical care of patients with cancer. CA Cancer J Clin. 2016;66(6):496–517.

34. Soares M, Bozza FA, Angus DC, Japiassu AM, Viana WM, Costa R, et al. Organizational characteristics, outcomes, and resource use in 78 Brazilian intensive care units: the ORCHESTRA study. Intensive Care Med. 2015;41(12):2149–60.

35. Soares M, Bozza FA, Azevedo LC, Silva UV, Correa TD, Colombari F, et al. Effects of organizational characteristics on outcomes and resource use in patients with cancer admitted to intensive care units. J Clin Oncol. 2016;34(27):3315–24.

36. Solberg BC, Dirksen CD, Nieman FH, van Merode G, Ramsay G, Roekarts P, et al. Introducing an integrated intermediate care unit improves ICU utilization: a prospective intervention study. BMC Anesthesiol. 2014;14:76.

37. Taccone FS, Artigas AA, Sprung CL, Moreno R, Sakr Y, Vincent JL. Characteristics and outcomes of cancer patients in European ICUs. Crit Care. 2009;13(1):R15.

38. Temel JS, Greer JA, Muzikansky A, Gallagher ER, Admane S, Jackson VA, et al. Early palliative care for patients with non- small- cell lung cancer. N Engl J Med. 2010;363(8):733–42.

39. Teno JM, Gozalo PL, Bynum JP, Leland NE, Miller SC, Morden NE, et al. Changes in end-of-life care for Medicare beneficiaries site of death, place of care and health care transitions in 2000, 2005 and 2009. JAMA. 2013;309(5):470–7.

40. The Joint Commission: Performance Measurement. Available at: http://www.jointcommission.org/performance_measurement.aspx. Accessed 17 Oct 2018.

41. Wallace SK, Rathi NK, Waller DK, Ensor JE, Haque SA, Price KJ, et al. Two decades of ICU utilization and hospital outcomes in a comprehensive cancer center. Crit Care Med. 2016;44(5):926–33.

42. Weled BJ, Adzhigirey LA, Hodgman TM, Brilli RJ, Spevetz A, Kline AM, et al. Critical care delivery: the importance of process of care and icu structure to improved outcomes: an update from the American College of Critical Care Medicine Task Force on models of critical care. Crit Care Med. 2015;43(7):1520–5.

43. Wunsch H, Angus DC, Harrison DA, Collange O, Fowler R, Hoste EA, et al. Variation in critical care services across North America and Western Europe. Crit Care Med. 2008;36(10):2787–93.

44. Wunsch H, Wagner J, Herlim M, Chong DH, Kramer AA, Halpern SD. ICU occupancy and mechanical ventilator use in the United States. Crit Care Med. 2013;41(12):2712–9.

45. Zimmerman JE, Wagner DP, Knaus WA, Williams JF, Kolakowski D, Draper EA. The use of risk predictions to identify candidates for intermediate care units: implications for intensive care utilization and cost. Chest. 1995;108(2):490–9.

46. Society of Critical Care Medicine. Critical care units: A descriptive analysis. 2nd Ed. Des Plainness, IL: Society of Critical Care Medicine; 2011.

Critical Care Admissions and Discharge Criteria in Cancer Patients

3

Ignacio Pujol Varela and Isidro Prieto del Portillo

Contents

Introduction 20
What Has Changed to Improve the Prognosis of Cancer Patients in ICUs? 20
Better Results, but at What Cost? 22
Organizational Aspects of the ICUs 22

Admission Criteria 24
The Patient and Their Characteristics 24
Tumor Type and Stage 26
Reason for Admission 26
New Strategies of ICU Admission 27

ICU Discharge 27

Summary 30

References 30

Abstract

More and more patients with solid or hematological tumors are admitted to the Intensive Care Units. The improvement in the physiopathological understanding of this group of patients, as well as the increasingly better and more targeted treatment options for their underlying disease, has led to a significant increase in their survival over the past two decades. We are living in an era in which we are defining the standards that offer the best way to care for them: From the organization and running of ICUs, the definition of clear admission criteria from the available evidence, and the development of new admission policies that expand the classic dichotomous view of whether or not they are candidates for admission to ICUs to analyzing the best treatment for them, avoiding excessive treatment, and, above all, respecting their principle of autonomy.

Keywords

Oncologic patients · Admission policies · Multidisciplinary care · Early response team · Critical care transition programs · Full code admission · ICU trial · Palliative care

I. Pujol Varela (✉) · I. P. del Portillo
Department of Critical Care, Hospital MD Anderson
Cancer Center, Madrid, Spain
e-mail: ipujol@mdanderson.es;
ignaciopujolvarela@yahoo.es; iprieto@mdanderson.es;
isidroprieto69@gmail.com

© Springer Nature Switzerland AG 2020
J. L. Nates, K. J. Price (eds.), *Oncologic Critical Care*,
https://doi.org/10.1007/978-3-319-74588-6_3

Introduction

Cancer patients are increasingly common in intensive care units around the world. One out of every six to eight patients admitted to intensive care units (ICUs) worldwide presents a neo-proliferative process [1, 3]. Those of us who treated this type of patient two decades ago in hospitals dedicated to cancer treatment were accused of using very expensive resources in patients with a short life expectancy. At the time, some scientific societies, such as the American College of Chest Physicians or the Society of Critical Care Medicine in its 1992 Consensus Conference, pointed out the futility of admitting oncology patients to Intensive Care Units, arguing that if they needed mechanical ventilation, cate-cholamine, or renal replacement therapies, their mortality rate of over 90% was not worth the therapeutic effort. At the time, the fact of being a cancer patient was an independent risk factor for refusing to admit the patient to the ICUs [2].

The incidence of cancer does not stop growing; diagnosis is made at an earlier stage, which increases the treatment and life expectancy of these patients; the social and healthcare level in developed countries increases, and we find ourselves with an increasingly aging population and therefore more prone to suffering mutations in genetic structure that make it develop a neo-formative process. The age-adjusted incidence of cancer is 533.8 cases (532.6–535.1) per 100,000 population with a 95% CI [3]. To give you an idea of its magnitude, in 2009 there were 1.4 million and 3.2 million newly diagnosed cases of cancer in the USA and Europe, respectively (100,000 and 230,000 cases of oncological blood disorders in the same period). And this increase in the number of cases leads to more and more people being admitted to Intensive Care Units. During the first 100 days after the diagnosis of cancer, the risk of entering the ICU is considerably high and this exponential growth is subsequently reduced. Nearly 5.2% of all cancer patients develop a complication requiring ICU admission within 2 years of diagnosis [4]. If we are talking about patients with allogeneic hematopoietic stem cell transplantation (HSCT), up to 20% of them will require ICU admission after their procedure.

This whole process is underpinned by scientific research. While the first studies on cancer patients in the 1990s were rare and merely observational about their occurrence and survival (mainly developed in France, Brazil, and the USA), today, on the other hand, there is a proliferation of articles written all across the world by single-unit ICUs, general ICUs, including multi-centric ICUs that bring together large numbers of patients. Contributions include retrospective or prospective articles aimed both at describing the experience of specialized centers with regard to their patients, for example with lung cancer [5] or after cytoreductive surgery Mogal et al. [51], and above all, studies aimed at reviewing signs of admission, studies that assess factors that influence their short- and long-term prognosis or those aimed at finding the best organization of units to treat them [6]. The societies of Intensive Care and Oncology seek meeting points and create work units to improve the outcome for their patients, as is the case with the SEOM and SEMICYUC in Spain [7]. A section within the new working guidelines [8] on admission, discharge criteria, and patient triage from the Society of Critical Care Medicine (SCCCM) has included a section on the admission criteria for cancer patients.

What Has Changed to Improve the Prognosis of Cancer Patients in ICUs?

Comparative mortality studies have shown a significant improvement in the life expectancy of cancer patients in ICUs in recent years. Of these, the systematic reviews of Puxty et al. [4] and Soubani [9] are noteworthy. The first one deals with the review of 48 articles between 1997 and 2011 with a total of 74,061 patients with solid tumors in which the overall mortality in ICU was 31.2% and in hospitalized patients 38.2%, but with such a wide range of intra-Intensive Care Unit mortality between 4.5% and 85% due to the great heterogeneity of the sample. Soubani [9] compares studies from the 1980s and 1990s where mortality of patients with cancer and mechanical ventilation was around 80–90%, while more recent studies describe mortalities between 27% and 30% in solid tumors, 40% in autologous transplants, and around 60% in allogeneic transplants.

The reasons for this improvement in outcome results are multifactorial and due to improvements and innovations in all fields of cancer research, diagnosis, and treatment, as well as intensive care.

In the field of Critical Care, the main change has been the return to the physiological understanding of the different pathologies and its application in their treatment. Understanding and using optimal peep, limiting plateau pressure or tidal volume, meaning of the response or non-response to volume administration during resuscitation, assessing weaning-related cardiac dysfunction, limiting airway pressure to optimize cardiovascular function, understanding why prone positioning minimizes lung damage and improves gas exchange, understanding that small changes in creatinine can lead to significant kidney damage, all of these are some examples of practices that we all develop today and whose basis is our physiology [10]. The use of noninvasive ventilation or high-flow systems capable of generating positive pressure has been shown to be effective in reducing intubation and mortality due to respiratory distress [11]. Improvements in sedation and analgesia techniques, with less depth in them and with periodic interruptions to improve weaning; being attentive to the psychological needs of the patient and the family, preventing and diagnosing delirium of our critical patients early; the daily use for bedside diagnosis or for safer techniques through ultrasound; the improvement of nutrition for critical patients; better understanding of common processes such as polyneuropathy or myopathy of the critically ill, etc., and thus small advances in all areas of intensive care have contributed to a more physiological and less aggressive management of our patients. From an organizational point of view, the systematic work carried out using operating protocols, the progressive distribution of our Intensive Care Units and medium level units according to the need for monitoring, the complexity of each

patient, and the nursing care ratios allow us to attend to each of our patients with a specific level of priority, thereby being more cost-effective.

In the field of Oncology, surgery is becoming more and more sophisticated, more advanced supplemented before, after, and even at the same time with chemotherapy or radiotherapy. Other developments include advances in conventional RT or brachytherapy, improving optimal doses and minimizing damage to healthy tissues, development, and augmentation of proton RT indications. Furthermore, we have the increasingly physiological hormone therapy in those dependent tumors and the great advancement in immunotherapy. Regarding chemotherapy, on the one hand, the use of intensive schemes that allow a greater response or cure and, on the other, the development of therapies directed at certain genetic and biological targets.

Just as important as these advances are, there is also the development of a better and earlier supportive treatment: nutritional, psychological, and pharmacological; the importance of a correct nutritional and psychological assessment to prepare the patient for treatment. Other factors include pharmacological development with potent antiemetics, granulocyte stimulators that decrease the duration of neutropenia, and new bisphosphonates or recombinant rasburicase that decrease the toxicity of chemotherapy.

Nowadays, early diagnosis of infections is fundamental through the systematic use of b-D glucan, galactomannan, PCR, or procalcitonin tests [12] as well as the use of noninvasive ventilation (NIV) or high-flow devices to perform fibrobronchoscopies and thus obtain samples for culture. Also the early use of better targeted antibiotics and the development of new antifungals and antibiotics after a long period without new patents have caused mortality around the treatment to decrease. Because of all this, from the 1990s to the present day, mortality from cancer has fallen by 23% [13].

But multidisciplinary collaboration and patient care decisions between oncologists, hematologists, and Intensive Care specialists have undoubtedly been fundamental, as demonstrated in numerous articles such as Soares et al. [6]. Primary care physicians are able to inform us of the prognosis, treatment options, and adverse effects of the traditional and new chemotherapy regimens. Intensivists can make the overall situation about the patient be understood from the real expectation of the medical situation that is being developed. And together, a plan can be agreed on in terms of time, in terms of limiting efforts, and together informing the patient and the family. The inclusion of other specialists such as pharmacists in cancer patient care has been shown to be beneficial because of the combination of polymedication and potential toxicity and interactions [6].

Better Results, but at What Cost?

The cost of this improvement in survival rates entails not only economic costs, even though this is very high (the cost of intensive care beds amounts to between 16.9% and 38.4% of hospital costs; approximately 200 billion dollars per year) but also more and more sick people those are dying in our units. A US review of Medicare of over 85,000,000 patients shows that the percentage of patients who were in ICU in their last month of life increased [14], rising from 24.3% in 2000 to 29.2% in 2009. Because of this, it has come to be considered as a quality measurement factor in many health care systems. Although the majority of cancer patients would prefer to die at home, the truth is that in the USA 40% of citizens die in hospital and nearly 60% do so after being admitted to the ICUs. One in five Americans dies in our units.

Organizational Aspects of the ICUs

In the following points, we will describe what organizational characteristics of our Intensive Care Units have proven to be beneficial in the treatment of cancer patients.

Oncologic vs General ICUs: Volume of Cases

With the first studies there seemed to be a difference in mortality in favour of ICUs specialising in cancer, mainly due to the large volume of admissions to intensive care. Patients with cancer and ARDS or septic shock had a mortality rate of between 34% and 50% when they were managed in oncology specialized ICUs while it raise to 66–68% in general ICUs [15]. Little by little, due to the transmission of knowledge and the monitoring of standardized protocols, this gap is gradually narrowing to practically the same level. Soares et al. [6] in a study of 9,946 patients with solid tumors could not demonstrate that the higher number of cases or the specialization of the ICU were determining factors for improving outcomes in these patients.

Multidisciplinary Care

Each day the ICUs are becoming less closed off and there is greater collaboration with a large number of specialists: oncologists, hematologists, specialists in infectious diseases, nephrologists, cardiologists, pneumologists, pharmacologists, etc. Although the daily burden of decision-making lies with the intensivist, there is more and more joint work with these specialists, both in terms of carrying out complementary tests and for consulting on specific problems or the progression of the illness. The development of working protocols in ICUs has also been shown to decrease the mortality of our patients, including general protocols for infection prevention, initiating early enteral nutrition, developing protective mechanical ventilation, using intermittent sedation, beginning physiotherapy and early mobilization, etc.

When deciding on admission to the ICU, several studies ([16]; Nasir et al. [17]) have shown that although a joint assessment by several specialists may be useful, it is the intensivist, due to his global assessment of the patient and experience in making such decisions, who is best placed to approach the reality of the process and who can best prevent inappropriate admissions (up to 37% according to Nasir et al. [17]), avoiding both aggressive procedures, family and patient stress, as well as delaying access to quality palliative care.

Joint daily sessions between intensivists and oncologists/hematologists for decision-making and the presence of a clinical pharmacologist on the rounds are associated with a reduction in mortality in critical oncology patients [6]. In addition, the presence of palliative care specialists on the rounds helps to improve patient comfort, improve symptom control, communication, and family participation in decisions.

Early Warning and Admissions

The importance of early detection of multi-organic dysfunction outside intensive care units has been noted for some time now; for this reason, "out of wall" ICU strategies have been developed over years to recognize this early dysfunction by means of early intervention teams or the active assessment of frail patients by intensivists. Song et al. [52] demonstrated in a general hospital that those patients who are transferred to the ICU early (four-hour cut-off point) have significantly lower mortality rates, lower costs, and significantly shorter hospital stays. Oncohematological patients are fragile patients, their immunological and nutritional status and the toxicity of their treatments make them particularly sensitive to a rapid deterioration in their physical functioning if something happens that makes them unstable. Therefore, early intervention in these patients is perhaps more important and evident than in the case of other sufferers. Recent studies carried out in Seoul [18] show that prompt care (<1.5 h after detecting the anomaly and assessing it) with respect to late care (>1.5 h) was accompanied by lower mortality in ICU (18.1% vs. 42.4%) and for hospital care (29% vs. 55.3%). Late care was also accompanied by increased need for vasoactive drugs, more severe neutropenia, and documented infection data.

Two multicentric studies in hematological [19] or oncological patients undergoing shock [20] show that delaying their admission to ICUs is an independent mortality factor.

The benefit is clearly associated with aggressive and early treatment of multi-organ dysfunction and prevention of organ failure. And within this group, tests or risk procedures would be performed on our patients in a safer and more controlled environment such as our ICUs.

Admission Policies

The decision to admit a patient to the ICU has always had a certain interpersonal and variable component; this is even more evident with cancer patients because of an ICU doctor's memory of not admitting them.

A study by Thiery et al. [21] showed that in a tertiary hospital, when cancer patients were referred to the ICU, 50% of them were rejected, with the label "cancer" being the main reason for their rejection. The 20% who were not admitted because they were "too well to be admitted" died before leaving the hospital and the 25% of patients who were initially rejected and subsequently admitted to the ICU left the hospital alive. This shows how difficult it is to get the admission decision right.

For all these reasons, admission policies in Intensive Care are changing and recommendations are being sought based on best practices and available evidence. All of them have a low level of evidence except the high-intensity ICU model characterized by the intensivist being responsible for day-to-day management of the patient in a closed ICU setting (level of evidence 1B) [8]. In the specific case of cancer patients, the SCCM recommends (no evidence available):

– Access to ICU on the basis established for all critical care patients, with careful consideration of their long-term prognosis
– These patients be reassessed and discussed with the patient, next of kin, legal representative, or power of attorney at regular intervals.

Given the difficulty of giving weight to these recommendations, new admission policies have been developed for cancer patients, and full code, ICU trial, or palliative care in ICU will be discussed in more detail at a later point.

As a summary of what is external to the patients themselves, Table 1 shows the factors that have been seen to have a positive influence on the care of the oncology patient in our Units.

Admission Criteria

The criteria that the intensivist must assess to admit a patient into the unit should include:

- The true indication or need for management in the ICU
- Presence of a trained specialist in the field
- Prioritizing depending on the patient's condition

Table 1 Hospital organizational factors that improve care

Hospital organizational factors that improve care
A high-intensity ICU model characterized by the intensivist being responsible for day-to-day management of the patient in a closed ICU setting
ICU's relationship and collaboration with other services
Joint daily decision-making between critical care physicians, hematologists, and oncologists
Participation in medical rounds made by other specialists such as palliative care physicians or clinical pharmacologists
Drawing up protocols for routine care and procedures in intensive care as well as the provision of clinical guidelines
Strategies for the early detection of multiorganic dysfunction, either by means of early intervention teams, through alarms in clinical information systems, or with the help of rounds by intensive care physicians assessing the frail patients at the request of their treating physicians
Dissemination of the knowledge and facts about the cancer patients in triage for admission to hospital
Introducing early palliative care for critical ill cancer patients
Structure and equipment so as to offer the necessary care in the different admission policies: Full code, ICU trial, exceptional admissions, or palliative care in ICU

- Reason for admission
- Bed availability
- Objective vital data
- Patient prognosis
- Potential benefit of interventions performed on the patient

This is really what is done every day when patients are assessed. According to the beds available in the unit, the patient is assessed, taking into account his/her background, prognosis, acute condition, and whether or not his/her needs can be met in the ICU.

There are four pillars of assessment (Fig. 1) when it comes to determining whether to admit a cancer patient to the ICU from the patient's perspective.

In the following paragraphs, what factors within each of these pillars will be explained and how they can and should affect our decision when deciding to admit a cancer patient.

The Patient and Their Characteristics

The cancer patient presents some differentiating characteristics in comparison with other patients. This does not mean that different measures are taken to restrict their access to the ICU; moreover, because they are cancer patients, they should not have fewer opportunities for admission than others.

Among the characteristics **that should not influence** us when deciding on their admission are age, the presence of neutropenia, as well

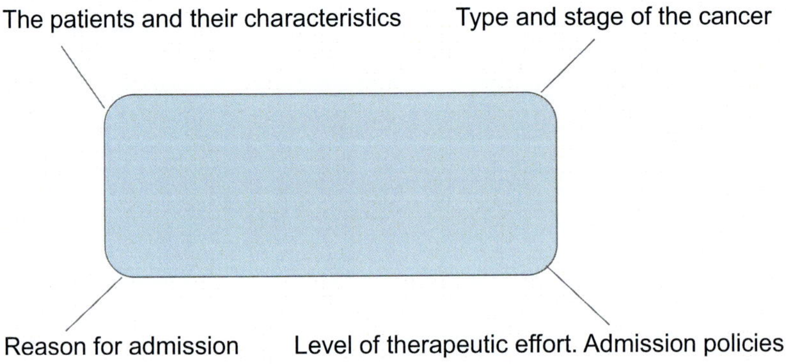

Fig. 1 Pillars of assessment

The patients and their characteristics   Type and stage of the cancer

Reason for admission   Level of therapeutic effort. Admission policies as hematological disease with autologous transplants.

It has already been demonstrated in numerous articles that access to intensive care units is not restricted for the elderly. Recommendation 2c of the SCCM guidelines is to assess the comorbidities of patients, their physical functional status, and the severity of the process coupled with their opinion rather than the chronological age in patients over the age of 80. Specifically in our patients, a review of Auclin et al. [22] found no difference in the subgroup of older cancer patients (75 +/− 6.7 years) with those who did not have tumor disease (33.6% vs. 32.6%).

Neutropenia in cancer patients is not a risk factor for them. Bouteloup et al. [23] in a systematic review of 6,054 cancer patients of whom 2,097 had neutropenia in studies between 2005 and 2015 found that neutropenia when adjusted for patient severity did not affect patient mortality.

Patients with blood disorders, who have undergone autologous bone marrow transplantation, due to the intensity of chemotherapy and the increased frequency of neutropenia and organ failure have typically presented slightly higher mortality rates; but advances in supportive care and ICU treatments have made it similar to that of any patient in general intensive care units today [24].

Among the factors that **marginally affect** their prognosis are admission severity scores (which actually tell us about the patient's multi-organ dysfunction) as well as excessive comorbidity.

All the clinical scoring commonly used in ICUs at admission (MPM, APACHE, or SAPS) overestimate the severity of the cancer patients' condition by considerably increasing the probability of having tumor disease [25]. For all these reasons, other more specific indices (HCT-CI or Cancer Mortality Model CMM) ([26, 53]) have been developed and are pending validation through multicenter trials. SOFA does appear to have a good discriminatory capacity to predict mortality rates in ICUs and hospitals of oncology patients admitted for medical reasons, rather than for surgical procedures, according to a review by Cárdenas-Turanzas et al. [27] of a population of 6,645 patients admitted to an oncology ICU. Aygencel et al. [28] found a SOFA value of 9 or higher in patients with solid tumors or 10 or higher in patients with hematological tumors as the highest mortality indicator in critical oncological patients. More important than the number of organ failures on admission of our patients is their response to treatment during the first few days of their stay in our units. The persistence or worsening of this multi-organ dysfunction is clearly associated with mortality in ICU. This is the basis of the ICU trial that will be discussed below.

Other factors, which should be taken into account, are their previous quality of life, their performance status, personal and family decisions regarding their decision to be admitted to the ICU, and the appearance of complications in an allogeneic transplant.

The patient's previous quality of life as measured by the performance status (PS) is a simple scale that assesses the patient's physical functionality and quality of life (Table 2). It is useful for predicting mortality in all critical patients and has been corroborated by numerous studies in critical cancer patients. A PS 3–4 is associated with an increase in ICU mortality of four to seven times in patients with a PS 0–2 [4]. Only those situations in which the deterioration of the patient's condition is due to a recent diagnosis of the tumor or a potentially reversible cause would be significantly improved with aggressive treatment.

Table 2 ECOG performance status

Grade	ECOG performance status
	Description
0	Fully active, able to carry out all pre-disease performance without restriction
1	Restricted in physically strenuous activity but ambulatory and able to carry out work of a light or sedentary nature
2	Ambulatory and capable of all self-care but unable to carry out any work activities. Up and about more than 50% of waking hours
3	Capable of only limited self-care, confined to bed or chair more than 50% of waking hours
4	Completely disabled. Cannot carry out any self-care. Totally confined to bed or chair
5	Dead

According to the 5th International Consensus Conference on Intensive Care, the decision to limit treatment in the ICU should be based on the principle of patient autonomy.

Because that only 5% of the patients admitted to our units have the capacity to make decisions about their illness intact [29], prior consensus between the patient, family members, and treating physicians is essential. When this does not occur, the patient receives more aggressive measures and usually loses the possibility of receiving quality palliative care. For all these reasons, it is essential to advance along the path of dynamic decision-making during the course of the disease [30]. The oncologist's continuous, immediate, and clear communication, the patient's functional status, as well as the therapeutic options at all times must be weighed against each other in order to clearly understand the transition from curative to palliative care. But we still find that even in cancer centers, many patients are not sure of the essential measures they need to take with their oncologists, such as non-resuscitation [31].

The need for intensive care admission for allogeneic transplant patients has decreased by 8% over the past two decades; mortality has also decreased from 80% in the 1990s to 60% today [32]. Although infections are common in these patients, the main cause of death is severe respiratory failure requiring mechanical ventilation of a noninfectious origin. In spite of the high mortality rate, admission is still recommended for its management, especially if complications appear in the immediate post-transplant period. But the appearance of multi-organ failure in these patients, especially in the midst of anti-graft disease, should prompt us to reconsider the decision to go ahead.

Intensivist cannot base the decision of admission to the ICU on the stage of the tumor. This has been inconsistently associated with increased mortality. Thus, while some studies showed that patients with stage IV or metastatic tumors were more likely to die in hospital [33, 34], other more recent studies with a greater number of patients ([22, 35]) did not find a link between disseminated disease and short-term outcomes (ICU and hospital mortality).

Provided there are therapeutic options, the failure of any treatment line should not be a reason to refuse admission [11]. Yes, tumor progression without treatment options is associated with poor prognosis.

The origin and histological classification of the tumor is not related to prognosis in the ICU, although it does influence long-term outcomes. Typically, hemato-oncological diseases have had worse outcomes than solid tumors, but these differences have been disappearing over the years in ICU and hospital mortality outcomes [36, 37]. However there are groups of patients in whom mortality has remained virtually unchanged and remains extremely high and whose admission must be considered; these bone marrow transplant patients with severe graft-versus-host disease (GVHD) do not respond to immunosuppressive therapy. Also, these are the patients who exhibit solid tumors with severe complications such as acute respiratory failure due to lymphangitis, meningeal carcinomatosis, and coma or when they infiltrate and produce spinal cord failure.

With regard to tumor disease, it is believed that the following indications (Table 3) are shown in and are usually accepted in any cancer center.

Tumor Type and Stage

Cancer patients are an extremely heterogeneous group of patients. There are many and very different types of tumors, each one of them with a different evolution according to its genetics and biology; with different answers for the same treatment depending on the evolutionary stage of the disease and even in each individual.

Reason for Admission

Each hospital has its own particular caseload regarding the reasons for admission of oncohematological patients to its ICUs; this will depend on whether we are in an oncology hospital, in a privately or publicly managed hospital, and the ratio of ICU beds to the patient reference population.

Table 3 Admission criteria from the perspective of the disease

Admission criteria from the perspective of the disease
Patients in complete remission
Newly diagnosed patients of less than 3 months and with a life expectancy of more than 6 months
Patient with failure of one or more treatment lines but with future options (transplant, clinical trial) without malignant involvement of vital organs
Patients with treatment toxicity, complications of this treatment or of procedures related to its process
Patients in clinical trials whose aggravation may be related to the treatment
Patients in whom it is essential to reduce tumor pressure, which is responsible for complications and organ failure. QT is safe in the ICU and its administration does not worsen the prognosis [11]

We will now look at the main reasons for admission to our units Soubani [9] and the advances and changes that have led to improved survival of clinical profiles (Table 4).

New Strategies of ICU Admission

There are four scenarios in which cancer patients have a place depending on all the variables previously analyzed (Fig. 2):

- *Full code management*: This would be treatment with curative intent and without restrictions, similar to any other critical care patient.
- *ICU trial*: An increasingly accepted admission policy that began with a study of hematological patients with respiratory failure by Lecuyer et al. [42]. All oncohematological patients (except bedridden patients, those who refused admission and palliative care patients) were admitted to the ICU for 3 days without restrictions in terms of techniques, treatments (including QT), and resources. It was observed that all patients who worsened in terms of their organ dysfunction (by measuring the SOFA) by day three of admission showed a clearly unfavorable development with those who improved in terms of their organ dysfunction by the third day of admission. All those patients who required mechanical ventilation,

vasopressors, or dialysis after the third day died. This unrestricted ICU test is currently the path being followed in most intensive care units when faced with the admission of an oncology patient [43, 44]. Recent studies attempt to establish the optimal trial period such as Shrime et al. [45] concluding that trials of ICU care lasting 1–4 days may be sufficient in patients with poor-prognosis solid tumors, whereas patients with hematologic malignant neoplasms or less severe illness seem to benefit from longer trials of intensive care.

- *No ICU admission* and no intensive care treatment: No indication of admission or use of intensive care therapy such as renal clearance techniques or noninvasive ventilation.
- *ICU admission outside of routine indications*: Here there would be prophylactic admissions, exceptional admissions, as well as palliative care administration.

ICU Discharge

Related literature in the last few years is full of admission criteria, patient and disease characteristics, causes for admission, and its policies, but few articles evaluate the reasons, timing, and follow-up of ICU discharges, especially in relation to cancer patients.

A meta-analysis of Hosein et al. [46] on the discharge from ICU of almost two million patients found that, of every 100 patients discharged alive from ICU, between 4 and 6 are re-admitted and 3–7 die before being discharged again from hospital. This has led to the search for safety predictors in patients discharged from the ICUs, as well as to the enabling of discharge or follow-up policies that reduce these complications.

The discharge APACHE II score and hospital length of stay before ICU admission are significant independent factors in predicting post-ICU mortality and is superior to the admission APACHEII score in predicting early ICU readmission in surgical ICU patients.

On the other hand, seeing how the rapid response teams have demonstrated their

Table 4 Improvement areas depending cause of admission

Causes of admission (%)	Improvement areas
Postoperative elective or emergency 50–60%	Increased specialization in surgery, as well as in case management, and fast track recovery management
Severe sepsis and septic shock 16–18%	Early recognition of sepsis and rapid implementation of sepsis bundles Better understanding and management of multiorgan failure Use of biomarkers to diagnostic

Respiratory failure 10%
   Infectious
   Noninfectious: ARDS secondary to polytransfusion, underlying disease, treatment and/or toxicity of same
	Early NIV may be harmful
	High-flow oxygen has demonstrated survival benefits compared to NIV [38, 39]
	Compared to BAL, noninvasive tests have the same diagnostic and therapeutic fields
	Do not delay mechanical ventilation if indicated
	Protective lung ventilation

Change in level of consciousness 5%
   Metabolic
   Sepsis
   Cerebral LOE versus bleeding
   Posterior reversible encephalopathy
	Daily interruption of sedation
	New sedative agents
	Sedation based on analgesia

Oncological emergencies: 3%
   Tumor lysis syndrome (TLS)
   Superior vena cava syndrome (SVCS)
   Cardiac tamponade
   Airway obstruction
   Hypercalcemia
	Early admission of cancer patients at risk of tumor lysis syndrome or renal failure has been shown to improve survival
	Use of ultrasound at the bedside

Bleeding from leakage, coagulopathy, thrombopenia 2%	The values of Hb without active bleeding are considered safe around 7 g/dl except in postoperative major surgery which should be greater than 9 g/dl [40] The dysfunction of platelet aggregation and the alteration of vascular integrity means that we should not look only at the number of platelets to indicate their transfusion
Concomitant medical processes: ischemic heart disease, COPD, PTE, liver failure, renal failure, etc. 2%	The increasing knowledge of the adverse effects of cancer treatments helps us to focus on the dysfunction of the affected organ
Administration of QT in fragile patients or patients with an allergy to QT 1%	Providing it in the safe environment of the ICU reduces complications and has better results. Associated sepsis or need for life support at the same time is not a contraindication to administer it [41]
PostRCP	Survival is <2% and ICU care after resuscitation may be considered futile
Multiple readmissions for organic dysfunction after ICU admission	Hospital mortality is multiplied by 11 and cancer treatment is not usually continued, so continued readmissions can be considered futile

usefulness in reducing the mortality of cancer patients in ICUs by detecting their organic dysfunction early, an attempt has been made to transfer this model to close monitoring by intensive care doctors, nurses, and respiratory specialists of those patients who are discharged from ICUs during the first 48–72 h. These Critical care transition programs have been widely assessed by Stelfox et al. [47]. After analyzing 32,234 patients over 10 years in eight hospitals, he has observed that, although there is a certain trend towards a decrease in readmissions in the patients followed by these teams compared to the control group (also described in the meta-analysis by Niven et al. for the NHS), a significant difference in mortality cannot be determined for both groups.

The SCCM in its guidelines on admission and discharge policy for ICUs recommends a series of

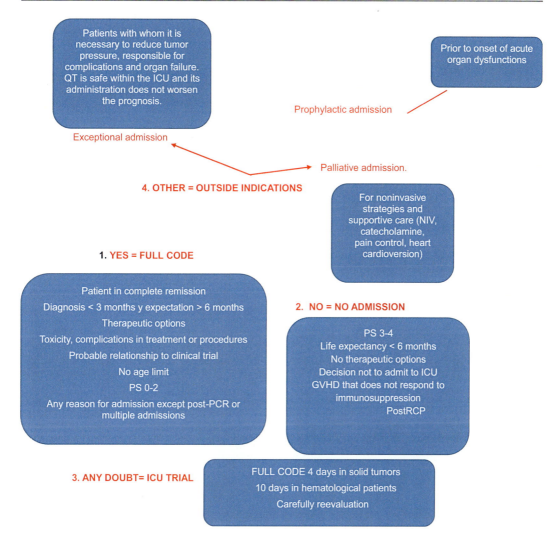

Fig. 2 Admission policies

actions, most of them lacking any compelling evidence, but which are widely accepted and usually carried out by the majority of intensive care physicians.

– Discharge patients when they are physiologically stable and do not require monitoring or their own intensive care treatment.
– Discharge patients at a lower level of acute care depending on patient disposition, prognosis, stability, or the need for patient interventions.
– Taking into account, as we discussed previously APACHE II at discharge, the rates as an aid in identifying those patients at high risk

of deterioration following discharge from the ICU.
– Whenever possible, especially with frail patients, talk to the doctor receiving the patient to tell him/her about their progress, treatment, and management. This could reduce the frequency of readmissions.
– With level 2C, patients would not be discharged at night, hospital mortality has increased (OR1.31), but there is no difference between discharging them on weekdays and weekends.
– Also, with level 2C there would be the use of intermediate care units or long-stay hospitals

for those patients who are still fragile, either because of the severity of the disease, their multiple comorbidities, physiological instability, or because they still have the support of a vital organ at discharge.

Regarding the survival and quality of life outcomes of cancer patients, studies tend to focus on intra-ICU mortality, hospital mortality or mortality at 30–90 days. Such short results do not give us valid conclusions as to the actual benefits and overall cost-effectiveness of ICU care in cancer patients. Fifteen years ago, the one-year survival rate for cancer and hematological patients was 25% [48], whereas more recent studies place it between 18 and 64% [49].

In general, it seems to be shown that the long-term survival of cancer patients does not depend on the severity of the process or the time spent in the ICUs, but rather on the prognosis of the tumor disease [50].

Summary

The progressive increase in the incidence of cancer cases (mainly solids), the technological advance, the accumulated experience, and, above all, the better knowledge of the etiopathogenesis of the neoformative processes have sparked interest in this type of patients from all areas. The ICUs are not alien to this interest, seeing in these patients the possibilities that they did not see before, considering this group of patients in a similar way to another subgroup of severe diseases. But not everything goes, sensibly they have been developing guidelines of action or strategies against them according to the moment of the diagnosis and treatment options, with special attention to the moment in which they develop failure of some organ and evaluating each day this dysfunction. This careful monitoring within a multidisciplinary team, far from the usual loneliness of the intensivist, has brought the possibilities of survival in our units closer to that of any other type of seriously ill patient. Today we can say that no cancer patient should have fewer opportunities for treatment than another critical patient, always respecting personal autonomy.

References

1. Soares M, Carusi P, Silva E, et al. Characteristics and outcomes of patients with cancer requiring admission to intensive care units: a prospective multicenter study. Crit Care Med. 2010;38(1):9–15.
2. Azoulay E, Alberti C, Bornstain C, et al. Improved survival in cancer patients requiring mechanical ventilation support: impact of noninvasive mechanical support. Crit Care Med. 2001;29(3):519–25.
3. Taccone FS, Artigas AA, Sprung CL, Moreno R, Sakr Y, Vincent JL. Characteristics and outcomes of cancer patients in European ICUs. Crit Care 2009;13(1):R15.
4. Puxty K, McLoone P, Quasim T, et al. Survival in solid cancer patients following intensive care unit admission. Intensive Care Med. 2014;40(10):1409–28.
5. Toffart AC, Pizarro C, Schwebel C, et al. Selection criteria for intensive care unit referral of lung cancer patients: a pilot study. Eur Respir J. 2015;45:491–500.
6. Soares M, Bozza FA, Azevedo CP, et al. Effects of organizational characteristics on outcomes and resource use in patients with cancer admitted to intensive care units. J Clin Oncol. 2016;34:3315–24.
7. Carmona-Bayonas A, Gordo F, Beato C, et al. Intensive care in cancer patients in the age of immunotherapy and molecular therapies: commitment of the SEOM-SEMICYUC. Med Intensiva. 2018;42:363.
8. Nates JL, Nunnally M, Kleinpell R, Blosser S, Goldner J, Birriel B, Fowler CS, Byrum D, Miles WS, Bailey H, Sprung CL. ICU admission, discharge, and triage guidelines: a framework to enhance clinical operations, development of institutional policies, and further research. Crit Care Med. 2016;44(8):1553–602.
9. Soubani O. Critical care prognosis and outcomes in patients with cancer. Clin Chest Med. 2017;38(2): 333–353.
10. Pinsky MR, Brochard L, Kellum JA. Ten recent advances that could not have come about without applying physiology. Intensive Care Med. 2015. https://doi.org/10.1007/s00134-015-3746-9. Online print 25th March.
11. Azoulay E, Pene F, Darmon M, et al. Managing critically ill hematology patients: time to think differently. Blood Rev. 2015;29(6):359–67.
12. Sbrana A, Torchio M, Comolli G, et al. Use of procalcitonin in clinical oncology: a literature review. New Microbiol. 2016;39(3):174–80.
13. Miller KD, Siegel RL, Lin CC, et al. Cancer treatment and survivorship statistics. CA Cancer J Clin. 2016;66: 271–89.
14. Teno JM, Gozalo PL, Bynum J, et al. Change in end-of-life care for Medicare beneficiaries: site of dead, place

of care, and health care transitions in 2000, 2005 and 2009. JAMA. 2009;309(5):470–7.

15. Benoit DD, Soares M, Azoulay E. Has survival increased in cancer patients admitted to the ICU? We are not sure. Intensive Care Med. 2014;40(10):1576–9.

16. Soubani AO, Decruyenaere J. Improved outcome of critically ill patients with hematological malignancies: what is next? Intensive Care Med. 2014;40(9):1377–8.

17. Nasir SS, Muthiad M, Ryder K, et al. ICU deaths in patients with advanced cancer: reasonable criteria to decrease potentially inappropriate admissions and lack of benefit of advance planning discussions. Am J Hosp Palliat Med. 2017;34(2):173–179.

18. Suh GY, Ryu JA, Chung CR, et al. Effect of early intervention on long term outcomes of critically ill cancer patients admitted to ICUs. Crit Care Med. 2015;43(7):1439–48.

19. Azoulay E, Mokart D, Péne E, et al. Outcomes of critically ill patients with hematological malignances prospective multicenter data from France and Belgium. J Clin Oncol. 2013;31(22):2810–8.

20. de Monmollin E, Tandjaoui-Lambiotte Y, Legrand M, et al. Outcome in critically ill cancer patients with septic shock of pulmonary origin. Shock. 2013;39(3):250–4.

21. Thiery G, Azoulay E, Darmon M, et al. Outcome of cancer patients considered for intensive care unit admission: a hospital-wide prospective study. J Clin Oncol. 2005;23(19):4406–13.

22. Auclin E, Charles-Nelson A, Abbar B, et al. Outcomes in elderly patients admitted to the intensive care unit with solid tumors. Ann Intensive Care. 2017;7:26.

23. Bouteloup M, Perinel S, Bourmaud A, et al. Outcomes in adult critically ill cancer patients with and without neutropenia: a systematic review and meta-analysis of the Groupe de Recherche en Réanimation Respiratoire du patient d'Onco-Hématologie (GRRR-OH). Oncotarget. 2017;8(1):1860–70.

24. Al-Zubaidi N, Soubani AO. Predictors of mortality in patients with hematologic malignancies admitted to the ICU- a prospective observational study. Am J Respir Crit Care Med. 2016;193:A3657.

25. Soares M, Fontes F, Dantas J, et al. Performance of six severity-of-illness scores in cancer patients requiring admission to the intensive care unit: a prospective observational study. Crit Care Med. 2004;8(4):R194–203.

26. Bayraktar UD, Shpall EJ, Liu P, et al. Hematopoietic cell transplantation specific comorbidity index predicts inpatient mortality and survival in patients who received allogeneic transplantation admitted to the intensive care unit. J Clin Oncol. 2013;31(33):4207–14.

27. Cárdenas-Turanzas M, Ensor J, Wakefield C, et al. Cross-validation of a Sequential Organ Failure Assessment score-based model to predict mortality in patients with cancer admitted to the intensive care unit. J Crit Care. 2012;27(6):673–80.

28. Aygencel G, Turkoglu M, Turkoz Sucak G, et al. Prognostic factors in critically ill cancer patients admitted to the intensive care unit. J Crit Care. 2014;29:618–26.

29. Prendergast TJ, Luce JM. Increasing incidence of withholding and withdrawal of life support from the critically ill. Am J Respir Crit Care Med. 1997;155(1):15–20.

30. Kostakou E, Rovina N, Kyriakopoulou M, et al. Critically ill cancer patient in intensive care unit: issues that arise. J Crit Care. 2014;29:817–22.

31. Keating NL, Landrum MB, Rogers SO, et al. Physician factors associated with discussions about end-of-life care. Cancer. 2010;116(4):998–1006.

32. Afessa B, Azoulay E. Critical care of the hematopoietic stem cell transplant recipient. Crit Care Med. 2010;26(1):133–50.

33. Mendoza V, Lee A, Mark PE. The hospital survival and prognostic factors of patients with solid tumors admitted to an ICU. Am J Hosp Palliat Care. 2008;25:240–3.

34. Soares M, Salluh JL, Spector N, Rocco JR. Characteristics and outcomes of cancer patients requiring mechanical ventilatory support for >24 hrs. Crit Care Med. 2005;33:520–6.

35. Maccariello E, Valente C, Nogueira L, et al. Outcomes of cancer and non-cancer patients with acute kidney injury and need of renal replacement therapy admitted to general intensive care units. Nephrol Dial Transplant. 2011;26:537–43.

36. Benoit DD, Vandewoude KH, Decruyenaere JM, et al. Outcome and early prognostic indicators in patients with a hematologic malignancy admitted to the ICU for a life-threatening complication. Crit Care Med. 2003;31(1):104–12.

37. Shimabukuro-Vornhagen A, Boll B, Kochanek M, et al. Critical care of patients with cancer. CA Cancer J Clin. 2016;66:496–517.

38. Frat JP, Thile AW, Mercat A, et al. High flow oxygen through nasal cannula in acute hypoxemic respiratory failure. N Engl J Med. 2015;372:2186–96.

39. Mokart D, Geay C, Chow-Chine L, et al. High flow oxygen therapy in cancer patients with acute respiratory failure. Intensive Care Med. 2015;41:2008–10.

40. de Almeida JP, Vincent JL, Galas FR, et al. Transfusion requirements in surgical oncology patients: a prospective randomized controlled trial. Anesthesiology. 2015;122:29–38.

41. Azoulay E, Schellongowski P, Darmon M, et al. The Intensive Care Medicine research agenda on critically ill oncology and hematology patients. Intensive Care Med. 2017;43:1366–82.

42. Lecuyer L, Chevret S, Guidet B, et al. The ICU trial: a new admission policy for cancer patients requiring mechanical ventilation. Crit Care Med. 2007;35(3):808–14.

43. Azoulay E, Afessa B. The intensive care support of patients with malignance: do everything that can be done. Intensive Care Med. 2006;32:3–5.

44. Suhag V, Sunita BS, Sarin A, et al. Intensive care for cancer patients, an overview. Asian Australas J Anim. 2014;13:193–201.

45. Shrime MG, Ferket BS, Scott DJ, et al. Time-limited trials of intensive care for critically ill patients with

cancer: how long is long enough? JAMA Oncol. 2016;2:76–83.

46. Hosein FS, Roberts DJ, Turin TC, et al. A meta-analysis to derive literature-based benchmarks for readmission and hospital mortality after patient discharge from intensive care. Crit Care. 2014;18 (6):715.

47. Stelfox HT, Bastos J, Niven DJ, et al. Critical care transition programs and the risk of readmission or death after discharge from ICU. Intensive Care Med. 2016;42(3):401–10.

48. Staudinger T, Stoiser B, Mullner M, et al. Outcome and prognostic factors in critically ill cancer patients admitted to the intensive care unit. Crit Care Med. 2000;28:1322–1328.

49. Wohlfarth P, Staudinger T, Sperr W, et al. Prognostic factors, long term survival, and outcome of cancer patients receiving chemotherapy. Ann Hematol. 2014;93:1629–1636.

50. Wohlfarth P, Beutel G, Lebiedz P, et al. Characteristics and outcome of patients after allogenic sterm cell transplantation treated with extracorporeal membrane oxygenation for acute respiratory distress syndrome. Crit care Med. 2017;45:e500–e507.

51. Mogal HD, Levine E, Fino N, et al. Routine Admission to Intensive Care Unit after cytoreductive surgery and heated intraperitoneal chemotherapy: not always a requirement. Ann Surg Oncol. 2015;23:1486–1495.

52. Song JU, Suh GY, Park HY, et al. Early intervention on the outcomes in critically ill cancer patients admitted to intensive care unit. Intensive Care Med. 2012;38(9):1505–13. https://doi.org/10.1007/s00134-012-2594-0

53. Soares M, Fontes F, Dantas J, et al. Performance of six severity-of-illness scores in cancer patients requiring admission to the intensive care unit: a prospective observational study. Crit Care Med. 2004;8(4):R194–203.

ICU Staffing, Models, and Outcomes

4

Karen Chen and Joseph L. Nates

Contents

Introduction 34

Open Versus Closed ICUs 34

Leapfrog Group Standards 35

Staffing Models 35

Associated Costs in Various Models 37

Associated Outcomes with 24-Hour In-house Intensivists 38

Patient Ratios 38

Burnout Syndrome in Intensivists 39

Summary 40

References 41

Abstract

As one of the most expensive resources in the healthcare system, the intensive care units (ICUs) are closely monitored for appropriate utilization and adequate staffing. The latter, considered one of the most challenging and controversial, is extensively discussed in this chapter. Optimal staffing of an ICU is highly dependent on multiple factors including, but not limited to availability of trained personnel, educational trainees, acuity of patients, size of ICU, and economic constraints. Therefore, staffing models need to be carefully selected and implemented based on the local setting. The key commodity in ICU staffing is the availability of specialty trained personnel, namely the intensivists and ICU nurses. Thus, in order to efficiently staff the ICU, attracting and retaining the intensivists, requires creative models which may focus on time off and lifestyle factors. The benefits of open versus closed units, high-intensity versus low-intensity models, and the classic academic and 24-h models are explored to provide the reader with a clear understanding of the benefits of these complex options and associated outcomes.

K. Chen · J. L. Nates (✉)
Department of Critical Care and Respiratory Care, The University of Texas MD Anderson Cancer Center, Houston, TX, USA
e-mail: kachen@mdanderson.org; jlnates@mdanderson.org

© Springer Nature Switzerland AG 2020
J. L. Nates, K. J. Price (eds.), *Oncologic Critical Care*,
https://doi.org/10.1007/978-3-319-74588-6_2

Keywords

ICU staffing · ICU beds · Leapfrog Group ·
ICU models · Open ICU · Closed ICU ·
Moonlighting · Telemedicine · Advance
practice providers · Hospitalists · Intensivists

Introduction

Intensive care is one of the most expensive aspects of health care in the United States. By some estimates, it has exceeded 108 billion dollars in 2010 [1]. Although ICU beds usually comprise approximately only 10% of the hospital beds, its associated costs are around 30% of the hospital budget [2]. As the population ages, associated healthcare costs and ICU utilization will increase. Thus, ICU staffing with its impact on outcomes and costs will need to be clearly evaluated.

The patients in the ICU utilize specially trained personnel in order to implement effective processes and perform specialized procedures in order to improve mortality and length of stay (LOS) [2]. Due to the limitation of resources along with its associated costs, staffing of the ICU in the United States varies widely throughout the nation.

The sentinel paper affecting ICU physician staffing was published in 2002 by Pronovost et al. [2]. In this landmark study, critical care staffing came into the forefront. The ICU groups were classified into high-intensity (mandatory intensivist consultation or closed ICU, where all care was directed by the intensivists) versus low-intensity (no intensivist involvement or elective intensivist consultation). In this study, high-intensity ICU physician staffing reduced hospital and ICU mortality as well as hospital and ICU LOS [2]. At the time of the study, it was estimated that only about one third of the ICUs in the United States utilized a high-intensity staffing model [3]. This contrasts to the predominantly closed ICU staffing model utilized throughout Europe and Australia.

Open Versus Closed ICUs

A basic premise in staffing a critical care unit first depends on a closed versus an open ICU system. In a closed ICU, only critical care staff admits and manages the critically ill patient. The primary service becomes a consultant on these patients. All decisions in a closed ICU are made by the critical care team, taking into consideration the advice as provided by the consultants. All issues are addressed by the critical care team and admission to and discharge from the ICU is determined by the critical care staff. In terms of ICU staffing, this is usually the most labor intensive as it requires a dedicated ICU team to provide consistent care and efficiently triage patients in and out of the ICU around the clock. This is the predominant staffing model utilized in Europe and in Australia. Although it is not widely implemented in the United States, when it is used, it is most commonly found in major academic medical centers due to the significant amount of resources required.

On the other hand, an open ICU allows anyone with hospital admission privileges to admit and treat with or without the involvement of the ICU team. In essence, ICU admission, management, and subsequent discharge are at the discretion of the admitting physician. Essentially, the ICU provides nursing care, monitoring, and certain therapies that may be limited to ICU utilization (i.e., vasopressors, invasive monitoring) without requiring ICU attending consultation or input.

Many current ICU models utilize a system which is a hybrid between the two. These ICUs are considered either semi-closed or semi-open. By definition, the semi-closed ICU is one in which anyone can admit a patient to the ICU, but the critical care team is automatically consulted and comanages all patients. Whereas in the semi-open unit, anyone can admit a patient to the ICU and the critical care team is consulted but not all patients are comanaged.

Thus utilizing these definitions, the closed and semi-closed ICUs would be considered high-intensity staffing versus the open and semi-open ICUs which would be considered the low-intensity staffing as defined by the Pronovost study in JAMA [4].

Leapfrog Group Standards

New ICU staffing models were proposed after the Institute of Medicine published a report in 1999 showing a high rate of preventable medical errors [37]. In addition, it was noted many ICUs had an unacceptably high rate of mortality with an exorbitant cost structure. Due to this financial burden, health care purchasers became involved [5]. Most notably, the Leapfrog Group, a consortium representing large employers who are purchasers of health care, proposed regulatory guidelines in ICU physician staffing (IPS) to improve the quality of care and with associated cost containment thus increasing value in the healthcare system [6].

As noted in the Leapfrog-ICU Physician Staffing (IPS) factsheet, over 200,000 patients die in US ICUs each year [7]. Unfortunately, the quality varies widely across hospitals [8]. Thus, in order to improve the quality of care, certain requirements were placed on IPS by the Leapfrog Group. The two major components affecting the quality of care include whether "intensivists" are providing care and how the staff is organized in the ICU (open vs. closed ICUs) [6].

By the Leapfrog IPS standard, the definition of "intensivists" must satisfy one of the following: board-certified physicians who are additionally certified in the subspecialty of critical care medicine or physicians who are board-certified in medicine, anesthesiology, pediatrics, emergency medicine, or surgery who have completed training prior to the availability of a subspecialty certification in critical care and provide at least 6 weeks of full-time ICU care each year [6]. Neurointensivists are an approved alternative to intensivists as well.

The Leapfrog IPS safety standard requires intensivists who are present during daytime hours and provide clinical care exclusively in the ICU and when not present on-site or via telemedicine, returns notification alerts at least 95% of the time within 5 min, and arranges for a physician, physician assistant, nurse practitioner, or a FCCS-certified nurse to reach ICU patients within 5 min [6].

Many challenges have come out of meeting the Leapfrog IPS standards. Some of these include: some nonintensivist physicians unwilling to relinquish care to intensivists, lack of intensivists due to shortage of available personnel, decreased sizes of training programs in critical care, many board-certified intensivists choose not to work in the ICU [9], and small hospitals may lack the economies of scale to support full-time intensivists thus necessitating consolidation of these units or introduction of telemedicine into these units [6].

Various models need to incentivize the commodity, which currently is the skilled labor force, which namely consists of the critical care intensivist and/or physician extenders. As noted by studies published by the major professional societies representing critical care, namely SCCM and ATS, these shortfalls will continue to worsen as the need for critical care services increases as the workforce cannot keep up with these demands and provide due to multiple reasons [10, 11].

A report to Congress by Duke also noted this shortfall to continue through 2020 though not predicted to be at the same pace as per the methodology of the COMPACCS study [12].

Staffing Models

As there has been tremendous growth in the number, size, and occupancy of ICU beds, but not a commensurate growth in critical care physicians, there is a workforce shortage to staff these ICUs [13]. Multiple issues have led to the shortfall in the workforce. This includes lack of critical care intensivists, lack of resident and fellow trainees due to restricted work hours, and lack of critical care nursing staff. In addition, the cost of care in an ICU along with decreased reimbursements as well as the 24–7 coverage needed, whether in-house or readily available, adds an additional layer of complexity to ICU staffing. Although "society invests billions in the development of new drugs and technologies but comparatively little in the fidelity of health care, that is, improving systems to ensure delivery of care to all patients in need" [14]. Due to the various factors as outlined earlier, novel models for staffing critical care units will need to be utilized in order to deliver effective care. This chapter will focus on the staffing of the critical care unit as it applies to intensivists, house staff, and other licensed allied providers. It will not discuss nurse staffing for the ICU.

In order to bridge the gap, various models to staff the ICUs have been utilized. There are advantages and disadvantages to each of these models, which are described in further below.

Historically, the academic model with 24-h coverage has been the default model in most critical care units. This model traditionally utilizes residents, fellows, and medical students led by an attending physician. Challenges in staffing this model include poor work–life balance, limited availability of trainees due to duty hour and length of shift restrictions, as well as limited attending faculty available to work nights, weekends, and holidays. This strictly academic in-house intensivist model is resource heavy and extremely costly. A recent meta-analysis has shown that in-house nighttime intensivist staffing has not resulted in improved patient outcomes [15]. In addition, in many institutions this has become nonviable due to lack of residents and fellows or due to the duty hour restrictions on them. Furthermore, as critical care is a subspecialty with all providers first having primary training in surgery, anesthesiology, pulmonary, internal or emergency medicine, many trainees choose or resort back to their primary specialties due to the better quality of life or financial incentives offered in the primary specialty. Thus, the available resource pool to staff this model is highly restrictive.

A variation of this model would be the modified academic model, which may provide 24-h in-house coverage with fundamentals of critical care support (FCCS) certified providers in-house with backup from an attending physician available 24 h a day. This has been typically utilized due to the limited availability of trainees to fill this role in house 24 h a day. In this model, instead of or in addition to the trainees, advanced practice providers (APPs) such as physician assistants (PA) or advanced practice registered nurses who are FCCS certified supervised by an attending physician provide care in the ICU. Many ICUs throughout the nation are using advanced practice providers (APPs) including nurse practitioner (NP) and PAs to cover the shortfall in meeting ICU workforce demands [16, 17]. A comprehensive review of the literature by Kleinpell et al. concluded that the literature supports the value of APPs in patient management, reinforcement of practice guidelines, education of patients, families and ICU staff as well as quality and research initiatives in the acute and critical care setting. Research studies that address the utilization of the advanced practice provider in the acute care setting as it relates to patient outcomes still need to be conducted. In addition, successful models of multidisciplinary ICU care utilizing the advanced practice providers need to be widely distributed to optimally utilize these resources for ICU staffing [18]. In this model, the APPs are trained and maintain competency in certain frequently performed procedures such as ventilator management, central and arterial line placements, and possibly some unit-specific procedures, such as lumbar punctures in neurointensive care units. Some high-risk procedures such as intubations or chest tube placement need to have in-house support, often by other specialists namely anesthesiologists or emergency physicians.

Further modification of this model may include in-house "moonlighting physician" supervision of the advance practice providers. For instance, pulmonary critical care fellows or oncology fellows, who are board certified in internal medicine with adequate ICU experience, could be utilized to work in conjunction and supervise these advanced practice providers. In this model, the attending faculty intensivist remains available for emergency phone consultation. The major drawback in this model is the lack of consistency and additional costs incurred in the employment of these "moonlighting physicians." Also, if the scheduling of these moonlighters is on a voluntary basis, there may be holes in the schedules or last minute vacancies. Thus, contingency plans must be made in order to fulfill patient care needs.

Due to the difficulty attracting and retaining intensivists, there has been a shortage in these qualified specialists. Thus, other models have been explored and utilized. The following models are not compliant with Leapfrog standards for IPS.

One staffing model which has grown in popularity recently (though usually not compliant with Leapfrog standards) due to the shortfall of intensivists is one in which advanced practice providers fully provide the care in the ICU. In this model, a team of advanced practice providers provide 24-h in-house coverage of the patients. There are a few abstracts which have demonstrated that this model does not have any worse outcomes than the traditional academic (attending and resident/fellow) or modified academic (attending and APPs) models. The advantages to this model is that there is no need for an intensivist, who is in short supply, and is much more easily accomplished as there has been a tremendous growth in programs training APPs with critical care expertise. In addition, this care model is significantly less costly.

Another model consists of utilizing hospitalists to staff or also cover the ICU. In a study published more than a decade, 83% of hospitalists provided care in the ICU [19]. Furthermore, a study conducted in medical ICUs in a community hospital published in 2012 demonstrated similar outcomes between an ICU staffed predominantly with hospitalists and a companion ICU with an intensivist model [20]. Therefore, more collaboration between hospitalists and intensivists will likely continue to occur and the results of these endeavors are still to be determined.

Other models which have been utilized include an intensivist staffing during the day with FCCS trained nurses, or a full open ICU where anyone can admit to the ICU, consult an intensivist if and when desired, and then be managed by the bedside registered nurse and/or "moonlighting coverage" physician, of various specialty training. Oftentimes, these physicians may be house staff or trainees from nearby training programs. Patient outcomes in these models have not been studied against the Leapfrog IPS standards. As healthcare evolves, further exploration into newer staffing models may be necessary due to ongoing skilled personnel shortages.

With improvements in technology, ICU telemedicine plays a role in improving outcomes while limiting costs by more effective resource utilization. In a multicenter case-control study published in 2016, ICU telemedicine facilities had a small but statistically significant relative overall mortality reduction, with large-volume urban setting hospitals achieving the largest decrease in mortality [21].

In conclusion, APPs and hospitalists are likely to contribute significantly to ICU staffing in the future. Of utmost importance, is ensuring their adequate critical care training, establishing competency, and credentialing, in order to effectively collaborate with the intensivists in providing multidisciplinary care [17]. These providers should be considered complementary, not a substitute, to the intensivist.

Associated Costs in Various Models

Although costs vary, personnel compensation costs comprise a large proportion of critical care costs. In the classic academic model, the attending intensivist's, residents', and fellows' compensation must be calculated. Although actual dollar values are not compared, the relative costs based on current market compensation of each of these individual roles will be utilized. For example, attending intensivists cost more than hospitalists, who cost significantly more than advanced practice providers (physician assistants and nurse practitioners), who cost more than fellows and residents. In addition, what is the staffing ratio necessary to provide optimal care in this model? Another question, especially for attending physicians, is the differential for night coverage for which one must be compensated either through time or money. Does the additional cost of delivery of care in this model improve the patient outcomes? Does patient satisfaction and experience improve by having the availability of an attending 24 h a day in the ICU? These questions will be analyzed in this chapter.

In the modified academic model, the substitution of APPs for the residents/fellows slightly increases the costs as these salaries in the current market environment are higher than the cost of house staff. On the other hand, could the APPs require less supervision and manage certain ICU patients independently and thus bill individually, therefore offsetting the cost of their salaries?

In a fully open model, often utilizing the private practice model, the costs of care in these patients are variable. The patient is billed by the consulting intensivist who gives recommendations and is available by telephone for questions. The intensivists usually do not take over the care of these patients and ensure that the recommended treatment is carried out in a timely fashion, trying to shorten the length of stay in these critically ill patients.

As technology has improved, telemedicine has become a viable alternative. Present day, the cost of telemedicine varies from $50,000 to 123,000 per day [22]. In the implementation of this model, the cost of staffing the telemedicine with qualified personnel is a large component of the costs. In addition, this does not account for the costs incurred for the on-site personnel, which is necessary to perform procedures or provide physical contact/examination of the patients.

Associated Outcomes with 24-Hour In-house Intensivists

Initially, in the classic Pronovost study as utilized in the Leapfrog IPS recommendations, high-intensity ICU physician staffing improves outcomes [4]. Thus, these results were extrapolated to a 24-h in-house intensivists model which significantly increased costs. Unfortunately, most studies with Mandatory 24-h staffing by

intensivists did not affect ICU or hospital mortality [15, 17].

Although initially in 2003, SCCM and Leapfrog Group endorsed a 24-h intensivist staffing model [23]; the economic constraints and limitations of resources may not justify this. In addition, further studies did not show a mortality or hospital or ICU LOS benefit in a 24-h intensivist model [15, 17]. Wilcox et al. in 2013 concluded in a systematic review and meta-analysis that "High-intensity staffing is associated with reduced ICU and hospital mortality. Within a high-intensity model, 24-h in-hospital intensivist coverage did not reduce hospital, or ICU, mortality" [24]. The 24-h intensivist model had more benefit in surgical or mixed medical-surgical ICUs versus medical ICUs [24]. In addition, a recent ATS systematic review and meta-analysis concluded that nighttime intensivist staffing is not associated with ICU patient mortality [15].

Patient Ratios

There are multiple scholarly articles that discuss the negative impact of poor nurse to patient ratios but as previously stated this will not be covered in this chapter. Unfortunately, there is less evidence for optimal staffing ratios for intensivist to patient.

Matching healthcare personnel resources with patient acuity and needs is essential to maintain safe care in ICUs. Adequate patient-to-nurse (P/N) and patient-to-physician (P/P) ratios may be associated with higher survival rates and a lower risk of failure to rescue [25]. However, the optimal ratio, or the level above which outcomes worsen, have not been established. In addition, these ratios have been determined by panels of experts and not scientifically validated [17].

As noted in the Leapfrog IPS factsheet, outcomes are better in ICUs staffed by intensivists. Unfortunately, the optimal intensivist–patient ratio is not specified and unknown [26]. The intensivist–patient ratio is likely to be influenced by several factors including, but not limited to the patients' acute severity of illness and comorbidities, other available physician specialists, and other allied healthcare professional support as well as nonhuman resources such as medical equipment or information technology [17, 26].

A recent statement from the society of critical care medicine on ICU staffing in closed ICUs concluded that "while advocating a specific maximum number of patients cared for is unrealistic, an approach that considers the following principles is essential: (1) proper staffing impacts patient care; (2) large caseloads should not preclude rounding in a timely fashion; (3) staffing decisions should factor surge capacity and nondirect patient care activities; (4) institutions should regularly reassess their staffing; (5) high staff turnover or decreases in quality-of-care indicators in an ICU may be markers of overload; (6) telemedicine, advanced practice professionals, or nonintensivist medical staff may be useful to alleviate overburdening the intensivist, but should be evaluated using rigorous methods; (7) in teaching institutions, feedback from faculty and trainees should be sought to understand the implications of potential understaffing on medical education; and (8) in academic medical ICUs, there is evidence that intensivist/patient ratios less favorable than 1:14 negatively impact education, staff well-being, and patient care" [17]. In this Task Force Statement, there is a proposed intensivist–patient ratio staffing tool as noted in Appendix 1 in this paper. This roughly calculates the intensivist's direct patient care time taking into account the number of patients and acuity of illness as well as nondirect patient care activities, which may include administrative duties, family meetings, teaching responsibilities, sign out, or curbside consultations [17].

Other supporting evidence includes a multicenter study done over 1 year that demonstrated an associated risk of mortality in nurse to patient ratio of greater than 1: 2.5 and a provider to patient ratio of greater than 1: 14. Interestingly, the times associated with nursing shortage was scattered but more commonly on weekends, and for intensivist's nighttime hours. Provider ratios were as low as 3.6 patients per physician during the day versus 8.5 during the night [27].

In conclusion, a high-intensity model where intensivists manage patients either during the day or at night improves outcomes but the 24-h intensivist model does not show additional benefit in outcomes but does incur additional costs. Adequate management with performance improvement processes and structured rounds with implementation of daily care plans improves outcomes [28].

An official American Thoracic Society systematic review of current literature and meta-analysis, published in 2017, suggested that nighttime intensivist staffing is not associated with reduced ICU patient mortality [15]. In addition, minimal or no difference was noted in the ICU or hospital length of stay. Other outcomes and alternative staffing models should be evaluated to further guide staffing decisions [15].

These models included use of residents, fellows, nurse practitioners, or physician assistants. It included general or specialty ICUs as well as academic or community settings [15].

Burnout Syndrome in Intensivists

In a 2007 study, a high level of burnout among intensivists was noted. The results showed approximately one-half of respondents showed professional burnout [29]. A major challenge in ICU staffing needs a balance between continuity of care for patient care versus avoidance of burnout by allowing for uninterrupted time off clinically. Geva et al. utilized a computer simulation model to create a shared service schedule to best balance these opposing factors [30].

Working in a stressful workplace, especially in an environment like the ICU, precipitates burnout in the workforce [31]. In this systematic review, the following factors were associated with burnout: age, sex, marital status, personality traits, work experience in an ICU, work environment, workload and shift work, ethical issues, and end-of-life decision-making. Of note, younger age, male, single and childless, and those who work night shifts and longer than 36 h shifts as well as frequent end-of-life decision-making including decision to withdraw or withhold life support were positively correlated with burnout [31].

Also, patient-centric care has become a driving force impacting payment models. Thus, patient preferences must also be factored into the ICU staffing model as this affects reimbursement.

Most staffing model research has focused on patient-related outcomes; as a result, little is known about the consequences of work schedules in intensive care on intensivists themselves. In some studies, there is no patient outcome differences in continuous intensivist scheduling versus cross coverage by intensivists for the weekend, but in the second scenario providers showed less burnout and improved work–life balance [32].

Due to the shortage of intensivists, other models utilizing APPs or other specialists such as hospitalists or family practice physicians will need to be studied for its effects on outcomes, costs, and overall value in health care as it pertains to ICU staffing. Furthermore, hospital administration and leadership need to be engaged to provide work environments that better support intensivists and critical care staff [33].

Summary

As advocated by the Leapfrog Group based on the initial study by Pronovost, daytime intensivists staffing has been associated with improved outcomes for patients admitted to the intensive care units [4]. This was further extrapolated by experts to extend 24-h around-the-clock care by an in-house intensivist in the ICU in an attempt to improve outcomes. This was an expensive endeavor due to the costs and shortage of intensivists. In addition, depending on the daytime staffing model this did not necessarily improve outcomes and incurred additional costs [15, 17].

The results showed that In ICUs with optional consultation with an intensivist, nighttime intensivist staffing was associated with a reduction in risk-adjusted in-hospital mortality. This may be due to more timely resuscitation or less medical errors. In ICUs with high-intensity daytime staffing defined as those which mandated an intensivist consultation or transfer of care to the intensivist, nighttime intensivist staffing conferred no benefit with respect to risk-adjusted in-hospital mortality [34]. Furthermore, a randomized study done at a large academic medical center published in 2013 in the NEJM by Kerlin showed no improvement of in-hospital intensivists on ICU or hospital mortality or length of stay [35]. Further studies, as noted by the Checkley study group, states that a 24-h staffing model by intensivists or a closed ICU does not improve ICU patient mortality [28].

Is there a difference in outcomes for the surgical patient population? This question was explored by Van del Wilden et al. They published a study in the surgical ICU population that showed no difference of the addition of an in-house intensivist on ICU or hospital mortality, ventilation days, complications, or readmission rates [36]. The addition of an in-house nighttime intensivist did decrease utilization of blood products and imaging studies, but it increased relative value units per full time equivalent (RVU/FTE) as the intensivists increased billing when present on-site [36]. Thus, based on the value equation of outcome–cost, overall health care value may be decreased in this model.

Optimal staffing of an ICU is highly dependent on multiple factors including, but not limited to availability of trained personnel, educational trainees, acuity of patients, size of ICU, and economic constraints. Therefore, staffing models need to be carefully selected and implemented based on the local setting. In addition, modifications may need to be made as these factors frequently change. The key commodity in ICU staffing is the availability of specialty trained personnel, namely the intensivists and ICU nurses. Thus, in order to efficiently staff the ICU, attracting and retaining the intensivist requires creative models which may focus on time off and lifestyle factors. These may also vary depending on the locale of the ICU and individual characteristics of the members of the group. Striking a balance between the needs of the ICU staffing model and the intensivists' lifestyle with avoidance of burnout is paramount to success.

References

1. Halpern NA, Pastores SM. Critical care medicine beds, use, occupancy and costs in the United States: a methodological review. Crit Care Med. 2015;43(11):2452–9.
2. Halpern NA, Pastores SM. Critical care medicine in the United States 2000–2005: an analysis of bed numbers, occupancy rates, payer mix, and costs. Crit Care Med. 2010;38:65–7.
3. Schmitz, et al. Needs in pulmonary and critical care medicine. Cambridge, MA: ABT Associates; 1999.
4. Pronovost PJ, Angus DC, Dorman T, et al. Physician staffing patterns and clinical outcomes in critically ill patients: a systematic review. JAMA. 2002;288(17):2151–62.
5. Milstein A, Galvin RS, Delbanco SF, Salber P, Buck CR Jr. Improving the safety of health care: the Leapfrog initiative. Eff Clin Pract. 2000;3:313–6.
6. The Leapfrog Group for Patient Safety. Fact sheet: ICU physician staffing (IPS). Available at http://www.leapfroggroup.org/media/file/Leapfrog-ICU_Physician_Staffing_Fact_Sheet.pdf. Accessed 27 Apr 2018.
7. Lwin AK, Shepard DS. Estimating lives and dollars saved from universal adoption of the Leapfrog safety and quality standards: 2008 update. Washington, DC: The Leapfrog Group; 2008.
8. Knaus WA, Wagner DP, Zimmerman JE, Draper EA. Variations in mortality and length of stay in intensive care units. Ann Intern Med. 1993;118:753–61.
9. Angus DC, Kelly M, Schmitz R, White A, Popovich J. Current and projected workforce requirements for care of the critically ill and patients with pulmonary disease: can we meet the requirements of an aging population? JAMA. 2000;284:2762–70.
10. Angus DC, Shorr AF, White A, Dremsizov TT, Schmitz RJ, Kelley MA, Committee on Manpower for Pulmonary and Critical Care Societies (COMPACCS). Critical care delivery in the United States: distribution of services and compliance with the Leapfrog recommendations. Crit Care Med. 2006;34(4):1016–24.
11. Kelley MA, Angus D, Chalfin DB, et al. The critical care crisis in the United States: a report from the profession. Chest. 2004;125:1514–7.
12. Duke EM. The study of supply and demand for critical care physicians. Senate Report 108–81, Senate Report 109–103 and House Report 109–143, US Dept. of Health and Human Services, Health Resources and Services Administration, 2006.
13. US Department of Health and Human Services, Health Resources and Services Administration. Report to Congress. The critical care workforce: a study of the supply and demand for critical care physicians.

May 2006. http://bhpr.hrsa.gov/healthworkforce/reports/studycriticalcarephys.pdf. Accessed 23 Oct 2015.
14. Woolf SH, Johnson RE. The break-even point: when medical advances are less important than improving the fidelity with which they are delivered. Ann Fam Med. 2005;3(6):545–52.
15. Kerlin MP, Adhikari NK, Rose L, et al. An official American thoracic society systematic review: the effect of nighttime intensivist staffing on mortality and length of stay among intensive care unit patients. Am J Respir Crit Care Med. 2017;195(3):383–93.
16. Pastores SM, O'Connor MF, Kleinpell RM, et al. The ACGME resident duty-hour new standards: history, changes, and impact on staffing of intensive care units. Crit Care Med. 2012;39:2540–9.
17. Ward NS, Afessa B, Kleinpell R. Intensivist/patient ratios in closed ICUs: a statement from the Society of Critical Care Medicine Taskforce on ICU Staffing. Crit Care Med. 2013;41(2):638–45.
18. Kleinpell RM, Ely EW, Grabenkort R. Nurse practitioners and physician assistants in the ICU: an evidence based review. Crit Care Med. 2008;36(10):2888–97.
19. Lindenauer PK, Pantilat SZ, Katz PP, et al. Hospitalists and the practice of inpatient medicine: results of a survey of the National Association of Inpatient Physicians. Ann Intern Med. 1999;130(4 Pt 2):343–9.
20. Wise KR, Akopov VA, Williams BR Jr, et al. Hospitalists and intensivists in the medical ICU: a prospective observational study comparing mortality and length of stay between two staffing models. J Hosp Med. 2012;7:183–9.
21. Kahn JM, Le TQ, Barnato AE. ICU telemedicine and critical care mortality: a national effectiveness study. Med Care. 2016;54(3):319–25.
22. Kumar G, Falk DM, Bonello RS, Kahn JM, Perencevich E, Cram P. The costs of critical care telemedicine programs: a systematic review and analysis. Chest. 2013;143(1):19–29.
23. Haupt MT, Bekes CE, Brilli RJ, Carl LC, Gray AW, Jastremski MS, Naylor DF, PharmD MR, Md AS, Wedel SK, Md MH, Task Force of the American College of Critical Care Medicine, Society of Critical Care Medicine. Guidelines on critical care services and personnel: recommendations based on a system of categorization of three levels of care. Crit Care Med. 2003;31(11):2677–83.
24. Wilcox ME, Chong CA, Niven DJ, Rubenfeld GD, Rowan KM, Wunsch H, Fan E. Do intensivist staffing patterns influence hospital mortality following ICU admission? A systematic review and meta-analyses. Crit Care Med. 2013;41(10):2253–74.
25. West E, Barron DN, Harrison D, et al. Nurse staffing, medical staffing and mortality in intensive care: an observational study. Int J Nurs Stud. 2014;51:781–94.
26. Afessa B. Intensive care unit physician staffing: Seven days a week, 24 hours a day. Crit Care Med. 2006;34:894–5.
27. Neuraz A, Guérin C, Payet C, Polazzi S, Aubrun F, Dailler F, Lehot JJ, Piriou V, Neidecker J, Rimmelé T,

Schott AM, Duclos A. Patient mortality is associated with staff resources and workload in the ICU: a multicenter observational study. Crit Care Med. 2015;43(8):1587–94.

28. Checkley W, Martin GS, Brown SM, Chang SY, Dabbagh O, Fremont RD, Girard TD, Rice TW, Howell MD, Johnson SB, O'Brien J, Park PK, Pastores SM, Patil NT, Pietropaoli AP, Putman M, Rotello L, Siner J, Sajid S, Murphy DJ, Sevransky JE, United States Critical Illness and Injury Trials Group Critical Illness Outcomes Study Investigators. Structure, process, and annual ICU mortality across 69 centers: United States Critical Illness and Injury Trials Group Critical Illness Outcomes Study. Crit Care Med. 2014;42(2):344–56.

29. Embriaco N, Azoulay E, Barrau K, Kentish N, Pochard F, Loundou A, Papazian L. High level of burnout in intensivists: prevalence and associated factors. Am J Respir Crit Care Med. 2007;175(7):686–92.

30. Geva A, Landrigan CP, van der Velden MG, Randolph AG. Simulation of a novel schedule for intensivist staffing to improve continuity of patient care and reduce physician burnout. Crit Care Med. 2017;45(7):1138–44.

31. Chuang CH, Tseng PC, Lin CY, Lin KH, Chen YY. Burnout in the intensive care unit professionals: a systematic review. Medicine (Baltimore). 2016;95(50):e5629.

32. Ali NA, Hammersley J, Hoffmann SP, O'Brien JM Jr, Phillips GS, Rashkin M, Warren E, Garland A, Midwest Critical Care Consortium. Continuity of care in intensive care units: a cluster-randomized trial of intensivist staffing. Am J Respir Crit Care Med. 2011;184:803–8.

33. Addressing burnout in ICU clinicians: strategies for prevention from a national summit. SSCM 47th Critical Care Congress.

34. Wallace DJ, Angus DC, Barnato AE, Kramer AA, Kahn JM. Nighttime intensivist staffing and mortality among critically ill patients. N Engl J Med. 2012;366 (22):2093–101.

35. Kerlin MP, Small DS, Cooney E, Fuchs BD, Bellini LM, Mikkelsen ME, Schweickert WD, Bakhru RN, Gabler NB, Harhay MO, Hansen-Flaschen J, Halpern SD. A randomized trial of nighttime physician staffing in an intensive care unit. N Engl J Med. 2013;368(23):2201–9.

36. van der Wilden GM, Schmidt U, Chang Y, Bittner EA, Cobb JP, Velmahos GC, Alam HB, de Moya MA, King DR. Implementation of 24/7 intensivist presence in the SICU: effect on processes of care. J Trauma Acute Care Surg. 2013;74(2):563–7.

37. Kohn LT, Corrigan JM, Donaldson MS. To err is human: building a safer health system. Washington, DC: National Academy Press; 1999.

Multidisciplinary Care of Critically Ill Cancer Patients

Ninotchka Brydges, Brandi McCall, and Tiffany Mundie

Contents

Introduction 44

Nursing 44
Reasons for ICU Admission 45
Complications of the Oncologic Critical Care Patient 45
Compassion Fatigue 46

Nutrition 47
Nutrition Screening and Assessment 48
Malnutrition Interventions 49
Feeding Tube Placement in the Setting of Thrombocytopenia 50

Physical and Occupational Therapy 51
Early Mobility in the ICU 51

Patient Support in the Oncologic ICU 52
Patient Support 52
Routine ICU Care 53

Social Work and Patient Advocacy 54
Role of the Social Worker in the Intensive Care Unit 54
Social Worker Training 55
Activities and Barriers 55
Role of the Patient Advocate in the Intensive Care Unit 55
Patient Advocate Training 56

Chaplaincy 57
History of the Chaplain 57
Professional Training 57
Role of the Chaplain 58
Assessment Tools 58
Outcomes and Efficacy of Chaplaincy 59

N. Brydges (✉) · B. McCall · T. Mundie
Department of Critical Care and Respiratory Care, The
University of Texas MD Anderson Cancer Center,
Houston, TX, USA
e-mail: nbrydges@mdanderson.org;
bmmccall@mdanderson.org; tamundie@mdanderson.org

© Springer Nature Switzerland AG 2020
J. L. Nates, K. J. Price (eds.), *Oncologic Critical Care*,
https://doi.org/10.1007/978-3-319-74588-6_10

Conclusion   60

References   60

Abstract

Critically ill cancer patients have complex physical and emotional needs that are best met by utilizing a multidisciplinary care approach. Physicians, advanced practice providers, nurses, clinical pharmacists, dieticians, physical therapists, occupational therapists, patient advocates, social workers, and chaplains are essential members of the multidisciplinary team working together to achieve a patient-centered approach when caring cancer patients in the intensive care unit (ICU). This chapter focuses on six different areas of the multidisciplinary team and discusses how each group is utilized to support the critically ill cancer patient. Oncologic considerations and challenges in regard to nursing, nutrition, physical and occupational therapy, patient support, advocacy and social work, and chaplaincy are thoroughly reviewed in relation to the critically ill oncologic patient.

Keywords

Intensive care unit · Critical care · Oncology nurse · Compassion fatigue · Enteral nutrition · Parenteral nutrition · Malnutrition · Nutrition screening · Nutrition assessment · Physical therapy · Occupational therapy · Mobility · Acquired weakness · Delirium · Early mobility · Patient support · Chaplain · Chaplaincy · Spiritual care · Communication · Advocacy · Patient advocate · Social worker

of physicians, advanced practice providers (APPs), nurses, respiratory therapists, and clinical pharmacists. In addition to these core team members, dieticians or nutritionists, social workers, patient advocates, physical therapists, occupational therapists, and chaplains can provide invaluable support and expertise that improves the overall care and satisfaction of the patient and their family members. Studies have also shown that using a multidisciplinary team approach is associated with decreased mortality in clinical ICU patients [32]. Working together, each member of the team provides their expertise and suggestion for the care of the patient, and the team leader, typically the physician, finalizes the patient's plan of care. Once the plan of care is established, each member carries out their part. By recognizing and addressing both physical and emotional needs of the patient, the team is providing holistic care that results in improved patient satisfaction and outcomes. This chapter will discuss some of the unique roles and functions of various members of the multidisciplinary care team and how their actions can benefit the outcome of critically ill cancer patients. It will discuss barriers faced in caring for this complicated patient population and strategies to help overcome these difficulties. These techniques can be applied not only to critically ill cancer patients, but also to critically ill patients without cancer as well as complex patients who may be hospitalized but not necessarily require intensive care unit (ICU) care.

Introduction

Care of critically ill patients in general is complex. The addition of cancer, immunocompromised systems, bleeding tendencies, and therapy-related organ failure makes for a challenging patient population. The best approach to care for both critically ill patients and those with cancer involves a multidisciplinary care team consisting

Nursing

Nurses in oncologic critical care settings are specifically trained to care for patients with various kinds of cancer throughout all stages of the disease process. Oncology nurses must learn specific skills beyond that required of a basic nursing program, including chemotherapy administration, immunosuppression and chemotherapy side effects, and complications of chemotherapy, radiation, and investigational treatments. Many oncology nurses undergo rigorous testing to acquire oncology-specific certification through national cancer nursing organizations such as the Oncology Nursing Certification Corporation (ONCC), who offers many different cancer-specific certifications including OCN (Oncology Certified Nurse), AOCNP (Advanced Oncology Certified Nurse Practitioner), AOCN (Advanced Oncology Certified Nurse), and more [43]. Oncology certification ensures that the nurse has met minimum standards to provide safe effective care to the oncology patient. In addition to oncology and chemotherapy administration certification, nurses can undergo testing to receive specialized critical care certification. Although not required to work in any ICU, critical care certification through a national critical care nursing body is highly recommended for all ICU nurses, as it attests to the nurse's ability to provide proficient care for the critically ill patient. The American Association of Critical Care Nurses (AACN) offers a nationally recognized critical care specialty certification, the CCRN, which identifies nurses who have demonstrated mastery in the field of critical care nursing. By undergoing certification, nurses show their commitment to delivering high-quality expert care to the critically ill cancer patient.

Reasons for ICU Admission

Cancer patients are at risk for a multitude of complications including many that are not related to their malignancy. Studies have shown that roughly 5% of patients with solid tumors and 15% of patients with hematologic malignancies require ICU admission during the early phases of their illness [47, 48]. The retrospective observational study conducted by Puxty et al. [47] found that of 118,541 patients with solid malignancies, 14.1% of them died in the ICU and 24.6% of them died during their hospital stay. In a study performed by Pene et al. [46], patients with malignancies admitted to the ICU with septic shock had 30 day-mortality rates of 55.5% between 1998 and 2000, which had actually improved when compared to 79.4% between 1995 and 1997. Because of this improvement, various adjuvant therapies for both septic shock and general ICU care, which resulted to form the basis of recommendations of the Surviving Sepsis Campaign. However, with such high death rates and concern for lack of resources, practitioners should be diligent in their ICU admission criteria particularly when the cancer patient is considered end-stage or there are no further treatment therapy options.

It is well-known that immunosuppressed cancer patients are at risk for requiring higher level of care and interventions that can only be performed in an ICU. Some common examples of reasons for ICU admission include drug reaction, infectious complications after immunotherapy or chemotherapy, organ dysfunction due to the physical size or location of a tumor, post-stem cell transplantation complications, tumor lysis syndrome, hyperleukocytosis, thrombotic events, and severe electrolyte abnormalities [49]. The top reasons for ICU admission of the cancer patient have consistently been respiratory failure and sepsis [49]. Nurses caring for critically ill oncology patients must familiarize themselves with the expert treatment of the most commonly seen ICU admission diagnoses. The ICU nurse is at the bedside more frequently than the clinical provider, thus it is the nurse's responsibility to promptly recognize worsening of the patient's status and intervene as needed. Oncology critical care nurses should know common side effects and complications of frequently used chemotherapies and immunotherapies administered in their institution as well as common solid and liquid tumor complications. Table 1 identifies common causes of ICU admission that the oncology nurse must be aware of and competent to manage.

Complications of the Oncologic Critical Care Patient

Patients with cancer who have undergone chemotherapy or immunotherapy are at increased risk of

Table 1 Common reasons for ICU admission of the cancer patient

Admission reason	Example
Infection	Pneumonia, sepsis, cellulitis, abscess
Oncologic emergencies	Superior vena cava syndrome, tumor lysis syndrome, hypercalcemia, pulmonary embolism, gastrointestinal bleed, disseminated intravascular coagulation (DIC), severe mucositis
Acute respiratory failure	Transfusion-related acute lung injury (TRALI), transfusion-associated circulatory overload (TACO), pneumonitis, diffuse alveolar hemorrhage, malignant pleural effusion, acute respiratory distress syndrome (ARDS), flash pulmonary edema
Surgical complications	Post-op monitoring, bleeding complications, hemodynamic instability, multistage surgeries
Adverse drug reactions	Anaphylaxis, cytokine release syndrome, all-trans retinoic acid (ATRA) syndrome, thrombotic microangiopathy
Neurologic complications	Seizures, posterior reversible encephalopathy syndrome (PRES), altered mental status, metabolic encephalopathy, neurotoxicity
Cardiovascular complications	Myocardial infarction, congestive heart failure, arrhythmias, pulmonary thromboembolism, hypotension
Stem cell transplant complications	Graft-versus-host-disease (GVHD), organ damage

Adapted from Shimabukuro-Vornhagen et al. [53]

decompensation due to infection, organ failure, and decreased overall strength. Nurses caring for cancer patients in the critical care setting must be aware of common complications and adverse reactions specific to this patient population. They should be able to detect early signs of organ dysfunction or treatment toxicity and promptly notify the appropriate provider to help manage these complications. Cancer patients are specifically at increased risk of infection, sepsis, and respiratory failure. Many patients with malignancy will be at risk for either excessive bleeding or clotting, or both. Patients with hematologic malignancies such as acute myeloid leukemia may require frequent blood product transfusions and these patients should be monitored closely for transfusion reaction and volume overload. Care must also be taken to reduce the risk of nosocomial infection in the immunocompromised patient; thus nurses and other providers entering the room of an ICU patient, particularly those who are neutropenic, should strictly adhere to hand hygiene practices.

Nurses administering chemotherapy are specifically trained in the safe handling of such medications and how to handle chemotherapy spills. Hospitals have customized protocols regarding cleanup of hazardous medications, depending on the size of the spill. Oncology nurses are responsible for protecting not only themselves but also those around them from the harmful effects of chemotherapy. Chemotherapy and immunotherapy safety administration training is typically required upon hiring and renewed annually to provide a safe environment for these harmful medications.

The ICU mortality rate of cancer patients remains high and many patients and their families will prompt discussions regarding end-of-life with the bedside nurse, since they typically spend the most time throughout the day attending to the patient. Oncology critical care nurses should be prepared to discuss death and dying with their patients and their family members. Nurses can seek out educational opportunities within their institution or online to better equip themselves with the tools needed to empathetically and effectively discuss the dying process.

Compassion Fatigue

Working in the clinical field can be emotionally draining, particularly in the case of oncology patients, as a moderate percentage of those encountered in the ICU are in the terminal stages of cancer. One study has shown the mortality rate of cancer patients admitted to the ICU to be 46.6%

[1]. Oncology critical care nurses must be able to handle the stress of frequent patient deaths while maintaining their compassion and empathy for all of their patients. They should be a source of hope and support to their patients and families, but also realistic in goals of care. The physical and emotional distress of caring for chronically ill cancer patients puts nurses at risk for developing poor quality of life as well as compassion fatigue, also known as burnout.

To help prevent burnout, some ICUs have committees that focus on debriefing and stress reduction therapies. For example, some units have routine "Stress Buster" sessions in which all of the nurses are invited to participate in stress reducing activities for about 15 min, such as massage, dance, games, or comedy. Other committees may focus on regularly scheduled debriefing sessions to discuss in a group setting tough cases and allow nurses to share their feelings about those cases. Unit social workers can be excellent resources to help facilitate these stress-relieving sessions and provide guided council that can help decrease burnout. Team building activities, particularly those done outside of the unit or off campus, can promote comradery among colleagues and reduce stress. A systematic review performed by Toh et al. [56] found that oncology nurses who worked in units with inadequate staffing had higher levels of job dissatisfaction, stress, and burnout. It is imperative that nursing administration provides adequate nursing coverage for ICU oncology units to ensure a safe environment and decrease the risk of compassion fatigue and burnout.

Oncologic critical care nursing requires compassion, empathy, intelligence, awareness, and autonomy. Additional institutional and online training specific to the care of the critically ill oncology patient is advised to provide expert nursing care to this unique subspecialty of patients. Burnout and compassion fatigue can be significantly reduced by the actions of nursing management when adequate nursing coverage is established and a culture of safety is promoted. Routine training on common ICU admission diagnoses and treatment as well as training on support of the patient's emotional needs can greatly increase the satisfaction of patients' and families' experiences in the ICU. Adequate training along with regularly scheduled stress-relieving activities and debriefing sessions will promote a culture of healing and purpose and provide a healthier environment overall for the management of acutely ill oncology patients.

Nutrition

Critically ill cancer patients are at increased risk of malnutrition, weight loss, cachexia, and sarcopenia that can result in increased hospital length of stay, poor quality of life, and increased mortality. The American Society for Parenteral and Enteral Nutrition (ASPEN) define malnutrition as "an acute, subacute or chronic state of nutrition, in which a combination of varying degrees of overnutrition or undernutrition with or without inflammatory activity have led to a change in body composition and diminished function" [6]. Cachexia in the cancer patient is defined as weight loss greater than 5% within the last 6 months, or weight loss greater than 2% in persons already showing body mass index (BMI) depletion or sarcopenia (muscle mass loss) [21]. Weight loss can be the presenting symptom in many different types of cancer, among other nonspecific complaints, such as nausea, vomiting, and fatigue. Up to 40% of patients in general have had some sort of weight loss at the time of their cancer diagnosis [60]. The prevalence of weight loss can be remarkably higher in specific cancers such as pancreas cancer, in which up to 85% of those patients present with weight loss at the time of their diagnosis [9]. As cancer progresses, malnutrition often worsens, resulting in severe weight loss in about 80% of those with advanced disease [60]. Although prompt intervention cannot always reverse malnutrition, it may be able to prevent progression and improve quality of life.

Preventing further weight loss and malnutrition in the critically ill cancer patient begins with nutrition screening and assessment. Specific tools are available to screen all patients for malnutrition. These tools help identify at-risk patients, who then undergo a full nutrition assessment.

The results of a nutrition assessment guide the practitioner to develop a patient-specific nutrition intervention plan, which may include oral supplements, a specific diet, enteral nutrition feeding, parenteral nutrition feeding, or a combination of these. Early nutritional intervention aims to improve function and quality of life, decrease frequency and length of hospital stay, reduce overall healthcare costs, and decrease morbidity and mortality [63]. Adult malnutrition is so important that in 1996, The Joint Commission began requiring inpatient nutritional screening within 24 h of admission [63]. This brought awareness to the frequently unrecognized condition of malnutrition and promoted prompt identification of the problem, resulting in earlier intervention. Today, nutrition and malnutrition are commonly discussed topics during inpatient rounds and many hospitals have developed malnutrition intervention strategies that involve using registered dieticians and nutritionists as regular members of multidisciplinary care teams, who guide providers in appropriate intervention strategies developed specifically for individual patient needs.

Nutrition Screening and Assessment

Nutrition screening is the first step in identifying cancer patients with malnutrition and those at risk for malnutrition. Screening should be performed on all cancer patients at the time of admission by using tests that have been validated and found to be reliable. Patients should be reassessed frequently throughout the disease course to increase the likelihood of early recognition and intervention. There are many different tools available to assist in screening patients for nutritional deficits, although a single gold standard tool has not been found. ASPEN and the Society of Critical Care Medicine (SCCM) recently updated their guidelines for the provision and assessment of nutrition support therapy in the critically ill adult patient. These guidelines are what many ICUs use across the country to direct nutritional care of adult patients who are expected to require 3 or more days of clinical ICU or surgical ICU care. The ASPEN

guidelines for nutrition assessment in the critically ill adult patient are discussed in Table 2.

In addition to national guidelines, validated nutrition screening tools allow for quick identification of patients who would benefit from a full nutritional assessment. Table 3 lists nutrition screening tools that have been validated for use in the oncology critical care population. The Nutrition Risk in the Critically Ill (NUTRIC) and Nutrition Risk Screening (NRS-2002) tools are ideal for use in the critically ill cancer patient because they take into account the severity of illness. Although the NUTRIC screening has many variables, most of these can be obtained from electronic clinical records if the ICU patient is mechanically ventilated or cannot participate in the screening due to mentation [34]. The malnutrition screening tool (MST) is commonly used for adult cancer patients due to its simplicity, reliability, and validity [60]. The MST is a three-question screening tool that identifies recent weight loss and poor appetite and can be done quickly within 24 h of hospital admission. The malnutrition universal screening tool (MUST) is more complex, but can predict length of hospital stay, discharge destination, and mortality after controlling for age [7]. The mini nutritional assessment (MNA) is used to assess nutrition in the geriatric population and assesses a subjective clinical nutrition status evaluation and objective lab, anthropometric, and dietary evaluation [7]. The MNA comes in

Table 2 ASPEN guidelines for nutrition assessment in the adult critically ill patient

Determination of nutrition risk should be performed on all patients admitted to the ICU for whom voluntary per os (PO) intake is anticipated to be insufficient
Nutritional assessment should include an evaluation of comorbid conditions, gastrointestinal tract function, and risk of aspiration
Nutritional assessment should not include traditional nutrition indicators or surrogate markers
Indirect calorimetry should be used when available to determine energy requirements
If indirect calorimetry is not available, a weight-based calculation (25–30 kcal/kg/day) or a published predictive equation may be used to evaluate energy requirements
Adequate protein intake should be evaluated frequently

Adapted from McClave et al. [38]

Table 3 Validated nutritional screening tools for the oncology population

Screening tool	Abbr.	Patient population	Parameters
Malnutrition Screening Tool	MST	Inpatient, outpatient	Recent weight loss, recent poor intake
Malnutrition Screening Tool for Cancer Patients	MSTC	Inpatient	Change in intake, weight loss, performance status, BMI
Patient-Generated Subjective Global Assessment	PG-SGA	Inpatient, outpatient	Weight, food intake, nutrition-related symptoms, function and activities, physical exam
Malnutrition Universal Screening Tool	MUST	Inpatient, outpatient	BMI, unintentional weight loss >5% over last 3–6 months, decreased oral intake for >5 days
Nutrition Risk in the Critically Ill	NUTRIC	Inpatient, ICU	Age, baseline severity of illness (APACHE II and SOFA), comorbidities, days from hospital admission to ICU admission, BMI <20 kg/m^2, estimated percentage oral intake in the week prior, weight loss in last 3 months, serum interleukin 6, procalcitonin, CRP
Nutrition Risk Screening	NRS-2002	Inpatient, ICU	BMI, weight loss within 3 months, reduced dietary intake of the past week, severity of illness
Subjective Global Assessment	SGA	Inpatient, outpatient	Clinical history, physical exam
Mini Nutritional Assessment	MNA	Geriatric inpatient, outpatient	BMI, weight loss, arm and calf circumference, lifestyle, medication, mobility, presence of depression or dementia, dietary assessment, number of meals, fluid/food intake, autonomy of feeding, self-perception of health and nutrition
Mini Nutritional Assessment Short Form	MNA-SF	Geriatric inpatient, outpatient	Food intake, weight loss, mobility, psychological stress or acute disease, presence of depression or dementia, BMI, calf circumference

Adapted from Lach and Peterson [34] and Anthony [7]

a short form (MNA-SF) and full form and takes anywhere from 5 to 15 min to complete. Low MNA scores indicate that a patient is at risk of adverse outcomes, prolonged length of stay, discharge to a nursing home, and increased mortality [7]. While the MNA can accurately predict early risk of malnutrition, it should not be used on patients who cannot provide a reliable self-assessment or for patients being fed via enteral feeding tubes.

Malnutrition Interventions

Once a patient is identified as having malnutrition, interventions to halt and potentially reverse the damage are initiated. Patients with malnutrition have been found to have more complications, longer hospitalizations, more infectious and non-infectious complications, and greater mortality [40]. Average protein and energy requirements

of the cancer patient are similar to those of healthy people. Cancer patients should seek to consume 25–30 kcal/kg/day and 1–1.5 g/kg/day of protein [60]. Protein goals need to be adjusted if there is protein catabolism or acute or chronic renal failure. Sodium and water intake may also need to be monitored, particularly if the patient has peritoneal carcinomatosis with obstruction or ascites, as excess sodium intake can lead to fluid overload and third spacing [8].

Initial interventions revolve around providing nutrition via the least invasive route. Ideally, the patient would be administered the appropriate type and amount of per os (PO) food, possibly aided by oral supplements or additional snacks. If the patient is not able or willing to take food by mouth, enteral nutrition should be considered. The European Society for Clinical Nutrition and Metabolism (ESPEN) guidelines on nutrition in cancer patients states that "artificial nutrition is indicated if patients are unable to eat adequately (e.g., no food for more than 1 week or less than 60% of requirement for more than 1–2 weeks)" [8]. Artificial nutrition begins with enteral nutrition, more commonly known as "tube feeds." Benefits of enteral nutrition include decreased intestinal permeability, lower risk of hyperglycemia, improved nitrogen balance, weight gain, improved wound healing, maintenance of gut integrity, and decreased ICU length of stay [40]. Enteral nutrition can also improve functional status or quality of life in some patients as well as provide comfort [19].

When enteral nutrition is not an option, parenteral nutrition can be considered. Enteral nutrition may be contraindicated if the patient has a persistent ileus, gut ischemia, severe malabsorption, intestinal obstruction, active gastrointestinal hemorrhage, or hemodynamic instability [52]. Parenteral nutrition is indicated in patients with moderate to severe malnutrition in which enteral feeding is contraindicated for a period of 7–10 days or greater [34]. The risks of using parenteral nutrition should be weighed against the benefit to the patient. Parenteral nutrition can cause increased infections, increased surgical complications, liver dysfunction, electrolyte and blood glucose abnormalities, volume overload, and metabolic bone disease [34]. Parenteral nutrition is expensive and should be considered only after less invasive methods have been exhausted.

The various formulas of enteral and parenteral nutrition are abundant and an evaluation of each is beyond the scope of this text. It is important to know that formulas should be adjusted to account for existing comorbidities or acute conditions, such as diabetes, acute renal failure, and acute or chronic liver dysfunction. Registered dieticians are valuable members of the multidisciplinary critical care team as they can help determine the appropriate formula for each individual patient. In addition to enteral and parenteral formulas, modular products such as protein and fiber supplements can be used to support the patient with malnutrition. Dieticians and nutritionists can also assess and modify nutrition plans for patients taking PO and can recommend supplemental drinks or snacks that can improve the overall nutritional state of those patients.

Feeding Tube Placement in the Setting of Thrombocytopenia

Thrombocytopenia is characteristic among patients with cancer and those who are critically ill, and this can be a concern when considering nasoenteric feeding tube insertion. Studies have shown that the incidence of thrombocytopenia varies widely, but up to 67% of patients have thrombocytopenia upon ICU admission, and up to 44% of patients develop thrombocytopenia during the course of their ICU stay [30]. Patients with cancer, particularly those with liquid tumors such as leukemia, are at high risk for developing thrombocytopenia. Very little data exists regarding the risk of placing nasoenteric feeding tubes in cancer patients with thrombocytopenia. One study evaluated bleeding outcomes in patients admitted to an oncology ICU and found no difference amongst patients with and without thrombocytopenia in total, overt, or clinically significant bleeding complications within 72 h of attempted feeding tube placement [44]. Of note, blood products had been transfused 24 h prior to insertion in 86% of the patients with thrombocytopenia. A comparison of bleeding events in thrombocytopenic patients who received blood products versus thrombocytopenic patients who did not receive blood was not done. The study concluded, however, that critically ill thrombocytopenic oncology patients did not have an increased risk of bleeding complications with nasoenteric feeding tube insertion. Professional judgment and risk versus benefit should be used when deciding to place a nasoenteric tube in the thrombocytopenic patient. In patients with grade 4 thrombocytopenia ($<25,000/\mu L$ platelets), platelets can be transfused before, during, or immediately after tube insertion to decrease the risk and severity of bleeding.

Malnutrition in the critically ill cancer patient can be a complex problem to manage. Most sources agree that nutrition should be assessed quickly so that interventions can be immediately implemented to prevent further deterioration of the patient. ASPEN, ESPEN, and SCCM guidelines are available online to guide the practitioner in appropriate management of the patient with malnutrition. Initiation of nutritional support should start with the least invasive method and progress to enteral and parenteral feeding when needed. Efforts should be made to minimize enteral and parenteral interruptions once initiated. Nutrition should be progressively reevaluated and adjusted intermittently and on an ongoing basis by licensed dieticians or nutritionists. By having a proactive stance on treating malnutrition, the provider will likely see improved outcomes, improved quality of life, and decreased mortality in the complex critically ill cancer patient.

Physical and Occupational Therapy

Patients in the ICU often experience complications related to prolonged bedrest, mechanical ventilation, sedation, and delirium. ICUs are typically loud environments due to patient monitoring alarms frequently going off, and multiple providers, including consultants, constantly going in and out of patient rooms. ICU rooms are often made of at least one glass wall that allows for better visualization of the critically ill patient and life-supporting machinery, but also decreases patient privacy and increases the amount of light filtered into the room, particularly at nighttime. Increased monitoring and alarms in the ICU and increased nighttime lighting can contribute to the disruptions of sleep–wake cycles often resulting in delirium of the ICU patient. In addition to delirium, patients on mechanical ventilators undergo prolonged bedrest and receive continuous sedation and analgesia medications that can worsen delirium and result in profound muscular weakness. Critical care patients should be proactively assessed for beginning physical and occupational rehabilitation early on, regardless of the presence of mechanical ventilation. The following paragraphs will briefly discuss physical therapy and occupational therapy for patients in the critical care environment as it relates to early mobility.

Early Mobility in the ICU

Physical therapists (PTs) "promote the ability to move, reduce pain, restore function, and prevent disability" [5]. Occupational therapists (OTs) assess patients' needs related to cognition, emotional, and physical symptoms and provide interventions which aim to "improve functional status and safety" [4]. PTs and OTs work in a variety of settings, such as home health, outpatient, nursing homes, and inpatient acute care settings, including ICUs. The rehab needs of patients in the ICU can present complex obstacles to overcome related to the effects of prolonged bedrest, sedation, and mechanical ventilation. These patients are at risk for development of ICU-acquired weakness. ICU-acquired weakness is a phenomenon that occurs when a patient develops more weakness than expected from prolonged bedrest. This is usually coupled with organ dysfunction and may be more common in patients who have been mechanically ventilated. Weakness associated with an ICU stay can be so severe that it significantly limits patients from performing basic activities, such as walking, dressing themselves, or having grip strength. Unfortunately, ICU-acquired weakness can still be present upon hospital discharge, with some patients reporting weakness of several months to years post-critical illness [42]. Patients who are mechanically ventilated can show signs of ICU-acquired weakness beginning at days 4–7 of mechanical ventilation [42].

The concept of early mobility is well-known in the ICU. Years ago, rehabilitation began after the cessation of invasive therapies like mechanical ventilation. With a movement toward early mobility, rehabilitation of ICU patients now occurs alongside of these processes and can start as early as 24–48 h after ICU admission [50]. The primary goal of early ICU mobility is to improve patient outcomes. Because these patients are critically ill; however, patient safety must be assessed prior to working with PT or OT. Each patient should be individually assessed to determine if they are safe and stable enough to be a part of early mobility. Some factors that could limit or restrict rehab for a critically ill cancer patient include extremes in heart rate (severe tachycardia or bradycardia), blood pressure (hypotension or hypertension), respiratory rate (typically tachypnea), inability to maintain oxygenation, high FiO2 requirements (>60%), increased intracranial pressure, acute myocardial ischemia, unsecure airway, extreme agitation, uncontrolled seizures, and ventilator dysynchrony [51, 29]. This is not an all-inclusive list as the individual patient situation can be assessed and deemed by the primary team as cautionary or contraindicated to proceed with early mobility. The skill level of clinicians and availability of resources should also be considered.

Early mobility requires a multidisciplinary approach that includes physicians, APPs, bedside registered nurses, respiratory therapists, physical therapists, and occupational therapists. The mobility effort is collaborative as it requires initiation of orders for PT/OT by a provider. Patients who are mechanically ventilated and sedated are at risk for the development of delirium. Consequences of delirium in the ICU include an increase in ventilator days, prolonged ICU and hospital stay, and increased mortality [51]. Nonpharmacologic approaches to the prevention of delirium in the ICU include daily sedation holidays as well as early mobilization [3]. Collaboration with the bedside nurse allows for daily sedation holiday and coordination to begin the therapy session for the day. The respiratory therapist must also be included in the mobility plan for the day, to meet the respiratory needs of the patient. The patient may require a transport ventilator while walking the unit, a high-flow oxygen setup while getting out of bed to the chair, or some other apparatus that only the respiratory therapist can manage. Patients may have increase work of breathing or hypoxia after working with PT/OT and respiratory therapists can assess the patient's oxygenation needs before, during, and after therapy and adjust oxygen delivery as needed.

The goal of physical and occupational therapy interventions is to improve functional status of the patient. Wahab et al. [61] described primary PT and OT patient interventions as ambulation, passive range of motion, physical transfers (e.g., bed to chair), and those related to ADLs such as feeding, dressing, and toileting. Not all patients will tolerate these interventions and will require careful assessment and gradual increase as tolerated in the level of therapy. The safety of early mobilization programs has been documented in recent literature. According to Hodgson et al. [29], adverse events that occurred as a result of early mobilization were low at <4%.

The institution of early mobility protocols in the ICU setting can positively impact patient care. Early mobility has been proven to be safe and is a result of collaborative care amongst the multidisciplinary ICU team. Physical and occupational therapy play a key role in the utilization of early mobility measures that have been shown to improve functional status, combat delirium in the ICU, and reduce length of ICU stay as well as number of ventilator days. Patients should undergo PT/OT evaluation within 24–48 h of admission to the ICU, even if they are receiving mechanical ventilation. Bedside nurses and respiratory therapists can help the physical or occupational therapist to determine if the patient is stable enough to start therapy, and can assist the PT/OT in providing a safe environment when therapy is underway. By working with PT and OT on a daily basis, ICU patients benefit from improved mobility, fewer pressure sores, and decreased delirium.

Patient Support in the Oncologic ICU

The critical care environment is often a scene of emotional and physical stress that can affect patients, family, personal caregivers, and staff members. The care of a critically ill patient in the ICU can present a time of crisis where life and death decisions and clinical interventions must happen quickly. This requires ongoing collaboration, discussion, and orchestration between the members of the multidisciplinary team, ICU staff, patients, family members, and care givers. All staff members who are involved in the patient's management from ICU admission to discharge contribute to the support of the patient in the ICU setting. The following paragraphs will discuss the impact of general caregivers on patient support in the oncologic ICU setting.

Patient Support

Cancer patients are admitted to the ICU for several reasons which can include treatment and disease-related complications. This can prove stressful for the patient and family or caregivers, therefore support of the patient starts at ICU admission. Patient-centered care is promoted by the Institute of Medicine (IOM), which defines six characteristics that patient care should have [57]. The IOM states that patient-centered care must: "(1) be respectful to patients' values, preferences and expressed needs; (2) be coordinated and integrated; (3) provide information, communication, and education; (4) ensure physical comfort; (5) provide emotional support – relieving fear and anxiety; and (6) involve family and friends" [57]. Patient-centered care is a collaborative effort by all ICU staff.

The bedside staff of physicians, APPs, nurses, and patient care technicians are usually the first to meet the patient and priority is given to the patient's immediate physical and emotional needs to stabilize the patient. Because the bedside clinicians need to focus on the patient's needs, they may at first require assistance with family members and caregivers. The unit clerk or patient service coordinator can assist with the family and caregivers by orienting them to the ICU through an information brochure, showing them the waiting room, and briefly overviewing the visitation policies. They cannot answer questions specific to the patient's clinical treatment, but can locate the appropriate clinician to address the family's concerns. The bedside clinicians support patients at admission with clinical interventions, but also with education and discussion regarding their current clinical issues and plan of care. The family members and caregivers are also updated on the current status and plan of care.

Family members and caregivers are imperative to the support systems of the patient. Cancer patients often have long-term support systems which have traveled the journey of cancer treatment with them and are deeply involved in their care. Because of this, they may need increased support to cope with a decline in the patient's status. The integration of additional disciplines such as chaplain services and social work may be needed.

Social workers in the oncology setting have knowledge of cancer care and are able to provide psychosocial services across the spectrum of the disease. As part of their role, social workers provide counseling and education to patients and families, as well as participate in treatment and/or goals of care discussions [10]. The social worker also works with the patient and family to identify the clinical power of attorney (MPOA) or legal decision maker in the event the patient becomes unable to make their own decisions. Social workers in the ICU are involved throughout the ICU stay and often participate in goals of care discussions alongside physicians and APPs. Chaplains are often called to the ICU for spiritual support of the patient and family at various intervals of the ICU stay including on admission, decline in status, or for the dying patient. Involving chaplains in spiritual care contributes to providing multidisciplinary and holistic care and it has been reported that family satisfaction with spiritual care in the ICU leads to increased overall patient satisfaction [15].

Routine ICU Care

Patient support occurs throughout the ICU stay. This support includes the patient and family remaining updated on the current plan of care. These updates can occur during the multidisciplinary rounding process or after rounds, when the provider may have more time to spend with the patient and their family. According to a study by Allen et al. [2], participation of family during ICU daily rounds promotes patient- and family-centered care and allows an opportunity for questions to be addressed. Family and/or patient involvement in multidisciplinary rounds is not always feasible, and therefore, each discipline seeing the patient should provide a daily update to the patient and family regarding their particular role upon examining the patient. For example, if the patient and/or family has concerns regarding a new medication that has been added to the treatment regimen, the clinical pharmacist can address the question. If the patient has questions about their cancer treatment plan or future chemotherapy or radiation plans, the best team to address these concerns is the oncology team. Each clinical team rounding on the patient should off time for the patient and family to ask questions when they are examining the patient, as this makes the patient feel like they are contributing to their own care and understanding the whole plan of care.

Ancillary staff in the ICU contribute to patient support via their contribution to family support and ICU workflow. The unit clerk or patient service coordinator is usually the frontline person who greets the family and assists them with non-clinical issues such as obtaining contact numbers, showing them the waiting room, notifying them of visitation hours, and helping them navigate the hospital. Unit clerks and patient service coordinators provide patient support through assisting the bedside staff with paging consultants and teams, stocking clinical supplies, and ensuring equipment issues such as computer malfunctions are addressed in a timely manner.

Patient care technicians, also known as nurse assistants, are imperative to patient support in the ICU setting. They are available to complete nurse-delegated tasks such as blood glucose checks, feeding patients, assistance with positioning and patient mobility, and bathing and skin care. Cancer patients in the ICU often require multiple lab draws throughout the day. Phlebotomists in the cancer ICU can be utilized to efficiently and effectively draw blood for lab tests. These tests allow for the timely identification of changes in patient's status, and providers use this information to adjust the plan of care accordingly.

Social Work and Patient Advocacy

Healthcare social workers and patient advocates work closely with patients, their families, physicians, nurses, and others to help determine educational and logistical needs of the patient and provide them with resources to meet those needs. In the ICU, social workers provide many services, including helping patients and families cope with the present critical illness. Patient advocates can be utilized when a patient or their family member has a grievance against the hospital or a staff member, or when the patient needs additional logistical support that the social worker cannot provide. The ICU can be a stressful environment for any patient, especially if their stay is prolonged for several days or weeks. Social workers can assist patients and families by providing community and hospital-based resources specific to the patient's needs. In a study performed by Hartman-Shea et al., 74% of social workers stated that their most frequent service performed was talking about family members' feelings [24]. Social workers themselves felt more satisfied in their work when they were able to meet family needs [39]. Patient advocates can help support a strong relationship between caregivers and their patients, and can provide additional resources for families in need.

Role of the Social Worker in the Intensive Care Unit

The role of the social worker in the ICU is multifaceted and can include facilitating communication, supportive interventions, hospitality, and counseling [18]. Additional interventions include crisis intervention, psychosocial assessment, staff support, end of life care, and family education [24]. Social workers are available to talk with families, listen to their concerns, and help provide a solution for most needs. The social worker then communicates needs to the healthcare team as necessary, resulting in improved overall communication, which can lead to increased patient and family experience satisfaction. If further clarification of the goals of care is needed or if the patient or family has several questions for the clinical team, the social worker helps to coordinate a family meeting in which key members of the clinical team meet with the patient and their family at an allotted time where all questions can be discussed and answered. The social worker often attends these meetings with the family if possible, to act as a liaison between the patient and provider, ensuring the plan of care is clear to everyone and that all questions have been answered. The social worker also provides emotional support during family meetings as needed.

In addition to offering traditional services, social workers are often the primary deliverer of psychosocial services in the oncology patient [17]. Psychosocial problems of the cancer patient can include among other things, depression and inadequate coping skills. Oncology social workers are trained in effective communication with and support of the cancer patient, and can offer high-quality psychosocial care that is evidence-based [64]. Multiple studies have shown that psychosocial care of cancer patients leads to enhanced patient outcomes and improved quality of life. One method that social workers use to help cancer patients and their families cope with their current situation is family-focused grief therapy. Family-focused grief therapy is a grief counseling model developed by Kissane et al. in which "the functioning of the family is screened routinely when the patient is admitted to a service in order to identify families at risk of morbid psychosocial outcome as a result of how members relate together" [33]. This type of counseling has been shown to reduce distress, depression, complications of bereavement, and pathological grief amongst family members of deceased cancer patients (Kissane et al 2006).

Social Worker Training

Social workers are trained in individual and family human behavior, active listening, social perceptiveness, and critical thinking. Social workers typically achieve a Bachelor of Social Work or Masters of Social Work degree via a program accredited by the Council on Social Work Education. Postgraduate licensure requirements vary by state. The National Association of Social Workers (NASW) provides practice standards and guidelines that describe in detail the various responsibilities of social workers. Standards vary depending on the focus population and environment. The standards are aligned with the NASW Code of Ethics and are meant to "guide decision-making and everyday professional conduct of social workers" [42]. They offer the new social worker a foundation on which to base their interventions and can provide seasoned social workers with ongoing references as needed. These standards are readily accessible via the NASW website and are updated as changes in practice are recommended.

Activities and Barriers

The stress of being in the ICU with a cancer diagnosis can lead to increased tension and/or grief that can affect the relationship between the patient, their family, and the clinical providers. Social workers in the ICU are a valuable resource to help reassure or comfort patients and families during a stressful time, provide education regarding how the ICU works and different provider role dynamics, and improve communication between all parties. Social workers perform many different duties in the ICU and in doing so, they recognize several barriers to care. In an effort to determine the primary social worker activities and barriers faced in the ICU, McCormick et al. performed a study at a Level I trauma center in the northwestern USA that surveyed social workers who had participated in care of patients who died in the ICU [39]. Social workers completed three different questionnaires and results were summarized into two categories: activities and barriers. The most commonly identified activities for communication and barriers to care that social workers faced are listed in Table 4. Heavy caseloads contributed to decreased social worker satisfaction since this required them to spend less time dedicated to counseling [39]. Overall, social workers seem to be most satisfied when barriers are limited and they have enough time to spend speaking with and offering counseling to patients and their families.

Role of the Patient Advocate in the Intensive Care Unit

Patient advocates typically work for a hospital but on behalf of the patient and can help promote patient autonomy and empowerment. Patient advocates are valuable resources to the multidisciplinary team and can be requested by either the healthcare worker or the patient and their family. If a patient feels that an issue is not getting resolved or they have a grievance against the hospital or a staff member, a patient advocate can provide an unbiased opinion of the situation and provide resources to help resolve the conflict. Patient advocates may help patients make sense of

Table 4 Social worker identified activities for communication and barriers to care

Activities
Discuss feelings with family members
Support patient care decisions made by family members
Discuss patient's live values
Reminisce with the patient and family
Discuss spiritual and religious needs
Review the patient's wishes regarding care or what they would have wanted if the patient is not able to discuss themselves
Facilitate room privacy (e.g., family conference room)
Attend and provide support during family care conferences
Encourage family to talk to and touch their loved one
Discuss cultural needs
Mediate family disagreement
Barriers
Severity of patient illness
Inability of patient to interact with family (e.g., sedation, breathing tube)
Understaffing
Minimal family interactions or visits
Lack of communication between care team
Unrealistic patient or family expectations of clinical treatment or prognosis
Family anger
Lack of privacy
Language barriers
Lack of support for family communication
Lack of staff communication
Topics outside the scope of practice of the social worker
Personality difficulties between staff and family

Adapted from McCormick et al. [39]

insurance issues, costs of procedures, or may simply be a trusted unbiased confidant in whom the patient can express frustrations or worries. In the ICU, strong emotions such as fear, anxiety, worry, and anger can arise and the patient may have difficulty discussing these with their immediate care takers. By involving the patient advocate, the patient is likely to immediately feel some relief because they recognize that the term "advocate" means that that person is going to support them and their best interest. Patient advocates can aid in goals of care or end of life discussions and can follow-up with the patient in private after these meetings or discussions have completed to answer any further questions that the patient may have had. Patient advocates both patient and staff experiences and are a valuable member of the multidisciplinary approach to patient care.

Patient Advocate Training

Until recently, there were no set national standards or certifications required to become a patient advocate. By definition, anyone who acts on behalf of the patient, with their best interest in mind, is a patient advocate. Physicians, APPs, nurses, and others can all be considered patient advocates. However, it is beneficial to have a designated employee whose title is Patient Advocate as this allows this person to solely focus on the unbiased support of patients and their families. Traditionally, patient advocates have come from a variety of backgrounds and held anywhere from a high school diploma up to a master's degree. In March of 2018, the Patient Advocate Certification Board (PACB) began offering the first nationally recognized patient advocate certification in which successful applicants earned the title "Board Certified Patient Advocate (BCPA)" [46]. PACB's certification is the first step to developing national standards and practice guidelines for patient advocates in the USA. Currently the BCPA certification does not have a minimum education or experience requirement, however they will potentially require this in the future.

Social workers are an invaluable resource to have as a member of a critical care interdisciplinary team. Their work with families improves patient satisfaction and supports the role of the clinical provider by improving communication and overall patient well-being. Social workers are trained to assess patients and their loved ones for barriers to communication and decision-making, and can individualize counseling based on their assessments. They provide community resources when needed, such as transportation, financial, and emotional support agencies and often follow up with patients and/or their families after the patient is discharged from the ICU. Although many barriers to care have been identified, social workers are adequately trained to react to these barriers and provide problem-solving solutions. Their work has a positive effect over the patient's overall ICU experience, resulting in improved quality of life.

Chaplaincy

The word "cancer" can invoke fear, anxiety, and grief in those patients and their families diagnosed with it. A survey published in 2011 by Harris Interactive [23] found that cancer is the most feared disease in the USA, with 41% of respondents listing it as their primary feared disease. Cancer is the second leading cause of death in the USA, with nearly 600,000 deaths reported per year, accounting for one in every four deaths [27]. A cancer diagnosis conjures a measure of uncertainty due to a lack of knowledge and may forge a list of questions wondering what the treatment plan, duration, and outcomes will be. It can cause emotional distress and lead some to turn to spirituality or religion for support [28]. Spirituality is defined as a sensitivity or attachment to religious values or the quality or state of being spiritual [54]. Spirituality can refer to one's connection with others or beliefs about the meaning and purpose of life, and does not necessarily include religion. Religion refers to a specific set of beliefs, attitudes, or practices, typically involving worship of a supernatural being or god that may also revolve around certain rituals or the following of sacred texts. People are often drawn closer to their spirituality or religion during times of distress and may seek out assistance in the form of a priest or chaplain to help answer questions, find meaning, and cope with their situation. Hospital chaplains are an integral part of a multidisciplinary team, attending to the spiritual and religious needs of patients and their families, which has been shown to improve patient satisfaction outcomes [28].

History of the Chaplain

The modern-day chaplain originated in the fourth century and comes from the legend of Martin of Tours [26]. Legend states that Martin, a Roman soldier who had been born to a pagan family in the Roman Province Pannonia, was passing by the gates of Amiens in Gaul (current day France) when he saw an unclothed beggar freezing on the side of the road. Moved by compassion, Martin used his sword to cut his own cape in half, giving one half to the beggar and keeping the other half for himself. Martin later had a vision in which he recalled the event and believed the beggar to be Christ himself. From that time on, Martin followed the Christian faith and eventually left the army to devote himself to the church. After his death, the remaining half of his cape was kept in a shrine and its location took on the name of the cape, "chapele" in French. Custodial priests carried the cape into battles on behalf of kings, as a sign that God was with them. The guardian of the capellanus (cape) was termed "chapelain" in Old French, and this is the word that "chaplain" stems from [26]. Since this time, chaplains have been used in various hospitals and healthcare settings. Over the last several decades, their presence has continued to increase, with 54–64% of US hospitals offering chaplaincy services between 1980 and 2003 [26].

The Joint Commission on the Accreditation of Healthcare Organizations (JCAHO) is a nonprofit organization who accredits healthcare organizations throughout the USA, certifying them on quality and the ability to meet certain performance standards [55]. JCAHO states that "Patients have a fundamental right to considerate care that safeguards their personal dignity and respects their cultural, psychosocial, and spiritual values" [35]. Healthcare settings, including hospitals, are required by JCAHO to perform and document a spiritual assessment on patients, which addresses questions like "How does the patient express their spirituality?" and "What type of spiritual/religious support does the patient desire?" [55]. Integrating clinically trained chaplains into the multidisciplinary care team is one way to integrate spirituality into the care of patients and address these basic patient rights [16].

Professional Training

Clinical chaplains are highly trained professionals who offer spiritual care for patients, their families, and staff [31]. Although board certification is not required for chaplains to practice in the hospital setting, it can improve competence, qualification, and ability to function as a professional chaplain [16]. The Board of Chaplaincy Certification, Inc. [14] states that board certification requires a master degree with graduate-level theological education, clinical pastoral education (CPE), endorsement from a recognized faith group, and demonstrated competency in functioning as a chaplain. CPE teaches chaplain students how to effectively listen to patients, engage their loved ones, establish rapport, and respond to verbal and nonverbal communications [25]. Like many other subspecialties in healthcare, board certified chaplains must complete at least 50 h of continuing education yearly [16]. This keeps them up to date on evolving spiritual care and improves their effectiveness in chaplaincy skills.

Role of the Chaplain

The role of the chaplain in the hospital is expansive. Chaplains attend to the spiritual and religious needs of any person who seeks them, whether religious or not, without proselytizing. They reaffirm religious beliefs and faith, listen to people's concerns and distress, provide grief and loss counseling, conflict resolution, assistance with decision-making, and facilitate communication between patients and staff [28]. They are often involved with end-of-life discussions for advanced cancer or chronically ill patients. A study performed by Flannely et al. [22] found the availability of chaplaincy services were associated with significantly lower rates of hospital deaths and higher rates of hospice enrollment compared to hospitals that did not offer chaplaincy services. Chaplains are able to help patients align their care plans with their values, which may lead to less aggressive care at the end-of-life and a shift to focusing on comfort [37]. Chaplains provide many other services, as discussed in Table 5.

Although their primary function may be to assist patients and their families during stressful situations, chaplains also attend to the spiritual needs of healthcare staff. Chaplains offer similar services, such as prayer and counseling and may perform special rituals like "Blessing of the Hands" in which chaplains pray over healthcare workers'

Table 5 Services provided by chaplains in the hospital setting

Religious
Reaffirm religious beliefs and faith
Spiritual assessment and risk screening
Lead religious ceremonies of worship and ritual
Offer religious materials and prayers
Conduct special holiday services
Provide Holy Communion
Counseling
Actively listen and try to understand client's distress
Assist with decision-making
Provide grief and loss care
Participate in patient care conferences and end of life discussions
Conflict resolution
Provide advice pertaining to healthcare ethics
Educate the healthcare team and community on spiritual issues
Mediate or reconcile parties
Facilitate finding meaning or purpose
Facilitation of spiritual issues related to organ/tissue donation
Advocacy
Communicate with caregivers
Facilitate staff communication
Enable existential empowerment
Support
Staff support relative to personal crises or work stress
Institutional support during organizational change or crisis
Critical incident stress debriefing
Provide emotional support
Referral to internal and external resources
Help patients prepare for death
Facilitate memorial services and funerals

Adapted from Ho et al. [28] and VandeCreek and Burton [59]

hands asking God to bless them as they are used to help others. The effects of spiritual care of employees have not been extensively studied, but it may decrease staff burnout by helping healthcare workers cope with the stress of patient care.

Assessment Tools

Various tools exist to assist the chaplain and other healthcare providers screen persons for spiritual risks. Some techniques that any member of the healthcare team can use are ask open-ended questions, listen actively, focus on nonbioclinical concerns and needs, and provide empathetic responses [28]. The Faith and belief, Importance and influence, Community, and Address in care (FICA) spiritual care assessment tool is typically used in the outpatient setting but can be used in inpatient settings as well. The FICA acronym guides the interviewer's questioning to elicit information about the patient's spiritual preferences and beliefs and can open up dialogue between the patient, their family, and the provider as well as ease anxiety or fear.

When patients require higher level of care, such as in the intensive care unit (ICU), there may be factors limiting their interactions with providers, particularly if they are intubated on mechanical ventilation or sedated. Mechanical ventilation can induce emotional distress and fear that is compounded by the inability to verbally communicate to others while an endotracheal tube is in place. Attempts at reading handwriting or lips of the mechanically ventilated patient are often futile and can cause the patient to become frustrated. In an effort to improve spiritual assessments of intubated patients, a chaplain at an urban tertiary care clinical center developed an illustrated spiritual care communication card to help awake and alert mechanically ventilated patients interact with spiritual care providers. The communication card enabled the patient to identify spiritual or religious affiliations, express a range of feelings, and rate spiritual pain [13]. Using the communication card, the patient could also request various interventions offered by the chaplain, such as prayer, blessing, song, communion, and more. Anxiety was measured immediately before and after chaplain-led, picture-guided spiritual care using a 100-mm visual analog scale (VAS). Patient encounters with chaplains using the communication card displayed a 20-point reduction in the mean (SD) VAS score, showing a significant reduction in patients' anxiety post-interaction. Other benefits of using the communication card included patients feeling more capable of dealing with their hospitalization (81%), an increased sense of peace (81%), and an increased

sense of connection to something sacred (71%) [13]. Although this study had a small sample size ($n = 50$), the findings suggest that patients benefit significantly from the utilization of communication cards in the mechanically ventilated patient by improving communication and decreasing anxiety and stress.

Outcomes and Efficacy of Chaplaincy

Many studies have shown the positive impacts that inhospital chaplaincy has on patient outcomes and patient satisfaction. Astrow et al. [11] found 73% of patients interviewed identified at least one spiritual need and they had significantly higher satisfaction and quality of care scores if their spiritual need was addressed during their visit. VandeCreek [58] studied 1440 patients at 14 US hospitals showed that patients felt chaplain visits met their spiritual needs and helped them use their faith, belief, and values to cope with their situation. One prospective study of 8978 patients discharged from a tertiary care hospital found patients who were visited by the chaplain were more likely to recommend the hospital to others and endorse the staff that met their spiritual and emotional needs [36]. In the same study, chaplain visits accounted for improved patient satisfaction scores on both the Press Ganey survey and Hospital Consumer Assessment of Healthcare Providers and Systems survey.

Despite outcomes supporting the use of chaplains in the hospital setting, spiritual care is infrequently provided, and chaplaincy consults are requested even less. A cross-sectional cohort study performed at Harvard Clinical School explored among other things the frequency of spiritual care provided to seriously ill advanced cancer patients [20]. Overall, only 10% of patients underwent a spiritual history and 16% of patients had a chaplain referral. The most common type of spiritual care provided was encouragement or affirming beliefs. The Coping With Cancer study published in 2007 was a multi-institutional investigation of advanced cancer patients and their unpaid caregivers that looked at religiousness and spiritual support, religious coping, and quality of life [12]. Seventy-two percent of the study population ($n = 230$) felt their spiritual needs were supported only minimally or not at all by the clinical system.

One of the factors accounting for low chaplaincy utilization rates is the fact the referrals tend to be more common when the patient is actively dying, rather than proactively. A cross-sectional retrospective chart review over a 6-month period performed at Duke University Hospital found that of 4169 admissions to adult ICUs, only 248 patients (5.9%) had documented chaplaincy services during their stay in the ICU [15]. Most of the chaplain visits occurred within the last 24–48 h of life. Despite the late referrals, studies have shown that family satisfaction is improved when spiritual care is provided during the last 24 h of life [62]. Other barriers to chaplaincy utilization include lack of time and training of physicians to conduct a thorough spiritual assessment, poor communication between the multidisciplinary team regarding spiritual needs, and infrequent physician–chaplain interactions [28]. One way to improve chaplain utilization would be to increase physician, nursing, and other clinical professional training in regards to spiritual care. Typically, the spiritual assessment is documented once, upon admission. Increasing the required frequency of this documentation could potentially increase chaplain referrals and utilization, resulting in high patient satisfaction.

There is clear evidence that inhospital chaplains are beneficial to the satisfaction and overall emotional well-being of patients. Physicians, advanced practice providers, and nurses are often too busy with tasks to consistently sit down with patients and assess their spiritual needs thoroughly. Chaplains have the ability and special training to perform spiritual needs assessments and intervene as needed. They help bridge communication between patients, their families, and healthcare providers, and assist with end-of-life discussions and needs. Their involvement improves patient satisfaction, particularly if utilized in the last 24 h of life. There is room for improvement in the frequency in which chaplains are consulted and in the spiritual care training

provided for nonchaplain healthcare workers such as physicians and nurses. By providing these services, organizations are committing to the holistic care and overall well-being of their patients, which results in happier patients and improved quality of life.

Conclusion

In all clinical settings, the concept of patient-centered care requires multiple teams of clinical, supportive, and ancillary services to work together for the benefit of the patient. Each department has a unique and vital role in promoting the well-being of patients. This multidisciplinary approach addresses the physical, mental, and spiritual aspects of the whole body. Patients and their families are typically more satisfied with the multidisciplinary approach because of the wide range of services offered to them. Caution must be taken, however, to ensure that each member of the team is portraying the same plan of care message to the patient. When the multidisciplinary team does not communicate with each other effectively, mixed messages can be sent to the patient and their family regarding plan of care and even prognosis. This can result in patient dissatisfaction and confusion, which can lead to increased anxiety and poor patient outcomes. Overall, the multidisciplinary approach appears to be the best approach to patient-centered care, as long as communication amongst the members is a top priority.

References

1. Aksoy Y, Kaydu A, Sahin OF, Kacar CK. Analysis of cancer patients admitted to intensive care unit. North Clin Istanb. 2016;3(3):217–21.
2. Allen SR, Pascual J, Martin N, Reilly P, Luckianow G, Datner E, . . ., Kaplan LJ. A novel method of optimizing patient- and family-centered care in the ICU. J Trauma Acute Care Surg. 2017;82(3):582–86.
3. Álvarez EA, Garrido MA, Tobar EA, Prieto SA, Vergara SO, Briceño CD, González FJ. Occupational therapy for delirium management in elderly patients without mechanical ventilation in an intensive care unit: a pilot randomized clinical trial. J Crit Care. 2017;37:85–90.

4. American Occupational Therapy Association, Inc. Occupational therapy in acute care. 2017. https://www.aota.org/About-Occupational-Therapy/Professionals/RDP/AcuteCare.aspx. Accessed 20 Apr 2018.

5. American Physical Therapy Association. Role of a physical therapist. 2016. http://www.apta.org/PTCareers/RoleofaPT/. Accessed 20 Apr 2018.

6. American Society for Parenteral and Enteral Nutrition (ASPEN). Board of directors and clinical practice committee: definition of terms, style and conventions used in ASPEN board of directors-approved documents. 2012. http://www.nutritioncare.org/uploadedFiles/Home/Guidelines_and_Clinical_Practice/DefinitionsStyleConventions.pdf. Accessed 17 Apr 2018.

7. Anthony PS. Nutrition screening tools for hospitalized patients. Nutr Clin Pract. 2008;23(4):373–82.

8. Arends J, Bachmann P, Baracos V, Barthelemy N, Bertz H, Bozzetti F, et al. ESPEN guidelines on nutrition in cancer patients. Clin Nutr. 2017;36(1):11–48.

9. Argiles JM. Cancer-associated malnutrition. Eur J Oncol Nurs. 2005;9:S39–50.

10. Association of Oncology Social Work (AOSW). Oncology social work standards of practice. 2012. http://www.aosw.org/professional-development/standards-of-practice/. Accessed 18 Apr 2018.

11. Astrow AB, Wexler A, Texeira K, Kai He M, Sulmasy DP. Is failure to meet spiritual needs associated with cancer patients' perceptions of quality of care and their satisfaction of care? J Clin Oncol. 2007;25(36):5753–7.

12. Balboni TA, Vanderwerker LC, Block SD, Paulk ME, Lathan CS, Peteet JR, Prigerson HG. Religiousness and spiritual support among advanced cancer patients and associations with end-of-life treatment preferences and quality of life. J Clin Oncol. 2007;25(5):555–60.

13. Berning JN, Poor AD, Buckley SM, Patel KR, Lederer DJ, Goldstein NE, Brodie D, Baldwin MR. A novel picture guide to improve spiritual care and reduce anxiety in mechanically ventilated adults in the intensive care unit. Ann Am Thorac Soc. 2016;13(8):1333–42.

14. Board of Chaplaincy Certification, Inc. Certification frequently asked questions. 2018. http://bcci.professionalchaplains.org/content.asp?pl=25&contentid=26. Accessed 26 Mar 2018.

15. Choi PJ, Curlin FA, Cox CE. The patient is dying, please call the chaplain: the activities of chaplains in one clinical center's intensive care units. J Pain Symptom Manag. 2015;50(4):501–6.

16. Cunningham CJL, Panda M, Lambert J, Daniel G, DeMars K. Perceptions of chaplains' value and impact within hospital care teams. J Relig Health. 2017;56(4):1231–47.

17. Deshields T, Zebrack B, Kennedy V. The state of psychosocial services in cancer care in the United States. Psycho-Oncology. 2013;22(3):699–703.

18. Dowling J, Wang B. Impact on family satisfaction: the critical care family assistance program. Chest. 2005;128(3):76S–80S.

19. Dy SM. Enteral and parenteral nutrition in terminally ill cancer patients: a review of literature. Am J Hosp Palliat Care. 2006;23(5):369–77.

20. Epstein-Peterson ZD, Sullivan AJ, Enzinger AC, Trevino KM, Zollfrank AA, Balboni MJ, VanderWeele TJ, Balboni TA. Examining forms of spiritual care provided in the advanced cancer setting. Am J Hosp Palliat Care. 2015;32(7):750–7.

21. Fearon K, Strasser F, Anker SD, Bosaeus I, Bruera E, Fainsinger RL, Jatoi A, Loprinzi C, MacDonald N, Mantovani G, Davis M. Definition and classification of cancer cachexia: an international consensus. Lancet Oncol. 2011;12(5):489–95.

22. Flannelly KJ, Emanuel LL, Handzo GF, Galek K, Silton NR, Carlson M. A national study of chaplaincy services and end-of-life outcomes. BMC Palliat Care. 2012;11:10.

23. Harris Interactive. What America thinks: MetLife Foundation Alzheimer's survey. 2011. https://www.metlife.com/assets/cao/foundation/alzheimers-2011.pdf. Accessed 23 Mar 2018.

24. Hartman-Shea K, Hahn AP, Kraus JF, Cordts G, Sevransky J. The role of the social worker in the adult critical care unit: a systematic review of the literature. Soc Work Health Care. 2011;50(2):143–57.

25. HealthCare Chaplaincy Network. Clinical pastoral education. 2018. https://healthcarechaplaincy.org/clinical-pastoral-education.html. Accessed 26 Mar 2018.

26. Healthcare Chaplains Ministry Association. History of healthcare chaplaincy and HCMA. 2018. http://www.hcmachaplains.org/history-of-healthcare-chaplaincy-and-hcma/. Accessed 26 Mar 2018.

27. Heron M. Death: leading causes for 2015. Natl Vital Stat Rep. 2017;66(5):1–75.

28. Ho JQ, Nguyen CD, Lopes R, Ezeji-Okoye SC, Kuschner WG. Spiritual care in the intensive care unit: a narrative review. J Intensive Care Med. 2017;33:279–87.

29. Hodgson CL, Stiller K, Needham DM, Tipping CJ, Harrold M, Baldwin CE, . . ., Green M. Expert consensus and recommendations on safety criteria for active mobilization of mechanically ventilated critically ill adults. Crit Care. 2014;18(6):658.

30. Hui P, Cook DJ, Lim W, Fraser GA, Arnold DM. The frequency and clinical significance of thrombocytopenia complicating critical illness: a systematic review. Chest. 2011;139(2):271–8.

31. Jacobs MR. What are we doing here? Chaplains in contemporary health care. Hastings Cent Rep. 2008;38(6):15–8.

32. Kim MM, Barnato AE, Angus DC, Fleisher LF, Kahn JM. The effect of multidisciplinary care teams on intensive care unit mortality. Arch Intern Med. 2010;170(4):369–76.

33. Kissane DW, McKenzie M, Block S, Moskowitz C, McKenzie D, O'Neill I. Family focused grief therapy: a randomized controlled trial in palliative care and bereavement. Am J Psychiatr. 2006;163(7):1208–18.

34. Lach K, Peterson SJ. Nutrition support for critically ill patients with cancer. Nutr Clin Pract. 2017;32(5):578–86.

35. LaPierre LL. JCAHO safeguards spiritual care. Holist Nurs Pract. 2003;17(4):219.

36. Marin DB, Sharma V, Sosunov E, Egorova N, Goldstein R, Handzo GF. Relationship between chaplain visits and patient satisfaction. J Health Care Chaplain. 2015;21(1):14–24.

37. Massey K, Barnes MJD, Villines D, Goldstein JD, Pierson ALH, Scherer C, Laan BV, Summerfelt WT. What do I do? Developing a taxonomy of chaplaincy activities and interventions of spiritual care in intensive care unit palliative care. BMC Palliat Care. 2015;14:10.

38. McClave SA, Taylor BE, Martindale RG, Warren MM, Johnson DR, …, Compher C. Guidelines for the provision and assessment of nutrition support therapy in the adult critically ill patient: Society of Critical Care Medicine (SCCM), and American Society for Parenteral and Enteral Nutrition (ASPEN). J Parenter Enteral Nutr. 2016;40:159–211.

39. McCormick AJ, Engelberg R, Curtis JR. Social workers in palliative care: assessing activities and barriers in the intensive care unit. J Palliat Med. 2007;10(4):929–37.

40. Mueller C, Compher C, Ellen DM, American Society for Parenteral and Enteral Nutrition (ASPEN) Board of Directors. Nutrition screening, assessment, and intervention in adults. J Parenter Enter Nutr. 2011;35(1):16–24.

41. National Association of Social Workers (NASW). Code of ethics. 2018. https://www.socialworkers.org/about/ethics/code-of-ethics. Accessed 1 May 2018.

42. Nordon-Craft A, Moss M, Quan D, Schenkman M. Intensive care unit-acquired weakness: implications for physical therapist management. Phys Ther. 2012;92(12):1494–506.

43. Oncology Nursing Certification Cooperation (ONCC). Certifications. 2018. https://www.oncc.org/certifications. Accessed 19 Apr 2018.

44. Patel RP, Canada TW, Nates JL. Bleeding associated with feeding tube placement in critically ill oncology patients with thrombocytopenia. Nutr Clin Pract. 2016;31(1):111–5.

45. Patient Advocate Certification Board (PACB). Frequently asked questions. 2018. https://pacboard.org/questions/. Accessed 12 Sept 2018.

46. Pène, F., Percheron, S., Lemiale, V., Viallon, V., Claessens, Y. E., Marqué, S., … & Mira, J. P. (2008). Temporal changes in management and outcome of septic shock in patients with malignancies in the intensive care unit. Critical care medicine, 36(3), 690–696

47. Puxty K, McLoone P, Quasim T, Sloan B, Kinsella J, Morrison DS. Risk of critical illness among patients with solid cancers: a population-based observational study. JAMA Oncol. 2015;1(8):1078–85.

48. Schellongowski P, Staudinger T, Kundi M, Laczika K, Locker GJ, Bojic A, Robak O, Fuhrmann V, Valent P, Sperr WR. Prognostic factors for intensive care unit admission, intensive care outcome, and post-intensive care survival in patients with de novo acute myeloid leukemia: a single center experience. Haematologica. 2011;96(2):231–7.

49. Schellongowski P, Sperr WR, Wohlfarth P, Knoebl P, Rabitsch W, Watzke HH, Staudinger T, Working Group for Hemato-Oncologic Intensive Care Medicine of the Austrian Society of Clinical and General Intensive Care Medicine and Emergency Medicine (OEGIAIN). Critically ill patients with cancer: chances and limitations of intensive care medicine – a narrative review. ESMO Open. 2016;1(5):e000018. http://esmoopen.bmj.com/content/esmoopen/1/5/e000018.full.pdf. Accessed 18 Apr 2018

50. Schober AE, Thornton KC. Early mobilization in the intensive care unit. Curr Anesthesiol Rep. 2013;3(2):73–8.

51. Schweickert WD, Pohlman MC, Pohlman AS, Nigos C, Pawlik AJ, Esbrook CL, …, Schmidt GA. Early physical and occupational therapy in mechanically ventilated, critically ill patients: a randomized controlled trial. Lancet. 2009;373(9678):1874–82.

52. Seron-Arbeloa C, Zamora-Elson M, Labarta-Monzon L, Mallor-Bonet T. Enteral nutrition in critical care. J Clin Med Res. 2013;5(1):1–11.

53. Shimabukuro-Vornhagen A, Böll B, Kochanek M, Azoulay É, von Bergwelt-Baildon MS. Critical care of patients with cancer. CA Cancer J Clin. 2016;66:496–517. https://doi.org/10.3322/caac.21351.

54. "Spirituality" Merriam-Webster. https://www.merriam-webster.com/dictionary/spirituality. 2017. Accessed 25 Mar 2018.

55. The Joint Commission. Clinical record – spiritual assessment. 2018. https://www.jointcommission.org/mobile/standards_information/jcfaqdetails.aspx?StandardsFAQId=1492&StandardsFAQChapterId=31&ProgramId=0&ChapterId=0&IsFeatured=False&IsNew=False&Keyword=. Accessed 9 Sept 2018.

56. Toh SG, Ang E, Devi MK. Systematic review on the relationship between the nursing shortage and job satisfaction, stress and burnout levels among nurses in oncology/haematology settings. Int J Evid Based Healthc. 2012;10(2):126–41.

57. Tzelepis F, Sanson-Fisher RW, Zucca AC, Fradgley EA. Measuring the quality of patient-centered care: why patient-reported measures are critical to reliable assessment. Patient Prefer Adherence. 2015;9:831.

58. VandeCreek L. How satisfied are patients with the ministry of chaplains? J Pastoral Care Counsel. 2004;58(4):335–42.

59. VandeCreek L, Burton L. Professional chaplaincy: its role and importance in healthcare. J Pastoral Care. 2001;55(1):81–97.

60. Virizuela JA, Camblor-Alvarez M, Luengo-Perez LM, Grande E, Alvarez-Hernandez J, Sendros-Madrono MJ, Jimenez-Fonseca P, Cervera-Peris M, Ocon-Breton MJ. Nutritional support and parenteral nutrition in cancer patients: an expert consensus report. Clin Transl Oncol. 2017;20(5):619–29.

61. Wahab R, Yip NH, Chandra S, Nguyen M, Pavlovich KH, Benson T, …, Perez-Mir E. The

implementation of an early rehabilitation program is associated with reduced length of stay: a multi-ICU study. J Intensive Care Soc. 2016;17(1):2–11.

62. Wall RJ, Engelberg RA, Gries CJ, Glavan B, Curtis JR. Spiritual care of families in the intensive care unit. Crit Care Med. 2007;35(4):1084–90.

63. White JV, Guenter P, Jensen G, Malone A, Schofield M, Academy Malnutrition Work Group, ASPEN Malnutrition Task Force, ASPEN Board of Directors. Consensus statement: Academy of Nutrition and Dietetics and American Society for Parenteral and Enteral Nutrition: characteristics recommended for the identification and documentation of adult malnutrition (undernutrition). J Parenter Enter Nutr. 2012;36(3):275–83.

64. Zebrack B, Kayser K, Oktay J, Sundstrom L, Sachs AM. The Association of Oncology Social Work's project to assure quality cancer care (APAQCC). J Psychosoc Oncol. 2018;36(1):19–30.

Advanced Practice Providers in the Oncologic Intensive Care Unit

6

Ninotchka Brydges, Tiffany Mundie, and Garry Brydges

Contents

Introduction 66

Evolution of APP Role in the ICU 66

APP Role in the Oncological ICU 67

Outcomes of APP Role in ICU 68

Advanced Practice Nursing and Professional Regulatory Requirements 68
Credentialing 68
Privileging 69
Competency 70

Implications to Clinical Practice 71

Conclusion 72

References 72

Abstract

In most organizations, health-care workforce is comprised of advanced practice registered nurses (APRNs) and physician assistants, which they are collectively called as advanced practice providers (APPs). APPs can provide care in various settings depending on their education, training, and population focus. The role of APPs was originally intended to address access to primary care in underserved areas and eventually extended to the critical care environment. In critical care, APP is proven to be beneficial in providing safe and effective care especially in oncological intensive care environment. In order for the APP to establish clinical practice, essential standardized processes must be attained. Credentialing and privileging are standardized processes ensuring that APPs have the necessary qualifications to provide direct safe patient clinical care. These processes will provide the highest level

N. Brydges (✉) · T. Mundie
Department of Critical Care and Respiratory Care, The University of Texas MD Anderson Cancer Center, Houston, TX, USA
e-mail: nbrydges@mdanderson.org;
tamundie@mdanderson.org

G. Brydges
Anesthesiology – CRNA Support, The University of Texas MD Anderson Cancer Center, Houston, TX, USA

Division of Anesthesia, Critical Care and Pain Medicine, Department of Anesthesiology, The University of Texas MD Anderson Cancer Center, Houston, TX, USA
e-mail: gbrydges@mdanderson.org

© Springer Nature Switzerland AG 2020
J. L. Nates, K. J. Price (eds.), *Oncologic Critical Care*,
https://doi.org/10.1007/978-3-319-74588-6_17

of reliability that the APP is providing safe competent care.

Keywords

Nurse practitioners · Advanced practice provider · Acute care setting · Acute care nurse practitioner · APP role · Physician assistants · Credentialing · Privileging · Critical care · Oncologic ICU · Intensive care unit · Intubation · Invasive procedures · Multidisciplinary team

Introduction

Advanced practice providers (APPs) include advanced practice nurses and physician assistants and other specialized advanced practices. APPs can provide care in various settings depending on their education, training, and population focus. The role of APPs was originally intended to address access to primary care in underserved areas and patient populations but has since extended to the critical care environment. APPs have also proven to be a beneficial addition to the critical care team to provide consistent safe and effective patient care. In oncology, APPs are integral members to interdisciplinary care [3]. The employment of APPs in oncology practice has been shown to contribute greatly in cancer care in response to aging population and the projected physician shortage.

The credentialing and privileging are two distinct processes, which APPs must complete on an initial hire and biannually within hospital systems. The credentialing process is a comprehensive professional background review of the provider. Credentials are documented evidence of licensures, education, training, experience, and other qualifications required by health-care organizations (www.jointcommission.org). The privileging process is a structured review and documentation of the practice aspects of the advance practice providers' role within a facility. The advanced practice providers' privileges are granted by the organization within their scope of practice that is governed by state regulations and licensure practice acts. In many institutions, the advanced practice providers comprise of advanced practice registered nurses (APRNs) and physician assistants (PAs). Although, APRNs and PAs differ in terms of education, clinical training, licensing, and certification, these advanced practice providers follow similar credentialing and privileging process in most organizations. These mechanisms will provide high level of reliability that APP is providing safe competent care [22].

Evolution of APP Role in the ICU

The role of nurse practitioners (NPs) and physician assistants (PAs) has evolved over time. NPs and PAs had their beginnings in the primary care setting and have progressed to include different population-focused NP roles. Nurse practitioners (NP), certified registered nurse anesthetists (CRNAs), certified midwives, clinical nurse specialist, and physician assistants (PAs) are grouped into a category known as advanced practice providers. APPs have minimum of a graduate degree and obtain national certification in their specialty. The role of NPs was initially established in 1965 to prepare registered nurses to practice in a primary care setting to combat the shortage of access of pediatric health care and primary health care in underserved communities [5, 6]. The PA role was first developed in 1965 to train former military medics to work with physicians to increase availability of primary medical care to underserved areas [5].

APPs have now been integrated into today's critical care environment. The quality of their care has been compared and proven similar to that of the traditional physician-only model. The addition of APPs to the ICU team has provided increased availability of consistent 24-h coverage of the critically ill patient. The oncologic ICU setting presents its own set of unique patient complications and challenges which requires the APP working in this type of ICU to be confident and comfortable in managing these situations as well as participating in difficult discussions with families and caregivers.

Over time, the role of NPs and PAs has expanded into the critical care environment. Multiple factors influenced the addition of APPs to the critical care team. In 2003, the American College of Graduate Medical Education (ACGME) restricted the working hours of a physician resident, and this along with the shortage of board-certified critical care physicians hindered the 24-h availability of critical care coverage [23]. McCarthy et al. [13] also described the aging population and increased the need for critical care as providing an opportunity to integrate APPs as part of the ICU team.

In the mid-1990s, the certification of acute care nurse practitioners (ACNP) was developed to prepare experienced registered nurses to manage patients in the adult acute and critical care environment [6]. Physician assistants are educated in medical care that encompasses all ages/levels of care and are able to complete postgraduate training programs in critical care [4]. The integration of advanced practice providers (APP) as part of the multidisciplinary team is common in today's critical care environment. It has been reported that 70% of ACNPs and 24% of PAs work in an ICU setting as members of the critical care team [6].

An APP in the ICU setting is either an ACNP or PA that works collaboratively with a physician-led ICU team to care for critically ill patients. In general, the critical care APP role includes obtaining history and physicals, reviewing relevant lab and imaging data, patient rounds, care coordination, prescribing treatment, developing plan of care, patient and family education, and performing invasive procedures [5, 6]. Common types of procedures performed by ICU APPs are endotracheal intubation and insertion of chest tubes, central lines and arterial lines, lumbar puncture, and feeding tube insertion [5, 6]. Additional invasive procedures can be performed by ICU APPs depending on unit-specific needs while maintaining competence of APPs.

The critical care APP is the front line for addressing acute changes in a patient's condition. They can manage a wide variety of conditions which commonly include but not limited to respiratory distress/failure, cardiac arrhythmias, hypo-/hypertension, septic shock, altered mental status, and delirium. APPs also have opportunities in their role to educate patients, families, and other member of the critical care staff such as the bedside nurses. Coordination of care is important in the ICU setting, and APPs act as liaisons between ICU team, consultants, primary team, and ancillary services such as social work and case management.

APP Role in the Oncological ICU

The care of patients in the oncologic setting present unique circumstances for the APP and ICU care team. Cancer patients may need transfer to the ICU for management of the effects of cancer treatment modalities such as reaction to chemotherapy or immunotherapy, complications of stem cell transplant, and the effects of the cancer itself affecting organ function [18]. Reasons for ICU admission specific to the cancer patient can include airway obstruction from tumor, diffuse alveolar hemorrhage, tumor lysis syndrome, cytokine release syndrome, hyperleukocytosis, electrolyte derangements, and complications from thrombocytopenia and coagulopathies. The APP caring for patients in the oncologic ICU setting requires a knowledge base on management of these oncologic-related disorders but also the usual MICU patient presentation such as respiratory failure, acute kidney injury, septic shock, etc. The management of cancer patients in the ICU requires close collaboration with the primary oncology team and other members of the multidisciplinary ICU team.

The APP in the oncologic ICU functions similarly to the traditional ICU APP in non-cancer ICUs but has additional facets to their role. One aspect is admitting or transferring patients to the ICU. As a member of the critical care team, the APP collaborates with the critical care attending and primary oncologic team to determine a patient's suitability for ICU admission. Prognosis related to cancer diagnosis and treatment as well as quality of life is considered prior to ICU admission [18]. The cancer ICU APP can also encounter challenges when performing invasive procedures such as refractory thrombocytopenia, enlarged lymph nodes, and skin abnormalities related to cancer treatment or to the cancer diagnosis such as graft versus host disease or cutaneous T-cell lymphoma.

In the oncologic ICU, families and caregiver support is imperative. Cancer patients under intense, long-term treatments and their support system have usually experience the journey alongside the patient and are actively involved in their care. The care of the families and caregivers includes updating them on the daily plan of care, allowing them to ask questions, and also listening to and addressing their concerns. In order to ensure the families and caregivers are supported, the APP collaborates with other members of the multidisciplinary team for assistance and support. These multidisciplinary members can include social work, case management, patient advocacy, nutrition, PT/OT, and pharmacy. Goals of care and end-of-life discussions are part of the care of oncologic ICU patients. The APP along with the attending physician and other members of the multidisciplinary team such as social work and patient advocacy participate in these types of discussions with the patients and caregivers.

Outcomes of APP Role in ICU

The addition of APPs to the critical care team has been compared in recent studies to the use of the resident model in the university setting. [19] found that when compared to resident-staffed medical intensive care unit (MICU), the nurse practitioner-staffed MICU did not show a significant difference in the rates of 48-h readmission rates or ICU mortality rate. Another study by Kawar and DiGiovine [9] found there was no significant difference between the PA-staffed MICU and resident-staffed MICU in regard to ICU mortality, readmission rates, and hospital length of stay. The trend of APP practice resulting in similar outcomes continues in a retrospective review by [20] in which they compared the complication rates of invasive procedures done by residents and those done by NPs and PAs in a trauma and surgical intensive care unit setting. The study found the complication rate for both groups to be the same at 2%. A study by Kapu et al. [7] showed a reduction in the length of stay and hospital charges when NPs were added to the critical care team.

The care provided by APPs is not only comparable to the resident model but benefits other aspects of care provided. APPs are a constant compared to the resident physician who is part of the team for a short period of time, typically 1 month. Advantages of the constant presence of the APP are continuity of care, improved hand-off between providers, and also care team members having a familiarity with each other, which can help build a culture of safety [4]. Several studies found that acute care NP practices result to significantly improved patient service and family satisfaction including cost-effectiveness and efficiency as measured by length of stay [13]. There were no significant differences in the ICU procedures performed by acute care NPs compared with same procedures done by trauma surgeons. Hospital mortality, length of stay, and hospital discharge measure patient outcomes found no significant differences in the care provided by critical care APPs and a house staff-based team. Kapu et al. [8] stated that one of the key components to the success of the critical care NP program has been the relationship, insight, and commitment of physician champions. Because of the physician champions, the role of the advanced practice providers has progressed as partner, collaborator, and provider.

Advanced Practice Nursing and Professional Regulatory Requirements

Credentialing

By definition, credentialing is a process that enables the institution to evaluate qualifications of each advance practice nurse to determine the appropriateness for a position as an advanced practice registered nurse at a given facility. Credentialing is a term used to processes designating that individual, program, institution, or product has met established standards set by an agent and recognized as qualified to carry out the task [22]. Licensure, registration, accreditation, approval, certification, recognition, or endorsement may be used to describe different credentialing methods; however, this may not consistently apply across different settings or countries. In some states, a comprehensive standardized credentialing form is utilized for advanced practice providers. For example, in the state of Texas, Texas Standardized Credentialing Application is used by facilities across the state in an effort to standardize the process of credentialing advanced practice providers. In addition to standardized credentialing application, a medical staff office performs primary source verification on each provider. Primary source verification is performed on every advanced practice registered nurses' education, licenses, certifications, authorizations, professional experience, and any related data from state and federal regulatory agency databases. Licensure is one of the credentialing processes by which the agency of state government grants permission to individuals accountable for the practice of a profession and prohibits all other from legally doing so [22]. The main purpose of this process is to protect the public by ensuring a minimum level of professional competence, while certification is the process by which nongovernment agency or association grants recognition to an individual who has met certain predetermined qualification specified by an agency or association with the purpose of ensuring the public that an individual has a mastered body of knowledge and acquired skills based on the specialty. Certification can be mandatory or voluntary.

Further, it is very important to understand the difference between the categories of advanced practice registered nurses [2]. There are four categories of advanced practice registered nurses (APRNs) including nurse midwives, clinical nurse specialists, nurse practitioners, and certified registered nurse anesthetists. Each category of APRNs has very different credentialing and privileging requirements based on their subspecialty. For example, endotracheal intubation is not the same privilege for an acute care nurse practitioner compared to a certified registered nurse anesthetist. Endotracheal intubation is a basic skill for a certified registered nurse anesthetist and an advanced privilege for a nurse practitioner. This highlights the importance of understanding the differentiation between the four APRNs and their unique scope of practice within their specialty. Hospitals employ APRNs in their various clinical settings such inpatient units, outpatient clinics, emergency departments, and acute care units. Credentials must be periodically renewed to assure continued quality, and they may be removed when standards of competence or behavior are not met [22].

Privileging

By definition, privileging is the process where health-care institutions grant authority to APRNs to provide certain patient care and treatment services. When a privilege is granted by the facility, the patient care or treatment service must be consistent with the scope of practice, licensure, and certification. APRN privileges within an organization are usually broken into three classifications: core, class I, and class II privileges. The core privileges are the services provided by an APRN based on education, training, certification, and or licensure that do not require any form of delegated medical authority [8]. Basic examples include obtaining a medical history, performing a physical examination, and ordering basic laboratory and diagnostic imaging. These core privileges apply across advanced practice providers.

Class I privileges are services provided by an APRN that require delegated medical authority and are unique to his/her patient population and consistent with state board of nursing authorization, rules and regulations, training, and experience. Examples include procedures that require a correspondingly increased degree of expertise and skill. Class II privileges require supervised training and require verification of competency. These privileges may be requested at any point as patient care needs and technologies evolve. Class II privileges may not be required by all APRNs. For example, invasive procedures in acute care settings such as ultrasound-guided arterial line insertion, central venous catheter placement in different locations fiber-optic bronchoscopy, dialysis catheter insertions, and other invasive procedures. These invasive procedures require competency and expertise [20]. It is noted that procedural proficiency often requires a learning curve, and inadequate training can result to adverse outcomes. These adverse outcomes may impact patients' morbidity, mortality, and length of ICU stay.

It is important to note that each state has a wide variability on how class II privileges are granted. For example, states that have fully implemented the APRN consensus model do not require delegated medical authority. For example, Alaska, Hawaii, Washington, Oregon, Nevada, Arizona, New Mexico, Colorado, Utah, Wyoming, Idaho, Montana, North Dakota, South Dakota, Nebraska, Oklahoma, Arkansas, Iowa, Minnesota, Wisconsin, Michigan, Kentucky, West Virginia, Delaware, Maryland, New Hampshire, Vermont, Rhode Island, and Connecticut have full APRN consensus model implementation, which define the advance practice registered nurse as independent providers and do not require written collaborative agreements, supervision, or conditions for practice (www.ncsbn.org, 2018; [15]). The APRN consensus model establishes national standards for education and training for all categories of APRNs and would extend to consumers in all states access to comprehensive care by APRNs [2, 20].

Competency

Competency standards are widely used in health care as benchmark for entry to work practice [14]. Advanced practice provider service, specifically NP, is being implemented internally to improve timely access in the health care across a range of settings. Therefore competencies are useful and necessary for definition and education of practice-based professional. It is recognized that competencies are designed for practice in stable environments with familiar problems [14]. When translating competencies to practice to guide NP, it enables the development of theory-driven standards that accommodate the complex and cognitive domain. The cognitive domain encompasses the capacity to master skills and tasks and incorporating effective processes and critical thinking

for complex situations. In most organizations, orientation program is used to provide standard process, establish clear expectations of orientation, improve accountability for oversight and orientation structure, and streamline the workload for the leadership team and preceptors [21]. The specialty competency-based assessment tool includes knowledge, systems, procedural skills, communication, professionalism, and performance improvement competencies.

Professional Processes and Evaluation of APP Practice

Hospitals and other health-care facilities grant APRNs authority to practice after comprehensive verification of education, license, clinical training, and certification. APRN prescriptive authority, title recognition, education requirements, and licensing must be addressed during credentialing and privileging processes to reflect state statutes, rules, and regulations. The Joint Commission requires health-care institutions to have a credentialing and privileging process to systematically review applicant's qualifications [10]. Credentialing and privileging for the APPs (APRNs and PAs) are largely similar to physicians and dictated by the institution's governing documents [8].

Medical staff and credentialing services play a critical role in the credentialing and privileging of physicians and advanced practice providers. One of its most important responsibilities is preparing applications for appointment, reappointment, and privileging for review of appropriate individuals and groups. However, other organizational disciplines such as division of nursing, advance practice providers group (APRNs and PAs), and human resource department have important roles in the process. In some institutions, a committee-based credentialing and privileging process comprises of advanced practice providers. The committee reviews the medical staff credentialing process primary findings and forwards recommendations to the nursing and medical executives. Specifically, the credentialing committee formulates policies, procedures, and practices related to the APRN credentialing process and forwards recommendations to the entire APRN membership and chief nursing officer that then will be forwarded to final review of chair of medical staff.

The credentialing and privileging process include completion of standardized application form with evidence of education, training, state licensure and certification, professional resume or curriculum vitae, and other essential information required by the institution. After application is submitted, primary source verification is performed including criminal background check, and a query to the National Practitioner Data Bank is made to evaluate occurrence of licensure disciplinary action, malpractice payments, or adverse action affecting professional membership [10]. Also, medical staff professionals must keep abreast of requirements of state licensing authorities, Centers for Medicare & Medicaid Services (CMS), Occupational Safety and Health Administration (OSHA), The Joint Commission, National Committee for Quality Assurance (NCQA), and insurance and managed care companies.

In addition, hospitals and other health-care institutions have specific bylaws, which include credentialing and privileging process, policies and governance procedures, and rules and regulations. Every hospital or health-care institutions has different credentialing and privileging process such as initial, recredentialing, transfer to different department, and requesting additional privileges. In addition, hospital bylaws include professional practice evaluation as mandated by the Joint Commission. The professional practice evaluation comprised of ongoing professional practice evaluation (OPPE) and focused professional practice evaluation (FPPE). OPPE is a continuous evaluation of providers' clinical competence and professional behavior that impact quality, patient safety, and maintaining existing privileges [12]. The FPPE process verifies new hire's competency and when applying new privileges. FPPE also serves as a means to identify providers with poor technical skills, poor judgment, age-related limitations, or other professional performance issues that affect patient safety. FPPE can be triggered during an OPPE [8]. The FPPE process should be clearly defined and consistently implemented.

FPPE can be performed in several methods such as chart review, evaluating practice patterns, peer review, and involving in multidisciplinary discussions.

Implications to Clinical Practice

Because of the US aging population and ongoing health reform, there is an increasing demand of advanced practice providers (APPs) and a projection of hematologists/oncologists shortage [3, 13, 16]. APPs are essential to interdisciplinary care of oncologic patients [16]. The APP scope of practice permits for major contributions across the different stages cancer disease trajectory, health promotion and prevention, diagnosis and treatment, and palliative care. Collaborative oncology practice promotes high satisfaction to APPs and physicians including patients and families. Aside from the clinical and educational contributions, APP can also be an instrument in quality improvement initiatives, research efforts, and exploring innovative ways to improve quality and safe health-care delivery in oncological patients [16].

Advanced provider practice is focused on clinical decision, collaboration among disciplines, reimbursement, quality indicators, patient satisfaction, and incorporating evidence-based decision-making into clinical practice [1]. The core functions of APPs include education, professional development and coaching, practice development and innovation, and regulatory processes. The study of Bruinooge et al. [3] provides baseline data indicating that the APPs spend a majority of their time in patient care and conduct wide array of patient care services ranging from new patient visits to follow-up care to more specialized services such as genetic counseling, surgery first assists, and procedures.

A comprehensive literature review of acute care NP practices examined 47 studies relevant to ICU practice and found that measures of patient service and family satisfaction were significantly improved including cost-effectiveness and efficiency as measured by length of stay [13]. In addition, ICU procedures performed by acute care NPs compared with same procedures done by trauma surgeons were found no significant differences. Hospital mortality, length of stay, and hospital discharge measure patient outcomes found no significant differences in providing care by critical care APPs and a traditional, house staff-based team.

Credentialing and privileging are essential processes to APRN practice in acute care settings [10]. The processes ensure that APRNs are providing safe patient care based on education, training, and licensure. Credentialing and privileging promote practice accountability, adhere to professional standards, and authorize qualified health-care providers to communicate scope of practice to other clinicians. In addition to standard care provision, APRNs have expanded role such as case management, medication management, admitting, and discharge planning [11]. Thus, credentialing and privileging processes evaluate scope of practice and compliance with federal and state laws [10, 11]. The translation from competencies to practice standards to define and guide APRN (including APPs) practice and education facilitates theory-driven standard development that adapts the complex and cognitive domain [14].

Conclusion

APPs are integral members of the health-care workforce. Given the projected deficit of critical care physicians, and oncologists, it is expected that acute care APPs will play a major role to many critical care units [13]. APP's practice model has shown similar in relation to better patient outcomes when compared to the care provided by physicians. Because outcomes are similar, it makes sense to incorporate official training of the APP to practice to the full extent of their scope, including performing all major invasive procedures after being credentialed, and demonstrate competency. The practice environment and patient acuity level should dictate which procedures the APP is trained to perform while continuing to measure patient outcomes and support the expanding roles and APP utilization in critical care settings.

Credentialing and privileging are interrelated processes that promote patient safety and offer another layer regarding advanced practice [22]. The processes ensure that clinical providers have the necessary qualifications to direct quality patient care in hospitals and other health-care settings. Streamlining the process of credentialing and privileging will not only address the increasing number of APRNs and other primary care providers but also provide solution to the increased number of the insured population seeking health care [2, 17]. The projected shortage of physicians warrants preparation and strategies to train advanced practice providers to meet patient care demands.

References

1. Ackerman MH, Mick D, Witzel P. Creating an organizational model to support advanced practice. J Nurs Adm. 2010;40(2):63–8.
2. Brassard A, Smolenski MC. Removing barriers to advanced practice registered nurse care: hospital privileges. Washington, DC: AARP Public Policy Institute; 2011.
3. Bruinooge SS, Pickard TA, Vogel W, Hanley A, Schenkel C, Garrett-Mayer E, …, Smith N. Understanding the role of advanced practice providers in oncology in the United States. J Oncol Pract 2018;14(9):e518–e532.
4. Gershengorn HB, Johnson MP, Factor P. The use of nonphysician providers in adult intensive care units. Am J Respir Crit Care Med. 2012;185(6):600–5.
5. Grabenkort WR, Meissen HH, Gregg SR, Coopersmith CM. Acute care nurse practitioners and physician assistants in critical care: transforming education and practice. Crit Care Med. 2017;45(7):1111–4.
6. Hoffman LA, Guttendorf J. Preparation and evolving role of the acute care nurse practitioner. Chest. 2017;152(6):1339–45.
7. Kapu AN, Kleinpell R, Pilon B. Quality and financial impact of adding nurse practitioners to inpatient care teams. J Nurs Adm. 2014;44(2):87–96.
8. Kapu AN, Thomson-Smith C, Jones P. NPs in the ICU: the Vanderbilt initiative. Nurse Pract. 2012;37(8):46–52.
9. Kawar E, DiGiovine B. MICU care delivered by PAs versus residents: do PAs measure up? J Am Acad Physician Assist. 2011;24(1):36–41.
10. Kleinpell RM, Hravnak M, Hinch B, Llewellyn J. Developing an advanced practice nursing credentialing model for acute care facilities. Nurs Adm Q. 2008;32(4):279–87.

11. Klein T. Credentialing the nurse practitioner in your workplace: evaluating scope for safe practice. Nurs Adm Q. 2008;32(4):273–8.

12. Makary MA, Wick E, Freischlag JA. PPE, OPPE, and FPPE: complying with the new alphabet soup of credentialing. Arch Surg. 2011;146(6):642–4.

13. McCarthy C, O'rourke NC, Madison JM. Integrating advanced practice providers into medical critical care teams. Chest. 2013;143(3):847–50.

14. O'Connell J, Gardner G, Coyer F. Beyond competencies: using a capability framework in developing practice standards for advanced practice nursing. J Adv Nurs. 2014;70(12):2728–35.

15. Phillips SJ. APRN consensus model implementation and planning. Nurse Pract. 2012;37(1):22–45.

16. Reynolds RB, McCoy K. The role of advanced practice providers in interdisciplinary oncology care in the United States. Chin Clin Oncol. 2016;5(3):44.

17. Trepanier S, Duran P, Lawson L. The use of advanced practice nurses in the acute care setting. Nurse Lead. 2013;11(1):45.

18. Schellongowski P, Sperr WR, Wohlfarth P, Knoebl P, Rabitsch W, Watzke HH, Staudinger T. Critically ill patients with cancer: chances and limitations of intensive care medicine – a narrative review. ESMO Open. 2016;1(5):e000018.

19. Scherzer R, Dennis MP, Swan BA, Kavuru MS, Oxman DA. A comparison of usage and outcomes between nurse practitioner and resident-staffed medical ICUs. Crit Care Med. 2017;45(2):e132–7.

20. Sirleaf M, Jefferson B, Christmas AB, Sing RF, Thomason MH, Huynh TT. Comparison of procedural complications between resident physicians and advanced clinical providers. J Trauma Acute Care Surg. 2014;77(1):143–7.

21. Simone S, McComiskey CA, Andersen B. Integrating nurse practitioners into intensive care units. Crit Care Nurse. 2016;36(6):59–69.

22. Smolenski MC. Credentialing, certification, and competence: issues for new and seasoned nurse practitioners. J Am Acad Nurse Pract. 2005;17(6):201–4.

23. Ulmer C, Miller Wolman D, Johns MME. Resident duty hours: enhancing sleep, supervision, and safety. Institute of Medicine (US) committee on optimizing graduate medical trainee (resident) hours and work schedule to improve patient safety. Washington, DC: National Academies Press (US); 2009. Accessed 12 Apr 2018

Early Warning Systems and Oncological Critical Care Units

7

Michelle O'Mahony and Tim Wigmore

Contents

Introduction 76

Principles of Early Warning Systems 76

Evolution of Early Warning Systems 78

Evidence for Early Warning Systems 78
Predictive Value 78
Weighted Vital Sign Prediction 78
Outcomes 79

Human Factors and Infrastructure 79
Familiarity 79
Hierarchy and Division of Labor 79
Infrastructure 80

Early Warning Systems in an Oncology Population 80

Immunotherapy 81

Chemotherapy 83

Conclusion 84

References 84

Abstract

In the late twentieth century, it was increasingly recognized that up to three-quarters of all patients who suffer an inhospital cardiac arrest and/or require rescue transfer to a higher level of care have worsening physiological parameters in the antecedent hours prior to critical demise. This recognition highlighted the need for early identification of these patients to facilitate timely intervention and provide the appropriate language for escalation of care. Subsequent development and implementation of early warning systems became a global healthcare initiative, and while there are multiple derivations, the vast majority of hospitals now utilize some form of track and trigger system to facilitate early identification of patients at risk of clinical demise.

M. O'Mahony (✉) · T. Wigmore
Department of Anaesthesia, Critical Care and Pain Medicine, Royal Marsden Hospital, London, UK
e-mail: Michelle.O'Mahony@rmh.nhs.uk; timothy.wigmore@rmh.nhs.uk

© Springer Nature Switzerland AG 2020
J. L. Nates, K. J. Price (eds.), *Oncologic Critical Care*,
https://doi.org/10.1007/978-3-319-74588-6_7

Oncology patients are at risk of clinical deterioration due to the neoplastic state, complications of antitumor therapies, and noncancer-related comorbidities. Early identification of at-risk oncology patients would prove particularly beneficial to facilitate early and appropriate discussions for treatment goals, ceilings of care, and multidisciplinary team input. At present, generic early warning systems have not been validated in this population and fail to account for a persistent deranged physiology which may represent a new baseline in these patients.

In this chapter we discuss the fundamental principles of early warning systems and their position within modern medicine, their strengths and limitations, the associated infrastructures, and the particular challenges facing early warning systems in oncological patients.

Keywords

Early warning systems · Rapid response teams · Track and trigger

Introduction

Medical early warning systems (EWSs) are a tool to preempt imminent physiological collapse and initiate timely health interventions to optimize patient outcomes. The systems track and record patient deviations from healthy physiological baselines to increasing abnormalities which may precipitate critical events. The fundamental principle of EWSs is objective and accurate collection of patient vital signs, assignment of exponential points based on deviations from normal baseline, calculation of a total EWS score, and escalation of care based on the cumulative score. Proposed benefits are an objective measure which is cheap and easy to implement as well as being noninvasive with early identification of potentially sick patients. In this chapter, we will discuss the basic principles of EWSs, the evolution of these systems within medicine, the evidence for their use, the associated human factors and necessary infrastructures, and finally the

value of these systems within an oncology population.

Principles of Early Warning Systems

Early warning systems have evolved as a means for early identification of physiologically deteriorating patients and escalation of care prior to a critical event. The impetus for these track and trigger systems was initially driven by the recognition that up to 72% of ward patients who suffer an inhospital cardiac arrest or require rescue transfer to a higher level of care have worsening abnormalities in their bedside observations several hours prior to these events [25, 27]. It was postulated if these deteriorating patients could be flagged to the appropriate healthcare professionals in a timely manner; outcomes such as 30 day mortality, hospital length of stay, and critical care unit admission may be improved. In the intervening decades, EWSs have developed throughout medicine and now form an integral component of the end of bed observations. In fact, the National Institute for Health and Clinical Excellence mandates the use of physiological track and trigger systems for all adult patients in acute hospital settings [2]. Early warning points are appointed based on degrees of aberrancy (scoring 1–3) from normal physiological parameters (scoring 0), and then care is directed according to the cumulative early warning score in an exponential manner, i.e., the greater the physiological aberrancy, the greater the early warning score, the more time critical the medical review by an increasing seniority of healthcare professional.

Although early warning systems are based on an cumulative score based on predominantly objectively collected parameters, the scores can be modified based on the patient cohort to account for physiological differences in some demographics, i.e., obstetrics and pediatrics. The standard ward-based early warning systems use between four to seven vital signs parameters although there are many more derivations consisting of single parameter systems, multi-parameter systems, and complex computer-based algorithms. In order to lend uniformity to the

Physiological Parameters	3	2	1	0	1	2	3
Respiration Rate	</= 8		9-11	12-20		21-24	>/=25
Oxygen Saturations	</= 91	92-93	94-95	>/= 96			
Any Supplemental Oxygen		Yes		No			
Temperature	</= 35.0		35.1 – 36.0	36.1 – 38.0	38.1 – 39.0	>/= 39.1	
Systolic BP	</= 90	91 - 100	101 - 110	111 - 219			>/= 220
Pulse	</= 40		41 - 50	51 - 90	91 - 110	111 - 130	>/= 131
Consciousness				A			V, P or U

NEWS Score	Frequency of Monitoring	Clinical Response
0	Minimum 12 hourly	Continue routine NEWS monitoring with every set of observations
Total 1 - 3	Minimum 4 hourly	-Inform registered nurse who must assess the patient. - Registered nurse to decide if increased frequency of monitoring and/or escalation of clinical care is required.
Total 4 or more OR 3 in one parameter	Minimum 1 hourly	- Registered nurse to **urgently** inform the medical team and nurse in charge. - Urgent assessment by medical team/surgical/critical care outreach team. - Consider clinical care in an environment with monitoring facilities; if appropriate.
Total 6 or more	Continuous monitoring of vital signs	-Registered nurse to **immediately** inform the medical team caring for the patient – this should potentially be at least a specialist registrar. - Emergency assessment by critical care outreach team or clinical site practitioner. - Consider transfer of clinical care to a level 2 or 3 care facility, i.e. HDU or ICU -If patient is at risk of imminent cardiac arrest, call crash code.

Fig. 1 National early warning score parameters and triggers

recording and interpretation of patient vital signs and the triggered responses, the Royal College of Physicians introduced a National Early Warning Score (NEWS) in 2012 which was standardized across all hospitals, recently updated and endorsed by NHS England [50] (Fig. 1).

Evolution of Early Warning Systems

The first early warning system was implemented toward the end of the twentieth century [42] using an aggregate system of weighted physiological variables to produce an algorithm of timely healthcare escalations. These scoring systems were not devised with a predictive model in mind but more a pathway for escalation and communication in the face of serious antecedents. Since then, multiple variations of these aggregate weighted track and trigger systems (AWTTS) have developed ranging from paper-based simple scoring systems to complex computer-based software algorithms which direct healthcare interventions [28]. In the early years, one of the biggest challenges to the widespread applicability of EWSs was differences in population-specific physiological baselines particularly the pediatric and maternity patient cohorts.

The 2006 Confidential Enquiry into Maternal and Child Health [11] identified that one in five children who have inhospital mortality have avoidable factors preceding terminal events and made recommendations for early identification of these factors in a pediatric population. The application of an early warning system in a pediatric healthcare setting has posed its own difficulties due to variations in normal physiological parameters according to age, robust pediatric compensatory mechanisms, and often hindered verbal communication with children [22]. Currently there are many different adaptations of pediatric early warning tools in use which have been validated in tertiary pediatric centers [3, 4, 7]. However, a recent systematic review examining PEWS has reported an absence of a standardized PEWs across international settings making reviews of standardized outcomes inconclusive at best [30].

Evidence for Early Warning Systems

While early warning tools provide the right language for escalation of care, evidence of benefit needs further analysis. Early warning systems can be evaluated under a number of criteria.

Predictive Value

The predictive value of early warning scores has previously been evaluated based on outcomes of cardiac arrest and death within 48 h. For mortality prediction, one large study of over 75,000 patients using the Vitalpac Early Warning Score (ViEWS) had an AUROC of 0.89 (95% CI 0.85–0.92) for death within 48 h [47]. Similar results were found in the same patient cohort using the National Early Warning System [53] for death within 24 h with AUROC of 0.89 (95% CI 0.89–0.90). These results would suggest both ViEWS and NEWS are useful for mortality prediction.

Early warning systems have shown similarly high discriminative value at cardiac arrest prediction with a ViEWS AUROC for cardiac arrest within 24 h of 0.74 (95% CI 0.72–0.75) and a NEWS AUROC for cardiac arrest within 24 h of 0.857 (95% CI 0.847–0.868) [47, 53]. For both death and cardiac arrest prediction, there is a clinically significant trade off in sensitivity and specificity with specificity usually in the range of 90% being balanced with lower sensitivities in the mid-50–70% range [28].

Weighted Vital Sign Prediction

Is there a single vital sign parameter that is most associated with clinical deterioration? A 2010 case control study of 580 patients found a respiratory rate of >35 (OR 31.1, 95% CI 7.5–129.6) or requirement for 100% supplemental oxygen (OR 13.7, 95% CI 5.4–35) to be most associated with a life-threatening clinical deterioration [49]. The results of this have led to adaptations of some early warning systems with a greater focus on respiratory monitoring, as previous studies have questioned the interobserver reliability for end of bed measured respiratory rates [44, 46]. Following on from respiratory parameters, a tachycardia of >140 bpm (OR 8, CI 95% 2.4–27.5) was next most associated with serious clinical demise [49].

Outcomes

There is a paucity of evidence showing significant improvement in mortality following the introduction of track and trigger systems. While the systems have good discriminative power for detecting patients at risk of clinical deterioration, the subsequent escalation of care does not appear to have an overall mortality benefit at 30 days [6, 21].

The impact of early warning systems on cardiac arrests has shown mixed results, but the majority of studies have reported a decrease in the number of cardiac arrests per adult admission following EWS implementation [17, 41].

One of the largest trials in this area was the 2005 MERIT trial which was a cluster-randomized trial studying the use of medical emergency teams following a track and trigger system in 23 hospitals in Australia to determine if the MET system could reduce the incidence of cardiac arrests, unplanned admissions to intensive units, and deaths among general ward patients [39]. The outcome of the study as summarized by the investigators stated "The MET system greatly increases emergency team calling, but does not substantially affect the incidence of cardiac arrest, unplanned ICU admissions, or unexpected death."

Human Factors and Infrastructure

While the standardized national early warning system is now mandatory in all NHS hospitals, there is significant heterogeneity between the responsible personnel, the planned rapid response, and the governance of these practices. The barriers to successful implementation of early warning systems are multifactorial, and the involved human factors may be related to traditional hierarchical models of care and organizational cultures that can lead to a degree of institutional inertia [9].

A common criticism of track and trigger systems is delayed activation of the rapid response or medical emergency team [36, 51, 56]. The MERIT trial, which to date, is the largest multicenter randomized controlled trial for medical emergency teams reported delayed activation of a triggered response in 70% of cases. These results were reproduced in a 2011 study which examined 575 patients with trigger failure in 22.8% [54]. Thus, one must question what are the barriers to successful rapid response system activations?

Familiarity

Inadequate training, inaccurate recording, and misinterpretation of the results can all lead to failures of the triggering system. There are currently over 33 different early warning systems in use worldwide. Lack of familiarity with the system can lead to reduced compliance, increased recording errors, and a cognitive failure in recognition of high triggers. Awareness of the system, education sessions for staff, and frequent auditing and training would enhance accuracy of recording and interpretation of results.

Hierarchy and Division of Labor

Early warning systems at their core require the recording of patient vital signs. This is recognized as a fundamental practice across all spectrums of patient assessment; however, it is also seen as a basic task that can be delegated down the hierarchical chain. Historically, vital signs were recorded for each patient by their assigned nurse. However, given the increasing demands on hospital staff and disproportionately high patient to nursing ratios, it is becoming increasingly difficult for bedside observations to remain a core nursing duty. More frequently, it is assigned to a nursing student or healthcare assistant to record bedside observations. This has been driven by reforms within the nursing workforce sector which has seen nurses take on more complex roles of drug administration, discharge planning, and managerial roles, leading to delegation of more fundamental tasks to other personnel [5]. However, while some vital signs such as blood pressure and heart rate are measured objectively, there can be a greater degree of subjectivity with respiratory rate [44, 46] and levels of consciousness [18] leading to potential inaccuracies in recording. Even if the mechanistic activity of recording is accurate, it still needs to be interpreted within a clinical context and appropriate responses triggered. Early warning systems in some part obviate the need for clinical interpretation as it is a score-directed algorithm; however, studies have shown that the recorded variables have at times been manipulated to accommodate the recorders perceptions [33]. Similarly, if clinical concerns are not addressed within the limits of the early warning system, such as subtle changes in patient color or distended abdomen, it could lead to nullification of genuine clinical acumen [34].

One proposed advantage of early warning systems is providing nurses and junior physicians the clinical autonomy to bypass traditional hierarchical models of care and escalate clinical situations to senior personnel based on the early warning scores. However, studies have shown that there is still a reluctance to activate these systems due to fear of reprimand and persistent professional hierarchical barriers [13].

Infrastructure

Acknowledging the impediments to successful EWS implementation informs us to the necessary infrastructure for these systems. Early warning systems are a single component of a multifaceted patient safety pathway within an organizational framework. This pathway includes recognition

of at-risk patients, triggering a response, continuous auditing, quality control, and improvement of the practice. Ultimately, leadership and governance are required to drive and implement the policy and prioritize patient safety. To surmount the human factors and embedded system barriers requires an invested program of awareness campaigns, staff education, implementation of policies, and auditing of practices by early warning system teams or assigned leads [9].

The triggered response and escalation pathway needs to be predetermined within the staffing, economic, and clinical availabilities of that institution. Staffing for a medical emergency team can be considered based on cost and the expected number of MET calls. There may be a freestanding full-time MET team, or it may be composed of individuals with concurrent duties elsewhere in the hospital. The cost of running a MET team may be offset against the cost of preventing or reducing unplanned ICU admissions [8] (Fig. 2).

Early Warning Systems in an Oncology Population

Cancer patients are at risk of inhospital clinical deterioration due to either the neoplastic disease, complications of cancer treatment, or unrelated medical comorbidities.

Fig. 2 Patient safety pathway with afferent and efferent limbs, quality control, and governance

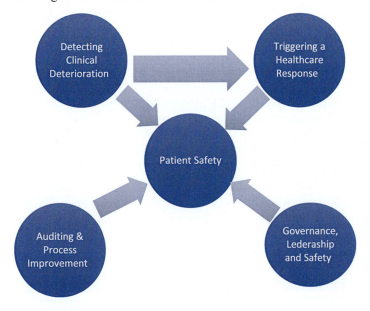

Cancer treatment falls broadly into chemotherapy, radiotherapy, and surgery with many patients having some combination of all three.

Early identification of clinically deteriorating oncology patients is valuable not only to augment timely interventions but also to allow discussion of appropriate treatments, potential ceilings of care and cardiopulmonary resuscitation, involvement of multidisciplinary teams including critical care and palliative care, as appropriate, and potential end of life planning. As cancer treatments improve, it is likely that in the future there will be increased demands on critical care beds for oncology patients. Historically, intensive care units have not always been open to cancer patients as it was deemed to be an expensive intervention for patients with a terminal prognosis. However, since the late 1990s, with improvements in cancer treatments and prolonged disease-free states, these perceptions have been challenged with the new concept of cancer as a chronic illness [37]. Increasingly, ICU doors are being opened to oncology patients with many studies showing similar outcomes to noncancer medical patients for acute illnesses [40, 57].

The use of early warning systems which have good discriminative value for predicting oncology patients at high risk of inhospital cardiac arrest, CCU admission and 30-day mortality would be of particular benefit in this cohort. Unfortunately, the generic early warning systems available seem to be less predictive in oncology patients and do not incorporate clinical signs which may have higher prognostic value in this cohort. A disease-specific early warning system for oncology may be of more benefit and includes parameters such as capillary refill time, FiO2, and type of malignancy (solid organ or hematological) [12]. A recent retrospective multicenter study of inhospital survival of critically ill solid organ cancer patients demonstrated medical patients with cancer had a 30.4% ICU mortality versus 16.2% ICU mortality for noncancer medical patients. The authors of this developed an "OncoScore" yet to be validated, which is a prognostic score for 4-month mortality in critically ill solid organ cancers and may be useful in determining ICU triage and could be considered in conjunction with an early warning system. The components of the OncoScore are (i) type of cancer, (ii) presence of distant metastasis, and (iii) type of organ support received in the intensive care unit [55].

A potential challenge of early warning systems in the oncology population is the recognition that some oncology patients will always have a degree of physiological aberrancy with associated high early warning scores despite being systemically well. These generalized physiological perturbations are a consequence of localized tumor effects. Neoplastic fever is a cytokine-driven pyrexia in the absence of infection or drug reactions. All fevers in oncology patients should be investigated for occult sepsis and treated, but after 1–2 weeks of a persistent pyrexia of unknown origin, with negative cultures and systemically well, neoplastic fever could be considered as a diagnosis of exclusion [58]. Hepatobiliary and gynecological cancers are both associated with ascites with a resultant increase in intra-abdominal pressure and subsequent reduction in venous return clinically manifesting as hypotension [19]. A compensatory tachycardia may ensue to preserve cardiac output. Large retroperitoneal tumors invading the IVC may further compromise venous return with subsequent hypotension. A multifactorial anemia is common in cancer [43] both at diagnosis (39%) and during treatment (67%) [32]. This may manifest clinically as hypotension, tachycardia, or tachypnea.

This would suggest that trends in early warning scores or vital signs rather than the absolute number may be of greater importance in assessing acute illness in oncology patients.

Similar perturbations may result from cancer treatment modalities. The use of both chemo and more specifically immunotherapy can lead to marked physiological abnormalities.

Immunotherapy

As the treatment for many cancers improve, an important consideration is the use of immunotherapy which utilizes the body's own immune system to target tumor cells. Immune evasion is a key component to tumor survival, and targeting tumor proteins such as the cytotoxic T-lymphocyte antigen 4 (CTLA-4) and programmed death receptor-1 (PD-1) by immune checkpoint inhibitors has significantly improved cancer survivorship [15, 24, 48] (Table 1).

Despite the beneficial results of immunotherapy in cancer treatments, immune checkpoint inhibitors (ICIs) can lead to autoimmunity and the development of immune-related adverse events (IRAE) with significant morbidity. These ICI toxicities pose a particular clinical challenge as symptoms may be diverse based on the mechanism of action of distinct therapies. The commonest toxicities are dermatological 44%, autoimmune colitis 35%, and endocrinopathies 6% [38]. In general, there is a higher incidence of IRAEs with CTLA-4 inhibitors than with PD-1 or PD-L1 inhibitors [31], and there is also greater therapy with combined therapy compared to monotherapy [14] (Table 2).

While the incidence of these toxicities is wide ranging, between 10% and 15% of patients develop grade 3–4 (severe – life-threatening) morbidities [29], and a further 25% of these suffer long-term sequelae with most of the endocrinopathies requiring permanent hormone replacement [1]. The treatment of immunotherapy-related toxicity is largely supportive but may require discontinuation ICI therapy, NSAIDs, steroid therapy, TNF-alpha inhibitors, tacrolimus, and mycophenolate [16].

Aside from checkpoint inhibitors which enable the body to target tumor cells, CAR T-cell immunotherapy goes even further and allows reprogramming of the body's immune system to target tumorigenesis. Chimeric antigen receptor (CAR) T-cell is an adoptive cellular immunotherapy. It involves extraction of the patient's own endogenous T-cells, laboratory engineering of the T-cells to target tumor cells, and injection of the newly modified T-cells back to the patient where they will go on to direct polyclonal T-cells toward tumor-specific surface antigens and facilitate elimination. CAR T-cell immunotherapy was awarded the American Society of Clinical Oncology's Cancer Advance of the Year Award for 2018. Although there is potential for huge benefit, side effects include a cytokine release

Table 1 Currently approved cancer immunotherapy agents and their targets

Antibody	Target	Treatment
Atezolizumab	PD-L1	Bladder cancer
Avelumab	PD-L1	Metastatic Merkel cell cancer
Ipilimumab	CTLA-4	Metastatic melanoma
Nivolumab	PD-1	Metastatic melanoma
		Squamous non-small cell lung cancer
		Renal cell cancer
		Hodgkin lymphoma
Pembrolizumab	PD-1	Metastatic melanoma
Durvalumab	PD-L1	Bladder cancer
		Non-small cell lung cancer

Table 2 Commonest agent-specific toxicities

ICI therapy	Adverse events (decreasing frequency)
Ipilimumab	Colitis, hepatitis, pancreatitis (39.7%)
	Endocrinopathies (29.1%)
	Ophthalmic, neurologic, hematologic, autoimmune (less frequent)
Pembrolizumab	Cutaneous reactions (30%)
Nivolumab	Endocrinopathies (42.9%)
	Pneumonitis (42.9%)

syndrome (CRS) which results in inflammatory turbulence and hemodynamic instability which may require invasive support. CRS is classified from a grade 1 constitutional illness of fever, arthralgia, tachycardia, gastrointestinal upset, hyponatremia, hypokalemia, hypomagnesaemia, hypophosphatemia, and mild degrees of renal and liver dysfunction to a progressively deteriorating grade 4 state of severe systemic multiorgan failure requiring invasive mechanical support. As the utilization of CAR T-cell therapy continues to proliferate, it is essential for intensivists to be cognizant of these impending signs of toxicity as the clinical presentation in conjunction with indices of CRP, ferritin, and serum cytokine levels will aid diagnosis. A monoclonal antibody to interleukin-6, tocilizumab has recently been approved for treatment of CRS [35]. Neurological toxicities are also common across a spectrum of mild inattention, tremor, dysgraphia and dyskinesia (grade 1) to severe global aphasia, severe dyskinesia, coma, status epilepticus, complete loss of motor power, and advanced cerebral edema which may present with clinical signs of herniation (grade 4). While neurotoxicity seems to be self-limiting for the majority, once present it can progress rapidly despite interventions; therefore close monitoring and a low index of suspicion are essential in safely treating these patients. A recent review by Gutierrez et al. proposed an algorithm for management of CRS and neurotoxicity, advocating initial symptom grading with continuous re-evaluation as a system for triaging patients to appropriate levels of care and determining further escalations in treatment. ICU admission was proposed for all grade 3 CRS and/or neurotoxicity; however, it should be considered for grade 2 toxicities, and management includes supportive organ failure care in conjunction with anti-interleukin 6 therapy +/− corticosteroids for CRS and corticosteroids for neurotoxicity [20]. For now the future is bright for CAR T-cells, but questions remain as to their long-term benefit and if the same impressive results which to date have been limited to hematological malignancies be replicated in solid organ malignancies. Whether or not success is limited to one cohort of malignancies, their proliferating use is likely to continue and with that increasing incidences of toxicity which will mandate early critical care intervention for completion of successful treatment.

As the use of immunotherapy is becoming more prevalent and the market for immunotherapy agents increases, a keen knowledge of their mechanism of action and expected toxicities and treatments will be required to appropriately triage these patients and manage associated morbidities.

Chemotherapy

Chemotherapeutic agents are systemic non-targeted toxic agents that not only affect the cancer but all mitotically dividing cells. Rapidly dividing cells such as those in the gut, bone marrow, and hair are particularly susceptible to chemotherapeutic agents, and thus common side effects include mucositis, immunosuppression, and alopecia. Knowledge of agent-specific toxicities is essential in assessing these patients and directing treatment. Commonly encountered chemotherapy-induced toxicities include:

Bleomycin Pulmonary Toxicity [10]: Bleomycin is an antibiotic that generates oxygen-free radicals with resultant DNA separation. Bleomycin may cause pneumonitis in up to 40% of patients and may progress to pulmonary fibrosis in a small cohort [52] which may be worsened by high inspired oxygen concentrations. It is primarily used in the treatment of germ cell tumors as part of the BEP regime (bleomycin, etoposide, Cisplatin) [23].

Ifosfamide Neurotoxicity: Ifosfamide is an alkylating agent used in the treatment of ovarian, breast, and lung cancer. It causes an encephalopathy in up to 27% of patients due to its metabolites of chloroacetaldehyde and dicarboxylic acid. It usually improves following discontinuation of treatment and has previously been treated with methylene blue [45].

Anthracycline Cardiotoxicity: Anthracyclines are antibiotics derived from *Streptomyces* bacteria and include doxorubicin, daunorubicin, and epirubicin. Their main mechanism of action is inhibition of DNA and RNA synthesis as well as free radical generation. Anthracyclines are a common cancer therapy in the breast, stomach, lung, and ovary and have improved cancer survivorship but increased later-life cardiovascular morbidity which may manifest as cardiac arrhythmias to heart failure requiring the full spectrum of treatment [26].

A knowledge of the different chemotherapy toxicities and their management will aid in the treatment of these patients and will add to the end of bed assessment in the context of interpreting high early warning scores and associated physiological derangements.

Conclusion

Although, the evidence for early warning systems is inconclusive at best, it would seem intuitive that early intervention for patients with physiological abnormalities is not only paramount to best possible patient care but also a paradigm of patient safety. The oncology population is unique not only due to their neoplastic state but also as a consequence of their cancer treatments which can lead to a penumbra of physiological derangements which require significant treatment-specific knowledge to minimize further clinical demise. A disease-specific early warning score which incorporates type of malignancy, systemic treatments, and potentially neutropenia may be useful in this cohort.

References

1. Abdel-Wahab N, Shah M, Suarez-Almazor ME. Adverse events associated with immune checkpoint blockade in patients with cancer: a systematic review of case reports. PLoS One. 2016;11(7): e0160221.
2. National Institute for Health and Care Excellence. Acutely ill patients in hospital. Recognition of and response to acute illness in adults in hospital. NICE Clinical Guidelines, No. 50. 2007; https://www.nice. org.uk/Guidance/CG50.
3. Agulnik A, Forbes PW, Stenquist N, Rodriguez-Galindo C, Kleinman M. Validation of a pediatric early warning score in hospitalised pediatric oncology and hematopoietic stem cell transplant patients. Pediatr Crit Care Med. 2016;17:e146–53.
4. Akre M, Finkelstein M, Erickson M, Liu M, Vanderbilt L, Billman G. Sensitivity of the pediatric early warning score to identify patient deterioration. Pediatrics. 2010;215:2763–9.
5. Bach S, Kessler I, Heron P. Nursing a grievance? The role of healthcare assistants in a modernized national health service. Gender Work Organ. 2009;19(2). https://doi.org/10.1111/j.1468-0432.2009.00502.x.
6. Bailey TC, Chen Y, Mao Y, Lu C, Hackmann G, Micek ST, Heard KM, Faulkner KM, Kollef MH. A trial of a real-time alert for clinical deterioration in patients hospitalized on general medical wards. J Hosp Med. 2013;8:236–42.
7. Bell D, Mac A, Ochoa Y, Gordon M, Gregurich MA, Taylor T. The Texas Children's Hospital Pediatric Advanced Warning Score as a predictor of clinical deterioration in hospitalized infants and children: a

8. Bonafide CP, Localio AR, Song L, Roberts KE, Nadkarni VM, Priestley M, Paine CW, Zander M, Lutts M, Brady PW, Keren R. Cost-benefit analysis of a medical emergency team in a children's hospital. Pediatrics. 2014;134(2):235–41.
9. Chua W, See M, Legio-Quigley H, Jones D, Tee A, Liaw S. Factors influencing the activation of the rapid response system for clinically deteriorating patients by frontline ward clinicians: a systematic review. Int J Qual Health Care. 2017;29(8):981–98.
10. Comis RL, Kuppinger MS, Ginsberg SJ, Crooke ST, Gilbert R, Auchincloss JH, Prestayko AW. Role of single-breath carbon monoxide-diffusing capacity in monitoring the pulmonary effects of bleomycin in germ cell tumor patients. Cancer Res. 1979;39:5076–80.
11. Confidential Enquiry into Maternal and Child Health (CEMACH). Why children die – a pilot study 2006. London: CEMACH; 2008.
12. Cooksley T, Kitlowski E, Haji-Michael P. Effectiveness of Modified Early Warning Score in predicting outcomes in oncology patients. Qjm Int J Med. 2012;105(11):1083–8.
13. Douglas C, Osborne S, Windsor C, Fox R, Booker C, Jones L, Gardner G. Nursing and medical perceptions of a hospital rapid response system: new process but same old game? J Nurs Care Qual. 2016;31:E1–10.
14. Dyck L, Mills KHG. Immune checkpoints and their inhibition in cancer and infectious diseases. Eur J Immunol. 2017;47:765–79.
15. Eggermont AM, Chiarion-Sileni V, Grob JJ, Dummer R, Wolchok J, Schmidt H, Hamid O, Robert C, Ascierto PA, Richards JM, Lebbe C, Ferraresi V, et al. Prolonged survival in stage III melanoma with ipilimumab adjuvant therapy. N Engl J Med. 2016;375:1845–55. https://doi.org/10.1056/ NEJMoa1611299.
16. Friedman CF, Proverbs-Singh TA, Postow MA. Treatment of the immune-related adverse effects of immune checkpoint inhibitors: a review. JAMA Oncol. 2016;2:1346–53. https://doi.org/10.1001/jamaoncol. 2016.1051.
17. Green AL, Williams A. An evaluation of an early warning clinical marker referral tool. Intensive Crit Care Nurs. 2006;22:274–82.
18. Gill MR, Reiley DG, Green SM. Interrater reliability of Glasgow Coma Scale scores in the emergency department. Ann Emerg Med. 2004;43(2):215–23.
19. Guazzi M, Polese A, Magrini F, Fiorentini C, Olivari MT. Negative influences of ascites on the cardiac function of cirrhotic patients. Am J Med. 1975;59(2): 165–70.
20. Gutierrez C, McEvoy C, Mead E, Stephens RS, Munshi L, Detsky ME, Pastores SM, Nates JL. Management of the critically ill adult chimeric antigen receptor-T cell therapy patient: a critical care

modification of the PEWS tool. J Pediatr Nurs. 2013;28:e2–9.

perspective. Crit Care Med. 2018; https://doi.org/10.1097/CCM.0000000000003258. [Epub ahead of print]

21. Haegdorens F, Van Bogaert P, Roelant E, De Meester K, Misselyn M, Wouters K, Monsieurs KG. The introduction of a rapid response system in acute hospitals: a pragmatic stepped wedge cluster randomised controlled trial. Resuscitation. 2018;129:127–34.

22. Haines C, Perrott M, Weir P. Promoting care for acutely ill children—development and evaluation of a paediatric early warning tool. Intensive Crit Care Nurs. 2006;22:73–81. https://doi.org/10.1016/j.iccn.2005.09.

23. Haugnes H, Oldenburg J, Bremnes R. Pulmonary and cardiovascular toxicity in long-term testicular cancer survivors. Urol Oncol. 2015;33(9):399–406.

24. Herbst RS, Baas P, Kim DW, Felip E, Pérez-Gracia JL, Han JY, Molina J, Kim JH, Arvis CD, Ahn MJ, Majem M, Fidler MJ, de Castro G Jr, Garrido M, Lubiniecki GM, Shentu Y, Im E, Dolled-Filhart M, Garon EB. Pembrolizumab versus docetaxel for previously treated, PD-L1-positive, advanced non-small-cell lung cancer: a randomised controlled trial. Lancet. 2016;387:1540–50. https://doi.org/10.1016/S0140-6736(15)01281-7.

25. Hillman KM, Bristow PJ, Chey T, Daffurn K, Jacques T, Norman SL, Bishop GF, Simmons G. Duration of life-threatening antecedents prior to intensive care admission. Intensive Care Med. 2002;28:1629–34.

26. Horan PG, McMullin MF, McKeown PP. Anthracycline cardiotoxicity. Eur Heart J. 2006;27(10):1137–8. Epub 2006 Apr 12

27. Kause J, Smith G, Prytherch D, Parr M, Flabouris A, Hillman K, Intensive Care Society (UK), Australian and New Zealand Intensive Care Society Clinical Trials Group. A comparison of antecedents to cardiac arrests, deaths and emergency intensive care admissions in Australia and New Zealand, and the United Kingdom – the ACADEMIA study. Resuscitation. 2004;62:275–82.

28. Kellett J, Kim A. Validation of an abbreviated VitalPAC™ Early Warning Score (ViEWS) in 75,419 consecutive admissions to a Canadian regional hospital. Resuscitation. 2012;83:297–302.

29. Kumar V, Chaudhary N, Garg M, Floudas CS, Soni P, Chandra AB. Current diagnosis and management of immune related adverse events (irAEs) induced by immune checkpoint inhibitor therapy. Front Pharmacol. 2017;8:49.

30. Lambert V, Matthews A, MacDonell R, Fitzsimons J. Paediatric early warning systems for detecting and responding to clinical deterioration in children: a systematic review. BMJ Open. 2017;7:e014497. https://doi.org/10.1136/bmjopen-2016-014497.

31. Larkin J, Chiarion-Sileni V, Gonzalez R, Grob JJ, Cowey CL, Lao CD, Schadendorf D, Dummer R, Smylie M, Rutkowski P, Ferrucci PF, Hill A, Wagstaff J, Carlino MS, Haanen JB, Maio M, Marquez-Rodas I, McArthur GA, Ascierto PA, Long GV, Callahan MK, Postow MA, Grossmann K, Sznol M, Dreno B, Bastholt L, Yang A, Rollin LM, Horak C, Hodi FS, Wolchok JD. Combined nivolumab and ipilimumab or monotherapy in untreated melanoma. N Engl J Med. 2015;373:23–34.

32. Ludwig H, Van Belle S, Barrett-Lee P, Birgegård G, Bokemeyer C, Gascón P. The European Cancer Anaemia Survey (ECAS): a large, multinational, prospective survey defining the prevalence, incidence, and treatment of anaemia in cancer patients. Eur J Cancer. 2004;40(15):2293–306.

33. Mackintosh N, Humphrey C, Sandall J. The habitus of 'rescue' and its significance for implementation of rapid response systems in acute health care. Soc Sci Med. 2014;120:233–42.

34. Mackintosh N, Sandall J. Overcoming gendered and professional hierarchies in order to facilitate escalation of care in emergency situations: the role of standardised communication protocols. Soc Sci Med. 2010;71:1683–6.

35. Magee MS, Snook AE. Challenges to chimeric antigen receptor (CAR)-T cell therapy for cancer. Discov Med. 2014;18(100):265–71.

36. Maharaj R, Stelfox HT. Rapid response teams improve outcomes: no. Intensive Care Med. 2016;42:596–8.

37. McCorkle R, Ercolano E, Lazenby M, Schulman-Green D, Schilling LS, Lorig K, Wagner EH. Self-management: enabling and empowering patients living with cancer as a chronic illness. CA Cancer J Clin. 2011;61(1):50–62. https://doi.org/10.3322/caac.20093.

38. Menzies AM, Johnson DB, Ramanujam S, Atkinson VG, Wong ANM, Park JJ, McQuade JL, Shoushtari AN, Tsai KK, Eroglu Z, Klein O, Hassel JC, Sosman JA, Guminski A, Sullivan RJ, Ribas A, Carlino MS, Davies MA, Sandhu SK, Long GV. Anti-PD-1 therapy in patients with advanced melanoma and preexisting autoimmune disorders or major toxicity with ipilimumab. Ann Oncol. 2017;28:368–76.

39. MERIT study investigators. Introduction of the medical emergency team (MET) system: a cluster-randomised controlled trial. Lancet. 2005;365(9477):2091–7.

40. Miller KD, Siegel RL, Lin CC, Mariotto AB, Kramer JL, Rowland JH, Stein KD, Alteri R, Jemal A. Cancer treatment and survivorship statistics, 2016. CA Cancer J Clin. 2016;66:271–89.

41. Moon A, Cosgrove JF, Lea D, Fairs A, Cressey DM. An eight year audit before and after the introduction of modified early warning score (MEWS) charts, of patients admitted to a tertiary referral intensive care unit after CPR. Resuscitation. 2011;82:150–4.

42. Morgan RJM, Williams F, Wright MM. An early warning scoring system for detecting developing critical illness. Clin Intensive Care. 1997;8:100.

43. Naoum FA. Iron deficiency in cancer patients. Rev Bras Hematol Hemoter. 2016;38(4):325–30. https://doi.org/10.1016/j.bjhh.2016.05.009.

44. Nielsen LG, Folkestad L, Brodersen JB, Brabrand M. Inter-observer agreement in measuring respiratory rate. PLoS One. 2015;10(6):E0129493.

45. Pelgrims J, De Vos F, Van den Brande J, Schrijvers D, Prové A, Vermorken JB. Methylene blue in the treatment and prevention of ifosfamide-induced encephalopathy: report of 12 cases and a review of the literature. Br J Cancer. 2000;82(2):291–4.

46. Philip K, Richardson R, Cohen M. Staff perceptions of respiratory rate measurement in a general hospital. Br J Nurs. 2013;22(10):570–4.

47. Prytherch DR, Smith GB, Schmidt PE, Featherstone PI. ViEWS – towards a national early warning score for detecting adult inpatient deterioration. Resuscitation. 2010;81:932–7.

48. Robert C, Long GV, Brady B, Dutriaux C, Maio M, Mortier L, Hassel JC, Rutkowski P, McNeil C, Kalinka-Warzocha E, Savage KJ, Hernberg MM, Lebbé C, Charles J, Mihalcioiu C, Chiarion-Sileni V, Mauch C, Cognetti F, Arance A, Schmidt H, Schadendorf D, Gogas H, Lundgren-Eriksson L, Horak C, Sharkey B, Waxman IM, Atkinson V, Ascierto PA. Nivolumab in previously untreated melanoma without BRAF mutation. N Engl J Med. 2015;372:320–30. https://doi.org/10.1056/NEJMoa1412082.

49. Rothschild JM, Gandara E, Woolf S, Williams DH, Bates DW. Single-parameter early warning criteria to predict life-threatening adverse events. J Patient Saf. 2010;6:97–101.

50. Royal College of Physicians. National Early Warning Score (NEWS) 2: standardising the assessment of acute-illness severity in the NHS, Updated report of a working party. London: RCP; 2017.

51. Sandroni C, Cavallaro F. Failure of the afferent limb: a persistent problem in rapid response systems. Resuscitation. 2011;82:797–8.

52. Simpson AB, Paul J, Graham J, Kaye SB. Fatal bleomycin toxicity in the west of Scotland 1991–1995: a review of patients with germ cell tumours. Br J Cancer. 1998;78:1061–6.

53. Smith GB, Prytherch DR, Meredith P, Schmidt PE, Featherstone PI. The ability of the National Early Warning Score (NEWS) to discriminate patients at risk of early cardiac arrest, unanticipated intensive care unit admission, and death. Resuscitation. 2013;8(4):465–70.

54. Trinkle RM, Flabouris A. Documenting Rapid Response System afferent limb failure and associated patient outcomes. Resuscitation. 2011;82(7):810–4.

55. Vincent F, Soares M, Mokart D, Lemiale V, Bruneel F, Boubaya M, Gonzalez F, Cohen Y, Azoulay E, Darmon M. In-hospital and day-120 survival of critically ill solid cancer patients after discharge of the intensive care units: results of a retrospective multicenter study – a Groupe de recherche respiratoire en réanimation en Onco–Hématologie (Grrr-OH) study. Ann Intensive Care. 2018;8(1):1–8.

56. Wendon J, Hodgson C, Bellomo R. Rapid response teams improve outcomes: we are not sure. Intensive Care Med. 2016;42:599–601.

57. Wigmore T, Farquhar-Smith P. Outcomes for critically ill cancer patients in the ICU: current trends and prediction. Int Anesthesiol Clin. 2016;54:e62–75.

58. Zell JA, Chang JC. Neoplastic fever: a neglected paraneoplastic syndrome. Support Care Cancer. 2005;13(11):870–7.

Rapid Response Team (RRT) in Critical Care

8

Ninotchka Brydges and Tiffany Mundie

Contents

Introduction 88

Evolution of Rapid Response Teams (RRTs) 88

Rapid Response Team and Its Components 89
Implementation of Rapid Response Team 89
Subset of Rapid Response Team 90

Oncologic Considerations 91

Implications to Clinical Practice 92

Conclusion 93

References 93

Abstract

Rapid response teams (RTTs) were initially established in the mid-1990s and expanded to the Institute for Health Improvement's 100,000 lives campaign and a Joint Commission's national patient safety goal. The aim of implementing RTT in any organizations was to improve patient safety and quality of care through identifying deterioration in patient status and intervening to stabilize the patient in a timely manner. Members of the RRT include multidisciplinary healthcare professionals who are trained in critical care and capable to provide advanced assessment and interventions and facilitate communication with the primary team. The RRT is called for specific physiologic changes or for a more generalized concern raised by bedside nurses, other providers, or even family members. More recently specialized subsets of RRTs have developed, including sepsis teams and pulmonary embolism response team, in which responders to a specific situation are experts in related field. In the oncologic setting, the RRTs face unique challenges related to this patient population's underlying malignancy, specified treatments and complications, as well as comorbidities.

N. Brydges (✉)
Division of Anesthesia, Critical Care and Pain Medicine, Department of Critical Care and Respiratory Care, The University of Texas MD Anderson Cancer Center, Houston, TX, USA
e-mail: nbrydges@mdanderson.org

T. Mundie
Department of Critical Care and Respiratory Care, The University of Texas MD Anderson Cancer Center, Houston, TX, USA
e-mail: tamundie@mdanderson.org

© Springer Nature Switzerland AG 2020
J. L. Nates, K. J. Price (eds.), *Oncologic Critical Care*,
https://doi.org/10.1007/978-3-319-74588-6_9

Keywords

Rapid response team · Medical emergency
response team · Sepsis · Pulmonary embolism
response team · Acute care nurse practitioners ·
Nursing · Early resuscitation

Introduction

Rapid response teams (RRTs) have been introduced to intervene in the care of patients with
unexpected clinical deterioration. The key functions of RRTs are responding to critical situations
which evidently missed or "failure to rescue"
with available clinical services, leading to serious
adverse events [14]. A serious adverse event may
be defined as an unintended injury due to delayed
or incorrect medical management resulting to
increased risk of patient's death and results in
measurable disability. Rapid response teams differ from traditional code teams (TCTs) in several
ways including criteria of calling the team, conditions that the team assesses and treats, team
composition, call rate, and inhospital mortality
[14]. TCTs are called due to no recordable pulse
and blood pressure, absence of respiratory effort,
and unresponsive related to cardiopulmonary
arrest and airway obstruction. While RRTs are
called due to vital changes such as low blood
pressure, rapid or slow heart rate, respiratory
distress, and altered mental status, conditions
that RRT typically respond are commonly associated with failure to rescue including acute respiratory failure, acute changes in consciousness,
hypotension, arrhythmias, pulmonary edema,
and sepsis. TCT is typically composed of physicians specialized in anesthesia and intensive care
unit (ICU), internal medicine house staff, and
ICU nurse. RRTs are composed of ICU trained
healthcare professionals only (ICU physician,
nurse), and other institution includes internal
medicine staff. RRT has a primary goal of identifying an acute deterioration in a patient's status
and intervene in a timely manner. RRTs have
higher call rates than TCTs. In addition, the mortality rate of TCT ranges from 70% to 90%, while
RRT has significantly lower mortality rate ranging from 0% to 20% [14]. RRTs are also known as

medical emergency response teams (MET) and
medical early response intervention and therapy
(MERIT).

Evolution of Rapid Response Teams (RRTs)

The response teams began being discussed in
literature in the mid-1990s. Lee et al. [19] describe
the evolution and utilization of a MET in 1990 at a
South Western Sydney hospital. Further, a study
in 1993 reviewed MET team calls over an
11-month period which showed that the RRTs
were frequently called due to physiological
changes such as sudden change or decreased
level of consciousness and changes in blood pressure and heart rate. In regard to specific conditions, the MET team most frequently intervened in
cases of acute respiratory failure and status
epilepticus [19]. Goldhill et al. [9] also describe
the use of a "patient at risk team" (PART) in
a 1997 study at a London hospital which showed
a statistically significant decrease in the rates of
cardiopulmonary resuscitation (CPR) in the
patient group that was assessed by the
PART team.

In 2004, the Institute of Healthcare Improvement (IHI) began the 100,000 Lives Campaign.
The campaign took place over an 18-month
period and was composed of six interventions
that were aimed at saving lives by focusing on
patient safety and ensuring quality patient care
[6]. Many hospitals subsequently developed
RRTs, in part motivated by the recommendation
from the IHI's 100,000 Lives Campaign as one of
the six strategies to reduce preventable inpatient
deaths [29]. One of the interventions was the
deployment of rapid response teams [6]. The use
of RRTs to improve the recognition and response
to change in patient's condition was also a Joint
Commission National Patient Safety Goal in 2006
[22, 29]). The IHI continued to support the use of
RRTs through their 5 Million Lives Campaign
from December 2006 to December 2008 [13].
Since the inception of the 100,000 lives campaign
and 2008 Joint Commission National Patient
Safety Goal, the presence of RRTs is

commonplace, and as of 2011, approximately 3700 hospitals in the United States are incorporating RRTs [4]. The use of these teams has yielded positive results for patients. In a systematic review by Jones et al. [15], RRTs show a decrease in the number cardiac arrests, reduced adverse events following major surgery, as well as effectively address end-of-life care.

Rapid Response Team and Its Components

Rapid response teams (RRTs) are group of healthcare providers implemented by hospitals to respond to patients who are distressed in the hospital wards [8]. The RRTs are composed of clinicians typically with critical care training and allied healthcare professionals who respond immediately to hospital patients manifesting objective or subjective signs of clinical deterioration. The patients assessed by RRTs may require admission in the intensive care unit (ICU). Composition of the RRT varies between institutions to meet the needs of their patient population. Members of the team are certified in the Advanced Cardiac Life Support (ACLS) and can consist of a provider such as an intensivist, hospitalist, nurse practitioner or physician's assistant, an ICU or ED nurse, and a respiratory therapist (Sundararajan et al. 2016; [12]). The team can also solely be an ICU Nurse and Respiratory Therapist [2]. Activation of the RRT occurs when a staff member is concerned or worried about the patient's condition or notes a specific change such as abnormal vital signs, increased respiratory effort, airway compromise, altered mental status, seizures, and severe bleeding ([14, 15]). The RRT's focus is to provide further assessment, interventions to stabilize the patient, information gathering and facilitating communication with patient's physician, expert consultation, as well as utilizing the opportunity to provide education to non-ICU staff regarding the current patient situation [3, 12]. Common interventions performed by the team are fluid resuscitation, obtaining stat lab results, airway management, and facilitating transfer to the ICU. At times, the team can respond to a patient who has an acute change or decline status in the setting of a life-limiting disease and is approaching end of life. In this instance, the RRT members can play a role in goals of care and code status discussions which may result in a change in code status to do-not-resuscitate (DNR) and/or limiting specified medical therapies.

Most of the literature has focused on the responding team; however, there are four components in rapid response system including afferent limb, efferent limb, patient safety and quality improvement, and administrative or governance [14]. The afferent limb component is designed to trigger a response when clinical deterioration is identified. The second component, the efferent limb, consists of personnel and the equipment brought to the patient. Patient safety and quality improvement is considered as the third component, which provides a feedback loop through data collection and analysis taken from events in order to improve prevention and response. This component reviews data from the rapid response team calls and the patient outcomes in an attempt to develop strategies for clinical deterioration prevention meeting the rapid response criteria to optimize patient outcomes by RRTs. The administrative or governance component constitutes the fourth component that coordinates resources to improve care, overseeing the appointment of responding team staff and the purchase of equipment and coordinating the education of hospital staff regarding the rapid response process. The composition of the RRT is tailored to align with institutional goals, aims of the team, severity of patients' illnesses, and resources availability.

Implementation of Rapid Response Team

Careful and coordinated strategies must be considered to avoid implementation failure [14]. Introducing a rapid response team (RRT) can present challenges to various aspects of patient care and operation including logistic, political, anthropologic, social, and medical. Thus, the support of hospital leaders, including senior medical and nursing personnel, is imperative in order for RRT to succeed. First year of implementation may require the continuous explanation of the concept of the RRT while obtaining support from key stakeholders. The role of RRT and its positive outcomes need to be emphasized, clarifying the goal of providing rapid second opinion rather than to take over patient care. It is important that the team must have adequate resources in relation to both staffing and resources and the ability to manage critical care events. Hospital-wide staff education must be instituted for the system's afferent limb to be functional. It is crucial to provide frontline providers cyclical and multimodal education. The better the staff understand how to work with an RRT, the better the outcomes for the patient [17]. Educating physicians and nurses by highlighting RRT and staff responsibilities and emphasizing the timely disposition will produce positive change and significant help when RRT responds to staff calls. Improved outcomes of RTT are dependent on the afferent and efferent limbs [8]. Further, the ICU-leading physician or member of the RRT should reach out to the other team to expedite ICU transfer as well as facilitating end-of-life issues care planning. In order to provide and safe intervention, good training is vital. Simulation training improves team performances as well as providing team structured method in managing clinical deterioration in patients. In addition, regular audits are essential to assess contributing factors of rapid response system's activation and failures and to guide quality improvement activities [14].

The development of rapid response system (RRS) is a hospital-wide approach to manage patients at risk of unexpected death and cardiopulmonary arrest by early recognition of clinical deterioration and early resuscitation [11]. The innovation involves the creation of medical emergency team (MET), rapid response team, and a critical care outreach team. Despite of various models for activating MET, the calling criteria in the afferent limb are frequently comprised of similar vital signs. Also, there is a significant gap between knowledge of critical need for MET activation and how it is actually utilized by clinicians. Thus, Huh and colleagues introduced a modified

MET with both an afferent limb, which was triggered by 24-h electronic medical recording (EMR), and an efferent limb which was responsible to provide early goal-directed therapy for shock, respiratory care comprising of advanced airway management, and cardiopulmonary resuscitation [11]. Huh and colleagues observed that that the ICU admission rate for patients when MET activation was triggered by the EMR-based screening criteria was lower than patients with MET activation triggered by traditional calling criteria. Patient cases triggered by call were more frequently urgent or needed an emergency treatment such as difficult airway management or cardiopulmonary arrest, whereas surgical patients showed better outcomes in the EMR-triggered group. Several models for RRS have been developed and the implementation varies throughout hospitals and worldwide. The most common models are the physician – led team and nurse led teams. Another model of the team consists of critical care trained nurses who have an expanded role and improve outcomes of RRS through patient follow-up [11]. The study of Kapu et al. [18] described that including acute care nurse practitioners (ACNPs) to existing RRTs allowed the teams to provide diagnostic and therapeutic interventions outside the scope of the original RRTs. Because some calls required critical care management and/or procedures, therefore adding ACNP to the mix was the correct choice. Further, the charge nurses were surveyed and showed high satisfaction with the addition of ACNPs to the RRTs. The qualitative results supported that an ACNP could provide immediate diagnosis and treatment, enhance communication between the primary physician and the ICU team, and facilitate transfers to the ICU.

Subset of Rapid Response Team

Pulmonary Embolism Team

Pulmonary Embolism Response Teams (PERT) were developed to have 24-h on-call access to expert consultation and the ability to provide advanced treatment and interventions beyond the standard treatment of anticoagulation to patients newly diagnosed with high-risk pulmonary embolism [16]. It is a multidisciplinary team with representation from anesthesiology, cardiology, thoracic and cardiovascular surgery, echocardiography, pharmacy, emergency medicine, hematology, pulmonary medicine, critical care, radiology, interventional radiology, and vascular medicine [16, 20]. The team is activated by a referring physician and will review the patient's data, make recommendations, and possibly intervene on a patient who has a confirmed diagnosis of a high-risk pulmonary embolism. Interventions provided by the PERT team can include catheter-directed thrombolysis, percutaneous thromboaspiration, surgical procedures, and extracorporeal membrane oxygenation (ECMO) [16].

Sepsis Response

It is well-known that early recognition and treatment of sepsis improves patient outcomes. RRTs have been incorporated into hospital initiatives which focus on identifying and intervening during early sepsis and have been described in current literature. In a study by Guirgis et al. [10], the RRT was part of a hospital-wide sepsis program in which the team became aware of suspected septic patients by rounding on high-risk patients, notification by the bedside nurse if a patient met predetermined sepsis criteria, and also an electronic health record automated screening tool. These notifications along with staff education and timely intervention decrease sepsis-related mortality, ICU and hospital length of stay, need for mechanical ventilation, and financial burden to institution [10].

Oncologic Considerations

The oncologic patient population is complex in nature due to their underlying disease process, comorbidities, and treatment-related complications which can present unique challenges for the RRT beginning with the frequency of RRT calls. Early studies have shown that the mortality rates for patients with cancer were substantially higher than those patients without cancer suggesting that the presence of malignancy could be classified as a gloomy prognostic factor in the critical care environment [24]. In their study, Parmar et al. [21] found the number of medical emergency team activations (MET) of patients with newly diagnosed acute myeloid leukemia (AML) to be 6.9 times higher than that of non-AML patients with a quarter of these patients requiring more than one interaction with the MET. The authors report the most common reasons for MET team activation were respiratory distress and hemodynamic instability and 73% of the patients who were admitted to ICU were placed in ICU due to respiratory failure and majority of those patients required mechanical ventilation [21].

According to a study by Austin et al. [4] on RRT in a comprehensive cancer center, the oncology patient population has a high level of acuity and increased hospital mortality rate vs. non-oncology medical patients. The study also identifies the cancer patient population on longer hospital stays versus the non-oncology patients prior to MET activation which could lead to increased risk of infection given their immunocompromised status. Because of the increased acuity and complexity of the oncologic patent population, it is recommended to increase the resources allocated to RRT caring for unique patient population [4].

The RRT in the oncologic environment has to consider situations specific to the cancer patient population. A RRT can be activated because of a patient's reaction to their chemotherapy, immunotherapy, or Car T-cell therapy which may require further consultation with the patient's oncologist for assistance with management. Cancer patients may also be thrombocytopenic putting them at increased risk for bleeding that can present spontaneously and could include hemoptysis, GI bleed, or intracranial hemorrhage.

As noted previously, the oncologic patient population has a higher hospital mortality rate when compared to patients without a cancer diagnosis. Therefore addressing death and the dying patient is a very real situation for RRT staff caring a patient with a cancer diagnosis. It is important for the MET to recognize when the decline in patient status is due to a problem which can be resolved and when the decline is related to the process of dying [7]. During a rapid response call, depending on the patient's overall status including cancer prognosis, the RRT/MET team may have initiative goals of care discussion with the patient and/or family that can result in do-not-resuscitate orders, orders for limiting medical therapies, and/or involving palliative care services.

Implications to Clinical Practice

The rapid response teams have been associated with various benefits including reduced incidence of inhospital cardiac arrest, improved overall hospital mortality, and early end-of-life care involvement [8]. Although the challenge of early identification of patients at risk of clinical deterioration and repeat medical emergency team (MET) activation on the hospital wards is a major area of concern [8, 26], there are few reliable indicators that may be identified prospectively when it comes to patients at risk of recurrent deterioration. In addition patients with recurrent deterioration had similar characteristics to those with a single activation and more likely to have particular comorbidities, there were no significant differences in other patient characteristics, laboratory values, or vital signs. Delays in RRT activation have been shown to be associated with negative outcomes.

Rapid response teams (RRTs) typically include the critical care staff and respiratory staff but noted that these teams provide no education for bedside nurses caring for patients with clinical education [17]. Therefore, empowering and getting frontline clinicians such as bedside nurses to be a part of the team make a significant difference in getting the response and disposition streamlined. Developing a structure RRT for patient's safety empowers staff to function at a higher competence level [27]. The authors noted that most nurses have an intrinsic desire to function at a higher level. RRTs are nurse-driven, self-directed, and self-managed working teams to promote safe and efficient patient care within the hospital.

Data collected from RRT calls including activation and failure rapid responses can be used to develop a preemptive management algorithm which might facilitate administration of therapy to a specific group of patients with hypotension [5]. The implementation of the algorithm suggested its administration would be associated with a reduction of medical emergency team (MET) without compromising patient outcomes. In response to early adoption of MET and an increasing workload, implementation of the preemptive algorithm demonstrates system redesign and safe resource allocation. One of the potential advantages of implementing preemptive management algorithm is to avoid delay. The study of Aneman et al. [1] demonstrated that the introduction of a two-tier response to clinical deterioration increased ICU admission triggered by cardiorespiratory criteria, while admissions triggered by more subjective criteria decreased. A two-tier system to respond to patients who are at risk was introduced in New South Wales, Australia. In this system, the primary clinical team responds to less serious first-tier criteria, and the rapid response system (RRS) is activated when patient required the more serious second-tier criteria. Overall, the ICU mortality for patient admitted following MET review decreased indicating that two-tier system resulted to earlier recognition of reversible pathology or a decision of non-escalation of level of care.

Repeat medical emergency team (MET) calls due to recurrence of clinical deterioration of patients are noted to be common and associated with increased risk of subsequent ICU admission, prolonged hospital stay, and increased hospital mortality [26]. In addition, patient, provider, and institutional characteristics were associated with the risk of patients experiencing recurrent clinical deterioration and repeat MET calls. It was found in the study of Stelfox et al. [26] that patients who received airway suctioning, noninvasive mechanical ventilation, or with central venous catheters were high risk of repeat MET activation. Thus, consequences of recurrent clinical deterioration and repeat MET activation are significantly crucial to warrant efforts to identify patients at risk of clinical deterioration recurrence. The study of Reardon et al. [23] has shown that delays were common when deterioration was secondary to respiratory distress and hypotension, but complaints such as dysrhythmias or altered level of consciousness were noted with fewer delays. The fewer delay can be associated with feasibility of treatment for some of these conditions such as initiating supplemental oxygen for desaturation or fluid resuscitation for hypotension. However, treatment that stabilizes vital signs may defer the diagnosis of dangerous condition underlying condition. Dysrhythmia such as atrial fibrillation with rapid ventricular response may require specific treatment and monitoring necessitating RRT. In addition, nonsurgical services have increased number of delays in activating rapid response team compared to surgical services. The delays in the RRT activation may be related to the effect of nonsurgical services having readily available personnel to respond to a patient's clinical deterioration without activating the RRT. A qualitative study by Sheary and colleagues [25] described one of the most common reasons for not activating the RRT was the floor staff felt they were able to provide the necessary patient care with their own resources. Evidence is limited regarding these delays, therefore, it warrants further study.

Conclusion

Rapid response teams (RRTs) were developed out of a nationwide initiative to improve patient safety and quality of care and have since been fully integrated into the current hospital landscape. Despite a lack of level 1 evidence that demonstrates their effectiveness, rapid response systems have been introduced at hospitals in many countries [14]. RRTs activations can have diverse results depending on the patient situation. The use of RRTs can efficiently facilitate transferring a patient to the ICU for further management but, on the other hand, can be involved in code discussions or conversations regarding the limitation of medical treatment [28]. Adding acute care nurse practitioners can provide diagnostic and therapeutic interventions as well as high satisfaction to nurses [18]. The rationale that early intervention is beneficial in almost all medical emergencies has also provided support for the introduction of rapid response systems. Moreover,

such systems are considered to be consistent with the concept that taking critical care expertise and skills out of the ICU to the patient's bedside as rapidly as possible is physiologically and clinically sound [14]. Delays in RRT activation on the hospital wards is associated with increased mortality, ICU admissions, and hospital length of stay [23]. Delays and clinical deterioration in non-surgical services are more common secondary to respiratory complaints and hypotension. Early RRT activation is warranted in these conditions to facilitate timely diagnosis and management by the treating team. In the oncologic setting, RRTs must be aware of the complexity of this patient population and recognize the complications specific to those who are receiving active cancer therapies. Further, improving communication among multidisciplinary oncology and critical care teams can offer timely and complete vital support for those patients with a reasonable baseline prognosis [24].

References

1. Aneman A, Frost SA, Parr MJ, Hillman KM. Characteristics and outcomes of patients admitted to ICU following activation of the medical emergency team: impact of introducing a two-tier response system. Crit Care Med. 2015;43(4):765–73.
2. Angel M, Ghneim M, Song J, Brocker J, Tipton PH, Davis M. The effects of a rapid response team on decreasing cardiac arrest rates and improving outcomes for cardiac arrests outside critical care areas. Medsurg Nurs. 2016;25(3):153–9.
3. Astroth K, Woith WM, Stapleton SJ, Degitz RJ, Jenkins SH. Qualitative exploration of nurses' decisions to activate rapid response teams. J Clin Nurs. 2013;22(19–20):2876–82.
4. Austin CA, Hanzaker C, Stafford R, Mayer C, Culp L, Lin FC, Chang L. Utilization of rapid response resources and outcomes in a comprehensive cancer center. Crit Care Med. 2014;42(4):905–9.
5. Bergmeir C, Bilgrami I, Bain C, Webb GI, Orosz J, Pilcher D. Designing a more efficient, effective and safe Medical Emergency Team (MET) service using data analysis. PLoS One. 2017;12(12):e0188688.
6. Berwick DM, Calkins DR, McCannon CJ, Hackbarth AD. The 100 000 lives campaign: setting a goal and a deadline for improving health care quality. JAMA. 2006;295(3):324–7.
7. Brown C, Drosdowsky A, Krishnasamy M. An exploration of medical emergency team intervention at the

end of life for people with advanced cancer. Eur J Oncol Nurs. 2017;31:77–83.

8. Fernando SM, Reardon PM, Scales DC, Murphy K, Tanuseputro P, Heyland DK, Kyeremanteng K. Prevalence, risk factors, and clinical consequences of recurrent activation of a rapid response team: a multicenter observational study. J Intensive Care Med. 2018; https://doi.org/10.1177/0885066618773735.

9. Goldhill DR, Worthington L, Mulcahy A, Tarling M, Sumner A. The patient-at-risk team: identifying and managing seriously ill ward patients. Anaesthesia.-LONDON. 1999;54:853–60.

10. Guirgis FW, Jones L, Esma R, Weiss A, McCurdy K, Ferreira J, … Gerdik C. Managing sepsis: electronic recognition, rapid response teams, and standardized care save lives. J Crit Care. 2017;40:296–302.

11. Huh JW, Lim CM, Koh Y, Lee J, Jung YK, Seo HS, Hong SB. Activation of a medical emergency team using an electronic medical recording–based screening system. Crit Care Med. 2014;42(4):801–8.

12. Institute for Healthcare Improvement. How to guide: deploy Rapid Response teams. 2008. Available at: https://www.ihi.org. Accessed 27 Mar 2018.

13. Institute for Healthcare Improvement. 5 million lives campaign. Last modified 2015. Available at: https://www.ihi.org/Enagage/Initiatives/Completed/5MillionLivesCampaign. Accessed 28 Mar 2018.

14. Jones DA, DeVita MA, Bellomo R. Rapid-response teams. N Engl J Med. 2011;365(2):139–46.

15. Jones D, Rubulotta F, Welch J. Rapid response teams improve outcomes: yes. Intensive Care Med. 2016;42:593–5.

16. Kabrhel C, Rosovsky R, Channick R, Jaff MR, Weinberg I, Sundt T, … Chang Y. A multidisciplinary pulmonary embolism response team: initial 30-month experience with a novel approach to delivery of care to patients with submassive and massive pulmonary embolism. Chest. 2016;150(2):384–93.

17. Kim R, Passev J. Nursing education improves RRT team efficiency. Hosp Peer Rev. 2017;42(6):67–9.

18. Kapu AN, Wheeler AP, Lee B. Addition of acute care nurse practitioners to medical and surgical rapid response teams: a pilot project. Crit Care Nurse. 2014;34(1):51–9.

19. Lee A, Bishop G, Hillman KM, Daffurn K. The medical emergency team. Anesth Intensive Care. 1995;23(2):183–6.

20. MD Anderson Cancer Center. Pulmonary embolism response team (PERT). 2017. Available at: http://inside.mdanderson.org/departments/acute-care-services/pulmonary-embolism-response-team.html. Accessed 28 Mar 2018.

21. Parmar A, Richardson H, McKinlay D, Gibney RN, Bagshaw SM. Medical emergency team involvement in patients hospitalized with acute myeloid leukemia. Leuk Lymphoma. 2013;54(10):2236–42.

22. Revere A, Eldridge N, Joint Commission on Accreditation of Healthcare Organizations. National patient safety goals for 2008. Top Patient Saf. 2008;12:1–4.

23. Reardon PM, Fernando SM, Murphy K, Rosenberg E, Kyeremanteng K. Factors associated with delayed rapid response team activation. J Crit Care. 2018;46:73–8.

24. Rosa RG, Tonietto TF, Duso BA, Maccari JG, de Oliveira RP, Rutzen W, … Cremonese RV. Mortality of adult critically ill subjects with cancer. Respir Care. 2017. https://doi.org/10.4187/respcare.05210.

25. Shearer B, Marshall S, Buist MD, Finnigan M, Kitto S, Hore T, … Ramsay W. What stops hospital clinical staff from following protocols? An analysis of the incidence and factors behind the failure of bedside clinical staff to activate the rapid response system in a multi-campus Australian metropolitan healthcare service. BMJ Qual Saf. 2012. https://doi.org/10.1136/bmjqs-2011-000692.

26. Stelfox HT, Bagshaw SM, Gao S. Characteristics and outcomes for hospitalized patients with recurrent clinical deterioration and repeat medical emergency team activation. Crit Care Med. 2014;42(7):1601–9.

27. Thomas K, Force MV, Rasmussen D, Dodd D, Whildin S. Rapid response team challenges, solutions, benefits. Crit Care Nurse. 2007;27(1):20–7.

28. Tirkkonen J, Tamminen T, Skrifvars MB. Outcome of adult patients attended by rapid response teams: a systematic review of the literature. Resuscitation. 2017;112:43–52.

29. Wunderink RG, Diederich ER, Caramez MP, Donnelly HK, Norwood SD, Kho A, Reed KD. Rapid response team-triggered procalcitonin measurement predicts infectious intensive care unit transfers. Crit Care Med. 2012;40(7):2090–5.

Quality Assurance and Improvement in the Intensive Care Unit

9

Mary Lou Warren

Contents

Introduction 96

Methods/Models to Improve Care 96
Use of Evidence-Based Practice 96
The Plan, Do, Study, Act (PDSA) Conceptual Framework 97
Additional Quality Improvement Models 97
Use of Safety Reporting 98

Agencies to Evaluate Quality and Safety 99
General Programs 99
Oncology Programs 100
ICU Specific Programs 100

Identifying ICU Performance Metrics 101

Conducting Quality Improvement 102

Summary 104

References 104

Abstract

Quality of care is defined as care which produces the greatest expected improvement in health status. Major strides towards quality and safety initiatives were made after the Institute of Medicine published the report: To Err Is Human, in 2000. Although innumerous quality and safety initiatives have been implemented and some improvements in health care delivery and outcomes have been demonstrated, gaps still exist. This chapter will describe methods and conceptual frameworks used to improve processes and outcomes in the care of critically ill patients. Agencies involved in evaluating quality and offering assistance to health care providers, institutions, and systems will also be discussed. Finally, performance measures specific to the intensive care unit will be outlined.

Keywords

Quality improvement · Patient safety · Performance indicators · Health outcomes · Critical care · Quality models

M. L. Warren (✉)
Department of Critical Care, UT MD Anderson Cancer Center, Houston, TX, USA
e-mail: mlwarren@mdanderson.org

© Springer Nature Switzerland AG 2020
J. L. Nates, K. J. Price (eds.), *Oncologic Critical Care*,
https://doi.org/10.1007/978-3-319-74588-6_4

Introduction

Although quality of care and the potential for harm to the hospitalized patient had been identified as early as the 1960s, the concept of quality of care in the intensive care unit (ICU) has only recently been defined. Quality of care is defined as care which produces the greatest expected improvement in health status [9]. Organizations such as the Institute of Medicine (IOM), National Quality Forum (NQF), the Joint Commission, Institute for Health Care Improvement (IHI), and the Agency for Healthcare Research and Quality (AHRQ) have been driving forces behind the quality movement in the ICU. The IOM defines quality as the degree to which health services for individuals and populations increase the likelihood of desired health outcomes and are consistent with current professional knowledge [22]. Major strides towards quality and safety initiatives were made after the IOM published the report: To Err Is Human, in 2000. The report estimated that up to 98,000 deaths per year were attributed to preventable medical errors. More astounding is the comparison of the IOM figures to a jet crash resulting in the deaths of 130–330 passengers per day [17].

The IOM has also published a report specific to cancer care. Ensuring Quality Cancer Care was published in 1999 and outlined the delivery of cancer care in the United States [13]. The report also described the ideal system for delivering cancer care and established ten recommendations to increase understanding of quality cancer care, improve quality cancer care, and decrease the barriers to achieving quality cancer care. The recommendations focused on implementing guidelines based on best available evidence, improving access to care, ensuring quality and timeliness of care at end of life, conducting research to answer questions related to cancer care, and developing data bases to establish quality benchmarks.

Although innumerous quality and safety initiatives have been implemented and some improvements in health care delivery and outcomes have been demonstrated, gaps still exist. The National Patient Safety Foundation (NPSF) issued a follow up report 15 years after the initial IOM To Err Is Human report. Free from Harm: Accelerating Patient Safety Improvement Fifteen Years after To Err Is Human [28] again calls for a systems approach to safety and creating a culture in which the government, regulators, health care professionals, patients, and families prioritize patient safety through research and implementation.

Methods/Models to Improve Care

Use of Evidence-Based Practice

Evidence-based practice is defined as the integrated use of clinical research through systematic review and clinical expertise [34]. As clinicians, practice decisions should be based on both research and expertise. However, science is not always available to answer clinical questions and hence other sources of evidence must be used. Practice decisions can also be based on consensus panels, data from internal databases, and quality improvement data. Regardless of the origin of the evidence, practitioners need to ensure that the evidence is reliable and of good quality. The development of systematic reviews and meta-analyses, which provide a summary of the best available evidence, has facilitated the use of evidence-based medicine into actual practice. However, practitioners must look at the evidence in the context of the individual patient. This involves the integration of the evidence with clinical expertise as it applies to the individual patient. The triad of evidence, clinical practice, and the individual patient is a common approach in the critically ill oncology patient.

Key to implementing evidence based practice is a culture that promotes seeking out the evidence and developing tools to standardize care-based evidence and clinical practice. These tools may include guidelines, order sets, algorithms, and protocols. The National Comprehensive Cancer Network (NCCN) as well as the American Society of Clinical Oncology (ASCO) have coordinated the development of numerous cancer care guidelines which have been adopted nationally. Additionally, many critical care organizations such as the Society of Critical Care Medicine (SCCM) and the American Association of Critical-Care Nurses (AACN) promote the use of evidence-based practices and provide resources to critical care practitioners.

The IHI has incorporated the use of bundles to help promote aspects of care that have been shown to improve patient outcomes. The IHI defines bundles as, "a group of interventions related to a disease process that, when executed together, result in better outcomes than when implemented individually." Bundles have been developed to facilitate the care for patients with sepsis as well as to prevent infections related to central lines and invasive mechanical ventilation. The IHI provides resources and tools to assist ICUs in the implementation and monitoring of the bundles. The bundle approach has been adopted in many ICUs and, with good adherence, has been shown to be effective in improving patient outcomes.

The Plan, Do, Study, Act (PDSA) Conceptual Framework

The PDSA cycle has been used as a model for improvement since 1993. The model developed over time from concepts of pragmatism developed by Charles Peirce and William James in 1872 and Clarence I. Lewis in 1929. Walter A. Shewhart first published a straight line, three-step process based on the steps in the scientific method to acquire knowledge [35]. The three steps included specification, production, and inspection which corresponded to hypothesis development, experimentation, and hypothesis testing. Shewhart later constructed the straight line process into a cyclical concept to emphasize the dynamic process of acquiring new knowledge. W. Edwards Deming modified the Shewhart cycle in 1950 while in Japan to add the fourth step of redesigning through marketing research. The revised cycle was known as the Deming wheel. The Japanese later presented the Deming wheel as the Plan, Do, Check, Act (PDCA) cycle and incorporated concepts of establishing standards to prevent errors [15]. The Japanese continued to modify the PDCA cycle to stress the concepts of goal development, formulation of methods to attain the goals, training, and education [18]. Principles of quality control and improvement using the PDCA cycle continued to be developed in Japan and are currently used today.

In 1986, Deming re-introduced the Shewhart cycle and discouraged the use of PDCA because of the English connotation of check meaning to hold back [7]. Finally, in 1994, the PDSA cycle was established to replace check with study [8]. The study phase emphasizes the examination of results to evaluate lessons learned. The Model of Improvement which encompasses three questions to supplement the PDSA cycle was later established [20]. The three questions center on the identification of the specific aim of the project or what the team is trying to accomplish; the established measures of the project or how the team will know the project led to an improvement; and whether or not changes to the project are needed to result in an improvement.

The PDSA cycle was developed as an approach to implement change in real practice and to evaluate if improvements have been achieved. The cycle involves planning, implementing, evaluating, and then acting upon the results. The action may lead to modification of the original plan which is then again implemented, evaluated, and acted upon based on the results. If an improvement was seen, the action may involve spreading the change throughout an organization or system.

Additional Quality Improvement Models

Six Sigma was developed by Motorola Corporation and further enhanced by General Electric Corporation [26]. The model centers on improving outcomes by eliminating variation within a process. The goal of Six Sigma is to lower the defect rate to at least the sixth standard deviation which reflects 3.4 million defects per million events. A higher sigma indicates a lower defect rate. Several tools within the Six Sigma methodology guide teams to achieve quality improvement goals through identifying defects in the system and working to eliminate them.

The Lean methodology was established by the Toyota Motor Company in the 1980s [21] to streamline processes and eliminate waste in order to offer improved value to the customer. Lean focuses on identifying the steps involved in a process in order to identify areas to improve efficiency, reliability, and reproducibility. Application of the Lean principles in healthcare have led to improvement in processes and systems including fast-track programs in the Emergency Department, improvement in lab, and other diagnostic turnaround time, and realignment of resources and space to improve efficiency. Lean has also been applied in the critical care setting with improvement demonstrated with carrying out patient care rounds.

Health care also has looked towards the aviation industry to understand improvement in safety through standardization of processes. Standardization of processes has been a consistent theme in improving quality and safety in health care. However, adoption of additional aviation methodologies has further advanced achieving safe quality care. The use of checklists, improving teamwork and communication, and utilizing scientific methods to collaboratively identify and eliminate risks are proven interventions to reduce error [44]. Checklists have been effectively implemented in the operating room to ensure that the right procedure is being done on the right patient and have also demonstrated a reduction in blood stream infections when utilized for central line insertions.

Use of Safety Reporting

Traditional methods of reviewing incidents have been through morbidity and mortality committees and medical malpractice claims or through retrospective chart reviews. These methods are time consuming and costly. According to AHRQ, the use of an incident reporting system, which identifies incidents prospectively, is an effective method of capturing error and adverse event data. However, studies reveal that incident reporting systems often underestimate the number of errors [10, 33]. Despite the promotion of a culture of safety, healthcare providers continue to under report. One survey of nurses on barriers to reporting medication errors identified the two top barriers as the time needed to complete the report and fear of repercussion [33]. Other identified barriers to reporting include a lack of understanding of what constitutes an incident, lack of feedback, lack of time, and dissatisfaction with the process [10].

One strategy developed to increase the reporting of incidents and promote patient safety was the incorporation of potential errors [25]. These programs commonly called close calls, near misses or good catches, are now integrated into incident reporting systems but can also act as a separate system which clearly delineates incidents that actually reached the patients from incidents that were caught prior to reaching the patients. Close call reporting allows for anonymous reporting that focuses on system issues rather than individual performance. Attaching positive feedback or rewards to reporting close calls and incorporating reporting at the end of each shift has led to increase reporting [25].

Tracking of adverse events is an additional method of identifying medical errors. The IHI has identified a model of tracking adverse events through the use of trigger modules. Triggers act as tools to identify adverse events. The IHI Global Trigger Tool for Measuring Adverse Events include clusters of triggers that could possibly result in adverse events related to general hospital care, medications, surgical care, ICU care, perinatal, and emergency care. The methodology is a retrospective review which includes the identification of the triggers in a randomized selection of patient encounters. After a trigger is identified, a review of the medical record is conducted to evaluate if the trigger was the result of an adverse event. The methodology is not meant to identify every adverse event but rather to allow for trending of information. The IHI recommends the tracking of three measures: adverse events per 1,000 patient days, percent of admissions with an adverse event, and adverse events per 100 admissions [16].

Medication Errors

Medication errors account for 78% of serious medical errors in the ICU [19, 32]. Common medication errors leading to adverse events involve error of omission, wrong dose, wrong drug, and wrong administration technique [19]. Improving medication systems help reduce the incidence of medication errors and prevent harm to patients. Strategies to improve medication safety include medication standardization, use of bar coding technology, computerized order entry technology, use of "smart" intravenous administration pumps, and medication reconciliation [1]. Other strategies involve the role of the clinical pharmacist, specifically in the ICU. In a subgroup analysis of a meta-analysis of four observational studies, pharmacist intervention significantly reduced preventable adverse drug events (ADEs) and prescribing errors [43]. Timely recommendations to physicians and nurses as well as monitoring of adverse drug events in the ICU are key functions of the clinical pharmacist. Including pharmacists on patient care rounds, having pharmacists available on call, as well as having a pharmacist review medication orders prior to the first dose are recommended by several quality organizations.

Identifying high-risk medications, such as anticoagulants and insulin, and implementing processes to reduce errors associated with high-risk medications are currently mandated by The Joint Commission (2018) [36]. Outlining a process of medication reconciliation has been identified as one of the Patient Safety Goals established by The Joint Commission (2018). Medication reconciliation should occur at every transition within the hospital system and includes transfers to and from the ICU. Despite the IHI recommending specific outcome measures for reporting medication errors and ADEs, considerable variability in reporting exists. In one systematic review of the incidence of medical errors in critical care units, the incidence of ADEs ranged widely and were reported in multiple units from 1 to 96.5 per 1000 patient days; 1.3 to 21.1 ADEs per 100 admissions; 34.1% of patients; and 0.16 per 100 medication orders [23]. Standard reporting metrics should assist in evaluating improvement in medication

processes resulting in a reduction in human error and the chance of harm to the patient.

Agencies to Evaluate Quality and Safety

Several agencies and organizations have established programs for evaluating and rewarding healthcare institutions and providers based on performance. Through these programs, data have become available to the public on performance at the hospital and practitioner level. Many of these programs were originated to promote best practices and improve outcomes; however, studies to evaluate the impact of some of these programs have not demonstrated any improvement in outcomes [24]. Although most of these programs do not evaluate the performance of ICUs alone, more recent work has produced ICU specific benchmarking. The following section will discuss both general, oncology, and ICU specific programs.

General Programs

The Center for Medicare and Medicaid Services (CMS) offers a pay-for-performance program for hospitals through the Reporting Hospital Quality Data for Annual Payment Update [40]. Data include process of care indicators including timely and effective access to care, outcomes indicators including complications and unexpected mortality, and patient experience indicators. The data are available free of charge at the Hospital Compare website. Consumers have the ability to select and compare hospitals and view the data in a variety of formats. One limitation to the data is the inclusion of only Medicare certified hospitals and Medicare beneficiaries. Additionally, data include the value of care provided by each hospital. These data are derived by first comparing the hospital's average payment to the national average payment and then again comparing the hospital's unexpected mortality rate with the national average. This information is provided to promote and encourage the reduction of waste and unnecessary care while maintaining high quality care.

The Joint Commission (2018) offers data on process of care indicators free of charge through the Joint Commission website [37]. The Joint Commission indicators are similar to the CMS indicators but include all patients and not just Medicare beneficiaries. Hospitals are required to submit data on nine performance measures focusing on timely and efficient care. These indicators involve the Emergency Centers/Departments, inpatient floors, and the ICUs. Recently, the Joint Commission established an electronic submission process for the majority of the quality indicators as well as a recognition program to encourage the use of the electronic process. These data are available to institutions for internal benchmarking and quality improvement as well to the public through their website.

The Leapfrog Group [38] offers an annual report of hospitals who volunteer to participate. The performance indicators reported are endorsed by NQF and include process and outcome indicators. Process indicators include use of physician order entry systems, adequacy of physician staffing in the intensive care unit, and the presence of processes which reflect safe practices. Outcome indicators include device-related infections and surgical-site infections. Comparisons between participating hospitals are available to the public and basic benchmarking data are available to hospitals. For a fee, more detailed benchmarking of the safe practices indicators, the computer order entry indicators, and other custom reports are available to hospitals. Over 1900 hospitals reported information to the Leapfrog Group in 2017.

Healthgrades [12] is an independent health care ratings organization which provides a comparative reporting system offering data on both hospital and physician practices. Consumers are able to evaluate the ratings for an individual hospital or may choose a procedure, condition, or diagnosis and compare hospital ratings. The ratings are based on the application of risk-adjusted models to administrative hospital discharge data. Healthgrades offers an award program for excellent performance based on selected AHRQ patient safety initiatives, risk-adjusted mortality and complication measures, and patient experience surveys. Most of the data are based on CMS data; however, some all payer data are available. The ratings are updated annually, and basic data can be accessed for free by consumers and hospitals. More detailed information is available for a fee.

US News and World Report [41] surveys physicians to evaluate the reputation of hospitals and hospital services. In addition to the reputation of the hospital, the ranking is based on Medicare patient volume, mortality, nurse to patient ratios, and recognition by the American Nurses Credentialing Centers as a Magnet hospital. Provision of advanced technologies and provision of specialized patient services such as genetic testing and comprehensive pain management are also utilized to rank the hospitals. Use of intensivists and success in meeting specific indicators utilized to measure patient safety are additional components of the overall ranking. Rankings are provided by specialty including cancer care.

Oncology Programs

ASCO offers a quality program for outpatient practices which focuses on over 190 metrics specific to cancer. Oncology practices can participate and report on identified core metrics along with disease specific metrics. The metrics were established to evaluate comprehensive oncology care including palliative and end of life care. The Commission on Cancer® (CoC) [4] is a program of the American College of Surgeons (ACoS), which also recognizes comprehensive cancer care programs. Participants can report metrics to aid in benchmarking. The CoC also provides an accreditation to participants who meet established standards in cancer care. Although not specific to critical care, these programs offer benchmarking to compare care related to oncology.

ICU Specific Programs

In 2011, the Critical Care Societies Collaborative [5] convened a task force to generate critical care performance measures with the intent of providing these measures to NQF. The collaborative consists of SCCM, AACN, American College of Chest Physicians, and the American Thoracic Society. The task force recommended seven performance measures to help bridge the gap in performance measures specific to the ICU: management of sepsis, overuse in blood transfusions, ventilator-associated pneumonia and mechanical ventilation, risk adjusted ICU outcomes, therapeutic hypothermia, daily chest radiographs in ICU patients, and screening of acute lung injury (ALI)/ARDS. NQF subsequently endorsed 13 measures associated with pulmonary and critical care including six measures specific to critical care. Three of the six measures address pediatric patients, two address adults, and one addresses both populations [29] (see Table 1).

The NQF promotes publicizing the data to increase awareness and encourage improvement in health outcomes. However, many believe that ICU LOS and mortality data are skewed based on transfer practices, differences in case mix and demographics, and other structural and process variabilities and should not be utilized as performance metrics or publicly reported [3, 39]. Others feel that ICU LOS and mortality are only short-term outcomes and do not reflect the patients' overall health status [39]. Because of the continued challenges and debate on the rationale for selection and supporting evidence for use, no one set of established metrics has been identified for the ICU. Instead institutions and critical care units have individually chosen metrics and formulated individual quality plans. Until consensus is established, critical care metrics will continue to be variable; however, some research and summary data are available to guide critical care leaders.

Identifying ICU Performance Metrics

In a recent publication, researchers from Canada identified quality indicators specific to critical care as reported by key critical care and quality and safety organizations [42]. The researchers found 127 unique quality indicators and evaluated each indicator for its rationale of use and supporting evidence as well as for implementation. The authors found that only 27 (21.2%) of the 127 unique indicators had reported formal grading of supporting evidence and only four organizations reported results of implementation. Indicators with the highest level of evidence were associated with mechanical ventilation bundles including ventilator-associated pneumonia bundle, elevation of the head of the bed, oral care, and daily sedation vacation and assessment of readiness to extubate. Central line insertion bundle and central line care bundles and bundles associated with sepsis management and

Table 1 National Quality Forum critical care performance measures

Population	Performance measure	Description
Pediatric	Severity-adjusted length of stay	Number of days between ICU admission and discharge
Pediatric	Unplanned readmission rate	Total number of patients requiring unscheduled readmission to the ICU within 24 h of transfer or discharge
Pediatric	Standardized mortality ratio	Ratio of actual deaths over predicted deaths
Adult	Ultrasound guidance for internal jugular central venous catheter placement	Percent of patients with an internal jugular venous catheter placed in the emergency department under ultrasound guidance
Adult	Hospital mortality rate	Percentage of patients admitted to the ICU whose hospital outcome is death. Both observed and risk-adjusted mortality reported with predicted LOS
Both	ICU length of stay	Total duration of time spent in the ICU until time of discharge for all patients admitted to the ICU. Both observed and risk-adjusted LOS reported with the predicted LOS

ICU Intensive care unit, *LOS* length of stay

resuscitation also had the highest grades of supporting evidence. The authors also found supporting evidence for several structural performance metrics including having pharmacists available on rounds, use of rapid response teams, and increasing nurse to patient staffing ratios.

Additional structural and process measures can be identified through focusing on the value care of care being delivered. The Choosing Wisely® campaign was established by the American Board of Internal Medicine to encourage communication between providers and patients in the avoidance of unnecessary tests, treatments, and procedures. The CCSC endorsed the campaign through the publication of the top five recommendations critical care providers could follow to avoid waste and improve the value of care for critically ill patients [11] (see Table 2). These five recommendations are supported by evidence including data that demonstrate the risk of additional harm to the patient when overuse occurs.

Table 2 Critical Care Societies Collaborative top five recommendations for choosing Wisely®

Topic	Recommendation
Diagnostics	Do not order diagnostic tests at regular intervals (such as every day) but rather in response to specific clinical questions
Transfusions	Do not transfuse red blood cells in hemodynamically stable, nonbleeding ICU patients with an Hb concentration greater than 7 g/dl
Nutrition	Do not use parenteral nutrition in adequately nourished critically ill patients within the first 7 days of an ICU stay
Sedation	Do not deeply sedate mechanically ventilated patients without a specific indication and without daily attempts to lighten sedation
End-of-Life Care	Do not continue life support for patients at high risk for death or severely impaired functional recovery without offering patients and their families the alternative of care focused entirely on comfort

ICU Intensive care unit, *Hb* hemoglobin, *g/dl* grams per deciliter

In a review article targeting ICU Directors to assist in identifying performance metrics, Murphy et al. [27] utilized both Donabedian's model of structure, process, and outcomes as well as the IOM's six domains of health care quality to highlight potential metrics. The six domains include safe, effective, patient-centered, timely, efficient, and equitable. Valiani et al. [42] also used these frameworks when identifying the quality indicators with the highest level of evidence of implementation. Engaging multidisciplinary team members including key senior leadership will assist in the development and improve implementation of quality metrics. Once the metrics have been identified, a model such as the PDSA cycle supports the evaluation of current processes and outcomes and identifies interventions to improve. Table 3 illustrates proposed ICU metrics supported in the literature and organized by Donabedian's model of structure, process, and outcomes.

Conducting Quality Improvement

The Hastings Center published a report, The Ethics of Using QI Methods to Improve Health Care Quality and Safety and defined quality improvement (QI) as "systematic, data-guided activities designed to bring about immediate, positive changes in the delivery of health care in particular settings" [2]. This definition has been used throughout the quality improvement literature and incorporated into QI programs nationally. The report addressed the questions of whether or not QI is considered human subjects research, requires Institutional Review Board (IRB) approval, and requires informed consent. The authors first outline ethical considerations in conducting QI activities and offer insights on the differences between research and QI. Research activities were defined as those that "are designed to learn something enduring about nature and function of human beings and their environment" [2]. The primary aims of research and quality improvement differ in that research establishes a hypothesis to generate new knowledge whereas

Table 3 Proposed ICU performance metrics

Metric type	Metric
Structure	Establishment of rapid-response teams
	Staffing ratios: increasing nurse to patient ratio
	Involvement of clinical pharmacist on rounds
	Isolation of patients with resistant infections
	Simulation training
	Transfusion policies
	Antibiotic stewardship programs
	Glycemic control protocols
Process	Ventilator-associated pneumonia bundle
	Elevation of head of bed
	Daily sedation vacation and assessment of readiness to extubate
	Stress ulcer prophylaxis
	Oral care with chlorhexidine
	Prevention of venous thromboembolism
	Central line insertion bundle
	Maximal barrier precautions
	Chlorhexidine skin antisepsis
	Hand hygiene
	Optimal catheter type and site selection
	Central line care bundle
	Daily review of line necessity
	Aseptic lumen access
	Catheter site and tubing care
	Ultrasound guidance for central venous catheter insertion
	Sepsis management bundle
	Steroids
	Adequate glycemic control
	Protective lung strategies
	Sepsis resuscitation bundle
	Serum lactate levels
	Blood culture drawn before antibiotics administered
	Adequate fluid resuscitation
	Maintain adequate central venous oxygen saturation
	Timely antibiotic administration
	Apply vasopressors for ongoing hypotension
	Glycemic control
	Documentation of goals of care
	Highest level of mobility
	Medication reconciliation by a pharmacist
	Hand hygiene compliance
Outcomes	Mortality
	Observed
	Risk-adjusted
	Length of stay
	Delayed ICU admissions
	Pressure ulcer prevalence
	Patient falls and falls with harm
	Patient/family satisfaction
	Delirium prevalence
	Length of time on the ventilator
	Central line-associated blood stream infections
	Catheter related urinary tract infections
	Probable ventilator-associated pneumonia
	Newly diagnosed venous thromboembolism

ICU Intensive care unit

quality improvement is applying current knowledge to improve processes and evaluate change [14, 30].

The Hastings report concluded that QI is not typically considered human subjects research and thus does not require IRB approval or formal consent. The report did acknowledge that, at times, QI overlaps with research and in those cases, should meet the requirements for human subject research. The report also concluded that the intent to publish QI activities does not label the activity as research and does not require IRB review. QI review boards have been established at the institutional level to assist with evaluating QI activities. Often times, these boards have IRB representation to clarify any questions of research activities. To promote QI activities, review boards and institutional departments of quality improvement have also established educational programs and processes including the use of the PDSA cycle and Model of Improvement [20] to assist employees. Databases have also been established to track QI activities and their sustainability.

Dissemination of QI activities is crucial so that healthcare institutions can adopt new processes in order to improve care. QI activities promote implementation of best practices and aids in improved quality of care and experience for patients and families. The publication of QI activities in peer review journals have become more widely accepted and encouraged. Guidelines to evaluate the strength of QI activities were established in 2005 to close the gap on the publication and appraisal of QI activities. This draft proposal for evaluation criteria was built upon earlier guidelines published in 1999 and evolved further in 2008 when the Standards for Quality Improvement Reporting Excellence (SQUIRE) Guidelines were published [6]. The SQUIRE guidelines have since been updated [31] and continue to provide a structure for publication and evaluation of quality improvement activities. Application of the guidelines is intended for system level initiatives using methods to establish that the observed outcomes were due to the intervention being evaluated.

Summary

The health care system, especially ICUs, has been described as a tightly coupled and complex adaptive system. Systems that are loosely coupled may tolerate delays and/or variations to the sequences. However, tightly coupled systems are intolerant of delays and deviations and are at an increased risk of errors and accidents. Adopting proven quality and safety methods are no longer optional. ICUs must utilize a multidisciplinary approach in improving quality of care for critically ill patients. Promoting a culture of patient safety includes the use of evidence-based practice and error reporting systems such as incident and close call reporting. Utilizing models, such as the PDSA cycle, can assist practitioners in creating continuous quality improvement within the ICU. Multiple professional and government organizations promote patient safety and quality of care and serve as resources to assist individuals and institutions in creating a safe environment for patients. Conducting and publishing QI activities are crucial to improving health care processes and outcomes.

References

1. Aspden P, Wolcott JA, Bootman JL, et al., editors. Preventing medication errors. Washington, DC. 2007. https://psnet.ahrq.gov/resources/resource/4053/preventing-medication-errors-quality-chasm-series
2. Baily MA, Bottrell M, Lynn J, et al. The ethics of using QI methods to improve health care quality and safety. Hastings Cent Rep. 2006;36(4):S1.
3. Churpek MM, Hall JB. Measuring and rewarding quality in the ICU: the yardstick is not as straight as we wish. Am J Respir Crit Care Med. 2012;185(1):3. https://doi.org/10.1164/rccm.201110-1813ED.
4. Commission on Cancer®. 2018. https://www.facs.org/quality-programs/cancer/coc
5. Critical Care Societies Collaborative (CCSC). NQF measures. 2018. http://ccsconline.org/high-value-care/nqf-measures
6. Davidoff F, Batalden PB, Stevens DP, et al. Development of the SQUIRE Publication Guidelines: evolution of the SQUIRE project. BMJ Qual Saf. 2008;34: 681–7.
7. Deming WE. Out of the crisis. Cambridge, Mass: Massachusetts Institute of Technology, Center for Advanced Engineering Study, 1986.

8. Deming WE. The new economics for industry, government & education. Cambridge, MA: Massachusetts Institute of Technology, Center for Advanced Engineering Study, 1994.

9. Donabedian A. The quality of care: how can it be assessed? JAMA. 1988;260(12):1743–8. https://doi.org/10.1001/jama.260.12.1743.

10. Evans SM, Berry JG, Smith BJ, et al. Attitudes and barriers to incident reporting: a collaborative hospital study. Qual Saf Health Care. 2006;15(1):39–43. https://doi.org/10.1136/qshc.2004.012559.

11. Halpern SD, Becker D, Curtis JR, et al. An official American Thoracic Society/American Association of Critical-Care Nurses/American College of Chest Physicians/Society of Critical Care Medicine policy statement: the Choosing Wisely® top 5 list in critical care medicine. Am J Respir Crit Care Med. 2014;190(7):818–26. https://doi.org/10.1164/rccm.201407-1317ST.

12. HealthGrades. 2018. http://www.healthgrades.com/

13. Hewitt M, Simone JV, editors. Ensuring quality cancer care. Washington, DC: Institute of Medicine National Research Council, National Academy Press; 1999.

14. Holm M, Selvan M, Smith M, et al. Quality improvement or research: defining and supervising QI at the University of Texas M.D. Anderson Cancer Center. In: Jennings B, et al., editors. Health Care Quality Improvement: ethical and regulatory issues. New York: The Hastings Center; 2006. p. 145–69.

15. Imai M. Kaizen (Ky'Zen), the key to Japan's competitive success. New York: Random House Business Division, 1986.

16. Institute for Healthcare Improvement. How to improve. 2018. http://www.ihi.org/IHI/Topics/Improvement/ImprovementMethods/HowToImprove

17. Kohn LT, Corrigan J, Donaldson MS. To err is humans: Building a safe health system. Washington, DC, National Academy Press; 2000.

18. Ishikawa K. What is total quality control? The Japanese way. Englewood Cliffs, N.J.: Prentice-Hall, 1985.

19. Kopp BJ, Erstad BL, Allen ME, et al. Medication errors and adverse drug events in an intensive care unit: direct observation approach for detection. Crit Care Med. 2006;34(2):415–25.

20. Langley GJ, Nolan KM, Nolan TW, et al. The improvement guide: a practical approach to enhancing organizational performance. San Francisco, CA: Jossey-Bass Publishers, 2009.

21. Lean Enterprise Institute. What is Lean? 2018. https://www.lean.org/WhatsLean/

22. Institute of Medicine (U.S.). Division of Health Care Services, Lohr KN, United States. Health Care Financing Administration, Institute of Medicine (U.S.). Committee to Design a Strategy for Quality Review and Assurance in Medicare. Medicare: a strategy for quality assurance. Washington, DC: National Academy Press; 1990.

23. MacFie CC, Baudouin SV, Messer PB. An integrative review of drug errors in critical care. JICS. 2015;17(1):63–72.

24. Mendelson A, Kondo K, Damberg C, et al. The effects of pay-for-performance programs on health, health care use, and processes of care: a systematic review. Ann Intern Med. 2017;166(5):341–53. https://doi.org/10.7326/M16-1881.

25. Mick JM, Wood GL, Massey RL. The good catch pilot program: increasing potential error reporting. J Nurs Adm. 2007;37(11):499–503.

26. Munro RA, Ramu G, Zyrmiac DJ. The certified six sigma green belt handbook, 2nd ed., Milwaukee, Wisconsin: ASQ Quality Press, 2015.

27. Murphy DJ, Ogbu OC, Coopersmith CM. ICU director data using data to assess value, inform local change, and relate to the external world. Chest. 2015;147(4): 1168–78.

28. National Patient Safety Foundation. Free from harm: accelerating patient safety improvement fifteen years after to err is human. Boston, MA: National Patient Safety Foundation, 2015.

29. National Quality Forum (NQF). Pulmonary and critical care 2015–2016 technical report. 2016. Accessed 24 July 2018. http://www.qualityforum.org/Publications/2016/10/Pulmonary_and_Critical_Care_2015-2016_Final_Report.aspx

30. Newhouse RP, Pettit JC, Poe S, et al. The slippery slope: differentiating between quality improvement and research. JONA. 2006;36(4):211–9.

31. Ogrinc G, Davies L, Goodman D, et al. SQUIRE 2.0 (Standards for Quality Improvement Reporting Excellence): revised publication guidelines from a detailed consensus process. BMJ Qual Saf. 2015;0:1–7. https://doi.org/10.1136/bmjqs-2015-004411.

32. Rothschild JP, Landrigan CP, Cronin JW, et al. The critical care safety study: the incidence and nature of adverse events and serious medical errors in intensive care. Crit Care Med. 2005;33(8):1694–700.

33. Rutledge DN, Retrosi T, Ostrowski G. Barriers to medication error reporting among hospital nurses. J Clin Nurs. 2018;27:1941–9. https://doi.org/10.1111/jocn.14335.

34. Sackett DL, Rosenberg WMC, Gray JA, et al. Evidence based medicine: what it is and what it isn't. BMJ. 1996;312:7023.

35. Shewhart WA Deming WE. Statistical method from the viewpoint of quality control. Washington: The Graduate School, The Dept. of Agriculture, 1939.

36. The Joint Commission. 2018 Hospital national patient safety goals. 2018a. https://www.jointcommission.org/assets/1/6/2018_HAP_NPSG_goals_final.pdf

37. The Joint Commission. Measures. 2018b. https://www.jointcommission.org/core_measure_sets.aspx

38. The Leapfrog Group. The Leapfrog hospital safety grade. 2018. http://www.leapfroggroup.org/cp

39. Timmers TK, Verhofstad MHJ, Moons KGM, et al. Intensive care performance: how should we monitor performance in the future? World J Crit Care Med. 2014;3(4):74–9.

40. U.S. Department of Health and Human Service. Hospital compare. 2018. https://www.medicare.gov/hospitalcompare/search.html

41. U.S. News and World Reports. Health hospitals. 2018. http://health.usnews.com/best-hospitals

42. Valiani S, Rigal R, Stelfox HT, et al. An environmental scan of quality indicators in critical care. CMAJ Open. 2017;5(2):E488–95. https://doi.org/10.9778/cmajo.20150139.

43. Wang T, Benedict N, Olsen KM. Effect of critical care pharmacist's intervention on medication errors: a systematic review and meta-analysis of observational studies. J Crit Care. 2015;30 (5):1101–6.

44. Weiser T, Haynes A, Lashoher A, et al. Perspectives in quality: designing the WHO surgical safety checklist. Int J Qual Health Care. 2010;22:365–70. https://doi.org/10.1093/intqhc/mzq039.

Patient Risk Prediction Model

10

Severity of Illness Scores

Michelle O'Mahony and Tim Wigmore

Contents

Introduction 108

Unique Characteristics of Cancer Patients 108

Outcome Prognosticators 110

System-Specific Factors 110
Critical Care Improvements 110
Case Volume Mix and Admission Policies 110
Multidisciplinary Approach 111

Patient-Specific Factors 111
Age 111
Performance Status 111

Cancer-Specific Factors 111
Neoplastic Disease and Treatment 111
Acute Respiratory Failure and Mechanical Ventilation 112
Organ Failure 112
Neutropenia 113
Solid Organ Versus Hematological Malignancy 113
Repeated Critical Care Admissions 113
The ICU Trial 113

Outcome Prediction Models 114
Outcomes Following Elective Cancer Surgery 115
Long-Term Quality of Life and Morbidity 116

Conclusions 116

References 117

M. O'Mahony (✉) · T. Wigmore
Department of Anaesthesia, Critical Care and Pain
Medicine, Royal Marsden Hospital, London, UK
e-mail: Michelle.O'Mahony@rmh.nhs.uk; timothy.
wigmore@rmh.nhs.uk

Abstract

Historically, oncology patients have been refused critical care admission due to pessimistic perceptions of outcomes in the context of terminal illness. This refusal was advocated by some critical care colleges who stated patients with metastatic cancers would be poor

© Springer Nature Switzerland AG 2020
J. L. Nates, K. J. Price (eds.), *Oncologic Critical Care*,
https://doi.org/10.1007/978-3-319-74588-6_8

candidates for intensive care unit (ICU) admission. More contemporaneously, tremendous advances in antitumor therapies have evolved, and critically unwell cancer patients have demonstrated comparable survival rates to critically unwell non-cancer patients. This has revolutionized medical attitudes, opening the previously closed doors of ICU in facilitating the management of these complex patients.

As with all critically unwell patients, early identification of patients at risk of deleterious outcomes facilitates timely and appropriate therapeutic interventions, directs necessary discussions with multidisciplinary teams and supports frank and open communications with patients and their relatives. In the oncological population, there is a wealth of evidence to support the prognostic value of individual physiological derangements as superior outcome predictors to cancer stage or type. Despite this, general medical attitudes have retained some antiquated nihilism, and in the absence of specialized multidisciplinary teams, risk prediction models specific to oncological patients in ICU would prove to redirect attitudes and better inform of predicted outcomes.

In this chapter, we discuss independent predictors of outcomes in this patient cohort, the challenges of risk prediction in such a vastly heterogeneous population, specific illness severity scoring systems, outcomes following elective surgery, solid organ versus hematological malignancy, therapeutic complications, and long-term sequelae of cancer treatments.

Keywords

Outcome prognosticators · Organ failure · ICU trial · Outcome prediction models

Introduction

Since the start of the twenty-first century, the landscape of oncological critical care has changed significantly. A previously nihilistic approach has gradually been challenged by improved antitumor therapies and a more holistic approach to patient care. Enhanced disease-free survival has led to a re-evaluation of outcomes in these patients, and recent evidence supports non-inferior outcomes for critically unwell cancer patients compared to non-cancer patients for acute illness [6, 55]. Despite this evidence, cancer patients as a whole are a heterogeneous cohort with varying outcomes based on type of malignancy (hematological vs solid organ), elective postsurgical versus emergency admission, treatment toxicities, and neoplastic or other non-cancer comorbidities. In this chapter, we will discuss the unique characteristics of cancer patients related to their intensive care admissions, hematological versus solid organ malignancies, various scoring systems and outcome predictors in this population, and the usefulness of an ICU trial in predicting outcomes.

Unique Characteristics of Cancer Patients

Historically, cancer patients have tended toward dismal outcomes associated with ICU admissions with mortality rates as high as 80% for hematological malignancy often cited [11, 46]. In 2005, a prospective multicenter observational study in France reported metastatic cancer as the second leading factor for refusal of admission to ICU behind only functionally dependent patients [18]. This refusal of ICU admission was advocated by The American College of Critical Care in 1999 who stated that patients with hematological or metastasized solid organ malignancies were poor candidates for ICU. More recently, with an expanding repertoire of novel cancer treatments and more comprehensive critical care interventions, there has been a shifting medical paradigm from a previously terminal diagnosis to a chronic illness which can be managed with a selection of surgical resection, chemotherapy, radiotherapy, and immunotherapy. This has led to increased availability of critical care services to the oncological population, in recognition of outcomes which are no longer predominantly based on the cancer diagnosis but rather the degree of physiological derangement.

Current practice no longer deems metastatic disease as a contraindication to critical care admission, and there has been a global annual increase in the incidence of ICU admissions for cancer patients [57, 60]. Essentially, two types of cancer patients are admitted to intensive care units – elective admissions post-palliative or curative surgical resection and emergency admissions for cancer-related morbidities, therapeutic toxicities, or deterioration of non-cancer comorbidities (Table 1).

Oncological emergencies frequently warrant critical care intervention and require prompt diagnosis and management in order to avoid devastating sequelae for the patient. The commonest acute complications of cancer and/or its management include febrile neutropenia, hypercalcemia of malignancy, superior vena cava obstruction, metastatic spinal cord compression, and tumor lysis syndrome.

Table 1 Common causes of ICU admission in oncological population

Postsurgical care
Elective
Emergency
Oncological emergencies
Febrile neutropenia
Hypercalcemia of malignancy
Superior vena cava obstruction
Spinal cord compression
Tumor lysis syndrome
Chemotherapeutic toxicities
Cardiomyopathy and arrhythmias
Pneumonitis
Encephalopathy
Immunotherapeutic toxicities
Colitis and hepatitis
Endocrinopathy
Pneumonitis
Ophthalmic and neurologic
Cutaneous
Organ failure
Acute respiratory failure
Fluid refractory hypotension
Renal failure
Sepsis
Comorbid disease

Therapeutic toxicities are related to the side effect profiles of various chemotherapy, radiotherapy, and immunotherapy treatments. Knowledge of these agent-specific toxicities facilitates a more focused patient assessment and instigation of appropriate treatment.

Systemic toxicities of chemotherapeutic agents include:

– Cardiovascular: Anthracyclines are frequently implicated in chemotherapy-induced cardiomyopathy. Anthracyclines are antibiotics derived from *Streptomyces* bacteria and include doxorubicin, daunorubicin, and epirubicin. Their main mechanism of action is inhibition of DNA and RNA synthesis as well as free radical generation. They are a common cancer therapy in the breast, stomach, lung, and ovary and have improved disease-free survival but increased later life cardiovascular morbidity which may manifest as cardiac arrhythmias to heart failure requiring the full spectrum of treatment [25].
– Respiratory: Bleomycin is an antibiotic that generates oxygen-free radicals with resultant DNA separation and pulmonary toxicity. Bleomycin may cause pneumonitis in up to 40% of patients and may progress to pulmonary fibrosis in a small cohort [50] which may be worsened by high inspired oxygen concentrations. It is primarily used in the treatment of germ cell tumors as part of the BEP regime (Bleomycin, Etoposide, Cisplatin) [21].
– Neurological: Ifosfamide is an alkylating agent used in the treatment of ovarian, breast, and lung cancer which has previously been implicated in neurotoxicity. It causes an encephalopathy in up to 27% of patients due to its metabolites of chloroacetaldehyde and dicarboxylic acid. It usually improves following discontinuation of treatment and has previously been treated with methylene blue [37].

While chemotherapy and radiotherapy are well-established treatment modalities with recognized toxicities, immunotherapy is a relatively new regimen which has proven to significantly improve cancer prognosis but at a cost of significant systemic toxicities. Effective immuno-therapy regimens include immune checkpoint inhibition and adoptive cellular responses such as CAR T-cell immunotherapy which have reinvigorated the field of cancer immunotherapy.

CAR T-cell immunotherapy involves extrac-tion of the patient's T cells, reengineering to target specific tumor cells, and delivering the T cells back to the patient where they direct poly-clonal T cells to target specific tumor surface antigens [34]. Increasing recognition of CAR T-cell toxicities includes cytokine release syn-drome (CRS) characterized by an inflammatory storm with sequelae of hemodynamic instability often requiring invasive organ support and potential fatalities. There does not appear to be any correlation between the severity of CRS and disease response to immunotherapy although risk factors appear to be disease burden, the administered dose of active agent, and the strength of T-cell activation. The diagnosis of CRS can be challenging due to the array of non-specific symptoms and diagnosis requires a high degree of clinical acumen [48].

Outcome Prognosticators

Irrespective of hematological or solid organ malignancy, the past two decades have demon-strated significant improvements in all cancer out-comes in ICU. A recent extensive systematic review of the literature reported an average ICU mortality for solid organ malignancy of 31.2% (95% CI 24–39%) and overall hospital mortality of 38.2% (95% CI 33.8–42.7%) [39]. The same group then carried out a population-based obser-vational study looking at 118,541 patients with solid organ malignancies and reported an ICU mortality of 14.1% and hospital mortality of 24.6% [40]. These outcome improvements have been attributed to fundamental changes in critical care attitudes toward the oncology population as well as improved anticancer therapies. Within the oncological and critical care communities, various factors contributing toward successful or deleterious ICU admissions have become apparent. These factors can be separated into

system-specific, patient-specific, and cancer-specific factors, and not all are equally weighted.

System-Specific Factors

Critical Care Improvements

General advances in critical care medicine such as the early use of noninvasive ventilation, care bun-dles including timely sepsis management, increased awareness of infection control and asso-ciated practices, and wider availability of supports and technologies for management of multi-organ failure have led to an overall expansion and improvement in critical care medicine. This has directly benefitted all critically unwell patients but particularly oncology patients who are commonly deconditioned and immunocompromised with little physiological reserve to sustain wellbeing in the face of complex opportunistic infections and therapeutic toxicities as well as concurrent illnesses [54].

Case Volume Mix and Admission Policies

Increased cancer case volume and the develop-ment of specialty cancer centers have been shown to improve outcomes for these patients [63]. These high-volume centers tend to have greater experience in managing critically unwell oncolog-ical patients with well-established protocols and admission policies in place. They also maintain a familiarity with the complexities of oncological patients which serves as a stable foundation in managing such a heterogeneous population.

High-volume centers tend to have cancer-friendly critical care units whereby the presence of disseminated disease or multiple lines of treat-ment is not automatic refusals for admission. Determining precise admission policies will remain controversial, and clinical evaluation is often challenging in this cohort with a previous study showing 21% of patients dying at day 30 who had on clinical assessment been consid-ered too well and refused critical care admission

[59]. However, given the overall improved survival in outcomes in cancer patients, guidelines for ICU admission should be based on the same parameters that are used for non-cancer patients and implemented accordingly.

Timing of critical care admission is paramount with several studies reporting increased mortality with delayed admissions [32, 53].

Multidisciplinary Approach

Optimal care for critically unwell cancer patients mandates multidisciplinary input. The repertoire of anticancer treatments and their associated toxicities continues to grow, challenging the most fastidious of oncologists. Antimicrobial stewardship, infection control, nutritional requirements in a catabolic state, and management of organ dysfunction require the full spectrum of intensivists, microbiologists, pharmacists, dieticians, and physiotherapists. Multidisciplinary input in high-intensity critical care units has previously been shown to reduce mortality in acutely unwell patients [27].

Patient-Specific Factors

Age

As the global population continues to increase, there has been a fundamental change within population characteristics and a rightward shift of the bell curve indicating more people living longer and an increased elderly population, particularly, in the developed world. This is of significance to the oncological community as half of all cancers occur in individuals aged greater than 70 years [10]. In general, age has not been shown to be a poor prognostic factor in cancer outcomes [51]. However, in the context of a critically unwell oncological patient, age does play a role due to the association with increased numbers of comorbidities [22], polypharmacy often reflecting underlying physiological pathology and the likelihood of viable and meaningful outcomes such as the quality-adjusted life years. Recognition of

these age-related factors often mandates early discussion of treatment goals and alterations in the therapeutic pathway accordingly.

Performance Status

Functional performance status is a measure of a patient's ability to independently perform certain activities of daily living. The two commonest measures of performance status are the Eastern Cooperative Oncology Group (ECOG) scale and the Karnofsky scale. ECOG performance status is a scale from 0 to 4 with 0 being fully independent and asymptomatic and 4 being bedridden. ECOG scores of $>/=1$ have previously been associated with overall worse cancer outcomes compared to scores of 0 as demonstrated in pancreatic cancer [58], bladder cancer [24], lung cancer [49], and ovarian cancer [43]. The Karnofsky scale ranges from 100 to 10 with 100 being completely independent and 10 being moribund. Performance status is routinely measured in clinical assessment of oncology patients as a marker of baseline function, tolerance to therapy, and eligibility to certain clinical trials [62].

Poor performance status may be irreversible due to a combination of advanced age and severe comorbid illness, or it may be a potentially reversible phenomenon related to symptomatic neoplastic disease, treatment toxicities, and suboptimal pain management. When considering performance status as a predictor of critical care outcomes, it is essential to optimize any reversibility to fully reflect the patient's true functional ability.

Cancer-Specific Factors

Neoplastic Disease and Treatment

As previously discussed, hematological malignancies have nearly always been associated with worse critical care outcomes than solid organ malignancies. When associated with organ failure, particularly the requirement for mechanical ventilation, this differential cancer-type prognosticator is less well-defined with some studies showing no difference in outcomes. Despite this, the usual cancer characteristics of cancer type, stage, and remission status seem to have little impact on short-term critical care outcomes [31, 45, 52]. While the unique features of the underlying malignancy are poor indicators of short-term critical care outcomes, the availability of treatment is of relevance in determining benefit of critical care admission. One of the primary goals of oncological critical care is to return patients to a physiological state of wellbeing which can withstand the rigors of further systemic treatments. If the malignancy has remained refractory to all lines of treatment including potential trial therapies, then early discussion is warranted as to treatment goals to avoid invasive but potentially futile critical care interventions.

Acute Respiratory Failure and Mechanical Ventilation

Acute respiratory failure is the commonest reason for emergency referral of a cancer patient to critical care. Among oncology patients, 10–50% will develop respiratory failure requiring critical care admission and some form of mechanical ventilation [36]. Traditionally, requirement for mechanical ventilation has been the most ominous predictor of oncological critical care outcomes with mortality rates ranging from 67% to 90% [4, 38]. Among patients with hematological malignancies, worsening severity of hypoxemia prior to intubation and prolonged durations of mechanical ventilation are poor prognostic indicators. The causes of acute respiratory failure in cancer patients include infection [5], neutropenia associated with acute respiratory distress syndrome, pulmonary and cardiac comorbidities, therapeutic pulmonary toxicities, and pulmonary involvement of the underlying malignancy.

Recent advances in the management of respiratory insufficiency have somewhat ameliorated outcomes in these patients with lower thresholds for commencing and wider availability of noninvasive ventilation including high-flow nasal cannula [3, 23, 61]. However, the true benefit of these noninvasive techniques has yet to be widely validated in this group. A recent multicenter trial of 374 patients examined traditional noninvasive ventilation compared to oxygen-only therapy in immunocompromised patients with hypoxemic respiratory failure and showed no demonstrable superiority [29]. While the evidence for noninvasive ventilation is questionable, there has been increasing clinical application of high-flow nasal cannula techniques which have shown improved outcomes compared to traditional noninvasive ventilation. Noninvasive ventilation has been shown to be an independent risk factor for endotracheal intubation and mortality compared to oxygen therapy alone or high-flow nasal cannula oxygen therapy in immunocompromised patients [17, 33].

Organ Failure

Organ failures are major negative predictive factors for critical care outcomes with increasing numbers of failing organs associated with increasing mortality [13]. A prospective study by Gordon et al. in 2005 reported a 100% mortality rate for oncology patients with four or more organ failures [19]. Data from the Intensive Care National Audit and Research Centre (ICNARC) database has shown exponential increase in mortality with involved organ failures with one, three, and five organ failures having 50%, 84%, and 98% mortality, respectively. Despite these harbingers of doom, early and aggressive management of unwell patients with organ failure through comprehensive critical care interventions has led to improved although still poor outcomes in this cohort [12]. This has been facilitated through the widespread implementation of track and trigger systems to identify unwell patients, improvements in our pathophysiological knowledge base and technological innovations and developments to support or replace primary organ functions for extended periods in order to permit physiological recuperation.

As identified earlier, the type of organ dysfunction has prognostic implications with acute respiratory failure and mechanical ventilation the largest contributor toward poor outcomes.

Renal replacement therapy for acute renal failure is associated with increased mortality with a prospective cohort study of 773 patients receiving renal replacement therapy reporting an increased mortality of 78% versus 68% ($p = 0.042$), and mortality was higher with those in whom there was a delay in commencing renal therapy [30].

It is apparent the underlying degree of organ dysfunction may have greater prognostic importance than any individual cancer type or stage.

Neutropenia

Neutropenia is an abnormally low level of neutrophils in the blood which can predispose to increased risk of infection, with severe neutropenia classified as a neutrophil count of $<0.5 \times 10^9$/L. It is common in oncology patients due to sequelae of systemic chemotherapeutic agents. Neutropenia has classically been associated with poor critical care outcomes [7], and growth factors such as granulocyte-colony stimulating factor have commonly been used to shorten the duration of neutropenia with no demonstrable survival benefit. Studies have shown that it is not the presence of neutropenia which modifies mortality outcomes in cases of sepsis but the presence of respiratory and/or hepatic dysfunction [41]. This supports evidence from organ failure studies and oncological critical care outcomes and echoes the importance of the physiological derangement rather than the cancer entity in determining outcomes [16].

Solid Organ Versus Hematological Malignancy

Historically hematological malignancies have been associated with worse critical care outcomes and higher mortality than solid organ malignancy; however, these outcomes have been improving. A French-Belgium multicenter prospective observational analysis looking at critical care outcomes for 1011 patients with hematological malignancy showed ICU mortality of 27.6% and an overall hospital mortality of 39.3% [6]. This evidence of improved outcomes has been reproduced in other studies with data reporting hospital mortality rates as low as 22.8–45.3% [2]. Within the hematological malignancy cohort, outcomes vary between transplant and non-transplanted groups with post-transplant groups faring worse and can be further divided into outcomes based on autologous versus allogenic hematopoietic stem cell transplant. Autologous HSCT has an inhospital mortality ranging from 18.8% to 40%, whereas allogenic HSCT continues to have a high but improved mortality of 60% [2]. A major contributory factor to mortality in these groups is the requirement for mechanical ventilation [26]. When considering the outcome data for hematological malignancies post-HSCT, it is important to contextualize the evidence distinguishing allogenic or autologous transplant as reported data often underestimates the risk profile in allogenic transplants due to pooling.

Repeated Critical Care Admissions

Similar to non-cancer patients, frequent readmissions to critical units are associated with an overall worse prognosis and higher inhospital mortality [15]. A large retrospective study looking at critical care admissions in 247,103 patients in Australia reported an inhospital mortality rate $5\times$ times higher with repeated critical care readmission compared to a single admission [42]. Situations, such as these, necessitate a multidisciplinary approach with expertise in oncology, intensive care, and palliative care, to discuss the potential benefits and limitations of further critical care.

The ICU Trial

Physiological derangements and severity and number of organ failures are key predictors of critical care outcomes. Recent evidence supports the use of these key parameters as prognostic factors; however, it has been shown there is an element of differential survivorship in organ failure based on response to treatment [28].

Fundamentally, two patients with multi-organ failure and similar cancers may not have the same treatment outcomes despite an equally poor prognosis. A trial of critical care may be warranted to assess reversibility and response to interventions. The ICU trial would provide appropriate critical care management for a specified and limited duration with frequent reassessment of the patient in whom there are further lifespan improving therapeutic options available. This strategy enables individualized dynamic real-time evaluation of treatment benefit, and further care can be planned accordingly. The evidence of optimal duration for time-limited trials is lacking. The initial Lecuyer study recommended 6 days, but a recent simulation study reported trial lengths of 4 days for solid organ malignancy and longer to assess response in hematological malignancy [47].

The inherent advantage of the ICU trial is a departure from population-derived indices to individualized assessment based on response to treatment. Disadvantages include a default expectation of ICU admission regardless of benefit of ICU therapies or the patients' baseline performance status. A specified duration for assessment may be inappropriate with inevitable outcomes becoming apparent quicker in some patients such as poor prognosis solid organ malignancies or requiring longer trials of treatment to demonstrate response in hematological malignancies and less acutely unwell patients (Fig. 1).

Outcome Prediction Models

Several challenging issues underscore the need for reliable and valid outcome prediction scoring systems in this population. There is a plethora of evidence to support the strong prognostic value of individual physiological derangements rather than the cancer type or stage. However, this evidence is not widely recognized beyond the fields of oncology and oncological critical care, and many physicians retain a pessimistic view on outcomes for critically unwell cancer patients. In the absence of a multidisciplinary approach, specialist knowledge relevant to short-term critical care

and long-term cancer outcomes can be lacking potentially leading to ill-informed decisions, inappropriate patient selection, and widespread variations in care packages.

Illness severity scoring systems are commonly used in general critical care units to predict population-based outcomes. These scoring systems do not predict individual patient outcomes and tend to perform poorly in the oncological population due to the heterogeneous nature of the patients [14]. The general prognostic models of the APACHE (Acute Physiology and Chronic Health Evaluation), SAPS (Simplified Acute Physiology Score), and MPM (Mortality Prediction Model) have been shown to underestimate mortality in oncology patients. This is a significant limitation as these scoring systems can be a useful tool in communication with patients and families to help make informed decisions regarding invasive critical care treatments based on risk and prognosis.

Oncology-specific illness severity scoring systems have been developed such as the ICMM (ICU Cancer Mortality Model) which is a disease-specific logistic regression model that scores 16 variables to assess hospital mortality in critically unwell oncology patients [20]. However, this model has been shown to overestimate mortality and would benefit from reconfiguration to reflect contemporaneous improvements in treatments [8, 44].

The lack of a highly discriminative risk prediction scoring system in critically unwell cancer patients may reflect the heterogeneous disease nature as seen in the disparate outcomes between solid organ and hematological malignancies. The scoring systems tend to rely on a number of physiological variables; however oncology patients may have an altered baseline due to the disease spectrum and its selected treatments resulting in persistently aberrant physiological parameters which may confound any prediction scores.

As reflected in an ICU trial strategy, the initial assessment of a critically unwell cancer patient is not always reflective of future response to treatment. This is evident in a 2005 study examining outcomes for patients considered for critical care admission. Of the 54 patients considered to be too

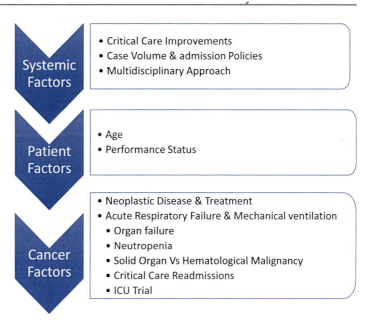

Fig. 1 Interplay of systemic-, patient-, and cancer-specific factors affecting short-term critical care outcomes

Systemic Factors
- Critical Care Improvements
- Case Volume & admission Policies
- Multidisciplinary Approach

Patient Factors
- Age
- Performance Status

Cancer Factors
- Neoplastic Disease & Treatment
- Acute Respiratory Failure & Mechanical ventilation
  - Organ failure
  - Neutropenia
  - Solid Organ Vs Hematological Malignancy
  - Critical Care Readmissions
  - ICU Trial

unwell for admission, 26% were still alive at day 30 and 17% at 6 months compared to the 54% and 32% still alive following critical care admission. Of those deemed too well for admission, only 79% were still alive at day 30 [59]. This exemplifies the challenges of outcome prediction in these patients even for short-term outcomes.

As previously stated, the degree of physiological derangement is strongly associated with ICU mortality. The ICNARC case mix analysis for 1995–2007 reported a linear association between the number of organ failures and hospital mortality in hematological malignancy with one organ failure having an associated mortality of 50% and five organ failures having a mortality of 98%.

Outcomes Following Elective Cancer Surgery

The global burden of cancer surgery is continuing to increase with an estimated 45 million cancer surgeries to be required annually by 2030. Current estimates report 80% of all cancer patients require some surgical intervention be it diagnostic, curative, palliative, or reconstructive [56]. Elective cancer surgeries encompass a deluge of procedures within the different surgical specialties ranging from minor to major complex surgeries mandating increasingly comprehensive infrastructures and dedicated postoperative environments. For solid organ malignancies, many surgeries provide localized resection with curative potential, thus providing the impetus for these surgeries to be performed in an increasingly complex population of elderly multi-morbid patients. These major surgical resections in complex high-risk patients clearly identify an obligation for appropriate postoperative care within a continuum of oncological management.

A recent multicenter observational study analyzed all ICU admissions in the Netherlands following elective cancer surgery over a 5-year period. Twenty-eight thousand and nine hundred seventy-three patients were admitted following elective cancer surgery, representing 9% of all ICU admissions in that time frame and reflective of the contribution of this cohort to the ICU workload. The commonest surgical procedures were for colorectal and lung cancers. The commonest comorbidities were diabetes mellitus and chronic obstructive pulmonary disease (COPD). Almost one-tenth of all patients were considered immunosuppressed based on non-surgical oncological treatments. Approximately 25% of patients required mechanical ventilation postoperatively, and this was most frequent in esophageal cancers and head and neck cancers. Twenty percent of patients had a vasopressor requirement in the first 24 h again most commonly in esophageal cancers. The median ICU stay was 0.9 days with the longest median length of stay, stratified by cancer type, of 2.0 days for esophageal cancers. The median hospital length of stay was 12 days with longest stays for hepatobiliary, head and neck, and bladder cancers. ICU mortality was 1.4% following all surgery and 4.7% hospital mortality. Gastrointestinal cancer had the highest ICU and hospital mortality. Standardized mortality ratios were <1.0 for most types of cancer surgery indicating better than expected outcomes based on APACHE IV prognostic models. This is one of the first studies to look at outcomes in this cohort and is representative of more favorable outcomes than previously thought for elective major cancer surgery [9].

Long-Term Quality of Life and Morbidity

Within the general intensive care populations, there is an increasing recognition that traditional outcome measures such as 30-day mortality and hospital length of stay are inadequate to fully inform of patient long-term outcomes and direct future practice improvements. While overall cancer survivorship has improved, there is limited knowledge on long-term outcomes and quality of life following critical care discharge. In a recent single-center prospective study of 483 patients examining mortality and quality of life outcomes following critical care discharge, there was an increased overall mortality at 1 year compared to inhospital (41% vs. 16%). This may reflect neoplastic disease progression or post-critical care complications such as frailty. It does strengthen the argument for a robust post-critical care discharge program extending beyond the hospital architecture. Quality of life decreased post-critical care discharge with a nadir at 3 months although still lower at 1 year compared to baseline. The improvement in quality of life from 3 months to 12 months was primarily in the mental domains,

and this may reflect a degree of psychological acceptance of a reduced performance status, while physical limitations continued to account for ongoing limiting functional compromise. Interestingly, while most patients reported a reduction in quality of life, the vast majority would opt for a further readmission to critical care if further deterioration warranted such an intervention [35].

Further studies are necessitated in this area to facilitate dissemination of appropriate outcome expectations to patients, their families and oncological specialties alike. Complications following critical care discharge can have significant sequelae with delays in return to intended oncological treatment (RIOT). Surgical resections of tumors are often followed by a planned course of adjuvant systemic treatment within a specified window of opportunity. Delays in RIOT have been shown to result in shorter periods of disease-free survival and reduced overall survival. Aloia in 2014 reported inability to RIOT following open surgery for colorectal liver metastasis was associated with shorter disease-free and overall survivals ($P < 0.001$, HR = 2.16; and $P = 0.005$, HR = 2.07, respectively) [1].

Conclusions

Cancer has evolved from a previously terminal uncontrollable disease to a chronic illness managed through a selection of systemic and surgical treatments. Critical care forms a fundamental continuum of treatment in the management of critically unwell cancer patients. The unique characteristics of cancer as a disease state and its associated therapies require specialist knowledge to ensure an integrated and collaborative framework for delivery of high-quality care. The ongoing improvements in cancer treatments and prolonged disease-free states, inevitably, will lead to increased oncological critical care admissions, and the use of outcome prognosticators and risk prediction models will facilitate targeted and appropriate care in these patients. While the evolution of cancer critical care is likely to continue, areas of future research include evaluation of long-term outcomes following critical care, methods of enhancing patient selection for benefit, and managing death in the unit.

References

1. Aloia TA, Zimmitti G, Conrad C, Gottumukalla V, Kopetz S, Vauthey JN. Return to intended oncologic treatment (RIOT): a novel metric for evaluating the quality of oncosurgical therapy for malignancy. J Surg Oncol. 2014;110(2):107–14. https://doi.org/10.1002/jso.23626.

2. Al-Zubaidi N, Soubani AO. Predictors of mortality in patients with hematologic malignancies admitted to the ICU – a prospective observational study. Am J Respir Crit Care Med. 2016;193:A3657.

3. Antonelli M, Conti G, Bufi M, Costa M, Lappa A, Rocco M, Gasparetto A, Meduri GU. Noninvasive ventilation for treatment of acute respiratory failure in patients undergoing solid organ transplantation: a randomized trial. JAMA. 2000;283(2):235–41.

4. Azevedo LC, Caruso P, Silva UV, Torelly AP, Silva E, Rezende E, Netto JJ, Piras C, Lobo SMA, Knibel MF, Teles JM, Lima RA, Ferreira BS, Friedman G, Rea-Neto A, Dal-Pizzol F, Bozza FA, Salluh JIF, Soares M, Brazilian Research in Intensive Care Network (BRICNet). Outcomes for patients with cancer admitted to the ICU requiring ventilatory support: results from a prospective multicenter study. Chest. 2014;146:257–66.

5. Azoulay E, Lemiale V, Mokart D, Pène F, Kouatchet A, Perez P, Vincent F, Mayaux J, Benoit D, Bruneel F, Meert AP, Nyunga M, Rabbat A, Darmon M. Acute respiratory distress syndrome in patients with malignancies. Intensive Care Med. 2014;40:1106–14.

6. Azoulay E, Mokart D, Pene F, Lambert J, Kouatchet A, Mayaux J, Vincent F, Nyunga M, Bruneel F, Laisne LM, Rabbat A, Lebert C, Perez P, Chaize M, Renault A, Meert AP, Benoit D, Hamidfar R, Jourdain M, Darmon M, Schlemmer B, Chevret S, Lemiale V. Outcomes of critically ill patients with hematologic malignancies: prospective multicenter data from France and Belgium–a Groupe de Recherche Respiratoire en Reanimation Onco-Hematologique study. J Clin Oncol. 2013;31(22):2810–8.

7. Benoit DD, Vandewoude KH, Decruyenaere JM, Hoste EA, Colardyn FA. Outcome and early prognostic indicators in patients with a hematologic malignancy admitted to the intensive care unit for a life-threatening complication. Crit Care Med. 2003;31(1):104–12.

8. Berghmans T, Paesmans M, Sculier JP. Is a specific oncological scoring system better at predicting the prognosis of cancer patients admitted for an acute medical complication in an intensive care unit than general gravity scores? Support Care Cancer. 2004;12(4):234–9.

9. Bos M, Bakhshi-Raiez F, De Keizer J, Dekker N, De Jonge E. Outcomes of intensive care unit admissions after elective cancer surgery. Eur J Surg Oncol. 2013;39(6):584–92.

10. Cancer Research UK. 2016.

11. Crawford SW, Schwartz DA, Petersen FB, Clark JG. Mechanical ventilation after marrow transplantation. Risk factors and clinical outcome. Am Rev Respir Dis. 1988;137(3):682–7.

12. Cubitt J, Smythe J, O'Gara G, Farquhar-Smith WP. Examination of risk factors for mortality of patients with haematological malignancies admitted to intensive care. Eur J Cancer Suppl. 2007;5(4):351.

13. Darmon M, Thiery G, Ciroldi M, De Miranda S, Galicier L, Raffoux E, Le Gall JR, Schlemmer B, Azoulay E. Intensive care in patients with newly diagnosed malignancies and a need for cancer chemotherapy. Crit Care Med. 2005;33(11):2488–93.

14. Den Boer S, De Keizer NF, De Jonge E. Performance of prognostic models in critically ill cancer patients – a review. Crit Care. 2005;9(4):R458–63. https://doi.org/10.1186/cc3765.

15. Elliott M, Worrall-Carter L, Page K. Intensive care readmission: a contemporary review of the literature. Intensive Crit Care Nurs. 2014;30(3):121–37.

16. Farquhar-Smith PW, Wigmore T. Outcomes for cancer patients in critical care. Curr Anaesth Crit Care. 2008;19(2):91–5.

17. Frat JP, Ragot S, Girault C, Perbet S, Prat G, Boulain T, Demoule A, Ricard JD, Coudroy R, Robert R, Mercat A, Brochard L, Thille AW, REVA network. Effect of non-invasive oxygenation strategies in immunocompromised patients with severe acute respiratory failure: a post-hoc analysis of a randomised trial. Lancet Respir Med. 2016;4(8):646–52.

18. Garrouste-Orgeas M, Montuclard L, Timsit J, Reignier J, Desmettre T, Karoubi P, Moreau D, Montesino L, Duguet A, Boussat S, Ede C, Monseau Y, Paule T, Misset B, Carlet J, French ADMISSIONREA Study Group. Predictors of intensive care unit refusal in French intensive care units: a multiple-center study. Crit Care Med. 2005;33(4): 750–5.

19. Gordon AC, Oakervee HE, Kaya B, Thomas JM, Barnett MJ, Rohatiner AZ, Lister TA, Cavenagh JD, Hinds CJ. Incidence and outcome of critical illness amongst hospitalised patients with haematological malignancy: a prospective observational study of ward and intensive care unit based care. Anaesthesia. 2005;60(4):340–7.

20. Groeger JS, Lemeshow S, Price K, Nierman DM, White P Jr, Klar J, Granovsky S, Horak D, Kish SK. Multicenter outcome study of cancer patients admitted to the intensive care unit: a probability of mortality model. J Clin Oncol. 1998;16(2):761–70.

21. Haugnes H, Oldenburg J, Bremnes R. Pulmonary and cardiovascular toxicity in long-term testicular cancer survivors. Urol Oncol Semin Orig Investig. 2015;33(9):399–406.

22. Hermosillo-Rodriguez J, Anaya DA, Sada Y, Walder A, Amspoker AB, Berger DH, Naik AD. The effect of age and comorbidity on patient-centered health outcomes in patients receiving adjuvant chemotherapy for colon cancer. J Geriatr Oncol. 2013;4(2):99–106. https://doi.org/10.1016/j.jgo.2012.12.004.

23. Hilbert G, Gruson D, Vargas F, Valentino R, Gbikpi-Benissan G, Dupon M, Reiffers J, Cardinaud JP. Non-invasive ventilation in immunosuppressed patients with pulmonary infiltrates, fever, and acute respiratory failure. N Engl J Med. 2001;344(7):481–7.

24. Hinata N, Miyake H, Miyazaki A, Nishikawa M, Tei H, Fujisawa M. Performance status as a significant prognostic predictor in patients with urothelial carcinoma of the bladder who underwent radical cystectomy. Int J Urol. 2015;22(8):742–6. https://doi.org/10.1111/iju.12804.

25. Horan P, McMullin M, McKeown P. Anthracycline cardiotoxicity. Eur Heart J. 2006;27(10):1137–8.

26. Jackson SR, Tweeddale MG, Barnett MJ, Spinelli JJ, Sutherland HJ, Reece DE, Klingemann HG, Nantel SH, Fung HC, Toze CL, Phillips GL, Shepherd JD. Admission of bone marrow transplant recipients to the intensive care unit: outcome, survival and prognostic factors. Bone Marrow Transplant. 1998;21(7):697–704.

27. Kim JM, Barnato AE, Angus DC, Fleisher LF, Kahn JM. The effect of multidisciplinary care teams on intensive care unit mortality. Arch Intern Med. 2010;170:369–76.

28. Lecuyer L, Chevret S, Thiery G, Darmon M, Schlemmer B, Azoulay E. The ICU trial: a new admission policy for cancer patients requiring mechanical ventilation. Crit Care Med. 2007;35(3):808–14.

29. Lemiale V, Mokart D, Resche-Rigon M, Pène F, Mayaux J, Faucher E, Nyunga M, Girault C, Perez P, Guitton C, Ekpe K, Kouatchet A, Théodose I, Benoit D, Canet E, Barbier F, Rabbat A, Bruneel F, Vincent F, Klouche K, Loay K, Mariotte E, Bouadma L, Moreau AS, Seguin A, Meert AP, Reignier J, Papazian L, Mehzari I, Cohen Y, Schenck M, Hamidfar R, Darmon M, Demoule A, Chevret S, Azoulay E. Effect of noninvasive ventilation vs oxygen therapy on mortality among immunocompromised patients with acute respiratory failure: a randomized clinical trial. JAMA J Am Med Assoc. 2015;314(16):1711–9.

30. Maccariello E, Valente C, Nogueira L, Bonomo H Jr, Ismael M, Machado JE, Baldotto F, Godinho M, Rocha E, Soares M. Outcomes of cancer and non-cancer patients with acute kidney injury and need of renal replacement therapy admitted to general intensive care units. Nephrol Dial Transplant. 2011;26(2):537–43.

31. McGrath S, Chatterjee F, Whiteley C, Ostermann M. ICU and 6-month outcome of oncology patients in the intensive care unit. QJM Int J Med. 2010;103(6):397–403.

32. Mokart D, Lambert J, Schnell D, Fouché L, Rabbat A, Kouatchet A, Lemiale V, Vincent F, Lengliné E, Bruneel F, Pene F, Chevret S, Azoulay E. Delayed intensive care unit admission is associated with increased mortality in patients with cancer with acute respiratory failure. Leuk Lymphoma. 2013;54(8):1724–9.

33. Neuschwander A, Lemiale V, Darmon M, Pène F, Kouatchet A, Perez P, Vincent F, Mayaux J, Benoit D, Bruneel F, Meert AP, Nyunga M, Rabbat A, Mokart D, Azoulay E. Noninvasive ventilation during acute respiratory distress syndrome in patients with cancer: trends in use and outcome. J Crit Care. 2017;38(C):295–9.

34. Newick K, O'Brien S, Moon E, Albelda SM. CAR T cell therapy for solid tumors. Annu Rev Med. 2017;68(1):139–52.

35. Oeyen SG, Benoit DD, Annemans L, Depuydt PO, Van Belle SJ, Troisi RI, Noens LA, Pattyn P, Decruyenaere JM. Long-term outcomes and quality of life in critically ill patients with hematological or solid malignancies: a single center study. Intensive Care Med. 2013;39:889. https://doi.org/10.1007/s00134-012-2791-x.

36. Pastores SM, Voigt LP. Acute respiratory failure in the patient with cancer: diagnostic and management strategies. Crit Care Clin. 2010;26(1):21–40.

37. Pelgrims J, De Vos F, Van Den Brande J, Schrijvers D, Prové A, Vermorken JB. Methylene blue in the treatment and prevention of ifosfamide-induced encephalopathy: report of 12 cases and a review of the literature. Br J Cancer. 1999;82(2):291–4.

38. Peters SG, Meadows JA 3rd, Gracey DR. Outcome of respiratory failure in hematologic malignancy. Chest. 1988;94(1):99–102.

39. Puxty K, McLoone P, Quasim T, Kinsella J, Morrison D. Survival in solid cancer patients following intensive care unit admission. Intensive Care Med. 2014;40(10):1409–28.

40. Puxty K, McLoone P, Quasim T, Sloan B, Kinsella J, Morrison DS. Risk of critical illness among patients with solid cancers: a population-based observational study. JAMA Oncol. 2015;1(8):1078–85.

41. Regazzoni CJ, Irrazabal C, Luna CM, Poderoso JJ. Cancer patients with septic shock: mortality predictors and neutropenia. Support Care Cancer. 2004;12(12):833–9.

42. Renton J, Pilcher D, Santamaria J, Stow P, Bailey M, Hart G, Duke G. Factors associated with increased risk of readmission to intensive care in Australia. Intensive Care Med. 2011;37(11):1800–8.

43. Sabatier R, Calderon B Jr, Lambaudie E, Chereau E, Provansal M, Cappiello MA, Viens P, Rousseau F. Prognostic factors for ovarian epithelial cancer in the elderly: a case-control study. Int J Gynecol Cancer. 2015;25(5):815–22. https://doi.org/10.1097/IGC.0000000000000418.

44. Schellongowski P, Benesch M, Lang T, Traunmuller F, Zauner C, Laczika K, Locker GJ, Frass M,

Staudinger T. Comparison of three severity scores for critically ill cancer patients. Intensive Care Med. 2004;30(3):430–6.

45. Schellongowski P, Sperr WR, Wohlfarth P, on behalf of Working Group for Hemato-Oncologic Intensive Care Medicine of the Austrian Society of Medical and General Intensive Care Medicine and Emergency Medicine (OEGIAIN), et al. Critically ill patients with cancer: chances and limitations of intensive care medicine – a narrative review. ESMOOpen. 2016;1:e000018. https://doi.org/10.1136/esmoopen-2015-000018.

46. Schuster DP, Marion JM. Precedents for meaningful recovery during treatment in a medical intensive care unit. Outcome in patients with hematologic malignancy. Am J Med. 1983;75(3):402–8.

47. Shrime MG, Ferket BS, Scott DJ, Lee J, Barragan-Bradford D, Pollard T, Arabi YM, Al-Dorzi HM, Baron RM, Hunink MG, Celi LA, Lai PS. Time-limited trials of intensive care for critically ill patients with cancer: how long is long enough? JAMA Oncol. 2016;2:76–83.

48. Shimabukuro-Vornhagen AA, Gödel PS, Schlößer HJ, Von Bergwelt-Baildon M, Kochanek M, Böll B, Schlaak M. Cytokine release syndrome. J Immunol Ther Cancer. 2018;6:56. https://doi.org/10.1186/s40425-018-0343-9.

49. Simmons CP, Koinis F, Fallon MT, Fearon KC, Bowden J, Solheim TS, Gronberg BH, McMillan DC, Gioulbasanis I, Laird BJ. Prognosis in advanced lung cancer – a prospective study examining key clinicopathological factors. Lung Cancer. 2015;88(3):304–9. https://doi.org/10.1016/j.lungcan.2015.03.020.

50. Simpson AB, Paul J, Graham J, Kaye SB. Fatal bleomycin pulmonary toxicity in the west of Scotland 1991–95: a review of patients with germ cell tumours. Br J Cancer. 1998;78(8):1061–6.

51. Soares M, Carvalho MS, Salluh JI, Ferreira CG, Luiz RR, Rocco JR, Spector N. Effect of age on survival of critically ill patients with cancer. Crit Care Med. 2006;34(3):715–21.

52. Soares M, Salluh JIF, Torres VBL, Leal JVR, Spector N. Short- and long-term outcomes of critically ill patients with cancer and prolonged ICU length of stay. Chest. 2008;134(3):520–6. https://doi.org/10.1378/chest.08-0359.

53. Song JU, Suh GY, Park HY, Lim SY, Han SG, Kang YR, Kwon OJ, Woo S, Jeon K. Early intervention on the outcomes in critically ill cancer patients admitted to intensive care units. Intensive Care Med. 2012;38(9):1505–13.

54. Soubani AO. Critical care prognosis and outcomes in patients with cancer. Clin Chest Med. 2017;38:333–53. https://doi.org/10.1016/j.ccm.2016.12.011.

55. Staudinger T, Stoiser B, Mullner M, Locker GJ, Laczika K, Knapp S, Burgmann H, Wilfing A, Kofler J, Thalhammer F, Frass M. Outcome and prognostic factors in critically ill cancer patients admitted to the intensive care unit. Crit Care Med. 2000;28(5):1322–8.

56. Sullivan R, Alatise OI, Anderson BO, Audisio R, Autier P, Aggarwal A, Balch C, Brennan MF, Dare A, D'Cruz A, Eggermont AM, Fleming K, Gueye SM, Hagander L, Herrera CA, Holmer H, Ilbawi AM, Jarnheimer A, Ji JF, Kingham TP, Liberman J, Leather AJ, Meara JG, Mukhopadhyay S, Murthy SS, Omar S, Parham GP, Pramesh CS, Riviello R, Rodin D, Santini L, Shrikhande SV, Shrime M, Thomas R, Tsunoda AT, van de Velde C, Veronesi U, Vijaykumar DK, Watters D, Wang S, Wu YL, Zeiton M, Purushotham A. Global cancer surgery: delivering safe, affordable, and timely cancer surgery. Lancet Oncol. 2015;16(11):1193–224.

57. Taccone FS, Artigas AA, Sprung CL, Moreno R, Sakr Y, Vincent JL. Characteristics and outcomes of cancer patients in European ICUs. Crit Care. 2009;13(1):R15.

58. Tas F, Sen F, Odabas H, Kilic L, Keskin S, Yildiz I. Performance status of patients is the major prognostic factor at all stages of pancreatic cancer. Int J Clin Oncol. 2013;18:839. https://doi.org/10.1007/s10147-012-0474-9.

59. Thiery G, Azoulay E, Darmon M, Ciroldi M, De Miranda S, Le'vy V, Fieux F, Moreau D, Le Gall JR, Schlemmer B. Outcome of cancer patients considered for intensive care unit admission: a hospital-wide prospective study. J Clin Oncol. 2005;23(19):4406–13.

60. Van Vliet M, Verburg IW, van den Boogaard M, de Keizer NF, Peek N, Blijlevens NM, Pickkers P. Trends in admission prevalence, illness severity and survival of haematological patients treated in Dutch intensive care units. Intensive Care Med. 2014;40(9):1275–84.

61. Walkey AJ, Wiener RS. Use of noninvasive ventilation in patients with acute respiratory failure, 2000–2009: a population-based study. Ann Am Thorac Soc. 2013;10:10–7. https://doi.org/10.1513/AnnalsATS.201206-034OC.

62. West H, Jin JO. Performance status in patients with cancer. JAMA Oncol. 2015;1(7):998. https://doi.org/10.1001/jamaoncol.2015.3113.

63. Zuber B, Tran TC, Aegerter P, Grimaldi D, Charpentier J, Guidet B, Mira JP, Pène F. Impact of case volume on survival of septic shock in patients with malignancies. Crit Care Med. 2012;40(1):55–62.

Outcomes in Critically Ill Oncologic Patients

11

Silvio A. Ñamendys-Silva

Contents

Introduction 122

Outcomes of Critically Ill Patients with Solid Tumors 122

Outcome of Critically Ill Patients with Hematological Malignancies 122

Admission of Patients with Cancer to the Intensive Care Unit 123

Early ICU Admission 124

Impact of Chemotherapy in Critically Ill Patients with HMs 124

Conclusion 125

References 125

Abstract

Cancer is the second leading cause of death globally, responsible for 8.8 million deaths in 2015. Globally, nearly 1 in 6 deaths is due to cancer. The introduction of new treatments for cancer and advances in the intensive care of critically ill cancer patients has improved the prognosis and survival. In recent years, classical intensive care unit (ICU) admission comorbidity criteria have been discouraging in this group of patients because the risk factors for death that have been studied, primarily the number of organ failures, allow us to understand the determinants of the prognosis inside the ICU. The number of cancer patients needing ICU care has increased both for cancer-related complications and for treatment-associated side effects. Approximately 13–22% of cancer patients will need admission to a general ICU, and only the 27% of ICU admissions are directly linked with cancer. Survival rates for patients with cancer who are admitted to the ICU have improved; therefore, admission should not be denied to patients only on the basis of their cancer diagnosis. Specialists who treat

S. A. Ñamendys-Silva (✉)
Department of Critical Care Medicine, Medica Sur Clinic and Foundation, Mexico City, Mexico

Department of Critical Care Medicine, Instituto Nacional de Cancerología, Mexico City, Mexico

Department of Critical Care Medicine, Instituto Nacional de Ciencias Médicas y Nutrición Salvador Zubirán, Mexico City, Mexico
e-mail: snamendyss@medicasur.org.mx;
snamendys@gmail.com

© Springer Nature Switzerland AG 2020
J. L. Nates, K. J. Price (eds.), *Oncologic Critical Care*,
https://doi.org/10.1007/978-3-319-74588-6_145

critically ill cancer patients should implement preventive measures to avoid in-hospital death of cancer patients, identifying them at an earlier stage of organ failures. ICU admission should help to prevent, detect, and treat organ dysfunction when offering full support to those cancer patients who are candidates for ICU admission to impact their final outcome. At present, treatment of these patients presents challenges for the oncologist, hematologist, surgical oncologist, and critical care specialist.

Keywords

Cancer patients · Oncologic patients · Solid tumors · Hematological malignancies · Intensive care unit · Critical care · Outcomes

Introduction

Cancer is the second leading cause of death globally, responsible for 8.8 million deaths in 2015. Globally, nearly 1 in 6 deaths is due to cancer [39]. The introduction of new treatments for cancer and advances in the intensive care of critically ill cancer patients has improved the prognosis and survival. In recent years, classical intensive care unit (ICU) admission comorbidity criteria have been discouraging in this group of patients because the risk factors for death that have been studied, primarily the number of organ failures, allow us to understand the determinants of the prognosis inside the ICU [29]. The number of cancer patients needing ICU care has increased both for cancer-related complications and for treatment-associated side effects [20]. Approximately 13–22% of cancer patients will need admission to a general ICU, and only the 27% of ICU admissions are directly linked with cancer [5].

Outcomes of Critically Ill Patients with Solid Tumors

The reported ICU and hospital mortalies for patients with solid tumors varies from 5% to 85% and 5% to 77%, respectively [32]. This variation reflects the substantial heterogeneity between studies and patients, with various tumors at different stages, and reasons for admission to the ICU. Patients with solid tumors are frequently admitted to the ICU for routine postoperative care after undergoing definitive surgical treatment of their underlying malignancy. Cancer patients with unplanned admission to the ICU had a hospital survival of 69% and a 180-day survival rate of 48% [14]. The 1-year and 2-year survival rates survival rates of patients with metastatic solid cancer admitted to the ICU due to emergencies were 12% and 2.4%, respectively [8]. The probability of leaving the hospital alive was greater for patients with solid tumors without established organ failure on admission to ICU [14]. In a cohort study of 25,017 surgical admissions to general ICUs in the West of Scotland, cancer was a common morbidity at 21.8% of all admissions. ICU and hospital mortality were lower in the group of ICU patients with cancer [12.2% (95% CI, 11.3–13.1%) vs. 16.8% (95% CI, 16.3–17.4%) (P <0.001) and 22.9% (95% CI, 21.8–24.1%) vs. 28.1% (95% CI, 27.4–28.7%) (P <0.001)]; however, this survival advantage had reversed by 6 months [33]. Mortality was higher in the cancer group for patients admitted to the hospital electively (14.8%, 95% CI, 13.6–16.1%; vs. 12.8%, 95% CI, 11.7–13.9%; P = 0.010) and for patients admitted to the hospital as an emergency (32.7%, 95% CI, 30.7–34.7%; vs. 29.1%, 95% CI, 28.4–29.9%; P = 0.001). The factor with the greatest association with hospital mortality was severity of illness (APACHE II score, $\geq$20; OR, 4.67; 95% CI, 4.34–5.01) followed by age 65 years or older (OR, 2.14; 95% CI, 2.01–2.29) and emergency hospitalization (OR, 2.86; 95% CI, 2.62–3.12) [33].

Outcome of Critically Ill Patients with Hematological Malignancies

The prognosis for patients with hematological malignances (HM) admitted to the ICU is poor. Despite advances in the treatments of patients with HM [4, 7], recent reports indicated that the

ICU mortality for critically ill patients with HMs ranges from 24% to 57% [2, 10, 11, 13, 17, 18, 26]. The main reasons for ICU admission in this group of patients include acute respiratory failure, sepsis or septic shock, and postoperative care. Nevertheless, the use of intensive chemotherapy protocols can lead to complications requiring ICU admission [26]. Bone marrow transplant recipients staying in the ICU during subsequent hospitalizations have a high mortality. A study of 2653 consecutive patients undergoing bone marrow transplant over a decade in Ontario reported that ICU admission during subsequent hospitalizations is associated with high mortality (67%). Death rates at 1 year were highest among patients requiring aggressive ICU treatments including as mechanical ventilation (87%), pulmonary artery catheterization (91%), and hemodialysis (94%) [35]. The outcomes of critically ill patients with HMs primarily depend on the number of organ failures [38]. Taccone et al. [38] reported that more than 75% of cancer patients with three organs failing died compared with 50% of patients without cancer. Patients with a SOFA score ≥ 10 at the time of ICU admission had higher probability of dying during the hospital stay [26]. Critically ill patients affected by HMs with acute respiratory failure who required invasive mechanical ventilation had high mortality [27, 30]. The need for vasopressors was an independent predictor of hospital mortality [15, 21, 26]. Cárdenas-Turanzas et al. [9] validated the performance of the SOFA score to predict death of critically ill patients with cancer. The authors reported overall ICU and in-hospital mortality rates of 11% and 17%, respectively. Medical patients had higher ICU and in-hospital mortality rates (25% and 37%, respectively) than did surgical patients (2% and 4%) [9]. Despite advances in critical care and hematology, bone marrow transplant (BMT) recipients have not shown improved survival in the ICU. Unfortunately, the development of organ failure after BMT, especially respiratory failure and kidney failure, remains associated with a high risk of death. High mortality rates have been reported at 1 year in BMT recipients requiring advanced and aggressive organ support in the ICU, mechanical ventilation (87%), monitoring

with pulmonary artery flotation catheter (91%), and hemodialysis (94%) [35]. Patients with graft-versus-host disease requiring immunosuppression with steroids (≥ 0.5 mg/kg of prednisone daily), in addition to having a high risk of infectious complications, presented a higher risk of hospital death (HR: 1.60, 95% CI: 1.09–2.34, $p = 0.010$) [31]. Gilbert et al. [16] reported 100% mortality in hematopoietic stem cell transplant recipients requiring mechanical ventilation and hemodialysis or mechanical ventilation with hepatic dysfunction (bilirubin ≥ 2 mg/dL). Thus, the medical team and the patient should always consider the poor prognosis of BMT recipients associated with the need for advanced organ support in the ICU. The decision to provide treatment in the ICU to this group of patients remains complex and difficult; therefore medical groups in the ICU who treat patients with HMs who are potential candidates for BMT must maintain constant and objective communication in relation to prognosis.

Admission of Patients with Cancer to the Intensive Care Unit

Cancer patients, in particular those with hematologic malignancies, are often considered poor candidates for ICU admission because of their historic high mortality rates, and their access to critical care services may be limited. The decision as to whether or not to admit a critically ill patient with cancer to the ICU should be based on already established criteria [28]. Admission policies for ICUs should take into account improvements in the prognosis of critically ill patients with cancer over the last two decades. Admission to the ICU of critically ill cancer patients should be decided on the basis of their severity of illness and long-term prognosis, which rapidly and continuously changes, rather than on the basis of the presence of a malignancy or metastasis [35].

Cancer patients who benefit of ICU admission have the following characteristics [26, 28, 29]:

1. Less than three organ failures.
2. Recent diagnosis of hemato-oncological disease.

3. Treatment of medical emergencies related to cancer or its treatment; tumor lysis syndrome, pulmonary infiltrates in patients with leukemia or leukostasis as the initial manifestation of leukemia.
4. The likelihood of a cure or probable disease control.
5. Performance status (Eastern Cooperative Oncology Group scale) between 0 and 1.
6. Postoperative intensive care for patients undergoing complex surgical procedures who require hemodynamic monitoring and/or mechanical ventilation.

ICU admission should not be considered in the following scenarios:

1. The patient or responsible family members do not accept admission to the ICU.
2. Patients in palliative care as the only treatment option.
3. Poor quality of life before the acute event.

When there is no certainty of the potential benefit of admitting the patient to the ICU, admission is suggested to ensure that the patient has a chance to recover from an acute complication [37].

Early ICU Admission

Overall, patients admitted late and those who are never admitted to the ICU present with higher Acute Physiology and Chronic Health disease Classification System II (APACHE II) and a higher risk of death compared to patients admitted immediately [36]. Early intervention for physiological derangement that developed during hospitalization and led to ICU admission was independently associated with improved short-term and long-term outcomes in critically ill cancer patients [23]. Lee et al. [23] reported that early intervention within 1.5 h of physiological derangement reduced the relative risk of 1-year mortality by 16% compared with late intervention after 1.5 h [23]. Early ICU admission increased the chance of survival; in particular, a period of less than 24 h from hospital entry to ICU admission was associated with improved survival in patients with HMs (OR: 0.94, 95% CI: 0.89–0.99, $p = 0.020$) [1]. These results suggest that patients with cancer should be admitted early to the ICU, with fewer resulting organ failures [1, 23, 24, 26]. Organ failure over the first hours or days of full life-support treatment could be a simple and objective tool for oncologists and intensivists group to identify patients who should be admitted earlier to the ICU [25].

Impact of Chemotherapy in Critically Ill Patients with HMs

Many patients with newly diagnosed HMs who have not yet received chemotherapy present with acute complications requiring ICU admission. Clinicians should consider that the administration of chemotherapy in the ICU is feasible, and the prognosis depends mainly on the number and severity of organ failures. Moreover, in patients with HMs and serious conditions such as severe sepsis or septic shock, recent treatment with chemotherapy was not associated with an increased risk of death [40]. Furthermore, Darmon et al. [12] described 100 patients with newly diagnosed HMs and organ failures requiring chemotherapy to control HM, and the mortality rates at 30 and 180 days were 40% and 51%, respectively. The administration of urgently indicated CT in selected ICU cancer patients with acute organ failure was effective and was associated with considerable long-term survival, as well as long-term disease-free survival [41].

Patients with neutropenia are at high risk for infection. Several studies have suggested that the presence of neutropenia in patients with cancer admitted to the ICU was associated with worse outcomes [3, 19, 26]; however, it remains unclear whether neutropenia is a risk factor for death in critically ill cancer patients. A recent systematic review suggested a higher risk of death of 10% (6–14%) in neutropenic critically ill cancer patients [6]. Nevertheless, the prognosis of patients with neutropenia and severe sepsis or septic shock has improved. Regazzoni et al. [34] reported the prognosis of 73 patients with cancer and septic shock and showed that neutropenia was not associated with increased mortality (56%) or longer stays in the ICU (6.6 days), compared to patients without neutropenia (52.1%, and 6.8 days). Namendys-Silva et al. [26] reported that neutropenia was one of the independent prognostic factors for hospital death among patients with HMs (OR: 4.24, 95% CI: 1.36–13.19, $p = 0.012$), and hospital mortality was 46.8%. This result was similar to that reported by Legrand et al. [22], who reported 43% mortality in patients with neutropenia and severe sepsis or septic shock. This improvement in survival is likely related to developments in the treatment of chemotherapy-induced neutropenia; severely ill patients with neutropenia should have the same opportunity to receive intensive care as patients with normal leukocyte counts.

Conclusion

Survival rates for patients with cancer who are admitted to the ICU have improved; therefore, admission should not be denied to patients only on the basis of their cancer diagnosis. Specialists who treat critically ill cancer patients should implement preventive measures to avoid in-hospital death of cancer patients, identifying them at an earlier stage of organ failures. ICU admission should help to prevent, detect, and treat organ dysfunction when offering full support to those cancer patients who are candidates for ICU admission to impact their final outcome. At present, treatment of these patients presents challenges for the oncologist, hematologist, surgical oncologist, and critical care specialist.

References

1. Azoulay E, Mokart D, Pène F, et al. Outcomes of critically ill patients with hematologic malignancies: prospective multicenter data from France and Belgium – a Groupe de Recherche Respiratoire en Reanimation Onco-Hematologique study. J Clin Oncol. 2013;31(22):2810–8.
2. Al-Zubaidi N, Shehada E, Alshabani K, ZazaDitYafawi J, Kingah P, Soubani AO. Predictors of outcome in patients with hematologic malignancies admitted to the intensive care unit. Hematol Oncol Stem Cell Ther. 2018;11:206. pii: S1658-3876(18) 30028-1 [Epub ahead of print].
3. Benoit DD, Vandewoude KH, Decruyenaere JM, et al. Outcome and early prognostic indicators in patients with a hematologic malignancy admitted to the intensive care unit for a life-threatening complication. Crit Care Med. 2003;31(1):104–12.
4. Bird GT, Farquhar-Smith P, Wigmore T, Potter M, Gruber PC. Outcomes and prognostic factors in patients with haematological malignancy admitted to a specialist cancer intensive care unit: a 5 yr study. Br J Anaesth. 2012;108(3):452–9.
5. Bos MM, Verburg IW, Dumaij I, et al. Intensive care admission of cancer patients: a comparative analysis. Cancer Med. 2015;4(7):966–76.
6. Bouteloup M, Perinel S, Bourmaud A, et al. Outcomes in adult critically ill cancer patients with and without neutropenia: a systematic review and meta-analysis of the Groupe de Recherche en Réanimation Respiratoire du patient d'Onco-Hématologie (GRRR-OH). Oncotarget. 2017;8(1):1860–70.
7. Coiffier B, Lepage E, Briere J, et al. CHOP chemotherapy plus rituximab compared with CHOP alone in elderly patients with diffuse large-B-cell lymphoma. N Engl J Med. 2002;346(4):235–42.
8. Caruso P, Ferreira AC, Laurienzo CE, et al. Short- and long-term survival of patients with metastatic solid cancer admitted to the intensive care unit: prognostic factors. Eur J Cancer Care (Engl). 2010;19 (2):260–6.
9. Cárdenas-Turanzas M, Ensor J, Wakefield C, et al. Cross-validation of a sequential organ failure assessment score-based model to predict mortality in patients with cancer admitted to the intensive care unit. J Crit Care. 2012;27(6):673–80.
10. Cornish M, Butler MB, Green RS. Predictors of poor outcomes in critically ill adults with hematologic malignancy. Can Respir J. 2016;2016:9431385.
11. Contejean A, Lemiale V, Resche-Rigon M, et al. Increased mortality in hematological malignancy patients with acute respiratory failure from undetermined etiology: a Groupe de Recherche en Réanimation Respiratoire en Onco-Hématologique (Grrr-OH) study. Ann Intensive Care. 2016;6(1):102.
12. Darmon M, Thiery G, Ciroldi M, et al. Intensive care in patients with newly diagnosed malignancies and a need for cancer chemotherapy. Crit Care Med. 2005;33(11): 2488–93.
13. Darmon M, Vincent F, Canet E, et al. Acute kidney injury in critically ill patients with haematological malignancies: results of a multicentre cohort study from the Groupe de Recherche en Réanimation Respiratoire en Onco-Hématologie. Nephrol Dial Transplant. 2015;30(12):2006–13.
14. Fisher R, Dangoisse C, Crichton S, et al. Short-term and medium-term survival of critically ill patients with solid tumours admitted to the intensive care unit: a retrospective analysis. BMJ Open. 2016;6(10): e011363.

15. Geerse DA, Span LF, Pinto-Sietsma SJ, van Mook WN. Prognosis of patients with haematological malignancies admitted to the intensive care unit: sequential organ failure assessment (SOFA) trend is a powerful predictor of mortality. Eur J Intern Med. 2011;22(1):57–61.

16. Gilbert C, Vasu TS, Baram M. Use of mechanical ventilation and renal replacement therapy in critically ill hematopoietic stem cell transplant recipients. Biol Blood Marrow Transplant. 2013;19(2):321–4.

17. Grgić Medić M, Gornik I, Gašparović V. Hematologic malignancies in the medical intensive care unit–outcomes and prognostic factors. Hematology. 2015;20(5):247–53.

18. Irie H, Otake T, Kawai K, et al. Prognostic factors in critically ill patients with hematological malignancy admitted to the general intensive care unit: a single-center experience in Japan. J Anesth. 2017;31(5): 736–43.

19. Jackson K, Mollee P, Morris K, et al. Outcomes and prognostic factors for patients with acute myeloid leukemia admitted to the intensive care unit. Leuk Lymphoma. 2014;55(1):97–104.

20. Koutsoukou A. Admission of critically ill patients with cancer to the ICU: many uncertainties remain. ESMO Open. 2017;2(4):e000105.

21. Lamia B, Hellot MF, Girault C, et al. Changes in severity and organ failure scores as prognostic factors in onco-hematological malignancy patients admitted to the ICU. Intensive Care Med. 2006;32(10):1560–8.

22. Legrand M, Max A, Peigne V, et al. Survival in neutropenic patients with severe sepsis or septic shock. Crit Care Med. 2012;40(1):43–9.

23. Lee DS, Suh GY, Ryu JA, et al. Effect of early intervention on long-term outcomes of critically ill Cancer patients admitted to ICUs. Crit Care Med. 2015;43(7):1439–48.

24. Mokart D, Lambert J, Schnell D, et al. Delayed intensive care unit admission is associated with increased mortality in patients with cancer with acute respiratory failure. Leuk Lymphoma. 2013;54(8):1724–9.

25. Namendys-Silva SA, Herrera-Gómez A. Organ dysfunction in patients with cancer admitted to the intensive care unit. Crit Care Med. 2010;38(4):1232–3.

26. Namendys-Silva SA, González-Herrera MO, García-Guillén FJ, et al. Outcome of critically ill patients with hematological malignancies. Ann Hematol. 2013;92(5):699–705.

27. Namendys-Silva SA, Jarquin-Badiola YD, García-Guillén FJ, et al. Mechanical ventilation in critically ill cancer patients. Heart Lung. 2015;44(1):85–6.

28. Nates JL, Nunnally M, Kleinpell R, et al. ICU admission, discharge, and triage guidelines: a framework to enhance clinical operations, development of institutional policies, and further research. Crit Care Med. 2016;44 (8):1553–602.

29. Ñamendys-Silva SA, Plata-Menchaca EP, Rivero-Sigarroa E, Herrera-Gómez A. Opening the doors of the intensive care unit to cancer patients: a current perspective. World J Crit Care Med. 2015;4(3):159–62.

30. Owczuk R, Wujtewicz MA, Sawicka W, Wadrzyk A, Wujtewicz M. Patients with haematological malignancies requiring invasive mechanical ventilation: differences between survivors and non-survivors in intensive care unit. Support Care Cancer. 2005;13(5):332–8.

31. Pène F, Aubron C, Azoulay E, et al. Outcome of critically ill allogeneic hematopoietic stem-cell transplantation recipients: a reappraisal of indications for organ failure supports. J Clin Oncol. 2006;24(4): 643–9.

32. Puxty K, McLoone P, Quasim T, Kinsella J, Morrison D. Survival in solid cancer patients following intensive care unit admission. Intensive Care Med. 2014;40(10):1409–28.

33. Puxty K, McLoone P, Quasim T, et al. Characteristics and outcomes of surgical patients with solid cancers admitted to the intensive care unit. JAMA Surg. 2018;153(9):834–40.

34. Regazzoni CJ, Irrazabal C, Luna CM, Poderoso JJ. Cancer patients with septic shock: mortality predictors and neutropenia. Support Care Cancer. 2004;12(12): 833–9.

35. Scales DC, Thiruchelvam D, Kiss A, Sibbald WJ, Redelmeier DA. Intensive care outcomes in bone marrow transplant recipients: a population-based cohort analysis. Crit Care. 2008;12(3):R77.

36. Sprung CL, Geber D, Eidelman LA, et al. Evaluation of triage decisions for intensive care admission. Crit Care Med. 1999;27(6):1073–9.

37. Thiéry G, Azoulay E, Darmon M, et al. Outcome of cancer patients considered for intensive care unit admission: a hospital-wide prospective study. J Clin Oncol. 2005;23:4406–13.

38. Taccone FS, Artigas AA, Sprung CL, et al. Characteristics and outcomes of cancer patients in European ICUs. Crit Care. 2009;13(1):R15.

39. The World Health Organization. Cancer. 2018. http:// www.who.int/news-room/fact-sheets/detail/cancer Accessed 31 Oct 2018.

40. Vandijck DM, Benoit DD, Depuydt PO, et al. Impact of recent intravenous chemotherapy on outcome in severe sepsis and septic shock patients with hematological malignancies. Intensive Care Med. 2008;34(5): 847–55.

41. Wohlfarth P, Staudinger T, Sperr WR, et al. Prognostic factors, long-term survival, and outcome of cancer patients receiving chemotherapy in the intensive care unit. Ann Hematol. 2014;93(10):1629–36.

Part II

Pharmacologic Considerations for the ICU Cancer Patient

Role of the Clinical Pharmacist in the Oncologic Intensive Care Unit

12

Brian M. Dee

Contents

Introduction 129

Roles and Responsibilities of the Critical Care Clinical Pharmacist 130

Impact of Clinical Pharmacy Services in the ICU 130

Considerations in Critically Ill Oncology Patients 133

Conclusion 134

References 134

Abstract

A clinical pharmacist is an essential and valuable member of the multidisciplinary ICU team. The impact of ICU clinical pharmacy services is well documented in the primary literature, with positive outcomes in areas such as adverse drug events, drug-drug interactions, antimicrobial therapy, anticoagulant therapy, sedation/analgesia therapy, and provision of advanced cardiac life support. Recent research has shown that the presence of clinical pharmacists in ICUs that care for critically ill oncology patients is associated with decreased mortality. Critical care clinical pharmacists who practice in oncology ICUs often face a unique set of circumstances, including high level of patient acuity, complex pharmacotherapeutic regimens, and high volume of medication use. These practitioners should be familiar with the management of oncology-specific disease states and the complications associated with the treatment of malignancy. The integration of clinical pharmacists and clinical pharmacy services in oncology ICUs is imperative.

Keywords

Intensive care unit · Critical care · Pharmacy · Clinical pharmacist · Clinical pharmacy services · Oncology

Introduction

The provision of pharmacy services to critically ill patients has evolved and expanded rapidly over the past several decades, as the paradigm of care within the intensive care unit (ICU) has shifted to a multidisciplinary approach. The growing

B. M. Dee (✉)
The University of Texas MD Anderson Cancer Center, Houston, TX, USA
e-mail: bmdee@mdanderson.org

complexity of pharmacotherapeutic regimens that critically ill patients require during acute illness has led to the clinical pharmacist becoming an integral member of the ICU team [3, 6, 14]. The importance of a clinical pharmacist's expertise may be even more vital in an oncology ICU, where acute illness may be combined with significant preexisting comorbidities, chronic immunosuppression, chemotherapy, and complications associated with medical and/or surgical intervention for cancer [7, 16]. This chapter will review the roles and responsibilities of the critical care clinical pharmacist, highlight the literature supporting the impact of clinical pharmacy services in critically ill patients, and provide practical considerations in oncology patients.

Roles and Responsibilities of the Critical Care Clinical Pharmacist

The model for critical care pharmacy services was first outlined in a position paper published by the Society of Critical Care Medicine and the American College of Clinical Pharmacy [15]. The authors defined three categories of pharmacist responsibilities and department of pharmacy services: fundamental, desirable, and optimal. Fundamental activities are functions considered vital in order to provide safe pharmaceutical care to critically ill patients. Desirable activities describe the provision of higher-level, specialized clinical pharmacotherapeutic services. Optimal activities reflect a fully cohesive model of critical care pharmacy services that aim to optimize patient outcomes through the highest level of pharmacy practice. Examples of fundamental, desirable, and optimal critical care pharmacist services are provided in Table 1. Multidisciplinary professional organizations have recognized the value a clinical pharmacist can provide to the care of critically ill patients and have recommended the incorporation of a devoted clinical pharmacist into the ICU team [2].

Despite this recommendation, provision of clinical pharmacy services in the ICU may be inconsistent. Results of a survey published by MacLaren et al. [10] summarized clinical pharmacy services provided in ICUs in the US hospitals. A total of 382 hospitals responded (11.8% response rate), comprising 1034 ICUs. Approximately two-thirds (62.2%) of respondents indicated they provided direct clinical pharmacy services to the ICU, with pharmacists attending patient care rounds a mean of 4.4 days/week. During a typical work week, activities included direct patient care (43% of work hours), drug distribution (26.2%), administrative activities (12.6%), education (10.9%), and scholarly activities (7.3%). Fundamental activities that were performed at least 75% of ICU patient days included answering drug information questions, prospectively evaluating and intervening on pharmacotherapeutic regimens, performing therapeutic drug monitoring, and educating other health care providers. The majority of desirable and optimal activities were provided less than 50% of ICU patient days. This data indicates the potential for continued expansion and optimization of clinical pharmacy services in the ICU.

Impact of Clinical Pharmacy Services in the ICU

The impact provided by clinical pharmacy services in the ICU is well documented in the medical literature. Positive outcomes have been shown in a variety of areas, including adverse drug events (ADEs) [8], drug-drug interactions [13], antimicrobial therapy [11], anticoagulant therapy [9], sedation/analgesia therapy [12], and provision of advanced cardiac life support (ACLS) [1, 5].

One of the landmark trials demonstrating the benefit a clinical pharmacist can provide through incorporation into a multidisciplinary ICU team examined the rate of preventable ADEs due to prescribing errors [8]. The study utilized a before-after intervention design following the integration of a clinical pharmacist into a medical ICU (MICU). A coronary ICU that lacked clinical pharmacy support served as a control unit. The rate of preventable ADEs due to prescribing errors in the MICU decreased from 10.4 to 3.5 per 1000 patient-days pre- versus postintervention

Table 1 Fundamental, desirable, and optimal critical care pharmacist services [15]

	Patient care	Administrative	Educational	Scholarly
Fundamental	• Prospectively evaluate medication regimens • Monitor medication regimens for effectiveness and safety • Intervene to change medication regimens • Evaluate and modify parenteral nutrition regimens • Document clinical interventions • Perform pharmacokinetic monitoring • Answer drug information and IV compatibility questions	• Identify, manage, and report ADEs • Implement and maintain policies and procedures related to medication therapy • Prepare ICU for Joint Commission surveys • Consult with institutional committees as necessary	• Provide education regarding medication therapy to ICU team • Provide education regarding medication-related policies and procedures to health care professionals	• Contribute to institutional newsletters and drug monographs
Desirable	• Round regularly with multidisciplinary ICU team • Perform medication histories to determine necessary maintenance medications • Provide formal nutrition consults with clinical dietitian • Respond to adult and pediatric ACLS events	• Develop and implement medication therapy protocols • Document economic and clinical impact of interventions • Participate on institutional and ICU committees	• Provide lectures to health care professional students • Precept pharmacy students, residents, and fellows	• Conduct clinical research • Publish case reports, case series, and letters to the editor
Optimal	• Aid physicians with patient care discussions	• Develop and implement pharmacy training programs for ICU personnel • Evaluate impact of medication therapy protocols utilized in ICU • Develop and implement new critical care-related pharmacy services	• Provide pharmacy accredited educational programs • Teach ACLS courses • Oversee critical care pharmacy residencies and fellowships • Educate community members regarding role of pharmacists on multidisciplinary ICU teams	• Secure clinical research grants and funding • Conduct pharmacoeconomic analyses • Present results of clinical research at professional meetings • Publish clinical research in peer-reviewed journals

Abbreviations: IV, intravenous; ADEs, adverse drug events; ICU, intensive care unit; ACLS, advanced cardiac life support

(p <0.001). By comparison, the rate of preventable ADEs due to prescribing errors in the coronary ICU remained consistent during the same period, 10.9 and 12.4 per 1000 patient-days ($p = 0.76$). Of note, the pharmacist in the MICU made 366 recommendations during the 9-month postintervention period, of which 362 (99%) were accepted by the ICU team.

An important, but oftentimes overlooked, function of a clinical pharmacist in the ICU is monitoring for drug-drug interactions. A trial published by Ng et al. [13] studied the impact of clinical pharmacist monitoring for corrected QT (QTc) interval prolongation using an algorithm versus a standard care group lacking such support in a mixed MICU and step-down unit population. One hundred forty-nine patients receiving QTc prolonging medications (amiodarone, procainamide, levofloxacin, erythromycin, and/or haloperidol) were included in the study. The primary endpoint, a composite of QTc interval greater than 500 msec or an increase in the QTc interval of 60 msec or more from baseline, was statistically lower in the intervention group versus the standard care group (19% vs. 39%, $p = 0.006$). The composite outcome was primarily driven by a lower incidence of QTc interval greater than 500 msec in the intervention group (13%) versus the standard care group (33%, $p = 0.003$). Overall, 70% of the recommendations generated from the clinical pharmacist's algorithm were accepted by the medical team.

Arguably, one of the most significant contributions a critical care clinical pharmacist can provide is the management of complex antimicrobial regimens. Outcomes associated with clinical pharmacist involvement in caring for critically ill patients with infections were examined by cross-referencing data from the previously described survey of critical care clinical pharmacy services [10], the International Classification of Disease, Ninth Revision, Clinical Modification codes, and the Centers for Medicare and Medicaid Services [11]. This retrospective study compared clinical outcomes between critically ill patients in ICUs with and without clinical pharmacist coverage with regards to nosocomial infections, community-acquired infections, and sepsis. In ICUs with clinical pharmacist coverage, mortality was significantly lower in nosocomial infections (14.6% vs. 18.1%, p <0.001), community-acquired infections (11.4% vs. 13.3%, $p = 0.008$), and sepsis (18.5% vs. 19.4%, $p = 0.008$). Additionally, in ICUs with clinical pharmacist coverage, mean ICU length of stay was significantly lower in nosocomial infections (16.1 ± 15.6 days vs. 17.4 ± 19.7 days, p <0.001), community-acquired infections (12 ± 12.5 days vs. 12.7 ± 19.5 days, $p = 0.03$), and sepsis (12.6 ± 13.2 days vs. 13.4 ± 16 days, p <0.001).

A similarly designed study was conducted in critically ill patients who were retrospectively identified as experiencing thromboembolic and infarction-related events (TIE), as well as critically ill patients experiencing TIE with bleeding complications [9]. In ICUs with clinical pharmacist coverage, mortality was significantly lower in TIE patients (7.6% versus 10.4%, p <0.0001) and TIE patients with bleeding (5.8% vs. 7.6%, p <0.001). Additionally, in ICUs with clinical pharmacist coverage, mean ICU length of stay was significantly lower in TIE patients (6.3 ± 7.8 days vs. 7.3 ± 8.2 days, p <0.0001) and TIE patients with bleeding (10.7 ± 9.5 days vs. 12.4 ± 13.3 days, $p = 0.008$). TIE patients experiencing bleeding complications in ICUs with clinical pharmacy coverage also had statistically lower bleeding rates and transfusion requirements.

Pain, agitation, and delirium management is another area of critical care where a clinical pharmacist's involvement can be instrumental in optimizing patient care. A trial designed as a before-after intervention study evaluated the impact of a clinical pharmacist's presence during patient care rounds in an MICU, specifically aimed at optimizing sedative therapy and guideline adherence in mechanically ventilated patients [12]. Data were collected prospectively on 78 intervention patients and compared with data collected retrospectively on 78 control patients. The mean duration of mechanical ventilation was statistically lower in the intervention patients (178.1 ± 177.9 h) versus the control patients (338.4 ± 344.7 h, $p = 0.0004$). Additionally,

ICU length of stay, hospital length of stay, average daily dose of fentanyl equivalents, and average daily dose of midazolam were all statistically lower in the intervention patients. During the 3-month intervention period, 192 of the 210 pharmacist recommendations (91%) were accepted by the MICU team.

Pharmacist participation during emergency response, in particular cardiopulmonary arrest, has been associated with improved compliance with ACLS guidelines [5]. The study, completed at a 350-bed community teaching hospital, retrospectively analyzed 74 consecutive in-hospital arrests. Approximately one-third of the arrests were attended by a pharmacist. A total of 650 total treatment interventions were analyzed, of which 581 (89.4%) were considered compliant with ACLS guidelines. The authors found that strict compliance with ACLS guidelines during an arrest was statistically more likely when a pharmacist was present (16/27 [59.3%] vs. 15/47 [31.9%], $p = 0.03$). Additional research has also shown decreased in-hospital mortality with pharmacist participation on resuscitation teams [1].

Although there is a relative paucity of data specifically in critically ill oncology patients, recent literature indicates the provision of clinical pharmacy services to this patient population might be of vital importance [16]. A retrospective cohort study analyzed organizational characteristics of 70 ICUs in Brazil that admitted 9946 patients with cancer in 2013. After adjusting for baseline patient characteristics using multivariate logistic regression, three characteristics were associated with lower mortality: implementation of clinical protocols (odds ratio [OR] 0.92, 95% confidence interval [CI] 0.87–0.98); daily meetings between intensivist and oncologist for patient care coordination (OR 0.69, 95% CI 0.52–0.91); and presence of clinical pharmacists in the ICU (OR 0.67, 95% CI 0.49–0.90). Interestingly, an a priori subgroup analysis found the beneficial effects of a clinical pharmacist's presence were most pronounced in MICU patients and patients with the highest acuity of illness based on the Simplified Acute Physiology Score. This study highlights the potential impact of providing formalized clinical pharmacy services to critically ill oncology patients, as well as the need for further research.

Considerations in Critically Ill Oncology Patients

The University of Texas MD Anderson Cancer Center (MD Anderson), a 680-bed comprehensive cancer center in Houston, Texas, contains an 18-bed surgical ICU and a 34-bed MICU. Both ICUs utilize an open-unit concept, with multidisciplinary ICU teams and primary hematology/oncology teams co-managing patients. Specialized consultant teams (e.g., cardiology, infectious diseases, nephrology, etc.) are also available when necessary. Core members of the ICU team include attending physicians, advanced practice providers (e.g., physician assistants and/or nurse practitioners), medical trainees, and clinical pharmacists. Other allied health professionals involved in the care of ICU patients include dietitians, respiratory therapists, physical therapists, social workers, and case managers. Patient care rounds are conducted on a daily basis utilizing an academic model. Although the ICU and hematology/oncology teams round separately, a large degree of communication and coordination of care occurs. As such, the critical care clinical pharmacist and the oncology clinical pharmacist work together to optimize pharmacotherapeutic and monitoring plans.

One of the key functions of the critical care clinical pharmacist in the oncology ICU is serving as the pharmacotherapy expert. This function is paramount, given the high level of patient acuity, complexity of pharmacotherapeutic regimens, and high volume of medications utilized. Research has shown that patients in the ICU receive nearly twice as many medications per day as patients in general care units (15 ± 4.7 versus 9.3 ± 4.3, $p < 0.0001$) [4]. Patients in an oncology ICU may require even more medications per day, with a typical MICU patient at MD Anderson averaging 25 active medication orders per day (i.e., scheduled, continuous infusions, and as needed). Accordingly, screening patient medication profiles for preventable ADEs and drug-drug interactions is a fundamental task. Antimicrobial regimens for critically ill oncology patients can be particularly complex, as patients may require empiric and/or targeted therapy for multidrug resistant gram-positive and gram-negative microorganisms, as well as fungal and viral pathogens. The critical care clinical pharmacist often functions in the dual role of infectious disease clinical pharmacist for these patients. Pancytopenia is oftentimes present, either as a consequence of underlying malignancy and/or chemotherapeutic regimens. Thrombocytopenia and anemia become problematic when patients require prophylactic or therapeutic anticoagulation and/or antiplatelet therapy. Additionally, underlying end-organ dysfunction, hemodynamic instability, and overall respiratory function may severely limit sedation, analgesia, and delirium pharmacotherapeutic options. Consequently, effectively applying evidence-based medicine when critically ill oncology patients do not precisely match patient populations studied in the published literature is one important way a critical care clinical pharmacist can impact overall care.

Although most critical care clinical pharmacists who practice in an oncology ICU may not be experts in the management of primary malignancies, these practitioners should have a foundational knowledge of unique disease states encountered in these patients. Febrile neutropenia, tumor lysis syndrome, hypercalcemia of malignancy, posterior reversible encephalopathy syndrome, diffuse alveolar hemorrhage, veno-occlusive disease, hemophagocytic lymphohistiocytosis, anemia of inflammation and chronic disease, spinal cord compression, and pathological fractures are just a few of the complications associated with malignancy and/or chemotherapeutic regimens that critical care clinical pharmacists may encounter on a routine basis in the oncology ICU. As the use of chemotherapy becomes more prevalent in oncology ICUs, these practitioners should also be familiar with identifying and managing toxicities associated with commonly used chemotherapeutic regimens. This is of particular importance with emerging cancer immunotherapies and chimeric antigen receptor (CAR) T-cells, which can result in treatment-related toxicities including cytokine release syndrome and neurotoxicity that may necessitate ICU admission.

Conclusion

As the care of critically ill patients has shifted towards a multidisciplinary approach, the clinical pharmacist has become an essential member of the ICU team. The clinical pharmacist's highly specialized skillset carves out a unique role in the care of critically ill patients. Primary literature has demonstrated the positive impact of clinical pharmacy services in the ICU in a variety of areas, including but not limited to preventable ADEs, drug-drug interactions, antimicrobial therapy, anticoagulant therapy, sedation/analgesia management, and provision of ACLS. Recent research has also demonstrated the presence of clinical pharmacists in ICUs that care for critically ill oncology patients decreases mortality. Critical care clinical pharmacists who practice in oncology ICUs often face a distinctive set of circumstances, including high patient acuity, complex pharmacotherapeutic regimens, and high volume of medication use. These practitioners should be well versed in the management of oncology-specific disease states and complications associated with the treatment of malignancy. The importance of clinical pharmacists and clinical pharmacy services integration in ICUs caring for critically ill oncology patients cannot be overemphasized.

References

1. Bond CA, Raehl CL. Clinical pharmacy services, pharmacy staffing, and hospital mortality rates. Pharmacotherapy. 2007;27:481–93.
2. Brilli RJ, et al. Critical care delivery in the intensive care unit: defining clinical roles and the best practice model. Crit Care Med. 2001;29:2007–19.
3. Chant C, Dewhurst NF, Friedrich JO. Do we need a pharmacist in the ICU? Intensive Care Med. 2015;41:1314–20.
4. Cullen DJ, Sweitzer BJ, Bates DW, Burdick E, Edmondson A, Leape LL. Preventable adverse drug events in hospitalized patients: a comparative study of

intensive care and general care units. Crit Care Med. 1997;25:1289–97.

5. Draper HM, Eppert JA. Association of pharmacist presence on compliance with advanced cardiac life support guidelines during in-hospital cardiac arrest. Ann Pharmacother. 2008;42:469–74.

6. Erstad BL, Haas CE, O'Keeffe T, Hokula CA, Parrinello K, Theodorou AA. Interdisciplinary patient care in the intensive care unit: focus on the pharmacist. Pharmacotherapy. 2011;31:128–37.

7. Koch A, Checkley W. Do hospitals need oncological critical care units? J Thorac Dis. 2017;9:E304–9.

8. Leape LL, Cullen DJ, Clapp MD, Burdick E, Demonaco HJ, Erickson JI, Bates DW. Pharmacist participation on physician rounds and adverse drug events in the intensive care unit. JAMA. 1999;282:267–70.

9. MacLaren R, Bond CA. Effects of pharmacist participation in intensive care units on clinical and economic outcomes of critically ill patients with thromboembolic or infarction-related events. Pharmacotherapy. 2009;29:761–8.

10. MacLaren R, Devlin JW, Martin SJ, Dasta JF, Rudis MI, Bond CA. Critical care pharmacy services in United States hospitals. Ann Pharmacother. 2006;40:612–8.

11. MacLaren R, Bond CA, Martin SJ, Fike D. Clinical and economic outcomes of involving pharmacists in the direct care of critically ill patients with infections. Crit Care Med. 2008;36:3184–9.

12. Marshall J, Finn CA, Theodore AC. Impact of a clinical pharmacist-enforced intensive care unit sedation protocol on duration of mechanical ventilation and hospital stay. Crit Care Med. 2008;36:427–33.

13. Ng TM, et al. Pharmacist monitoring of QTc interval-prolonging medications in critically ill medical patients: a pilot study. Ann Pharmacother. 2008;42:475–82.

14. Preslaski CR, Lat I, MacLaren R, Poston J. Pharmacist contributions as members of the multidisciplinary ICU team. Chest. 2013;144:1687–95.

15. Rudis MI, Brandl KM. Position paper on critical care pharmacy services. Society of Critical Care Medicine and American College of Clinical Pharmacy Task Force on Critical Care Pharmacy Services. Crit Care Med. 2000;28:3746–50.

16. Soares M, et al. Effects of organizational characteristics on outcomes and resource use in patients with cancer admitted to intensive care units. J Clin Oncol. 2016;34:3315–24.

Stress Ulcer Prophylaxis in the Critically Ill Oncology Population

13

Reagan D. Collins

Contents

Introduction 138

Incidence of Clinically Important Bleeding 138

Risk Factors for Clinically Important Bleeding 139
Clinical Considerations in the Critically Ill Oncology Population 139

Pharmacological Management 140
PPIs Versus H2RAs: Efficacy 140
PPIs Versus H2RAs: Safety 141

Clinical Controversies with SUP 145
Acid Suppressive Therapy Versus Placebo in Patients Receiving Early Enteral
Nutrition 145

Current Guideline Recommendations 148

Conclusion 148

References 148

Abstract

Stress-related mucosal disease in the critically ill population can lead to clinically important gastrointestinal bleeding. Common risk factors for the development of clinically important bleeding include invasive mechanical ventilation for greater than 48 h, coagulopathy, and multiorgan failure. Gastric acid suppression with proton pump inhibitors or histamine-2 receptor antagonists are commonly prescribed in intensive care units for stress ulcer prophylaxis. However, use of stress ulcer prophylaxis is not without risk and has been associated with *Clostridium difficile* infection and pneumonia. Factors inherent to malignancy and/or treatment may pose additional risk for clinically important bleeding as well as infection in the critically ill oncology population. This chapter will provide an evidence-based review of stress ulcer prophylaxis as well as considerations in the critically ill oncology population.

R. D. Collins (✉)
Critical Care/Nutrition Support, Division of Pharmacy,
The University of Texas MD Anderson Cancer Center,
Houston, TX, USA
e-mail: RDCollins@mdanderson.org

© This is a U.S. government work and not under copyright protection in the U.S.;
foreign copyright protection may apply 2020
J. L. Nates, K. J. Price (eds.), *Oncologic Critical Care*,
https://doi.org/10.1007/978-3-319-74588-6_28

Keywords
Stress ulcer prophylaxis · Proton pump
inhibitor · Histamine-2 receptor antagonist ·
Critically ill · Oncology

Introduction

Stress ulcers or stress-related mucosal disease
(SRMD) can develop in critically ill patients due
to physiological disorders, such as gastric hypoperfusion, often seen in this patient population
[56]. SRMD may lead to clinically important
bleeding (CIB), which has been associated with
increased morbidity and mortality [22, 23]. Stress
ulcer prophylaxis (SUP) is commonly prescribed
in general intensive care units (ICU) around the
world to prevent CIB. This chapter will provide
an evidence-based review of SUP as well as
considerations in the critically ill oncology
population.

Incidence of Clinically Important Bleeding

SRMD may manifest as an overt bleed or CIB.
Overt gastrointestinal (GI) bleeding is marked by
hematemesis, blood in nasogastric aspirate,
hematochezia, or melena [22]. Although variations exist in the literature, CIB is classically
defined as overt bleeding plus one of the following within 24 h of bleeding onset: decrease in
systolic blood pressure (SBP) by more than
20 mmHg; an increase of more than 20 beats per
minute in heart rate or a decrease of more than
10 mmHg in SBP measured upon sitting up; or a
decrease in the hemoglobin level of more than 2 g
per deciliter requiring subsequent transfusion
[22]. The overall incidence of CIB varies in the
literature but appears to be low, ranging from
0.6% to 3.5% (Table 1) [13, 22, 23, 28, 34, 62].
CIB is of concern given the associated increase in
mortality as well as length of ICU stay [22,
23]. Limitations with reporting the incidence of
CIB include varying study definitions, varying
methods of SUP, and competing risks for development of an upper GI bleed. It is theorized that
the current incidence of CIB among critically ill
patients is even lower than that historically
reported given advancements in resuscitation
and increased emphasis on early enteral nutrition.
Limited data exists specifically describing CIB in
the critically ill oncology population. To date,
there has been one, single-center, observational
study in an exclusive critically ill oncology population (Table 1) [13] in which 1% (1/100) of
patients experienced CIB.

Table 1 Incidence of overt bleeding and clinically important bleeding (CIB) among critically ill patients

		Population		Overall Incidence	
Study	Design	Overall (n)	Oncology (n)	Overt Bleed (%)	CIB (%)
Zandstra and Stoutenbeek [62]	P, SC, Cohort	167; Med-Surg ICU on MV[a]	NA	7.7	0.6
Cook et al. [22]	P, MC, Cohort	2252; Med-Surg ICUs[b]	NA	4.4	1.5
Cook et al. [23]	P, MC, Cohort	1666; Med-Surg ICUs on MV[b]	NA	NA	3.5
Faisy et al. [28]	R, SC, observational	737; Med-Surg ICU[a]	NA	1.6	1.1
Bruno et al. [13]	P, SC, observational	100; Med-Surg ICUs[c]	100	3	1
Krag et al. [34]	P, MC, Cohort	1034; mixed ICUs[b]	82	4.7	2.6

P prospective, *SC* single-center, *Med* medical, *Surg* Surgical, *ICU* intensive care unit, *MV* mechanical ventilation, *NA* not available, *MC* multicenter, *R* retrospective, *SUP* stress ulcer prophylaxis
[a]Did not receive SUP
[b]Patients included with and without SUP use
[c]All patients received SUP

Risk Factors for Clinically Important Bleeding

Risk factors for the development of CIB in critical illness have been identified via observational studies (Table 2) [21, 22, 34]. Overall, critically ill patients at highest risk of CIB include those requiring invasive mechanical ventilation, coagulopathic, and/or in multiorgan failure. The impact of noninvasive mechanical ventilation on the risk of CIB is unknown.

Clinical Considerations in the Critically Ill Oncology Population

There are a number of considerations in the critically ill oncology population that may increase the risk of CIB and warrant provision of SUP. These considerations may be inherent to malignancy and/or treatment-related and include prolonged and severe thrombocytopenia, use of high-dose corticosteroids (greater than hydrocortisone 250 mg/day equivalent), and GI mucosal injury (e.g., chemotherapy-induced or radiation-induced).

Table 2 Risk factors for development of CIB noted in observational studies

Respiratory failure[a] [22]
Coagulopathy[b] [22, 34]
Chronic liver disease [34]
Maximum SCr[c] [21]
Renal replacement therapy on first day of ICU admission [34]
Multiorgan dysfunction [34]
Greater than or equal to 3 comorbid conditions [34][d]

CIB clinically important bleed, *SCr* serum creatinine, *ICU* intensive care unit
[a]Defined as a need for mechanical ventilation for at least 48 h
[b]Defined as a platelet count <50,000 per cubic millimeter, an international normalized ratio of >1.5, or a partial-thromboplastin time > 2 times the control value
[c]Maximum SCr noted during study period
[d]Comorbid conditions may include: chronic lung disease, previous myocardial infarction, chronic heart failure, chronic renal failure, chronic liver disease, metastatic cancer, hematological cancer, acquired immune deficiency syndrome, immunosuppression, coagulopathy

Prolonged/Severe Thrombocytopenia

Although coagulopathy, inclusive of a platelet count less than 50,000 per cubic millimeter, is an established independent risk factor for CIB in critically ill patients [22], emphasis is warranted in the oncology population given the potential for prolonged and severe thrombocytopenia. In one observational study, 65% of critically ill oncology patients had a coagulopathy [13], which is significantly higher than that seen in past trials of general critically ill populations [18, 22]. Thrombocytopenia is a well-established cause of spontaneous bleeding in patients with malignancies [6], particularly when the platelet count is less than 20,000 per cubic millimeter. There are a number of potential causes of thrombocytopenia in oncology patients, including but not limited to: (1) decreased production due to myelosuppressive effects of chemotherapy, radiation therapy, and/or malignancy infiltration into bone marrow, (2) splenic sequestration, (3) diffuse intravascular coagulation, or (4) immune-mediated thrombocytopenia [6]. In a review of 451 patients with a hematologic malignancy, 22 (4.9%) patients had 25 episodes of an upper GI bleed over a 6-year period [55], and 82% of these patients had a platelet count of less than 20,000 per cubic millimeter at the time of bleed. Comorbidities, such as organ failure (4 episodes) and sepsis (7 episodes), were also present at the time of bleed, indicating some of these patients were critically ill.

Corticosteroid Use

A concern with the use of corticosteroids is the risk of peptic ulcer disease leading to GI bleed and/or perforation [17, 42, 46]. A meta-analysis completed in 2014 that included 159 trials evaluated if the use of systemic corticosteroids (regardless of drug, dose, or frequency) was associated with an increased risk of GI bleed or perforation in a mixed population (N = 33,253; included adult and pediatric patients, hospitalized and ambulatory, critically ill and noncritically ill) [42]. The odds ratio (OR) of GI bleed or perforation was significantly increased with the use of corticosteroids versus placebo, specifically if patients were hospitalized (OR 1.42, 95% CI 1.22–1.66). In the critically ill population, Cook et al. [22] completed a prospective, multicenter, cohort study evaluting risk factors for CIB in the critically ill population (n = 2256) and did not find glucocorticoid administration (200 mg/day or more of hydrocortisone equivalent) as an independent risk factor via multivariate analysis. However, the average daily hydrocortisone equivalent dose received and for what duration was not reported for patients in this trial, making interpretation difficult. The American Society of Health-System Pharmacist's (ASHP) Guidelines on SUP [5] suggest use in critically ill patients with at least two of the following: sepsis, ICU stay of greater than 1 week, occult or overt bleeding for greater than or equal to 6 days, or corticosteroid therapy equivalent of greater than 250 mg/day hydrocortisone, based on the expert opinion of panel members.

Focusing on the oncology ICU population, in a single-center, prospective, observational study of 100 critically ill oncology patients all receiving SUP [13], 51 (51%) of patients received corticosteroids with a median hydrocortisone equivalent dose of 500 (range 50–10,000) mg/day, doses up to 50 times greater than that evaluated by Cook et al. There is some literature available to support that corticosteroid-induced gastric mucosal damage may be dose-related [24, 27, 60]. As such, concern exists given that methylprednisolone doses of 1–2 mg/kg/day (i.e., hydrocortisone equivalent of 5–10 mg/kg/day) or more are utilized in the critically ill population for management of disorders such as immunotherapy-related toxicities [48], diffuse alveolar hemorrhage [49], graft-versus-host disease, and intracranial metastasis. Collectively, there is no convincing literature at this time to justify SUP in critically ill oncology patients solely based on corticosteroid therapy; however, SUP should be a consideration based on the risk-benefit profile for each patient, particularly when corticosteroid regimens are more aggressive than those evaluated in the literature.

Chemotherapy or Radiation-Induced Upper GI Mucosal Injury

Multiple chemotherapeutic agents have been associated with gastric mucosal damage [43]. The use of acid suppressive therapy may prevent GI mucosal damage and reduce symptoms (e.g.,

acid reflux). In fact, omeprazole used prophylactically in noncritically ill patients receiving active chemotherapy has been found to reduce endoscopic-mucosal damage and improve symptom control versus ranitidine, misoprostol, and placebo [51, 52]. However, findings of endoscopic GI mucosal damage do not necessarily correlate with a clinically relevant outcome as no severe complications were reported [51, 52]. Given the acuity of a critically ill oncology patient, there are no trials evaluating the effects of chemotherapy and radiation-induced mucositis on CIB in these patients. Therefore, SUP at this time is only warranted in patients who have recently received chemotherapy and/or radiation that can induce GI mucosal injury in the presence of other risk factors for CIB.

Pharmacological Management

Acid suppressive therapy with proton pump inhibitors (PPIs) or histamine-2 receptor antagonists (H2RAs) represent the cornerstones of SUP in the ICU. Historically, sucralfate was utilized for SUP but use has significantly decreased after ranitidine demonstrated superiority in preventing CIB in a landmark, randomized, controlled trial (RCT) [20]. An international survey conducted in 97 adult ICUs in 11 countries reported that PPIs were the most common SUP agent prescribed, being utilized in 66% of ICUs [35]. This may be due to the superiority of PPIs for achieving and maintaining a gastric pH of greater than 4 [18], which is a surrogate goal due to inhibition of proteolytic activity (i.e., pepsin inhibition) [45]. Unfortunately, there is a lack of RCTs that have evaluated the efficacy and safety of SUP therapy in an exclusive critically ill oncology population. The following will provide a summary of the available pertinent literature evaluating SUP in the general critically ill population.

PPIs Versus H2RAs: Efficacy

There have been multiple trials evaluating PPIs versus H2RAs but only a few that evaluated CIB as a primary endpoint in a prospective fashion

Table 3 RCTs evaluating proton pump inhibitors versus histamine-2 receptor antagonists for SUP in critically ill patients

Study	Design	Population	Methods	Results
Levy et al. [38]	P, SC, RCT	n = 67 ICU patients with at least 1 risk factor[a] Oncology – NR	Omeprazole 40 mg PT/PO daily (n = 32) Ranitidine 150 mg daily by IVCI or 50 mg IV q8H (n = 35)	CIB, n (%): Omeprazole 2 (6%) Ranitidine 11 (31%) p-value = 0.013 Risk factors/patient, mean ± SD: Omeprazole 1.9 ± 1.0 Ranitidine 2.7 ± 1.8 $p < 0.05$
Kantorova et al. [32]	P, SC, RCT	n = 287 Trauma ICU/SICU with projected MV > 48 H or coagulopathy Oncology – NR	Omeprazole 40 mg IV daily (n = 72) Famotidine 40 mg IV q12H (n = 71) Sucralfate 1 g PT q6H (n = 69) Placebo (n = 75)	CIB, n (%): Omeprazole 1 (1) Famotidine 2 (3) Sucralfate 3 (4) Placebo 1 (1) p-value = NS
Conrad et al. [18]	P, DB, MC, RCT, noninferiority trial	n = 359 ICU patients with MV ≥ 48 H Oncology – NR	Omeprazole 40 mg PT q6h × 2 then 40 mg PT daily (n = 178) Cimetidine 300 mg IV × 1, then 50 mg/H (n = 181)	CIB, n (%): Omeprazole 7 (3.9) Cimetidine 10 (5.5) Noninferiority analysis: Upper bound of one-sided 97.5% CI for the difference in bleeding rates was 2.8%, demonstrating omeprazole is no less effective than cimetidine
Solouki et al. [54]	P, SC, DB, RCT	N = 129 ICU patients with MV ≥ 48 H Oncology – NR	Omeprazole 20 mg PT BID (n = 61) Ranitidine 50 mg IV BID (n = 68)	CIB, n (%): Omeprazole 1 (1.6) Ranitidine 4 (5.9) p-value = NS

SUP stress ulcer prophylaxis, *P* prospective, *SC* single-center, *RCT* randomized controlled trial, *ICU* intensive care unit, *NR* not reported, *mg* milligram, *PT* per tube, *PO* by mouth, *IVCI* intravenous continuous infusion, *IV* intravenous, *q* every, *H* hour, *CIB* clinically important bleeding, *SD* standard deviation, *SICU* surgical intensive care unit, *MV* mechanical ventilation, *NS* not significant, *DB* double-blind, *MC* multicenter, *CI* confidence interval, *BID* twice daily
[a]Burns, coagulopathy, acute hepatic failure, major neurologic insult, acute renal failure, respiratory failure, sepsis, shock, or trauma

(Table 3) [18, 32, 38, 54]. Overall, all but one of these trials reported no difference in CIB among patients receiving PPIs versus H2RAs [18, 32, 54]. In a study of 67 ICU patients with at least one risk factor for CIB, Levy and colleagues [38] found that 11 (31%) versus 2 (6%) of patients receiving ranitidine versus omeprazole, respectively, developed a CIB (p = 0.013); however, patients in the ranitidine arm had more risk factors for the development of SRMD. The results of this trial have yet to be replicated in subsequent studies with larger sample sizes. A number of meta-analyses have evaluated the impact of PPIs versus H2RAs on the clinical endpoint of CIB (Table 4) [1, 2, 4, 8]. In summary, the results from these meta-analyses were relatively consistent, indicating PPIs are more effective than H2RAs in preventing CIB, but in all meta-analyses, there were a high number of trials with an unclear or high risk of bias. Of interest, Alhazzani and colleagues [1] did not find a difference in CIB between the use of PPIs versus H2RAs when only trials with low risk of bias were evaluated.

PPIs Versus H2RAs: Safety

Concerns have been raised about the use of acid suppression and risk of infection, particularly *Clostridium difficile* (Table 5) [10, 14, 39] and pneumonia. Decreased gastric acidity may lead to bacterial overgrowth, bacterial translocation, decreased gastric mucus viscosity, and GI flora changes, which may impair gastric host defenses [9].

Table 4 Meta-analyses evaluating SUP in critically ill patients

Study	Inclusion criteria	Results	Discussion
Barkun et al. [8]	RCTs comparing PPIs, H2RAs up to 9/2011 (regardless of drug, dose, or route) 13 RCTs (5 abstracts) n = 1587	Reported as pooled OR (95% CI) of PPIs vs. H2RAs: CIB (13 trials, n = 1587) OR 0.3 (0.17–0.54) Nosocomial pneumonia (7 trials, n = 1017) OR 1.05 (0.69–1.62) Mortality (8 trials, n = 1260) OR 1.19 (0.84–1.68) Days in ICU (3 trials, n = 339) OR − 0.12 (−1.9–1.66)	Cochrane risk of bias tool (1 low/1 high/11 unclear) Results did not change based on sensitivity analysis for CIB: Definition of bleeding included: OR 0.39 (0.19–0.77), Fully published trials: OR 0.35 (0.18–0.68), Patients receiving enteral feeding or with a naso(oro)gastric tube: OR 0.33 (0.18–0.6)
Alhazzani et al. [1]	RCTs comparing PPIs, H2RAs up to 3/2012 (regardless of drug, dose, or route) 14 RCTs n = 1720	Reported as pooled RR (95% CI) of PPIs vs. H2RAs: CIB (12 trials, n = 1614) RR 0.36 (0.19–0.68) Nosocomial pneumonia (8 trials, n = 1100) RR 1.06 (0.73–1.52) Mortality (8 trials, n = 1196) RR 1.01 (0.83–1.24) ICU Length of Stay (5 trials, n = 555) Mean difference −0.54 days (−2.2 − 1.13)	Cochrane risk of bias tool (3 low/6 high/5 unclear) Subgroup analysis of low risk of bias vs. high or unclear risk of bias for CIB lost treatment effect: RR 0.6 (0.27–1.35)
Alshamsi et al. [4]	RCTs comparing PPIs, H2RAs up to 11/2015 (regardless of drug, dose, or route) 19 RCTs (6 abstracts) n = 2117	Reported as pooled RR (95% CI) of PPIs vs. H2RAs: CIB (14 trials, n = 1679) RR 0.39 (0.21–0.71) Pneumonia (13 trials, n = 1571) RR 1.12 (0.86–1.46) Mortality (11 trials, n = 1487) RR 1.05 (0.87–1.27) ICU Length of Stay (7 trials, n = 744) Mean difference − 0.38 days (−1.49–0.74)	Cochrane risk of bias tool (3 low/10 high/6 unclear) Subgroup analysis between magnitude of effect and risk of bias found no significant interaction Sensitivity analysis excluding abstracts (n = 6) yielded similar results for CIB: RR 0.42 (0.21–0.82)

Alhazzani et al. [2]	NMA evaluating RCTs comparing PPIs, H2RAs, sucralfate, or no SUP up to 5/2017 (regardless of drug, dose, or route)
	57 RCTs
	n = 7293
		Reported as pooled OR (95% CI)
		CIB (NMA estimate, moderate quality of evidence)
		  PPI vs. H2RA (14 RCTs)
		    OR 0.38 (0.2–0.73)
		  PPI vs. placebo (4 RCTs)
		    OR 0.24 (0.1–0.6)
		  H2RA vs. placebo (7 RCTs)
		    OR 0.64 (0.32–1.3)
		  PPI vs. sucralfate (1 RCT)
		    OR 0.3 (0.13–0.69)
		  H2RA vs. sucralfate (12 RCTs)
		    OR 0.8 (0.46–1.4)
		Pneumonia (NMA estimate, moderate quality of evidence)
			Cochrane risk of bias tool (16 low/30 high/11 unclear)
			Adherence to PRISMA guidelines for reporting a NMA
			Limitations:
			  Differences in study definitions

(continued)

Table 4 (continued)

Study	Inclusion criteria	Results	Discussion
		PPI vs. H2RA (13 RCTs)	
		OR 1.27 (0.96–1.68)	
		PPI vs. placebo (3 RCTs)	
		OR 1.52 (0.95–2.42)	
		H2RA vs. placebo (8 RCTs)	
		OR 1.19 (0.8–1.78)	
		PPI vs. sucralfate (4 RCTs)	
		OR 1.65 (1.2–2.27)	
		H2RA vs. sucralfate (16 RCTs)	
		OR 1.3 (1.08–1.58)	
		Mortality (NMA estimate, moderate quality of evidence)	
		H2RA vs. PPI (11 RCTs)	
		OR 0.83 (0.63–1.1)	
		Placebo vs. PPI (4 RCTs)	
		OR 0.86 (0.62–1.18)	
		H2RA vs. placebo (17 RCTs)	
		OR 0.97 (0.77–1.23)	
		Sucralfate vs. PPI (1 RCT)	
		OR 0.8 (0.58–1.1)	
		Sucralfate vs. H2RA (12 RCTs)	
		OR 0.96 (0.79–1.16)	

SUP stress ulcer prophylaxis, *RCTs* randomized controlled trials, *PPIs* proton pump inhibitors, *H2RAs* histamine-2 receptor antagonists, *OR* odds ratio, *CI* confidence interval, *vs.* versus, *CIB* clinically important bleeding, *ICU* intensive care unit, *RR* risk ratio, *NMA* network meta-analysis, *PRISMA* Preferred Reporting Items for Systematic Reviews and Meta-Analyses

The rate of gastric bacterial overgrowth has been shown to be higher with PPIs compared to H2RAs, likely due to greater gastric acid inhibition [59]. In a critically ill oncology population, the potential infectious risk associated with acid suppressive therapy may be greater due to immunosuppression (at times, prolonged and severe) related to chemotherapy or the malignancy itself.

Clostridium difficile Infection (CDI)

Multiple meta-analyses of noncritically ill patients have demonstrated an association with acid suppressive therapy (either PPIs, H2RAs, or both) and the development of CDI [7, 36, 37, 58]. In these analyses of mainly observational data, the association appears to be stronger with the use PPIs, although the risk was also seen with H2RAs. Similarly, in the critically ill population, large observational trials have indicated a potential association between acid suppressive therapy, particularly PPIs, and CDI (Table 5) [10, 14, 39]. Practitioners should exhibit caution in interpreting such findings given limitations inherent to observational studies. The association with the use of acid suppressive therapy, whether it be PPIs or H2RAs, and CDI has not been confirmed in prospective, RCTs. The 2017 Infectious Diseases Society of America Clinical Practice Guidelines for CDI state that there is insufficient evidence for discontinuation of PPIs as a measure to prevent CDI, and as such, no recommendation is provided [41]. However, since CDI is associated with significant morbidity and mortality [14, 33], it is important to evaluate the risk versus benefit of acid suppressive therapy for SUP, particularly with PPIs. This may be of even greater consideration in the oncology population, as this population has frequent healthcare and antimicrobial exposure, both of which are established risk factors for the development of CDI [11, 16].

Pneumonia

Recent large observational studies have demonstrated a possible association between PPIs and pneumonia [12, 39]; however, meta analyses

Table 5 Observational studies evaluating the use of SUP and association with CDI

Study	Design	Population	Intervention	Results for CDI
MacLaren et al. [39]	R, pharmaco-epidemiologic study, Premier Perspective Database	n = 35,312 adult ICU patients on MV ≥ 24 H and SUP ≥ 48 H 0.5% with neutropenia	PPI – 61.9% H2RA – 38.1%	Reported as adjusted OR (95% CI): PPI vs. H2RA[a]: 1.29 (1.04–1.59) With neutropenia[a]: 1.08 (0.48–2.43)
Buendgens et al. [14]	R, SC, observational, cohort	n = 3286 MICU patients 53% on MV 15.3% malignancy	PPI – 72.6% H2RA – 18.4% No SUP – 8.7%	Reported as OR (95% CI): PPI[a]: 3.11 (1.11–8.74) H2RA: NSS via univariate analysis Malignancy[a]: 1.59 (0.91–2.76)
Barletta and Sclar [10]	R, case-control, MIMIC II Database	n = 408 adult patients with CDI in ICU ≥ 48 H 6% malignancy 30% immuno- suppression	PPI – 81% (78% use ≥2 days) H2RA – 34% (28% use ≥2 days)	Reported as OR (95% CI): PPI use ≥2 days[a]: 2.19 (1.27–3.78) H2RA[a]: 1.12 (0.70–1.79) Immunosuppression[a]: 0.79 (0.51–1.23)

SUP stress ulcer prophylaxis, *CDI Clostridium difficile* infection, *R* retrospective, *ICU* intensive care unit, *H* hour, *MV* mechanical ventilation, *NSS* not statistically significant, *PPI* proton pump inhibitor, *H2RA* histamine-2 receptor antagonist, *OR* odds ratio, *CI* confidence interval, *vs.*: versus, *SC* single-center, *MICU* medical intensive care unit
[a]Results determined via multivariable analysis

evaluating PPIs versus H2RAs for SUP in critically ill patients have not demonstrated differences in pneumonia incidence (Table 4). Similarly, recent exploratory RCTs evaluating PPIs versus placebo for SUP have not identified differences in pneumonia rates [3, 53]. A recent meta-analysis evaluated 5 RCTs (n = 759) [30] comparing SUP (regardless of drug, dose, frequency, duration) versus placebo or no SUP and found that patients who received SUP had an increased risk of hospital-acquired pneumonia (HAP) [Risk ratio 1.53 (95% CI 1.04–2.27)]; this difference was not corroborated with ventilator-associated pneumonia (VAP) [3 studies, n = 425; Risk ratio 1.24, (95% CI 0.72–2.15)]. The RCTs included in this meta-analysis to evaluate HAP spanned over 20 years with varying definitions of pneumonia; therefore, the results should be interpreted cautiously.

Thrombocytopenia

Thrombocytopenia has been reported to occur in up to 15–58% of critically ill patients [47]. There are multiple risk factors for thrombocytopenia development, including sepsis, hepatic insufficiency, hemodynamic instability, and certain medications (e.g., chemotherapy) [61]. Thrombocytopenia is more common among the medical oncologic critically ill population given disease and/or treatment-related factors. The use of H2RAs and PPIs have been associated with thrombocytopenia, albeit only in case reports and case studies [31, 47, 61]. There is not a clear recommendation or guidance on how to manage SUP in patients with thrombocytopenia or those that develop it while on therapy. In these situations, all other causes of thrombocytopenia should be ruled out prior to therapy modification. Although sucralfate is not as protective in preventing CIB [2, 20], it may be considered an alternative therapy as it does not carry the risk of thrombocytopenia [57].

Clinical Controversies with SUP

Acid Suppressive Therapy Versus Placebo in Patients Receiving Early Enteral Nutrition

Due to the overall low incidence of CIB as well as concerns for CDI and/or pneumonia associated with acid suppressive therapy, recent literature has evaluated the use of pantoprazole versus placebo for SUP in patients receiving early enteral nutrition (EN) (Table 6) [3, 25, 53]. EN may be protective against SRMD [15, 26, 44] by augmenting intramucosal pH and distribution of GI blood flow [19, 30]. Invasive mechanical ventilation for greater than 24–48 h was an inclusion criteria in these studies, denoting all patients had at least one risk factor

for development of CIB. Overall, there were no differences in the incidence of CIB between pantoprazole or placebo in patients receiving early EN. Huang et al. [30] evaluated 7 RCTs (n = 889) in which greater than 50% of enrolled patients in each trial had to have received EN. In this meta-analysis, there was no difference found in GI bleeding [Risk ratio 0.8 (95% CI 0.49–1.31)] in patients who received SUP (regardless of drug, dose, frequency, or duration) versus no prophylaxis. CIB (n = 725) was evaluated via sensitivity analysis and no difference was identified between groups [Risk ratio 0.63 (95% CI 0.2–1.37)]. The body of literature evaluating the omission of SUP in at risk critically ill patients who receive EN has demonstrated positive results but remains hypothesis-generating in nature given the limited number of patients enrolled in these studies. Furthermore, it should be emphasized that extrapolation of the results of these exploratory trials is only prudent in patients that resemble those fulfilling study enrollment criteria (i.e., mechanically ventilated

Table 6 Trials comparing pantoprazole versus placebo in patients receiving early enteral nutrition

Study	Design	Population	Methods	Results
Selvanderan et al. [53]	P, R, DB, SC, parallel-group trial	n = 214 adult patients with MV > 24 H + EN w/i 48 H Oncology – 6 patients (2.8%)	Pantoprazole 40 mg IV daily (n = 106) Placebo (n = 108)	CIB, n (%): PPI 0 (0) vs. Plac 0 (0) # of patients who received EN, n (%): PPI 88 (83) vs. Plac 94 (87), p = 0.41
Alhazzani et al. [3]	DB, MC, RCT, parallel-group, pilot trial	n = 91 adult patients with MV ≥ 48 H Oncology – 6 patients (6.6%)	Pantoprazole 40 mg IV daily (n = 49) Placebo (n = 42)	CIB, n (%): PPI 3 (6.1) vs. Plac 2 (4.8), p = 1.0 # of patients who received EN w/i first 3 days, n (%): 81 (89)
El-Kersh et al. [25]	P, DB, MC, RCT	n = 102 adult patients with MV > 48 H with no contraindication to volume-based EN w/i 24 H of ICU admission Oncology – NR	Pantoprazole 40 mg IV daily + EN (n = 55) Placebo + EN (n = 47)	CIB, n (%): PPI 1 (1.82) vs. Plac 1 (2.13), p = 0.99% of goal volume EN delivered, median (IQR) PPI 55 (36.625–66.43) vs. Plac 64.38 (40.2–69.42), p = 0.26

P prospective, *R* randomized, *DB* double-blind, *SC* single-center, *MV* mechanical ventilation, *h* hour, *EN* enteral nutrition, *w/i* within, *IV* intravenous, *CIB* clinically important bleed, *PPI* pantoprazole, *vs.* versus, *Plac* placebo, *MC* multicenter, *RCT* randomized controlled trial, *ICU* intensive care unit, *NR* not reported, *IQR* interquartile range

Table 7 SUP recommendations from published evidence-based guidelines

Organization	Level of evidence definitions	SUP indications	Treatment recommendations
ASHP Therapeutic Guidelines on Stress Ulcer Prophylaxis. ASHP Commission on Therapeutics and approved by the ASHP Board of Directors on November 14, 1998	Category A: Level I+, I, I- Category B: Level II+, II, II- Category C: Level III+, III, IV+, IV, V Category D: Expert opinion of panel members	MV for more than 48 h or coagulopathy (LOE = C) Patients with history of GI ulceration or bleeding within 1 year before admission (LOE = D) ICU patients with: Head injury with GCS $\leq$ 10 (LOE = B) Thermal injury >35% of BSA (LOE = B) Partial hepatectomy (LOE = C) Hepatic or renal transplant (LOE = D) Hepatic failure (LOE = D) Trauma with ISS $\geq$ 16 (LOE = D) SCI (LOE = D) Presence of at least two of the following (LOE = D): Sepsis ICU stay >1 week Occult or overt bleeding $\geq$6 days Corticosteroid therapy (> 250 mg/day HC)	Choice of H2RAs, antacids, sucralfate should be made on an institution-specific basis (LOE = A) Insufficient data on misoprostol or PPIs are available to allow any recommendation about these agents.
Guillamondegui et al. [29]	Level of recommendations derived from Class I, II, and III evidence. Level I: Strongest evidence for effectiveness and represent principles of patient management that reflect a high degree of clinical certainty Level II: Moderate degree of clinical certainty Level III: Degree of clinical certainty is not established	Level 1: MV Coagulopathy TBI Major burn injury Level 2: Multitrauma Sepsis Acute renal failure Level 3: ISS > 15 Corticosteroid therapy (> 250 mg/day HC)	Level 1: There is no difference between H2RAs, cytoprotective agents, some PPIs. Antacids should not be used. Level 2: Aluminum containing compounds should not be used in dialysis patients. Level 3: Enteral feeding alone may be insufficient SUP.

| Madsen et al. [40] | GRADE | Recommend not using SUP routinely for adult critically ill patients in the ICU (grade 1C). There is insufficient evidence to make any recommendation on SUP and enteral nutrition. There is insufficient evidence to make any recommendation on SUP in ICU subpopulations: trauma, burn, septic, and cardiothoracic patients. | We suggest using PPIs when SUP is indicated in adult critically ill patients in the ICU (grade 2C). |
| Rhodes et al. [50] | GRADE | Recommend that SUP be given to patients with sepsis or septic shock who have risk factors for GI bleeding (strong recommendation, low quality of evidence). Recommend against SUP in patients without risk factors for GI bleeding. | Suggest using either PPIs or H2RAs when SUP is indicated (weak recommendation, low quality of evidence). |

SUP stress ulcer prophylaxis, *MV* mechanical ventilation, *LOE* level of evidence, *GI* gastrointestinal, *ICU* intensive care unit, *GCS* Glasgow coma score, *BSA* body surface area, *ISS* injury severity score, *SCI* spinal cord injury, *mg* milligram, *HC* hydrocortisone, *H2RAs* histamine-2 receptor antagonists, *PPIs* proton pump inhibitors, *TBI* traumatic brain injury, *GRADE* Grading of Recommendations Assessment

patients who were initiated on early EN within 48 h of ICU admission).

Current Guideline Recommendations

Table 7 summarizes the current guidelines recommendations for the use of SUP in critically ill patients [5, 29, 40, 50]. In addition to these guideline recommendations, the risk-benefit profile of SUP should be considered on a case by case basis in critically ill oncology patients who are receiving high-dose corticosteroid therapy and/or those currently experiencing chemotherapy- or radiation-induced GI mucosal injury.

Conclusion

The incidence of stress-related CIB in critically ill patients appears low. SUP is recommended to prevent CIB in critically ill patients with risk factors related to severity of illness (e.g., invasive mechanical ventilation, coagulopathy, number of comorbid conditions, etc.). It is not clear which class of agents (if any), H2RAs or PPIs, is superior in preventing CIB as data is limited and predominantly consists of trials with a high or unclear risk of bias. Infectious risk, inclusive of pneumonia and CDI, associated with SUP therapy, particularly the use of PPIs, has been demonstrated in observational studies and deserves further evaluation in large prospective RCTs. Potential SUP-associated infectious complications should be of concern in all critically ill patients, and even more so in the critically ill oncologic subset. Overall, prescribing of SUP in the oncologic critically ill subset should be guided by the same principles as the general critically ill population. Other considerations in the oncology population include prolonged and severe thrombocytopenia, the use of high dose corticosteroids, and treatment-related GI mucosal injury. Although promising data is emerging for withholding SUP in at risk critically ill patients receiving early EN, larger RCTs are needed to elucidate the true impact of such practice on the incidence of CIB.

References

1. Alhazzani W, Alenezi F, Jaeschke RZ, Moayyedi P, Cook DJ. Proton pump inhibitors versus histamine 2 receptor antagonists for stress ulcer prophylaxis in critically ill patients: a systematic review and meta-analysis. Crit Care Med. 2013;41(3):693–705. https://doi.org/10.1097/CCM.0b013e3182758734.
2. Alhazzani W, Alshamsi F, Belley-Cote E, Heels-Ansdell D, Brignardello-Petersen R, Alquraini M, Perner A, Moller MH, Krag M, Almenawer S, Rochwerg B, Dionne J, Jaeschke R, Alshahrani M, Deane A, Perri D, Thebane L, Al-Omari A, Finfer S, Cook D, Guyatt G. Efficacy and safety of stress ulcer prophylaxis in critically ill patients: a network meta-analysis of randomized trials. Intensive Care Med. 2018;44(1):1–11. https://doi.org/10.1007/s00134-017-5005-8.
3. Alhazzani W, Guyatt G, Alshahrani M, Deane AM, Marshall JC, Hall R, Muscedere J, English SW, Lauzier F, Thabane L, Arabi YM, Karachi T, Rochwerg B, Finfer S, Daneman N, Alshamsi F, Zytaruk N, Heel-Ansdell D, Cook D. Withholding Pantoprazole for Stress Ulcer Prophylaxis in critically Ill patients: a pilot randomized clinical trial and meta-analysis. Crit Care Med. 2017;45(7):1121–9. https://doi.org/10.1097/ccm.0000000000002461.
4. Alshamsi F, Belley-Cote E, Cook D, Almenawer SA, Alqahtani Z, Perri D, Thabane L, Al-Omari A, Lewis K, Guyatt G, Alhazzani W. Efficacy and safety of proton pump inhibitors for stress ulcer prophylaxis in critically ill patients: a systematic review and meta-analysis of randomized trials. Crit Care (London). 2016;20(1):120. https://doi.org/10.1186/s13054-016-1305-6.
5. ASHP Therapeutic Guidelines on Stress Ulcer Prophylaxis. ASHP Commission on Therapeutics and approved by the ASHP Board of Directors on November 14, 1998. Am J Health Syst Pharm. 1999;56(4):347–79.
6. Avvisati G, Tirindelli MC, Annibali O. Thrombocytopenia and hemorrhagic risk in cancer patients. Crit Rev Oncol Hematol. 2003;48(Suppl):S13–6.
7. Azab M, Doo L, Doo DH, Elmofti Y, Ahmed M, Cadavona JJ, Liu XB, Shafi A, Joo MK, Yoo JW. Comparison of the Hospital-Acquired Clostridium difficile infection risk of using proton pump inhibitors versus histamine-2 receptor antagonists for prophylaxis and treatment of stress ulcers: a systematic review and meta-analysis. Gut Liver. 2017;11(6):781–8. https://doi.org/10.5009/gnl16568.
8. Barkun AN, Bardou M, Pham CQ, Martel M. Proton pump inhibitors vs. histamine 2 receptor antagonists for stress-related mucosal bleeding prophylaxis in critically ill patients: a meta-analysis. Am J Gastroenterol. 2012;107(4):507–20; quiz 521. https://doi.org/10.1038/ajg.2011.474.
9. Barletta JF, Bruno JJ, Buckley MS, Cook DJ. Stress Ulcer Prophylaxis. Crit Care Med. 2016;44

(7):1395–405. https://doi.org/10.1097/ccm.00000000 00001872.

10. Barletta JF, Sclar DA. Proton pump inhibitors increase the risk for hospital-acquired Clostridium difficile infection in critically ill patients. Crit Care (London). 2014;18(6):714. https://doi.org/10.1186/s13054-014-0714-7.

11. Bartlett JG. Historical perspectives on studies of Clostridium difficile and C. difficile infection. Clin Infect Dis. 2008;1:S4–11. https://doi.org/10.1086/521865.

12. Bateman BT, Bykov K, Choudhry NK, Schneeweiss S, Gagne JJ, Polinski JM, Franklin JM, Doherty M, Fischer MA, Rassen JA. Type of stress ulcer prophylaxis and risk of nosocomial pneumonia in cardiac surgical patients: cohort study. BMJ (Clin Res ed). 2013;347:f5416. https://doi.org/10.1136/bmj.f5416.

13. Bruno JJ, Canada TW, Wakefield CD, Nates JL. Stress-related mucosal bleeding in critically ill oncology patients. J Oncol Pharm Pract. 2009;15(1):9–16. https://doi.org/10.1177/1078155208094122.

14. Buendgens L, Bruensing J, Matthes M, Duckers H, Luedde T, Trautwein C, Tacke F, Koch A. Administration of proton pump inhibitors in critically ill medical patients is associated with increased risk of developing Clostridium difficile-associated diarrhea. J Crit Care. 2014;29(4):696.e611–95. https://doi.org/10.1016/j.jcrc.2014.03.002.

15. Canada T. Does enteral nutrition provide stress ulcer prophylaxis in critically ill patients? Nutr Clin Pract. 1998;13(4):177.

16. Chitnis AS, Holzbauer SM, Belflower RM, Winston LG, Bamberg WM, Lyons C, Farley MM, Dumyati GK, Wilson LE, Beldavs ZG, Dunn JR, Gould LH, MacCannell DR, Gerding DN, McDonald LC, Lessa FC. Epidemiology of community-associated Clostridium difficile infection, 2009 through 2011. JAMA Intern Med. 2013;173(14):1359–67. https://doi.org/10.1001/jamainternmed.2013.7056.

17. Conn HO, Poynard T. Corticosteroids and peptic ulcer: meta-analysis of adverse events during steroid therapy. J Intern Med. 1994;236(6):619–32.

18. Conrad SA, Gabrielli A, Margolis B, Quartin A, Hata JS, Frank WO, Bagin RG, Rock JA, Hepburn B, Laine L. Randomized, double-blind comparison of immediate-release omeprazole oral suspension versus intravenous cimetidine for the prevention of upper gastrointestinal bleeding in critically ill patients. Crit Care Med. 2005;33(4):760–5.

19. Cook D, Guyatt G. Prophylaxis against upper gastrointestinal bleeding in hospitalized patients. N Engl J Med. 2018;378(26):2506–16. https://doi.org/10.1056/NEJMra1605507.

20. Cook D, Guyatt G, Marshall J, Leasa D, Fuller H, Hall R, Peters S, Rutledge F, Griffith L, McLellan A, Wood G, Kirby A. A comparison of sucralfate and ranitidine for the prevention of upper gastrointestinal bleeding in patients requiring mechanical ventilation. Canadian Critical Care Trials Group. N Engl J Med. 1998;338(12):791–7. https://doi.org/10.1056/nejm199803193381203.

21. Cook D, Heyland D, Griffith L, Cook R, Marshall J, Pagliarello J. Risk factors for clinically important upper gastrointestinal bleeding in patients requiring mechanical ventilation. Canadian Critical Care Trials Group. Crit Care Med. 1999;27(12):2812–7.

22. Cook DJ, Fuller HD, Guyatt GH, Marshall JC, Leasa D, Hall R, Winton TL, Rutledge F, Todd TJ, Roy P, et al. Risk factors for gastrointestinal bleeding in critically ill patients. Canadian Critical Care Trials Group. N Engl J Med. 1994;330(6):377–81. https://doi.org/10.1056/nejm199402103300601.

23. Cook DJ, Griffith LE, Walter SD, Guyatt GH, Meade MO, Heyland DK, Kirby A, Tryba M. The attributable mortality and length of intensive care unit stay of clinically important gastrointestinal bleeding in critically ill patients. Crit Care. 2001;5(6):368–75.

24. Dayton MT, Kleckner SC, Brown DK. Peptic ulcer perforation associated with steroid use. Arch Surg (Chicago: 1960). 1987;122(3):376–80.

25. El-Kersh K, Jalil B, McClave SA, Cavallazzi R, Guardiola J, Guilkey K, Persaud AK, Furmanek SP, Guinn BE, Wiemken TL, Alhariri BC, Kellie SP, Saad M. Enteral nutrition as stress ulcer prophylaxis in critically ill patients: A randomized controlled exploratory study. J Crit Care. 2018;43:108–13. https://doi.org/10.1016/j.jcrc.2017.08.036.

26. Ephgrave KS, Kleiman-Wexler RL, Adair CG. Enteral nutrients prevent stress ulceration and increase intragastric volume. Crit Care Med. 1990;18(6):621–4.

27. Estruch R, Pedrol E, Castells A, Masanes F, Marrades RM, Urbano-Marquez A. Prophylaxis of gastrointestinal tract bleeding with magaldrate in patients admitted to a general hospital ward. Scand J Gastroenterol. 1991;26(8):819–26.

28. Faisy C, Guerot E, Diehl JL, Iftimovici E, Fagon JY. Clinically significant gastrointestinal bleeding in critically ill patients with and without stress-ulcer prophylaxis. Intensive Care Med. 2003;29(8):1306–13. https://doi.org/10.1007/s00134-003-1863-3.

29. Guillamondegui OD, Gunter J, Oliver L., Bonadies JA, Coates JE, Kurek SJ, De Moya MA, Sing RF, Sori AJ. Practice management guidelines for stress ulcer prophylaxis. 2008. http://www.east.org/tpg/archive/html/stressulcer.html.

30. Huang HB, Jiang W, Wang CY, Qin HY, Du B. Stress ulcer prophylaxis in intensive care unit patients receiving enteral nutrition: a systematic review and meta-analysis. Crit Care (London). 2018;22(1):20. https://doi.org/10.1186/s13054-017-1937-1.

31. Kallam A, Singla A, Silberstein P. Proton pump induced thrombocytopenia: a case report and review of literature. Platelets. 2015;26(6):598–601. https://doi.org/10.3109/09537104.2014.953045.

32. Kantorova I, Svoboda P, Scheer P, Doubek J, Rehorkova D, Bosakova H, Ochmann J. Stress ulcer prophylaxis in critically ill patients: a randomized controlled trial. Hepato-Gastroenterology. 2004;51(57):757–61.

33. Kenneally C, Rosini JM, Skrupky LP, Doherty JA, Hollands JM, Martinez E, McKinzie WE, Murphy T,

Smith JR, Micek ST, Kollef MH. Analysis of 30-day mortality for clostridium difficile-associated disease in the ICU setting. Chest. 2007;132(2):418–24. https://doi.org/10.1378/chest.07-0202.

34. Krag M, Perner A, Wetterslev J, Wise MP, Borthwick M, Bendel S, McArthur C, Cook D, Nielsen N, Pelosi P, Keus F, Guttormsen AB, Moller AD, Moller MH. Prevalence and outcome of gastrointestinal bleeding and use of acid suppressants in acutely ill adult intensive care patients. Intensive Care Med. 2015a;41(5):833–45. https://doi.org/10.1007/s00134-015-3725-1.

35. Krag M, Perner A, Wetterslev J, Wise MP, Borthwick M, Bendel S, McArthur C, Cook D, Nielsen N, Pelosi P, Keus F, Guttormsen AB, Moller AD, Moller MH. Stress ulcer prophylaxis in the intensive care unit: an international survey of 97 units in 11 countries. Acta Anaesthesiol Scand. 2015b;59(5):576–85. https://doi.org/10.1111/aas.12508.

36. Kwok CS, Arthur AK, Anibueze CI, Singh S, Cavallazzi R, Loke YK. Risk of Clostridium difficile infection with acid suppressing drugs and antibiotics: meta-analysis. Am J Gastroenterol. 2012;107 (7):1011–9. https://doi.org/10.1038/ajg.2012.108.

37. Leonard J, Marshall JK, Moayyedi P. Systematic review of the risk of enteric infection in patients taking acid suppression. Am J Gastroenterol. 2007;102(9): 2047–56; quiz 2057. https://doi.org/10.1111/j.1572-0241.2007.01275.x.

38. Levy MJ, Seelig CB, Robinson NJ, Ranney JE. Comparison of omeprazole and ranitidine for stress ulcer prophylaxis. Dig Dis Sci. 1997;42(6):1255–9.

39. MacLaren R, Reynolds PM, Allen RR. Histamine-2 receptor antagonists vs proton pump inhibitors on gastrointestinal tract hemorrhage and infectious complications in the intensive care unit. JAMA Intern Med. 2014;174(4):564–74. https://doi.org/10.1001/jamainternmed.2013.14673.

40. Madsen KR, Lorentzen K, Clausen N, Oberg E, Kirkegaard PR, Maymann-Holler N, Moller MH. Guideline for stress ulcer prophylaxis in the intensive care unit. Dan Med J. 2014;61(3):C4811.

41. McDonald LC, Gerding DN, Johnson S, Bakken JS, Carroll KC, Coffin SE, Dubberke ER, Garey KW, Gould CV, Kelly C, Loo V, Shaklee Sammons J, Sandora TJ, Wilcox MH. Clinical Practice Guidelines for Clostridium difficile Infection in Adults and Children: 2017 Update by the Infectious Diseases Society of America (IDSA) and Society for Healthcare Epidemiology of America (SHEA). Clin Infect Dis. 2018;66 (7):987–94. https://doi.org/10.1093/cid/ciy149.

42. Narum S, Westergren T, Klemp M. Corticosteroids and risk of gastrointestinal bleeding: a systematic review and meta-analysis. BMJ Open. 2014;4(5):e004587. https://doi.org/10.1136/bmjopen-2013-004587.

43. Numico G, Fusco V, Franco P, Roila F. Proton Pump Inhibitors in cancer patients: How useful they are? A review of the most common indications for their use. Crit Rev Oncol Hematol. 2017;111:144–51. https://doi.org/10.1016/j.critrevonc.2017.01.014.

44. Pingleton SK, Hadzima SK. Enteral alimentation and gastrointestinal bleeding in mechanically ventilated patients. Crit Care Med. 1983;11(1):13–6.

45. Piper DW, Fenton BH. pH stability and activity curves of pepsin with special reference to their clinical importance. Gut. 1965;6(5):506–8.

46. Piper JM, Ray WA, Daugherty JR, Griffin MR. Corticosteroid use and peptic ulcer disease: role of nonsteroidal anti-inflammatory drugs. Ann Intern Med. 1991;114(9):735–40.

47. Priziola JL, Smythe MA, Dager WE. Drug-induced thrombocytopenia in critically ill patients. Crit Care Med. 2010;38(6 Suppl):S145–54. https://doi.org/10.1097/CCM.0b013e3181de0b88.

48. Puzanov I, Diab A, Abdallah K, Bingham CO 3rd, Brogdon C, Dadu R, Hamad L, Kim S, Lacouture ME, LeBoeuf NR, Lenihan D, Onofrei C, Shannon V, Sharma R, Silk AW, Skondra D, Suarez-Almazor ME, Wang Y, Wiley K, Kaufman HL, Ernstoff MS. Managing toxicities associated with immune checkpoint inhibitors: consensus recommendations from the Society for Immunotherapy of Cancer (SITC) Toxicity Management Working Group. J Immunother Cancer. 2017;5(1):95. https://doi.org/10.1186/s40425-017-0300-z.

49. Rathi NK, Tanner AR, Dinh A, Dong W, Feng L, Ensor J, Wallace SK, Haque SA, Rondon G, Price KJ, Popat U, Nates JL. Low-, medium- and high-dose steroids with or without aminocaproic acid in adult hematopoietic SCT patients with diffuse alveolar hemorrhage. Bone Marrow Transplant. 2015;50:420.

50. Rhodes A, Evans LE, Alhazzani W, Levy MM, Antonelli M, Ferrer R, Kumar A, Sevransky JE, Sprung CL, Nunnally ME, Rochwerg B, Rubenfeld GD, Angus DC, Annane D, Beale RJ, Bellinghan GJ, Bernard GR, Chiche JD, Coopersmith C, De Backer DP, French CJ, Fujishima S, Gerlach H, Hidalgo JL, Hollenberg SM, Jones AE, Karnad DR, Kleinpell RM, Koh Y, Lisboa TC, Machado FR, Marini JJ, Marshall JC, Mazuski JE, McIntyre LA, McLean AS, Mehta S, Moreno RP, Myburgh J, Navalesi P, Nishida O, Osborn TM, Perner A, Plunkett CM, Ranieri M, Schorr CA, Seckel MA, Seymour CW, Shieh L, Shukri KA, Simpson SQ, Singer M, Thompson BT, Townsend SR, Van der Poll T, Vincent JL, Wiersinga WJ, Zimmerman JL, Dellinger RP. Surviving sepsis campaign: international guidelines for management of sepsis and septic shock: 2016. Crit Care Med. 2017;45(3):486–552. https://doi.org/10.1097/ccm.0000000000002255.

51. Sartori S, Trevisani L, Nielsen I, Tassinari D, Abbasciano V. Misoprostol and omeprazole in the prevention of chemotherapy-induced acute gastroduodenal mucosal injury. A randomized, placebo-controlled pilot study. Cancer. 1996;78(7):1477–82.

52. Sartori S, Trevisani L, Nielsen I, Tassinari D, Panzini I, Abbasciano V. Randomized trial of omeprazole or ranitidine versus placebo in the prevention of chemotherapy-induced gastroduodenal injury. J Clin Oncol Off J Am Soc Clin Oncol. 2000;18(3):463–7. https://doi.org/10.1200/jco.2000.18.3.463.

53. Selvanderan SP, Summers MJ, Finnis ME, Plummer MP, Ali Abdelhamid Y, Anderson MB, Chapman MJ, Rayner CK, Deane AM. Pantoprazole or Placebo for Stress Ulcer Prophylaxis (POP-UP): randomized double-blind exploratory study. Crit Care Med. 2016;44(10):1842–50. https://doi.org/10.1097/ccm.00 00000000001819.

54. Solouki M, Marashian SM, Kouchak M, Mokhtari M, Nasiri E. Comparison between the preventive effects of ranitidineand omeprazole on upper gastrointestinal bleeding among ICU patients. Tanaffos. 2009;8(4): 37–42.

55. Soylu AR, Buyukasik Y, Cetiner D, Buyukasik NS, Koca E, Haznedaroglu IC, Ozcebe OI, Simsek H. Overt gastrointestinal bleeding in haematologic neoplasms. Dig Liver Dis. 2005;37(12):917–22. https://doi.org/10.1016/j.dld.2005.07.017.

56. Stollman N, Metz DC. Pathophysiology and prophylaxis of stress ulcer in intensive care unit patients. J Crit Care. 2005;20(1):35–45.

57. Teva Pharmaceuticals Inc. (2017) Sucralfate [package insert]. North Wales, PA.

58. Tariq R, Singh S, Gupta A, Pardi DS, Khanna S. Association of gastric acid suppression with recurrent clostridium difficile infection: a systematic review and meta-analysis. JAMA Intern Med. 2017;177(6):784–91. https://doi.org/10.1001/jamainternmed.2017.0212.

59. Thorens J, Froehlich F, Schwizer W, Saraga E, Bille J, Gyr K, Duroux P, Nicolet M, Pignatelli B, Blum AL, Gonvers JJ, Fried M. Bacterial overgrowth during treatment with omeprazole compared with cimetidine: a prospective randomised double blind study. Gut. 1996;39(1):54–9.

60. Tseng CL, Chen YT, Huang CJ, Luo JC, Peng YL, Huang DF, Hou MC, Lin HC, Lee FY. Short-term use of glucocorticoids and risk of peptic ulcer bleeding: a nationwide population-based case-crossover study. Aliment Pharmacol Ther. 2015;42(5):599–606. https://doi.org/10.1111/apt.13298.

61. Wade EE, Rebuck JA, Healey MA, Rogers FB. H (2) antagonist-induced thrombocytopenia: is this a real phenomenon? Intensive Care Med. 2002;28 (4):459–65. https://doi.org/10.1007/s00134-002-1233-6.

62. Zandstra DF, Stoutenbeek CP. The virtual absence of stress-ulceration related bleeding in ICU patients receiving prolonged mechanical ventilation without any prophylaxis. A prospective cohort study. Intensive Care Med. 1994;20(5):335–40.

Antimicrobial Prophylaxis in High-Risk Oncology Patients

14

Jeffrey J. Bruno and Frank P. Tverdek

Contents

Introduction 153

Antimicrobial Prophylaxis in Surgery 154

Antimicrobial Prophylaxis Considerations in the Oncologic Critically
Ill Patient 160

Conclusion 164

References 164

Abstract

Oncology patients are often vulnerable to the development of infection. Accordingly, antimicrobial prophylaxis may be necessary. In caring for oncology patients, critical care providers should be astute at determining the risk of infection, identifying patients appropriate for antimicrobial prophylaxis, and assessing the risk-benefit profile of available prophylactic options. Using best available evidence and current guidelines (when applicable), this chapter will provide a framework to guide the critical care clinician in addressing the above considerations for both the surgical population and those with malignancy and/or treatment-related immune compromise. In regard to surgical patients, emphasis will be placed on the prevention of surgical site infections following procedures for the management of malignancy and for which postoperative admission to the intensive care unit may be necessary. The remainder of the chapter will highlight principles for the prevention of bacterial, fungal, and viral infections among the immunocompromised oncology population.

Keywords

Surgical procedures · Antimicrobial prophylaxis · Surgical site infection · Immunocompromised · Fungal infection · Bacterial infection · Pneumocystis · Hepatitis · Viral infection

J. J. Bruno (✉) · F. P. Tverdek
The University of Texas MD Anderson Cancer Center,
Houston, TX, USA
e-mail: jjbruno@mdanderson.org;
fptverdek@mdanderson.org

© Springer Nature Switzerland AG 2020
J. L. Nates, K. J. Price (eds.), *Oncologic Critical Care*,
https://doi.org/10.1007/978-3-319-74588-6_27

Introduction

In the oncologic intensive care unit (ICU), there will be a diverse population of patients at risk of infection. Infection risk may be attributable to malignancy and/or treatment-related (e.g., chemotherapy, stem cell transplantation) immune compromise, interventions provided (e.g., surgical procedures), or a combination of such factors. Given that infection is especially deadly in this population, diligence must be demonstrated to prevent and detect the development of infection.

Oncology patients in the ICU will typically have multiple teams coordinating care, necessitating many hand-offs among providers [2]. This is especially true when factoring in surgery and anesthesia teams in patients undergoing surgical intervention [30]. While ICU practice may vary from site to site with regard to critical care team responsibility (i.e., primary vs. a consulting service), critical care clinicians should serve as stewards to identify appropriate antimicrobial prophylaxis opportunities in critically ill oncology patients. The critical care clinician should be able to determine the risk of infection, identify the need for antimicrobial prophylaxis, and assess the risk-benefit profile of available prophylactic options. This chapter will guide the ICU clinician in assessing infection risk and determining evidence-based prophylactic strategies among patients undergoing surgical intervention and those with treatment and/or malignancy-related immune compromise.

Antimicrobial Prophylaxis in Surgery

This section provides an overview of the use of antimicrobial agents for the prevention of postoperative infections (POI), particularly surgical site infections (SSI), in adult cancer patients undergoing surgical procedures. This section is not intended to be all inclusive, but rather functions to highlight (1) the fundamental principles regarding provision of antimicrobial prophylaxis prior to surgery, with (2) an emphasis on surgical procedures that are utilized for the management of

malignancy and for which postoperative admission to the ICU may be necessary. The goal is to provide practical information for the bedside ICU clinician. For a more comprehensive review, practitioners are encouraged to read the 2013 clinical practice guideline for antimicrobial prophylaxis in surgery [9], the 2017 Centers for Disease Control and Prevention guideline for the prevention of SSI [6], and organization-based guidelines for specific practice areas, as available (e.g., American Urological Association, Urologic Surgery Antimicrobial Prophylaxis) [62].

SSI can be defined as infections of the surgical incision (superficial vs. deep) or of the organ/space that is manipulated during the operative procedure [11]. In 2008, SSI were estimated to account for 36% of healthcare-associated infections in the United States, with an attributable cost of $3.3 billion to the healthcare system [63]. Furthermore, the impact of SSI on patient morbidity can be devastating, including the potential for delayed wound healing, sepsis, and repeat surgical procedures. Although many factors (e.g., infection control strategies, preoperative patient care, etc.) may impact the rate of SSI postoperatively, appropriate antimicrobial prophylaxis plays a pivotal role [9].

Antimicrobial regimens utilized for prophylaxis against SSI should encompass the following five characteristics: (1) activity against the predominant surgical site pathogens (the narrowest spectrum of sufficient activity is preferred over excessively "broad" activity); (2) the administered dose(s) should be sufficient to achieve adequate serum and tissue concentrations (see Table 1); (3) the timing of the initial dose and if necessary, repeat doses, should be sufficient for the start and duration of the operative period (see Table 1); (4) minimal adverse effects; and (5) the shortest possible duration of therapy to facilitate effectiveness while minimizing risk (i.e., adverse events, antimicrobial resistance, and cost) [9]. In most cases, the intravenous route of administration is utilized/most feasible for antimicrobial prophylaxis. For the initial dose, current guidelines recommend beginning antimicrobial administration within 60 min of surgical incision (within 120 min for vancomycin and fluoroquinolones

Table 1 Antimicrobial doses and intraoperative re-dosing intervals for surgical prophylaxis

Antimicrobial	Adult dose	Re-dosing interval[a, b] (from initial preoperative dose)
Ampicillin-sulbactam	3 g	2 h
Aztreonam	2 g	4 h
Cefazolin	2 g (3 g if actual BW ≥ 120 kg)	4 h
Cefuroxime	1.5 g	4 h
Cefoxitin	2 g	2 h
Cefotetan	2 g	6 h
Ceftriaxone	2 g	N/A
Ciprofloxacin[c]	400 mg	N/A
Clindamycin	900 mg	6 h
Ertapenem	1 g	N/A
Gentamicin[d]	5 mg/kg (actual BW; use adjusted BW if ≥120% IBW)	N/A
Levofloxacin[c]	500 mg	N/A
Metronidazole	500 mg	N/A
Vancomycin[e]	15 mg/kg	N/A

BW body weight, *IBW* ideal body weight

[a]Re-dosing intervals represent approximately two times the half-life of the agent in patients with normal renal function; patients with impaired renal function need individualized re-dosing intervals

[b]NA (not applicable) for re-dosing based on typical surgical case length, but re-dosing may be needed for long procedures

[c]Fluoroquinolones have been associated with an increased risk of tendonitis/tendon rupture; single dose use is generally deemed safe

[d]Gentamicin should be limited to a single-dose preoperatively given the risk of unexpected accumulation/nephrotoxicity with elevated serum trough levels

[e]Vancomycin prophylaxis should be considered for patients with known MRSA colonization or at high risk for MRSA colonization in the absence of surveillance data

due to prolonged administration times) [9]. Comparatively, majority of data demonstrates an increased risk of SSI when prophylactic antimicrobial administration begins sooner than 60 min prior to incision; of interest, some studies suggest a reduced incidence of SSI when antimicrobial administration begins within 30 min of incision, but this is still under debate. Given most beta-lactam agents (e.g., cefazolin) are administered over a 30 min period, the currently recommended 60 min window will facilitate administration of the entire dose and initial tissue distribution prior to incision [9]. Intraoperative re-dosing is recommended at intervals equivalent to two times the half-life of the antimicrobial agent (from the time of first dose administration) or if intraoperative blood loss exceeds 1500 mL ([9, 53, 42].

Table 2 provides a summary of appropriate antimicrobial prophylactic regimens organized by the type of surgical procedure and the presence or absence of a penicillin allergy (i.e., immunoglobulin E-mediated reaction). Antimicrobial prophylaxis is of most benefit to patients undergoing clean-contaminated (i.e., entry into the respiratory, alimentary, genital, or urinary tracts under controlled conditions) or contaminated procedures (i.e., break in sterile technique, spillage from the gastrointestinal tract); in addition, antimicrobial prophylaxis may be of benefit in clean procedures in which SSI carry severe consequences (e.g., neurosurgical and spinal procedures) [9, 11]. Table 2 provides overarching information regarding antimicrobial prophylaxis in adult patients for each surgical procedure category, followed by specifics regarding management of the cancer patient, if available. Given the scope of this chapter (surgical procedures for management of malignancy and/or malignancy-related complications and for which postoperative

Table 2 Surgical antimicrobial prophylaxis in adult patients

Surgical procedure type	Predominant organisms of concern	Appropriate first-line prophylaxis[a]	Alternative prophylaxis (i.e., Ig-E-mediated penicillin allergy)[b]	Comments
Neurosurgical				
• Craniotomy, CSF shunting, spinal procedures (e.g., decompression) • Endoscopic endonasal pituitary and skull base surgery	• *Staphylococcus* spp., skin flora (e.g., *Propionibacterium acnes*) • For sinonasal endoscopic procedures, nasal flora includes *Staphylococcus* and *Streptococcus* spp.	Cefazolin (<24 h)	Clindamycin (<24 h)	• An ~2% incidence of SSI following craniotomy for intracranial neoplasm has been reported [38] • With EVDs, there is uncertainty regarding the need and duration of antimicrobial prophylaxis [37]; the Neurocritical Care Society recommends one dose of antimicrobials prior to EVD placement and recommends against prophylaxis for the duration of EVD placement [15] • For endoscopic endonasal skull-based surgery, a duration of prophylaxis of 24–48 hrs is often reported [10, 24]
Head and neck				
Procedures involving incision through the oral or pharyngeal mucosa +/− flap reconstruction	• Usually polymicrobial • Oropharyngeal flora: *Streptococcus, Staphylococcus, Peptostreptococcus, Prevotella, Fusobacterium, Veillonella,* and *Bacteroides* spp. (not *B. fragilis*), plus *Enterobacteriaceae* • Nasal flora: *Staphylococcus* and *Streptococcus* spp.	Cefazolin plus metronidazole or cefuroxime plus metronidazole or ampicillin–sulbactam (<24 h)	Clindamycin or levofloxacin plus metronidazole (<24 h)	• Historical data indicates an incidence of SSI up to 87% in clean-contaminated procedures without antibiotic prophylaxis [25] • With flap reconstruction, uncertainties remain regarding the benefit/risk of prophylaxis for greater than 24 h [40, 49] • Use of clindamycin has been associated with an increased risk of SSI and/or POI compared to standard prophylaxis (i.e., cefazolin or ampicillin-sulbactam [40, 43, 45, 49] • Lack of postoperative gram-negative coverage has also been associated with SSI [59] • Despite limited literature, alternatives to clindamycin, such as levofloxacin plus metronidazole, can be considered in cases of beta-lactam allergy

Thoracic (non-cardiac)				
Pneumonectomy, lobectomy, lung resection, thoracotomy	• SSI: *Staphylococcus* spp. • Pneumonia/empyema: variable, inclusive of gram-positive and gram-negative pathogens	Cefazolin, cefuroxime, or ampicillin-sulbactam x 24–48 h	Clindamycin or levofloxacin x 24–48 h	• Prophylactic agent, duration of therapy, and endpoints (e.g., prevention of SSI, pneumonia, empyema, or a combination) varied widely in clinical trials [5, 8, 44, 57] • Antibiotic prophylaxis recommended regardless of surgical method: thoracotomy vs. VATS [9]
Gastrointestinal				
• Gastrectomy (total or partial) • Small bowel procedures (e.g., small bowel resection, bypass) • Procedures involving biliary reconstruction (e.g., pancreaticoduodenectomy, extended hepatectomy)	• *Staphylococcus* spp., *Streptococcus* spp., *Enterococcus* spp., enteric gram-negatives (*Enterobacter* spp., *E. coli, Klebsiella pneumoniae, Citrobacter* spp.) • In the setting of SBO, anaerobes (in addition to the above pathogens) become of greater concern (i.e., *Bacteroides fragilis*)	• Cefotetan or cefoxitin or cefazolin or ertapenem (<24 h) • With small bowel obstruction: If cefazolin is utilized, add metronidazole for anaerobic coverage	• Levofloxacin or clindamycin plus ciprofloxacin or clindamycin plus gentamicin or clindamycin plus aztreonam (<24 h) • With small bowel obstruction: If levofloxacin is utilized, add metronidazole for anaerobic coverage	• Trials evaluating gastric cancer patients undergoing a partial or total gastrectomy did not demonstrate a higher incidence of SSI with intraoperative only vs. extended durations (48–96 hrs) of antimicrobial prophylaxis [20, 22, 41] • Ertapenem has not been shown to be superior to non-ertapenem prophylaxis (e.g., cefoxitin) in cancer patients undergoing intra-abdominal surgery, with the exception of colorectal surgery [33]
Colorectal[c]	*E. coli* and *Bacteroides fragilis*	Ertapenem or cefotetan or cefoxitin or cefazolin plus metronidazole or ceftriaxone plus metronidazole (<24 h)	Ciprofloxacin plus metronidazole or levofloxacin plus metronidazole or clindamycin plus gentamicin or clindamycin plus aztreonam (<24 h)	• In patients undergoing elective colorectal surgery, ertapenem has been shown to be superior to cefotetan for the prevention of SSI [23] • In cancer patients undergoing colorectal surgery, ertapenem has been associated with a lower rate of SSI in comparison to non-ertapenem regimens [33] • For institutions with a high prevalence of *E. coli* resistance to 1st- and 2nd-generation cephalosporins, some experts recommend ceftriaxone plus metronidazole over ertapenem in attempt to minimize the risk of promoting carbapenem resistance [9]

(*continued*)

Table 2 (continued)

Surgical procedure type	Predominant organisms of concern	Appropriate first-line prophylaxis[a]	Alternative prophylaxis (i.e., Ig-E-mediated penicillin allergy)[b]	Comments
Urologic				
• Procedures involving entry into the urinary tract (e.g., prostatectomy, cystectomy, nephrectomy) • Procedures involving entry into the intestinal lumen (e.g., ileal conduit creation)	• Staphylococcus spp., Streptococcus spp., Enterococcus spp., E. coli • In addition to the pathogens above, other enteric gram-negatives (Enterobacter spp., Klebsiella pneumoniae, Bacteroides fragilis) are of concern in procedures that involve the ileum	• Cefazolin (<24 h) • Intestinal procedures: cefotetan or cefoxitin or cefazolin plus metronidazole or ceftriaxone plus metronidazole or ertapenem (<24 h)	• Ciprofloxacin or levofloxacin or gentamicin +/− clindamycin (<24 h) • Intestinal procedures: Ciprofloxacin plus metronidazole or levofloxacin plus metronidazole or clindamycin plus gentamicin or clindamycin plus aztreonam (<24 h)	• Goal is to prevent SSI in addition to postoperative UTI • Available literature supports single dose or less than 24 h of antibiotic prophylaxis [54, 56, 62] • Antibiotic duration should not be based on presence of urinary catheters [9]
Gynecologic				
Hysterectomy (vaginal or abdominal)	• Polymicrobial (for both abdominal and vaginal approach) • Staphylococcus spp., Streptococcus spp., Enterococcus spp., enteric gram-negatives (Enterobacter spp., E. coli, Klebsiella pneumoniae, Bacteroides fragilis)	Cefazolin or cefotetan or cefoxitin or ampicillin-sulbactam (<24 h)	Clindamycin plus ciprofloxacin or clindamycin/ metronidazole plus levofloxacin or clindamycin plus gentamicin or clindamycin plus aztreonam (<24 h)	• Cephalosporins are most frequently studied as prophylaxis for vaginal/abdominal hysterectomy [9] • If GI manipulation is likely, anaerobic coverage should be provided

Orthopedic				
• Spinal procedures, with or without instrumentation (e.g., fusions, laminectomies) • Hip fracture, internal fixation (e.g., long-bone fracture) • Joint replacement (e.g., knee or hip arthroplasty) • Long-bone tumor resection with endoprosthetic reconstruction (e.g., sarcomas) • Pelvic bone resection	• *Staphylococcus* spp., *Streptococcus* spp. +/− gram-negative bacilli • In the setting of pelvic bone resection for primary malignancy, gram-negative bacilli appear as prevalent as gram-positive pathogens in SSI	• Cefazolin (single dose or <24 h) • 2nd- (e.g., cefuroxime) and 3rd-generation cephalosporins (e.g., ceftriaxone) have also been studied, but advantages over cefazolin remain debatable • 3rd-generation cephalosporins (e.g., ceftriaxone) may be preferred for pelvic bone resections	• Clindamycin (single dose or <24 h) • For pelvic bone resection, gram-negative coverage should be considered via addition of levofloxacin, ciprofloxacin, gentamicin, or aztreonam	• Antibiotic prophylaxis is not recommended for clean orthopedic procedures involving the hands, knees, or feet unless there is instrumentation or implantation of foreign materials • In cancer patients undergoing long-bone primary tumor surgery with endoprosthetic reconstruction (deep SSI rate of ~10%) [47] or pelvic bone resection (SSI rate of 10–47%) [51], a duration of antibiotic prophylaxis greater than 24 h has been proposed

− Patients scheduled for surgery should have the selected antimicrobial prophylactic agent(s) ordered prior to the procedure; administration should be initiated within 60 min of the initial incision (vancomycin and ciprofloxacin should be initiated within 120 min of incision) with intraoperative re-dosing as indicated (see Table 1).

− The duration of prophylaxis should be less than 24 h, unless otherwise noted.

− Local resistance patterns for *E. coli* with regard to fluoroquinolones and ampicillin/sulbactam should be reviewed before choosing these agents as prophylaxis.

[a]Vancomycin prophylaxis should be considered for patients with known MRSA colonization or at high risk for MRSA colonization in the absence of surveillance data.

[b]Allergy history should be carefully evaluated prior to use of alternative agents − patients who report penicillin allergies that are not Ig-E mediated may be able to safely receive a cephalosporin or carbapenem.

[c]Patients undergoing colorectal resection should be considered for preoperative mechanical (e.g., polyethylene glycol) and oral antibiotic (e.g., neomycin plus erythromycin) bowel preparation.

CSF cerebrospinal fluid, *EVD* external ventricular drain, *GI* gastrointestinal, *Ig-E* immunoglobulin E, *POI* postoperative infection, *SBO* small bowel obstruction, *SSI* surgical site infection, *UTI* urinary tract infection, *VATS* video-assisted thoracoscopic surgery

admission to the ICU may be necessary), the following surgical procedures are not presented: coronary artery bypass, appendectomy, hernia repair, breast cancer procedures, cesarean delivery, ophthalmic procedures, and solid organ transplantation.

It should be noted that a great portion of the literature regarding antimicrobial prophylaxis, particularly in regard to cancer patients, is limited to single-center and retrospective trials. As described in current guidelines, antimicrobial prophylaxis recommendations are based on best available evidence, expert opinion, and the risk-benefit profile of alternative options for the predominant pathogens of concern [9]. With a few exceptions and/or areas of uncertainty (as noted in the comments section of Table 2), the recommended duration of antimicrobial prophylaxis is less than 24 h.

Routine use of vancomycin as antimicrobial prophylaxis is not recommended for any surgical procedure, including as an alternative agent in the setting of a penicillin allergy. Use of vancomycin for antimicrobial prophylaxis should be reserved for patients known to be colonized with methicillin-resistant *Staphylococcus aureus* (MRSA) or, in the absence of surveillance data, patients considered to be at high risk of MRSA colonization [9]. Individual institutions are encouraged to maintain surveillance data regarding SSI cases attributable to MRSA (e.g., to identify patterns and/or clusters) as well as to develop guidelines governing and limiting use of vancomycin for surgical antimicrobial prophylaxis.

Antimicrobial Prophylaxis Considerations in the Oncologic Critically Ill Patient

With the myriad of malignancy effects as well as treatment-related effects employed to combat cancer, it can be daunting to determine what risk a patient may be at for infection and, furthermore, which patients are at such high risk that antimicrobial prophylaxis is warranted. The National Cancer Care Network (NCCN) and the Infectious Diseases Society of America (IDSA)/American Society of Clinical Oncology (ASCO) have comprehensive evidence-based documents that detail the role of prophylaxis in cancer patients [4, 55]. This section is a distillation of that literature and recommendations as they apply to critically ill patients.

A general approach to assessing the need for antimicrobial prophylaxis in the cancer patient starts with an assessment of cancer type and treatment status. These factors will provide insight into the degree of immune compromise and ultimately the need for prophylaxis. Typically, malignancy and/or treatment-related neutropenia puts patients at risk for bacterial infections [7]. Patients expected to be neutropenic more than 7 days are candidates for bacterial prophylaxis as they are considered at high risk for infection [55]. If neutropenia is prolonged, more than 14 days, then fungal prophylaxis should also be considered [55]. Lymphopenia often exists concomitant to neutropenia and puts patients at further risk for viral and/or other unique pathogens, such as *Pneumocystis jirovecii*. Even in the absence of neutropenia and lymphopenia, certain drugs effecting cellular immunity may increase the risk of infection (e.g., corticosteroids.). Table 3 provides an overview of antimicrobial prophylaxis considerations in cancer patients, organized by pathogen type. Within each pathogen class, key demographics associated with infection risk are identified, and the primary choice of prophylaxis is highlighted. Additionally, detail is provided regarding alternative agents in the case that the drug of choice is not feasible due to one or more factors (e.g., organ system compromise, comorbidities, drug-drug interactions, lack of enteral access or tolerance).

Bacterial prophylaxis in patients with cancer is based on a risk-stratified approach with a focus on the duration of neutropenia. In general, patients receiving chemotherapy for hematologic malignancy will be expected to have a duration of neutropenia longer than 7 days, similarly true for patients receiving hematopoietic stem cell transplantation. Conversely, most solid tumor chemotherapy regimens will result in shorter durations of neutropenia, and as such, prophylaxis is not recommended as the risk of infection is low.

Table 3 Antimicrobial prophylaxis in high-risk patients

Pathogen class	Pathogen	Indications for prophylaxis	Prophylaxis choice	Alternative prophylaxis	Comments
Bacteria	Gram-positive *(Streptococci spp., Staphylococci spp.)*, gram-negative *(E.coli, K. pneumoniae, P. aeruginosa, E. cloacae)*	AML/MDS, ALL, CLL, HSCT, lymphoma, multiple myeloma, purine analog therapy (e.g., fludarabine, cladribine) other malignancy/ treatment causing neutropenia for greater than 7 days	Levofloxacin 500 mg daily (IV/PO/PT)	Trimethoprim/ sulfamethoxazole 160 mg (TMP) daily (IV/PO/PT), cefpodoxime 200 mg q12h (PO/PT)	Continue prophylaxis until neutropenia resolves or if superseded by active antimicrobial therapy
Fungal	*Candida* spp., *Aspergillus* spp., *Mucormycetes*, endemic fungi (*histoplasmosis*, *blastomycosis*, *Cryptococcus* spp.)	Auto SCT, ALL, and allogeneic SCT w/o GVHD	Fluconazole 200 mg daily (IV/PO/ PT) or echinocandin (IV)	Voriconazole 200 mg q12h (IV/PO/PT), posaconazole 300 mg daily (IV/PO), amphotericin formulations (IV)	Continue prophylaxis until neutropenia resolves
	Candida spp., *Aspergillus* spp., *Mucormycetes*, endemic fungi (*histoplasmosis*, *blastomycosis*, *Cryptococcus* spp.)	AML/MDS treated patients and allogeneic HSCT w/GVHD, neutropenia greater than 14 days	Posaconazole 300 mg daily (IV/PO)	Voriconazole 200 mg q12h (IV/PO/PT), echinocandins (IV), amphotericin formulations (IV)	Continue prophylaxis until neutropenia resolves
	Pneumocystis jirovecii	AML, MDS, autologous SCT w/mucositis, allogeneic SCT, lymphopenia, corticosteroids with prednisone equivalent >20 mg/day	Trimethoprim/ sulfamethoxazole 160mg (TMP) Daily (IV/PO/PT)	Dapsone 100 mg Daily (PO/PT), atovaquone 1500 mg daily (PO/PT), pentamidine 4 mg/kg IV or 300 mg inhaled every 3-4 weeks	Continue prophylaxis during immunosuppressive therapy and/or until CD4 count >200 cells/mm^3
Viral	Herpes simplex virus, varicella zoster virus	AML/MDS, ALL, CLL, HSCT, lymphoma, multiple myeloma, purine analog therapy (fludarabine, cladribine), proteasome inhibitors (bortezomib, carfilzomib, ixazomib), alemtuzumab, corticosteroid therapy	Valacyclovir 500 mg q12h (PO/PT)	Acyclovir 400 mg q12h (IV/PO/PT), famciclovir 500 mg q12h (PO/PT)	Prophylaxis should continue during active chemotherapy, during periods of neutropenia, for at least 2 months with CD4 count above 200 for alemtuzumab treated patients, and at least 1 year after allogeneic HSCT. May consider longer duration of prophylaxis if using as secondary prophylaxis.

(*continued*)

Table 3 (continued)

Pathogen class	Pathogen	Indications for prophylaxis	Prophylaxis choice	Alternative prophylaxis	Comments
	Cytomegalovirus	CMV seropositive allogeneic HSCT patients	Letermovir 480 mg daily (IV/PO)	None, consider regular screening with preemptive treatment strategy	Prophylaxis to continue through day 100 post stem cell transplant
	Hepatitis B virus	HBsAg-positive patients, history of resolved HepB infection undergoing chemotherapy. Increasing HepB viral load prior to HSCT, anti-CD20 or anti-CD52 monoclonal antibody therapy	Entecavir 0.5 mg once daily (PO/PT) or tenofovir 300 mg daily (PO/PT)	Lamivudine 100 mg daily (PO/PT)	During period of treatment of malignancy and 6–12 months beyond; entecavir dosing may be increased to 1 mg daily if decompensated liver disease or history of hepatitis B viremia while receiving lamivudine

ALL acute lymphocytic leukemia, *AML* acute myelogenous leukemia, *CLL* chronic lymphocytic leukemia, *CMV* cytomegalovirus, *GVHD* graft-versus-host disease, *HBsAg* hepatitis B surface antigen, *HSCT* hematopoietic stem cell transplant, *IV* intravenous, *MDS* myelodysplastic syndrome, *PO* by mouth, *PT* per enteral feeding tube, *SCT* stem cell transplant

Trimethoprim/sulfamethoxazole was one of the initial agents considered for bacterial prophylaxis. However, bacterial prophylaxis with fluoroquinolones, during neutropenia, has been demonstrated to consistently decrease overall infection rate and all-cause mortality as compared to placebo or trimethoprim/sulfamethoxazole [16]. Specifically, antipseudomonal, respiratory fluoroquinolones (i.e., ciprofloxacin and levofloxacin) are the primary agents considered appropriate for prophylaxis in this setting. The fluoroquinolones are particularly useful in the critically ill patient as their excellent bioavailability allows for transitioning between oral and intravenous formulations seamlessly. It is important to note that enteral fluoroquinolone administration should be avoided in critically ill patients receiving continuous tube feeding due to decreased absorption secondary to chelation with cations; IV administration would be preferred in such cases. Other important considerations exist that fluoroquinolones have been implicated in prolonging the QT interval, CNS excitability, as well as other adverse effects. Despite increasing fluoroquinolone resistance worldwide, there still appears to be benefit of prophylaxis in decreasing overall infection rate and preventing infection-related mortality [27]. It is important to note that despite prophylaxis, some patients will still develop an infection. Often, the infection will manifest with a pathogen with reduced susceptibility to typical neutropenic fever agents [14]. As such, these patients should receive aggressive and broad-spectrum therapy with consideration of local patterns of resistance. In the critically ill patient who is receiving antibacterial treatment with broad-spectrum beta-lactams (i.e., cefepime, piperacillin/tazobactam, or carbapenems), additional bacterial prophylaxis is not warranted.

Initiation of fungal prophylaxis should be considered in a more restrictive subset of neutropenic patients. Specifically, it is warranted for patients who will have prolonged periods of neutropenia (beyond 14 days) or in those receiving allogeneic hematopoietic stem cell transplantation, especially those undergoing immunosuppressive treatment for graft-versus-host disease (GVHD). Azole antifungals are the class of choice for fungal prophylaxis. Fluconazole was the initial antifungal demonstrating promise as a prophylactic agent, with efficacy in decreasing fungal infection and related mortality in patients treated for leukemia as well as following autologous hematopoietic stem cell transplant [48]. However, prolonged neutropenia is a risk for infection with not only pathogenic yeasts but also molds. Ideally, prophylactic agents would protect against infection with clinically relevant yeasts (*Candida* spp.) and molds (*Aspergillus spp., Mucorales, and Fusarium* spp.). Voriconazole, having activity against most *Aspergillus* spp., was compared to fluconazole for fungal prophylaxis in allogeneic hematopoietic stem cell transplantation patients. A decrease in invasive fungal infections was demonstrated; however the results did not reach statistical significance, nor did the study demonstrate a survival benefit [60]. More recently, posaconazole, with anti-mold and anti-candida activity, has demonstrated improved prophylactic efficacy as compared to fluconazole in reducing invasive fungal infections as well varied benefits on infection-related mortality [13, 60]. These studies were performed with the suspension formulation, which is notorious for absorption issues. Newer formulations of posaconazole have improved the logistics of prophylaxing patients with enteral absorption issues [26]. Azole antifungals are implicated in many drug-drug interactions as they often are substrates and inhibitors of CYP450 enzymes. In addition they are associated with hepatic toxicity and QTc prolongation, which may hinder use in the critically ill patient [32]. Echinocandin antifungals are a safer alternative to azoles and have a much more limited role in drug-drug interactions; however, they are generally considered inferior to the anti-mold azoles for prophylaxis [19]. It is generally accepted that the echinocandins are interchangeable as a class of drugs with respect to prophylactic efficacy, though only micafungin was demonstrated to be superior to fluconazole for decreasing invasive candida infection [58]. Amphotericin products may be as effective as fluconazole for fungal prophylaxis; however, the increased risk of nephrotoxicity limits their use, especially in the critically ill patient who may have multiple nephrotoxic agents present [28, 34, 61].

Pneumocystis jirovecii is a fungal organism that causes significant and serious pulmonary infection in patients with impaired cell-mediated immunity, particularly common in patients with chemotherapies targeting lymphocytes [3]. The prophylaxis of choice is trimethoprim/sulfamethoxazole. Most literature exploring alternative prophylactic strategies are extrapolated from the HIV-infected population, with use of atovaquone, dapsone, and pentamidine. These drugs are considered inferior prophylactic agents as compared to trimethoprim/sulfamethoxazole or in the case of dapsone, more toxic [36]. Atovaquone is only available as a liquid for enteral administration with no IV formulation. Pentamidine is available as an IV infusion to be given every 3 weeks or as an inhalation, with inhalation being the least effective prophylaxis strategy [36].

Viral pathogens are also of concern in patients with impaired cellular immunity (see specific risk groups in Table 3). Prophylactic strategies focus on the herpes family of viruses as they are the most common viral pathogens implicated in clinically relevant infections, and consequently there are systemic antivirals with activity against them [46]. Herpes simplex virus (HSV) is a common virus that is latent in many adults. In an immunocompromised patient, HSV can manifest as localized disease, but may also cause more systemic and life-threatening infection in rare instances (e.g., encephalitis). As such, patients at risk are typically prophylaxed with an anti-HSV therapy [17, 18]. Valacyclovir, a prodrug of acyclovir, is the ideal oral agent given its excellent bioavailability. Patients unable to tolerate oral medications can instead receive intravenous acyclovir. Oral acyclovir is typically thought of as a less desirable option given its poor bioavailability, though has demonstrated a beneficial prophylactic effect as compared to placebo in hematologic malignancy patients at risk for HSV infection [46]. Ganciclovir, foscarnet, and cidofovir are active against HSV, but toxicities preclude their use as prophylactic agents. Varicella zoster virus (VZV) is also an important viral pathogen, responsible for more serious manifestations of the infection (e.g., multiple dermatomes, neurologic) in patients with impaired lymphocyte function [50]. Risk factors and treatment options parallel those of HSV, as does the prophylactic strategy. In the cancer patient, cytomegalovirus (CMV) is also a concern as it can manifest from simple viremia to serious retinitis, colitis, and pneumonitis. However, given the toxicity of active agents (i.e., foscarnet, ganciclovir, cidofovir), CMV has traditionally been dealt with via a screening and preemptive treatment strategy in oncology patients, especially those at highest risk receiving allogeneic stem cell transplant [39]. More recently, there is a prophylactic option in letermovir. Prophylactic use of letermovir has resulted in a decreased CMV infection rate in allogeneic stem cell transplant patients compared to placebo [12, 35]. Of note, letermovir does not have activity against HSV or VZV; therefore, additional viral prophylaxis should be considered for those viruses. Of the hepatitis viruses, hepatitis B virus is the one virus for which prophylaxis should be considered as patients with previous unresolved infection or exposure are at risk for reactivation during times of immunosuppression [31]. Specific risk factors are listed in Table 3. Tenofovir and entecavir are preferred prophylactic agents over lamivudine due to a lower barrier of resistance with lamivudine [52]. Unfortunately, the current prophylaxis options are available only in oral formulations, thus limiting utility for critically ill patients who lack enteral access.

Conclusion

As highlighted in this chapter, there are numerous considerations for the prevention of infection in oncology patients undergoing surgical procedures as well as for those immunocompromised secondary to malignancy and/or treatment-related factors. For patients undergoing clean-contaminated or contaminated procedures, the prevention of bacterial postoperative SSI remains the primary goal, with cephalosporins or penicillins as the preferred agent in most cases. Antimicrobial prophylaxis should be administered within 60 min of surgical incision, re-dosed intraoperatively when indicated, limited in scope to the likely pathogens, and in most cases, limited to a duration of less than 24 hours. Among the immunocompromised oncology population, concern exists for the development of bacterial, fungal, viral, or multi-

pathogen infections, largely attributable to the degree and duration of neutropenia as well as other concomitant factors (e.g., prolonged corticosteroid therapy).

References

1. Alotaibi AF, et al. The efficacy of antibacterial prophylaxis against the development of meningitis after craniotomy: a meta-analysis. World Neurosurg. 2016;90:597–603 e591. https://doi.org/10.1016/j.wneu.2016.02.048.
2. Ancker JS, Witteman HO, Hafeez B, Provencher T, Van de Graaf M, Wei E. The invisible work of personal health information management among people with multiple chronic conditions: qualitative interview study among patients and providers. J Med Internet Res. 2015;17:e137. https://doi.org/10.2196/jmir.4381.
3. Avino LJ, Naylor SM, Roecker AM. Pneumocystis jirovecii pneumonia in the non-HIV-infected population. Ann Pharmacother. 2016;50:673–9. https://doi.org/10.1177/1060028016650107.
4. Baden LR, et al. Prevention and treatment of cancer-related infections, version 2.2016, NCCN clinical practice guidelines in oncology. J Natl Compr Cancer Netw. 2016;14:882–913.
5. Bernard A, Pillet M, Goudet P, Viard H. Antibiotic prophylaxis in pulmonary surgery. A prospective randomized double-blind trial of flash cefuroxime versus forty-eight-hour cefuroxime. J Thorac Cardiovasc Surg. 1994;107:896–900.
6. Berrios-Torres SI, et al. Centers for disease control and prevention guideline for the prevention of surgical site infection, 2017. JAMA Surg. 2017;152:784–91. https://doi.org/10.1001/jamasurg.2017.0904.
7. Bodey GP, Buckley M, Sathe YS, Freireich EJ. Quantitative relationships between circulating leukocytes and infection in patients with acute leukemia. Ann Intern Med. 1966;64:328–40.
8. Boldt J, Piper S, Uphus D, Fussle R, Hempelmann G. Preoperative microbiologic screening and antibiotic prophylaxis in pulmonary resection operations. Ann Thorac Surg. 1999;68:208–11.
9. Bratzler DW, et al. Clinical practice guidelines for antimicrobial prophylaxis in surgery. Am J Health Syst Pharm. 2013;70:195–283. https://doi.org/10.2146/ajhp120568.
10. Brown SM, Anand VK, Tabaee A, Schwartz TH. Role of perioperative antibiotics in endoscopic skull base surgery. Laryngoscope 2007;117(9):1528–1532.
11. Centers for Disease Control C. Procedure-associated Module SSI. 2018. http://www.cdc.gov/nhsn/pdfs/pscmanual/9pscssicurrent.pdf. Accessed 24 Sept 2018.
12. Chemaly RF, et al. Letermovir for cytomegalovirus prophylaxis in hematopoietic-cell transplantation. N Engl J Med. 2014;370:1781–9. https://doi.org/10.1056/NEJMoa1309533.

13. Cornely OA, et al. Posaconazole vs. fluconazole or itraconazole prophylaxis in patients with neutropenia. N Engl J Med. 2007;356:348–59. https://doi.org/10.1056/NEJMoa061094.

14. Eleutherakis-Papaiakovou E, et al. Prophylactic antibiotics for the prevention of neutropenic fever in patients undergoing autologous stem-cell transplantation: results of a single institution, randomized phase 2 trial. Am J Hematol. 2010;85:863–7. https://doi.org/10.1002/ajh.21855.

15. Fried HI, et al. The insertion and management of external ventricular drains: an evidence-based consensus statement: a statement for healthcare professionals from the neurocritical care society. Neurocrit Care. 2016;24:61–81. https://doi.org/10.1007/s12028-015-0224-8.

16. Gafter-Gvili A, et al. Antibiotic prophylaxis for bacterial infections in afebrile neutropenic patients following chemotherapy. Cochrane Database Syst Rev. 2012;1:CD004386. https://doi.org/10.1002/14651858.CD004386.pub3.

17. Glenny AM, Fernandez Mauleffinch LM, Pavitt S, Walsh T. Interventions for the prevention and treatment of herpes simplex virus in patients being treated for cancer. Cochrane Database Syst Rev. 2009; https://doi.org/10.1002/14651858.CD006706.pub2.

18. Gold D, Corey L. Acyclovir prophylaxis for herpes simplex virus infection. Antimicrob Agents Chemother. 1987;31:361–7.

19. Gomes MZ, Jiang Y, Mulanovich VE, Lewis RE, Kontoyiannis DP. Effectiveness of primary anti-aspergillus prophylaxis during remission induction chemotherapy of acute myeloid leukemia. Antimicrob Agents Chemother. 2014;58:2775–80. https://doi.org/10.1128/AAC.01527-13.

20. Haga N, Ishida H, Ishiguro T, Kumamoto K, Ishibashi K, Tsuji Y, Miyazaki T. A prospective randomized study to assess the optimal duration of intravenous antimicrobial prophylaxis in elective gastric cancer surgery. Int Surg. 2012;97:169–76. https://doi.org/10.9738/CC91.1.

21. Haines SJ, Walters BC. Antibiotic prophylaxis for cerebrospinal fluid shunts: a meta-analysis. Neurosurgery. 1994;34:87–92.

22. Imamura H, et al. Intraoperative versus extended antimicrobial prophylaxis after gastric cancer surgery: a phase 3, open-label, randomised controlled, noninferiority trial. Lancet Infect Dis. 2012;12:381–7. https://doi.org/10.1016/S1473-3099(11)70370-X.

23. Itani KM, Wilson SE, Awad SS, Jensen EH, Finn TS, Abramson MA. Ertapenem versus cefotetan prophylaxis in elective colorectal surgery. N Engl J Med. 2006;355:2640–51. https://doi.org/10.1056/NEJMoa054408.

24. Johans SJ, Burkett DJ, Swong KN, Patel CR, Germanwala AV. Antibiotic prophylaxis and infection prevention for endoscopic endonasal skull base surgery: our protocol, results and review of the literature. J Clin Neurosci 2018;47:249–253.

25. Johnson JT, Myers EN, Thearle PB, Sigler BA, Schramm VL Jr. Antimicrobial prophylaxis for contaminated head and neck surgery. Laryngoscope. 1984;94:46–51.

26. Jung DS, Tverdek FP, Kontoyiannis DP. Switching from posaconazole suspension to tablets increases serum drug levels in leukemia patients without clinically relevant hepatotoxicity. Antimicrob Agents Chemother. 2014;58:6993–5. https://doi.org/10.1128/AAC.04035-14.

27. Kern WV, et al. Fluoroquinolone resistance of Escherichia coli at a cancer center: epidemiologic evolution and effects of discontinuing prophylactic fluoroquinolone use in neutropenic patients with leukemia. Eur J Clin Microbiol Infect Dis. 2005;24:111–8. https://doi.org/10.1007/s10096-005-1278-x.

28. Koh LP, Kurup A, Goh YT, Fook-Chong SM, Tan PH. Randomized trial of fluconazole versus low-dose amphotericin B in prophylaxis against fungal infections in patients undergoing hematopoietic stem cell transplantation. Am J Hematol. 2002;71:260–7. https://doi.org/10.1002/ajh.10234.

29. Korinek AM, Golmard JL, Elcheick A, Bismuth R, van Effenterre R, Coriat P, Puybasset L. Risk factors for neurosurgical site infections after craniotomy: a critical reappraisal of antibiotic prophylaxis on 4,578 patients. Br J Neurosurg. 2005;19:155–62. https://doi.org/10.1080/02688690500145639.

30. Lane-Fall MB, et al. Developing a standard handoff process for operating room-to-ICU transitions: multidisciplinary clinician perspectives from the handoffs and transitions in critical care (HATRICC) Study. Jt Comm J Qual Patient Saf. 2018;44:514–25. https://doi.org/10.1016/j.jcjq.2018.02.004.

31. Law MF, et al. Prevention and management of hepatitis B virus reactivation in patients with hematological malignancies treated with anticancer therapy. World J Gastroenterol. 2016;22:6484–500. https://doi.org/10.3748/wjg.v22.i28.6484.

32. Lewis RE. Current concepts in antifungal pharmacology. Mayo Clin Proc. 2011;86:805–17. https://doi.org/10.4065/mcp.2011.0247.

33. Mahajan SN, Ariza-Heredia EJ, Rolston KV, Graviss LS, Feig BW, Aloia TA, Chemaly RF. Perioperative antimicrobial prophylaxis for intra-abdominal surgery in patients with cancer: a retrospective study comparing ertapenem and nonertapenem antibiotics. Ann Surg Oncol. 2014;21:513–9. https://doi.org/10.1245/s10434-013-3294-x.

34. Marr KA, et al. Itraconazole versus fluconazole for prevention of fungal infections in patients receiving allogeneic stem cell transplants. Blood. 2004;103:1527–33. https://doi.org/10.1182/blood-2003-08-2644.

35. Marty FM, et al. Letermovir prophylaxis for cytomegalovirus in hematopoietic-cell transplantation. N Engl J Med. 2017;377:2433–44. https://doi.org/10.1056/NEJMoa1706640.

36. Masur H, et al. Prevention and treatment of opportunistic infections in HIV-infected adults and adolescents: updated guidelines from the Centers for Disease Control and Prevention, National Institutes of

Health, and HIV Medicine Association of the Infectious Diseases Society of America. Clin Infect Dis. 2014;58:1308–11. https://doi.org/10.1093/cid/ciu094.

37. McCarthy PJ, Patil S, Conrad SA, Scott LK. International and specialty trends in the use of prophylactic antibiotics to prevent infectious complications after insertion of external ventricular drainage devices. Neurocrit Care. 2010;12:220–4. https://doi.org/10.1007/s12028-009-9284-y.

38. McCutcheon BA, et al. Predictors of surgical site infection following craniotomy for intracranial neoplasms: an analysis of prospectively collected data in the American college of surgeons national surgical quality improvement program database. World Neurosurg. 2016;88:350–8. https://doi.org/10.1016/j.wneu.2015.12.068.

39. Meijer E, Boland GJ, Verdonck LF. Prevention of cytomegalovirus disease in recipients of allogeneic stem cell transplants. Clin Microbiol Rev. 2003;16:647–57.

40. Mitchell RM, Mendez E, Schmitt NC, Bhrany AD, Futran ND. Antibiotic prophylaxis in patients undergoing head and neck free flap reconstruction. JAMA Otolaryngol Head Neck Surg. 2015;141:1096–103. https://doi.org/10.1001/jamaoto.2015.0513.

41. Mohri Y, Tonouchi H, Kobayashi M, Nakai K, Kusunoki M, Mie Surgical Infection Research G. Randomized clinical trial of single- versus multiple-dose antimicrobial prophylaxis in gastric cancer surgery. Br J Surg. 2007;94:683–8. https://doi.org/10.1002/bjs.5837.

42. Morita S, Nishisho I, Nomura T, Fukushima Y, Morimoto T, Hiraoka N, Shibata N. The significance of the intraoperative repeated dosing of antimicrobials for preventing surgical wound infection in colorectal surgery. Surg Today 2005;35:732–738.

43. Murphy J, Isaiah A, Dyalram D, Lubek JE. Surgical site infections in patients receiving osteomyocutaneous free flaps to the head and neck. Does choice of antibiotic prophylaxis matter? J Oral Maxillofac Surg. 2017;75:2223–9. https://doi.org/10.1016/j.joms.2017.02.006.

44. Olak J, Jeyasingham K, Forrester-Wood C, Hutter J, Al-Zeerah M, Brown E. Randomized trial of one-dose versus six-dose cefazolin prophylaxis in elective general thoracic surgery. Ann Thorac Surg. 1991;51:956–8.

45. Pool C, et al. Increased surgical site infection rates following clindamycin use in head and neck free tissue transfer. Otolaryngol Head Neck Surg. 2016;154:272–8. https://doi.org/10.1177/0194599815617129.

46. Poole CL, James SH. Antiviral therapies for herpesviruses: current agents and new directions. Clin Ther. 2018;40:1282–98. https://doi.org/10.1016/j.clinthera.2018.07.006.

47. Racano A, Pazionis T, Farrokhyar F, Deheshi B, Ghert M. High infection rate outcomes in long-bone tumor surgery with endoprosthetic reconstruction in adults: a systematic review. Clin Orthop Relat Res. 2013;471:2017–27. https://doi.org/10.1007/s11999-013-2842-9.

48. Rotstein C, Bow EJ, Laverdiere M, Ioannou S, Carr D, Moghaddam N. Randomized placebo-controlled trial of fluconazole prophylaxis for neutropenic cancer patients: benefit based on purpose and intensity of cytotoxic therapy. The Canadian Fluconazole Prophylaxis Study Group. Clin Infect Dis. 1999;28:331–40. https://doi.org/10.1086/515128.

49. Saunders S, Reese S, Lam J, Wulu J, Jalisi S, Ezzat W. Extended use of perioperative antibiotics in head and neck microvascular reconstruction. Am J Otolaryngol. 2017;38:204–7. https://doi.org/10.1016/j.amjoto.2017.01.009.

50. Schroder C, Enders D, Schink T, Riedel O. Incidence of herpes zoster amongst adults varies by severity of immunosuppression. J Infect. 2017;75:207–15. https://doi.org/10.1016/j.jinf.2017.06.010.

51. Severyns M, Briand S, Waast D, Touchais S, Hamel A, Gouin F. Postoperative infections after limb-sparing surgery for primary bone tumors of the pelvis: incidence, characterization and functional impact. Surg Oncol. 2017;26:171–7. https://doi.org/10.1016/j.suronc.2017.03.005.

52. Siyahian A, et al. Prophylaxis for hepatitis B virus reactivation after allogeneic stem cell transplantation in the era of drug resistance and newer antivirals: a systematic review and meta-analysis. Biol Blood Marrow Transplant. 2018;24:1483–9. https://doi.org/10.1016/j.bbmt.2018.02.027.

53. Swoboda SM, Merz C, Kostuik J, Trentler B, Lipsett PA. Does intraoperative blood loss affect antibiotic serum and tissue concentrations? Arch Surg. 1996;131:1165–71; discussion 1171–1162

54. Takeyama K, Takahashi S, Maeda T, Mutoh M, Kunishima Y, Matsukawa M, Takagi Y. Comparison of 1-day, 2-day, and 3-day administration of antimicrobial prophylaxis in radical prostatectomy. J Infect Chemother: Off J Jpn Soc Chemother. 2007;13:320–3. https://doi.org/10.1007/s10156-007-0540-9.

55. Taplitz RA et al. Antimicrobial prophylaxis for adult patients with cancer-related immunosuppression: ASCO and IDSA clinical practice guideline update. J Clin Oncol. 2018;JCO1800374. https://doi.org/10.1200/JCO.18.00374.

56. Terai A, Ichioka K, Kohei N, Ueda N, Utsunomiya N, Inoue K. Antibiotic prophylaxis in radical prostatectomy: 1-day versus 4-day treatments. Int J Urol. 2006;13:1488–93. https://doi.org/10.1111/j.1442-2042.2006.01597.x.

57. Turna A, Kutlu CA, Ozalp T, Karamustafaoglu A, Mulazimoglu L, Bedirhan MA. Antibiotic prophylaxis in elective thoracic surgery: cefuroxime versus cefepime. Thorac Cardiovasc Surg. 2003;51:84–8. https://doi.org/10.1055/s-2003-38991.

58. van Burik JA, et al. Micafungin versus fluconazole for prophylaxis against invasive fungal infections during neutropenia in patients undergoing hematopoietic stem

cell transplantation. Clin Infect Dis. 2004;39:1407–16. https://doi.org/10.1086/422312.

59. Wagner JL, Kenney RM, Vazquez JA, Ghanem TA, Davis SL. Surgical prophylaxis with gram-negative activity for reduction of surgical site infections after microvascular reconstruction for head and neck cancer. Head Neck. 2016;38:1449–54. https://doi.org/10.1002/hed.24178.

60. Wingard JR, et al. Randomized, double-blind trial of fluconazole versus voriconazole for prevention of invasive fungal infection after allogeneic hematopoietic cell transplantation. Blood. 2010;116:5111–8. https://doi.org/10.1182/blood-2010-02-268151.

61. Winston DJ, et al. Intravenous and oral itraconazole versus intravenous and oral fluconazole for long-term antifungal prophylaxis in allogeneic hematopoietic stem-cell transplant recipients. A multicenter, randomized trial. Ann Intern Med. 2003;138:705–13.

62. Wolf JS Jr, Bennett CJ, Dmochowski RR, Hollenbeck BK, Pearle MS, Schaeffer AJ, Urologic Surgery Antimicrobial Prophylaxis Best Practice Policy P. Best practice policy statement on urologic surgery antimicrobial prophylaxis. J Urol. 2008;179:1379–90. https://doi.org/10.1016/j.juro.2008.01.068.

63. Zimlichman E, et al. Health care-associated infections: a meta-analysis of costs and financial impact on the US health care system. JAMA Intern Med. 2013;173:2039–46. https://doi.org/10.1001/jamainternmed.2013.9763.

Considerations for Medications Commonly Utilized in the Oncology Population in the Intensive Care Unit

15

Anne Rain Tanner Brown, Michelle Horng, and Terri Lynn Shigle

Contents

Introduction 170

Antimicrobial Agents 170
Gram Positive Agents 170
Gram Negative Agents 171
Antiviral Agents 171
Antifungal Agents 173
Pneumocystis Jiroveci Pneumonia 177

Antiepileptics 177

Immunosuppressants 181

Antifibrinolytic/Antihemophilic Agents 181
Diffuse Alveolar Hemorrhage (DAH) 181
Thrombocytopenia 184
Disseminated Intravascular Coagulation (DIC) 184
Gastrointestinal (GI) Bleeding 184

Thrombolytics 184

Uric Acid Reducing Agents 184

Hypercalcemia of Malignancy/Hypercalcemia Management 186

A. R. T. Brown (✉) · M. Horng
Critical Care/Nutrition Support, The University of Texas
MD Anderson Cancer Center, Houston, TX, USA
e-mail: artanner@mdanderson.org;
mhorng1@mdanderson.org

T. L. Shigle
Oncology, The University of Texas MD Anderson Cancer
Center, Houston, TX, USA

Stem Cell Transplantation and Cellular Therapy, The
University of Texas MD Anderson Cancer Center,
Houston, TX, USA
e-mail: tshigle@mdanderson.org

Interleukin-6 Receptor Antagonists 186

Growth Factors 186

Antidotes 193

References 193

Abstract

An increasing number of oncologic patients are presenting to the intensive care unit with complications from both their chronic disease states and cancer therapies due to improved survival rates. The management of these patients is complex due to immunosuppression (from the malignancy and/or treatment), metabolic complications, and diverse medication regimens with the potential for significant drug-drug interactions and overlapping adverse effects. This chapter will provide clinicians with an overview of non-chemotherapy medications frequently encountered in the critically ill oncologic patient, with a focus on practical considerations.

Keywords

Oncology · Critical care · Cancer · Drug interactions · Pharmacology · Intensive care · Critically ill · Drug monitoring · Adverse events · Immunocompromised

Introduction

As advances in cancer therapies continue to improve, a growing number of patients are living with cancer. As such, there is an increased probability for critical care providers to encounter cancer patients within the intensive care unit (ICU). Furthermore, oncologic patients require increased utilization of resources in the ICU due to disease-related complications and/or treatment-related adverse events [124]. Metabolic complications present difficult challenges in the management of critically ill cancer patients [72]. Immunosuppression, secondary to the cancer itself or cancer-related therapies (e.g., chemotherapy, corticosteroids, hematopoietic cell transplant, etc.), places patients at an increased risk for infection. In addition, many new chemotherapy and targeted therapies have

numerous adverse effects that not only increase the risk for ICU admission but require multiple other therapies to help manage these side effects.

Medication regimens for critically ill cancer patients are complex. Many patients require a large number of concomitant medications to manage the critical, oncologic, and supportive care issues encountered. Accordingly, avoidance and detection of drug-drug interactions and overlapping adverse effect profiles is of high concern. The intent of this chapter is to provide critical care practitioners with an overview of non-chemotherapy medications that are frequently encountered during the care of a critically ill cancer patient in hopes of increasing awareness of such therapy. It should be emphasized that this chapter is not all-inclusive in respect to the medications discussed and details provided, and clinicians are advised to seek additional information as applicable. In addition, medication doses are reflective of a patient with normal renal function and clinicians should refer to drug dosing references for organ dysfunction adjustments unless otherwise noted.

Antimicrobial Agents

Gram Positive Agents

Risk for methicillin resistant *staphylococcus aureus* (MRSA) and vancomycin resistant *enterococcus* (VRE) as shown in Table 1 may be heightened in the oncology population due to increased exposure to the healthcare setting and antimicrobials [11]. While initial therapy of patients with febrile neutropenia may not require coverage for MRSA, empiric antibiotic regimens for all patients progressing to sepsis or septic shock or those patients with additional risk factors should be broadened to include an agent targeting aerobic

Table 1 Considerations for MRSA/VRE coverage

MRSA	VRE
Vascular access devices	Previous VRE infection
Gram positive bacteremia prior to speciation	High rates of hospital endemicity
Known colonization or prior infection with MRSA	Known colonization
Clinical instability (hypotension or shock)	
Skin or soft tissue infection	
Pneumonia requiring ICU admission	
Penicillin resistant *Streptococcus pneumoniae*	
High rates of hospital endemicity	
Severe mucositis if FQ prophylaxis + ceftazidime is employed as empiric therapy	

MRSA methicillin resistant *staphylococcus aureus*, *VRE* vancomycin resistant enterococcus, *ICU* intensive care unit, *FQ* fluoroquinolone
Adapted from [11, 43]

gram positive cocci [102]. For MRSA, consider early addition of vancomycin, linezolid, or daptomycin. For VRE, consider early addition of linezolid or daptomycin. Selection of a specific agent should be based on patient-specific (e.g., end organ function) as well as an infection-specific factors (e.g., source of infection). As mentioned in Table 2, use of linezolid may compromise bone marrow function; this does not preclude use of linezolid in patients with pancytopenia or thrombocytopenia, but it does justify a risk-benefit analysis inclusive of alternative options prior to therapy initiation [126]. Consider an infectious diseases (ID) consult if MRSA or VRE is isolated in the context of systemic infection [11, 43]. Discontinuation of MRSA and/or VRE therapy should be considered if a pathogen is not identified within 48–72 h of obtaining all pertinent cultures.

Gram Negative Agents

Empiric intravenous (IV) antibiotics with anti-pseudomonal coverage should be initiated immediately in high-risk patients with febrile neutropenia and may include piperacillin/tazobactam, ceftazidime, cefepime, meropenem, or imipenem-cilastatin [11, 43]. Unfortunately, frequent exposure to antimicrobials and repeated hospitalization result in greater risk of acquiring resistant gram-negative organisms [114].

Oncology patients are at increased risk of infections with gram negative organisms from translocation from the gastrointestinal (GI) tract, particularly in patients with mucositis or graft versus host disease (GVHD). Risk of acquiring multi-drug resistant (MDR) gram negative organisms is increased by the use of prophylactic fluoroquinolones in patients with chemotherapy-induced neutropenia [33, 71, 78]. Initial empiric coverage of extended spectrum beta lactamase (ESBL) organisms and carbapenem resistant enterobacteraciae (CRE) should be based on patient-specific factors including prior exposure of antipseudomonal prophylaxis for febrile neutropenia patients and prior infections or microbiologic culture results. Double antipseudomonal gram-negative coverage may be warranted in patients with a history of *P. aeruginosa* or other MDR organism colonization or in hemodynamically unstable patients. Combination therapy with an aminoglycoside should be preferred in patients recently treated with fluoroquinolone prophylaxis (Table 2) [11]. Consider an infectious disease consult for patients with multidrug resistant organisms (MDRO).

Antiviral Agents

Oncology patients, particularly those with hematologic malignancy and/or history of HCT, are at risk for viral infections as a result of their underlying malignancy, chemotherapy, prolonged neutropenia, impaired cell-mediated immunity, and/or treatment complications (e.g., GVHD)

Table 2 Oncologic considerations for select antibiotics

Drug	Primary role in therapy	Dosing and administration	Monitoring, adverse events, and toxicities	Drug-drug interactions	Clinical pearls
Linezolid [67, 109]	Treatment of gram positive resistant organisms (MRSA, VRE)	**Dosing** PO, PT, IV: 600 mg q12h **Administration** PO, PT: Administer without regard to food IV: Administer over 30–120 min	**Monitoring** Obtain weekly CBC **AE/toxicities** Serotonin syndrome, lactic acidosis (rare) Bone marrow suppression (thrombocytopenia is the most common)	MAO inhibitors (caution with concurrent use or within 2 weeks)	• Prolonged therapy (≥ 2 weeks) may increase risk of serious hematologic toxicity • IV formulation contains 600 mL/day D5W (caution in fluid overload and/or hyponatremia) • Not a preferred agent in resistant *E. faecalis* infections susceptible to beta-lactams
Aminoglycosides [14, 51, 89, 92, 97, 99, 111]	MDROs, including pseudomonas and enterobacteriaceae	**Dosing** *Tobramycin/ Gentamicin* IV: 5–7 mg/kg/ dose *Amikacin* IV: 15–20 mg/ kg/dose Repeat dosing based on predicted trough	**Monitoring** Draw 4 h and 10 h random levels to calculate expected peak and trough Target peak for EIAD: *Tobramycin/Gentamicin* 40 mcg/mL; *Amikacin* 40 mcg/mL (For organisms with MICs of 2 mcg/mL and 4 mcg/mL, respectively) Target trough for EIAD: *Tobramycin/Gentamicin* < 2 mcg/mL, *Amikacin* < 4 mcg/mL **AE/toxicities** Ototoxicity Nephrotoxicity	Avoid/minimize concomitant use of neurotoxic and nephrotoxic medications	• EIAD approach aims to facilitate peak of 10 x MIC and minimize trough / probability of accumulation • Peak levels are associated with efficacy while trough concentrations are associated with nephrotoxicity • Nephrotoxicity is also exposure dependent and may develop with prolonged therapy despite EIAD approach • Use with caution in patients with neuromuscular disorders

MRSA methicillin resistant staphylococcus aureus, *VRE* vancomycin resistant enterococcus, *PO* by mouth, *PT* per enteral tube, *IV* intravenous, *CBC* complete blood count, *AE* adverse effects, *MAO* monoamine oxidase, *D5W* 5% dextrose in water, *MDROs* multidrug resistant organism, *EIAD* extended interval aminoglycoside dosing, *MIC* minimum inhibitor concentration

[136]. Infection with herpes simplex (HSV), herpes zoster (HZ), cytomegalovirus (CMV), and respiratory viruses (e.g., respiratory syncytial virus [RSV]) are of prominent concern. A review of the pharmacologic options for management of these infections is presented in Table 3.

Many oncology patients admitted in the ICU may already be receiving antiviral prophylaxis against herpes simplex virus (HSV) and herpes zoster (HZ) with acyclovir or valacyclovir. In addition to HSV/HZ, another common pathogen observed in patients with hematologic malignancy/post-HCT is cytomegalovirus (CMV). CMV is a beta herpes virus with a seroprevalence in the United States (US) of around 60% [130]. Typically, most people are asymptomatic when primary infection with CMV occurs and then the virus enters a latent infectious state in mononuclear leukocytes. Reactivation can occur in many instances, but in relation to the oncology patient population, this can be seen during times of immunosuppression (e.g., chemotherapy administration) and critical illness as well as in the elderly [34]. Prophylaxis against CMV is not routine, given the toxicity profile of traditional anti-CMV therapy (i.e., ganciclovir and foscarnet); rather a strategy of pre-emptive monitoring has been adopted with treatment reserved for patients with presumed or documented infection [136]. Recently, the Federal Drug Agency (FDA) approved letermovir for CMV prophylaxis in HCT CMV seropositive recipients. Given the more acceptable toxicity profile of this agent and the morbidity/mortality associated with CMV infection, use of letermovir will likely increase in hopes of preventing CMV reactivation [84].

Despite preventive strategies and increased awareness, respiratory viral infections may occur, with RSV, influenza, parainfluenza, and human metapneumovirus responsible for the majority of cases. Progression to lower respiratory tract infection often presents as dyspnea and hypoxia, which can prove fatal. Unfortunately, limited options currently exist for managing these viral infections (e.g., neuraminidase inhibitors for influenza, ribavirin for RSV) and therapy is primarily supportive. Studies are needed to further elucidate high-risk patients and determine efficacy of novel antiviral agents [23]. Other viruses that may be notable for complications in cancer patients include adenovirus, human herpesvirus 6 (HHV6), polyomaviruses (BK and JC), and Epstein-Barr virus (EBV).

Antifungal Agents

Antifungal coverage should be considered in febrile neutropenic patients on broad-spectrum antibiotics who have had a persistent fever for 4–7 days and no identified fever source [43]. Antifungal therapy should also be considered in critically ill ICU patients (regardless of the presence or absence of malignancy) with suspected infection who do not improve after 72 h of broad-spectrum antibiotics [110]. For empiric coverage of *Candida,* use of an echinocandin (anidulafungin, micafungin, or caspofungin) is preferred, especially in patients who have been recently treated with other antifungal agents, or if *Candida glabrata* or *Candida krusei* is suspected from previous culture data [47, 114].

Hematologic malignancy patients with prolonged neutropenia, status post allogeneic HCT, and/or chronic corticosteroid exposure (e.g., GVHD) are at risk for invasive aspergillosis infections [101]. Posaconazole or voriconazole are often utilized for prophylaxis against invasive aspergillosis in high-risk patients [29, 139, 146]. In the absence of contraindications (i.e., organ dysfunction, adverse effects) or development of a breakthrough infection, antifungal prophylactic regimens should be continued following ICU admission. For patients who develop breakthrough invasive aspergillosis while receiving prophylactic azole therapy, therapeutic drug monitoring (TDM) should be performed to assess adequacy of the current regimen, if available; however, the patient will likely need to be switched to another class of medications. Voriconazole remains the treatment of choice for *Aspergillus* infections (Table 4). However, if the patient is unable to tolerate voriconazole therapy, isavuconazonium or the liposomal formulation of Amphotericin B (AmB) are

Table 3 Oncologic considerations for select antivirals

Drug	Primary role in therapy	Dosing and administration	Monitoring, adverse events, and toxicities	Drug-drug interactions	Clinical pearls
Acyclovir [54, 136, 137]	HSV/HZ prophylaxis and treatment	**Dosing** Prophylaxis: PO, PT: 400–800 mg BID OR IV: 5 mg/kg or 2.5 mg/m2 q8–12 h (AdjBW) Treatment: IV: 10 mg/kg IBWq8h (Use adjBW for obese patients) **Administration** Administer over 1 h to reduce nephrotoxicity	**Monitoring** BUN, SCr, urine output **AE/toxicities** Nephrotoxicity	Monitor closely when used with other nephrotoxic medications	• Maintain adequate hydration • Avoid rapid infusion • Available as suspension for NG tube administration • Alternatively, valacyclovir, prodrug of acyclovir, may be utilized (not available IV)
Cidofovir [18, 53, 80]	Treatment of adenovirus Treatment of CMV	**Dosing** IV: 5 mg/kg q7 days OR 1 mg/kg 3x/week **Administration** High dose cidofovir must be given concomitantly with IV hydration and probenecid (2 gm PO 3 h prior to cidofovir dose, then 1 gm PO 2 and 8 h after completion of the infusion)	**Monitoring** SCr, urine output, and urine protein (at baseline and within 48 h of each dose), WBC **AE/toxicities** Nephrotoxicity Metabolic acidosis Neutropenia	Monitor closely when used with other nephrotoxic medications	• Inadequate HSV/HZ coverage when used as monotherapy – acyclovir/valacyclovir prophylaxis should be continued • Last line for CMV treatment given toxicity profile • Refer to package insert or [18] for renal dosage adjustment
Foscarnet [16, 38, 82]	Treatment of CMV	**Dosing** Induction: IV: 60 mg/kg q8h OR 90 mg/kg IV q12h Maintenance: IV: 90 mg/kg q24h Induction and maintenance is a minimum of 3 weeks; absolute duration also based on CMV PCR results **Administration** Administration rate not to exceed 1 mg/kg/minute. If given via peripheral IV, must be diluted not to exceed final concentration of 12 mg/mL	**Monitoring** CBC, SCr, urine output, electrolytes (Ca, Mg, K, Phos) Consider EKG **AE/toxicities** Nephrotoxicity, hypokalemia, hypomagnesemia, hypocalcemia, hypophosphatemia N/V/D Seizures (related to electrolyte imbalance)	Monitor closely when used with other nephrotoxic medications Monitor closely when used with other QTc prolonging medications	• Considered second line treatment for CMV if patient not responding/resistant to ganciclovir or as an alternative to avoid ganciclovir-associated myelosuppression • May be used to treat other viruses such as HHV6 • Provides HSV/HZ coverage-acyclovir/valacyclovir prophylaxis should be discontinued upon initiation of treatment • Use as prophylaxis has fallen out of favor given toxicity profile • Refer to package insert for renal dose

			Diabetes insipidus (nephrogenic) QTc prolongation Anemia Granulocytopenia		adjustment (See Fig. 1 for calculation of CrCL in mL/min/kg)
Ganciclovir [40]	Treatment of CMV	**Dosing** Induction: IV: 5 mg/kg q12h Maintenance: IV: 5 mg/kg q24h Induction and maintenance is a minimum of 3 weeks; absolute duration also based on CMV PCR results **Administration** Administer by slow IV infusion over at least 1 h	**Monitoring** CBC, SCr **AE/toxicities** Pancytopenia Nephrotoxicity – especially in elderly and with use of concomitant nephrotoxic agents	Monitor closely when used with other nephrotoxic medications	• Considered treatment of choice for CMV • Provides HSV/HZ coverage- acyclovir/valacyclovir prophylaxis should be discontinued upon initiation of treatment • Pancytopenia may occur at any time, but usually occurs during the first 1 to 2 weeks of treatment • May need to provide additional support with growth factors, red blood cell transfusion, or platelets • Use as prophylaxis has fallen out of favor given toxicity profile • Refer to package insert for renal dose adjustment
Letermovir [30, 84]	CMV prophylaxis	**Dosing** PO/IV: 480 mg daily PO/IV: 240 mg daily if patient also receiving cyclosporine Started between Day 0 and Day 28 after allogeneic HCT in CMV sero-positive recipients and continued through day 100	**Monitoring** CMV reactivation, SCr **AE/toxicities** Tachycardia Atrial fibrillation N/V/D Peripheral edema	Inhibits: CYP3A4 (moderate)	• Currently only FDA approved for prophylaxis of CMV • If patient unable to swallow tablet whole, use IV administration of letermovir (do not crush or administer via feeding tube). • With IV therapy, monitor serum creatinine closely in patients with CrCl <50 mL/min (IV vehicle, hydoxypropyl betadex, may accumulate leading to kidney injury)
Oseltamivir [21, 52]	Influenza	**Dosing** PO: 75 mg BID x 5–10 days Data in immunocompromised patients is lacking for dose and duration, but given prolonged viral shedding and increased risk for progression to LRTI,	**Monitoring** Signs/symptoms of unusual behavior – rare occurrence for neuropsychiatric events, SCr **AE/toxicities** Headache	N/A	• IDSA and CDC consider patients with malignancy and/or immunosuppressive therapy to be high risk for influenza progression to LRTI • Treatment should be initiated in symptomatic immunocompromised patients regardless of duration of

(continued)

Table 3 (continued)

Drug	Primary role in therapy	Dosing and administration	Monitoring, adverse events, and toxicities	Drug-drug interactions	Clinical pearls
		higher doses and longer duration may be considered	Vomiting Diarrhea/dyspepsia with suspension (contains sorbitol)		symptoms prior to diagnosis • Available as suspension for administration via feeding tube • Refer to package insert for renal dose adjustment
Ribavirin [22, 23, 42, 49, 58, 59, 60]	RSV treatment	**Dosing** Inhaled: 2 gm via SPAG unit over 3 h q8h x 5 days (Due to teratogenicity – must be administered in a scavenging tent) Two common PO / PT dosing strategies: 1. Fixed dose of 600 mg q8h 2. LD of 10 mg/kg followed by 20 mg/kg/day divided into three doses Optimal dose and duration of oral ribavirin not yet established	**Monitoring** Hemoglobin LFTs **AE/toxicities** Hemolytic anemia	N/A	• Due to short duration for treatment of RSV compared to Hepatitis C, adverse effects associated with long-term use not common • Ribavirin solution commercially available or can be compounded for administration via feeding tube • Recent increase in cost of inhaled ribavirin (~$30,000/day) –alternative methods for administration are being explored given lack of randomized controlled trials, concerns about occupational exposure, and high cost • Refer to [59] and [60] for dosing recommendations in renal dysfunction

HSV herpes simplex virus, *HZ* herpes zoster, *PO* by mouth, *PT* per enteral tube, *BID* twice daily, *IV* intravenous, *AdjBW* adjusted body weight, *IBW* ideal body weight, *BUN* blood urea nitrogen, *sCr* serum creatinine, *AE* Adverse effects, *N/A* not available, *NG* nasogastric, *CMV* cytomegalovirus, *SCr* serum creatinine, *WBC* white blood count, *PCR* polymerase chain reaction, *CBC* complete blood count, *Ca* calcium, *Mg* magnesium, *K* potassium, *Phos* phosphorus, *EKG* electrocardiogram, *N/V/D* nausea/vomiting/diarrhea, *HHV6* human herpesvirus 6, *CrCl* creatinine clearance, *HCT* hematopoietic cell transplant, *FDA* Food and Drug Administration, *LRTI* lower respiratory tract infection, *n/a* not applicable, *IDSA* Infectious Disease Society of America, *CDC* Center for Disease Control, *NG* nasogastric, *RSV* respiratory syncytial virus, *SPAG* small particle aerosol generator, *LD* loading dose, *LFTs* Liver function tests

$$[140 - age]/[\text{serum creatinine in mg/dL} \times 72]\ [\times\ 0.85\ \text{for females}] = ml/min/kg$$

Fig. 1 How to calculate CrCL as mL/min/kg with modified Cockcroft and Gault equation for Foscarnet dosing. (Reference: (1) Foscarnet package insert)

appropriate alternative options for initial therapy. Posaconazole can be considered for salvage therapy [101].

Severe and prolonged immunosuppression also places patients at risk for mucormycosis infections. Posaconazole has been shown to be the most effective antifungal for prophylaxis against mucormycosis; of note, voriconazole is not active against mucormycosis. Liposomal AmB is recommended by the guidelines as the treatment of choice for mucormycosis infections; however, isavuconazonium has recently been approved with the indication as well [10]. Posaconazole is reserved for salvage therapy. Surgical interventions combined with medical treatments have been associated with higher survival rates in patients with mucormycosis when compared to pharmacologic therapy alone [28].

Cancer patients are commonly on numerous medications and chemotherapies that may interact with concomitant azole therapy. Azoles are potent inhibitors and substrates of cytochrome p450 enzymes; therefore, clinicians must be diligent about evaluating for drug-drug interactions (DDIs). In addition, azoles can cause QTc prolongation. Clinicians should monitor closely and optimize electrolytes, particularly in patients on multiple QTc prolonging medications.

Pneumocystis Jiroveci Pneumonia

Prophylaxis and treatment for pneumocystis jiroveci pneumonia (PJP) should be considered in patients with risk factors (neutropenic, immunosuppressed, long-term or high-dose steroids) who are not improving on standard antimicrobial therapy. Prophylactic therapy is usually given to oncologic patients receiving certain types of chemotherapy (i.e., alemtuzumab, purine

analogs), HCT patients, or patients on immunosuppression with chronic and/or high-dose steroids. The choice of prophylaxis (e.g., sulfamethoxazole-trimethoprim [SMZ-TMP], pentamidine) is typically based on patient- and/or disease-specific factors (Table 5). Prophylaxis is usually continued until immunosuppression therapy has been discontinued and counts have recovered (absolute neutrophil count [ANC] >1000), CD4 > 200, or according to the specific chemotherapy regimens as noted on the package insert or protocol [32].

For treatment of PJP infection, sulfamethoxazole-trimethoprim (SMZ-TMP) remains the drug of choice (Table 5). However, certain circumstances preclude use of SMZ-TMP, such as an allergy to sulfa medications, the desire to avoid agents that may suppress the bone marrow (e.g., HCT patients pre-engraftment), or persistent SMZ-TMP-related hyperkalemia. In such situations, alternative agents such as clindamycin/primaquine should be considered.

Antiepileptics

Seizures are a common neurologic complication in oncologic patients, secondary to primary brain tumors, metastases, radiation toxicity, and metabolic abnormalities [57]. Selection of an antiepileptic drug (AED) warrants special consideration in the oncologic patient due to interactions with chemotherapy, side effects, and unique mechanisms of certain brain tumors. Enzyme inducing anticonvulsants such as phenytoin may lead to insufficient serum levels of concomitantly administered chemotherapy. Conversely, enzyme inhibiting anticonvulsants such as valproate may lead to toxic levels of chemotherapy [17]. AEDs that are substrates for P-gp (phenobarbital, carbamazepine, lamotrigine,

Table 4 Oncologic considerations for select antifungals

Drug	Primary role in therapy	Dosing and administration	Monitoring, adverse events, and toxicities	Drug-drug interactions	Clinical pearls
Voriconazole [8, 50, 98, 101, 120]	Prophylaxis against invasive Aspergillosis Antifungal of choice for invasive Aspergillosis Step-down oral therapy for candidiasis due to C. krusei or C. glabrata (as feasible, following initial treatment with an echinocandin)	**Dosing** **Treatment:** PO (IV, PO: 6 mg/kg ABW) IV: 6 mg/kg ABW* q12h x2 doses, then 4 mg/kg q12h **Prophylaxis:** PO: 200 mg q12h • Administer 1 h before or 1 h after a meal. • Avoid grapefruit juice *For obese patients:* use AdjBW	**Monitoring** Measure trough 2–5 days after initiation *Prophylaxis:* >1 mcg/mL *Treatment:* >1 mcg/mL Limited data, but target trough concentration< 5–6 mcg/mL to minimize toxicity **AE/Toxicities** Visual disturbances, hallucinations, skin reaction, neurotoxicity, QTc prolongation, hepatotoxicity	Inhibitor of CYP2C9, CYP3A4, and to a lesser extent, CYP2C19 P-gp inhibitor	• For subtherapeutic levels, increase IV therapy no more than 50% at a time (max 6 mg/kg twice daily). Increase PO therapy from 200 mg twice daily to 300 mg twice daily. Nonlinear pharmacokinetics result in unpredictable serum concentrations. • Caution with use of IV formulation in patients with renal dysfunction due to β-cyclodextrin solvent. Use PO therapy if feasible. • Suspension available for administration via feeding tube • Long-term use associated with rare cases of melanoma or squamous cell carcinoma • Long-term use associated with periostitis and skeletal disease due to elevated fluoride levels from triflourinated triazole chemical structure
Posaconazole [8, 56, 98, 101, 125]	Salvage therapy for invasive Aspergillosis Second line treatment for Mucormycosis	**Dosing** **Treatment:** IV/PO DR tablets: 300 mg q12h x2 doses, then 300 mg **Prophylaxis:** *DR tablets:* PO: 300 mg q12h x2 doses, then 300 mg q24h thereafter	**Monitoring** Measure trough 7 days after initiation *Prophylaxis:* >700 ng/mL *Treatment:* >1000 ng/mL Limited data on target trough concentration **AE/Toxicities** Nausea, vomiting, hepatotoxicity, QTc prolongation	Potent inhibitor of CYP3A4 Substrate and inhibitor of P-gp	• Long half-life of 26 to 31 h • The suspension form is *not* recommended. Variable bioavailability with food, fat, and acidity. *DR tablets:* • Not interchangeable with oral suspension due to increased absorption of tablet form. • Does not have to be administered with high-fat meal. • Can *not* be crushed for use in feeding tube. Use IV formulation in patients unable to swallow the tablet.
Isavuconazonium [41, 101, 119, 145]	Treatment for *Mucormycosis* Alternative primary therapy for invasive Aspergillosis	**Dosing** **Treatment dose:** IV/PO: 372 mg q8h x6 doses, then 372 mg q24h	**AE/Toxicities** Nausea, vomiting, diarrhea, skin reaction, hepatotoxicity	Substrate and moderate inhibitor of CYP3A4	• Limited data on isavuconazonium TDM. Does not need to be routinely monitored. • QTc shortening • IV formulation is β-cyclodextrin solvent free • Poor penetration to eyes, CNS, CSF fluid • Most well-tolerated anti-fungal from GI standpoint

IV intravenous, *ABW* actual body weight, *PO* oral, *AdjBW* adjusted body weight, *AE* adverse events, *P-gp* P-glycoprotein, *NG* nasogastric, *DR* delayed release, *PK* pharmacokinetics, *TDM* therapeutic drug monitoring, *CNS* central nervous system, *CSF* cerebral spinal fluid, *GI* gastrointestinal

Table 5 Oncologic considerations for Pneumocystis jiroveci pneumonia (PJP)

Drug	Primary role in therapy	Dosing and administration	Monitoring, adverse events, and toxicities	Drug-drug interactions	Clinical pearls
Sulfamethoxazole/ Trimethoprim [24, 32]	Drug of choice for treatment and prophylaxis of PJP	**Dosing** **Prophylaxis:** PO/PT: 80 mg TMP daily or 160 mg TMP three times weekly **Treatment:** IV/PO/PT: 15–20 mg/kg TMP given in divided doses 3–4x/day (usually 5 mg/kg q8h or q6h)	**Monitoring** CBC, LFTs, SCr/BUN **AE/toxicities** Agranulocytosis, hyperkalemia, nephrotoxicity, Stevens-Johnson syndrome, QTc prolongation	Inhibitor of CYP2C8 Substrate of P-gp	• PJP prophylaxis usually given for 3–12 months after last chemotherapy treatment • PJP prophylaxis in HCT starts at day +30 and continues for 6–12 months (or longer if still receiving immunosuppressive therapy) • IV formulation requires large volume of D5W as diluent (caution in fluid overload and/or hyponatremia) • High sorbitol content of oral suspension may contribute to diarrhea • Although treatment of choice for PJP, in hematologic malignancy/ HCT, alternative therapy may need to be considered given bone marrow suppressive effects and concomitant use with other nephrotoxic medications (risk vs. benefit analysis)
Clindamycin/ Primaquine [32]	Preferred alternative PJP treatment	**Dosing** **Treatment:** Clindamycin IV (600 mg q6h or 900 mg q8h) plus Primaquine 30 mg (base) PO/PT daily	**Monitoring** CBC, visual color check of urine, glucose, electrolytes **AE/toxicities** Primaquine- hemolytic anemia, methemoglobinemia, QTc prolongation Clindamycin – diarrhea (*C difficile* infection)	Clindamycin: Substrate CYP3A4 (minor) Primaquine: Substrate of CYP2D6 (major) and CYP3A4 (major)	• Primaquine is contraindicated in patients with known G6PD deficiency. • Primaquine can be compounded into a suspension for administration via a feeding tube • Preferred alternative therapy for patients unable to receive SMZ-TMP

(continued)

Table 5 (continued)

Drug	Primary role in therapy	Dosing and administration	Monitoring, adverse events, and toxicities	Drug-drug interactions	Clinical pearls
Pentamidine [32, 37]	Alternative PJP therapy	**Dosing** **Prophylaxis:** Nebulized pentamidine 300 mg every 28 days IV (limited data): 300 mg q21 days until patient able to tolerate oral alternative therapy **Treatment:** IV: 4 mg/kg every 24 h infused over at least 60 min for 21 days. May reduce dose to 3 mg/kg due to toxicities	**Monitoring** Glucose, CBC, EKG, LFTs **AE/toxicities** Bronchospasm, cough, fatigue, dizziness, fever, leukopenia, QTc prolongation, cardiac dysrhythmia		
Atovaquone [32]	Alternative PJP prophylaxis or treatment	**Dosing** **Prophylaxis:** PO/PT: 1500 mg daily with food **Treatment:** PO/PT: 750 mg BID with food Administer with high fat meal to enhance oral absorption	**AE/toxicities** Diarrhea, transaminase elevations	Do not co-administer with rifampin	• Substantially more expensive than alternative oral regimens • Not recommended for severe PJP infections • Only available as an oral suspension
Dapsone [32]	Alternative PJP prophylaxis	**Dosing** **Prophylaxis:** PO/PT: 100 mg daily or 50 mg BID	**Monitoring** CBC, LFTs, reticulocyte **AE/toxicities** Hemolytic anemia, methemoglobinemia, rash, serious dermatologic reactions (rare)		• Use with caution in patients with known G6PD deficiency • Use with caution with patients with hypersensitivity to sulfonamides

SMZ-TMP sulfamethoxazole-trimethoprim, *PJP* Pneumocystis jiroveci pneumonia, *PO* oral, *TMP* trimethoprim, *IV* intravenously, *CBC* complete blood count, *LFTs* liver function tests, *SCr* serum creatinine, *BUN* blood urea nitrogen, *AE* adverse effects, *P-gp* P-glycoprotein, *D5W* 5% dextrose in water, *HCT* hematopoietic cell transplant, *BID* twice daily, *G6PD* glucose-6-phosphate dehydrogenase, *NG* nasogastric, *EKG* electrocardiogram

topiramate, and felbamate) may result in insufficient intraparenchymal levels [88].

Patients with brain tumors are more prone to refractory epilepsy, requiring the use of multiple AEDs with different mechanisms. With the introduction of more well-tolerated AEDs, many practitioners are avoiding enzyme inducers as first-line agents [88]. While non-CYP-450 enzyme-inducing AEDs such as levetiracetam, gabapentin, and lamotrigine may be preferable in cancer patients receiving chemotherapy, levetiracetam may be preferred as an initial option in the ICU as it is available for IV administration, does not appear to be affected by P-gp expression, and has favorable pharmacokinetic properties (Table 6) [57, 142].

Corticosteroids are universally utilized immunosuppressants in oncology patients. Often times, corticosteroids are included in different chemotherapy regimens, especially to treat diseases such as diffuse large b-cell lymphoma or acute lymphoid leukemia. High-dose corticosteroids are also utilized to treat a wide range of complications in cancer patients, including but not limited to GVHD, diffuse alveolar hemorrhage (DAH), idiopathic pulmonary syndrome (IPS), and spinal cord compression (SCC) (Table 7). Collaboration between the oncology and critical care teams is recommended when initiating or stopping corticosteroids in the ICU to avoid untoward interactions with ongoing oncologic treatments.

Immunosuppressants

Recipients of a HCT, particularly allogeneic HCT, require immunosuppression to prevent GVHD [149]. Tacrolimus, sirolimus, or cyclosporine are often utilized for GVHD prophylaxis (Table 7). Similar to the approach in solid organ transplant patients, these medications are managed within a narrow therapeutic window in attempt to decrease both the risk of GVHD as well as toxicities of therapy. Additionally, practitioners should remain cognizant of DDIs with these agents [1].

Antifibrinolytic/Antihemophilic Agents

Diffuse Alveolar Hemorrhage (DAH)

Prognosis in patients with DAH secondary to cancer therapy or sepsis is poor [39]. Pulse dose corticosteroids (methylprednisolone 1–2 mg/kg/day) with or without antifibrinolytic therapy has been used in practice but has not been consistently associated with reductions in ICU or hospital mortality, ventilator days, or ICU and hospital

Table 6 Oncologic considerations for seizures

Drug	Primary role in therapy	Dosing and administration	Monitoring, adverse events, and toxicities	Drug-drug interactions	Clinical pearls
Levetiracetam [19, 138]	Prophylaxis or treatment of seizures	**Dosing** IV or PO/PT (immediate release tablet): 1000–3000 mg/day, divided doses q12h *max 4500 mg/day PO/PT: administer without regard to food **Administration** IV: 15 min, for SE, max 2–5 mg/kg/min	**AE/toxicities** CNS depression, toxic epidermal necrolysis, Stevens-Johnson syndrome, and aggression		• Dosing may be limited by somnolence • Prophylaxis may be warranted in patients receiving CAR T-cell therapy

IV intravenously, *PO* oral, *SE* status epilepticus, *AE* adverse events, *CNS* central nervous system, *CAR* chimeric antigen receptor

Table 7 Oncologic considerations for immunosuppressants

Drug	Primary role in therapy	Dosing and administration	Monitoring, adverse events, and toxicities	Drug-drug interactions	Clinical pearls
Tacrolimus [9, 104, 147, 148]	GVHD prevention	**Dosing** Starting dose CIVI: 0.03 mg/kg/day (age ≤50 y/o, no interacting medications) 0.015 mg/kg/day if one or more criteria met: age >50 y/o, renal dysfunction, interacting medication(e.g., voriconazole) Starting dose PO (in two divided doses): 0.12 mg/kg (age ≤50, no interacting medications) 0.06 mg/kg (age >50, renal dysfunction, interacting medication (e.g., voriconazole))	**Monitoring** Serum level: 5–15 ng/mL With continuous IV infusion can draw random level With PO dosing, should draw a trough 30 min prior to dose Wait at least 24–36 h after starting/adjusting dose for steady state **AE/toxicities** Neurotoxicity, PRES, nephrotoxicity, hypertension, diabetes, TMA-TTP, electrolyte imbalance (hypomagnesemia, hyper/hypokalemia), infection	Substrate of CYP3A4 (Major) Drug-food interaction: Avoid grapefruit and pomegranate	• IV to PO conversion is 1:3 or 1:4 • Dose based on IBW • Minimal renal excretion – no dose modification needed • Clearance lowered in patients with severe hepatic dysfunction – likely dose modifications needed • Dose reductions 50–75% required when used concomitantly with voriconazole or posaconazole • If unable to swallow capsules, content of capsule may be mixed with water and flushed through feeding tube • SL administration may be used by opening the contents of the capsule under the tongue – decrease dose in half if switching from PO to SL
Cyclosporine [93, 148]	GVHD prevention	**Dosing** Starting dose CIVI: 3 mg/kg/day Starting dose PO-in two divided doses: 10 mg/kg/day **Administration** Neoral®/Gengraf® and Sandimmune® are not bioequivalent and cannot be used interchangeably	**Monitoring** Goal: 200–400 ng/mL With continuous IV infusion can draw random level With PO dosing, should draw a trough 30 min prior to dose Wait at least 24–36 h after starting / adjusting dose for steady state **AE/toxicities** Neurotoxicity, PRES, nephrotoxicity, hypertension, hepatotoxicity, TMA-TTP, electrolyte imbalance (hypomagnesemia,	Substrate of CYP3A4 (Major) Drug-food interaction: Avoid grapefruit and pomegranate	• IV to PO is 1:2–3 or 1:4 conversion dependent upon formulation • Dose based on IBW • Minimal renal excretion – no dose modification needed • Clearance lowered in patients with severe hepatic dysfunction – likely dose modifications needed • Dose reductions 25–50% required when used concomitantly with

Drug	Indication	Dosing	Monitoring / AE/toxicities	Notes
			hyperkalemia), hyperuricemia, infection, gingival hyperplasia, malignancy	voriconazole or posaconazole • Suspension is available for administration via feeding tube
Sirolimus [1, 35, 108]	GVHD prevention	**Dosing** PO: 12 mg LD x1, then 4 mg daily OR 6 mg LD x1, then 2 mg daily	**Monitoring** Goal: 3–12 ng/mL Trough drawn 30 min prior to dose Due to long half-life, recommended to wait 3–4 days to check level after loading dose and reasonable to wait 1 week after dose adjustment **AE/toxicities** Hyperlipidemia, hypertriglyceridemia, hypertension, nephrotoxicity, hepatotoxicity (VOD), TMA-TTP	Substrate of CYP3A4 (Major) Drug-food interaction: Avoid grapefruit and pomegranate	• No IV formulation available • Suspension is commercially available for administration via feeding tube • Dose reductions 50–90% required when used concomitantly with voriconazole or posaconazole
Corticosteroids [2, 44, 45, 70, 79, 81, 85, 87, 106, 112, 113, 129, 135, 140, 141, 143]	GVHD treatment DAH IPS SCC	**Dosing** **GVHD treatment** Methylprednisolone 2 mg/kg IV in two divided doses followed by slow taper **DAH/IPS** Methylprednisolone 2 mg/kg IV in two to four divided doses followed by slow taper **Other dosing strategy for DAH** Methylprednisolone 500–1000 mg IV/day (in one to two divided doses) x 3–4 days, then taper to 1 mg/kg/day x 3 days followed by slow taper over 2–4 weeks **SCC** Dexamethasone 4–10 mg IV q6 h (doses range from 16 mg/day to 96 mg/day in four divided doses)	**Monitoring** Blood pressure, blood glucose, electrolytes, body weight, HPA axis suppression; IOP and bone mineral density (with long term use) **AE/toxicities** Hypertension, hyperglycemia, increased infection risk, steroid psychosis, myopathy, adrenal suppression, edema / fluid retention, electrolyte disturbances, visual impairment, increased IOP osteoporosis (Long term use)	Dexamethasone major CYP3A4 substrate and weak inducer of CYP3A4	• Concomitant use in patients receiving immune or cellular therapy should be avoided unless specifically treating toxicity related to treatment

GVHD graft *vs* host disease, *CIVI* continuous intravenous infusion, *PO* by mouth, *AE* adverse effects, *PRES* posterior reversible encephalopathy syndrome, *TMA-TTP* thrombotic microangiopathy-thrombotic thrombocytopenic purpura, *IBW* Ideal body weight, *NG* nasogastric, *SL* sublingual, *LD* loading dose, *IV* intravenous, *VOD* veno-occlusive disease, *DAH* Diffuse alveolar hemorrhage, *IPS* Idiopathic pulmonary syndrome, *SCC* Spinal cord compression, *IOP* intraocular pressure

length of stay in the literature [77, 113, 143]. Treatment with steroids or antifibrinolytic therapy can be considered in patients at high risk of rapid clinical deterioration or death (Table 8). Agents such as recombinant factor VIIa have been used to achieve hemostasis in non-hemophiliac patients with DAH [100]. Additionally, a case series of six patients successfully used intrapulmonary factor VII as adjunctive treatment for DAH with doses ranging from 30 to 60 mcg/kg [12]. The potential benefit of antifibrinolytic and antihemophilic therapies must be weighed against the risk of thrombotic events [150].

Thrombocytopenia

Spontaneous bleeding complications due to thrombocytopenia are common in the critically ill oncologic patient population [75]. Most patients can be managed by observation and supportive care alone. Use of antifibrinolytic agents have been used in emergency treatment of severe thrombocytopenia-associated bleeding to reduce transfusion requirements without increased risk in thromboembolic events (Table 8) but have not been shown to decrease mortality [7].

Disseminated Intravascular Coagulation (DIC)

Routine use of aminocaproic acid, tranexamic acid and recombinant FVIIa in patients with cancer-related DIC is not recommended. Practitioners may consider use of tranexamic acid in patients with therapy-resistant hyperfibrinolytic DIC bleeding (Table 8). Platelet transfusion to maintain platelets $>50 \times 10^3$/L, and transfusion of fresh frozen plasma (15–30 ml/kg) with careful monitoring, is the primary therapy in patients with DIC and active bleeding [134].

Gastrointestinal (GI) Bleeding

A large randomized control trial (RCT) is currently underway to examine the use of tranexamic acid for the treatment of GI bleeding [118].

Thrombolytics

Hepatic sinusoidal obstruction syndrome (SOS), previously referred to as veno-occlusive disease (VOD), is a potentially life-threatening complication with a wide-ranging incidence. Severe SOS is associated with a mortality rate greater than 80% [27]. SOS is characterized by a prothrombotic, hypofibrinolytic state as a result of endothelial damage and hepatocellular injury to sinusoidal endothelial cells. Hallmark symptoms include weight gain, painful hepatomegaly, fluid retention/ascites, and hyperbilirubinemia; the reported incidence varies in part due to variable definitions and evaluated populations [36]. SOS is a complication that occurs typically within 3 weeks of a myeloablative HCT but can also be observed in patients with risk factors of pre-existing liver disease, total body irradiation or abdominal/liver radiation, or exposure to certain hepatotoxic drugs, such as inotuzumab or gemtuzumab (list of VOD/SOS risk factors is not all-inclusive) [27, 36]. Defibrotide was FDA approved in the United States in 2016 for the treatment of severe hepatic SOS after publication of a pivotal phase III trial [117]. Its proposed mechanism of action is to reduce endothelial cell activation and injury and promote restoration of the thrombo-fibrinolytic balance [116]. Due to the severity of illness associated with SOS, many patients are transferred to the ICU for continued management and administration of defibrotide (Table 9).

Uric Acid Reducing Agents

Over 50% of oncologic patients with high-risk for tumor lysis syndrome (TLS) require ICU admission, and nearly 1/3 of those will present with acute kidney injury (AKI). Clinicians should be familiar with the management of hyperuricemia to help preserve renal function. Hyperuricemia results from the rapid release and catabolism of intracellular nucleic acids either spontaneously or in response to chemotherapy in patients with a high tumor burden. Patients who are considered high risk for TLS should receive rasburicase over allopurinol (Table 10) [25].

Table 8 Oncologic considerations for bleeding in the ICU

Drug	Primary role in therapy	Dosing and administration	Monitoring, adverse events, and toxicities	Drug-drug interactions	Clinical pearls
Aminocaproic acid [64, 113]	DAH, oral bleeding with thrombocytopenia	**Dosing** DAH: IV: 4 g over 1 h, followed by continuous infusion at 1 g/h **Topical for oral bleeding with thrombocytopenia:** Rinse with hydrogen peroxide, then rinse with saline, followed by a third rinse with 5 ml (1.25 g) aminocaproic acid syrup for 30 sec. Repeat q4h until bleeding controlled **Administration** Rapid IV administration can result in hypotension, bradycardia, and/or arrhythmias	**Monitoring** CPK, heart rate agranulocytosis, signs and symptoms of VTE **AE/toxicities** Bradycardia, arrhythmias, VTE		• May accumulate in renal failure. Specific guidelines for dosage adjustments are unavailable; dose should be modified based on clinical response and degree of renal impairment
Tranexamic acid [62, 105, 123]	DAH, thrombocytopenia-related bleeding	**Dosing** Minimal dosing recommendations *We recommend* IV/PO/PT: TXA 10–15 mg/kg q8-12 h *Alternate dosing regimens:* *Hemoptysis:* 250–500 mg TXA in 500 mg/5 mL solution nebulized via facemask over 15 min **Administration** Hypotension can occur when infusion rates exceed 100 mg/min	**AE/toxicities** VTE, abdominal pain, back pain, musculoskeletal pain, myalgia		• Accumulates in renal failure. Dose adjustment needed. See package insert.
Factor VIIa, recombinant [12, 63, 95, 100, 133]	Refractory bleeding	**Dosing** *Life-threatening bleeding:* IV: 35–120 mcg/kg q2h up to 4 doses per day. Usual starting dose was 75 mcg/kg	**Monitoring** aPTT, DIC **AE/toxicities** Thromboembolism		

DAH diffuse alveolar hemorrhage, *IV* intravenous, *PO* oral, *CPK* creatinine protein kinase, *VTE* venous thromboembolism, *TXA* tranexamic acid, *aPTT* activated partial thromboplastin time, *PTT* partial thromboplastin time, *DIC* disseminated intravascular coagulation, *PT* Prothrombin time

Table 9 Oncologic considerations for thrombolytics

Drug	Primary role in therapy	Dosing and administration	Monitoring, adverse events, and toxicities	Drug-drug interactions	Clinical pearls
Defibrotide [69, 117]	Hepatic SOS (VOD)	**Dosing** IV: 6.25 mg/kg q6h for at least 21 days and a maximum of 60 days (until SOS resolution or hospital discharge) Utilize baseline (dry) weight prior to stem cell transplant or initiation of chemotherapy **Administration** Administer over 2 h using 0.2 micron in-line filter via a dedicated line	**Monitoring** Platelets, INR, Fibrinogen **AE/Toxicities** Hemorrhage, Hypersensitivity reaction **CI** Active bleeding, hemodynamic instability requiring vasopressor support	Co-administration with systemic anticoagulation or fibrinolytic therapy is contraindicated	• For invasive procedures – discontinue defibrotide at least 2 h prior to procedure; resume treatment once the procedure-related risk of bleeding is resolved • Maintain platelets >30,000, INR <1.5, Fibrinogen >150 to decrease bleeding risk

SOS Sinusoidal obstruction syndrome, *VOD* Veno-occlusive disease, *IV* intravenous, *INR* International normalized ratio, *AE*: adverse effects, *CI* Contraindications

Hypercalcemia of Malignancy/ Hypercalcemia Management

All patients presenting with hypercalcemia of malignancy should be given IV crystalloids at 1–2 ml/kg/h to restore intravascular volume and promote calciuresis. For patients that are fluid restricted due to other co-morbidities (e.g., heart failure), consider concomitant diuresis with a loop diuretic if necessary. Symptomatic patients presenting with abdominal pain, confusion, weakness, and electrocardiogram (EKG) changes may require a bisphosphonate +/− calcitonin. Critical care practitioners should be cognizant of all prior therapy given in order to avoid duplicating therapy and the potential development of hypocalcemia (e.g., recent bisphosphonate or denosumab administration) (Table 11).

Interleukin-6 Receptor Antagonists

Chimeric antigen receptor (CAR) T-cell therapy induces rapid and durable clinical responses in many types of cancer but is associated with unique, acute toxicities that can be fatal. This includes both cytokine release syndrome (CRS) and cytokine-related encephalopathy syndrome (CRES). IL-6 therapy may be warranted in patients exhibiting signs and symptoms of toxicity, particularly those requiring ICU care. IL-6 receptor antagonists are indicated in patients with grade 2 and greater CRES and grade 3 and 4 CRS, and may be considered in those with grade 1 CRES and/or persistent grade 1 or 2 CRS [91]. See Table 12 for considerations for IL-6 therapy for CRS or CRES.

Growth Factors

Colony stimulating factors (CSF) are recommended to be administered in a prophylactic manner when the risk of febrile neutropenia (FN) with a given chemotherapy regimen is 20% or higher [127]. The American Society of Clinical Oncology (ASCO) and National Comprehensive Cancer Network (NCCN) recommend primary prophylaxis for FN with CSFs based on factors associated with the disease, chemotherapy regimen, patient risk, and treatment intent (curative vs. palliative). Secondary prophylaxis may be warranted in patients who have FN or a dose-

Table 10 Oncologic considerations for uric acid reduction

Drug	Primary role in therapy	Dosing and administration	Monitoring, adverse events, and toxicities	Drug-drug interactions	Clinical pearls
Allopurinol [144]	Prevention of hyperuricemia in TLS	**Dosing** PO/PT: 600–800 mg daily in one to three divided doses. IV: 200–400 mg/m^2 daily **Administration** Initiate 1–2 days before chemotherapy	**Monitoring** Serum uric acid levels, BUN, SCr HLA-B*5801 testing in high-risk patients (not typically feasible in acute setting) **AE/Toxicities** Dermatologic toxicities Hepatotoxicity (increased alkaline phosphatase) Nephrotoxicity	6-mercaptopurine, azathioprine, cyclophosphamide, thiazide, and loop diuretics, warfarin	• Preferred in patients with known G6PD deficiency • Does not lower existing uric acid levels • May require up to 72 h to effectively decrease uric acid levels • Does not warrant dose reductions in acute management of TLS • Caution in hypoxanthine/xanthine nephropathy
Rasburicase [20, 121]	Hyperuricemia associated with malignancy	**Dosing** IV: 3–6 mg x 1, may repeat **Administration** Infuse over 30 min to avoid reaction, dose 4 h prior to chemotherapy if possible	**Monitoring** Serum uric acid levels **AE/toxicities** Anaphylaxis CI: Patients with known hemolytic anemia, methemoglobinemia, and G6PD deficiency* *due to time sensitive administration, G6PD screening should not preclude administration of rasburicase acutely	N/A	• Initiate in patients with pre-existing hyperuricemia (Uric acid >7.5 mg/dL) or high-risk patients regardless of baseline uric acid levels • Achieves target uric acid lowering in ~ 4 h in most patients • Enzymatic degradation of uric acid in blood specimen will occur if left at room temperature; collect samples on ice and assay within 4 h

TLS tumor lysis syndrome, *PO* oral, *IV* intravenous, *AE* adverse events, *G6PD* glucose-6 phosphate dehydrogenase deficiency, *CI* contraindicated in, *N/A* not available

Table 11 Oncologic considerations for hypercalcemia of malignancy

Drug	Primary role in therapy	Dosing and administration	Monitoring, adverse events, and toxicities	Drug-drug interactions	Clinical pearls
Calcitonin [55, 90, 132]	Acute treatment for hypercalcemia of malignancy	**Dosing** SQ: 4–8 units/kg q12h Skin test should be performed in patients with sensitivity to salmon calcitonin	**AE/toxicities** Hypocalcemia, facial flushing, local injection site edema		• Onset within 2–4 h. Tachyphylaxis develops within 48–72 h • Not to be used as single agent • Bisphosphonate therapy can be prescribed on day 1 of calcitonin (overlap therapy to compensate for slow onset of bisphosphonate)
Pamidronate [13, 26, 55, 132]	Hypercalcemia of malignancy	**Dosing** IVPB: 60–90 mg x1 Dose can be repeated x1 after 7 days if inadequate response to initial treatment, then do not give more than once every 28 days due to risk of renal failure **Administration** Infuse over 2–24 h	**AE/toxicities** Hypocalcemia, nephrotoxicity Flu-like symptoms (fever, chills) Bone pain Osteonecrosis of the jaw (rare)		• Onset of action 2–4 days with response duration of 1–3 weeks • Not recommended in renal dysfunction. Dosage should be modified depending on degree of renal impairment and response, but no quantitative recommendations are available. Dose reduction generally not warranted unless SCr severely elevated >4.5 mg/dL
Zoledronic acid [26, 55, 94, 132]	Hypercalcemia of malignancy	**Dosing** 4 mg IVPB x1 Dose can be repeated x1 after 7 days if inadequate response to initial treatment, then do not give more than once every 28 days due to risk of renal failure **Administration** Can be infused over 15–30 min	**AE/toxicities** Hypocalcemia, nephrotoxicity Flu-like symptoms (fever, chills) Bone pain Osteonecrosis of the jaw (rare)		• Convenience of administration (IVPB over 15–30 min) for outpatients • Onset of action 2–4 days with response duration of 1–3 weeks • Not recommended in renal dysfunction. Dosage should be modified depending on degree of renal impairment, but no quantitative recommendations are available. Dose reduction generally not warranted unless SCr severely elevated >4.5 mg/dL
Denosumab [4, 55, 132]	Hypercalcemia refractory to bisphosphonates	**Dosing** 120 mg SQ weekly x4 weeks, then every 28 days **Administration** Denosumab should only be administered via the SQ route. Do not administer IV, IM, or ID	**AE/toxicities** Hypocalcemia Osteonecrosis of the jaw		• Onset of action 2–4 days. Terminal half-life of 25.4 days after single-dose administration

SQ subcutaneous, *AE* adverse effects, *IVPB* intravenous piggy back, *SCr* serum creatinine, *IV* intravenous, *IM* intramuscular, *ID* intradermal

Table 12 Oncologic considerations for treatment of cytokine release syndrome or cytokine related encephalopathy syndrome

Drug	Primary role in therapy	Dosing and administration	Monitoring, adverse events, and toxicities	Drug-drug interactions	Clinical pearls
Tocilizumab [48]	CRS CRES	**Dosing** IV: 8 mg/kg for up to 3 doses in a 24-h period (max 800 mg/dose) **Administration** Infuse over 1 h No premedications needed Have emergency medications immediately available in the event of hypersensitivity reaction	**Monitoring prior to therapy** Latent TB,CBC with diff, LFTs, lipid panel **AE/Toxicities** Infection, infusion reaction, anaphylaxis, GI perforation, CNS demyelinating disorders, increased cholesterol, increased LFTs, infusion reactions, neutropenia, thrombocytopenia	Theoretical increased metabolism of CYP 450 substrates	• May consider re-dosing in patients not responding or with worsening grade toxicities within 4 h.
Siltuximab [68]	CRS CRES	**Dosing** IV: 11 mg/kg once **Administration** Infuse over 1 h; complete infusion within 4 h of reconstitution No premedications needed Have emergency medications immediately available in the event of hypersensitivity reaction	**Monitoring prior to therapy** CBC prior to first dose **AE/Toxicities** Infection, infusion reaction, anaphylaxis, GI perforation, peripheral edema, fatigue (long-term exposure), pruritus, skin rash, weight gain, hyperuricemia, diarrhea, abdominal pain, arthralgia, URI, thrombocytopenia, hypertriglyceridemia	Theoretical increased metabolism of CYP 450 substrates	• Do not re-dose within 21 days • Consider in patients who fail to respond to 1–2 doses of tocilizumab

CRS cytokine release syndrome, *CRES* cytokine related encephalopathy syndrome, *IV* intravenous, *TB* tuberculosis, *CBC* complete blood count, *diff* differential, *LFTs* liver function tests, *AE* adverse effects, *GI* gastrointestinal, *CNS* cerebral nervous system, *CBC*: complete blood count, *URI* upper respiratory infection

limiting neutropenic event [31, 127]. Additionally, CSFs may be used to reduce the length of hospitalization and time to neutrophil recovery, for HCT mobilization, and to reduce the risk of infection in patients with intermittent/persistent neutropenia status post HCT. Of note, the medical record of oncology patients admitted to the ICU should be evaluated for prior CSF administration as such therapy my confound interpretation of leukocytosis (Table 13).

Thrombopoietin and thrombopoietin mimetics are FDA approved for the treatment of chronic immune thrombocytopenia; these agents may also be helpful off label to increase the platelet count in patients with thrombocytopenic disorders [66, 74, 76]. The management of thrombocytopenia in patients with increased bleeding risk (e.g., post-surgical), chemotherapy-induce thrombocytopenia, and/or promotion of platelet engraftment after HCT are

Table 13 Oncologic considerations for growth factors in the ICU

Drug	Primary role in therapy	Dosing and administration	Monitoring, adverse events, and toxicities	Drug-drug interactions	Clinical pearls
Filgrastim [6]	Increase WBC	**Dosing** 5 mcg/kg/day IV/SQ	**Monitoring** CBC with differential **AE/toxicities** Common: fatigue, bone/joint pain, peripheral edema/capillary leak syndrome, thrombocytopenia, headache, splenomegaly Serious: ARDS, pulmonary infiltrates, splenic rupture	N/A	• Higher doses may be used during mobilization for HCT • Onset of action, 24 h • Duration: Counts return to baseline within 4 days • Do not administer within 24 h (before or after) of cytotoxic chemotherapy
Pegfilgrastim [5]	Increase WBC	**Dosing** 6 mg SQ once per chemotherapy cycle, beginning at least 24 h after completion of chemotherapy	**Monitoring** CBC with differential **AE/toxicities** Common: bone/joint/muscle pain Serious: ARDS, pulmonary infiltrates, splenic rupture	N/A	• Onset of action is 96 h(delayed compared to filgrastim) • Pegylated formulation allows for prolonged duration of action (half-life 15–80 h) • Do not administer within 14 days before or 24 h after cytotoxic chemotherapy
Romiplostim [3]	Increase platelets in chronic ITP	**Dosing** 1 mcg/kg SQ once weekly; increasing by 1 mcg/kg/week increments to achieve platelet count $\geq$50,000/mm^3 (Max dose: 10 mcg/kg/week)	**Monitoring** CBC with differential **AE/toxicities** Common: headache, dizziness, abdominal pain, arthralgia, myalgia, increased circulating myeloblasts (MDA patients) Serious: angioedema, marrow fibrosis, VTE, hematology malignancy risk		• Onset of action between 4–9 days • Should be discontinued after 4 weeks if no response • Upon discontinuation of therapy, may see rebound thrombocytopenia and increased bleeding risk • May be used off label to increase platelet count if high risk for bleeding or for CIT

WBC white blood cell, *IV* intravenous, *SQ* subcutaneous, *CBC* complete blood count, *AE* adverse effects, *ARDS* acute respiratory distress syndrome, *ITP* idiopathic thrombocytopenia purpura, *VTE* venous thromboembolism, *CIT* chemotherapy-induced thrombocytopenia

Table 14 Antidotes for critically Ill oncologic patients

Drug	Primary role in therapy	Dosing and administration	Monitoring, adverse events, and toxicities	Drug-drug interactions	Clinical pearls
Sodium bicarbonate or sodium acetate [65]	Urinary alkalinization for methotrexate toxicity	**Dosing** **Dose:** IV: 50 meq/L to maximally tolerated rate ($\geq$3 L/m^2 per day) to maximize urine output and keep urine pH > 7	**AE/Toxicities** Metabolic alkalosis		• Limited compatibility with many other IV medications
Amifostine [122]	Cisplatin toxicity	**Dosing** **Dose:** IV: 910 mg/m^2 over 15 min once daily given 30 min prior to chemotherapy. Chemotherapy should be started 15 min after completion of amifostine infusion.	**Monitoring** BP every 3–5 min during infusion and decrease dose for severe decrease in SBP (see dosage adjustments from package insert). If full dose cannot be administered prior to cisplatin therapy, reduce amifostine dose to 740 mg/m^2 for subsequent cycles **AE/Toxicities** Hypotension, N/V	Patients should have antihypertensive therapy interrupted 24 h before receiving amifostine	• Cytoprotective detoxicant. Reduces ototoxicity, nephrotoxicity, and possible decrease in severity of peripheral neuropathy • Premedicate with antiemetics including dexamethasone and a serotonin 5HT$_3$ receptor antagonist
Dexrazoxane [107]	Extravasation Doxorubicin toxicity	**Dosing** First infusion should be started within 6 h after extravasation IV: Day 1: 1,000 mg/m2 (max 2000 mg/day) Day 2: 1,000 mg/m2 (Max: 2000 mg) Day 3: 500 mg/m2 (Max 1000 mg) Infusions on day 2 and 3 should start at the same hour ($\pm$ 3 h) as on the first day	**AE/Toxicities** myelosuppression		• Remove cooling procedures (e.g., ice packs) from area at least 15 min prior to administration to allow sufficient blood flow to area
Leucovorin [65]	Primary therapy for MTX toxicity	**Dosing** IV, IM, or PO: Initially 15 mg (10 mg/m^2), then 15 mg (10 mg/m^2) q6h until serum MTX <0.05 uM/L. Subsequent dosing based on follow-up MTX levels [65] If SCr $\geq$ 50% baseline 24 h post MTX, or if serum MTX > 5 uM/L, increase leucovorin to 100 mg/m^2 IV or q3h until serum MTX < 0.05 uM/L.	**AE/Toxicities** Dehydration, diarrhea		• Do *not* administer within 2 h before or after glucarpidase • Do not exceed infusion rate of 160 mg of leucovorin per minute due to calcium content of solution

(continued)

Table 14 (continued)

Drug	Primary role in therapy	Dosing and administration	Monitoring, adverse events, and toxicities	Drug-drug interactions	Clinical pearls
Glucarpidase [65]	MTX toxicity in patients with renal dysfunction	**Dosing** IV: 50 U/g over 5 min	**Monitoring** Serum MTX reduced by ≥97% within 15 min of dose administration		• MTX TDM is unreliable for at least 48 h following glucarpidase administration • No effect on intracellular MTX concentrations. Must be administered with high-dose leucovorin
Levocarnitine [15]	Pegaspargase-induced hepatotoxicity	**Dosing** IV LD: 50 mg/kg, followed by 50 mg/kg/day divided in six daily doses	**AE/Toxicities** Diarrhea, hypertension	Patients who are on antidiabetic agents may need dose adjustments for hypoglycemia	• Use with caution in patients with history of seizures
Methylene blue [103, 115]	Ifosfamide-induced neurotoxicity	**Dosing** IV: 50 mg infused up to six times daily	**AE/Toxicities** Contraindicated in patients with G6PD deficiency Dysgeusia, hot flashes	Avoid concomitant use with SSRIs, SNRIs, and MAOI therapy due to risk of serotonin syndrome	• Urine discoloration (blue or green) can occur due to oxidation when exposed to air
Thiamine [46, 61, 73, 131]	Ifosfamide toxicity Beriberi Wernicke's Encephalopathy	**Dosing** Limited data: IV: Ifosfamide toxicity: 100 mg q4h Beriberi: IV: 100 mg/day x7 days, followed by 10 mg/day orally until complete recovery Wernicke's Encephalopathy: IV: 200 mg TID x 5–7 days or until no further improvement in symptoms			• Consider thiamine for Wernicke in the malnourished and confused oncologic patient

IV intravenous, *AE* adverse effects, *BP* blood pressure, *SBP* systolic blood pressure, *N/V* nausea and vomiting, *MTX* methotrexate, *IM* intramuscular, *PO* by mouth, *q3h* every three hours, *TDM* therapeutic drug monitoring, *LD* loading dose, *TID* three times daily

some examples of off-label uses for thrombopoietin agents, such as romiplostim (Table 13) [83, 86, 96, 128].

Antidotes

The toxicity profiles of chemotherapy regimens are often severe and adversely affect patients' quality of life. Although most symptoms can be managed with supportive care (see Table 1 in ▶ Chap. 16, "Complications and Toxicities Associated with Cancer Therapies in the Intensive Care Unit"), there are times when treatment interruptions or reversal are necessary.

For reversal of toxicities or overdose, infusion of antidote should be started as soon as possible (Table 14).

References

1. Abouelnasr A, Roy J, Cohen S, Kiss T, Lachance S. Defining the role of sirolimus in the management of graft-versus-host disease: from prophylaxis to treatment. Biol Blood Marrow Transplant. 2013;19(1):12–21. https://doi.org/10.1016/j.bbmt.2012.06.020.
2. Afessa B, Tefferi A, Litzow MR, Peters SG. Outcome of diffuse alveolar hemorrhage in hematopoietic stem cell transplant recipients. Am J Respir Crit Care Med. 2002;166(10):1364–8. https://doi.org/10.1164/rccm.200208-792OC.
3. Amgen Inc. Nplate (romiplostim) [package insert]. Thousand Oaks; 2008.
4. Amgen Inc. Xgeva (denosumab) [package insert]. Thousand Oaks; 2013.
5. Amgen Inc. Neulasta (pegfilgrastim) [package insert]. Thousand Oaks; 2015a.
6. Amgen Inc. Neupogen (filgrastim) [package insert]. Thousand Oaks; 2015b.
7. Antun AG, Gleason S, Arellano M, Langston AA, McLemore ML, Gaddh M, el Rassi F, Bernal-Mizrachi L, Galipeau J, Heffner LT Jr, Winton EF, Khoury HJ. Epsilon aminocaproic acid prevents bleeding in severely thrombocytopenic patients with hematological malignancies. Cancer. 2013;119(21):3784–7. https://doi.org/10.1002/cncr.28253.
8. Ashbee HR, Barnes RA, Johnson EM, Richardson MD, Gorton R, Hope WW. Therapeutic drug monitoring (TDM) of antifungal agents: guidelines from the British Society for Medical Mycology. J Antimicrob Chemother. 2014;69(5):1162–76. https://doi.org/10.1093/jac/dkt508.
9. Astellas Pharma. Prograf (tacrolimus) [package insert]. Deerfield; 2012.
10. Astellas Pharma. Cresemba (Isavuconazonium sulfate) [package insert]. Northbrook; 2015.
11. Baden LR, Swaminathan S, Almyroudis NG, Angarone M, Blouin G, Camins BC, Cooper B, Dubberke ER, Engemann AM, Freifeld AG, Greene JN, Gregg K, Hakim H, Ito. IJ, Lustberg ME, Mones JV, Pergam S, Rolston K, Satyanarayana G, Schulz L, Seo SK, Shoham S, Taplitz R, Topal J, Wilson JW. Prevention and treatment of cancer-related infections, Version 1.2018. NCCN Clinical Practice Guidelines in Oncology; 2018.
12. Baker MS, Diab KJ, Carlos WG, Mathur P. Intrapulmonary recombinant factor VII as an effective treatment for diffuse alveolar hemorrhage: a case series. J Bronchol Intervent Pulmonol. 2016;23(3):255–8. https://doi.org/10.1097/lbr.0000000000000286.
13. Ben Venue Laboratories I. Aredia (pamidronate) [package insert]. Bedford; 2009.
14. Blackburn LM, Tverdek FP, Hernandez M, Bruno JJ. First-dose pharmacokinetics of aminoglycosides in critically ill haematological malignancy patients. Int J Antimicrob Agents. 2015;45(1):46–53. https://doi.org/10.1016/j.ijantimicag.2014.09.006.
15. Blackman A, Boutin A, Shimanovsky A, Baker WJ, Forcello N. Levocarnitine and vitamin B complex for the treatment of pegaspargase-induced hepatotoxicity: a case report and review of the literature. J Oncol Pharm Pract. 2017; https://doi.org/10.1177/1078155217710714.
16. Boeckh M, Ljungman P. How we treat cytomegalovirus in hematopoietic cell transplant recipients. Blood. 2009;113(23):5711–9. https://doi.org/10.1182/blood-2008-10-143560.
17. Brodie MJ, Mintzer S, Pack AM, Gidal BE, Vecht CJ, Schmidt D. Enzyme induction with antiepileptic drugs: cause for concern? Epilepsia. 2013;54(1):11–27. https://doi.org/10.1111/j.1528-1167.2012.03671.x.
18. Brody SR, Humphreys MH, Gambertoglio JG, Schoenfeld P, Cundy KC, Aweeka FT. Pharmacokinetics of cidofovir in renal insufficiency and in continuous ambulatory peritoneal dialysis or high-flux hemodialysis. Clin Pharmacol Ther. 1999;65(1):21–8. https://doi.org/10.1016/s0009-9236(99)70118-9.
19. Brophy GM, Bell R, Claassen J, Alldredge B, Bleck TP, Glauser T, Laroche SM, Riviello JJ Jr, Shutter L, Sperling MR, Treiman DM, Vespa PM. Guidelines for the evaluation and management of status epilepticus. Neurocrit Care. 2012;17(1):3–23. https://doi.org/10.1007/s12028-012-9695-z.
20. Cairo MS, Coiffier B, Reiter A, Younes A. Recommendations for the evaluation of risk and prophylaxis of tumour lysis syndrome (TLS) in adults and children with malignant diseases:

an expert TLS panel consensus. Br J Haematol. 2010;149(4):578–86. https://doi.org/10.1111/j.1365-2141.2010.08143.x.

21. Casper C, Englund J, Boeckh M. How I treat influenza in patients with hematologic malignancies. Blood. 2010;115(7):1331–42. https://doi.org/10.1182/blood-2009-11-255455.

22. Chemaly RF, Aitken SL, Wolfe CR, Jain R, Boeckh MJ. Aerosolized ribavirin: the most expensive drug for pneumonia. Transpl Infect Dis. 2016;18(4):634–6. https://doi.org/10.1111/tid.12551.

23. Chemaly RF, Shah DP, Boeckh MJ. Management of respiratory viral infections in hematopoietic cell transplant recipients and patients with hematologic malignancies. Clin Infect Dis. 2014;59(Suppl 5): S344–51. https://doi.org/10.1093/cid/ciu623.

24. Cho SY, Lee DG, Choi SM, Park C, Chun HS, Park YJ, Choi JK, Lee HJ, Park SH, Choi JH, Yoo JH. Stenotrophomonas maltophilia bloodstream infection in patients with hematologic malignancies: a retrospective study and in vitro activities of antimicrobial combinations. BMC Infect Dis. 2015;15:69. https://doi.org/10.1186/s12879-015-0801-7.

25. Coiffier B, Altman A, Pui CH, Younes A, Cairo MS. Guidelines for the management of pediatric and adult tumor lysis syndrome: an evidence-based review. J Clin Oncol. 2008;26(16):2767–78. https://doi.org/10.1200/jco.2007.15.0177.

26. Coleman R, Body JJ, Aapro M, Hadji P, Herrstedt J. Bone health in cancer patients: ESMO Clinical Practice Guidelines. Ann Oncol. 2014;25(Suppl 3):iii124–37. https://doi.org/10.1093/annonc/mdu103.

27. Coppell JA, Richardson PG, Soiffer R, Martin PL, Kernan NA, Chen A, Guinan E, Vogelsang G, Krishnan A, Giralt S, Revta C, Carreau NA, Iacobelli M, Carreras E, Ruutu T, Barbui T, Antin JH, Niederwieser D. Hepatic veno-occlusive disease following stem cell transplantation: incidence, clinical course, and outcome. Biol Blood Marrow Transplant. 2010;16(2):157–68. https://doi.org/10.1016/j.bbmt.2009.08.024.

28. Cornely OA, Arikan-Akdagli S, Dannaoui E, Groll AH, Lagrou K, Chakrabarti A, Lanternier F, Pagano L, Skiada A, Akova M, Arendrup MC, Boekhout T, Chowdhary A, Cuenca-Estrella M, Freiberger T, Guinea J, Guarro J, de Hoog S, Hope W, Johnson E, Kathuria S, Lackner M, Lass-Florl C, Lortholary O, Meis JF, Meletiadis J, Munoz P, Richardson M, Roilides E, Tortorano AM, Ullmann AJ, van Diepeningen A, Verweij P, Petrikkos G. ESCMID and ECMM joint clinical guidelines for the diagnosis and management of mucormycosis 2013. Clin Microbiol Infect. 2014;20(Suppl 3):5–26. https://doi.org/10.1111/1469-0691.12371.

29. Cornely OA, Maertens J, Winston DJ, Perfect J, Ullmann AJ, Walsh TJ, Helfgott D, Holowiecki J, Stockelberg D, Goh YT, Petrini M, Hardalo C, Suresh R, Angulo-Gonzalez D. Posaconazole vs. fluconazole or itraconazole prophylaxis in patients with neutropenia. N Engl J Med. 2007;356(4):348–59. https://doi.org/10.1056/NEJMoa061094.

30. Corp. MSD. Prevymis (letermovir) [package insert]. Whitehouse Station; 2017.

31. Crawford J, Becker PS, Armitage JO, Blayney DW, Chavez J, Curtin P, Dinner S, Fynan T, Gojo I, Griffiths EA, Hough S, Kloth DD, Kuter DJ, Lyman GH, Mably M, Mukherjee S, Patel S, Perez LE, Poust A, Rampal R, Roy V, Rugo HS, Saad AA, Schwartzberg LS, Shayani S, Talbott M, Vadhan-Raj S, Vasu S, Wadleigh M, Westervelt P, Burns JL, Pluchino L. Myeloid growth factors, Version 2.2017, NCCN Clinical Practice Guidelines in Oncology. J Natl Compr Cancer Netw. 2017;15(12):1520–41. https://doi.org/10.6004/jnccn.2017.0175.

32. Crothers K, Furrer H, Helweg-Larsen J, Huang L, Kovacs J, Miller R, Morris A (2017) Guidelines for the prevention and treatment of opportunistic infections in HIV-infected adults and adolescents: recommendations from the Centers for Disease Control and Prevention, the National Institutes of Health, and the HIV Medicine Association of the Infectious Diseases Society of America. Panel on Opportunistic Infections in HIV-Infected Adults and Adolescents. http://aidsinfo.nih.gov/contentfiles/lvguidelines/adult_oi.pdf. Accessed 19 Apr 2018.

33. Cruciani M, Rampazzo R, Malena M, Lazzarini L, Todeschini G, Messori A, Concia E. Prophylaxis with fluoroquinolones for bacterial infections in neutropenic patients: a meta-analysis. Clin Infect Dis. 1996;23(4):795–805.

34. Crumpacker C, Zhang J. Cytomegalovirus. In: Mandell G, Bennett J, Dolin R, editors. Mandell, Douglas, and Bennett's principles and practice of infectious diseases. 7th ed. Philadelphia: Elsevier; 2010. p. 1971–87.

35. Cutler C, Stevenson K, Kim HT, Richardson P, Ho VT, Linden E, Revta C, Ebert R, Warren D, Choi S, Koreth J, Armand P, Alyea E, Carter S, Horowitz M, Antin JH, Soiffer R. Sirolimus is associated with veno-occlusive disease of the liver after myeloablative allogeneic stem cell transplantation. Blood. 2008;112(12):4425–31. https://doi.org/10.1182/blood-2008-07-169342.

36. Dalle JH, Giralt SA. Hepatic veno-occlusive disease after hematopoietic stem cell transplantation: risk factors and stratification, prophylaxis, and treatment. Biol Blood Marrow Transplant. 2016;22(3):400–9. https://doi.org/10.1016/j.bbmt.2015.09.024.

37. Diri R, Anwer F, Yeager A, Krishnadasan R, McBride A. Retrospective review of intravenous pentamidine for Pneumocystis pneumonia prophylaxis in allogeneic hematopoietic stem cell transplantation. Transpl Infect Dis. 2016;18(1):63–9. https://doi.org/10.1111/tid.12486.

38. El Chaer F, Shah DP, Chemaly RF. How I treat resistant cytomegalovirus infection in hematopoietic cell transplantation recipients. Blood. 2016;128(23):2624–36. https://doi.org/10.1182/blood-2016-06-688432.

39. Escuissato DL, Warszawiak D, Marchiori E. Differential diagnosis of diffuse alveolar haemorrhage in immunocompromised patients. Curr Opin Infect Dis. 2015;28(4):337–42. https://doi.org/10.1097/qco.0000000000000181.

40. Exela Pharma Sciences. Ganciclovir [package insert]. Lenoir; 2017.

41. Falci DR, Pasqualotto AC. Profile of isavuconazole and its potential in the treatment of severe invasive fungal infections. Infect Drug Resist. 2013;6:163–74. https://doi.org/10.2147/idr.S51340.

42. Foolad F, Aitken S, Shigle T. Use of oral ribavirin for the treatment of RSV Infections in Hematopoietic Cell Transplant Recipients. Paper presented at the ID Week; 2017.

43. Freifeld AG, Bow EJ, Sepkowitz KA, Boeckh MJ, Ito JI, Mullen CA, Raad II, Rolston KV, Young JA, Wingard JR. Clinical practice guideline for the use of antimicrobial agents in neutropenic patients with cancer: 2010 update by the infectious diseases society of america. Clin Infect Dis. 2011;52(4):e56–93. https://doi.org/10.1093/cid/cir073.

44. Fresenius Kabi. Decadron (dexamethasone sodium phosphate) [package insert]. Lake Zurich; 2014.

45. Fukuda T, Hackman RC, Guthrie KA, Sandmaier BM, Boeckh M, Maris MB, Maloney DG, Deeg HJ, Martin PJ, Storb RF, Madtes DK. Risks and outcomes of idiopathic pneumonia syndrome after nonmyeloablative and conventional conditioning regimens for allogeneic hematopoietic stem cell transplantation. Blood. 2003;102(8):2777–85. https://doi.org/10.1182/blood-2003-05-1597.

46. Galvin R, Brathen G, Ivashynka A, Hillbom M, Tanasescu R, Leone MA. EFNS guidelines for diagnosis, therapy and prevention of Wernicke encephalopathy. Eur J Neurol. 2010;17(12):1408–18. https://doi.org/10.1111/j.1468-1331.2010.03153.x.

47. Garnacho-Montero J, Diaz-Martin A, Canton-Bulnes L, Ramirez P, Sierra R, Arias-Verdu D, Rodriguez-Delgado M, Loza-Vazquez A, Rodriguez-Gomez J, Gordon M, Estella A, Garcia-Garmendia JL. Initial antifungal strategy reduces mortality in critically ill patients with candidemia: a propensity score-adjusted analysis of a multicenter study. Crit Care Med. 2018;46(3):384–93. https://doi.org/10.1097/ccm.0000000000002867.

48. Genentech I. Actemra (tocilizumab) [package insert]. South San Francisco: Genentech, Inc; 2018.

49. Genentech USA I. Copegus (ribavirin) [package insert]. South San Francisco; 2011.

50. Gerber B, Guggenberger R, Fasler D, Nair G, Manz MG, Stussi G, Schanz U. Reversible skeletal disease and high fluoride serum levels in hematologic patients receiving voriconazole. Blood. 2012;120(12):2390–4. https://doi.org/10.1182/blood-2012-01-403030.

51. Gilbert D. Aminoglycosides. In: Mandell GLBJ, Dolin R, editors. Principles and practice of infectious diseases. 5th ed. New York: Churchill Livingston; 2000. p. 307–35.

52. Gilead Sciences I. Tamiflu (oseltamivir phosphate) [package insert]. Foster City; 2008.

53. Gilead Sciences I. Vistide (cidofovir injection) [package insert]. Foster City; 2010.

54. GlaxoSmithKline. Zovirax (acyclovir) [package insert]. Research Triangle Park; 2003.

55. Goldner W. Cancer-related hypercalcemia. J Oncol Pract. 2016;12(5):426–32. https://doi.org/10.1200/jop.2016.011155.

56. Greenberg RN, Mullane K, van Burik JA, Raad I, Abzug MJ, Anstead G, Herbrecht R, Langston A, Marr KA, Schiller G, Schuster M, Wingard JR, Gonzalez CE, Revankar SG, Corcoran G, Kryscio RJ, Hare R. Posaconazole as salvage therapy for zygomycosis. Antimicrob Agents Chemother. 2006;50(1):126–33. https://doi.org/10.1128/aac.50.1.126-133.2006.

57. Grewal J, Grewal HK, Forman AD. Seizures and epilepsy in cancer: etiologies, evaluation, and management. Curr Oncol Rep. 2008;10(1):63–71.

58. Gupta SK, Kantesaria B, Glue P. Pharmacokinetics, safety, and tolerability of ribavirin in hemodialysis-dependent patients. Eur J Clin Pharmacol. 2012;68(4):415–8. https://doi.org/10.1007/s00228-011-1137-x.

59. Gupta SK, Kantesaria B, Glue P. Pharmacokinetics and safety of single-dose ribavirin in patients with chronic renal impairment. Drug Discov Ther. 2013;7(4):158–63.

60. Gupta SK, Kantesaria B, Glue P. Exploring the influence of renal dysfunction on the pharmacokinetics of ribavirin after oral and intravenous dosing. Drug Discoveries & Therapeutics. 2014;8(2):89–95.

61. Hamadani M, Awan F. Role of thiamine in managing ifosfamide-induced encephalopathy. J Oncol Pharm Pract. 2006;12(4):237–9. https://doi.org/10.1177/1078155206073553.

62. Hankerson MJ, Raffetto B, Mallon WK, Shoenberger JM. Nebulized tranexamic acid as a noninvasive therapy for cancer-related hemoptysis. J Palliat Med. 2015;18(12):1060–2. https://doi.org/10.1089/jpm.2015.0167.

63. Holly P, Lisa L, Plamenova I, Dobrotova M, Kubisz P. Recombinant activated factor VII as an additional agent in the management of bleeding in patients with chemotherapy-induced thrombocytopenia. Blood transfus. 2013;11(3):466–8. https://doi.org/10.2450/2012.0077-12.

64. Hospira Inc. Amicar (aminocaproic acid) [package insert]. Lake Forest; 2017.

65. Howard SC, McCormick J, Pui CH, Buddington RK, Harvey RD. Preventing and managing toxicities of high-dose methotrexate. Oncologist. 2016;21(12):1471–82. https://doi.org/10.1634/theoncologist.2015-0164.

66. Imbach P, Crowther M. Thrombopoietin-receptor agonists for primary immune thrombocytopenia. N Engl J Med. 2011;365(8):734–41. https://doi.org/10.1056/NEJMct1014202.

67. Jaksic B, Martinelli G, Perez-Oteyza J, Hartman CS, Leonard LB, Tack KJ. Efficacy and safety of linezolid compared with vancomycin in a randomized, double-blind study of febrile neutropenic patients with cancer. Clin Infect Dis. 2006;42(5):597–607. https://doi.org/10.1086/500139.

68. Janssen Biotech I. Sylvant (siltuximab) [package insert]. Horsham; 2017.

69. Jazz Pharmaceuticals I. Defitelio (defibrotide) [package insert]. Palo Alto; 2016.

70. Kantrow SP, Hackman RC, Boeckh M, Myerson D, Crawford SW. Idiopathic pneumonia syndrome: changing spectrum of lung injury after marrow transplantation. Transplantation. 1997;63(8):1079–86.

71. Kim S-H, Kwon J-C, Choi S-M, Lee D-G, Park SH, Choi J-H, Yoo J-H, Cho B-S, Eom K-S, Kim Y-J, Kim H-J, Lee S, Min C-K, Cho S-G, Kim D-W, Lee J-W, Min W-S. Escherichia coli and Klebsiella pneumoniae bacteremia in patients with neutropenic fever: factors associated with extended-spectrum β-lactamase production and its impact on outcome. Ann Hematol. 2013;92(4):533–41. https://doi.org/10.1007/s00277-012-1631-y.

72. Kostakou E, Rovina N, Kyriakopoulou M, Koulouris NG, Koutsoukou A. Critically ill cancer patient in intensive care unit: issues that arise. J Crit Care. 2014;29(5):817–22. https://doi.org/10.1016/j.jcrc.2014.04.007.

73. Kuo SH, Debnam JM, Fuller GN, de Groot J. Wernicke's encephalopathy: an underrecognized and reversible cause of confusional state in cancer patients. Oncology. 2009;76(1):10–8. https://doi.org/10.1159/000174951.

74. Kuter DJ. Thrombopoietin and thrombopoietin mimetics in the treatment of thrombocytopenia. Annu Rev Med. 2009;60:193–206.

75. Kuter DJ. Managing thrombocytopenia associated with cancer chemotherapy. Oncology (Williston Park). 2015;29(4):282–94.

76. Kuter DJ, Bussel JB, Lyons RM, Pullarkat V, Gernsheimer TB, Senecal FM, Aledort LM, George JN, Kessler CM, Sanz MA, Liebman HA, Slovick FT, de Wolf JT, Bourgeois E, Guthrie TH Jr, Newland A, Wasser JS, Hamburg SI, Grande C, Lefrere F, Lichtin AE, Tarantino MD, Terebelo HR, Viallard JF, Cuevas FJ, Go RS, Henry DH, Redner RL, Rice L, Schipperus MR, Guo DM, Nichol JL. Efficacy of romiplostim in patients with chronic immune thrombocytopenic purpura: a double-blind randomised controlled trial. Lancet (London, England). 2008;371(9610):395–403. https://doi.org/10.1016/s0140-6736(08)60203-2.

77. Lara AR, Schwarz MI. Diffuse alveolar hemorrhage. Chest. 2010;137(5):1164–71. https://doi.org/10.1378/chest.08-2084.

78. Leibovici L, Paul M, Cullen M, Bucaneve G, Gafter-Gvili A, Fraser A, Kern WV. Antibiotic prophylaxis in neutropenic patients: new evidence, practical decisions. Cancer. 2006;107(8):1743–51. https://doi.org/10.1002/cncr.22205.

79. Lewis ID, DeFor T, Weisdorf DJ. Increasing incidence of diffuse alveolar hemorrhage following allogeneic bone marrow transplantation: cryptic etiology and uncertain therapy. Bone Marrow Transplant. 2000;26(5):539–43. https://doi.org/10.1038/sj.bmt.1702546.

80. Lindemans CA, Leen AM, Boelens JJ. How I treat adenovirus in hematopoietic stem cell transplant recipients. Blood. 2010;116(25):5476–85. https://doi.org/10.1182/blood-2010-04-259291.

81. Loblaw DA, Perry J, Chambers A, Laperriere NJ. Systematic review of the diagnosis and management of malignant extradural spinal cord compression: the Cancer Care Ontario Practice Guidelines Initiative's Neuro-Oncology Disease Site Group. J Clin Oncol. 2005;23(9):2028–37. https://doi.org/10.1200/jco.2005.00.067.

82. Ltd. CH. Foscavir (foscarnet sodium) [package insert]. DE14 2WW, UK; 2011.

83. Marshall AL, Goodarzi K, Kuter DJ. Romiplostim in the management of the thrombocytopenic surgical patient. Transfusion. 2015;55(10):2505–10. https://doi.org/10.1111/trf.13181.

84. Marty FM, Ljungman P, Chemaly RF, Maertens J, Dadwal SS, Duarte RF, Haider S, Ullmann AJ, Katayama Y, Brown J, Mullane KM, Boeckh M, Blumberg EA, Einsele H, Snydman DR, Kanda Y, DiNubile MJ, Teal VL, Wan H, Murata Y, Kartsonis NA, Leavitt RY, Badshah C. Letermovir prophylaxis for cytomegalovirus in hematopoietic-cell transplantation. N Engl J Med. 2017;377(25):2433–44. https://doi.org/10.1056/NEJMoa1706640.

85. Metcalf JP, Rennard SI, Reed EC, Haire WD, Sisson JH, Walter T, Robbins RA. Corticosteroids as adjunctive therapy for diffuse alveolar hemorrhage associated with bone marrow transplantation. University of Nebraska Medical Center Bone Marrow Transplant Group. Am J Med. 1994;96(4):327–34.

86. Miao J, Leblebjian H, Fowler-Scullion B, Parnes A. Single-center experience with Romiplostim for management of chemotherapy-induced thrombocytopenia (CIT). Blood. 2016;128:530.

87. Mielcarek M, Furlong T, Storer BE, Green ML, McDonald GB, Carpenter PA, Flowers ME, Storb R, Boeckh M, Martin PJ. Effectiveness and safety of lower dose prednisone for initial treatment of acute graft-versus-host disease: a randomized

controlled trial. Haematologica. 2015;100(6):842–8. https://doi.org/10.3324/haematol.2014.118471.

88. Mintzer S, Mattson RT. Should enzyme-inducing antiepileptic drugs be considered first-line agents? Epilepsia. 2009;50(Suppl 8):42–50. https://doi.org/10.1111/j.1528-1167.2009.02235.x.

89. Moore RD, Lietman PS, Smith CR. Clinical response to aminoglycoside therapy: importance of the ratio of peak concentration to minimal inhibitory concentration. J Infect Dis. 1987;155(1):93–9.

90. Mylan Institutional LLC. Miacalcin (calcitonin) [product insert]. Rockford; 2016.

91. Neelapu SS, Tummala S, Kebriaei P, Wierda W, Gutierrez C, Locke FL, Komanduri KV, Lin Y, Jain N, Daver N, Westin J, Gulbis AM, Loghin ME, de Groot JF, Adkins S, Davis SE, Rezvani K, Hwu P, Shpall EJ. Chimeric antigen receptor T-cell therapy – assessment and management of toxicities. Nat Rev Clin Oncol. 2018;15(1):47–62. https://doi.org/10.1038/nrclinonc.2017.148.

92. Nicolau DP, Freeman CD, Belliveau PP, Nightingale CH, Ross JW, Quintiliani R. Experience with a once-daily aminoglycoside program administered to 2,184 adult patients. Antimicrob Agents Chemother. 1995;39(3):650–5.

93. Novartis Pharmaceuticals Corporation. Sandimmune (cyclosporine capsules, oral solution, injection) [package insert]. East Hanover; 2015.

94. Novartis Pharmaceuticals Corporation. Zometa (zoledronic acid) [package insert]. East Hanover; 2016.

95. Novo Nordisk Inc. NovoSeven (coagulation factor VIIa) [package insert]. Princeton; 2006.

96. Ojeda E, Carca-Marco JA, Navarro B, Delalglesia A, Fores R, Bautista G, Krsnik I, Sanchez-Guerrero A, Sanjuan I, Regidor C, Gonzalo-Daganzo R, Martin-Donaire T, Sanchez R, Bravo G, Claros N, Cabero M, Beltran P, Cabrera JR. Use of romiplostim to facilitate platelet engraftment in allogeneic hematopoietic transplantation. Blood. 2011;118:1947.

97. Pagkalis S, Mantadakis E, Mavros MN, Ammari C, Falagas ME. Pharmacological considerations for the proper clinical use of aminoglycosides. Drugs. 2011;71(17):2277–94. https://doi.org/10.2165/11597020-000000000-00000.

98. Pappas PG, Kauffman CA, Andes DR, Clancy CJ, Marr KA, Ostrosky-Zeichner L, Reboli AC, Schuster MG, Vazquez JA, Walsh TJ, Zaoutis TE, Sobel JD. Clinical Practice Guideline for the Management of Candidiasis: 2016 update by the Infectious Diseases Society of America. Clin Infect Dis. 2016;62(4):e1–50. https://doi.org/10.1093/cid/civ933.

99. Paquette F, Bernier-Jean A, Brunette V, Ammann H, Lavergne V, Pichette V, Troyanov S, Bouchard J. Acute kidney injury and renal recovery with the use of aminoglycosides: a large retrospective study. Nephron. 2015;131(3):153–60. https://doi.org/10.1159/000440867.

100. Pathak V, Kuhn J, Gabriel D, Barrow J, Jennette JC, Henke DC. Use of activated factor VII in patients with diffuse alveolar hemorrhage: a 10 years institutional experience. Lung. 2015;193(3):375–9. https://doi.org/10.1007/s00408-015-9720-z.

101. Patterson TF, Thompson GR 3rd, Denning DW, Fishman JA, Hadley S, Herbrecht R, Kontoyiannis DP, Marr KA, Morrison VA, Nguyen MH, Segal BH, Steinbach WJ, Stevens DA, Walsh TJ, Wingard JR, Young JA, Bennett JE. Practice guidelines for the diagnosis and management of aspergillosis: 2016 update by the Infectious Diseases Society of America. Clin Infect Dis. 2016;63(4):e1–e60. https://doi.org/10.1093/cid/ciw326.

102. Paul M, Yahav D, Fraser A, Leibovici L. Empirical antibiotic monotherapy for febrile neutropenia: systematic review and meta-analysis of randomized controlled trials. J Antimicrob Chemother. 2006;57(2):176–89. https://doi.org/10.1093/jac/dki448.

103. Pelgrims J, De Vos F, Van den Brande J, Schrijvers D, Prove A, Vermorken JB. Methylene blue in the treatment and prevention of ifosfamide-induced encephalopathy: report of 12 cases and a review of the literature. Br J Cancer. 2000;82(2):291–4. https://doi.org/10.1054/bjoc.1999.0917.

104. Pennington CA, Park JM. Sublingual tacrolimus as an alternative to oral administration for solid organ transplant recipients. Am J Health Syst Pharm. 2015;72(4):277–84. https://doi.org/10.2146/ajhp140322.

105. Pfizer. Cyklokapron (tranexamic acid) [package insert]. New York; 2011a.

106. Pfizer. Solu-Medrol (methylprednisolone sodium succinate for injection) [package insert]. New York; 2011b.

107. Pfizer. Zinecard (dexrazoxane for injection) [package insert]. New York; 2012.

108. Pfizer Inc. Rapamune (sirolimus) [package insert]. Philadelphia; 2011.

109. Pharmacia & Upjohn Co. Zyvox (linezolid) [package insert]. New York; 2018.

110. Posteraro B, De Pascale G, Tumbarello M, Torelli R, Pennisi MA, Bello G, Maviglia R, Fadda G, Sanguinetti M, Antonelli M. Early diagnosis of candidemia in intensive care unit patients with sepsis: a prospective comparison of (1–>3)-beta-D-glucan assay, Candida score, and colonization index. Crit Care. 2011;15(5):R249. https://doi.org/10.1186/cc10507.

111. Radigan EA, Gilchrist NA, Miller MA. Management of aminoglycosides in the intensive care unit. J Intensive Care Med. 2010;25(6):327–42. https://doi.org/10.1177/0885066610377968.

112. Raptis A, Mavroudis D, Suffredini A, Molldrem J, Rhee FV, Childs R, Phang S, Barrett A. High-dose corticosteroid therapy for diffuse alveolar hemorrhage in allogeneic bone marrow stem cell transplant recipients. Bone Marrow Transplant.

1999;24(8):879–83. https://doi.org/10.1038/sj.bmt.1701995.

113. Rathi NK, Tanner AR, Dinh A, Dong W, Feng L, Ensor J, Wallace SK, Haque SA, Rondon G, Price KJ, Popat U, Nates JL. Low-, medium- and high-dose steroids with or without aminocaproic acid in adult hematopoietic SCT patients with diffuse alveolar hemorrhage. Bone Marrow Transplant. 2015;50(3):420–6. https://doi.org/10.1038/bmt.2014.287.

114. Rhodes A, Evans LE, Alhazzani W, Levy MM, Antonelli M, Ferrer R, Kumar A, Sevransky JE, Sprung CL, Nunnally ME, Rochwerg B, Rubenfeld GD, Angus DC, Annane D, Beale RJ, Bellinghan GJ, Bernard GR, Chiche JD, Coopersmith C, De Backer DP, French CJ, Fujishima S, Gerlach H, Hidalgo JL, Hollenberg SM, Jones AE, Karnad DR, Kleinpell RM, Koh Y, Lisboa TC, Machado FR, Marini JJ, Marshall JC, Mazuski JE, McIntyre LA, McLean AS, Mehta S, Moreno RP, Myburgh J, Navalesi P, Nishida O, Osborn TM, Perner A, Plunkett CM, Ranieri M, Schorr CA, Seckel MA, Seymour CW, Shieh L, Shukri KA, Simpson SQ, Singer M, Thompson BT, Townsend SR, Van der Poll T, Vincent JL, Wiersinga WJ, Zimmerman JL, Dellinger RP. Surviving Sepsis Campaign: International guidelines for management of sepsis and septic shock: 2016. Crit Care Med. 2017;45(3):486–552. https://doi.org/10.1097/ccm.0000000000002255.

115. Richards A, Marshall H, McQuary A. Evaluation of methylene blue, thiamine, and/or albumin in the prevention of ifosfamide-related neurotoxicity. J Oncol Pharm Pract. 2011;17(4):372–80. https://doi.org/10.1177/1078155210385159.

116. Richardson PG, Ho VT, Giralt S, Arai S, Mineishi S, Cutler C, Antin JH, Stavitzski N, Niederwieser D, Holler E, Carreras E, Soiffer R. Safety and efficacy of defibrotide for the treatment of severe hepatic veno-occlusive disease. Ther Adv Hematol. 2012;3(4):253–65. https://doi.org/10.1177/2040620712441943.

117. Richardson PG, Riches ML, Kernan NA, Brochstein JA, Mineishi S, Termuhlen AM, Arai S, Grupp SA, Guinan EC, Martin PL, Steinbach G, Krishnan A, Nemecek ER, Giralt S, Rodriguez T, Duerst R, Doyle J, Antin JH, Smith A, Lehmann L, Champlin R, Gillio A, Bajwa R, D'Agostino RB Sr, Massaro J, Warren D, Miloslavsky M, Hume RL, Iacobelli M, Nejadnik B, Hannah AL, Soiffer RJ. Phase 3 trial of defibrotide for the treatment of severe veno-occlusive disease and multi-organ failure. Blood. 2016;127(13):1656–65. https://doi.org/10.1182/blood-2015-10-676924.

118. Roberts I, Coats T, Edwards P, Gilmore I, Jairath V, Ker K, Manno D, Shakur H, Stanworth S, Veitch A. HALT-IT–tranexamic acid for the treatment of gastrointestinal bleeding: study protocol for a randomised controlled trial. Trials. 2014;15:450. https://doi.org/10.1186/1745-6215-15-450.

119. Rybak JM, Marx KR, Nishimoto AT, Rogers PD. Isavuconazole: pharmacology, pharmacodynamics, and current clinical experience with a new triazole antifungal agent. Pharmacotherapy. 2015;35(11):1037–51. https://doi.org/10.1002/phar.1652.

120. Sandherr M, Maschmeyer G. Pharmacology and metabolism of voriconazole and Posaconazole in the treatment of invasive aspergillosis: review of the literature. Eur J Med Res. 2011;16(4):139–44.

121. Sanofi-Aventis. Elitek (rasburicase) [package insert]. Bridgewater; 2017.

122. Santabarbara G, Maione P, Rossi A, Gridelli C. Pharmacotherapeutic options for treating adverse effects of Cisplatin chemotherapy. Expert Opin Pharmacother. 2016;17(4):561–70. https://doi.org/10.1517/14656566.2016.1122757.

123. Segrelles Calvo G, De Granda-Orive I, Lopez Padilla D. Inhaled tranexamic acid as an alternative for hemoptysis treatment. Chest. 2016;149(2):604. https://doi.org/10.1016/j.chest.2015.10.016.

124. Shimabukuro-Vornhagen A, Boll B, Kochanek M, Azoulay E, von Bergwelt-Baildon MS. Critical care of patients with cancer. CA Cancer J Clin. 2016; https://doi.org/10.3322/caac.21351.

125. Skiada A, Lanternier F, Groll AH, Pagano L, Zimmerli S, Herbrecht R, Lortholary O, Petrikkos GL. Diagnosis and treatment of mucormycosis in patients with hematological malignancies: guidelines from the 3rd European Conference on Infections in Leukemia (ECIL 3). Haematologica. 2013;98(4):492–504. https://doi.org/10.3324/haematol.2012.065110.

126. Smith PF, Birmingham MC, Noskin GA, Meagher AK, Forrest A, Rayner CR, Schentag JJ. Safety, efficacy and pharmacokinetics of linezolid for treatment of resistant Gram-positive infections in cancer patients with neutropenia. Ann Oncol. 2003;14(5):795–801.

127. Smith TJ, Bohlke K, Lyman GH, Carson KR, Crawford J, Cross SJ, Goldberg JM, Khatcheressian JL, Leighl NB, Perkins CL, Somlo G, Wade JL, Wozniak AJ, Armitage JO. Recommendations for the use of WBC growth factors: American Society of Clinical Oncology Clinical Practice Guideline update. J Clin Oncol. 2015;33(28):3199–212. https://doi.org/10.1200/jco.2015.62.3488.

128. Soff GA, Miao Y, Devlin SM, Mantha S, Mones JV, Li VJ, Abou-Alfa GK, Cercek A, Kemeny N, Parameswara R. Romiplostim for chemotherapy-induced thrombcytopenia (CIT). Results of a phase 2 trial. Blood. 2017;130:289.

129. Soubani AO, Pandya CM. The spectrum of non-infectious pulmonary complications following hematopoietic stem cell transplantation. Hematol Oncol Stem Cell Ther. 2010;3(3):143–57.

130. Staras SA, Dollard SC, Radford KW, Flanders WD, Pass RF, Cannon MJ. Seroprevalence of

cytomegalovirus infection in the United States, 1988–1994. Clin Infect Dis. 2006;43(9):1143–51. https://doi.org/10.1086/508173.

131. Steinberg A, Gorman E, Tannenbaum J. Thiamine deficiency in stem cell transplant patients: a case series with an accompanying review of the literature. Clin Lymphoma Myeloma Leuk. 2014;14(Suppl): S111–3. https://doi.org/10.1016/j.clml.2014.06.009.

132. Stewart AF. Clinical practice. Hypercalcemia associated with cancer. N Engl J Med. 2005;352(4):373–9. https://doi.org/10.1056/NEJMcp042806.

133. Tang Y, Wu Q, Wu X, Qiu H, Sun A, Ruan C, Wu D, Han Y. Use of recombinant factor VIIa in uncontrolled gastrointestinal bleeding after hematopoietic stem cell transplantation among patients with thrombocytopenia. Pak J Med Sci. 2015;31(6):1389–93. https://doi.org/10.12669/pjms.316.8357.

134. Thachil J, Falanga A, Levi M, Liebman H, Di Nisio M. Management of cancer-associated disseminated intravascular coagulation: guidance from the SSC of the ISTH. J Thromb Haemost. 2015;13(4):671–5. https://doi.org/10.1111/jth.12838.

135. Tizon R, Frey N, Heitjan DF, Tan KS, Goldstein SC, Hexner EO, Loren A, Luger SM, Reshef R, Tsai D, Vogl D, Davis J, Vozniak M, Fuchs B, Stadtmauer EA, Porter DL. High-dose corticosteroids with or without etanercept for the treatment of idiopathic pneumonia syndrome after allo-SCT. Bone Marrow Transplant. 2012;47(10):1332–7. https://doi.org/10.1038/bmt.2011.260.

136. Tomblyn M, Chiller T, Einsele H, Gress R, Sepkowitz K, Storek J, Wingard JR, Young J-A, Boeckh MJ. Guidelines for preventing infectious complications among hematopoietic cell transplant recipients: a global perspective. Bone Marrow Transplant. 2009;44(8):453–558.

137. Turner RB, Cumpston A, Sweet M, Briggs F, Slain D, Wen S, Craig M, Hamadani M, Petros W. Prospective, controlled study of acyclovir pharmacokinetics in obese patients. Antimicrob Agents Chemother. 2016;60(3):1830–3. https://doi.org/10.1128/aac.02010-15.

138. UCB I. Keppra (levetiracetam) [package insert]. Smyrna; 2017.

139. Ullmann AJ, Lipton JH, Vesole DH, Chandrasekar P, Langston A, Tarantolo SR, Greinix H, Morais de Azevedo W, Reddy V, Boparai N, Pedicone L, Patino H, Durrant S. Posaconazole or fluconazole for prophylaxis in severe graft-versus-host disease. N Engl J Med. 2007;356(4):335–47. https://doi.org/10.1056/NEJMoa061098.

140. Van Lint MT, Uderzo C, Locasciulli A, Majolino I, Scime R, Locatelli F, Giorgiani G, Arcese W, Iori AP, Falda M, Bosi A, Miniero R, Alessandrino P, Dini G, Rotoli B, Bacigalupo A. Early treatment of acute graft-versus-host disease with high- or low-dose 6-methylprednisolone: a multicenter randomized trial from the Italian Group for Bone Marrow Transplantation. Blood. 1998;92(7):2288–93.

141. Vecht CJ, Haaxma-Reiche H, van Putten WL, de Visser M, Vries EP, Twijnstra A. Initial bolus of conventional versus high-dose dexamethasone in metastatic spinal cord compression. Neurology. 1989;39(9):1255–7.

142. Vecht CJ, van Breemen M. Optimizing therapy of seizures in patients with brain tumors. Neurology. 2006;67(12 Suppl 4):S10–3.

143. Wanko SO, Broadwater G, Folz RJ, Chao NJ. Diffuse alveolar hemorrhage: retrospective review of clinical outcome in allogeneic transplant recipients treated with aminocaproic acid. Biol Blood Marrow Transplant. 2006;12(9):949–53. https://doi.org/10.1016/j.bbmt.2006.05.012.

144. West-Ward Pharmaceuticals. Allopurinol [package insert]. Eatontown; 2015.

145. Wilson DT, Dimondi VP, Johnson SW, Jones TM, Drew RH. Role of isavuconazole in the treatment of invasive fungal infections. Ther Clin Risk Manag. 2016;12:1197–206. https://doi.org/10.2147/tcrm.S90335.

146. Wingard JR, Carter SL, Walsh TJ, Kurtzberg J, Small TN, Baden LR, Gersten ID, Mendizabal AM, Leather HL, Confer DL, Maziarz RT, Stadtmauer EA, Bolanos-Meade J, Brown J, Dipersio JF, Boeckh M, Marr KA. Randomized, double-blind trial of fluconazole versus voriconazole for prevention of invasive fungal infection after allogeneic hematopoietic cell transplantation. Blood. 2010;116 (24):5111–8. https://doi.org/10.1182/blood-2010-02-268151.

147. Winter M. Basic and clinical pharmacokinetics. 5th ed. Philadelphia: Lippincott Williams and Wilkins; 2010. p. 263–70.

148. Woo M, Przepiorka D, Ippoliti C, Warkentin D, Khouri I, Fritsche H, Korbling M. Toxicities of tacrolimus and cyclosporin A after allogeneic blood stem cell transplantation. Bone Marrow Transplant. 1997;20(12):1095–8. https://doi.org/10.1038/sj.bmt.1701027.

149. Zeiser R, Blazar BR. Acute graft-versus-host disease – biologic process, prevention, and therapy. N Engl J Med. 2017;377(22):2167–79. https://doi.org/10.1056/NEJMra1609337.

150. Juhl RC, Roddy JVF, Wang TF, Li J, Elefritz JL (2018) Thromboembolic complications following aminocaproic acid use in patients with hematologic malignancies. Leukemia & lymphoma:1–6. https://doi.org/10.1080/10428194.2018.1434882.

Complications and Toxicities Associated with Cancer Therapies in the Intensive Care Unit

16

Melvin J. Rivera, Bryan Do, Jeffrey C. Bryan, Terri Lynn Shigle, and Rina Patel

Contents

Introduction 202
Toxicities of Anticancer Therapy 202
References 217

M. J. Rivera
Thoracic / Head and Neck Medicine, The University of Texas MD Anderson Cancer Center, Houston, TX, USA
e-mail: mjrivera@mdanderson.org

B. Do
Lymphoma and Myeloma, The University of Texas MD Anderson Cancer Center, Houston, TX, USA
e-mail: bdo@mdanderson.org

J. C. Bryan
Leukemia, The University of Texas MD Anderson Cancer Center, Houston, TX, USA
e-mail: jcbryan@mdanderson.org

T. L. Shigle
Oncology, The University of Texas MD Anderson Cancer Center, Houston, TX, USA

Stem Cell Transplantation and Cellular Therapy, The University of Texas MD Anderson Cancer Center, Houston, TX, USA
e-mail: tshigle@mdanderson.org

R. Patel (✉)
Critical Care / Nutrition Support, The University of Texas MD Anderson Cancer Center, Houston, TX, USA
e-mail: rppatel1@mdanderson.org

Abstract

Advances in the management of hematologic malignancies and solid tumors have given rise to diverse modalities to treat cancer other than cytotoxic chemotherapy, including targeted therapies, immunotherapies, and cellular therapies. Currently, there are over 175 FDA-approved antineoplastic agents in the United States, many with a diverse and profound toxicity profile. Complications of antineoplastic therapy may result in the need for intensive care unit (ICU) admission to provide acute symptom management. Accordingly, ICU providers caring for cancer patients should have a working knowledge of the toxicities and complications associated with antineoplastic therapy.

Keywords

Chemotherapy · Immunotherapy · Cancer · Toxicity · Oncology · Critical care · Intensive care · Complications · Adverse effects · Antineoplastic agents

© Springer Nature Switzerland AG 2020
J. L. Nates, K. J. Price (eds.), *Oncologic Critical Care*,
https://doi.org/10.1007/978-3-319-74588-6_21

Introduction

The prevalence of cancer has grown tremendously and with that so has the need for new or repurposed anticancer therapies. Advances in the management of hematologic malignancies and solid tumors have given rise to diverse modalities to treat cancer other than cytotoxic chemotherapy, including targeted therapies, immunotherapies, and cellular therapies. There are over 175 approved antineoplastic agents in the United States and more in development with unique toxicity profiles [163]. This has created a unique opportunity for critical care specialists to manage complications of critically ill cancer patients receiving anticancer therapies.

Toxicities of Anticancer Therapy

Tables 1A–H provides a list of antineoplastic agents and toxicities that may necessitate a higher level of care and/or impact care within the intensive care unit (ICU). These tables are not all-inclusive of every minor adverse effect of each agent. Instead, they focus on toxicities that are considered severe/life-threatening complications or clinically relevant (e.g., grade 3 or 4 adverse effects). Agents that did not meet the criteria for addition to Tables 1A–H include the following: azacitidine, cladarabine, decitabine, elotuzumab, hydroxyurea, ixazomib, lomustine, olaratumab, omacetaxine, procarbazine, talimogene, valrubicin, and venetoclax.

Table 1A

	Neuro		Cardiac						Pulmonary						Renal			GI				Endocrine				Miscellaneous						Notes
	Encephalopathy	Seizures	Heart failure	Thromboembolism	Arrhythmias	QT prolongation	Pericardial effusions	Severe hypertension	Pneumonitis	Pulmonary edema	Pulmonary hypertension	Pleural effusions	Organizing pneumonia	Diffuse alveolar hemorrhage	SIADH – hyponatremia	Renal failure	Hemorrhagic cystitis	Bowel perforation	Neutropenic colitis	Pancreatitis	Hepatotoxicity	Adrenal insufficiency	Hypophysitis	Hyperglycemia	Thyroid disorders	Cytokine release syndrome	Differentiation syndrome	Opportunistic infections	Bleeding (severe)	Rhabdomyolysis	Stevens – Johnson syndrome or Toxic epidermal necrolysis	
5-Fluorouracil (5-FU)	X	X	X		X					X																					X	See Note 1
Abemaciclib				X																	X											See Note 2
Acalabrutinib					X	X																						X	X			See Note 3
Ado-trastuzumab	X		X						X																				X			See Note 4
Afatinib			X						X							X					X										X	See Note 5
Aflibercept	X			X				X								X		X											X			See Note 6
Aldesleukin	X				X					X						X					X				X							See Note 7
Alectinib					X				X							X					X			X						X		See Note 8
Alemtuzumab																												X				See Note 9

[1] Cases of hyperammonemic encephalopathy have occurred within 72 h of infusion initiation. Most cases of hyperammonemic encephalopathy are treated with ammonia lowering therapies. Cases of acute cerebellar syndrome have also been reported. Higher incidence of cardiac toxicity with infusion vs bolus dosing of 5FU [60, 149, 151, 238]

[2] Delayed hepatotoxicity (ALT and AST elevations of grade 3 or greater) with median onset 2–6 months, generally resolving to less than grade 3 in 2 weeks with dose interruption, reduction, discontinuation, or delay [137, 225]

[3] Atrial fibrillation and flutter can occur. PJP prophylaxis and CMV monitoring are recommended. Major hemorrhage has been reported with BTK inhibitors. Consider withholding 3–7 days prior to procedures depending on risk of bleeding [13, 41]

[4] GI, CNS, and pulmonary bleeding have occurred in trials with some fatalities. Higher risk in patients on anticoagulants or antiplatelet therapy. Liver failure, hepatic encephalopathy, idiopathic noncirrhotic portal hypertension, and death have been reported [82]

[5] Hepatic impairment is rare but fatalities have been reported. Diarrhea can be severe and may lead to dehydration and subsequent renal failure [31]

[6] Hypertension onset is generally within the first two cycles. Proteinuria, nephrotic syndrome, and TMA have been associated with ziv-aflibercept [210]

[7] High-dose IL-2 has a black box warning for capillary leak syndrome, CNS toxicity, and increased risk for disseminated infection. Use should be restricted to patients with normal cardiac and pulmonary function. IL–2 should only be administered under the supervision of an experienced cancer chemotherapy physician in a facility with ICU facilities available. Consensus guidelines are available to provide criteria for safe administration and toxicity management [66, 196]

[8] Symptomatic bradycardia can occur. When treating hypertension use caution when administering antihypertensive agents that can cause bradycardia. Severe renal events are rare but fatal cases have been reported. The majority of hepatotoxicity occurs within the first 3 months of therapy. Monitor CPK and for signs or symptoms of muscle pain or weakness. Median time to grade 3 CPK elevations 14 days [86]

[9] PJP and HSV prophylaxis is recommended from initiation of treatment until 2 months following last dose or until CD4+ >200/mm^3 [91]

Table 1B

	Neuro		Cardiac						Pulmonary						Renal		GI					Endocrine				Miscellaneous						Notes
	Encephalopathy	Seizures	Heart failure	Thromboembolism	Arrhythmias	QT prolongation	Pericardial effusions	Severe hypertension	Pneumonitis	Pulmonary edema	Pulmonary hypertension	Pleural effusions	Organizing pneumonia	Diffuse alveolar hemorrhage	SIADH – hyponatremia	Renal failure	Hemorrhagic cystitis	Bowel perforation	Neutropenic colitis	Pancreatitis	Hepatotoxicity	Adrenal insufficiency	Hypophysitis	Hyperglycemia	Thyroid disorders	Cytokine release syndrome	Differentiation syndrome	Opportunistic infections	Bleeding (severe)	Rhabdomyolysis	Stevens–Johnson syndrome or Toxic epidermal necrolysis	Notes
Arsenic trioxide	X					X				X						X											X					See Note 10
Asparaginase Erwinia chrysanthemi	X			X																X	X			X								See Note 11
Atezolizumab	X		X						X						X	X				X	X	X	X	X	X					X	X	See Note 12
Avelumab	X		X		X		X		X						X	X				X	X	X	X	X	X					X	X	See Note 13
Axicabtagene ciloleucel	X	X	X																							X						See Note 14
Axitinib	X							X							X	X		X			X			X					X			See Note 15
Belinostat						X																										See Note 16
Bendamustine																															X	See Note 17
Bevacizumab	X		X	X				X						X		X		X											X			See Note 18
Bexarotene																				X	X				X							See Note 19
Bleomycin									X				X																			See Note 20
Blinatumomab	X	X																		X						X						See Note 21
Bortezomib	X		X						X		X										X											See Note 22
Bosutinib												X				X																See Note 23
Brentuximab vedotin																		X	X	X								X			X	See Note 24
Brigatinib					X				X											X				X								See Note 25
Busulfan		X							X				X								X											See Note 26
Cabazitaxel									X							X	X	X	X													See Note 27
Cabozantinib	X			X				X									X	X		X					X				X			See Note 28

[10]Differentiation syndrome usually occurs during the first cycle of arsenic, median onset 17 days (7–24 days) and is commonly associated with the development of hyperleukocytosis, pulmonary edema, generalized edema, headache, bone pain, and renal failure. Management includes steroids and/or discontinuation of arsenic depending on severity. Although QT prolongation is well described, clinically significant arrhythmias are rare when appropriately monitored and managed – maintain serum potassium levels above 4 mEq/L and magnesium levels above 1.8 mg/dL [201, 215]

[11]Similar to the other asparaginase formulations, pancreatitis, abnormal transaminases, coagulation abnormalities including thrombosis and hemorrhage, and hyperglycemia can occur [115]

[12]May cause severe immune-mediated adverse events including pneumonitis, median onset 3 months (3 days to 18.7 months) and median duration 2–6 weeks, up to 12.6 months or longer; severe diarrhea, median onset 3–7 weeks (12 days to 3.4 months); hepatitis, median onset 1 month; hypothyroidism, median onset 5 months (15 days to 31 months); hypophysitis, rare, two

case reports, onset 12–13 months. May aggravate underlying autoimmune disorders. Management includes holding therapy, systemic corticosteroids, +/− additional immunosuppressants (e.g., infliximab, mycophenolate, and vedolizumab). Consider PJP prophylaxis in patients with prolonged corticosteroid exposure [33, 89, 122, 160]

[13] May cause severe immune-mediated adverse events including pneumonitis, median onset: 2.5 months (3 days to 11 months); hepatitis, median onset 3.2 months (7 days to 15 months); colitis, median onset 2.1 months (2 days to 11 months); adrenal insufficiency, median onset 2.5 months; immune-mediated thyroid disorders, median onset for 2.8 months (2 weeks to 13 months). May aggravate underlying autoimmune disorders. Management includes holding therapy, systemic corticosteroids, +/− additional immunosuppressants (e.g., infliximab, mycophenolate, and vedolizumab). Consider PJP prophylaxis in patients with prolonged corticosteroid exposure [33, 73]

[14] ICANS: Median onset 4 days (1–43 days); median duration of neurologic toxicities 17 days. Most common neurological toxicities: encephalopathy, headache, tremor, dizziness, aphasia, delirium, insomnia, and anxiety. Fatal and serious cases of cerebral edema have occurred. Other serious events included leukoencephalopathy and seizures
CRS: Median onset 2 days (1–12 days); median duration 7 days (2–58 days). Key manifestations of CRS: fever, hypotension, tachycardia, hypoxia, and chills
Management of CRS depends on grading or severity but includes supportive care, interleukin-2 receptor antagonist tocilizumab, and/or systemic corticosteroids
Grade 2 or higher ICANS without CRS should be treated with supportive care and/or systemic corticosteroids as there is insufficient data with tocilizumab in this setting. Consider anti-seizure medicines (e.g., levetiracetam) for seizure prophylaxis for any grade 2 or higher neurologic toxicities
Cardiac arrhythmias (e.g., atrial fibrillation, ventricular tachycardia), cardiac failure, renal insufficiency, capillary leak syndrome, HLH/MAS can occur
Hypogammaglobulinemia secondary to B-cell aplasia may persist for up to 13 months and increase the risk for infections. PJP and HSV prophylaxis is recommended for at least 1 year after CAR-T cell therapy [128, 161, 221]

[15] Wound healing complications – hold for at least 24 h prior to surgery and restart when wound healed. RPLS is rare but serious. Monitor for headache, seizure, lethargy, and hypertension [187]

[16] QT prolongation is a class effect of HDAC inhibitors, although the incidence may be lower than initially reported. Optimize serum potassium and magnesium levels [205, 228]

[17] Severe cutaneous reactions including SJS, TEN, DRESS, and bullous pemphigoid have been reported [45, 131, 239]

[18] RPLS: onset of symptoms from 16 h to 1 year after the first dose. Monitor for headache, seizure, lethargy, and hypertension. Wound healing: if possible wait at least 4 weeks after bevacizumab discontinuation for major surgical procedures and do not restart for at least 4 weeks after surgery or until wound is fully healed. Cases of TMA have been reported. Higher incidence of GI perforation in patients with previous pelvic irradiation. Severe pulmonary hemorrhage reported in NSCLC [30, 75, 87, 107, 197, 218]

[19] Bexarotene induces significant lipid abnormalities, usually occurring within 2–4 weeks. Pancreatitis associated with hypertriglyceridemia has been reported. Interrupt treatment and evaluate if pancreatitis is suspected; triglycerides should be maintained <400 mg/dL utilizing HMG-CoA reductase inhibitors or fenofibrate. Gemfibrozil is not recommended due to increased bexarotene and triglyceride levels. Bexarotene rapidly suppresses TSH levels by directly inhibiting TSH secretion and thyroid hormone metabolism [98, 236]

[20] Bleomycin may cause pneumonitis leading to pulmonary fibrosis. Risk factors include age > 70 years, cumulative lifetime dose > 450 units, prior mantle radiation, renal impairment, oxygen exposure, smoking, and granulocyte-colony stimulating factor use [16, 37]

[21] Neurotoxicities include tremors, confusion, encephalopathy, aphasia, and seizures, which are reversible in most cases. Onset of symptoms usually occurs around day 7 of the first cycle of treatment. Management includes treatment with dexamethasone, with or without blinatumomab interruption, and anti-seizure medication as indicated. CRS is managed with dexamethasone, with or without blinatumomab interruption, and tocilizumab as indicated. Hepatotoxicity can present alone or in association with CRS [7, 242, 243]

[22] New onset or exacerbation of HF, pneumonitis, and pulmonary hypertension may occur. Acute liver failure and RPLS have been reported rarely with bortezomib. HSV/VZV prophylaxis is required during therapy due to risk of reactivation [150]

[23] Most common toxicities are GI (i.e., diarrhea, nausea, and vomiting). Pleural effusions may develop in patients with a prior history of pleural effusions and dasatinib exposure [125]

[24] Serious and fatal cases of GI complications (i.e., acute pancreatitis, hemorrhage, obstruction, perforation) and hepatotoxicity have been reported, with higher incidence in patients with GI or liver disease involvement. Cases of PML and death due to JC virus infection have occurred with median onset of 7 weeks after initiation (3–34 weeks) ([48], Seattle [217])

[25] Symptomatic bradycardia can occur. When treating hypertension, use caution when administering with antihypertensive agents that can cause bradycardia. Higher incidence and earlier onset of pneumonitis compared to other ALK inhibitors. ILD/pneumonitis typically occurs within 9 days of initiation – higher incidence with 180 mg/day vs 90 mg/day. Monitor CPK at baseline and periodically for signs or symptoms of muscle pain or weakness [9, 127].

[26] Anti-seizure prophylaxis required with administration of busulfan. VOD is a risk among patients receiving busulfan, but the incidence has decreased since the transition in standard of care from oral to IV busulfan and the use of PK for dosing. Avoid use of acetaminophen, metronidazole, or introduction of any medication that may inhibit/induce CYPA3A4 for at least 72 h before, during, and for 72 h after busulfan administration as these are major drug interactions that will affect PK dosing [52, 181]

[27] Case reports of hemorrhagic cystitis, which may be due to radiation recall in patients with history of pelvic irradiation. High rates of grade 3/4 neutropenia in clinical trials [97, 141, 213]

[28] RPLS has occurred rarely in trials. Monitor for headache, seizure, lethargy, and hypertension. Can impair wound healing – hold 28 days prior to surgery and resume once wound has healed [76]

Table 1C

	Neuro		Cardiac						Pulmonary						Renal			GI				Endocrine				Miscellaneous						Notes
	Encephalopathy	Seizures	Heart failure	Thromboembolism	Arrhythmias	QT prolongation	Pericardial effusions	Severe hypertension	Pneumonitis	Pulmonary edema	Pulmonary hypertension	Pleural effusions	Organizing pneumonia	Diffuse alveolar hemorrhage	SIADH – hyponatremia	Renal failure	Hemorrhagic cystitis	Bowel perforation	Neutropenic colitis	Pancreatitis	Hepatotoxicity	Adrenal insufficiency	Hypophysitis	Hyperglycemia	Thyroid disorders	Cytokine release syndrome	Differentiation syndrome	Opportunistic infections	Bleeding (severe)	Rhabdomyolysis	Stevens–Johnson syndrome or Toxic epidermal necrolysis	Notes
Capecitabine	X	X	X	X	X		X									X		X	X		X										X	See Note 29
Carboplatin	X			X											X				X													See Note 30
Carfilzomib	X		X	X				X	X							X													X			See Note 31
Carmustine									X			X																				See Note 32
Ceritinib					X	X	X	X	X											X	X			X							X	See Note 33
Cetuximab							X		X																						X	See Note 34
Chlorambucil		X		X																												See Note 35
Cisplatin	X	X													X	X																See Note 36
Clofarabine						X										X			X		X							X	X	X	X	See Note 37
Cobimetinib			X					X																				X	X	X		See Note 38
Copanlisib								X	X									X						X				X				See Note 39
Crizotinib					X	X			X						X						X			X								See Note 40
Cyclophosphamide	X		X		X		X		X	X					X		X				X											See Note 41
Cytarabine				X									X																			See Note 42
Dabrafenib						X			X												X			X					X			See Note 43
Dacarbazine																					X											See Note 44
Dactinomycin									X	X																					X	See Note 45
Daratumumab									X	X																						See Note 46
Dasatinib					X	X	X		X		X	X																	X		X	See Note 47
Daunorubicin			X																													See Note 48
Daunorubicin and cytarabine (liposomal)			X																													See Note 49

[29] Cardiotoxicity: lower incidence than 5FU, mechanism thought to be due to coronary vasospasm. Higher risk in patients with cardiac or renal comorbidities. Bowel perforation: higher incidence in colon/rectal cancer but cases also reported in breast cancer patients [57, 85, 207]

[30] Incidence of hypersensitivity reactions increases with repeated exposure. Rate of reactions increased from 1% to 27% in women with ovarian cancer who received >7 cycles. Desensitization may require ICU admission [109, 142]

[31] New onset or worsening HF, restrictive cardiomyopathy, pulmonary hypertension, myocardial ischemia, and infarction, including fatalities, may occur. Patients with prior cardiovascular disease or advanced age (>75 years of age) are at an increased risk. Acute kidney injury may be associated with progressive myeloma although prerenal insults, tumor lysis-like syndrome, ATN, and TMA have occurred. Acute liver failure and RPLS have been reported rarely with carfilzomib. Thromboembolism and hemorrhage risks are thought to be associated with disease-related processes or combination regimens containing immunomodulatory agents. Anticoagulation or antiplatelet therapy is not required for patients receiving carfilzomib monotherapy. HSV/VZV prophylaxis is required during therapy due to risk of reactivation [63, 178, 250]

[32] Black box warning for dose-related pulmonary toxicity, especially in patients receiving >1400 mg/m² cumulative dose. Pulmonary fibrosis may have delayed onset, occurring years after treatment, especially in children. Other risk factors, aside from cumulative dose, include history of lung disease and baseline FVC or DLCO <70% [101, 253]

[33] Symptomatic bradycardia can occur. When treating hypertension, use caution when administering antihypertensive agents that can cause bradycardia. Cases of grade 3 and 4 pancreatitis have been reported, including fatal ones. Monitor amylase/lipase at baseline, periodically during therapy and when clinically necessary [15, 167, 227]

[34] Cardiopulmonary arrest and/or sudden death in 2–3% of patients with squamous cell carcinoma of the head and neck treated with cetuximab-based therapy [69]

[35] Patients with a history of nephrotic syndrome and receiving high pulse doses of chlorambucil are at an increased risk of seizures [195, 208]

[36] RPLS has been reported. Monitor for headache, seizure, lethargy, and hypertension. Renal toxicity is dose-related and becomes more prolonged and severe with repeated courses. Hypocalcemia and hypomagnesemia-related tetany have been reported. Incidence of hypersensitivity reactions increases with repeated exposure, peaking after six cycles. Desensitization may require ICU admission [38, 229]

[37] Older age may correlate with decreased metabolic clearance of clofarabine or possibly decreased nonrenal excretion of the drug. Clofarabine may cause a capillary leak syndrome that can be prevented and managed with steroids. Consider PJP and fungal prophylaxis. Serious and fatal prophylaxis. Pneumonitis onset is generally within 3 months of treatment initiation. Severe cases of liver injury have been reported during the first 6 weeks of therapy. Fatal cases of ketoacidosis have been reported [190, 203, 223]

[38] Risk of GI perforation 0.3%. Median first onset of LVEF decline was 4 months (23 days to 13 months). Rhabdomyolysis: median time to first occurrence of grade 3 or 4 CPK elevations 16 days (12 days to 11 months) [84]

[39] PJP and noninfectious pneumonitis have been reported. PJP prophylaxis is recommended in patients with prior PJP infection or lymphopenia. Infusion-related hyperglycemia and hyperphosphatemia, including cerebral, GI, and pulmonary hemorrhage have occurred [77, 186]

[40] Symptomatic bradycardia can occur. When treating hypertension, use caution when administering antihypertensive agents that can cause bradycardia. Serum glucose levels typically peak 2 h post infusion [23]

[41] Cardiotoxicity is related to endothelial capillary damage. Risk is increased with higher doses, advanced age, prior radiation to the cardiac region, and/or prior use of other cardiotoxic agents. Reported cardiotoxicities include arrhythmias (atrial fibrillation, atrial flutter, and ventricular arrhythmias), HF, heart block, myocarditis (including hemorrhagic), pericarditis, and pericardial effusion (including cardiac tamponade). Late-onset pneumonitis (> 6 months) is associated with increased mortality. Hyperhydration plus/minus MESNA are utilized to help prevent hemorrhagic cystitis during the infusion of cyclophosphamide. VOD has been described with high doses of cyclophosphamide in combination with other agents, such as TBI or busulfan as part of a conditioning regimen for stem cell transplant [21, 62]

[42] Doses ≥3 g/m² every 12 h have been reported to cause an acute cerebellar syndrome in 10–25% of patients. Patients >40 years of age who have abnormal liver or renal function, underlying neurologic dysfunction, or who receive a total dose of >30 g, are particularly vulnerable to developing cerebellar toxicity [19, 102, 118, 226]

[43] Median onset of cardiomyopathy is 4 months when used alone or 8 months if used concurrently with trametinib. Fever is common with dabrafenib and trametinib and can lead to hypotension, dizziness, and kidney dysfunction if dehydration occurs [171, 255]

[44] Hepatotoxicity may be accompanied by hepatic vein thrombosis and hepatocellular necrosis [11]

[45] Increased risk of VOD in children <4 years of age [182]

[46] Infusion-related reactions including bronchospasm, pneumonitis, and pulmonary edema may occur. Combination regimens with corticosteroids and premedication with antihistamines and antipyretics have helped alleviate symptoms, although patients may still be at risk for delayed infusion reactions. Consider bronchodilators in patients with a history of COPD or FEV₁ < 80%. HSV prophylaxis should start within 1 week of initiation and continue for 3 months following treatment. May result in a false-positive Indirect Coombs test that may persist for up to 6 months after the last infusion [111]

[47] Optimize serum potassium and magnesium levels prior to and during therapy to reduce risk of cardiotoxicity. Pleural effusions can occur. Management of pleural effusions consists of temporary dose interruption, dose reductions, diuretics, and/or corticosteroids. Pulmonary arterial hypertension typically occurs after 8–48 months of exposure. Increased risk of bleeding in those with advanced disease and thrombocytopenia [28, 39, 55, 134, 152, 194, 220]

[48] Onset of cardiotoxic effects of anthracyclines can occur during or immediately after infusion (acute onset), within 1 year of exposure (early onset), and from 1–20 years (late onset) after initial exposure. Factors increasing the risk of cardiac toxicity include the extent of anthracycline exposure, higher doses, older age, pre-existing cardiac disease, concurrent or previous mediastinal radiation therapy, and concomitant administration of cardiotoxic chemotherapy regimens such as paclitaxel or trastuzumab. The incidence of cardiac toxicity increases after a total cumulative dose exceeding 400–550 mg/m² in adults, 300 mg/m² in children more than 2 years of age, or 10 mg/kg in children less than 2 years of age [27]

[49] Cardiotoxicity may occur due to the anthracycline component (daunorubicin) of the formulation. Observe the same risk factors for cardiotoxicity as with conventional anthracyclines. This formulation is not interchangeable with other formulations of daunorubicin and cytarabine [114, 132]

Table 1D

	Neuro		Cardiac						Pulmonary						Renal			GI			Endocrine					Miscellaneous						Notes
	Encephalopathy	Seizures	Heart failure	Thromboembolism	Arrhythmias	QT prolongation	Pericardial effusions	Severe hypertension	Pneumonitis	Pulmonary edema	Pulmonary hypertension	Pleural effusions	Organizing pneumonia	Diffuse alveolar hemorrhage	SIADH – hyponatremia	Renal failure	Hemorrhagic cystitis	Bowel perforation	Neutropenic colitis	Pancreatitis	Hepatotoxicity	Adrenal insufficiency	Hypophysitis	Hyperglycemia	Thyroid disorders	Cytokine release syndrome	Differentiation syndrome	Opportunistic infections	Bleeding (severe)	Rhabdomyolysis	Stevens – Johnson syndrome or Toxic epidermal necrolysis	
Dinutuximab	X														X	X					X			X					X			See Note 50
Docetaxel		X	X						X	X		X							X		X										X	See Note 51
Doxorubicin			X						X				X																			See Note 52
Doxorubicin liposomal			X						X	X			X																	X		See Note 53
Durvalumab									X						X	X				X	X	X	X	X	X							See Note 54
Enasidenib																											X					See Note 55
Epirubicin			X																													See Note 56
Erlotinib				X					X							X		X			X										X	See Note 57
Etoposide	X	X					X		X																						X	See Note 58
Everolimus	X								X			X		X		X								X				X				See Note 59
Fludarabine	X	X							X				X															X				See Note 60
Gefitinib									X									X			X											See Note 61
Gemcitabine	X								X	X				X		X					X										X	See Note 62
Gemtuzumab ozogamicin						X															X								X			See Note 63
Ibritumomab																															X	See Note 64
Ibrutinib					X	X																						X	X			See Note 65
Idarubicin			X																													See Note 66
Idelalisib									X				X					X			X							X			X	See Note 67

[50] Can cause capillary leak syndrome with hypotension, severe hypokalemia and hyponatremia, HUS, and subsequent renal failure. RPLS can occur – monitor for headache, seizure, lethargy, and hypertension [162, 199, 212]

[51] Fluid retention, due to capillary leakage, can lead to non-cardiogenic pulmonary edema or pleural effusions. Diuretics recommended for treatment [245]

[52] Onset of cardiotoxic effects of anthracyclines can occur during or immediately after infusion (acute onset), within 1 year of exposure (early onset), and from 1–20 years (late onset) after initial exposure. Factors increasing the risk of cardiac toxicity include the extent of anthracycline exposure, higher doses, older age, pre-existing cardiac disease, concurrent or previous mediastinal radiation therapy, and concomitant administration of cardiotoxic chemotherapy regimens such as paclitaxel or trastuzumab. Risk of cardiomyopathy is proportional to the cumulative exposure with incidences from 1% to 20% for cumulative doses of 300 mg/m^2–500 mg/m^2. At a cumulative dose of 400 mg/m^2, the risk of developing HF is 5% [26, 258]

[53] Onset of cardiotoxic effects of anthracyclines can occur during or immediately after infusion (acute onset), within 1 year of exposure (early onset), and from 1–20 years (late onset) after initial exposure. Factors increasing the risk of cardiac toxicity include the extent of anthracycline exposure, higher doses, older age, pre-existing cardiac disease, concurrent or previous mediastinal radiation therapy, and concomitant administration of cardiotoxic chemotherapy regimens such as paclitaxel or trastuzumab. Risk of cardiac toxicity has been reported to be 11% with cumulative doses between 450 and 550 mg/m^2 [113]

[54] May cause severe immune-mediated adverse events including pneumonitis, median onset 1.8 months; hepatitis, median onset ~52 days (2–45 weeks); and immune-mediated thyroid disorders, median onset 3 months (range: 2 weeks to 13 months). May aggravate underlying autoimmune disorders. Management includes holding therapy, systemic corticosteroids, +/– additional immunosuppressants (e.g., infliximab, mycophenolate and vedolizumab). Consider PJP prophylaxis in patients with prolonged corticosteroid exposure [12, 33]

[55] Differentiation syndrome is commonly associated with the development of hyperleukocytosis, pulmonary edema, generalized edema, headache, bone pain, and renal failure, with a median onset of 48 days (10–340 days). Management includes steroids and/or discontinuation of enasidenib depending on severity. For management, please refer to the package insert. Patients with leukocytosis can be managed with hydroxyurea [230]

[56] Onset of cardiotoxic effects of anthracyclines can occur during or immediately after infusion (acute onset), within 1 year of exposure (early onset), and from 1–20 years (late onset) after initial exposure. Factors increasing the risk of cardiac toxicity include the extent of anthracycline exposure, higher doses, older age, pre-existing cardiac disease, concurrent or previous mediastinal radiation therapy, and concomitant administration of cardiotoxic chemotherapy regimens such as paclitaxel or trastuzumab. Risk of cardiomyopathy is proportional to the cumulative exposure with incidences from 0.9% to 3.3% for cumulative doses from 550 mg/m^2–900 mg/m^2 [144]

[57] The risk of CVA is increased in patients with pancreatic cancer, with a higher incidence found in those receiving erlotinib + gemcitabine (2.5%) versus gemcitabine alone. Median onset of ILD symptoms is 39 days (5 days to more than 9 months) after initiating therapy. Renal failure may arise from exacerbation of underlying baseline hepatic impairment or severe dehydration. Rare incidence of renal failure in monotherapy (0.5%) and 1.4% when combined with gemcitabine.

[58] [2, 202]

[59] Noninfectious pneumonitis, PJP, and invasive fungal and viral infections have been reported. Administer prophylaxis for PJP when concomitant use of corticosteroids or other immunosuppressive agents are required [120, 164]

[60] Incidence of pulmonary toxicity 8.6%, more likely with CLL. Pneumonitis occurs days to weeks after therapy and may occur following the first cycle; management includes systemic corticosteroids. Fludarabine can also cause autoimmune hemolytic anemia (AIHA). Serious and sometimes fatal infections including opportunistic and reactivation of latent viral infections such as VZV, EBV, and JC virus have been reported [100, 231, 246]

[61] Median onset of ILD symptoms 3–6 weeks, with fatalities reported. Serum hepatic enzyme elevations typically occur after 4–12 weeks of treatment with a hepatocellular pattern [17]

[62] Associated with a range of pulmonary toxicities: interstitial pneumonitis, capillary leak, non-cardiogenic pulmonary edema, and pulmonary fibrosis; onset can be up to 2 weeks following the last dose. Potential for radiation recall. HUS has been reported, including fatalities or need for dialysis due to renal failure. Capillary leak syndrome and RPLS have been reported [46, 72, 206, 244]

[63] Optimize potassium and magnesium prior to and during therapy to reduce risk of cardiotoxicity. Increased risk for VOD. Median onset of hyperbilirubinemia and increases in AST and ALT 8 days and median duration 20 days following initiation of therapy [145, 224, 249]

[64] SJS may occur within days to 4 months following infusion [117]

[65] Arrhythmias (i.e., ventricular arrhythmias, atrial fibrillation, and flutter) have occurred, particularly in patients with cardiac risk factors, hypertension, acute infections, or history of arrhythmias. Cases of PJP have been reported with a median onset of 6 months (2–24 months). Invasive fungal infections (i.e., aspergillosis, cryptococcal, and mucor) have been reported. Consider PJP and fungal prophylaxis in patients with lymphopenia or prolonged corticosteroid exposure. Major hemorrhage (grade 3–4) has been reported with BTK inhibitors. Consider withholding for 3–7 days prior to procedures depending on the risk of bleeding [3, 20, 146, 176, 193, 219]

[66] Onset of cardiotoxic effects of anthracyclines can occur during or immediately after infusion (acute onset), within 1 year of exposure (early onset), and from 1–20 years (late onset) after initial exposure. Factors increasing the risk of cardiac toxicity include the extent of anthracycline exposure, higher doses, older age, pre-existing cardiac disease, concurrent or previous mediastinal radiation therapy, and concomitant administration of cardiotoxic chemotherapy regimens such as paclitaxel or trastuzumab. Estimated incidence of heart failure is 5–18% with doses >90 mg/m^2 [258]

[67] Pneumonitis and organizing pneumonia may occur 1–15 months after initiation of idelalisib and should be managed with corticosteroids. GI perforation typically preceded by moderate to severe diarrhea. Median onset of diarrhea 1.9 months (range, 0.0–29.8 months). Anti-motility drugs such as loperamide are not useful in the management of idelalisib-induced diarrhea, which is best managed with dose interruptions; the median time to resolution of diarrhea can be up to 1 month. Enteric budesonide or systemic corticosteroids may be considered for treatment of severe or unresolved diarrhea, leading to shorter time to resolution compared to interruption alone (1–2 weeks vs. 1 month). Elevations in ALT or AST >5 times ULN have been observed, usually occurring within the first 12 weeks of treatment. Most transaminase elevations were reversible with dose interruption. Median time to PJP event 4.5 months after initiation. Consider PJP prophylaxis and CMV monitoring [93]

Table 1E

	Neuro		Cardiac						Pulmonary						Renal			GI				Endocrine				Miscellaneous						Notes
	Encephalopathy	Seizures	Heart failure	Thromboembolism	Arrhythmias	QT prolongation	Pericardial effusions	Severe hypertension	Pneumonitis	Pulmonary edema	Pulmonary hypertension	Pleural effusions	Organizing pneumonia	Diffuse alveolar hemorrhage	SIADH – hyponatremia	Renal failure	Hemorrhagic cystitis	Bowel perforation	Neutropenic colitis	Pancreatitis	Hepatotoxicity	Adrenal insufficiency	Hypophysitis	Hyperglycemia	Thyroid disorders	Cytokine release syndrome	Differentiation syndrome	Opportunistic infections	Bleeding (severe)	Rhabdomyolysis	Stevens – Johnson syndrome or Toxic epidermal necrolysis	
Ifosfamide	X	X	X		X			X							X	X	X				X											See Note 68
Imatinib			X									X						X			X								X		X	See Note 69
Inotuzumab ozogamicin																					X											See Note 70
Ipilimumab	X		X						X				X			X		X		X	X	X	X		X						X	See Note 71
Irinotecan				X					X			X				X		X			X											See Note 72
Ixabepilone			X																		X											See Note 73
L-Asparaginase	X			X																X	X			X								See Note 74
Lapatinib			X			X		X													X										X	See Note 75
Lenalidomide				X					X												X				X						X	See Note 76
Lenvatinib	X		X			X		X								X		X		X	X				X				X			See Note 77
Lisocabtagene maraleucel	X	X	X		X											X										X		X				See Note 78
Mechlorethamine																												X				See Note 79
Melphalan									X						X						X											See Note 80
Methotrexate	X								X				X			X		X			X							X			X	See Note 81
Midostaurin									X															X								See Note 82
Mitomycin-C									X							X																See Note 83
Mitoxantrone									X																							See Note 84
Nab-paclitaxel			X	X																												See Note 85
Necitumumab			X	X																												See Note 86
Nelarabine	X	X																														See Note 87

68 Ifosfamide encephalopathy (ranging from mild somnolence to confusion and hallucinations to coma) may occur within hours to days after a dose. Risk factors for CNS toxicity include hypoalbuminemia, pre-existing renal dysfunction, concomitant use of aprepitant, and prior cisplatin exposure. IV albumin and thiamine supplementation are recommended for prevention. Encephalopathy typically resolves within 2–3 days after discontinuation; however, IV methylene blue may be considered as a treatment option. Cardiotoxicity including arrhythmias (i.e., SVT, atrial fibrillation, and pulseless ventricular tachycardia), heart failure with congestion and hypotension, pericardial effusion, fibrinous pericarditis, and epicardial fibrosis may occur. VOD has been reported in combination regimens [22, 183]

[69]Heart failure has been reported, although mostly in those with other comorbidities and risk factors, including advanced age and previous cardiac disease. Although rare, it is worth noting the reports of interstitial pneumonia. Median onset 7 weeks (1.5–40 weeks) and presentation includes low-grade fever, dry cough, and progressive dyspnea on exertion, with or without hypoxia. Management includes steroids and/or drug discontinuation of imatinib [175]

[70]VOD can occur during or after treatment. Median onset of VOD was 15 days (range, 3–57 days) for patients receiving stem cell transplant [123, 124]

[71]Pneumonitis: highest incidence when given with nivolumab (5–10% incidence) with median onset of symptoms 2.6 months following therapy initiation. Onset of GI symptoms is typically 6 weeks or more after initiating therapy. Moderate to severe endocrine disorders: median onset 2.2–2.5 months. Immune-mediated hepatitis (grade 3 or 4): median onset 2 months. Treat toxicities by holding ipilimumab and administering corticosteroids. Consider PJP and fungal prophylaxis in patients with prolonged corticosteroid exposure. Although rare, lethal myocarditis accompanied by myositis in patients treated with a combination of nivolumab and ipilimumab has been reported [34, 40, 42]

[72]Pulmonary toxicity more common with irinotecan than topotecan. Higher risk in patients with pre-existing lung disease, prior thoracic radiation, use of pneumotoxic drugs, and colony-stimulating factors. Severe/fatal diarrhea can occur with irinotecan. Early diarrhea (within 24 hrs) is accompanied by anticholinergic symptoms. Late diarrhea can occur more than 24 hrs following dose administration. Cases of megacolon and bowel perforation have been reported [192]

[73]MI and ventricular dysfunction have been reported [35]

[74]Noted complications typically occur after several weeks of treatment and often during the induction phase. Encephalopathy may be related to hyperammonemia and RPLS. Serious thrombotic events, including sagittal sinus thrombosis, have been reported [5, 78, 99, 125]

[75]Decreases in LVEF have been reported, usually within the first 3 months of treatment. Optimize serum potassium and magnesium levels prior to and during therapy. Case reports describe serious or fatal hepatotoxicity, usually 1–3 months following treatment initiation [165, 184, 185]

[76]Thromboprophylaxis with either aspirin or a LMWH should be considered for patients receiving lenalidomide in combination with chemotherapy and/or dexamethasone [140, 241]

[77]RPLS has been reported. Monitor for headache, seizure, lethargy, and hypertension. Median time to onset of new or worsening hypertension is 16–35 days. Can impair wound healing; should be held at least 6 days prior to surgical procedures [67]

[78]Lisocabtagene maraleucel is a CAR T-cell therapy undergoing FDA approval. Latest available data revealed a 1% incidence of severe CRS (35% any grade CRS) and 12% incidence of severe ICANS (19% any grade ICANS). Management of CRS and/or ICANS is grading dependent but may include supportive care, tocilizumab, and/or systemic corticosteroids. Anti-seizure, PJP, and HSV prophylaxis similar to other CAR T-cell therapies should be considered [119]

[79]PJP and CMV pneumonia have occurred due to severe and prolonged neutropenia. Consider PJP prophylaxis and CMV monitoring [43]

[80]GI toxicity, including grade 3/4 mucositis, has been reported with high-dose melphalan. Cryotherapy may help prevent/reduce mucositis severity [95]

[81]Glucarpidase may be considered for patients receiving high-dose methotrexate (HDMTX) with delayed clearance (serum methotrexate levels > 1 µmol/L beyond 42 h after the start of HDMTX infusion) and renal dysfunction (serum creatinine >1.3 mg/dL or > 50% increase from baseline). Leucovorin calcium should not be administered within 2 h of glucarpidase due to competing binding sites. Intrathecal methotrexate is commonly associated with aseptic meningitis characterized by fever, headache, and vomiting that can last several days. Generalized and focal seizures have been reported. Methotrexate may increase the risk of developing life-threatening opportunistic infections. Do not initiate penicillins, fluoroquinolones, sulfonamide antibiotics, nonsteroidal anti-inflammatory drugs, or proton pump inhibitors until methotrexate has cleared [80, 129]

[82]Fatal events involving pulmonary toxicity have occurred [232]

[83]Infrequent but severe pulmonary toxicity (e.g., ARDS) has been reported. HUS and subsequent renal failure have been reported. Dose-related pulmonary toxicity (>20 mg/m^2) [138, 177, 234, 248]

[84]Onset of cardiotoxic effects of anthracyclines can occur during or immediately after infusion (acute onset), within 1 year of exposure (early onset), and from 1–20 years (late onset) after initial exposure. Factors increasing the risk of cardiac toxicity include the extent of anthracycline exposure, higher doses, older age, pre-existing cardiac disease, concurrent or previous mediastinal radiation therapy, and concomitant administration of cardiotoxic chemotherapy regimens such as paclitaxel or trastuzumab. Estimated risk of CHF is 2.6% for doses up to 140 mg/m^2 [74]

[85][1]

[86]Cardiopulmonary arrest and/or sudden death has been reported in patients treated with necitumumab in combination with gemcitabine and cisplatin. Severe hypomagnesemia is common in those treated with necitumumab, gemcitabine, and cisplatin, with a median onset of 6 weeks. Optimize serum potassium, magnesium, and calcium during and for at least 8 weeks following administration. Cerebral stroke and MI have also been reported [68, 240]

[87]Most neurologic toxicities occur within 12 days of infusion or after successive cycles of therapy. The most common grade 3/4 neurologic adverse events reported include confusion, malaise, somnolence, ataxia, muscle weakness, and peripheral neuropathies [121, 130]

Table 1F

Drug	Neuro		Cardiac						Pulmonary						Renal		GI					Endocrine				Miscellaneous						Notes
	Encephalopathy	Seizures	Heart failure	Thromboembolism	Arrhythmias	QT prolongation	Pericardial effusions	Severe hypertension	Pneumonitis	Pulmonary edema	Pulmonary hypertension	Pleural effusions	Organizing pneumonia	Diffuse alveolar hemorrhage	SIADH – hyponatremia	Renal failure	Hemorrhagic cystitis	Bowel perforation	Neutropenic colitis	Pancreatitis	Hepatotoxicity	Adrenal insufficiency	Hypophysitis	Hyperglycemia	Thyroid disorders	Cytokine release syndrome	Differentiation syndrome	Opportunistic infections	Bleeding (severe)	Rhabdomyolysis	Stevens – Johnson syndrome or Toxic epidermal necrolysis	
Nilotinib						X	X			X		X								X	X			X					X		X	See Note 88
Niraparib								X																								See Note 89
Nivolumab	X								X						X	X				X	X	X	X	X	X					X	X	See Note 90
Obinutuzumab																												X			X	See Note 91
Ofatumumab																												X			X	See Note 92
Olaparib									X			X		X																		See Note 93
Osimertinib			X			X			X				X	X							X											See Note 94
Oxaliplatin	X	X			X	X		X	X																					X		See Note 95
Paclitaxel								X	X																						X	See Note 96
Palbociclib		X		X																												See Note 97
Panitumumab				X					X				X																		X	See Note 98
Panobinostat					X	X																										See Note 99
Pazopanib	X		X	X		X		X	X									X		X	X				X				X		X	See Note 100
PEG-asparaginase	X			X																X	X			X								See Note 101
Pembrolizumab	X								X				X		X	X				X	X	X	X	X	X						X	See Note 102
Pemetrexed								X	X							X															X	See Note 103
Pentostatin																X					X							X				See Note 104
Pertuzumab			X	X																												See Note 105
Pomalidomide								X	X												X				X						X	See Note 106
Ponatinib			X	X	X	X	X	X												X	X								X			See Note 107
Pralatrexate			X	X	X	X	X														X										X	See Note 108

88 Risk of QT prolongation warrants a baseline 12-lead EKG with repeat assessment after 7 days of therapy, following any dose change, and regularly during treatment. Optimize serum potassium and magnesium levels prior to and during therapy. Biochemical abnormalities are common (i.e., increased lipase, glucose, total bilirubin, ALT) [4, 94, 103, 135, 172, 198]

89 Hypertensive crisis has been reported [237]

90 May cause severe immune-mediated adverse events including pneumonitis, median onset 1.6–3.5 months (1 day to 22.3 months); nephritis, 2.7–4.6 months (9 days to 12.3 months); hepatitis, 2.1–3.3 months (6 days to 11 months); colitis, 1.6–5.3 months (2 days to 21 months); adrenal insufficiency (across several clinical trials), 3–4.3 months (15 days to 21 months);

hyperthyroidism, 23 days to 1.5 months (1 day to 14.2 months); hypothyroidism, 2–3 months (1 day to 16.6 months); and hypophysitis, 4.9 months (1.4–11 months). May aggravate underlying autoimmune disorders. Management includes holding therapy, systemic corticosteroids, and +/− additional immunosuppressants (e.g., infliximab, mycophenolate, and vedolizumab). Consider PJP prophylaxis in patients with prolonged corticosteroid exposure. Although rare, lethal myocarditis accompanied by myositis in patients treated with a combination of nivolumab and ipilimumab has been reported [33, 36, 116, 133, 159, 160]

[91]HBV reactivation may occur during and up to 24 months after discontinuation of anti-CD20 antibodies. Patients on antiviral prophylaxis should continue for 6–12 months after completing treatment. JC virus infection resulting in PML has been reported [32, 106]

[92]HBV reactivation may occur during and up to 24 months after discontinuation of anti-CD20 antibodies. Patients on antiviral prophylaxis should continue for 6–12 months after completing treatment. Fatal cases of PML have been reported [32, 106]

[93][14, 64]

[94][18]

[95]Ventricular arrhythmias, including fatal Torsades de Pointes, have been reported. RPLS has been reported. Monitor for headache, seizure, lethargy, and hypertension [154, 204, 211, 222]

[96][29, 162]

[97][191]

[98]Monitor for hypomagnesemia and hypocalcemia prior to, during and up to 8 weeks after therapy. Severe dermatologic complications may effect up to 15% of patients and can lead to life-threatening infectious complications such as necrotizing fasciitis and abscesses [8, 179]

[99]QT prolongation is a class effect of HDAC inhibitors, although the incidence may be lower than initially reported. Optimize serum potassium and magnesium levels prior to and during therapy [173, 205]

[100]RPLS is rare but serious. Monitor for headache, seizure, lethargy, and hypertension. Some fatal cases of hepatotoxicity have been reported. Serum hepatic enzyme elevations generally occur within 4–12 weeks. The most common hemorrhagic events were hematuria (4%), epistaxis (2%), hemoptysis (2%), and rectal hemorrhage. Rare cases of hypertensive crisis have been reported, most cases of hypertension within first 18 weeks of therapy. TMA including TTP and HUS can occur, generally within 3 months of treatment initiation [136, 158, 166, 209]

[101]Complications typically occur after several weeks of treatment during the induction phase. Clinical symptoms suggestive of pancreatitis have been reported to occur within 15 days of treatment [65]

[102]May cause severe immune-mediated adverse events including pneumonitis median onset 3.3 months (2 days to ~19 months) and is more common with prior thoracic radiation, hepatitis 1.3 months (8 days to 21.4 months), colitis 3.5 months (10 days to 16.2 months), autoimmune nephritis 5.1 months (12 days to 12.8 months), hyperthyroidism 1.4 months (1 day to ~22 months), and hypothyroidism 3.5 months (1 day to 19 months). May aggravate underlying autoimmune disorders. Management includes holding therapy, systemic corticosteroids, and +/− additional immunosuppressants (e.g., infliximab, mycophenolate, and vedolizumab). Consider PJP prophylaxis in patients with prolonged corticosteroid exposure [33, 148, 159, 160]

[103]Prophylactic folic acid and vitamin B12 supplementation should be provided while receiving pemetrexed to reduce the risk of hematologic toxicity. Renal damage ranges from acute to chronic kidney injury due to tubular and interstitial damage [70, 252]

[104]Consider HSV/VZV prophylaxis [105, 142]

[105]Prior anthracycline therapy or chest irradiation may increase the risk for cardiotoxicity (risk is lower than that seen with trastuzumab) [83, 235]

[106]Thromboprophylaxis with either aspirin or a LMWH should be considered for patients receiving pomalidomide in combination with chemotherapy and/or dexamethasone [49, 92].

[107]Vigilant monitoring for vascular events is recommended (i.e., MI, stroke, stenosis of large arterial vessels of the brain, severe peripheral vascular disease). Vascular occlusion/events can occur within weeks of starting therapy and is not dose dependent and requires interruption or permanent discontinuation of therapy. Arrhythmias, such as atrial fibrillation and symptomatic bradycardia, have been reported. Hypertension can be severe and should be managed as clinically indicated. Hepatotoxicity: median onset 3 months (range, less than 1 month to 47 months); may require treatment interruption or discontinuation. Bleeding can occur during therapy, particularly in patients with accelerated or blast phase disease and thrombocytopenia. RPLS has been reported. Monitor for headache, seizure, lethargy, and hypertension [53, 54, 139, 155, 247]

[108]Prophylactic folic acid and vitamin B12 supplementation are necessary to reduce hematologic toxicity [6]

Table 1G

Drug	Neuro		Cardiac						Pulmonary						Renal		GI					Endocrine				Miscellaneous						Notes
	Encephalopathy	Seizures	Heart failure	Thromboembolism	Arrhythmias	QT prolongation	Pericardial effusions	Severe hypertension	Pneumonitis	Pulmonary edema	Pulmonary hypertension	Pleural effusions	Organizing pneumonia	Diffuse alveolar hemorrhage	SIADH – hyponatremia	Renal failure	Hemorrhagic cystitis	Bowel perforation	Neutropenic colitis	Pancreatitis	Hepatotoxicity	Adrenal insufficiency	Hypophysitis	Hyperglycemia	Thyroid disorders	Cytokine release syndrome	Differentiation syndrome	Opportunistic infections	Bleeding (severe)	Rhabdomyolysis	Stevens–Johnson syndrome or Toxic epidermal necrolysis	Notes
Ramucirumab	X			X				X										X							X				X			See Note 109
Regorafenib	X							X										X			X								X		X	See Note 110
Ribociclib				X		X															X											See Note 111
Rituximab						X												X													X	See Note 112
Romidepsin					X																							X				See Note 113
Ruxolitinib																												X	X			See Note 114
Sipuleucel-T				X																				X								See Note 115
Sonidegib																X													X			See Note 116
Sorafenib	X		X	X		X		X	X									X		X	X				X				X		X	See Note 117
Sunitinib	X		X	X		X		X	X											X	X				X				X			See Note 118
Temozolomide									X												X							X			X	See Note 119
Thalidomide		X		X	X																				X							See Note 120
Thiotepa	X																				X									X	X	See Note 121
Tisagenlecleucel	X	X	X		X				X							X					X					X		X		X		See Note 122
Topotecan		X	X						X										X													See Note 123
Trabectedin			X	X														X			X									X		See Note 124
Trametinib			X			X		X	X			X	X											X					X	X		See Note 125
Trastuzumab			X		X			X	X			X	X																			See Note 126
Tretinoin (all-trans retinoic acid)										X						X					X						X		X			See Note 127

[109] Serious, sometimes fatal, MI, cardiac arrest, and CVA events have occurred in clinical trials. Can impair wound healing; therapy should be held prior to surgical procedures. Rates of hemorrhage or GI perforation unknown in patients on chronic NSAIDs or anticoagulation as many studies excluded these patients; therefore, use cautiously in combination with these agents [10, 71]

[110] Can impair wound healing. Discontinue 2 weeks prior to surgical procedures and resume once wound has healed. RPLS has been reported. Monitor for headache, seizure, lethargy, and hypertension [25, 158]

[111] Monitor and optimize serum potassium, calcium, phosphorus, and magnesium before and during therapy as electrolyte imbalances may occur to reduce risk of cardiotoxicity. Median onset of grade 3 or higher transaminase elevations ~2 months, with median time to resolution to grade 2 or lower of 24 days [104, 169]

[112]Abdominal pain, bowel obstruction, and perforation have been reported, with an average onset of symptoms ~6 days (1–77 days). JC virus infection resulting in PML has been reported. Median time to PML diagnosis 16 months following rituximab initiation and median time from last rituximab dose 5.5 months. HBV reactivation may occur during and up to 24 months after discontinuation of anti-CD20 antibodies. Patients on antiviral prophylaxis should continue for 6–12 months after completing treatment [32, 47, 106]

[113]QT prolongation is a class effect of HDAC inhibitors, although the incidence may be lower than initially reported. Optimize serum potassium, magnesium, and calcium levels prior to and during therapy. Viral reactivation has occurred during and within 30 days of initiation. Consider antiviral prophylaxis for patients with history of EBV or HBV [50, 205]

[114]Bacterial, mycobacterial, fungal, and viral infections have occurred including TB, PML, HSV/VZV and increased HBV viral load. Withdrawal syndrome can occur with abrupt discontinuation of treatment and is characterized by acute relapse of disease symptoms such as accelerated splenomegaly, worsening cytopenias, and sepsis-like syndrome. It can be managed with corticosteroids with a slow taper off [108]

[115]Vascular disorders including MI and stroke have been reported. Acute infusion reactions within 1 day of infusion have been reported [61].

[116]CPK elevations > grade 2 occur at a median of 13 weeks. CPK levels should be monitored at baseline and periodically during therapy. Rare cases of rhabdomyolysis have been reported [110, 233]

[117]HF, myocardial ischemia, and/or MI have been reported. Acute liver injury generally occurs a few days to up to 8 weeks after treatment initiation. Possible impaired wound healing. RPLS can rarely occur. Monitor for headache, seizure, lethargy, and hypertension [24, 216]

[118]RPLS can rarely occur. Case reports have occurred 1–34 weeks following treatment initiation. Monitor for headache, seizure, lethargy, and hypertension. Cardiac events including myocardial ischemia, MI, reductions in LVEF, and cardiac failure including death have occurred [56, 156, 158, 189]

[119]PJP prophylaxis is recommended [147]

[120]VTE, including ischemic heart disease, MI, and CVA have occurred in patients receiving thalidomide and dexamethasone. Thromboprophylaxis with either aspirin or a LMWH should be considered for patients receiving thalidomide in combination with chemotherapy and/or dexamethasone. Seizures and bradycardia have been reported in postmarketing data [51]

[121]Parent drug and/or metabolites may be partially excreted through the skin; severe blistering and desquamation can occur. As a result, patients should shower/bathe at least twice daily while receiving treatment and during the 48 h following therapy. Hepatotoxicity refers to VOD, which has been reported when high doses are used in combination with other chemotherapy as part of a conditioning regimen for stem cell transplant [58, 257]

[122]CRS: Median onset 3 days (1–22 days); median duration 8 days (1–36 days). Monitor for signs or symptoms of CRS for at least 4 weeks after treatment. Key manifestations include high fever, hypotension, and shortness of breath and may be associated with hepatic, renal, and cardiac dysfunction and coagulopathy. Risk factors for severe CRS are high pre-infusion tumor burden (>50% blasts in bone marrow), uncontrolled or accelerating tumor burden following lymphodepleting chemotherapy (fludarabine and cyclophosphamide), active infections, and/or inflammatory processes

ICANS: Most neurological toxicities occurred within 8 weeks and generally resolved within 12 days. Most common neurological toxicities include headache, encephalopathy, delirium, anxiety, and tremor. Fatal and serious cases of cerebral edema have occurred; other serious events included leukoencephalopathy and seizures.

Management of CRS with or without ICANS depends on grading or severity but includes supportive care, tocilizumab, and/or systemic corticosteroids. Grade 2 or higher ICANS without CRS should be treated with corticosteroids alone as there is insufficient data with tocilizumab in this setting. Other interleukin antagonists (e.g., siltuximab) and anti-T cell therapies are currently being evaluated.

Hypogammaglobulinemia secondary to B-cell aplasia may persist for up to 13 months and increase the risk for infections. PJP and HSV prophylaxis are recommended for at least 1 year after CAR-T cell therapy [143, 174]

[123]Post-marketing cases of ILD have been reported. Higher risk in patients with baseline interstitial lung disease, pulmonary fibrosis, lung cancer, thoracic exposure to radiation, use of pneumotoxic drugs, and/or colony-stimulating factors [168]

[124]Grade 3 or 4 CPK elevations have been reported with a median onset of 2 months and resolving in ~2 weeks with dose interruption, reduction, discontinuation, or delay. Capillary leak syndrome has been reported [112]

[125]Cardiomyopathy: median onset in melanoma patients for single-agent trametinib ~2 months (2–22 weeks) and ~8 months (~1–25 months) when used in combination with dabrafenib, in patients with NSCLC 6.7 months (1.4–14.1 months). Pneumonitis: median time to initial presentation in melanoma patients ~5 months (2 to ~6 months). Risk of GI perforation is 0.3% when administered with dabrafenib. Grade 3/4 hyperglycemia reported when used in combination with dabrafenib [170]

[126]Highest incidence of cardiomyopathy in patients receiving trastuzumab with an anthracycline. Reversible upon discontinuation of trastuzumab [81, 96]

[127]Differentiation syndrome is commonly associated with the development of hyperleukocytosis, pulmonary edema, generalized edema, headache, bone pain, and renal failure; bimodal with peaks occurring in the first and third weeks after the start of therapy. Management includes steroids, with or without diuretics, and possible discontinuation of tretinoin, depending on severity [59, 153]

Table 1H

	Encephalopathy (Neuro)	Seizures	Heart failure (Cardiac)	Thromboembolism	Arrhythmias	QT prolongation	Pericardial effusions	Severe hypertension	Pneumonitis (Pulmonary)	Pulmonary edema	Pulmonary hypertension	Pleural effusions	Organizing pneumonia	Diffuse alveolar hemorrhage	SIADH – hyponatremia (Renal)	Renal failure	Hemorrhagic cystitis (GI)	Bowel perforation	Neutropenic colitis	Pancreatitis	Hepatotoxicity	Adrenal insufficiency (Endocrine)	Hypophysitis	Hyperglycemia	Thyroid disorders	Cytokine release syndrome (Misc)	Differentiation syndrome	Opportunistic infections	Bleeding (severe)	Rhabdomyolysis	Stevens–Johnson syndrome or Toxic epidermal necrolysis	Notes
Vandetanib	X		X			X		X	X									X		X					X				X	X	X	See Note 128
Vemurafenib						X		X								X				X				X						X	X	See Note 129
Vinblastine															X																	See Note 130
Vincristine	X	X													X			X														See Note 131
Vinorelbine	X					X			X						X					X	X											See Note 132
Vismodegib				X											X															X		See Note 133
Vorinostat						X																		X								See Note 134

[128]ischemic cerebrovascular events have been reported – monitor for headache, seizure, lethargy, and hypertension. Optimize serum potassium, magnesium, and calcium levels prior to and during therapy. Rare cases of GI perforation. Due to long half-life (19 days), adverse reactions, including QT prolongation, may resolve slowly [214, 254]

[129]Optimize serum potassium, magnesium, and calcium levels prior to and during therapy to reduce risk of cardiotoxicity. AIN and ATN have been reported. Hypersensitivity: anaphylaxis and DRESS syndrome have been reported. Pancreatitis generally occurs within 2 weeks of treatment initiation [90, 157, 251, 255, 256]

[130]Paralytic ileus and obstruction may occur, although to a lesser extent than that observed with other vinca alkaloids

[131]Known to affect the cranial nerves resulting in ptosis, diplopia, and facial palsies. Paresthesias involving the hands and feet often occur within weeks of therapy and depending on severity and may require several months to resolve following drug discontinuation. Loss of motor involvement is possible as well (i.e., foot and hand drop, loss of deep tendon reflexes, weakness in the lower and upper extremities). Acute GI symptoms such as constipation and abdominal pain commonly occur within a few days of therapy, with more serious GI toxicities including adynamic ileus and bowel obstruction. SIADH-induced hyponatremia has led to seizures [200]

[132]May cause severe paralytic ileus [44, 188]

[133]May cause CPK elevations; rare occurrence of rhabdomyolysis [88]

[134]QT prolongation is a class effect of HDAC inhibitors, although the incidence may be lower than initially reported. Optimize serum potassium and magnesium levels prior to and during therapy [205]

5-FU, 5-fluorouracil; AIN, acute interstitial nephritis; ALK, anaplastic lymphoma kinase; ALT, alanine transaminase; AST, aspartate aminotransferase; ATN, acute tubular necrosis; BTK, Bruton's tyrosine kinase; CD4, cluster of differentiation 4; CLL, chronic lymphocytic leukemia; CMV, cytomegalovirus; CNS, central nervous system; COPD, chronic obstructive pulmonary disease; CPK, creatine phosphokinase; CRS, cytokine release syndrome; CVA, cerebrovascular accident; DLCO, diffusing capacity of carbon monoxide; DRESS, drug reaction with eosinophilia and systemic symptoms; EBV, Epstein-Barr virus; EKG, electrocardiogram; FVC, forced vital capacity; GI, gastrointestinal; HBV, hepatitis B virus; HDAC, histone deacetylase; HF, heart failure; HLH, hemophagocytic lymphohistiocytosis; HMG-CoA, hydroxymethylglutaryl coenzyme A; HUS, hemolytic uremic syndrome; ICANS, immune effector cell-associated neurotoxicity syndrome; ILD, interstitial lung disease; IV, intravenous; JC virus, John Cunningham virus; LMWH, low molecular weight heparin; LVEF, left ventricular ejection fraction; MAS, macrophage activation syndrome; MI, myocardial infarction; NSCLC, non-small cell lung cancer; PD-1, programmed cell death 1; PJP, Pneumocystis jiroveci pneumonia; PK, pharmacokinetics; PML, progressive multifocal leukoencephalopathy; REMS, risk evaluation and mitigation strategy; RPLS, reversible posterior leukoencephalopathy syndrome; SJS, Stevens-Johnson syndrome; TB, tuberculosis; TBI, total body irradiation; TEN, toxic epidermal necrolysis; TMA, thrombotic microangiopathy; TSH, thyroid-stimulating hormone; TTP, thrombotic thrombocytopenic purpura; ULN, upper limit of normal; VOD, veno-occlusive disease; VTE, venous thromboembolism; VZV, varicella zoster virus

References

1. Abraxis Bioscience LLC. Abraxane (paclitaxel protein-bound particles) [package insert]. Summit; 2017.
2. Accord Healthcare Inc. Toposar (etoposide) [package insert]. Durham; 2014.
3. Ahn IE, Jerussi T, Farooqui M, Tian X, Wiestner A, Gea-Banacloche J. Atypical Pneumocystis jirovecii pneumonia in previously untreated patients with CLL on single-agent ibrutinib. Blood. 2016;128 (15):1940–3. https://doi.org/10.1182/blood-2016-06-722991.
4. Aichberger KJ, Herndlhofer S, Schernthaner GH, Schillinger M, Mitterbauer-Hohendanner G, Sillaber C, Valent P. Progressive peripheral arterial occlusive disease and other vascular events during nilotinib therapy in CML. Am J Hematol. 2011; 86(7):533–9. https://doi.org/10.1002/ajh.22037.
5. Aldoss I, Douer D, Behrendt CE, Chaudhary P, Mohrbacher A, Vrona J, Pullarkat V. Toxicity profile of repeated doses of PEG-asparaginase incorporated into a pediatric-type regimen for adult acute lymphoblastic leukemia. Eur J Haematol. 2016;96(4): 375–80. https://doi.org/10.1111/ejh.12600.
6. Allos Therapeutics. Folotyn (pralatrexate) [package insert]. Westminister; 2009.
7. Amgen. Blincyto® (Blinatumomab) [package insert]. Thousand Oaks; 2017a.
8. Amgen. Vectibix (panitumumab) [package insert]. Thousand Oaks; 2017b.
9. Ariad Pharmaceuticals Inc. Alunbrig (brigatinib) [package insert]. Cambridge, MA; 2017.
10. Arnold D, Fuchs CS, Tabernero J, Ohtsu A, Zhu AX, Garon EB, Mackey JR, Paz-Ares L, Baron AD, Okusaka T, Yoshino T, Yoon HH, Das M, Ferry D, Zhang Y, Lin Y, Binder P, Sashegyi A, Chau I. Meta-analysis of individual patient safety data from six randomized, placebo-controlled trials with the anti-angiogenic VEGFR2-binding monoclonal antibody ramucirumab. Ann Oncol. 2017;28(12):2932–42. https://doi.org/10.1093/annonc/mdx514.
11. Asbury RF, Rosenthal SN, Descalzi ME, Ratcliffe RL, Arseneau JC. Hepatic veno-occlusive disease due to DTIC. Cancer. 1980;45(10):2670–4.
12. AstraZeneca. Imfinzi (durvalumab) [package insert]. Wilmington; 2016.
13. AstraZeneca Pharmaceuticals. Calquence (acalabrutinib) [package insert]. Wilmington; 2017a.
14. AstraZeneca Pharmaceuticals. Lynparza (olaparib) capsules [package insert]. Wilmington; 2017b.
15. Au TH, Cavalieri CC, Stenehjem DD. Ceritinib: a primer for pharmacists. J Oncol Pharm Pract. 2017;23(8): 602–14. https://doi.org/10.1177/1078155216672315.
16. Azambuja E, Fleck JF, Batista RG, Menna Barreto SS. Bleomycin lung toxicity: who are the patients with increased risk? Pulm Pharmacol Ther. 2005;18(5): 363–6. https://doi.org/10.1016/j.pupt.2005.01.007.
17. AztraZeneca Pharmaceuticals LP. Iressa (gefitinib) [package insert]. Wilmington; 2015.
18. AztraZeneca Pharmaceuticals LP. Tagrisso (osimertinib) [package insert]. Wilmington; 2017.
19. Baker WJ, Royer GL Jr, Weiss RB. Cytarabine and neurologic toxicity. J Clin Oncol. 1991;9(4):679–93. https://doi.org/10.1200/jco.1991.9.4.679.
20. Baron M, Zini JM, Challan Belval T, Vignon M, Denis B, Alanio A, Malphettes M. Fungal infections in patients treated with ibrutinib: two unusual cases of invasive aspergillosis and cryptococcal meningoencephalitis. Leuk Lymphoma. 2017;58(12):2981–2. https://doi.org/10.1080/10428194.2017.1320710.
21. Baxter. Cyclophosphamide Injection [package insert]. Deerfield; 2015.
22. Baxter Healthcare Corp. Ifex (ifosfamide) [prescribing information]. Deerfield; 2014.
23. Bayer Healthcare Pharmaceuticals Inc. Aliqopa (copanlisib) [package insert]. Whippany; 2017a.
24. Bayer Healthcare Pharmaceuticals Inc. Nexevar (sorafenib) [package insert]. Whippany; 2017b.
25. Bayer HealthCare Pharmaceuticals Inc. Stivarga (regorafenib) [package insert]. Whippany; 2017c.
26. Bedford Laboratories. Adriamycin (doxorubicin HCL) [package insert]. Bedford; 2012.
27. Bedford Laboratories. Daunorubicin hydrochloride injection [package insert]. Bedford; 2013.
28. Bergeron A, Rea D, Levy V, Picard C, Meignin V, Tamburini J, Bruzzoni-Giovanelli H, Calvo F, Tazi A, Rousselot P. Lung abnormalities after dasatinib treatment for chronic myeloid leukemia: a case series. Am J Respir Crit Care Med. 2007;176(8):814–8. https://doi.org/10.1164/rccm.200705-715CR.
29. Bielopolski D, Evron E, Moreh-Rahav O, Landes M, Stemmer SM, Salamon F. Paclitaxel-induced pneumonitis in patients with breast cancer: case series and review of the literature. J chemother (Florence, Italy). 2017;29(2):113–7. https://doi.org/10.1179/1973947 815y.0000000029.
30. Blake-Haskins JA, Lechleider RJ, Kreitman RJ. Thrombotic microangiopathy with targeted cancer agents. Clin Cancer Res. 2011;17(18):5858–66. https://doi.org/10.1158/1078-0432.Ccr-11-0804.
31. Boehringer-ingelheim. Gilotrif (afatinib) [package insert]. Ridgfield; 2018.
32. Bohra C, Sokol L, Dalia S. Progressive multifocal leukoencephalopathy and monoclonal antibodies: a review. Cancer Control. 2017;24(4): 1073274817729901. https://doi.org/10.1177/107327 4817729901.
33. Brahmer JR, Lacchetti C, Schneider BJ, Atkins MB, Brassil KJ, Caterino JM, Chau I, Ernstoff MS, Gardner JM, Ginex P, Hallmeyer S, Holter Chakrabarty J, Leighl NB, Mammen JS, McDermott DF, Naing A, Nastoupil LJ, Phillips T, Porter LD, Puzanov I, Reichner CA, Santomasso BD, Seigel C, Spira A, Suarez-Almazor ME, Wang Y, Weber JS, Wolchok JD, Thompson JA. Management of immune-related adverse events in patients treated with immune

checkpoint inhibitor therapy: American society of clinical oncology clinical practice guideline. J Clin Oncol. 2018a;36:1714–68. https://doi.org/10.1200/jco.2017.77.6385.

34. Brahmer JR, Lacchetti C, Schneider BJ, et al. Management of immune-related adverse events in patients treated with immune checkpoint inhibitor therapy: American society of clinical oncology clinical practice guideline. J Clin Oncol. 2018b;36:1714–68. (Published online: February 14, 2018).

35. Bristol-Myers Squibb. Ixempra (ixabepilone) [package insert]. Princeton; 2007.

36. Bristol-Myers Squibb. Opdivo (nivolumab) [package insert]. Princeton; 2018.

37. Bristol-Myers Squibb Company. Blenoxane (bleomycin) [package insert]. Princeton; 2010a.

38. Bristol-Myers Squibb Company. Platinol (cisplatin) [package insert]. Princeton; 2010b.

39. Bristol-Myers Squibb Company. Sprycel (dasatinib) [package insert]. Princeton; 2017a.

40. Bristol-Myers Squibb Company. Yervoy (ipilimumab) [package insert]. Princeton; 2017b.

41. Byrd JC, Harrington B, O'Brien S, Jones JA, Schuh A, Devereux S, Chaves J, Wierda WG, Awan FT, Brown JR, Hillmen P, Stephens DM, Ghia P, Barrientos JC, Pagel JM, Woyach J, Johnson D, Huang J, Wang X, Kaptein A, Lannutti BJ, Covey T, Fardis M, McGreivy J, Hamdy A, Rothbaum W, Izumi R, Diacovo TG, Johnson AJ, Furman RR. Acalabrutinib (ACP-196) in Relapsed Chronic Lymphocytic Leukemia. N Engl J Med. 2016;374(4):323–32. https://doi.org/10.1056/NEJMoa1509981.

42. Camacho LH. CTLA-4 blockade with ipilimumab: biology, safety, efficacy, and future considerations. Cancer Med. 2015;4(5):661–72. https://doi.org/10.1002/cam4.371.

43. Canellos GP, Anderson JR, Propert KJ, Nissen N, Cooper MR, Henderson ES, Green MR, Gottlieb A, Peterson BA. Chemotherapy of advanced Hodgkin's disease with MOPP, ABVD, or MOPP alternating with ABVD. N Engl J Med. 1992;327(21):1478–84. https://doi.org/10.1056/nejm199211193272102.

44. Canzler U, Schmidt-Gohrich UK, Bergmann S, Hanseroth K, Gatzweiler A, Distler W. Syndrome of inappropriate antidiuretic hormone secretion (SIADH) induced by vinorelbine treatment of metastatic breast cancer. Onkologie. 2007;30(8–9):455–6. https://doi.org/10.1159/000105143.

45. Carilli A, Favis G, Sundharkrishnan L, Hajdenberg J. Severe dermatologic reactions with bendamustine: a case series. Case Rep Oncol. 2014;7(2):465–70. https://doi.org/10.1159/000365324.

46. Carron PL, Cousin L, Caps T, Belle E, Pernet D, Neidhardt A, Capellier G. Gemcitabine-associated diffuse alveolar hemorrhage. Intensive Care Med. 2001;27(9):1554. https://doi.org/10.1007/s001340101037.

47. Carson KR, Evens AM, Richey EA, Habermann TM, Focosi D, Seymour JF, Laubach J, Bawn SD, Gordon LI, Winter JN, Furman RR, Vose JM, Zelenetz AD, Mamtani R, Raisch DW, Dorshimer GW, Rosen ST, Muro K, Gottardi-Littell NR, Talley RL, Sartor O, Green D, Major EO, Bennett CL. Progressive multifocal leukoencephalopathy after rituximab therapy in HIV-negative patients: a report of 57 cases from the Research on Adverse Drug Events and Reports project. Blood. 2009;113(20):4834–40. https://doi.org/10.1182/blood-2008-10-186999.

48. Carson KR, Newsome SD, Kim EJ, Wagner-Johnston ND, von Geldern G, Moskowitz CH, Moskowitz AJ, Rook AH, Jalan P, Loren AW, Landsburg D, Coyne T, Tsai D, Raisch DW, Norris LB, Bookstaver PB, Sartor O, Bennett CL. Progressive multifocal leukoencephalopathy associated with brentuximab vedotin therapy: a report of 5 cases from the Southern Network on Adverse Reactions (SONAR) project. Cancer. 2014;120(16):2464–71. https://doi.org/10.1002/cncr.28712.

49. Celegene Corporation. Pomalyst (pomalidomide) [package insert]. Summit; 2018.

50. Celgene Corporation. 2016 Istodax (romidepsin) [package insert]. Summit; 2018.

51. Celgene Corporation. Thalomid (thalidomide) [package insert]. Summit; 2017.

52. Ciurea SO, Andersson BS. Busulfan in hematopoietic stem cell transplantation. Biol Blood Marrow Transplant. 2009;15(5):523–36. https://doi.org/10.1016/j.bbmt.2008.12.489.

53. Cortes JE, Kantarjian H, Shah NP, Bixby D, Mauro MJ, Flinn I, O'Hare T, Hu S, Narasimhan NI, Rivera VM, Clackson T, Turner CD, Haluska FG, Druker BJ, Deininger MW, Talpaz M. Ponatinib in refractory Philadelphia chromosome-positive leukemias. N Engl J Med. 2012;367(22):2075–88. https://doi.org/10.1056/NEJMoa1205127.

54. Cortes JE, Kim DW, Pinilla-Ibarz J, le Coutre P, Paquette R, Chuah C, Nicolini FE, Apperley JF, Khoury HJ, Talpaz M, DiPersio J, DeAngelo DJ, Abruzzese E, Rea D, Baccarani M, Muller MC, Gambacorti-Passerini C, Wong S, Lustgarten S, Rivera VM, Clackson T, Turner CD, Haluska FG, Guilhot F, Deininger MW, Hochhaus A, Hughes T, Goldman JM, Shah NP, Kantarjian H. A phase 2 trial of ponatinib in Philadelphia chromosome-positive leukemias. N Engl J Med. 2013;369(19):1783–96. https://doi.org/10.1056/NEJMoa1306494.

55. Cortes JE, Saglio G, Kantarjian HM, Baccarani M, Mayer J, Boque C, Shah NP, Chuah C, Casanova L, Bradley-Garelik B, Manos G, Hochhaus A. Final 5-year study results of DASISION: the dasatinib versus imatinib study in treatment-naive chronic myeloid leukemia patients trial. J Clin Oncol. 2016;34(20):2333–40. https://doi.org/10.1200/jco.2015.64.8899.

56. Costa R, Costa R, Costa R, Junior GM, Cartaxo HQ, de Barros AC. Reversible posterior encephalopathy syndrome secondary to sunitinib. Case Rep Oncol Med. 2014;2014:952624. https://doi.org/10.1155/2014/952624.

57. Cowman S, Stebbing J, Tuthill M. Large bowel perforation associated with capecitabine treatment for breast cancer. Ann Oncol. 2008;19(8):1510–1. https://doi.org/10.1093/annonc/mdn397.

58. Dalle JH, Giralt SA. Hepatic veno-occlusive disease after hematopoietic stem cell transplantation: risk factors and stratification, prophylaxis, and treatment. Biol Blood Marrow Transplant. 2016;22(3):400–9. https://doi.org/10.1016/j.bbmt.2015.09.024.

59. De Botton S, Dombret H, Sanz M, Miguel JS, Caillot D, Zittoun R, Gardembas M, Stamatoulas A, Conde E, Guerci A, Gardin C, Geiser K, Makhoul DC, Reman O, de la Serna J, Lefrere F, Chomienne C, Chastang C, Degos L, Fenaux P. Incidence, clinical features, and outcome of all trans-retinoic acid syndrome in 413 cases of newly diagnosed acute promyelocytic leukemia. The European APL Group. Blood. 1998;92(8):2712–8.

60. de Forni M, Malet-Martino MC, Jaillais P, Shubinski RE, Bachaud JM, Lemaire L, Canal P, Chevreau C, Carrie D, Soulie P, et al. Cardiotoxicity of high-dose continuous infusion fluorouracil: a prospective clinical study. J Clin Oncol. 1992;10(11):1795–801. https://doi.org/10.1200/jco.1992.10.11.1795.

61. Dendreon Corporation. Provenge (sipuleucel-T) [package insert]. Seattle; 2014.

62. Dhesi S, Chu MP, Blevins G, Paterson I, Larratt L, Oudit GY, Kim DH. Cyclophosphamide-induced cardiomyopathy: a case report, review, and recommendations for management. J Invest Med High Impact Case Rep. 2013;1(1):2324709613480346. https://doi.org/10.1177/2324709613480346.

63. Dimopoulos MA, Roussou M, Gavriatopoulou M, Psimenou E, Ziogas D, Eleutherakis-Papaiakovou E, Fotiou D, Migkou M, Kanellias N, Panagiotidis I, Ntalianis A, Papadopoulou E, Stamatelopoulos K, Manios E, Pamboukas C, Kontogiannis S, Terpos E, Kastritis E. Cardiac and renal complications of carfilzomib in patients with multiple myeloma. Blood Adv. 2017;1(7):449–54. https://doi.org/10.1182/bloodadvances.2016003269.

64. Domchek SM, Aghajanian C, Shapira-Frommer R, Schmutzler RK, Audeh MW, Friedlander M, Balmana J, Mitchell G, Fried G, Stemmer SM, Hubert A, Rosengarten O, Loman N, Robertson JD, Mann H, Kaufman B. Efficacy and safety of olaparib monotherapy in germline BRCA1/2 mutation carriers with advanced ovarian cancer and three or more lines of prior therapy. Gynecol Oncol. 2016;140(2):199–203. https://doi.org/10.1016/j.ygyno.2015.12.020.

65. Douer D, Aldoss I, Lunning MA, Burke PW, Ramezani L, Mark L, Vrona J, Park JH, Tallman MS, Avramis VI, Pullarkat V, Mohrbacher AM. Pharmacokinetics-based integration of multiple doses of intravenous pegaspargase in a pediatric regimen for adults with newly diagnosed acute lymphoblastic leukemia. J Clin Oncol. 2014;32 (9):905–11. https://doi.org/10.1200/jco.2013.50.2708.

66. Dutcher JP, Schwartzentruber DJ, Kaufman HL, Agarwala SS, Tarhini AA, Lowder JN, Atkins MB. High dose interleukin-2 (Aldesleukin) – expert consensus on best management practices-2014. J Immuno Ther Cancer. 2014;2(1):26. https://doi.org/10.1186/s40425-014-0026-0.

67. Eisai Inc. Lenvima (lenvatinib) capsules [package insert]. Woodcliff Lake; 2017.

68. Eli Lilly and Company. Portrazza (necitumumab) [package insert]. Indianapolis; 2015.

69. Eli Lilly and Company. Erbitux (cetuximab) [package insert]. Indianapolis; 2016

70. Eli Lilly and Company. Alimta (pemetrexed) [package insert]. Indianapolis; 2017a.

71. Eli Lilly and Company. Cyramza (ramucirumab) [package insert]. Indianapolis; 2017b

72. Eli Lilly and Company. Gemzar (gemcitabine) [package insert]. Indianapolis; 2017c.

73. EMD Serono. Bavencio (avelumab) [package insert]. Rockland; 2017.

74. EMD Serono. Novantrone (Mitoxantrone) [package insert]. Rockland; 2008.

75. Eremina V, Jefferson JA, Kowalewska J, Hochster H, Haas M, Weisstuch J, Richardson C, Kopp JB, Kabir MG, Backx PH, Gerber HP, Ferrara N, Barisoni L, Alpers CE, Quaggin SE. VEGF inhibition and renal thrombotic microangiopathy. N Engl J Med. 2008;358(11):1129–36. https://doi.org/10.1056/NEJMoa0707330.

76. Exelixis Inc. Cometriq (cabozantinib) [package insert]. South San Francisco; 2017.

77. Faderl S, Ravandi F, Huang X, Garcia-Manero G, Ferrajoli A, Estrov Z, Borthakur G, Verstovsek S, Thomas DA, Kwari M, Kantarjian HM. A randomized study of clofarabine versus clofarabine plus low-dose cytarabine as front-line therapy for patients aged 60 years and older with acute myeloid leukemia and high-risk myelodysplastic syndrome. Blood. 2008;112(5):1638–45. https://doi.org/10.1182/blood-2007-11-124602.

78. Feinberg WM, Swenson MR. Cerebrovascular complications of L-asparaginase therapy. Neurology. 1988;38(1):127–33.

79. Gass-Jegu F, Gschwend A, Gairard-Dory AC, Mennecier B, Tebacher-Alt M, Gourieux B, Quoix E. Gastrointestinal perforations in patients treated with erlotinib: a report of two cases with fatal outcome and literature review. Lung Cancer (Amsterdam, Netherlands). 2016;99:76–8. https://doi.org/10.1016/j.lungcan.2016.06.012.

80. Geiser CF, Bishop Y, Jaffe N, Furman L, Traggis D, Frei E 3rd. Adverse effects of intrathecal methotrexate in children with acute leukemia in remission. Blood. 1975;45(2):189–95.

81. Genentech Inc. Herceptin (trastuzumab) [package insert]. South San Francisco; 2017a.

82. Genentech Inc. Kadcyla (ado-traztuzumab emtansine) [package insert]. South San Francisco; 2017b.

83. Genentech Inc. Perjeta (pertuzumab) [package insert]. South San Francisco; 2017c.

84. Genentech Inc. Cotellic (cobimetinib) [package insert]. South San Francisco; 2018.

85. Genentech USA Inc. Xeloda (capecitabine) [package insert]. South San Francisco; 2016

86. Genentech USA Inc. Alecensa (alectinib) [package insert] South San Francisco; 2017a.

87. Genentech USA Inc. Avastin (bevacizumab) [package insert]. South San Francisco; 2017b.

88. Genentech USA Inc. Erivedge (vismodegib) [package insert]. South San Francisco; 2017c.

89. Genentech USA Inc. Tecentriq (atezolizumab) [package insert]. South San Francisco; 2017d.

90. Genentech USA Inc. Zelboraf (vemurafenib) [package insert]. South San Francisco; 2017e.

91. Genzyme Corporation. Lemtrada (alemtuzumab) [package insert]. Cambridge, MA; 2017.

92. Geyer HL, Viggiano RW, Lacy MQ, Witzig TE, Leslie KO, Mikhael JR, Stewart K. Acute lung toxicity related to pomalidomide. Chest. 2011;140(2): 529–33. https://doi.org/10.1378/chest.10-2082.

93. Gilead Sciences. Zydelig (idelalisib) [package insert]. Foster City; 2016.

94. Giles FJ, Mauro MJ, Hong F, Ortmann CE, McNeill C, Woodman RC, Hochhaus A, le Coutre PD, Saglio G. Rates of peripheral arterial occlusive disease in patients with chronic myeloid leukemia in the chronic phase treated with imatinib, nilotinib, or non-tyrosine kinase therapy: a retrospective cohort analysis. Leukemia. 2013;27(6):1310–5. https://doi. org/10.1038/leu.2013.69.

95. GlaxoSmithKline. Alkeran®(melphalan) [package insert]. Research Triangle Park; 2012.

96. Goldhar HA, Yan AT, Ko DT, Earle CC, Tomlinson GA, Trudeau ME, Krahn MD, Krzyzanowska MK, Pal RS, Brezden-Masley C, Gavura S, Lien K, Chan KK. The temporal risk of heart failure associated with adjuvant trastuzumab in breast cancer patients: a population study. J Natl Cancer Inst. 2016;108(1). https:// doi.org/10.1093/jnci/djv301.

97. Grellety T, Houede N, Hoepffner JL, Riviere J, Merino C, Lieutenant V, Gross-Goupil M, Richaud P, Dupin C, Sargos P, Roubaud G. Hemorrhagic cystitis in patients treated with cabazitaxel: a radiation recall syndrome? Ann Oncol. 2014;25(6):1248–9. https:// doi.org/10.1093/annonc/mdu132.

98. Hamnvik OP, Larsen PR, Marqusee E. Thyroid dysfunction from antineoplastic agents. J Natl Cancer Inst. 2011;103(21):1572–87. https://doi.org/10.1093/ jnci/djr373.

99. Haskell CM, Canellos GP, Leventhal BG, Carbone PP, Block JB, Serpick AA, Selawry OS. L-asparaginase: therapeutic and toxic effects in patients with neoplastic disease. N Engl J Med. 1969;281(19):1028–34. https:// doi.org/10.1056/nejm196911062811902.

100. Helman DL Jr, Byrd JC, Ales NC, Shorr AF. Fludarabine-related pulmonary toxicity: a distinct clinical entity in chronic lymphoproliferative syndromes. Chest. 2002;122(3):785–90.

101. Heritage Pharmaceuticals. BiCNU (carmustine) [package insert]. Eatontown; 2017.

102. Herzig RH, Hines JD, Herzig GP, Wolff SN, Cassileth PA, Lazarus HM, Adelstein DJ, Brown RA, Coccia PF, Strandjord S, et al. Cerebellar toxicity with high-dose cytosine arabinoside. J Clin Oncol. 1987;5(6):927–32. https://doi.org/10.1200/jco.1987.5.6.927.

103. Hochhaus A, Saglio G, Hughes TP, Larson RA, Kim DW, Issaragrisil S, le Coutre PD, Etienne G, Dorlhiac-Llacer PE, Clark RE, Flinn IW, Nakamae H, Donohue B, Deng W, Dalal D, Menssen HD, Kantarjian HM. Long-term benefits and risks of front-line nilotinib vs imatinib for chronic myeloid leukemia in chronic phase: 5-year update of the randomized ENESTnd trial. Leukemia. 2016;30(5):1044–54. https://doi.org/10.1038/leu.2016.5.

104. Hortobagyi GN, Stemmer SM, Burris HA, Yap YS, Sonke GS, Paluch-Shimon S, Campone M, Blackwell KL, Andre F, Winer EP, Janni W, Verma S, Conte P, Arteaga CL, Cameron DA, Petrakova K, Hart LL, Villanueva C, Chan A, Jakobsen E, Nusch A, Burdaeva O, Grischke EM, Alba E, Wist E, Marschner N, Favret AM, Yardley D, Bachelot T, Tseng LM, Blau S, Xuan F, Souami F, Miller M, Germa C, Hirawat S, O'Shaughnessy J. Ribociclib as first-line therapy for HR-positive, advanced breast cancer. N Engl J Med. 2016;375(18):1738–48. https://doi.org/10.1056/NEJMoa1609709.

105. Hospira. Nipent (pentostatin for injection) [package insert]. Lake Forest; 2018.

106. Hwang JP, Somerfield MR, Alston-Johnson DE, Cryer DR, Feld JJ, Kramer BS, Sabichi AL, Wong SL, Artz AS. Hepatitis B virus screening for patients with cancer before therapy: American society of clinical oncology provisional clinical opinion update. J Clin Oncol. 2015;33(19):2212–20. https://doi.org/ 10.1200/jco.2015.61.3745.

107. Ikeda S, Sekine A, Kato T, Yoshida M, Ogata R, Baba T, Nagahama K, Okudela K, Ogura T. Diffuse alveolar hemorrhage as a fatal adverse effect of bevacizumab: an autopsy case. Jpn J Clin Oncol. 2014;44(5):497–500. https://doi.org/10.1093/jjco/ hyu023.

108. Incyte Corp. Jakafi (ruxolitinib) [package insert]. Wilmington; 2011.

109. Ingenus Pharmaceuticals. Carboplatin [package insert]. Orlando; 2017.

110. Jain S, Song R, Xie J. Sonidegib: mechanism of action, pharmacology, and clinical utility for advanced basal cell carcinomas. Onco Targets Ther. 2017;10:1645–53. https://doi.org/10.2147/ott.S130910.

111. Janssen Biotech. Darzalex (daratumumab) [package insert]. Horsham; 2017.

112. Janssen Products. Yondelis (trabectedin) [package insert]. Horsham; 2015.

113. Janssen Products. Doxil (doxorubicin HCl liposome injection) [package insert]. Horsahm; 2016.

114. Jazz Pharmaceuticals. VYXEOS (daunorubicin and cytarabine) liposome [package insert]. Palo Alto; 2018.

115. Jazz Pharmaceuticals. Erwinaze intramuscular injection, intravenous injection (asparaginase Erwinia

chrysanthemi intramuscular injection, intravenous injection) [package insert]. Palo Alto; 2016.

116. Johnson DB, Balko JM, Compton ML, Chalkias S, Gorham J, Xu Y, Hicks M, Puzanov I, Alexander MR, Bloomer TL, Becker JR, Slosky DA, Phillips EJ, Pilkinton MA, Craig-Owens L, Kola N, Plautz G, Reshef DS, Deutsch JS, Deering RP, Olenchock BA, Lichtman AH, Roden DM, Seidman CE, Koralnik IJ, Seidman JG, Hoffman RD, Taube JM, Diaz LA Jr, Anders RA, Sosman JA, Moslehi JJ. Fulminant myocarditis with combination immune checkpoint blockade. N Engl J Med. 2016;375(18):1749–55. https://doi.org/10.1056/NEJMoa1609214.

117. Johnston PB, Bondly C, Micallef IN. Ibritumomab tiuxetan for non-Hodgkin's lymphoma. Expert Rev Anticancer Ther. 2006;6(6):861–9. https://doi.org/10.1586/14737140.6.6.861.

118. Jolson HM, Bosco L, Bufton MG, Gerstman BB, Rinsler SS, Williams E, Flynn B, Simmons WD, Stadel BV, Faich GA, et al. Clustering of adverse drug events: analysis of risk factors for cerebellar toxicity with high-dose cytarabine. J Natl Cancer Inst. 1992;84(7):500–5.

119. June Therapeutics. Juno Therapeutics and Celgene corporation release additional data from TRANSCEND trial of JCAR017 in patients with relapsed or refractory aggressive B-cell non-Hodgkin lymphoma. 2017, viewed 11 March 2018. http://ir.celgene.com/releasedetail.cfm?releaseid=1051336

120. Junpaparp P, Sharma B, Samiappan A, Rhee JH, Young KR. Everolimus-induced severe pulmonary toxicity with diffuse alveolar hemorrhage. Ann Am Thorac Soc. 2013;10(6):727–9. https://doi.org/10.1513/AnnalsATS.201309-332LE.

121. Kadia TM, Gandhi V. Nelarabine in the treatment of pediatric and adult patients with T-cell acute lymphoblastic leukemia and lymphoma. Expert Rev Hematol. 2017;10(1):1–8. https://doi.org/10.1080/17474086.2017.1262757.

122. Kanie K, Iguchi G, Bando H, Fujita Y, Odake Y, Yoshida K, Matsumoto R, Fukuoka H, Ogawa W, Takahashi Y. Two cases of atezolizumab-induced hypophysitis. J Endocr Soc. 2018;2(1):91–5. https://doi.org/10.1210/js.2017-00414.

123. Kantarjian HM, DeAngelo DJ, Advani AS, Stelljes M, Kebriaei P, Cassaday RD, Merchant AA, Fujishima N, Uchida T, Calbacho M, Ejduk AA, O'Brien SM, Jabbour EJ, Zhang H, Sleight BJ, Vandendries ER, Marks DI. Hepatic adverse event profile of inotuzumab ozogamicin in adult patients with relapsed or refractory acute lymphoblastic leukaemia: results from the open-label, randomised, phase 3 INO-VATE study. Lancet Haematol. 2017;4(8):e387–98. https://doi.org/10.1016/s2352-3026(17)30103-5.

124. Kebriaei P, Wilhelm K, Ravandi F, Brandt M, de Lima M, Ciurea S, Worth L, O'Brien S, Thomas D, Champlin RE, Kantarjian H. Feasibility of allografting in patients with advanced acute lymphoblastic leukemia after salvage therapy with inotuzumab

ozogamicin. Clin Lymphoma Myeloma Leuk. 2013;13(3):296–301. https://doi.org/10.1016/j.clml.2012.12.003.

125. Khoury HJ, Cortes JE, Kantarjian HM, Gambacorti-Passerini C, Baccarani M, Kim DW, Zaritskey A, Countouriotis A, Besson N, Leip E, Kelly V, Brummendorf TH. Bosutinib is active in chronic phase chronic myeloid leukemia after imatinib and dasatinib and/or nilotinib therapy failure. Blood. 2012;119(15):3403–12. https://doi.org/10.1182/blood-2011-11-390120.

126. Kieslich M, Porto L, Lanfermann H, Jacobi G, Schwabe D, Bohles H. Cerebrovascular complications of L-asparaginase in the therapy of acute lymphoblastic leukemia. J Pediatr Hematol Oncol. 2003;25(6):484–7.

127. Kim DW, Tiseo M, Ahn MJ, Reckamp KL, Hansen KH, Kim SW, Huber RM, West HL, Groen HJM, Hochmair MJ, Leighl NB, Gettinger SN, Langer CJ, Paz-Ares Rodriguez LG, Smit EF, Kim ES, Reichmann W, Haluska FG, Kerstein D, Camidge DR. Brigatinib in patients with crizotinib-refractory anaplastic lymphoma kinase-positive non-small-cell lung cancer: a randomized, multicenter phase II trial. J Clin Oncol. 2017;35(22):2490–8. https://doi.org/10.1200/jco.2016.71.5904.

128. Kite Pharma Inc. Yescarta (axicabtagene ciloleucel) [package insert]. Santa Monica; 2017.

129. Krause AS, Weihrauch MR, Bode U, Fleischhack G, Elter T, Heuer T, Engert A, Diehl V, Josting A. Carboxypeptidase-G2 rescue in cancer patients with delayed methotrexate elimination after high-dose methotrexate therapy. Leuk Lymphoma. 2002;43(11):2139–43. https://doi.org/10.1080/1042819021000032953.

130. Kuhlen M, Bleckmann K, Moricke A, Schrappe M, Vieth S, Escherich G, Bronsema A, Vonalt A, Queudeville M, Zwaan CM, Ebinger M, Debatin KM, Klingebiel T, Koscielniak E, Rossig C, Burkhardt B, Kolb R, Eckert C, Borkhardt A, von Stackelberg A, Chen-Santel C. Neurotoxic side effects in children with refractory or relapsed T-cell malignancies treated with nelarabine based therapy. Br J Haematol. 2017;179(2):272–83. https://doi.org/10.1111/bjh.14877.

131. Lambertini M, Del Mastro L, Gardin G, Levaggi A, Bighin C, Giraudi S, Pronzato P. Stevens-Johnson syndrome after treatment with bendamustine. Leuk Res. 2012;36(7):e153–4. https://doi.org/10.1016/j.leukres.2012.03.006.

132. Lancet JE, Uy G, Cortes JE, Newell LF, Lin TL, Ritchie EK, Stuart RK, Strickland SA, Hogge D, Solomon SR, Stone RM, Bixby DL, Kolitz JE, Schiller GJ, Wieduwilt MJ, Ryan DH, Hoering A, Chiarella M, Louie AC, Medeiros BC (Abstract 7000) Final results of a phase III randomized trial of CPX-351 versus 7+3 in older patients with newly diagnosed high risk (secondary) AML. J Clin Oncol. 2016; 34(15 Suppl): p. 7000.

133. Larkin J, Chiarion-Sileni V, Gonzalez R, Grob JJ, Cowey CL, Lao CD, Schadendorf D, Dummer R,

Smylie M, Rutkowski P, Ferrucci PF, Hill A, Wagstaff J, Carlino MS, Haanen JB, Maio M, Marquez-Rodas I, McArthur GA, Ascierto PA, Long GV, Callahan MK, Postow MA, Grossmann K, Sznol M, Dreno B, Bastholt L, Yang A, Rollin LM, Horak C, Hodi FS, Wolchok JD. Combined Nivolumab and ipilimumab or monotherapy in untreated melanoma. N Engl J Med. 2015;373 (1):23–34. https://doi.org/10.1056/NEJMoa1504030.

134. Latagliata R, Breccia M, Fava C, Stagno F, Tiribelli M, Luciano L, Gozzini A, Gugliotta G, Annunziata M, Cavazzini F, Ferrero D, Musto P, Capodanno I, Iurlo A, Visani G, Crugnola M, Calistri E, Castagnetti F, Vigneri P, Alimena G. Incidence, risk factors and management of pleural effusions during dasatinib treatment in unselected elderly patients with chronic myelogenous leukaemia. Hematol Oncol. 2013;31(2):103–9. https://doi.org/10.1002/hon.2020.

135. Le Coutre P, Rea D, Abruzzese E, Dombret H, Trawinska MM, Herndlhofer S, Dorken B, Valent P. Severe peripheral arterial disease during nilotinib therapy. J Natl Cancer Inst. 2011;103(17):1347–8. https://doi.org/10.1093/jnci/djr292.

136. Lenihan DJ, Kowey PR. Overview and management of cardiac adverse events associated with tyrosine kinase inhibitors. Oncologist. 2013;18(8):900–8. https://doi.org/10.1634/theoncologist.2012-0466.

137. Lilly USA LLC. Verzenio (abemaciclib) [package insert]. Indianapolis; 2017.

138. Linette DC, McGee KH, McFarland JA. Mitomycin-induced pulmonary toxicity: case report and review of the literature. Ann Pharmacother. 1992;26(4):481–4. https://doi.org/10.1177/106002809202600404.

139. Lipton JH, Chuah C, Guerci-Bresler A, Rosti G, Simpson D, Assouline S, Etienne G, Nicolini FE, le Coutre P, Clark RE, Stenke L, Andorsky D, Oehler V, Lustgarten S, Rivera VM, Clackson T, Haluska FG, Baccarani M, Cortes JE, Guilhot F, Hochhaus A, Hughes T, Kantarjian HM, Shah NP, Talpaz M, Deininger MW. Ponatinib versus imatinib for newly diagnosed chronic myeloid leukaemia: an international, randomised, open-label, phase 3 trial. Lancet Oncol. 2016;17(5):612–21. https://doi.org/10.1016/s1470-2045(16)00080-2.

140. Lyman GH, Bohlke K, Khorana AA, Kuderer NM, Lee AY, Arcelus JI, Balaban EP, Clarke JM, Flowers CR, Francis CW, Gates LE, Kakkar AK, Key NS, Levine MN, Liebman HA, Tempero MA, Wong SL, Somerfield MR, Falanga A. Venous thromboembolism prophylaxis and treatment in patients with cancer: American society of clinical oncology clinical practice guideline update 2014. J Clin Oncol. 2015;33 (6):654–6. https://doi.org/10.1200/jco.2014.59.7351.

141. Malalagama GN, Chryssidis S, Parnis FX. CT findings in patients with Cabazitaxel induced pelvic pain and haematuria: a case series. Cancer Imaging. 2017;17(1):17. https://doi.org/10.1186/s40644-017-0119-3.

142. Markman M, Kennedy A, Webster K, Elson P, Peterson G, Kulp B, Belinson J. Clinical features of hypersensitivity reactions to carboplatin. J Clin Oncol. 1999;17(4):1141. https://doi.org/10.1200/jco.1999.17.4.1141.

143. Maude SL, Laetsch TW, Buechner J, Rives S, Boyer M, Bittencourt H, Bader P, Verneris MR, Stefanski HE, Myers GD, Qayed M, De Moerloose B, Hiramatsu H, Schlis K, Davis KL, Martin PL, Nemecek ER, Yanik GA, Peters C, Baruchel A, Boissel N, Mechinaud F, Balduzzi A, Krueger J, June CH, Levine BL, Wood P, Taran T, Leung M, Mueller KT, Zhang Y, Sen K, Lebwohl D, Pulsipher MA, Grupp SA. Tisagenlecleucel in children and young adults with B-Cell Lymphoblastic Leukemia. N Engl J Med. 2018;378(5):439–48. https://doi.org/10.1056/NEJMoa1709866.

144. Mayne Pharma Limited. Epirubicin hydrochloride [package insert]. Paramus; 2006.

145. McKoy JM, Angelotta C, Bennett CL, Tallman MS, Wadleigh M, Evens AM, Kuzel TM, Trifilio SM, Raisch DW, Kell J, DeAngelo DJ, Giles FJ. Gemtuzumab ozogamicin-associated sinusoidal obstructive syndrome (SOS): an overview from the research on adverse drug events and reports (RADAR) project. Leuk Res. 2007;31(5):599–604. https://doi.org/10.1016/j.leukres.2006.07.005.

146. McMullen JR, Boey EJ, Ooi JY, Seymour JF, Keating MJ, Tam CS. Ibrutinib increases the risk of atrial fibrillation, potentially through inhibition of cardiac PI3K-Akt signaling. Blood. 2014;124(25):3829–30. https://doi.org/10.1182/blood-2014-10-604272.

147. Merck & Co. Temodar (temozolomide) [package insert]. Whitehouse Station; 2017a.

148. Merck & Co. Keytruda (pembrolizumab) [package insert]. Whitehouse Station; 2017b.

149. Meyer CC, Calis KA, Burke LB, Walawander CA, Grasela TH. Symptomatic cardiotoxicity associated with 5-fluorouracil. Pharmacotherapy. 1997;17(4): 729–36.

150. Millennium Pharmaceuticals Inc. Velcade (bortezomib) [package insert]. Cambridge, MA; 2017.

151. Mitani S, Kadowaki S, Komori A, Sugiyama K, Narita Y, Taniguchi H, Ura T, Ando M, Sato Y, Yamaura H, Inaba Y, Ishihara M, Tanaka T, Tajika M, Muro K. Acute hyperammonemic encephalopathy after fluoropyrimidine-based chemotherapy: a case series and review of the literature. Medicine. 2017;96(22):e6874. https://doi.org/10.1097/md.0000000000006874.

152. Montani D, Bergot E, Gunther S, Savale L, Bergeron A, Bourdin A, Bouvaist H, Canuet M, Pison C, Macro M, Poubeau P, Girerd B, Natali D, Guignabert C, Perros F, O'Callaghan DS, Jais X, Tubert-Bitter P, Zalcman G, Sitbon O, Simonneau G, Humbert M. Pulmonary arterial hypertension in patients treated by dasatinib. Circulation. 2012;125(17):2128–37. https://doi.org/10.1161/circulationaha.111.079921.

153. Montesinos P, Bergua JM, Vellenga E, Rayon C, Parody R, de la Serna J, Leon A, Esteve J, Milone G, Deben G, Rivas C, Gonzalez M, Tormo M, Diaz-Mediavilla J, Gonzalez JD, Negri S, Amutio E, Brunet S, Lowenberg B, Sanz MA. Differentiation syndrome in patients with acute promyelocytic leukemia treated with all-trans retinoic acid and anthracycline chemotherapy: characteristics, outcome, and prognostic factors. Blood. 2009; 113(4):775–83. https://doi.org/10.1182/blood-2008-07-168617.

154. Moskovitz M, Wollner M, Haim N. Oxaliplatin-induced pulmonary toxicity in gastrointestinal malignancies: two case reports and review of the literature. Case Rep Oncol Med. 2015;2015:341064. https://doi.org/10.1155/2015/341064.

155. Moslehi JJ, Deininger M. Tyrosine Kinase Inhibitor-Associated Cardiovascular Toxicity in Chronic Myeloid Leukemia. J Clin Oncol. 2015;33(35):4210–8. https://doi.org/10.1200/jco.2015.62.4718.

156. Motzer RJ, Hutson TE, Olsen MR, Hudes GR, Burke JM, Edenfield WJ, Wilding G, Agarwal N, Thompson JA, Cella D, Bello A, Korytowsky B, Yuan J, Valota O, Martell B, Hariharan S, Figlin RA. Randomized phase II trial of sunitinib on an intermittent versus continuous dosing schedule as first-line therapy for advanced renal cell carcinoma. J Clin Oncol. 2012;30(12):1371–7. https://doi.org/10.1200/jco.2011.36.4133.

157. Munch M, Peuvrel L, Brocard A, Saint Jean M, Khammari A, Dreno B, Quereux G. Early-onset vemurafenib-induced DRESS syndrome. Dermatology (Basel, Switzerland). 2016;232(1):126–8. https://doi.org/10.1159/000439272.

158. Myint ZW, Sen JM, Watts NL, Druzgal TJ, Nathan BR, Ward MD, Boyer JE, Fracasso PM. Reversible posterior leukoencephalopathy syndrome during regorafenib treatment: a case report and literature review of reversible posterior leukoencephalopathy syndrome associated with multikinase inhibitors. Clin Colorectal Cancer. 2014;13(2):127–30. https://doi.org/10.1016/j.clcc.2013.12.003.

159. Naidoo J, Page DB, Li BT, Connell LC, Schindler K, Lacouture ME, Postow MA, Wolchok JD. Toxicities of the anti-PD-1 and anti-PD-L1 immune checkpoint antibodies. Ann Oncol. 2015;26(12):2375–91. https://doi.org/10.1093/annonc/mdv383.

160. Naidoo J, Wang X, Woo KM, Iyriboz T, Halpenny D, Cunningham J, Chaft JE, Segal NH, Callahan MK, Lesokhin AM, Rosenberg J, Voss MH, Rudin CM, Rizvi H, Hou X, Rodriguez K, Albano M, Gordon RA, Leduc C, Rekhtman N, Harris B, Menzies AM, Guminski AD, Carlino MS, Kong BY, Wolchok JD, Postow MA, Long GV, Hellmann MD. Pneumonitis in patients treated with anti-programmed death-1/programmed death ligand 1 therapy. J Clin Oncol. 2017; 35(7):709–17. https://doi.org/10.1200/jco.2016.68.2005.

161. Neelapu SS, Locke FL, Bartlett NL, Lekakis LJ, Miklos DB, Jacobson CA, Braunschweig I, Oluwole OO, Siddiqi T, Lin Y, Timmerman JM, Stiff PJ, Friedberg JW, Flinn IW, Goy A, Hill BT, Smith MR, Deol A, Farooq U, McSweeney P, Munoz J, Avivi I, Castro JE, Westin JR, Chavez JC, Ghobadi A, Komanduri KV, Levy R, Jacobsen ED, Witzig TE, Reagan P, Bot A, Rossi J, Navale L, Jiang Y, Aycock J, Elias M, Chang D, Wiezorek J, Go WY. Axicabtagene ciloleucel CAR T-Cell therapy in refractory large B-Cell lymphoma. N Engl J Med. 2017;377(26):2531–44. https://doi.org/10.1056/NEJMoa1707447.

162. Nesher L, Rolston KV. Neutropenic enterocolitis, a growing concern in the era of widespread use of aggressive chemotherapy. Clin Infect Dis. 2013;56 (5):711–7. https://doi.org/10.1093/cid/cis998.

163. NIH NCI. A to Z list of cancer drugs; 2018. Viewed 20 March 2018. https://www.cancer.gov/about-cancer/treatment/drugs

164. Novartis Pharmaceutical Co. Afinitor and Afinitor Disperz (everolimus) [package insert]. East Hanover; 2017a.

165. Novartis Pharmaceutical Co. Tykerb (Lapatinib) [package insert]. East Hanover; 2017b.

166. Novartis Pharmaceutical Co. Votrient (pazopanib) [package insert]. East Hanover; 2017c.

167. Novartis Pharmaceutical Co. Zykadia (ceritinib) [package insert] East Hanover; 2017d.

168. Novartis Pharmaceuticals. Hycamtin (topotecan oral capsules) [package insert]. East Hanover; 2016.

169. Novartis Pharmaceuticals. Kasqali (ribociclib) [package insert]. East Hanover; 2017a.

170. Novartis Pharmaceuticals. Mekinist (trametinib) [package insert]. East Hanover; 2017b.

171. Novartis Pharmaceuticals. Tafinlar (dabrafenib) [package insert]. East Hanover; 2017c.

172. Novartis Pharmaceuticals. Tasigna oral capsules, nilotinib oral capsules [package insert]. East Hanover; 2018.

173. Novartis Pharmaceuticals Corporation. Farydak (panobinostat) [package insert]. East Hanover; 2016.

174. Novartis Pharmaceuticals Corporation. Kymriah (tisagenlecleucel) [prescribing information]. East Hanover; 2017.

175. Ohnishi K, Sakai F, Kudoh S, Ohno R. Twenty-seven cases of drug-induced interstitial lung disease associated with imatinib mesylate. Leukemia. 2006;20(6): 1162–4. https://doi.org/10.1038/sj.leu.2404207.

176. Okamoto K, Proia LA, Demarais PL. Disseminated cryptococcal disease in a patient with chronic lymphocytic leukemia on ibrutinib. Case Rep Infect Dis. 2016;2016:4642831. https://doi.org/10.1155/2016/4642831.

177. Okuno SH, Frytak S. Mitomycin lung toxicity. Acute and chronic phases. Am J Clin Oncol. 1997;20(3): 282–4.

178. Onyx Pharmaceuticals Inc. Kyprolis (carfilzomib) [package insert]. Thousand Oaks; 2018.

179. Osawa M, Kudoh S, Sakai F, Endo M, Hamaguchi T, Ogino Y, Yoneoka M, Sakaguchi M, Nishimoto H,

Gemma A. Clinical features and risk factors of panitumumab-induced interstitial lung disease: a postmarketing all-case surveillance study. Int J Clin Oncol. 2015;20(6):1063–71. https://doi.org/10.1007/s10147-015-0834-3.

180. OSI Pharmaceuticals L, an affiliate of Astellas Pharma US, Inc. Tarceva (erlotinib) [package insert]. Northbrook; 2016.

181. Otsuka America Pharmaceutical. Busulfan [package insert]. Rockville; 2015.

182. Ovation Pharmaceuticals. Cosmegen (dactinomycin) [package insert]. Deerfield; 2008.

183. Patel PN. Methylene blue for management of Ifosfamide-induced encephalopathy. Ann Pharmacother. 2006;40(2):299–303. https://doi.org/10.1345/aph.1G114.

184. Perez EA, Koehler M, Byrne J, Preston AJ, Rappold E, Ewer MS. Cardiac safety of lapatinib: pooled analysis of 3689 patients enrolled in clinical trials. Mayo Clin Proc. 2008;83(6):679–86. https://doi.org/10.4065/83.6.679.

185. Peroukides S, Makatsoris T, Koutras A, Tsamandas A, Onyenadum A, Labropoulou-Karatza C, Kalofonos H. Lapatinib-induced hepatitis: a case report. World J Gastroenterol. 2011;17(18):2349–52. https://doi.org/10.3748/wjg.v17.i18.2349.

186. Petri CR, O'Donnell PH, Cao H, Artz AS, Stock W, Wickrema A, Hard M, van Besien K. Clofarabine-associated acute kidney injury in patients undergoing hematopoietic stem cell transplant. Leuk Lymphoma. 2014;55(12):2866–73. https://doi.org/10.3109/10428194.2014.897701.

187. Pfizer. Inlyta (axitinib) [package insert]. New York; 2014.

188. Pfizer. Navelbine (vinorelbine) [package insert]; Research Triangle Park; 2017a.

189. Pfizer. Sutent (sunitinib) [package insert]. New York; 2017b.

190. Pfizer Inc. Xalkori (crizotinib) [package insert]. New York; 2017.

191. Pfizer Labs. Ibrance (palbociclib) [package insert]. New York; 2017.

192. Pharmacia & Upjohn Camptosar (irinotecan) [package insert]. New York; 2016.

193. Pharmacyclics. Imbruvica (ibrutinib) [package insert]. Sunnyvale; 2017.

194. Porkka K, Khoury HJ, Paquette RL, Matloub Y, Sinha R, Cortes JE. Dasatinib 100 mg once daily minimizes the occurrence of pleural effusion in patients with chronic myeloid leukemia in chronic phase and efficacy is unaffected in patients who develop pleural effusion. Cancer. 2010;116(2):377–86. https://doi.org/10.1002/cncr.24734.

195. Prasco Laboratories. Leukeran (chlorambucil) [package insert]. Mason; 2017.

196. Prometheus Laboratories Inc. Proleukin (aldesleukin) [prescribing information]. San Diego; 2012.

197. Qi WX, Fu S, Zhang Q, Guo XM. Bevacizumab increases the risk of severe congestive heart failure in cancer patients: an up-to-date meta-analysis with a focus on different subgroups. Clin Drug Investig. 2014;34(10):681–90. https://doi.org/10.1007/s40261-014-0222-1.

198. Quintas-Cardama A, Kantarjian H, Cortes J. Nilotinib-associated vascular events. Clin Lymphoma Myeloma Leuk. 2012;12(5):337–40. https://doi.org/10.1016/j.clml.2012.04.005.

199. Read WL, Mortimer JE, Picus J. Severe interstitial pneumonitis associated with docetaxel administration. Cancer. 2002;94(3):847–53.

200. Robertson GL, Bhoopalam N, Zelkowitz LJ. Vincristine neurotoxicity and abnormal secretion of antidiuretic hormone. Arch Intern Med. 1973;132(5):717–20.

201. Roboz GJ, Ritchie EK, Carlin RF, Samuel M, Gale L, Provenzano-Gober JL, Curcio TJ, Feldman EJ, Kligfield PD. Prevalence, management, and clinical consequences of QT interval prolongation during treatment with arsenic trioxide. J Clin Oncol. 2014;32(33):3723–8. https://doi.org/10.1200/jco.2013.51.2913.

202. Rosen AC, Balagula Y, Raisch DW, Garg V, Nardone B, Larsen N, Sorrell J, West DP, Anadkat MJ, Lacouture ME. Life-threatening dermatologic adverse events in oncology. Anti-Cancer Drugs. 2014;25(2):225–34. https://doi.org/10.1097/cad.0000000000000032.

203. Rothenstein JM, Letarte N. Managing treatment-related adverse events associated with Alk inhibitors. Curr Oncol (Toronto, Ont). 2014;21(1):19–26. https://doi.org/10.3747/co.21.1740.

204. Rubbia-Brandt L, Audard V, Sartoretti P, Roth AD, Brezault C, Le Charpentier M, Dousset B, Morel P, Soubrane O, Chaussade S, Mentha G, Terris B. Severe hepatic sinusoidal obstruction associated with oxaliplatin-based chemotherapy in patients with metastatic colorectal cancer. Ann Oncol. 2004;15(3):460–6.

205. Sager PT, Balser B, Wolfson J, Nichols J, Pilot R, Jones S, Burris HA. Electrocardiographic effects of class 1 selective histone deacetylase inhibitor romidepsin. Cancer Med. 2015;4(8):1178–85. https://doi.org/10.1002/cam4.467.

206. Saif MW, McGee PJ. Hemolytic-uremic syndrome associated with gemcitabine: a case report and review of literature. J Pancreas. 2005;6(4):369–74.

207. Saif MW, Tomita M, Ledbetter L, Diasio RB. Capecitabine-related cardiotoxicity: recognition and management. J Support Oncol. 2008;6(1):41–8.

208. Salloum E, Khan KK, Cooper DL. Chlorambucil-induced seizures. Cancer. 1997;79(5):1009–13.

209. Sankhalla KK, Chawla NS, Syed I, Chawla SP. Management of toxicities with pazopanib in advanced soft tissue sarcoma. Sarcoma Res Int. 2016;3(2):1032–8.

210. Sanofi-Aventis. Zaltrapt (aflibercept) [package insert]. Bridgewater; 2016.

211. Sanofi-Aventis LLC. Eloxatin (oxaliplatin) [package insert]. Bridgewater; 2015.

212. Sanofi-Aventis U.S. LLC. Taxotere (docetaxel) [package insert]. Bridgewater; 2015.

213. Sanofi-Aventis U.S. LLC. Jevtana (cabazitaxel) [package insert]. Bridgewater; 2017.

214. Sanofi Genzyme Corp. Caprelsa (vandetanib) [package insert]. Cambridge, MA; 2016.

215. Sanz MA, Montesinos P. How we prevent and treat differentiation syndrome in patients with acute promyelocytic leukemia. Blood. 2014;123(18):2777–82. https://doi.org/10.1182/blood-2013-10-512640.

216. Schmidinger M, Zielinski CC, Vogl UM, Bojic A, Bojic M, Schukro C, Ruhsam M, Hejna M, Schmidinger H. Cardiac toxicity of sunitinib and sorafenib in patients with metastatic renal cell carcinoma. J Clin Oncol. 2008;26(32):5204–12. https://doi.org/10.1200/jco.2007.15.6331.

217. Seattle Genetics. Adcetris (brentuximab vedotin) [package insert]. Bothell; 2017.

218. Seet RC, Rabinstein AA. Clinical features and outcomes of posterior reversible encephalopathy syndrome following bevacizumab treatment. QJM. 2012;105(1):69–75. https://doi.org/10.1093/qjmed/hcr139.

219. Serota DP, Mehta AK, Phadke VK. Invasive fungal sinusitis due to Mucor species in a patient on ibrutinib. Clin Infect Dis. 2017; https://doi.org/10.1093/cid/cix1058.

220. Shah NP, Kantarjian HM, Kim DW, Rea D, Dorlhiac-Llacer PE, Milone JH, Vela-Ojeda J, Silver RT, Khoury HJ, Charbonnier A, Khoroshko N, Paquette RL, Deininger M, Collins RH, Otero I, Hughes T, Bleickardt E, Strauss L, Francis S, Hochhaus A. Intermittent target inhibition with dasatinib 100 mg once daily preserves efficacy and improves tolerability in imatinib-resistant and -intolerant chronic-phase chronic myeloid leukemia. J Clin Oncol. 2008;26(19):3204–12. https://doi.org/10.1200/jco.2007.14.9260.

221. Shank BR, Do B, Sevin A, Chen SE, Neelapu SS, Horowitz SB. Chimeric Antigen Receptor T Cells in Hematologic Malignancies. Pharmacotherapy. 2017;37(3):334–45. https://doi.org/10.1002/phar.1900.

222. Sharief U, Perry DJ. Delayed reversible posterior encephalopathy syndrome following chemotherapy with oxaliplatin. Clin Colorectal Cancer. 2009;8(3):163–5. https://doi.org/10.3816/CCC.2009.n.026.

223. Shaw AT, Kim DW, Nakagawa K, Seto T, Crino L, Ahn MJ, De Pas T, Besse B, Solomon BJ, Blackhall F, Wu YL, Thomas M, O'Byrne KJ, Moro-Sibilot D, Camidge DR, Mok T, Hirsh V, Riely GJ, Iyer S, Tassell V, Polli A, Wilner KD, Janne PA. Crizotinib versus chemotherapy in advanced ALK-positive lung cancer. N Engl J Med. 2013;368(25):2385–94. https://doi.org/10.1056/NEJMoa1214886.

224. Sievers EL, Larson RA, Stadtmauer EA, Estey E, Lowenberg B, Dombret H, Karanes C, Theobald M, Bennett JM, Sherman ML, Berger MS, Eten CB, Loken MR, van Dongen JJ, Bernstein ID, Appelbaum FR. Efficacy and safety of gemtuzumab ozogamicin in patients with CD33-positive acute myeloid leukemia in first relapse. J Clin Oncol. 2001;19(13):3244–54. https://doi.org/10.1200/jco.2001.19.13.3244.

225. Sledge GW Jr, Toi M, Neven P, Sohn J, Inoue K, Pivot X, Burdaeva O, Okera M, Masuda N, Kaufman PA, Koh H, Grischke EM, Frenzel M, Lin Y, Barriga S, Smith IC, Bourayou N, Llombart-Cussac A. MONARCH 2: abemaciclib in combination with fulvestrant in women with HR+/HER2- advanced breast cancer who had progressed while receiving endocrine therapy. J Clin Oncol. 2017;35(25):2875–84. https://doi.org/10.1200/jco.2017.73.7585.

226. Smith GA, Damon LE, Rugo HS, Ries CA, Linker CA. High-dose cytarabine dose modification reduces the incidence of neurotoxicity in patients with renal insufficiency. J Clin Oncol. 1997;15(2):833–9. https://doi.org/10.1200/jco.1997.15.2.833.

227. Soria JC, Tan DSW, Chiari R, Wu YL, Paz-Ares L, Wolf J, Geater SL, Orlov S, Cortinovis D, Yu CJ, Hochmair M, Cortot AB, Tsai CM, Moro-Sibilot D, Campelo RG, McCulloch T, Sen P, Dugan M, Pantano S, Branle F, Massacesi C, de Castro G Jr. First-line ceritinib versus platinum-based chemotherapy in advanced ALK-rearranged non-small-cell lung cancer (ASCEND-4): a randomised, open-label, phase 3 study. Lancet (London, England). 2017;389(10072):917–29. https://doi.org/10.1016/s0140-6736(17)30123-x.

228. Spectrum Pharmaceuticals Belcodaq (belinostat) [package insert]. Irvine; 2017.

229. Steeghs N, de Jongh FE, Sillevis Smitt PA, van den Bent MJ. Cisplatin-induced encephalopathy and seizures. Anti-Cancer Drugs. 2003;14(6):443–6. https://doi.org/10.1097/01.cad.0000078733.65608.38.

230. Stein EM, DiNardo CD, Pollyea DA, Fathi AT, Roboz GJ, Altman JK, Stone RM, DeAngelo DJ, Levine RL, Flinn IW, Kantarjian HM, Collins R, Patel MR, Frankel AE, Stein A, Sekeres MA, Swords RT, Medeiros BC, Willekens C, Vyas P, Tosolini A, Xu Q, Knight RD, Yen KE, Agresta S, de Botton S, Tallman MS. Enasidenib in mutant IDH2 relapsed or refractory acute myeloid leukemia. Blood. 2017;130(6):722–31. https://doi.org/10.1182/blood-2017-04-779405.

231. Stoica GS, Greenberg HE, Rossoff LJ. Corticosteroid responsive fludarabine pulmonary toxicity. Am J Clin Oncol. 2002;25(4):340–1.

232. Stone RM, DeAngelo DJ, Klimek V, Galinsky I, Estey E, Nimer SD, Grandin W, Lebwohl D, Wang Y, Cohen P, Fox EA, Neuberg D, Clark J, Gilliland DG, Griffin JD. Patients with acute myeloid leukemia and an activating mutation in FLT3 respond to a small-molecule FLT3 tyrosine kinase inhibitor, PKC412. Blood. 2005;105(1):54–60. https://doi.org/10.1182/blood-2004-03-0891.

233. Sun Pharmaceutical Industries. Odomzo (sonidegib) [package insert]. Cranbury; 2017.

234. SuperGen. Mitozytrex (mitomycin) [package insert]. Dublin; 2002.

235. Swain SM, Ewer MS, Cortes J, Amadori D, Miles D, Knott A, Clark E, Benyunes MC, Ross G, Baselga J. Cardiac tolerability of pertuzumab plus trastuzumab plus docetaxel in patients with HER2-positive metastatic breast cancer in CLEOPATRA: a randomized, double-blind, placebo-controlled phase III study. Oncologist. 2013;18(3):257–64. https://doi.org/10.1634/theoncologist.2012-0448.

236. Talpur R, Ward S, Apisarnthanarax N, Breuer-Mcham J, Duvic M. Optimizing bexarotene therapy for cutaneous T-cell lymphoma. J Am Acad Dermatol. 2002;47(5):672–84.

237. Tesaro Inc. Zejula (niraparib) [package insert]. Waltham; 2017.

238. Teva Pharmaceuticals Inc. Adrucil (fluorouracil injection) [package insert]. North Wales; 2017.

239. Teva Pharmaceuticals USA Inc. Bendeka (bendamustine hydrochloride) [package insert]. North Wales; 2017.

240. Thatcher N, Hirsch FR, Luft AV, Szczesna A, Ciuleanu TE, Dediu M, Ramlau R, Galiulin RK, Balint B, Losonczy G, Kazarnowicz A, Park K, Schumann C, Reck M, Depenbrock H, Nanda S, Kruljac-Letunic A, Kurek R, Paz-Ares L, Socinski MA. Necitumumab plus gemcitabine and cisplatin versus gemcitabine and cisplatin alone as first-line therapy in patients with stage IV squamous non-small-cell lung cancer (SQUIRE): an open-label, randomised, controlled phase 3 trial. Lancet Oncol. 2015;16(7):763–74. https://doi.org/10.1016/s1470-2045(15)00021-2.

241. Thornburg A, Abonour R, Smith P, Knox K, Twigg HL 3rd. Hypersensitivity pneumonitis-like syndrome associated with the use of lenalidomide. Chest. 2007; 131(5):1572–4. https://doi.org/10.1378/chest.06-1734.

242. Topp MS, Gokbuget N, Zugmaier G, Degenhard E, Goebeler ME, Klinger M, Neumann SA, Horst HA, Raff T, Viardot A, Stelljes M, Schaich M, Kohne-Volland R, Bruggemann M, Ottmann OG, Burmeister T, Baeuerle PA, Nagorsen D, Schmidt M, Einsele H, Riethmuller G, Kneba M, Hoelzer D, Kufer P, Bargou RC. Long-term follow-up of hematologic relapse-free survival in a phase 2 study of blinatumomab in patients with MRD in B-lineage all. Blood. 2012;120(26):5185–7. https://doi.org/10.1182/blood-2012-07-441030.

243. Topp MS, Gokbuget N, Zugmaier G, Klappers P, Stelljes M, Neumann S, Viardot A, Marks R, Diedrich H, Faul C, Reichle A, Horst HA, Bruggemann M, Wessiepe D, Holland C, Alekar S, Mergen N, Einsele H, Hoelzer D, Bargou RC. Phase II trial of the anti-CD19 bispecific T cell-engager blinatumomab shows hematologic and molecular remissions in patients with relapsed or refractory B-precursor acute lymphoblastic leukemia. J Clin

Oncol. 2014;32(36):4134–40. https://doi.org/10.1200/jco.2014.56.3247.

244. Umemura S, Yamane H, Suwaki T, Katoh T, Yano T, Shiote Y, Takigawa N, Kiura K, Kamei H. Interstitial lung disease associated with gemcitabine treatment in patients with non-small-cell lung cancer and pancreatic cancer. J Cancer Res Clin Oncol. 2011;137 (10):1469–75. https://doi.org/10.1007/s00432-011-1013-1.

245. United Therapeutics Corp. Unituxin (dinutuximab) [package insert]. Silver Spring; 2015.

246. Vahid B, Marik PE. Infiltrative lung diseases: complications of novel antineoplastic agents in patients with hematological malignancies. Can Respir J. 2008;15 (4):211–6.

247. Valent P, Hadzijusufovic E, Schernthaner GH, Wolf D, Rea D, le Coutre P. Vascular safety issues in CML patients treated with BCR/ABL1 kinase inhibitors. Blood. 2015;125(6):901–6. https://doi.org/10.1182/blood-2014-09-594432.

248. Verweij J, van Zanten T, Souren T, Golding R, Pinedo HM. Prospective study on the dose relationship of mitomycin C-induced interstitial pneumonitis. Cancer. 1987;60(4):756–61.

249. Wadleigh M, Richardson PG, Zahrieh D, Lee SJ, Cutler C, Ho V, Alyea EP, Antin JH, Stone RM, Soiffer RJ, DeAngelo DJ. Prior gemtuzumab ozogamicin exposure significantly increases the risk of veno-occlusive disease in patients who undergo myeloablative allogeneic stem cell transplantation. Blood. 2003;102(5):1578–82. https://doi.org/10.1182/blood-2003-01-0255.

250. Wanchoo R, Abudayyeh A, Doshi M, Edeani A, Glezerman IG, Monga D, Rosner M, Jhaveri KD. Renal toxicities of novel agents used for treatment of multiple myeloma. Clin J Am Soc Nephrol. 2017;12 (1):176–89. https://doi.org/10.2215/cjn.06100616.

251. Wanchoo R, Jhaveri KD, Deray G, Launay-Vacher V. Renal effects of BRAF inhibitors: a systematic review by the cancer and the Kidney International Network. Clin Kidney J. 2016;9(2):245–51. https://doi.org/10.1093/ckj/sfv149.

252. Waters MJ, Sukumaran S, Karapetis CS. Pemetrexed-Induced Interstitial pneumonitis: a case study and literature review. World J Oncol. 2014;5(5–6): 232–6. https://doi.org/10.14740/wjon845w.

253. Weiss RB, Poster DS, Penta JS. The nitrosoureas and pulmonary toxicity. Cancer Treat Rev. 1981;8(2): 111–25.

254. Wells SA Jr, Robinson BG, Gagel RF, Dralle H, Fagin JA, Santoro M, Baudin E, Elisei R, Jarzab B, Vasselli JR, Read J, Langmuir P, Ryan AJ, Schlumberger MJ. Vandetanib in patients with locally advanced or metastatic medullary thyroid cancer: a randomized, double-blind phase III trial. J Clin Oncol. 2012;30(2):134–41. https://doi.org/10.1200/jco.2011.35.5040.

255. Welsh SJ, Corrie PG. Management of BRAF and MEK inhibitor toxicities in patients with metastatic

melanoma. Ther Adv Med Oncol. 2015;7(2):122–36. https://doi.org/10.1177/1758834014566428.

256. Wenk KS, Pichard DC, Nasabzadeh T, Jang S, Venna SS. Vemurafenib-induced DRESS. JAMA Dermatol. 2013;149(10):1242–3. https://doi.org/10.1001/jamadermatol.2013.5278.

257. West-ward Pharmaceuticals. Thiotepa [package insert]. Eatontown; 2015.

258. Zamorano JL, Lancellotti P, Munoz DR, Aboyans V, Asteggiano R, Galderisi M, Habib G, Lenihan DJ, Lip GY, Lyon AR, Fernandez TL, Mohty D, Piepoli MF, Tamargo J, Torbicki A, Suter TM. 2016 ESC position paper on cancer treatments and cardiovascular toxicity developed under the auspices of the ESC committee for practice guidelines. Kardiol Pol. 2016;74(11): 1193–233. https://doi.org/10.5603/kp.2016.0156.

Supportive Care Considerations and Nutrition Support for Critically Ill Cancer Patients

17

Anne M. Tucker, Jacob W. Hall, Christine A. Mowatt-Larssen, and Todd W. Canada

Contents

Introduction 230

Nutrition Assessment 230

Refeeding Syndrome 233

Routes of Access 234

Enteral Nutrition 235
Common Indications 235
Enteral Formula Selection Considerations 235
Enteral Nutrition Protocols 236
Monitoring Enteral Nutrition 236
Complications of EN 237

Parenteral Nutrition and Supplemental Parenteral Nutrition 240
Complications of PN 242
Special Populations 243

Conclusion 243

References 244

Abstract

Protein-calorie malnutrition is frequently observed in elderly cancer patients admitted to the intensive care unit (ICU). The use of nutrition support in these patients is dictated through nutritional assessment and utilization of an available feeding access device, whether enteral or parenteral. Provision of hypocaloric regimens less than 20 kcal/kg/day with at least 1.2 g protein/kg/day is recommended in the 1st week of ICU care. Complications observed in the ICU cancer patient receiving nutrition support are primarily related to their underlying degree of malnutrition and comorbidities. The identification and management of hyperglycemia, electrolyte abnormalities, and vitamin deficiencies associated with refeeding syndrome in this ICU cancer population is of utmost importance.

A. M. Tucker · J. W. Hall · C. A. Mowatt-Larssen · T. W. Canada (✉)
Critical Care/Nutrition Support, The University of Texas MD Anderson Cancer Center, Houston, TX, USA
e-mail: amtucker@mdanderson.org; jhall1@mdanderson.org; cmowatt@mdanderson.org; tcanada@mdanderson.org

© Springer Nature Switzerland AG 2020
J. L. Nates, K. J. Price (eds.), *Oncologic Critical Care*,
https://doi.org/10.1007/978-3-319-74588-6_30

Keywords

Malnutrition · Enteral nutrition · Parenteral
nutrition · Refeeding syndrome · Vomiting ·
Diarrhea · Constipation · Aspiration ·
Hyperglycemia

Introduction

A recent review of almost 28 million non-
maternal and non-neonatal inpatient hospital
stays found that 2.2 million (8%) were related to
malnutrition [4]. Protein-calorie malnutrition
(PCM) occurred in 67% and is more frequently
observed in those over 65 years of age. The identification of PCM in critically ill cancer patients at
intensive care unit (ICU) admission is often
underappreciated and leads to longer lengths of
stay (LOS), higher costs, more comorbidities,
and, ultimately, greater mortality. The provision
of nutrition support to critically ill cancer patients
is considered a supportive care therapy given the
catabolic stress during an ICU stay on a patient's
lean body mass. This chapter focuses on critically
ill cancer patients and discusses important considerations when instituting nutrition support.

Nutrition Assessment

Malnutrition in cancer patients is common and
largely multifactorial. Metabolic changes related
to malignancy and reduced nutrient intake are the
major categories related to the etiology of cancer-
related malnutrition. Release of proinflammatory
cytokines associated with malignancy has been
related to alterations in resting energy expenditure, insulin resistance, and metabolism of carbo-
hydrates, protein, and lipids [34, 41]. Tumor-
related hormones such as proteolysis-inducing
factor and lipid-mobilizing factor may be released
leading to significant muscle and fat wasting [41].
Reduced nutrient intake can be due to primary
anorexia and secondary causes related to cancer-

directed treatments (e.g., nausea, vomiting, diarrhea, and gastrointestinal (GI) graft-versus-host
disease (GVHD)), malabsorption, surgical complications (e.g., high-output enterocutaneous fistula), and/or disease progression (e.g., chronic
malignant bowel obstruction). Regardless of the
exact cause, the result is a negative energy balance
and loss of lean body mass, both of which have
negative impacts on morbidity and mortality.
Inflammation related to critical illness has similar
negative effects on overall nutrition status and
patient outcomes occurring within a rapid time
period after insult or injury. This reinforces the
importance of appropriate nutrition screening,
assessment, and intervention of cancer patients
presenting to the ICU.

Assessment of patients at ICU admission is
critical specifically in regard to the timing and
goals of nutrition support. In 2016 the American
Society for Parenteral and Enteral Nutrition in
collaboration with the Society of Critical Care
Medicine updated the guidelines for nutrition
support in the critical care patient. Within these
guidelines, recommendations were made supporting the use of two nutritional risk screening
tools, the Nutritional Risk Score (NRS) 2002 and
Nutrition Risk in Critically Ill (NUTRIC) Score
[excluding interleukin-6 levels], for all ICU
patients "for whom volitional intake is anticipated
to be insufficient" [28]. Both scoring systems
relate nutritional status to severity of illness or
disease (see Table 1) and have been validated in
the ICU population [19, 20, 25]. High nutritional
risk is defined for both scoring systems as a score
greater than or equal to 5 [28]. In this group of
ICU patients, the provision of early enteral nutrition (EN) therapy has shown to decrease ICU
mortality, complications, and nosocomial infections [19, 22].

A full nutritional assessment should be
performed on all ICU patients to identify nutritional deficiencies and determine appropriate
nutritional requirements and interventions. The
components of such assessment should include a

Table 1 Nutritional risk scoring systems in the ICU

Nutritional Risk Score (NRS) 2002			Nutrition Risk in Critically Ill (NUTRIC) Score	
0	Absent	Normal nutritional status	0	Age <50
			1	Age 50–<75
			2	Age ≥75
1	Mild	Weight loss $>5\%$ in 3 months	APACHE II	
		OR	Score	Criteria
		Food intake below 50–75% normal requirement in previous week	0	<15
			1	15–<20
			2	20–<28
			3	≥28
2	Moderate	Weight loss $>5\%$ in 2 months	SOFA	
		OR	Score	Criteria
		BMI 18.5–20.5 kg/m^2 with impaired general condition	0	<6
			1	6–<10
		OR	2	≥10
		Food intake below 25–50% normal requirement in previous week		
3	Severe	Weight loss $>5\%$ in 1 month ($>15\%$ in 3 months)	Number of comorbidities	
		OR	Score	Criteria
		BMI <18.5 kg/m^2 with impaired general condition	0	0–1
		OR	1	≥2
		Food intake below 0–25% normal requirement in previous week		
Disease severity			Days from hospital to ICU admission	
Score	Description	Criteria	Score	Criteria
0	Absent	Normal nutritional requirements	0	0–<1
			1	≥1
1	Mild	Hip fracture	Interleukin-6 levels (commonly excluded)	
		Chronic patients, especially if acute complication (e.g., cirrhosis, COPD)	Score	Criteria
		ESRD requiring RRT	0	0–<400
		Diabetes mellitus	1	≥400
		Oncology/malignancy		
2	Moderate	Major abdominal surgery		
		Stroke		
		Severe pneumonia		
		Hematologic malignancy		
3	Severe	Head injury		
		Stem cell transplantation		
		Intensive care patient (APACHE II ≥10)		

(*continued*)

Table 1 (continued)

Nutritional Risk Score (NRS) 2002	Nutrition Risk in Critically Ill (NUTRIC) Score
To calculate the NRS 2002 score:	To calculate the NUTRIC score:
1. Determine score for impaired nutritional status (use the variable with the highest score)	1.1.1. Add up the scores for the above 5 categories (use the variable with the highest score)
2. Determine score for disease severity (use the variable with the highest score)	
3. Add the impaired nutritional status and disease severity scores	
4. Add 1 point if patient is ≥70 years of age to account for frailty of elderly	
NRS 2002 risk levels	NUTRIC risk levels
At risk: age-corrected score >3	High risk [excluding IL-6]: score ≥5
High risk: age-corrected score ≥5	High risk [including IL-6]: score >6

APACHE acute physiology and chronic health evaluation, *BMI* body mass index, *COPD* chronic obstructive pulmonary disease, *ESRD* end-stage renal disease, *IL* interleukin, *RRT* renal replacement therapy, *SOFA* sequential organ failure assessment

thorough history and physical exam to assess weight changes, dietary intake, social and cultural preferences, GI function, comorbid conditions, cancer type/stage, current and past cancer treatments (e.g., chemotherapy, radiation, surgery), and medications which could impact nutritional status. Use of historical nutritional markers such as serum albumin, prealbumin, and transferrin is no longer recommended as these are negative acute-phase proteins and have been found unreliable during inflammation and critical illness [28]. Caution should also be taken when evaluating weight measurements as fluid accumulation due to malignant ascites, edema, or fluid resuscitation may be present. In these instances, it is prudent for the ICU clinician to estimate dry weight (or ideal body weight (IBW) if unknown) for use in nutrition calculations and estimations. The use of ultrasonography and computed tomography to routinely assess body composition appears promising, but has yet to be validated in the critically ill and thus, has not been incorporated into clinical practice or guideline recommendations.

Identification of vitamin and trace element deficiencies in critically ill patients is primarily completed through physical exam and patient history as biochemical analysis of vitamins and trace elements are affected by the acute-phase and systemic inflammatory response. Serum levels of vitamin A, vitamin C, iron, zinc, and selenium are decreased during critical illness, while serum copper, ceruloplasmin, and ferritin are elevated [17]. Patients with large volume stool losses as seen with GI GVHD, malabsorptive syndromes (e.g., severe pancreatic exocrine insufficiency, short bowel syndrome), enterocutaneous fistulae, or ileostomy outputs greater than 2 L/day are at increased risk for zinc deficiency requiring supplementation. Zinc deficiencies can manifest as changes in taste, hair loss, poor wound healing, and skin changes, also referred to as acrodermatitis enteropathica. Copper losses through the GI tract can also produce deficiencies leading to microcytic anemia and neuropathy, both of which are common problems seen in cancer patients. Iron deficiency can also be an underlying cause of microcytic anemia in upper GI cancer patients; however, use of blood transfusions in the ICU may provide an alternative source of iron with approximately 1 mL of packed red blood cells providing 1 mg of iron. Macrocytic anemias from folate or cyanocobalamin deficiencies can also be seen commonly in cancer patients with prior gastric or ileal resections based upon tumor location. Unexplained cardiomyopathy and muscle weakness may be signs of selenium deficiency which may be observed during continuous renal replacement therapy (CRRT) or prolonged selenium-free parenteral nutrition (PN) solutions [9].

Accurate determination of energy needs in the critically ill is important in the prevention of feeding-associated adverse effects. Overfeeding, or the provision of energy above a patient's energy expenditure, can lead to hyperglycemia, hepatic dysfunction, and prolonged mechanical ventilation due to hypercarbia. On the contrary, underfeeding can also be detrimental contributing to malnutrition, muscle weakness, decreased wound healing, skin breakdown, and increased nosocomial infections, ICU LOS, and mortality.

Indirect calorimetry (IC) is considered the gold standard for assessment of energy expenditure and is supported by current guidelines [28]. However, it is not universally employed by many centers due to cost, lack of reimbursement, and need for dedicated respiratory therapists proficient to perform and interpret IC studies. Measurement of energy expenditure is accomplished through use of a metabolic cart or specialized ventilator with IC capabilities. The carbon dioxide produced (VCO_2) and oxygen consumption (VO_2) are obtained during a steady-state period (usually takes approximately 30 min) and used to calculate the measured energy expenditure and respiratory quotient. Careful selection of appropriate patients to perform IC is required to obtain accurate measurements. Contraindications to the use of IC can be found in Table 2. IC has been helpful in an attempt to better outline energy requirements for the cancer patient, but work remains to be done. It is known that altered metabolism exists for cancer patients; however, the extent and magnitude of

these to energy expenditure are not uniform among cancer types [15] nor found to correlate with disease extent, gender, nutritional status, or anthropometric assessments [24]. It is also unclear how the addition of critical illness affects energy expenditure in patients with cancer. Previous studies in critically ill cancer patients have shown poor correlation of measured energy expenditure to weight-based guideline estimations and commonly used estimation equations (e.g., Harris-Benedict equation) [36, 38]. When IC is not available, current guidelines recommend weight-based estimations [28]. See Table 3 for weight-based dosing guidelines.

Refeeding Syndrome

Refeeding syndrome (RFS) is a compilation of metabolic abnormalities occurring within the first 72 h of carbohydrate provision in the presence of prolonged inadequate nutritional intake. Profound depletion of phosphorus, potassium, and magnesium can occur during refeeding leading to respiratory failure, cardiac collapse, arrhythmias, hematological abnormalities, neuromuscular weakness, seizures, and coma. Hyponatremia may also ensue due to fluid retention related to hyperglycemia and hyperinsulinemia. Cancer patients are at increased risk for RFS due to reduced nutritional intake both prior to and during hospitalization or cancer treatment. Other patient populations and conditions placing patients at risk for RFS can be found in Table 4 [7]. Thiamine can become quickly depleted during early refeeding as cancer patients may have inadequate stores relative to the increased demand due to carbohydrate provision and metabolism, as thiamine is needed for conversion of pyruvate to acetyl coenzyme A and utilization of the citric acid cycle. During periods of thiamine deficiency, refractory lactic acidosis (i.e., from pyruvate conversion to lactate) and neurological complications, such as encephalopathy, may occur. Prevention strategies should be in place to identify those at risk of RFS. Initial caloric restriction with close monitoring of electrolytes, replacement of identified electrolyte abnormalities, and empiric thiamine

Table 2 Contraindications to indirect calorimetry

Fraction of inspired oxygen >0.5	Peak end expiratory pressure >10 mmHg
Respiratory rate >30 breaths per minute	Hemodynamic instability (heart rate >130 beats per minute, mean arterial pressure <60 mmHg)
During or within 3 h of blood transfusion	Continuous renal replacement therapy or intermittent hemodialysis within 3 h
Agitation	Hemoglobin <8 g/dL
Air leak within the ventilator circuit	Air leak around tracheal cuff
Air leak around chest tube	Untreated pneumothorax

Table 3 Parenteral nutrition dosing recommendations

Caloric recommendations	≤20 kcal/kg/day (or 80% of estimated energy needs) during first 7 days of ICU stay
	25–30 kcal/kg/day after first 7 days
	22–25 kcal/kg/day IBW for obese (BMI ≥30 kg/m^2)
	Discontinue when receiving >60% of target energy requirements from enteral nutrition
Protein (amino acids 4 kcal/g)	1.2–2 g/kg/day
	2–2.5 g/kg/day IBW for obese
	2.5 g/kg/day for patients receiving CRRT
Carbohydrate (dextrose 3.4 kcal/g)	Not to exceed 7 g/kg/day
Intravenous lipid emulsion *(recommended to be held during first 7 days of ICU stay unless malnourished)*	≤1 g/kg/day (100% soybean oil)
	1–2 g/kg/day (30% soybean oil, 30% medium chain triglycerides, 25% olive oil, 15% fish oil)
Electrolytes	
Sodium	1–2 mEq/kg/day
Potassium	1–2 mEq/kg/day
Phosphate	20–40 mmol/day
Magnesium	8–64 mEq/day
Calcium	10–15 mEq/day (dependent on phosphate content)
Acetate	As needed to maintain acid-based balance
Chloride	As needed to maintain acid-based balance

BMI body mass index, *CRRT* continuous renal replacement therapy, *IBW* ideal body weight, *ICU* intensive care unit

Table 4 Patient populations and conditions at increased risk for refeeding syndrome

Age >70 years	Intestinal failure
Bariatric surgery	Malabsorption (radiation enteritis, celiac disease)
Chronic alcoholism or drug abuse	Cancer
Chronic bowel obstruction	Neurologically impaired (stroke)
Chronic diarrhea	Postoperative patients
Dysphagia	Prolonged fasting/NPO status (>7 days)
Eating disorders (anorexia nervosa, bulimia)	Protracted vomiting
Failure to thrive	Severe malnutrition (BMI <18.5 kg/m^2)
Inflammatory bowel disease (Crohn's disease, ulcerative colitis)	

NPO nil per os, *BMI* body mass index

supplementation (100–300 mg daily) prior to and during the first 3–5 days of nutrition therapy is commonly employed in high-risk patients to prevent RFS complications [16]. Doig et al. conducted a study comparing caloric restriction of 20 kcal/h for at least 2 days versus standard nutrition therapy after the occurrence of RFS in critically ill adults. Their results did not find a decrease in the number of days alive after ICU discharge with the use of caloric restriction; however, significant improvements were noted for 60-day mortality and reductions in infectious morbidity [12].

Routes of Access

Selection of the most appropriate nutrition support feeding route involves an assessment of GI functionality and pre-existing enteral or venous access devices. Most cancer patients admitted to the ICU who have previously received chemotherapy will likely have a peripherally inserted central catheter or central venous catheter (e.g., tunneled, subcutaneous, or external) already in place, provided it is not a suspected source of infection and need to be removed in a neutropenic host. New placement of either an enteral or intravenous (IV) access device in the critically ill cancer patient is often met with relative contraindications including thrombocytopenia and shock.

Our institution has previously investigated the risks associated with placement of an oral or nasal feeding tube in critically ill thrombocytopenic cancer patients and did not find them to be at a higher risk of bleeding complications compared to patients without thrombocytopenia [35]. The choice to use the IV route because it already exists in a critically ill cancer patient with a functional GI tract is a matter of controversy as a recent meta-analysis showed no clear advantage of early EN over PN [39]. An important consideration if PN is to be utilized in the ICU cancer patient is the compatibility limitations when it comes to other IV drug administration as the use of certain drugs, such as acyclovir, amphotericin B, furosemide, and ganciclovir generally is incompatible with a wide range of other IV medications and may preclude PN use.

Enteral Nutrition

Common Indications

The multiple benefits of EN in critical illness support the functional integrity of the GI tract, stimulating blood flow and release of endogenous trophic mediators including gastrin, cholecystokinin, bombesin, and bile salts [28]. Ideally, the goal of care is to initiate EN within the first 24–48 h of an ICU stay anticipated to exceed 2–3 days. This is even more important in cancer patients who are often at high nutritional risk (NUTRIC score ≥5 or NRS 2002 ≥5) with cancer cachexia and prolonged poor intake prior to hospitalization and/or ICU admission. Common indications for use of EN in the ICU are listed in Table 5. Coexisting conditions of critical illness and cancer generate challenges for the initiation of EN including access placement (see section "Routes of Access") and feeding tolerance. Early EN initiation mitigates increased GI permeability and reduces infection rates, organ failure rates, and hospital LOS [28]. While there are clinical situations where EN is contraindicated (Table 6), practitioners are encouraged to evaluate medical histories, current diagnoses, and diagnostic imaging with physical assessments to see if enteral access may be safely established.

Table 5 Enteral nutrition trial encouraged

Head and neck cancer surgery patients
Upper gastrointestinal tumors (stented or distal enteral access)
Radiation enteritis
Failure to thrive
Esophageal motility disorder
Short bowel syndrome with >60 cm of small bowel with colon intact OR >120 cm of small bowel without colon
Enterocutaneous low output fistula (<500 mL/day)
Pancreatic fistula <200 mL/day
Pancreatitis (stable serum amylase/lipase, without complex fistula, infected phlegmon or pseudocyst)
Delayed gastric emptying
Acute respiratory failure, acute lung injury, diffuse alveolar hemorrhage
Sepsis
Neurologic impairment (altered mental status)

Table 6 Common barriers and limitations for enteral nutrition

Common barriers	Limitations
Prolonged ileus	Aspiration pneumonia
Intractable vomiting or diarrhea	
Gastrointestinal bleeding	
Major gastrointestinal ischemia	
Severe hemodynamic instability	
High-output fistulas (enterocutaneous >500 mL/day, pancreatic >200 mL/day)	
Malabsorption (severe pancreatic exocrine insufficiency)	
Short bowel syndrome	
Small or large bowel obstruction	
High-output ileostomy	
Severe mucositis	
Gastrointestinal graft-versus-host disease	

Enteral Formula Selection Considerations

Many EN formulations are available for use in critically ill patients. Standard, polymeric EN formulas are appropriate for most patients and are designed to mimic a normal diet. These formulas require normal GI digestion and absorption of nutrients. They are available as 1 kcal/mL, 1.2 kcal/mL, 1.5 kcal/mL, and 2 kcal/mL concentrations with selection depending on the fluid needs of the patient. Use of more concentrated EN formulas is indicated primarily for those ICU patients exhibiting fluid overload states such as end-stage renal disease, acute kidney injury without renal replacement therapy, and heart failure. Neurological surgery cancer patients may also require more concentrated EN formulas for fluid restriction. There are also instances where a non-fluid-restricted patient may require a more concentrated formula due to the need for multiple IV medications or abdominal intolerance of high rate 1 kcal/mL EN (e.g., >100 mL/h). A thorough medication review is needed to determine the total daily fluid content of all medications [13].

Several situations exist where selection of a non-polymeric or specific EN formula is desired. Switching to a semi-elemental or elemental EN formula may be appropriate if patients exhibit signs and symptoms of GI malabsorption or intolerance [13]. These formulas are composed of partially or completely hydrolyzed nutrients (e.g., protein as hydrolyzed casein or whey) and altered fats (e.g., fish oil, soybean oil) to reduce the need for full digestive capacity and maximization of nutrient absorption. Patients with renal dysfunction not undergoing CRRT therapy or patients with specific electrolyte abnormalities due to medications or comorbid conditions may require the use of a renal formula specifically designed to have reduced potassium, magnesium, and phosphorus concentrations [13].

Current guidelines recommend that clinicians consider the use of fiber or fiber-containing EN formulas in patients with persistent diarrhea. While these formulas may be beneficial in this subset of ICU patients, the guidelines strongly suggest against the use of both soluble and insoluble fiber in patients at risk for bowel ischemia and those exhibiting GI dysmotility [28]. Protein modular products (e.g., whey protein or glutamine) administered as bolus flushes are useful adjuncts to ensure adequate protein administration [13]. These products are especially useful for obese patients being fed via a hypocaloric and high-protein regimen, postoperative patients, and patients with large wounds where protein needs may exceed that found in commercially available formulations (e.g., generally 40–60 g protein/L).

Enteral Nutrition Protocols

Protocols for EN should be utilized in the critical care setting to improve delivery of nutrients to patients [11]. It has been shown that ICU or nursing-driven EN protocols can increase the percentage of goal calories that a patient receives and may reduce the incidence of nosocomial infections. Protocols involving EN therapy can include standardization through implementation of volume-based feedings, starting EN at goal, defined advancement rates, implementation of prokinetic agents, and feeding tube placement [28].

Monitoring Enteral Nutrition

EN should be monitored frequently for safety and efficacy. Laboratory monitoring of electrolytes, especially for those at risk for RFS (see Table 4) or other electrolyte abnormalities, should be performed at least daily. Monitoring of serum protein markers (i.e., albumin, prealbumin, retinol-binding protein) for sufficiency of nutrition support in the ICU is not recommended [28].

Tolerance to EN can be determined by GI passage of flatus and stool, abdominal radiologic evaluations, and absence of abdominal pain or distension. Intolerance to EN is generally defined as severe nausea, vomiting, abdominal discomfort or pain, high nasogastric (NG) or gastric output if utilizing an NG tube or transgastric jejunostomy feeding tube, diarrhea, or abnormal abdominal radiographs consistent with ileus or obstruction.

Gastric residual volumes (GRVs) have long been used in the critically ill population to denote EN intolerance. However, recent studies and current guidelines no longer support the practice of monitoring GRVs to assess EN tolerance as they have not been shown to reduce the incidence of pneumonia, regurgitation, or aspiration. In addition, the practice of checking GRVs may lead to clogging of the EN access device and lead to inappropriately holding of EN [28].

Complications of EN

Nausea/Vomiting

Nausea has been reported to occur in up to 20–25% of critically ill patients on EN [32]. Primary causes of nausea include delayed gastric emptying, constipation, cancer-directed therapies, surgery (e.g., pancreaticoduodenectomy, vagotomy), GI GVHD, and medication use. Specific medications associated with delayed gastric emptying in the ICU include opioids and medications with anticholinergic properties (e.g., scopolamine, antihistamines, atropine, hyoscyamine, and oxybutynin). Specific nutrition therapies have been associated with nausea including rapid infusion of EN, use of cold EN formulas, and formulas with high fat (e.g., >40%) and/or fiber contents. Treatment measures to alleviate nausea and vomiting include switching to a low-fat (e.g., 10% or less), low-fiber EN formula, slowing the EN infusion, changing to a postpyloric enteral feeding access device, use of antiemetics and/or prokinetic agents (e.g., metoclopramide or erythromycin), and limiting offending medications. Adequate hydration and use of a bowel regimen to prevent or limit constipation are also helpful in reducing nausea and vomiting with EN [26].

Constipation

Constipation can occur in critically ill patients due to multiple reasons. Overall causes of constipation include dehydration, inadequate dietary fiber, medications (e.g., opiates, anticholinergic agents, antiemetics), and physical inactivity. Attempts should be made to limit the use of offending medications while also providing adequate enteral water flushes and engaging the patient in physical therapy. As with nausea, a bowel regimen containing a stool softener plus or minus a laxative or enema should be instituted for all ICU patients to prevent constipation unless a contraindication such as abdominal distention or fecal impaction is present [26].

Diarrhea

Diarrhea in hospitalized patients is often defined as greater than 500 mL of stool output over 24 h or more than three stools per day for 2 consecutive days [26]. The incidence of diarrhea has been reported as high as 26% in critically ill patients and can have deleterious consequences if left untreated [2]. Causes of diarrhea include medications (e.g., sorbitol-containing as a sweetening agent), GI infection or disease, and less commonly EN. A systematic approach should be undertaken to determine the underlying cause of diarrhea in order to institute appropriate treatment and limit the development of dehydration, hypernatremia, hypokalemia, and other electrolyte imbalances.

Critically ill patients receive numerous medications during their ICU stay, many of which increase the risk of diarrhea (see Table 7). This includes commonly used medications such as antimicrobials, proton-pump inhibitors, and electrolyte replacements. Daily medication review should be completed to assess if de-escalation of therapy is clinically indicated in an effort to reduce diarrhea. The risk of diarrhea also increases especially when liquid medications are utilized, as many are hypertonic or contain sorbitol. Dilution of hypertonic medications prior to administration can limit diarrhea; however, this practice is not beneficial in the management of sorbitol-related diarrhea [43]. The provision of 10 or more grams of sorbitol per day through medication administration can lead to GI symptoms such as bloating, abdominal cramping, and diarrhea. The total sorbitol content should be calculated for critically ill cancer patients receiving multiple liquid medications, with considerations of alternative formulations when sorbitol content is high [8, 43].

Underlying conditions and diseases affecting the GI tract predispose patients to diarrhea (see Table 7). These include GI infections (e.g., enterotoxic organisms such as *Clostridium difficile*, *Escherichia coli*, *Salmonella*, *Shigella*, and *Campylobacter* species), inflammatory bowel disease, uncontrolled diabetes mellitus, celiac disease, fat malabsorption syndromes, stool impaction, and intestinal resections leading to end ileostomy or short bowel syndrome. Cancer-related causes include malignant carcinoid syndrome, villous adenoma of the colon, radiation

Table 7 Etiologies of diarrhea

Conditions and diseases	Medications	Enteral nutrition-related
Celiac disease	Antibiotics	Formula contamination
Diabetes mellitus, poorly controlled	Antineoplastics (e.g., irinotecan, 5-fluorouracil)	Hyperosmolar formulas (greater than 400 mOsm/kg)
Enteric infections (e.g., *C. difficile*, *E. coli*, *Salmonella*, *Shigella*, *Campylobacter*)	Digoxin	
	Histamine-2 receptor blockers	
Gastrointestinal graft-versus-host disease	Proton-pump inhibitors	
Fecal impaction	Laxatives	
Inflammatory bowel disease	Magnesium-containing antacids	
Malabsorption conditions	Metoclopramide	
Malignant carcinoid syndrome	Erythromycin (motilin receptor agonist)	
Pancreatic exocrine insufficiency	Oral potassium supplements	
Radiation enteritis	Oral phosphorus supplements	
Short bowel syndrome	Quinidine	
Villous adenoma of the colon	Sorbitol-containing medications	

enteritis, and GI GVHD [5]. Review of the medical history and appropriate diagnostic testing can aid the clinician in identifying such conditions in order to begin targeted treatments which can include surgery, chemotherapy, antimicrobials, systemic corticosteroids, dietary modifications, pancreatic enzyme replacement, and antidiarrheal agents (e.g., loperamide, diphenoxylate, codeine, and octreotide). Prior to antidiarrheal therapy, infectious diarrhea should be ruled out to prevent toxic megacolon [18].

When efforts to address medication therapy and concomitant conditions do not alleviate diarrhea, a focus on the EN formula is reasonable. Since critically ill patients typically receive continuous EN, diarrhea due to formula tonicity is less likely except in cases where hyperosmolar (e.g., >700 mOsm/kg) formulas are infused at high rates. Dilution of EN formulas to enhance GI tolerance is not indicated and can lead to inadequate nutritional provision, fluid overload, and formula contamination. Changing to an isotonic formula, semi-elemental or elemental peptide-based formula may be attempted in an effort to increase EN tolerance [13]. A trial of fiber supplements or fiber-containing EN formula is also an option, but only for stable critically ill patients

at low risk for bowel ischemia or dysmotility [28]. PN should be considered in cases where supplementation to EN is required to meet daily requirements, such as in severe, prolonged, and/or refractory diarrhea or when complete bowel rest is indicated (e.g., severe GI GVHD) [26].

Bowel Ischemia

Bowel ischemia is a rare, but potentially devastating complication, and all critically ill patients receiving EN should be closely monitored, especially those receiving vasopressor (e.g., norepinephrine) therapy. Risk factors include hypotension (mean arterial pressure <50 mmHg), initiation of vasopressor therapy, and need for escalating doses of vasopressor agents to maintain hemodynamics [28]. EN may be safely used, but with caution, in patients who are fully fluid-resuscitated, receiving stable, lower doses of vasopressors. In these situations, EN is associated with overall lower ICU and hospital mortality [23]. EN should be held or discontinued in patients exhibiting signs or symptoms of GI intolerance. These include abdominal distension, increasing NG or gastric output if utilizing an NG or transgastric jejunostomy feeding tube, reduced stool output or flatus, and increasing metabolic acidosis with or without base deficit. Those suspected to have bowel ischemia should be evaluated radiographically with surgical consultation to determine need for operative intervention [28].

Aspiration

Aspiration is the inspiration of fluid or foreign material, gastric contents, or food into the airways of the lung. Clinical manifestations of aspiration include dyspnea, tachypnea, wheezing, pneumonia, chemical pneumonitis, tachycardia, anxiety, hypoxia, and cyanosis. Patients at risk for aspiration include older age, EN administration, altered consciousness, gastroesophageal reflex disease, poor oral health, lack of oral care, misplaced enteral feeding access device, frequent movement or transfer of patient, and recumbent positioning [8, 26, 28].

Instituting measures to prevent aspiration should be the goal in critically ill patients receiving EN as many risk factors are frequently present. Radiographic verification of enteral access device placement should be completed prior to the commencement of EN to ensure appropriate placement. Elevating the head of the bed to at least 30° is a best practice supported by guidelines and employed within many ICU ventilator bundles. Other actions to reduce the risk of aspiration include regular monitoring for aspiration, minimizing the use of sedating medications and transportation of patients, use of post-pyloric feeding tubes, continuous EN infusion, and initiation of prokinetic agents (e.g., metoclopramide or erythromycin) in those illustrating delayed gastric emptying or regurgitation [8, 26, 28].

Use of GRVs to assess risk for aspiration is no longer recommended as this practice leads to unnecessary holding of EN and decreased nutrient provision and does not correlate to aspiration pneumonia or emesis rates. Current guidelines recommend that for institutions continuing to assess GRVs, holding of EN should not be done for GRVs less than 500 mL in those without clinical signs of feeding intolerance [28]. Detection of aspiration through blue dye administration and glucose oxidase testing is also no longer recommended due to reports of safety concerns and unreliable results [28].

Hyperglycemia

Stress-related hyperglycemia is common in critically ill cancer patients, especially in those receiving nutrition support therapy. Complex interactions between counterregulatory hormones and cytokines during illness or injury lead to hyperglycemia through increased glycogenolysis, enhanced gluconeogenesis, and insulin resistance. Risk factors for stress-related hyperglycemia include prior history of diabetes mellitus, occult diabetes, pancreatitis, cirrhosis, obesity, and use of systemic corticosteroids.

Endogenous insulin secretion in critically ill cancer patients is typically insufficient to prevent hyperglycemia necessitating exogenous insulin administration. Insulin therapy should be initiated in patients with persistent serum glucoses greater than 180 mg/dL. Validated, evidence-based insulin protocols should be employed for hyperglycemia management with a target glucose of 140–180 mg/dL. Continuous IV insulin infusion is the recommended method for achieving glycemic targets in critically ill patients as clinical conditions and pharmacotherapy lead to significant fluctuation in glucose values. Continuous IV insulin infusion is also highly effective in reducing hyperglycemia to goal levels within 24 h for most patients. Frequent glucose assessments and insulin infusion rate adjustments are required for optimal control of hyperglycemia and prevention of hypoglycemia. In cases where EN is to be discontinued or held for a given procedure or event, the insulin infusion should be held or decreased to a basal rate at least 30–60 min prior to the procedure or event. For chronic, stable ICU patients receiving continuous EN, conversion to a basal insulin and use of regular insulin bolus approach may be employed. Prolonged sole use of sliding-scale insulin therapy is not recommended as it is reactionary and does not mimic normal physiology [1, 31]. Close monitoring of renal function for patients receiving insulin is imperative, as insulin elimination is reduced in renal dysfunction and can lead to prolonged insulin effect with resultant hypoglycemia.

Additional strategies for hyperglycemia management include a thorough medication review to identify medications causing hyperglycemia, adjustment of medication regimens as medically appropriate, and compounding of IV medications in saline-containing diluents where possible due to compatibility. Medications that predispose patients to hyperglycemia include corticosteroids, catecholamines, diuretics, immunosuppressant agents (e.g., tacrolimus), and atypical antipsychotics (e.g., quetiapine). Prevention of overfeeding is important to minimize elevated glucose values. Use of diabetes-specific EN formulas is not recommended in critically ill patients [28].

Overfeeding

Provision of excess calories to patients during critical illness should be avoided as this has been shown to cause hepatic steatosis, hyperglycemia, hypercapnia, and cardiac arrhythmias. In addition, optimal caloric goals in critical illness may be less than a patient's typical needs especially in the 1st week of ICU stay, with higher caloric provision being associated with worse outcomes [10].

Parenteral Nutrition and Supplemental Parenteral Nutrition

PN is required for critically ill oncology patients when EN is not feasible or is not able to meet the patient's nutritional needs (e.g., <60% of target energy requirements from EN). For patients with a low nutritional risk (NRS 2002 ≤3 or NUTRIC score ≤5 [without interleukin-6]), PN should be withheld for the first 7 days after ICU admission in those who cannot receive EN. For patients with severe malnutrition or high nutrition risk (NRS 2002 ≥5 or NUTRIC score ≥5 [without interleukin 6]), PN should be initiated as soon as possible upon ICU admission [28].

Critically ill oncology patients are at risk for multiple barriers to fully tolerate EN, which may necessitate the use of PN. Common indications for PN can been seen in Table 8. Examples of those that may be unique to the oncology population include small or large bowel obstruction, GI GVHD, severe mucositis after hematopoietic stem cell transplantation (HSCT), neutropenic

Table 8 Common indications for parenteral nutrition

High-dose vasopressor use/hemodynamic instability
Paralytic or postoperative ileus
Open abdomen
Small or large bowel obstruction
Gastric outlet obstruction
Short bowel syndrome
Enterocutaneous fistula
Gastrointestinal graft-versus-host disease
Severe mucositis
Neutropenic colitis
Radiation enteritis

colitis, and radiation enteritis in which EN has failed [37].

Attempts to stabilize and resuscitate the critically ill patient should be made prior to initiating PN. It is recommended to withhold PN in patients with bacteremia and initially in those patients with septic shock [28]. Severe electrolyte abnormalities and hyperglycemia should be corrected prior to starting PN. In addition, volume overload is a relative contraindication for PN due to the volume required for adequate nutrition support. Available IV access may be limited by other needed interventions such as IV fluids, blood product administration, vasopressors, sedation, analgesia, antimicrobials, and CRRT, with PN requiring a dedicated line with limited data available on drug compatibility. Central IV access for PN is by far preferred over peripheral IV access in the critically ill due to the large volume required for adequate nutrition support due to the limited osmolarity of peripheral PN (<900 mOsm/L) [29].

The recommended dosing of macronutrients with PN in critically ill patients is similar to that of EN. A goal caloric intake of 25–30 kcal/kg/day is recommended. However, recent guidelines have recommended to limit caloric intake to less than or equal to 20 kcal/kg/day (no more than 80% of caloric goal) during the first 7 days after admission to the ICU, as this may reduce infectious complications and hyperglycemia [28]. A goal protein dose of 1.2–2 g/kg/day is recommended; however, studies indicate that a protein dose >1.2 g/kg/day may only result in a positive nitrogen balance, and it is unclear as to what dose of protein during critical illness is ideal

[21]. Higher-protein doses (i.e., 2.5 g/kg/day) are required in those patients requiring CRRT [28].

Intravenous lipid emulsion (ILE) is indicated for the provision of calories and prevention of essential fatty acid deficiency (EFAD) in patients requiring PN. While EFAD is a rare occurrence in the critically ill, it can occur in those cancer patients who are severely malnourished or who are receiving ILE-free PN for greater than 4 weeks [6]. In order to prevent EFAD, provision of at least 1–4% of daily caloric needs as linoleic acid is recommended. This may be provided as infrequently as a once-weekly dose of ILE high in linoleic acid (e.g., 50 g of 100% soybean oil). ILE in the critically ill is more often utilized for caloric provision due to its caloric density (10 kcal/g for a 20% ILE) and reduction in the need for dextrose as a nonprotein calorie source. Currently, there are only two ILEs available in the United States: (1) 100% soybean oil ILE and (2) a combination ILE consisting of 30% soybean oil, 30% medium chain triglycerides, 25% olive oil, and 15% fish oil (SMOF). Guidelines recommend to withhold or limit the use of ILE consisting of 100% soybean oil within the first 7 days of ICU stay based on a study indicating higher infection rates, longer hospital LOS, and longer duration of mechanical ventilation with 100% soybean oil ILE use [28]. ILE should be infused at a rate of less than 0.12 g/kg/h for 100% soybean oil ILE and at a rate of less than 0.15 g/kg/h for SMOF ILE to prevent worsening pulmonary hemodynamics and oxygenation index. According to the Centers for Disease Control and Prevention guidelines, ILE may only be infused for up to 12 h when infused separately from PN or up to 24 h when infusing within a PN as a total nutrient admixture [33].

Electrolyte dosing in PN will vary greatly in critically ill patients and must be individualized for each patient. General daily needs of electrolytes can be seen in Table 3 [30]. Multivitamins should be provided daily to patients requiring PN, and the amounts provided are included in Table 9 [42]. Trace elements should also be provided daily and are available either as individual components or in combination products [42]. Additional higher doses of selenium and other antioxidants have been studied in the critically ill, but no specific recommendations have been determined

Table 9 Parenteral vitamin and trace element recommendations

Multivitamin	Daily recommended dose	Content per 10 mL of Infuvite Adult™:
Vitamin A	3300 IU	3300 IU
Vitamin D	200 IU	200 IU
Vitamin E	10 IU	10 IU
Vitamin K	150 mcg	150 mcg
Vitamin B_1 (Thiamine)	6 mg	6 mg
Vitamin B_2 (Riboflavin)	3.6 mg	3.6 mg
Vitamin B_3 (Niacin)	40 mg	40 mg
Vitamin B_5 (Pantothenic acid)	15 mg	15 mg
Vitamin B_6 (Pyridoxine)	6 mg	6 mg
Vitamin B_{12} (Cyanocobalamin)	5 mcg	5 mcg
Vitamin C (Ascorbic acid)	200 mg	200 mg
Biotin	60 mcg	60 mcg
Folic acid	600 mcg	600 mcg
Trace elements	**Daily recommended dose**	**Amount in 3 mL of multitrace-5™:**
Copper	0.3–0.5 mg	1.2 mg
Chromium	10–15 mcg	12 mcg
Manganese	0.06–0.1 mg	0.3 mg
Zinc	2.5–5 mg	3 mg
Selenium	20–60 mcg	60 mcg

IU international units

regarding the optimal dose or regimen. Caution should be taken with providing excess copper and manganese in patients with liver dysfunction (e.g., direct bilirubin >2 mg/dL) as these are eliminated via the biliary system. Chromium and manganese are contaminates of PN components and IV fluids, so additional supplementation is not typically required in critically ill patients.

Complications of PN

The risk of RFS, overfeeding, and fluid overload are similar, if not increased, in patients receiving PN when compared to those receiving EN as most studies consistently show greater energy and protein intakes for PN over EN. Recommendations for the management of these conditions are similar to those receiving EN.

Hyperglycemia
PN is an independent risk factor for the development or worsening of hyperglycemia in both known diabetic and nondiabetic patients [44]. Since dextrose supplied through PN directly enters the systemic circulation bypassing intestinal regulators of glucose metabolism, insulin therapy is frequently required. To limit the development of hyperglycemia, dextrose infusion rates should not exceed 4 mg/kg/min (e.g., 20 kcal/kg/day). Provision of dextrose at lower rates may be necessary, especially in those with pre-existing diabetes mellitus, sepsis, and acute pancreatitis or during systemic corticosteroid therapy. As in critically ill patients receiving EN, IV insulin is the primary route of insulin administration. Use of continuous IV insulin infusions per standardized protocol remains the preferred method of insulin administration in critically ill cancer patients.

For stable patients, it may be appropriate to provide insulin via addition to the PN formulation. Initial insulin dosing is determined using the calculation of 0.1 unit of regular insulin for every gram of dextrose in the PN formulation (e.g., 250 g dextrose × 0.1 unit/g = 25 units of regular insulin) [30]. A higher ratio of insulin to infused dextrose (i.e., 0.1 unit of regular insulin per 0.5 g dextrose) is frequently required for obese (e.g., body mass index (BMI) >30 kg/m^2) patients and

those with significant insulin resistance [30]. PN dextrose advancement should not occur until blood glucose values are consistently less than 180 mg/dL. Concurrent subcutaneous administration of rapid- or short-acting regular insulin through use of a sliding-scale protocol is utilized to cover blood glucose values greater than 180 mg/dL. Daily adjustments of the PN insulin dose are made by adding two-thirds of the correction insulin needed from the previous 24 h to the PN. In clinical situations where glycemic control cannot be obtained or the clinical condition of the patient worsens, conversion to continuous IV insulin infusion is warranted. Close monitoring of medication changes affecting glucose control and changes in renal function is imperative to determine required insulin dose adjustments.

Parenteral Nutrition-Associated Liver Disease
PN-associated liver disease (PNALD) is a complication related to long-term (e.g., 4 weeks or more) use of PN. While it is more often diagnosed in children with intestinal failure, it can still manifest as cholestasis, hepatosteatosis, or cholelithiasis in adults. It can be definitively diagnosed via liver biopsy, but is more commonly diagnosed with an elevated direct bilirubin of >2 mg/dL, with elevated transaminases and no other obvious explanation for liver dysfunction. As it is a diagnosis of exclusion and is not seen immediately upon initiation of PN, it is rare for PN to be the sole cause of liver dysfunction in the critically ill cancer patient. Treatment and prevention of PNALD should be to utilize EN when possible, decrease caloric PN support, utilize cyclic PN, and provide ILE with omega-3 fatty acids [40].

Hypertriglyceridemia
Hypertriglyceridemia may occur as an adverse effect of the ILE provision within PN. Serum triglyceride levels should be monitored in patients receiving ILE at least weekly and ILE withheld if serum triglyceride levels exceed 400 mg/dL. Severe hypertriglyceridemia with levels >1000 mg/dL may result in acute pancreatitis. Critically ill cancer patients are at higher risk of developing elevated triglyceride levels due to altered hepatic lipid metabolism and provision of

medications requiring ILE vehicles (e.g., propofol, clevidipine) [30].

Central Line-Associated Bloodstream Infection

Central line-associated bloodstream infections (CLABSIs) remain a significant problem for cancer patients in the ICU. They are associated with increased mortality, LOS, and cost of hospitalization. Despite many advances that have decreased the rates of CLABSIs over the last few decades, PN still remains an independent risk factor for CLABSI. Clinicians must be diligent in monitoring for the development of CLABSI, and if bacteremia or fungemia develops, consider venous access removal if possible and temporary discontinuation of PN [14].

Special Populations

Renal Dysfunction

Acute kidney injury (AKI) is common in the critically ill patient, and providing appropriate nutrition in these patients comes with the concerns of significant electrolyte abnormalities, acid-base disturbances, and volume overload. The presence of renal replacement therapies (RRT) adds to the complexity of nutrient delivery in these patients. However, nutrition support should not be withheld in patients with AKI, and protein should not be limited as a strategy to prevent need for RRT. Adequate protein provision in patients with AKI may assist in recovery from AKI. Critically ill patients with AKI not receiving RRT should be provided standard dosing of macronutrients (Table 3). For patients receiving CRRT, additional protein is needed to supplement nitrogen losses at doses up to 2.5 g/kg/day [28].

Hepatic Dysfunction

Hepatic failure offers many challenges to appropriate nutrition therapy in the ICU as many of these patients have underlying malnutrition and loss of lean body mass. A patient's dry weight should be used to estimate their nutritional needs in the presence of ascites or anasarca. Additionally, protein restriction should be avoided for these patients receiving nutrition support. Higher branched-chain amino acid formulations, either enterally or parenterally, have not been shown to be superior to traditional formulations for hepatic failure patients in the ICU.

Stem Cell Transplantation

EN and PN may be required for cancer patients following HSCT. Consideration should be made for nutrition support therapy for patients undergoing HSCT who develop severe mucositis or GI GVHD. In this population, nutrition support therapy has been shown to provide various benefits including prevention of weight loss and reduction of mortality when compared to greater than 7 days of IV fluids or diet alone; however, PN was still found to be associated with significant risks, such as hyperglycemia, delayed engraftment, and bacteremia [3].

Obesity

Obesity is a known risk factor for the development of cancer. It is also associated with many comorbidities resulting in ICU admissions including sepsis, heart disease, and uncontrolled diabetes mellitus. Therefore, clinicians in the ICU face unique challenges in managing obese patients with cancer and critical illness. Nutrition support is an important intervention in the obese patient and should not be withheld due to an elevated BMI. The provision of higher-protein dosing based on a limited number of published studies in this population with decreased total caloric intake may lead to improved outcomes and less hyperglycemia [27]. Obese ICU patients should receive a nutrition support regimen of hypocaloric high-protein feeding as current guidelines recommend 11–14 kcal/kg/day of actual body weight for a BMI of 30–50 kg/m^2 and 22–25 kcal/kg/day of IBW for a BMI >50 kg/m^2. Additionally, the protein intake required is 2 g/kg/day of IBW for a BMI 30–40 kg/m^2 and 2.5 g/kg/day for a BMI >40 kg/m^2 [28].

Conclusion

Feeding the malnourished critically ill cancer patient represents a difficult clinical dilemma as the presence of multiple organ failure and hyperglycemia provides obstacles to optimal care. Nutrition support is generally accepted to have a supportive role in the ICU cancer patient; however, there is no universal agreement of which route of administration is best, how to provide optimally, and how long to continue. There are unanswered questions regarding what impact nutrition support has on functional status or quality of life after ICU discharge. Most clinical trials in ICU patients have excluded cancer patients leaving clinical guidelines for these patients unclear. However, these reasons should not be used for withholding nutrition support and safely providing it.

References

1. American Diabetes Association. Diabetes care in the hospital. 2016;39. https://doi.org/10.2337/dc16-S016.

2. Atasever AG, Ozcan PE, Kasali K, Abdullah T, Orhun G, Senturk E. The frequency, risk factors, and complications of gastrointestinal dysfunction during enteral nutrition in critically ill patients. Ther Clin Risk Manag. 2018;14:385–91. https://doi.org/10.21 47/tcrm.S158492.

3. August DA, Huhmann MB. A.S.P.E.N. clinical guidelines: nutrition support therapy during adult anticancer treatment and in hematopoietic cell transplantation. JPEN J Parenter Enteral Nutr. 2009;33:472–500. https://doi.org/10.1177/0148607109341804.

4. Barrett ML, BM, Owens PL. Non-maternal and non-neonatal inpatient stays in the United States involving malnutrition. 2018;2016:1–27. www.hcup-us.ahrq.gov/reports.jsp

5. Bisanz A, Tucker AM, Amin DM, Patel D, Calderon BB, Joseph MM, Curry EA 3rd. Summary of the causative and treatment factors of diarrhea and the use of a diarrhea assessment and treatment tool to improve patient outcomes. Gastroenterol Nurs. 2010;33: 268–81; quiz 282–263. https://doi.org/10.1097/SGA.0b013e3181e94307.

6. Bistrian BR. Clinical aspects of essential fatty acid metabolism: Jonathan Rhoads Lecture. JPEN J Parenter Enteral Nutr. 2003;27:168–75. https://doi.org/10.1177/0148607103027003168.

7. Boateng AA, Sriram K, Meguid MM, Crook M. Refeeding syndrome: treatment considerations based on collective analysis of literature case reports. Nutrition. 2010;26:156–67. https://doi.org/10.1016/j.nut.2009.11.017.

8. Boullata JI, et al. ASPEN safe practices for enteral nutrition therapy. JPEN J Parenter Enteral Nutr. 2017;41:15–103. https://doi.org/10.1177/0148607116673053.

9. Broman M, Bryland A, Carlsson O, Group TTAS. Trace elements in patients on continuous renal replacement therapy. Acta Anaesthesiol Scand. 2017;61: 650–9. https://doi.org/10.1111/aas.12909.

10. Dickerson RN, Drover JW. Monitoring nutrition therapy in the critically ill patient with obesity. JPEN J Parenter Enteral Nutr. 2011;35:44s–51s. https://doi.org/10.1177/0148607111413771.

11. Doig GS, Simpson F, Finfer S, Delaney A, Davies AR, Mitchell I, Dobb G. Effect of evidence-based feeding guidelines on mortality of critically ill adults: a cluster randomized controlled trial. JAMA. 2008;300:2731–41. https://doi.org/10.1001/jama.2008.826.

12. Doig GS, et al. Restricted versus continued standard caloric intake during the management of refeeding syndrome in critically ill adults: a randomised, parallel-group, multicentre, single-blind controlled trial. Lancet Respir Med. 2015;3:943–52. https://doi.org/10.1016/S2213-2600(15)00418-X.

13. Escuro AA, Hummell AC. Enteral formulas in nutrition support practice: is there a better choice for your patient? Nutr Clin Pract. 2016;31:709–22. https://doi.org/10.1177/0884533616668492.

14. Fonseca G, Burgermaster M, Larson E, Seres DS. The relationship between parenteral nutrition and central line-associated bloodstream infections: 2009–2014. JPEN J Parenter Enteral Nutr. 2018;42: 171–5. https://doi.org/10.1177/0148607116688437.

15. Fredrix EW, Soeters PB, Wouters EF, Deerenberg IM, von Meyenfeldt MF, Saris WH. Effect of different tumor types on resting energy expenditure. Cancer Res. 1991;51:6138–41.

16. Friedli N, et al. Management and prevention of refeeding syndrome in medical inpatients: an evidence-based and consensus-supported algorithm. Nutrition. 2018;47:13–20. https://doi.org/10.1016/j.nut.2017.09.007.

17. Galloway P, McMillan DC, Sattar N. Effect of the inflammatory response on trace element and vitamin status. Ann Clin Biochem. 2000;37(Pt 3):289–97. https://doi.org/10.1258/0004563001899429.

18. Greenwood J. Critical care nutrition at the clinical valuation research unit. Study tools: management of diarrhea algorithm. 2010. www.criticalcarenutrition.org/docs/tools/diarrhea.pdf. Accessed 6 June 2018.

19. Heyland DK, Dhaliwal R, Jiang X, Day AG. Identifying critically ill patients who benefit the most from nutrition therapy: the development and initial validation of a novel risk assessment tool. Crit Care. 2011;15: R268. https://doi.org/10.1186/cc10546.

20. Heyland DK, Dhaliwal R, Wang M, Day AG. The prevalence of iatrogenic underfeeding in the nutritionally 'at-risk' critically ill patient: results of an international, multicenter, prospective study. Clin Nutr. 2015;34:659–66. https://doi.org/10.1016/j.clnu.2014.07.008.

21. Heyland DK, Rooyakers O, Mourtzakis M, Stapleton RD. Proceedings of the 2016 clinical nutrition week research workshop-the optimal dose of protein provided to critically ill patients. JPEN J Parenter Enteral Nutr. 2017;41:208–16. https://doi.org/10.1177/0148607116682003.

22. Jie B, Jiang ZM, Nolan MT, Zhu SN, Yu K, Kondrup J. Impact of preoperative nutritional support on clinical outcome in abdominal surgical patients at nutritional risk. Nutrition. 2012;28:1022–7. https://doi.org/10.1016/j.nut.2012.01.017.
23. Khalid I, Doshi P, DiGiovine B. Early enteral nutrition and outcomes of critically ill patients treated with vasopressors and mechanical ventilation. Am J Crit Care. 2010;19:261–8. https://doi.org/10.4037/ajcc2010197.
24. Knox LS, Crosby LO, Feurer ID, Buzby GP, Miller CL, Mullen JL. Energy expenditure in malnourished cancer patients. Ann Surg. 1983;197:152–62.
25. Kondrup J, Rasmussen HH, Hamberg O, Stanga Z, Ad Hoc EWG. Nutritional risk screening (NRS 2002): a new method based on an analysis of controlled clinical trials. Clin Nutr. 2003;22:321–36.
26. Malone AM, Seres D, Lord LM. Complications of enteral nutrition. In: Mueller CM, editor. The ASPEN adult nutrition support core curriculum. 3rd ed. Silver Spring: American Society for Parenteral and Enteral Nutrition; 2017. p. 265–83.
27. McClave SA, et al. Nutrition therapy of the severely obese, critically ill patient: summation of conclusions and recommendations. JPEN J Parenter Enteral Nutr. 2011;35:88s–96s. https://doi.org/10.1177/0148607111415111.
28. McClave SA, et al. Guidelines for the provision and assessment of nutrition support therapy in the adult critically ill patient: Society of Critical Care Medicine (SCCM) and American Society for Parenteral and Enteral Nutrition (A.S.P.E.N.). JPEN J Parenter Enteral Nutr. 2016;40:159–211. https://doi.org/10.1177/0148607115621863.
29. Mirtallo J. Overview of parenteral nutrition. In: Gottschlich MM, editor. The A.S.P.E.N. Nutrition support core curriculum: a case-based approach – the adult patient. 2nd ed. Silver Spring: The American Society for Parenteral and Enteral Nutrition; 2007. p. 265–75.
30. Mirtallo J, et al. Safe practices for parenteral nutrition. JPEN J Parenter Enteral Nutr. 2004;28:S39–70.
31. Moghissi ES, et al. American Association of Clinical Endocrinologists and American Diabetes Association consensus statement on inpatient glycemic control. Diabetes Care. 2009;32:1119–31. https://doi.org/10.2337/dc09-9029.
32. Montejo JC, et al. Multicenter, prospective, randomized, single-blind study comparing the efficacy and gastrointestinal complications of early jejunal feeding with early gastric feeding in critically ill patients. Crit Care Med. 2002;30:796–800.
33. O'Grady NP, et al. Guidelines for the prevention of intravascular catheter-related infections. Centers for Disease Control and Prevention. MMWR Recomm Rep. 2002;51:1–29.
34. Palesty JA, Dudrick SJ. What we have learned about cachexia in gastrointestinal cancer. Dig Dis. 2003;21:198–213. https://doi.org/10.1159/000073337.
35. Patel RP, Canada TW, Nates JL. Bleeding associated with feeding tube placement in critically ill oncology patients with thrombocytopenia. Nutr Clin Pract. 2016;31:111–5. https://doi.org/10.1177/0884533615598964.
36. Pirat A, Tucker AM, Taylor KA, Jinnah R, Finch CG, Canada TD, Nates JL. Comparison of measured versus predicted energy requirements in critically ill cancer patients. Respir Care. 2009;54:487–94.
37. Roberts S, Mattox T. Cancer. In: Gottschlich MM, editor. The A.S.P.E.N. Nutrition support core curriculum: a case-based approach – the adult patient. 2nd ed. Silver Spring: American Society for Parenteral and Enteral Nutrition; 2007. p. 650–75.
38. Tajchman SK, Tucker AM, Cardenas-Turanzas M, Nates JL. Validation study of energy requirements in critically ill, obese cancer patients. JPEN J Parenter Enteral Nutr. 2016;40:806–13. https://doi.org/10.1177/0148607115574289.
39. Tian F, Heighes PT, Allingstrup MJ, Doig GS. Early enteral nutrition provided within 24 hours of ICU admission: a meta-analysis of randomized controlled trials. Crit Care Med. 2018;46:1049–56. https://doi.org/10.1097/ccm.0000000000003152.
40. Tillman EM. Review and clinical update on parenteral nutrition-associated liver disease. Nutr Clin Pract. 2013;28:30–9. https://doi.org/10.1177/0884533612462900.
41. Tisdale MJ. Pathogenesis of cancer cachexia. J Support Oncol. 2003;1:159–68.
42. Vanek VW, et al. A.S.P.E.N. position paper: recommendations for changes in commercially available parenteral multivitamin and multi-trace element products. Nutr Clin Pract. 2012;27:440–91. https://doi.org/10.1177/0884533612446706.
43. Williams NT. Medication administration through enteral feeding tubes. Am J Health Syst Pharm. 2008;65:2347–57. https://doi.org/10.2146/ajhp080155.
44. Ziegler TR. Parenteral nutrition in the critically ill patient. N Engl J Med. 2009;361:1088–97. https://doi.org/10.1056/NEJMct0806956.

Part III

Dermatologic Complications

Graft Versus Host Disease (GHVD) in Critically Ill Oncologic Patients

18

Ulas Darda Bayraktar

Contents

Introduction 250

Etiology and Pathophysiology 250

GVHD Clinical Features and Impact on Intensive Care 251
Acute GVHD 252
Chronic GVHD 253

GVHD Prevention/Treatment and Their Impact on Intensive Care 254
GVHD Prevention 254
GVHD Treatment 256
Immunosuppression Due to GVHD Treatment 258

Prognosis 259

References 259

Abstract

Graft-versus-host-disease (GVHD) is the most common life-threatening complication of allogeneic hematopoietic stem cell transplantation (ASCT). More than 40% of ASCT patients admitted to the intensive care unit (ICU) has GVHD, which has been reported to be associated with worsened ICU outcomes. GVHD commonly involves mucocutaneous tissues, gastrointestinal tract, and liver, manifesting itself in rash, diarrhea, anorexia, and cholestasis. Chronic GVHD may also involve lungs directly causing bronchiolitis obliterans

which may complicate mechanical ventilation. GVHD prophylaxis improves survival in ASCT patients. Calcineurin inhibitors are the backbone of GVHD prophylaxis and are frequently combined with methotrexate, mycophenolate mofetil, or sirolimus. While corticosteroids are used for the first-line treatment of GVHD, many options exist for steroid-refractory GVHD. Almost all GVHD agents suppress the immune system rendering patients susceptible to bacterial, viral, and fungal infections. The novel T cell selection methods used for GVHD prevention may cause less immunosuppression resulting in improved ICU outcomes. In this chapter, we will focus on the impact of GVHD and its treatment on the management of the critical care patient.

U. D. Bayraktar (✉)
Division of Hematology and Oncology, Aras Medical Center, Ankara, Turkey
e-mail: darda.bayraktar@lenfomadoktoru.com

© Springer Nature Switzerland AG 2020
J. L. Nates, K. J. Price (eds.), *Oncologic Critical Care*,
https://doi.org/10.1007/978-3-319-74588-6_31

Keywords

Graft-versus-host-disease · Bronchiolitis obliterans · T cells · Corticosteroids · Tacrolimus · Cyclosporine · Mycophenolate mofetil · Sirolimus · Methotrexate

increased worldwide use of high-risk transplants from haploidentical donors – related donors with mismatched HLAs – will likely increase the GVHD prevalence and GVHD prophylaxis/treatment intensity in ASCT patients admitted to ICU.

Introduction

Allogeneic hematopoietic stem cell transplantation (ASCT) is a potentially curative treatment of various hematological malignancies, bone marrow failure syndromes, and congenital diseases. Graft-versus-host-disease (GVHD) is the most common life-threatening complication of ASCT in which donated immune system (graft) reacts against the host body, particularly skin, gastrointestinal tract, liver, and lungs. GVHD is a syndrome of two distinct immune responses with similar pathogeneses but varying manifestations: acute and chronic GVHD. While acute GVHD (aGVHD) commonly emerges between posttransplant days 15 and 100 and affects skin, liver, and GI tract, chronic GVHD (cGVHD) occurs after day 100 and mimics autoimmune diseases such as scleroderma, primarily affecting skin, lungs, and GI tract. Whereas aGVHD progresses rapidly within days and weeks, cGVHD typically has a gradual onset. Clinical manifestations rather than the time of onset are used to differentiate between the two, as aGVHD may arise after or extend beyond posttransplant day 100. Additionally, chronic GVHD may overlap with or transform from aGVHD [1].

We previously reported that prevalence of grade II–IV aGVHD and cGVHD were 15% and 28%, respectively, in ASCT patients admitted to intensive care unit (ICU) [2]. Additionally, GVHD has been reported to be a poor prognostic factor for ASCT patients in ICU whose short-term mortality remains above 50% [3–5]. Accordingly, GVHD is of particular importance to the intensivists as: (a) it is frequently seen in patients admitted to ICU, (b) it often affects vital organ functions possibly worsening the patient survival and requiring management of the ensuing morbidities, and (c) GVHD treatment predisposes patients to potentially fatal infections. Finally,

Etiology and Pathophysiology

GVHD ensues if the transplanted donor immune system recognizes the host cells as foreign. Initially, conditioning chemotherapy/radiotherapy employed in ASCT to eliminate the malignant cells and clear an immunologic "space" for the new graft causes tissue injury, primarily in the intestines, releasing molecular patterns from damaged bowel wall and microbial luminal contents. These events activate antigen-presenting cells and initiate a torrent of proinflammatory cytokine release, which prime and activate donor T cells [6–11]. While donor helper and cytotoxic T cells are the primary mediators and effectors of GVHD, natural killer cells and regulatory T cells dampen GVHD [12–14]. Donor T cells can react to both host MHC or minor histocompatibility antigens [15].

Risk factors for GVHD are those that affect either initial tissue injury or donor immune cells' alloreactivity. Degree of major/minor histocompatibility disparity is the most important influencer of GVHD risk with the lowest GVHD incidence seen in syngeneic transplants – those between identical twins [16–19]. On the other hand, some antigen disparity between the donor and the host is generally desired to allow donor immune cells to react against host malignant cells. ASCT types can be sorted in order of GVHD risk as follows: syngeneic < HLA-matched related (sibling) < HLA-matched unrelated < HLA-mismatched unrelated ≅ haploidentical donors.

In addition to HLA disparity, gender disparity between donor and the recipient increases the GVHD risk, with female to male transplants bearing the highest risk [20, 21]. Graft type is another major determinant of GVHD risk. Number of T cells in peripheral blood grafts are significantly higher than those in bone marrow grafts, and hence, it is generally accepted that transplants from peripheral blood grafts carry a higher risk of GVHD compared to those from bone marrow graft [22]. It should be noted that most of the transplants worldwide are now being performed from peripheral blood grafts due to its convenience for the donors and the quicker recovery of neutrophils/platelets after the transplant. Meanwhile, immune cells in umbilical cord grafts are more "elastic" and tend to arouse less GVHD. Therefore, a greater degree of HLA disparity between the recipient and cord blood is allowed for ASCT [23].

Conditioning regimen intensity is another influencer of GVHD risk. Reduced intensity conditioning regimens, those typically including fludarabine, are associated with lower risk of GVHD compared to myeloablative regimens that result in complete ablation of host's hematopoietic and immune system along with more severe mucosal injury [16, 24]. Finally, presence of prior acute GVHD increases the risk of developing cGVHD [20, 25].

Almost all ASCT patients receive a prophylaxis for GVHD. Prophylaxis' type and intensity depends on the patient/transplant characteristics and the centers' standards of care. While more intense regimens, such as ex vivo T cell depletion of the graft [26] and high dose posttransplant cyclophosphamide [27], are generally reserved for ASCTs with

high risk for GVHD, calcineurin inhibitors with/ without methotrexate [28–30] or mycophenolate mofetil (MMF) [31, 32] are likely the most commonly used GVHD prophylaxis regimens for ASCT from HLA-matched donors. Regardless of their type, primary aim of GVHD prevention and treatment strategies is to deplete/suppress T cells, preferentially the ones with the potential to induce GVHD. In fact, the "holy grail" of ASCT is to achieve the selectivity between the GVHD-inducing and infection/malignancy fighting immune cells. This goal seems more reachable now with the selective T cell depletion strategies, such as αβ-T cell [33] and naïve T cell depletion [34].

GVHD Clinical Features and Impact on Intensive Care

GVHD, acute or chronic, is a spectrum of organ manifestations. Despite the widely varying presentations, most patients present with cutaneous and gastrointestinal (GI) manifestations in both aGVHD and cGVHD. Intensivists need to recognize the signs and symptoms promptly and manage the ensuing morbidities due to GVHD. Table 1 summarizes the important features of both acute and chronic GVHD along with their significances for intensive care management.

Table 1 Features of acute and chronic graft-versus-host-disease (GVHD) with their significance in intensive care unit

	Acute GVHD	Chronic GVHD
Mucocutaneous	Maculopapular rash and erythroderma => Third-spacing and bacterial superinfections	Sclerotic or lichen planus-like skin features Dry eyes and conjunctival hyperemia Oral ulcers, restriction of mouth opening Nail loss, onycholysis => Superinfections
Upper GI tract	Nausea, anorexia, epigastric pain => malnutrition, exclude infectious esophagitis	Esophageal webs/strictures, anorexia, and malabsorption => malnutrition
Lower GI tract	Secretory diarrhea => fluid loss, hypoalbuminemia, malnutrition. Increased risk of bacterial transposition. Exclude infections and drugs. Careful opioid therapy	Diarrhea => less frequent than in aGVHD
Liver	Elevated liver enzymes and bilirubin => exclude sinusoidal obstruction syndrome and drug toxicity. Drug dose modifications may be required	Similar to clinical picture of aGVHD and primary biliary cirrhosis
Lung	Rare direct involvement Increased diffuse alveolar hemorrhage risk	Bronchiolitis obliterans => obstructive changes, oxygenation and weaning difficult, increased pneumonia risk

Acute GVHD

Clinically significant aGVHD occurs in 10–60% of patients depending on the aforementioned risk factors [16, 35]. aGVHD classically presents in the early posttransplantation period and most commonly occurs around the time of neutrophil engraftment [24]. While acute and chronic GVHD used to be strictly defined based on their time of onset after ASCT (before and after day 100 posttransplant), NIH consensus criteria now uses clinical manifestations as onset of aGVHD can be delayed in some patients [1, 24]. Skin and the gastrointestinal tract are the most commonly involved organs in aGVHD [28].

In most patients, a maculopapular rash is the presenting sign of aGVHD. Classical erythematous maculopapular morbilliform eruptions generally start on the face, ears, palms, and soles. This may resemble a drug eruption or a viral exanthem requiring a histological confirmation with a punch skin biopsy [36]. Skin lesions may evolve to erythroderma with epidermolysis and extend to trunk. Oral mucosa is rarely involved [37]. Staging of cutaneous involvement depends on the extent and severity of rash [38] (Table 2). While mild cutaneous-only GVHD may be treated with

topical corticosteroids alone, most patients require systemic therapy. In addition to GVHD treatment, patients with nonintact skin require general wound care and antibiotics if deemed necessary. Extensive cutaneous involvement may lead to third-spacing increasing fluid requirements and predispose patients to cutaneous infections.

aGVHD commonly affects the GI tract, the lower being involved more frequently than the upper GI tract. The presenting symptom is usually secretory diarrhea that may reach more than 2 liters per day. In severe cases, gastrointestinal bleeding and ileus may occur, the latter being partly due to electrolyte imbalances and opioids used for pain management. Upper GI tract aGVHD may give rise to nausea, vomiting, and anorexia [39]. GI symptoms of aGVHD are not distinctive and may be seen with infectious colitis (with Clostridium difficile and cytomegalovirus (CMV) most commonly), drug toxicity, and neutropenic colitis after ASCT. Consequently, diagnosis of GI aGVHD is commonly based on excluding other causes clinically and histologically. CMV may need to be excluded by immunohistochemical staining of endoscopic biopsies [40]. Of note, rare pancreatic involvement with GVHD may lead to pancreatic exocrine

Table 2 Grading of acute graft-versus-host-disease

Organ	Stage	Description
Skin	1	Maculopapular rash over <25% of body area
	2	Maculopapular rash over 25–50% of body area
	3	Generalized erythroderma
	4	Generalized erythroderma with bullous formation and often with desquamation
Liver	1	Bilirubin 2–3 mg/dL; AST 150–750 IU
	2	Bilirubin 3.1–6.0 mg/dL
	3	Bilirubin 6.1–15.0 mg/dL
	4	Bilirubin >15 mg/dL
Gut	1	Diarrhea >500 mL/day
	2	Diarrhea >1000 mL/day
	3	Diarrhea >1500 mL/day
	4	Diarrhea >2000 mL/day; or severe abdominal pain with or without ileus

Glucksberg grade
I – Stage 1 or 2 skin involvement; no liver or gut involvement
II – Up to stage 3 skin involvement with stage 1 liver or gut involvement
III – Up to stage 4 liver, up to stage 3 skin or gut involvement
IV – Stage 4 skin or gut involvement, ECOG PS 4

Glucksberg et al. [38]

insufficiency and diarrhea. Staging of GI manifestations of aGVHD is based on the volume of diarrhea per day and presence of ileus (Table 2). In addition to the systemic aGVHD treatment, patients with GI aGVHD require carefully managed fluid resuscitation and, occasionally, parenteral protein/albumin supplementation. Caution is advised while using opioids for pain management due to the risk of ileus.

Although liver is involved in almost half of the patients, aGVHD rarely presents with sole hepatic impairment [28]. Typically, hepatic aGVHD manifests itself with a cholestatic picture with marked elevations in serum alkaline phosphatase and bilirubin levels accompanied by milder increases in alanine transaminase and aspartate transaminase levels. Patients may also develop painful hepatomegaly and fluid retention. The clinical picture may resemble that of sinusoidal obstruction syndrome (SOS), viral hepatitis, and cholestatic drug induced liver injury [41]. In a patient with no cutaneous and GI tract manifestations, a liver biopsy is required to diagnose aGVHD of liver and to exclude other causes of liver injury. On the other hand, a liver biopsy is not feasible in most patients early after ASCT due to thrombocytopenia [42, 43]. If required, the transjugular approach may be safer than the transcutaneous approach. The degree of liver involvement is determined based on the serum bilirubin level (Table 2). For the intensivist, it is important to suspect and recognize aGVHD in ASCT patients with a cholestatic picture. Furthermore, in those with liver enzyme elevations, dose adjustments may be needed for commonly used transplant medicines, i.e., tacrolimus and azole antifungals.

Less commonly, aGVHD may involve eyes causing photophobia and conjunctivitis; kidneys causing nephrotic/nephritic syndrome; lungs causing interstitial pneumonitis and hematopoietic system resulting in thymic atrophy, cytopenias, and hypogammaglobulinemia. Fortunately, direct pulmonary involvement with aGVHD is rarely seen. On the other hand, aGVHD may increase the risk of diffuse alveolar hemorrhage without causing direct lung injury [44].

Grading of aGVHD is important in determining its impact on prognosis, assessing treatment response, and for research purposes. Glucksberg grading system is commonly used and is based on the extent of cutaneous, GI tract, and hepatic involvements by aGVHD (Table 2).

Chronic GVHD

While their pathogeneses have similarities, and both depend primarily on donor T cell function, acute and chronic GVHD manifestations are distinctive. Chronic GVHD primarily occurs after the 100th day of the transplant, although it may start earlier and overlap with aGVHD. Whereas aGVHD is dominated by tissue necrosis and apoptosis, cGVHD resembles autoimmune diseases, i.e., scleroderma, and is primarily dominated by fibrosis.

cGVHD involves mucocutaneous tissues in two-thirds of the patients [45]. Skin involvement in cGVHD may present with sclerotic or nonsclerotic phenotypes. A lichen planus-like rash and poikiloderma with skin atrophy and pigmentary changes are the most commonly observed nonsclerotic manifestations. These may involve ears, face, palms, and soles [46]. Sclerotic manifestations are characterized by fibrosis mimicking scleroderma. Epidermal and dermal changes usually accompany each other with skin atrophy, hypo/hyperpigmentation, hair loss, and sweat impairment due to adnexal structure damage. Eyes may also be involved with dry eyes seen in half of the patients followed by cataracts and conjunctivitis. Additionally, nail dystrophy/loss, onycholysis, alopecia, and scaling of scalp may be observed [37]. cGVHD of skin is usually diagnosed clinically based on the diagnostic and distinctive features previously established by NIH Consensus Criteria [47] and may need to be confirmed histologically in some cases. Compared to the cutaneous manifestations seen in aGVHD, those of cGVHD tend to progress slowly and generally do not pose an acute problem for the intensivist, unless a skin ulcer develops with bacterial superinfection. In addition to systemic GVHD treatment, cutaneous lesions should be treated locally with topical steroids and/or topical tacrolimus. For resistant cases, phototherapy with psoralen and ultraviolet A (PUVA) may be used.

GI tract and oral mucosa is frequently involved with cGVHD. Xerostomia, hyperkeratotic plaques, and oral ulcers are seen in more than half of cGVHD patients [45]. Mouth opening may be restricted due to sclerosis which is diagnostic of cGVHD. Additionally, esophagus may be involved leading to esophageal webs and strictures that are also diagnostic of cGVHD. Nausea, anorexia, malabsorption, weight loss, and diarrhea may be seen with upper and lower GI involvement but are less commonly seen than in aGVHD. GI involvement may derail the nutrition of the patients in ICU but is usually not as dramatic as that with aGVHD.

Liver is involved in close to half of patients with cGVHD [45], commonly presenting with a cholestatic picture. Similar to aGVHD, serum alkaline phosphatase, bilirubin, ALT, and AST are elevated but typically progression is slower in cGVHD [41]. As in aGVHD, liver manifestations of cGVHD is nonspecific and other causes of hepatotoxicity, i.e., viral infections, drug toxicity, need to be excluded with a liver biopsy. Pathophysiology is thought to be similar to that of primary biliary cirrhosis with biliary cell necrosis [48]. Intensivists need to pay particular attention to the dosages of drugs metabolized in liver in patients with cGVHD with hepatic impairment.

Lungs are involved in up to half of patients with cGVHD and are of significant consequence for patients in ICU. cGVHD generally presents with mild airflow obstruction in the absence of infections and may lead to bronchiolitis obliterans (BO) characterized by small airways inflammation and narrowing due to fibrous scarring. BO is diagnosed after excluding infectious causes and with the aid of computerized tomography imaging and, occasionally, histological examination [49, 50]. BO causes moderate-to-severe airflow obstruction, predisposes patients to recurrent infections, and is diagnostic of cGVHD in ASCT patients. In addition to systemic GVHD treatment, cGVHD patients with BO will typically require inhaled corticosteroids, prophylactic antibiotics, and oral montelukast [51]. While azithromycin has historically been the preferred prophylactic

antibiotic for patients with BO based on the studies done in lung transplant patients [52], its use after ASCT has been associated with an increased disease relapse rate and a shortened survival [53]. Ventilatory support for patients with BO is particularly difficult to manage due to significant air trapping and fixed small airway obstruction [50].

Muscles and connective tissues may also be involved with cGVHD. Resulting fasciitis and myositis may cause contractures, joint stiffness, muscle weakness, and myalgia [54, 55]. Consequent functional dependencies may affect a patient's recovery from ICU and rare involvement of respiratory system muscles may prolong the weaning from mechanical ventilation.

GVHD Prevention/Treatment and Their Impact on Intensive Care

GVHD Prevention

All ASCT patients receive GVHD prophylaxis to avoid the GVHD-associated mortality/morbidity and the intense immunosuppression of GVHD treatment. The latter significantly increases the risk of infections and disease relapse. Moreover, GVHD may be refractory to the treatment and ultimately cause death. With prophylaxis, GVHD incidence is decreased improving survival after ASCT [29, 30].

There is not yet a globally accepted standard GVHD prevention scheme [56]. Instead, different transplant centers around the world use varying strategies based on the patient, donor, and transplant characteristics. GVHD prevention approaches are based on either inhibition of alloreactive T cells or ex vivo/in vivo T cell depletion. The following is a discussion of the commonly used agents and approaches for GVHD prophylaxis and their significance to the intensivists.

Most GVHD prophylaxis regimens place calcineurin inhibitors, cyclosporine, or tacrolimus as their backbone. Both drugs inhibit dephosphorylation and consequent nuclear translocation of nuclear factor of T-cell (NFAT), thereby suppressing transcription of IL-2 and T cell activation [57, 58]. Primary toxicity of cyclosporine and tacrolimus is renal function impairment as a result of afferent arteriole vasoconstriction [59]. Cyclosporine may also increase bilirubin levels. Other toxicities relevant to the intensivists include hypertension, hyperglycemia, and neurotoxicity. Neurotoxicity may present with mild tremor and progress to reversible posterior leukoencephalopathy syndrome characterized by severe headache, visual abnormalities, and seizures – similar to hypertensive encephalopathy [60]. Calcium channel blockers are considered the drugs of choice for hypertension. Calcineurin inhibitors may lower serum potassium and magnesium levels. Management of the latter can be particularly problematic in ASCT patients as magnesium supplementation can worsen diarrhea associated with GVHD. Thrombotic microangiopathy is another adverse effect of calcineurin inhibitors that is characterized by hemolytic anemia, thrombocytopenia, and presence of schistocytes in peripheral smear. Serum levels of tacrolimus and cyclosporine need to be monitored and managed according to the transplant team's target level that is commonly based on a patient's GVHD risk. Both tacrolimus and cyclosporine are metabolized extensively by the cytochrome p450 enzymes, rendering their serum levels labile to the patient medication changes.

Methotrexate is a folate antagonist that is used as a chemotherapeutic agent, an immunosuppressive for autoimmune diseases, and also a prophylactic agent for GVHD typically in combination with calcineurin inhibitors [30]. Methotrexate is typically given on days +1, +3, +6, and + 11 after ASCT and is thought to be particularly toxic to the donor T cells activated by the alloantigens. Its use after ASCT is limited by its toxicity to the mucosal membranes. Other than mucositis, methotrexate may lead to significant renal and hepatic toxicities. To accelerate its excretion and prevent its toxicities, urine needs to be alkalinized with sodium bicarbonate. Methotrexate should be avoided in patients with significant renal impairment or third-spacing since it can accumulate in extracellular fluid and then slowly leak back into the circulation, greatly increasing bone marrow suppression and nephrotoxicity. Leucovorin

rescue after Mtx administration may be considered in patients with significant mucositis [61].

Mycophenolate mofetil (MMF) inhibits inosine monophosphate dehydrogenase, a critical enzyme for de novo synthesis of purine nucleotides. Blockade of purine synthesis prevents activation of lymphocytes which are reliant on de novo production of purines [62]. MMF is synergistic with calcineurin inhibitors in ameliorating the residual host immune system after ASCT enhancing engraftment [63]. Clinical trials suggest MMF is as effective as methotrexate in GVHD prevention with reduced mucositis [31, 32]. Major side effects of MMF are bone marrow suppression and diarrhea, while it may also cause nephrotoxicity.

Sirolimus (rapamycin) inhibits mammalian target of rapamycin (mTOR) suppressing the cytokine-derived growth of T and B cells, rather sparing regulatory T cells, and hindering progression of cells from G1 into S phase [64]. Tacrolimus-sirolimus combination is another non-methotrexate GVHD prophylaxis regimen with similar efficacy and less mucositis compared to tacrolimus-methotrexate [65]. However, use of sirolimus for GVHD prevention is limited by associated SOS risk in patients who receive ablative doses of busulfan for transplant conditioning [66]. Sirolimus commonly affects GI tract causing diarrhea and liver enzyme elevations. Contrary to the calcineurin inhibitors, nephrotoxicity is rarely seen; however, bone marrow suppression is typically more pronounced hindering its use after ASCT. Sirolimus may cause interstitial pneumonitis that resembles bronchiolitis obliterans, complicating the cGVHD picture [67].

Cyclophosphamide is an alkylating chemotherapeutic agent that is commonly used in the treatment of lymphoproliferative malignancies. Similar to methotrexate, it is given early post-transplant on days +3 and + 4 at a dose of 50 mg/kg to deplete proliferating alloreactive T cells. Hematopoietic stem cells are mostly spared due to their high levels of intracellular aldehyde dehydrogenase enzyme [27, 68]. Posttransplant cyclophosphamide is commonly used for GVHD prophylaxis in haploidentical transplantation in combination with calcineurin inhibitors and MMF [69]. After haploidentical transplantation, patients commonly develop a short-lived fever the night of cyclophosphamide administration [70]. To prevent hemorrhagic cystitis, cyclophosphamide needs to be administered with vigorous hydration and intravenous mesna. Although rare, it may also cause early-onset pneumonitis and cardiotoxicity [71]. Prompt glucocorticoid initiation may resolve the pneumonitis with the caveat of ensuing immune suppression. Finally, cyclophosphamide-induced acute cardiotoxicity can be rapidly fatal progressing to acute heart failure and generally presents within 48 h of its administration [72].

Abatacept is a fusion protein that mimics CTLA-4 and inhibits T cell co-stimulation leading to immune tolerance [73]. Abatacept was recently reported to have significantly reduce GVHD rates when combined with a calcineurin inhibitor [74]. Its most common side effects are injection site/infusion reactions.

T cell depletion of the graft, ex vivo or in vivo, selective or not, may be the most efficacious method of GVHD prevention [75]. However, since donor T cells also play significant roles in engraftment, graft-versus-disease effect, and immune reconstitution after ASCT, T cell depletion may also increase the risk of graft failure, disease relapse, and posttransplant infections [76, 77]. Multiple studies did not demonstrate a difference in survival between patients who received GVHD prophylaxis based on T cell depletion versus calcineurin inhibitors [78, 79]. Traditional T cell depletion methods involve ex vivo depletion of T cells in the graft using immunoadsorbed magnetic beads or in vivo depletion by antibodies. The latter may be achieved with the use of polyclonal antithymocyte globulin (ATG) or monoclonal alemtuzumab (an anti-CD52 panlymphocytic antibody). These interventions are typically performed before or early after transplantation and intensivists rarely need to manage the associated acute side effects except that of ATG with resistant fever, serum sickness, and profound pancytopenia.

Selective depletion of unfavorable T cell subsets is a novel GVHD prevention strategy that is being evaluated particularly for the higher-risk haploidentical transplants. Depletion of naïve T cells – those never exposed to their cognate antigen and are thought to be the initiators of GVHD – while preserving memory T cells is currently being investigated in clinical trials [34]. Similarly, depleting T cells with αβ T cell receptor phenotype showed promising results [33]. Co-infusion of regulatory T cells that are protective against GVHD with cytotoxic T cells is another graft engineering method to prevent GVHD while preserving the graft-versus-leukemia effect [80]. If proven efficacious, these methods may transform the transplant practice and alter the intensive care requirements after ASCT. Importantly for the intensivists, transplant patients admitted to ICU may be less immunosuppressed in the near-future.

As an adjunct to the T-cell-directed therapies, interventions that target the cytokine release and antigen presentation to donor T cells are also being investigated for GVHD prevention. For instance, suppression or altercation of the intestinal microbiome may avert the first step of GVHD and lower its incidence [81].

GVHD Treatment

Although all the T cell suppressive drugs used for GVHD prevention can also be used for its treatment, the first-line therapy of GVHD is almost always with corticosteroids. Corticosteroids block proinflammatory gene transcription, while promoting anti-inflammatory gene transcription and blocking the function of nuclear factor-kappa-B [82–84]. Corticosteroids are seldom used for GVHD prevention since their addition to cyclosporine and methotrexate did not demonstrate a decrease in GVHD incidence [85] and also due to their side effects including severe immunosuppression, fluid retention, hyperglycemia, hypertension, and psychosis. The usual starting corticosteroid dose for acute or chronic GVHD treatment is 1–2 mg/kg/day of methylprednisolone. Different than the corticosteroid support for the shock treatment, prednisone or methylprednisolone is preferred over hydrocortisone due to their higher anti-inflammatory and lower mineralocorticoid effects. Upon improvement of symptoms, corticosteroids are very slowly tapered off. If there is a lack of response within a week, dose may be increased to 5–10 mg/kg/day and/or a second agent may be added to the regimen. Corticosteroids may also be used locally for GVHD affecting skin, GI tract (nonabsorbable budesonide or beclomethasone), eyes, oral mucosa, and lungs. In fact, limited and mild skin-only GVHD may be treated with topical corticosteroids alone.

For patients with corticosteroid resistant GVHD, there are various second- and third-line treatment options including calcineurin inhibitors, MMF, sirolimus, fusion proteins etanercept and abatacept, ruxolitinib, ibrutinib, pentostatin, and extracorporeal photopheresis. Specifically for steroid-refractory cutaneous cGVHD, PUVA is another alternative treatment. Most of these agents were discussed in the GVHD prevention section and will not be repeated.

Etanercept is a fusion protein inhibiting TNF-α, a cytokine which exacerbates GVHD through recruiting effector cells and instigating direct target organ injury [86, 87]. Etanercept may be used to treat both acute and chronic GVHD [88]. In addition to infusion/injection site reactions, etanercept may cause or worsen heart failure. Moreover, there are multiple reports of dismal survival in GVHD patients treated with etanercept due to infectious complications and progressive GVHD [86, 89].

Pentostatin, a purine analog, inhibits adenosine deaminase which is essential for lymphocyte proliferation [90]. In addition to the almost universally observed lymphopenia, pentostatin may also cause fever and a macular rash, similar to the rash of aGVHD. Late-onset infections are also increased after pentostatin use. Of note, a randomized trial of first-line aGVHD treatment suggested improved GVHD response rates and less toxicity with MMF compared to pentostatin and etanercept when combined with corticosteroids [91]. Therefore, MMF is generally prioritized over pentostatin and etanercept for the treatment of GVHD.

Ruxolitinib is a Janus kinase (jak) inhibitor primarily used to treat myeloproliferative disorders [92]. Jak inhibition disrupts signal transducer and activator of transcription (STAT) pathway which is associated with early cytokine storm [93] and inhibition of Tregs [94]. Ruxolitinib may be used for the treatment of both acute and chronic GVHD with mild-moderate toxicity including cytopenias, liver dysfunction, and neurological complaints [95]. Additionally, sudden discontinuation of ruxolitinib may cause withdrawal similar to systemic inflammatory response syndrome [96].

Ibrutinib is an inhibitor of Bruton's tyrosine kinase (btk) that is emerging as one of the most commonly used targeted anti-lymphoma agent [97]. It was also approved by FDA for the treatment of refractory cGVHD in 2017 [98]. After ASCT, most common side effects of ibrutinib are fatigue, diarrhea, muscle spasms, and nausea. More importantly to the intensivist, ibrutinib increases risks of major bleeding [99] and atrial fibrillation [100].

Extracorporeal photopheresis (ECP) involves administration of apheresed white blood cells after incubation with 8-methoxypsoralen and ultraviolet-irradiation. It is not completely understood how ECP ameliorates GVHD, but it seems to suppress activated T cells [101]. Hemodynamically stable patients may undergo while it is contraindicated for those with significant heart failure or renal insufficiency. A similar modality, PUVA may be used in patients with cGVHD and significant cutaneous involvement. Skin is irradiated with ultraviolet A light after psoralen administration [102].

In addition to the medical treatment, local supportive treatment of GVHD is essential. Cutaneous involvement by GVHD generally causes thinning and dryness of the skin that can be treated with emollients, topical steroids, and topical tacrolimus. Secondary skin infections may require topical and systemic antibiotic therapy. cGVHD may limit the ranges of motion of the mouth and joints requiring physical therapy in ICU. Oral mucosa frequently needs to be evaluated for superinfection with herpes simplex and fungi. Pulmonary GVHD needs to be treated with inhaled glucocorticoids in addition to the systemic ones and bronchodilators. Superimposed infections, bacterial, viral, and fungal need to be excluded in those with refractory pulmonary symptoms. Pancreatic exocrine deficiency is rare but requires oral/enteral pancreatic enzyme supplementation.

Immunosuppression Due to GVHD Treatment

The commonality to almost all GVHD drugs is the resulting immunosuppression and predisposition to opportunistic infections. However, the mechanisms of action and the characteristics of immunosuppression differ between these agents. Since multiple GVHD drugs are frequently used in combination, it is rather difficult to dissect each one's immunosuppressive effect. Below is a brief attempt to familiarize the intensivists with infectious propensities caused by the drugs used for GVHD treatment.

Corticosteroid administration causes neutrophilia and lymphopenia within a few hours at doses given for GVHD treatment. Neutrophilia is due to decreased neutrophil migration from blood into tissues that also results in decreased neutrophilic phagocytic responses and bactericidal activities. Monocyte migration into tissues as well as antigen presentation is also downregulated with glucocorticoids [103]. Corticosteroids also affect humoral immunity by lowering IgG and IgA levels by up to 20% [104]; however, their effect on cellular immunity is more pronounced. Corticosteroids produce a rapid depletion of circulating T cells, primarily the naïve T cells. This reduction is thought to be due to inhibition of IL-2 signaling, impaired release of lymphoid tissues, and apoptosis [105–108]. Corticosteroids also promote eosinophil apoptosis [109]. It is primarily because of corticosteroids' wide-ranging immunosuppressive effect that they are reserved for GVHD treatment rather than prevention. Risk of infection with bacterial, viral, and fungal pathogens increases early after their administration. Tuberculosis is also a concern for those who has been on corticosteroids for prolonged periods of time.

Calcineurin inhibitors, cyclosporine and tacrolimus, have been the backbone agents for GVHD prophylaxis/treatment after ASCT. They decrease the transcription of IL-2, TNF-alpha, CD40L, interferon-gamma in T lymphocytes [110, 111]. Calcineurin inhibitors primarily increase the risk of viral infections. Despite their similar mechanisms of action, CMV and BK virus infection rates may be higher with tacrolimus than cyclosporine [112–114]. BK virus-associated hemorrhagic cystitis is a significant cause of morbidity and mortality after ASCT, particularly after haploidentical ASCT [115], and may be worsened with high-dose cyclophosphamide [116]. While MMF suppresses both humoral and cellular immunity, it was shown to be protective against Pneumocystis infections [117].

Immunosuppressive effects of mTOR inhibition are diverse and not limited to T cells. mTOR inhibition is thought to prevent/treat GVHD primarily through inhibition of IL-2-induced proliferation of T cells [118]. However, it can also promote the development of memory T cells that are active against viruses [119]. In fact, various observational studies had suggested a protective effect of mTOR inhibitors from CMV infections after solid organ transplants [120–122]. Moreover, sirolimus may inhibit BK virus replication while tacrolimus may exert an opposite effect [123].

Abatacept mostly affects CD4+ T lymphocyte proliferation early after ASCT [73]. When used for GVHD prevention, abatacept is administered on days −1, +5, +14, and + 28 and its effect on T cell reconstitution is short-lived. Consequently, by day 60, circulating T cell numbers return almost to the expected levels limiting its effect on immune reconstitution minimized. Accordingly, first clinical studies demonstrated favorable rates of viral infections with abatacept [73, 74].

TNF-α is produced by macrophages and activated T cells playing important roles in macrophage differentiation/activation/recruitment, phagosome activation, and granuloma formation [124]. Correspondingly, etanercept, a TNF-αinhibitor, primarily increases the risk of bacterial and fungal infections, including late-onset mycobacterial infections [125]. On the other hand, viral infections are also frequently reported after etanercept use in GVHD [86].

Ibrutinib inhibits btk, a downstream messenger enzyme on the B cell receptor signaling cascade. While ibrutinib primarily affects humoral immunity, recent reports suggest increased rates of invasive Aspergillus and Pneumocystis infections in lymphoma/leukemia patients taking ibrutinib [126, 127]. This is likely due ibrutinib's inhibition of btk-dependent NFAT response in human macrophages during phagocytosis [128].

Antimicrobial prophylaxis is generally required during GVHD treatment. As cGVHD usually occurs during late postengraftment period when humoral immunity is particularly weak, cGVHD patients require antibiotics against encapsulated bacteria, i.e., penicillins, levofloxacin, and trimethoprim-sulfamethoxazole. Moreover, patients with severe GVHD are predisposed to invasive Aspergillus infections and may benefit from posaconazole or voriconazole [129]. Pneumocystis prophylaxis with trimethoprim-sulfamethoxazole should be continued during GVHD prevention and treatment [130]. GVHD patients also require prophylaxis against herpes-simplex and varicella zoster with acyclovir or valacyclovir. On the other hand, CMV primary prophylaxis with valganciclovir was not shown to improve outcomes compared to preemptive therapy alone in GVHD patients [131].

Prognosis

The most common reason for ICU admission after stem cell transplantation are respiratory failure and septic shock [3]. GVHD may increase the risk for ICU admissions as it can affect vital organ functions and predispose patients to infections. Accordingly, odds of ICU admission was found to be twice higher in patients with GVHD in a recent retrospective analysis [5]. On the other hand, some patients with severe GVHD may not receive critical care at some institutions as ICU admission criteria varies between different centers.

Prognosis of ASCT patients admitted to ICU is dismal with hospital mortality rates above 50%

despite the improvements made in intensive care in the last few decades. Organ failures, including mechanical ventilation requirement, vasopressor use, and hemodialysis, are the most commonly demonstrated poor prognostic factors [132]. Similarly, GVHD and its treatment may derail the course of an ASCT patient in ICU. While we did not find GVHD to be a prognostic factor for ASCT patients in ICU [2], others found presence of either GVHD [4] or refractory acute GVHD [5] to worsen survival of patients requiring intensive care. As GVHD has a wide clinical spectrum, skin-only to multiorgan involvement, and diverse treatment options, it is likely the severity and the treatment-refractoriness of GVHD that affect the ICU outcomes.

Finally, GVHD poses significant challenges to intensivists as it can involve multiple organs complicating an already complex clinical picture and also due to the toxicity of its treatment. Although transplant physicians are usually the ones responsible for the GVHD management, intensivists need to be well-informed in the disease itself and its treatment to anticipate and swiftly act upon their resulting morbidities.

References

1. Pavletic SZ, Vogelsang GB, Lee SJ. 2014 National Institutes of Health consensus development project on criteria for clinical trials in chronic graft-versus-host disease: preface to the series. Biol Blood Marrow Transplant. 2015;21:387–8. https://doi.org/10.1016/j.bbmt.2014.12.035.
2. Bayraktar UD, Milton DR, Shpall EJ, Rondon G, Price KJ, Champlin RE, Nates JL. Prognostic index for critically ill allogeneic transplantation patients. Biol Blood Marrow Transplant. 2017;23:991–6. https://doi.org/10.1016/j.bbmt.2017.03.003.
3. Bayraktar UD, Nates JL. Intensive care outcomes in adult hematopoietic stem cell transplantation patients. World J Clin Oncol. 2016;7:98–105. https://doi.org/10.5306/wjco.v7.i1.98.
4. Lengline E, et al. Changes in intensive care for allogeneic hematopoietic stem cell transplant recipients. Bone Marrow Transplant. 2015;50:840–5. https://doi.org/10.1038/bmt.2015.55.
5. Orvain C, et al. Different impact of the number of organ failures and graft-versus-host disease on the outcome of allogeneic stem cell transplantation recipients requiring intensive care. Transplantation.

2017;101:437–44. https://doi.org/10.1097/TP.00000 00000001143.

6. Choi SW, et al. Change in plasma tumor necrosis factor receptor 1 levels in the first week after myeloablative allogeneic transplantation correlates with severity and incidence of GVHD and survival. Blood. 2008;112:1539–42. https://doi.org/10.1182/blood-2008-02-138867.

7. Koyama M, et al. Recipient nonhematopoietic antigen-presenting cells are sufficient to induce lethal acute graft-versus-host disease. Nat Med. 2011;18: 135–42. https://doi.org/10.1038/nm.2597.

8. Mathewson ND, et al. Gut microbiome-derived metabolites modulate intestinal epithelial cell damage and mitigate graft-versus-host disease. Nat Immunol. 2016;17:505–13. https://doi.org/10.1038/ni.3400.

9. Schwab L, et al. Neutrophil granulocytes recruited upon translocation of intestinal bacteria enhance graft-versus-host disease via tissue damage. Nat Med. 2014;20:648–54. https://doi.org/10.1038/nm.3517.

10. Shalaby MR, Fendly B, Sheehan KC, Schreiber RD, Ammann AJ. Prevention of the graft-versus-host reaction in newborn mice by antibodies to tumor necrosis factor-alpha. Transplantation. 1989;47:1057–61.

11. Socie G, et al. Prognostic value of apoptotic cells and infiltrating neutrophils in graft-versus-host disease of the gastrointestinal tract in humans: TNF and Fas expression. Blood. 2004;103:50–7. https://doi.org/10.1182/blood-2003-03-0909.

12. Asai O, Longo DL, Tian ZG, Hornung RL, Taub DD, Ruscetti FW, Murphy WJ. Suppression of graft-versus-host disease and amplification of graft-versus-tumor effects by activated natural killer cells after allogeneic bone marrow transplantation. J Clin Invest. 1998;101:1835–42. https://doi.org/10.1172/JCI1268.

13. Palathumpat V, Dejbakhsh-Jones S, Holm B, Strober S. Different subsets of T cells in the adult mouse bone marrow and spleen induce or suppress acute graft-versus-host disease. J Immunol. 1992;149:808–17.

14. Ruggeri L, et al. Effectiveness of donor natural killer cell alloreactivity in mismatched hematopoietic transplants. Science. 2002;295:2097–100. https://doi.org/10.1126/science.1068440.

15. Zeiser R, Blazar BR. Acute graft-versus-host disease - biologic process, prevention, and therapy. N Engl J Med. 2017;377:2167–79. https://doi.org/10.1056/NEJMra1609337.

16. Jagasia M, et al. Risk factors for acute GVHD and survival after hematopoietic cell transplantation. Blood. 2012;119:296–307. https://doi.org/10.1182/blood-2011-06-364265.

17. Loiseau P, et al. HLA association with hematopoietic stem cell transplantation outcome: the number of mismatches at HLA-A, -B, -C, -DRB1, or -DQB1 is strongly associated with overall survival. Biol Blood Marrow Transplant. 2007;13:965–74. https://doi.org/10.1016/j.bbmt.2007.04.010.

18. Martin PJ, et al. Genome-wide minor histocompatibility matching as related to the risk of graft-versus-host disease. Blood. 2017;129:791–8. https://doi.org/10.1182/blood-2016-09-737700.

19. Santos N, et al. UGT2B17 minor histocompatibility mismatch and clinical outcome after HLA-identical sibling donor stem cell transplantation. Bone Marrow Transplant. 2016;51:79–82. https://doi.org/10.1038/bmt.2015.207.

20. Carlens S, et al. Risk factors for chronic graft-versus-host disease after bone marrow transplantation: a retrospective single centre analysis. Bone Marrow Transplant. 1998;22:755–61. https://doi.org/10.1038/sj.bmt.1701423.

21. Gratwohl A, et al. Gender and graft-versus-host disease after hematopoietic stem cell transplantation. Biol Blood Marrow Transplant. 2016;22:1145–6. https://doi.org/10.1016/j.bbmt.2016.03.020.

22. Chang YJ, Weng CL, Sun LX, Zhao YT. Allogeneic bone marrow transplantation compared to peripheral blood stem cell transplantation for the treatment of hematologic malignances: a meta-analysis based on time-to-event data from randomized controlled trials. Ann Hematol. 2012;91:427–37. https://doi.org/10.1007/s00277-011-1299-8.

23. Rocha V, Wagner JE Jr, Sobocinski KA, Klein JP, Zhang MJ, Horowitz MM, Gluckman E. Graft-versus-host disease in children who have received a cord-blood or bone marrow transplant from an HLA-identical sibling. Eurocord and International Bone Marrow Transplant Registry Working Committee on Alternative Donor and Stem Cell Sources. N Engl J Med. 2000;342:1846–54. https://doi.org/10.1056/NEJM200006223422501.

24. Mielcarek M, et al. Graft-versus-host disease after nonmyeloablative versus conventional hematopoietic stem cell transplantation. Blood. 2003;102:756–62. https://doi.org/10.1182/blood-2002-08-2628.

25. Przepiorka D, et al. Chronic graft-versus-host disease after allogeneic blood stem cell transplantation. Blood. 2001;98:1695–700.

26. Aversa F, et al. Full haplotype-mismatched hematopoietic stem-cell transplantation: a phase II study in patients with acute leukemia at high risk of relapse. J Clin Oncol. 2005;23:3447–54. https://doi.org/10.1200/JCO.2005.09.117.

27. Luznik L, Jalla S, Engstrom LW, Iannone R, Fuchs EJ. Durable engraftment of major histocompatibility complex-incompatible cells after nonmyeloablative conditioning with fludarabine, low-dose total body irradiation, and post-transplantation cyclophosphamide. Blood. 2001;98:3456–64. https://doi.org/10.1182/blood. V98.12.3 456.

28. Ratanatharathorn V, et al. Phase III study comparing methotrexate and tacrolimus (prograf, FK506) with methotrexate and cyclosporine for graft-versus-host disease prophylaxis after HLA-identical sibling bone marrow transplantation. Blood. 1998;92:2303–14.

29. Ringden O, Klaesson S, Sundberg B, Ljungman P, Lonnqvist B, Persson U. Decreased incidence of graft-versus-host disease and improved survival with methotrexate combined with cyclosporin compared with monotherapy in recipients of bone marrow from donors other than HLA identical siblings. Bone Marrow Transplant. 1992;9:19–25.

30. Storb R, et al. Methotrexate and cyclosporine compared with cyclosporine alone for prophylaxis of acute graft versus host disease after marrow transplantation for leukemia. N Engl J Med. 1986;314:729–35. https://doi.org/10.1056/NEJM198603203141201.

31. Bolwell B, Sobecks R, Pohlman B, Andresen S, Rybicki L, Kuczkowski E, Kalaycio M. A prospective randomized trial comparing cyclosporine and short course methotrexate with cyclosporine and mycophenolate mofetil for GVHD prophylaxis in myeloablative allogeneic bone marrow transplantation. Bone Marrow Transplant. 2004;34:621–5. https://doi.org/10.1038/sj.bmt.1704647.

32. Perkins J, et al. A randomized phase II trial comparing tacrolimus and mycophenolate mofetil to tacrolimus and methotrexate for acute graft-versus-host disease prophylaxis. Biol Blood Marrow Transplant. 2010;16:937–47. https://doi.org/10.1016/j.bbmt.2010.01.010.

33. Locatelli F, et al. Outcome of children with acute leukemia given HLA-haploidentical HSCT after alphabeta T-cell and B-cell depletion. Blood. 2017;130:677–85. https://doi.org/10.1182/blood-2017-04-779769.

34. Shook DR, Triplett BM, Eldridge PW, Kang G, Srinivasan A, Leung W. Haploidentical stem cell transplantation augmented by CD45RA negative lymphocytes provides rapid engraftment and excellent tolerability. Pediatr Blood Cancer. 2015;62:666–73. https://doi.org/10.1002/pbc.25352.

35. Lee SE, et al. Risk and prognostic factors for acute GVHD based on NIH consensus criteria. Bone Marrow Transplant. 2013;48:587–92. https://doi.org/10.1038/bmt.2012.187.

36. Kitamura K, et al. Relationship among human herpesvirus 6 reactivation, serum interleukin 10 levels, and rash/graft-versus-host disease after allogeneic stem cell transplantation. J Am Acad Dermatol. 2008;58:802–9. https://doi.org/10.1016/j.jaad.2008.01.005.

37. Strong Rodrigues K, Oliveira-Ribeiro C, de Abreu Fiuza Gomes S, Knobler R. Cutaneous graft-versus-host disease: diagnosis and treatment. Am J Clin Dermatol. 2018;19:33–50. https://doi.org/10.1007/s40257-017-0306-9.

38. Glucksberg H, et al. Clinical manifestations of graft-versus-host disease in human recipients of marrow from HL-A-matched sibling donors. Transplantation. 1974;18:295–304.

39. Malard F, Mohty M. New insight for the diagnosis of gastrointestinal acute graft-versus-host disease. Mediat Inflamm. 2014;2014:701013. https://doi.org/10.1155/2014/701013.

40. Liao X, Reed SL, Lin GY. Immunostaining detection of cytomegalovirus in gastrointestinal biopsies: clinicopathological correlation at a large academic health system. Gastroenterol Res. 2016;9:92–8. https://doi.org/10.14740/gr725e.

41. Matsukuma KE, Wei D, Sun K, Ramsamooj R, Chen M. Diagnosis and differential diagnosis of hepatic graft versus host disease (GVHD). J Gastrointest Oncol. 2016;7:S21–31. https://doi.org/10.3978/j.issn.2078-6891.2015.036.

42. Akpek G, et al. Hepatitic variant of graft-versus-host disease after donor lymphocyte infusion. Blood. 2002;100:3903–7. https://doi.org/10.1182/blood-2002-03-0857.

43. Snover DC, Weisdorf SA, Ramsay NK, McGlave P, Kersey JH. Hepatic graft versus host disease: a study of the predictive value of liver biopsy in diagnosis. Hepatology. 1984;4:123–30.

44. Agusti C, et al. Diffuse alveolar hemorrhage in allogeneic bone marrow transplantation. A postmortem study. Am J Respir Crit Care Med. 1995;151:1006–10. https://doi.org/10.1164/ajrccm/151.4.1006.

45. Jacobsohn DA, et al. Correlation between NIH composite skin score, patient-reported skin score, and outcome: results from the Chronic GVHD Consortium. Blood. 2012;120:2545–52; quiz 2774. https://doi.org/10.1182/blood-2012-04-424135.

46. Aractingi S, Chosidow O. Cutaneous graft-versus-host disease. Arch Dermatol. 1998;134:602–12.

47. Jagasia MH, et al. National Institutes of Health consensus development project on criteria for clinical trials in chronic graft-versus-host disease: I. The 2014 diagnosis and staging working group report. Biol Blood Marrow Transplant. 2015;21:389–401. e381. https://doi.org/10.1016/j.bbmt.2014.12.001.

48. Epstein O, Thomas HC, Sherlock S. Primary biliary cirrhosis is a dry gland syndrome with features of chronic graft-versus-host disease. Lancet. 1980;1:1166–8.

49. Song I, Yi CA, Han J, Kim DH, Lee KS, Kim TS, Chung MJ. CT findings of late-onset noninfectious pulmonary complications in patients with pathologically proven graft-versus-host disease after allogeneic stem cell transplant. AJR Am J Roentgenol. 2012;199:581–7. https://doi.org/10.2214/AJR.11.7165.

50. Williams KM. How I treat bronchiolitis obliterans syndrome after hematopoietic stem cell transplantation. Blood. 2017;129:448–55. https://doi.org/10.1182/blood-2016-08-693507.

51. Williams KM, et al. Fluticasone, azithromycin, and montelukast treatment for new-onset bronchiolitis obliterans syndrome after hematopoietic cell transplantation. Biol Blood Marrow Transplant. 2016;22:710–6. https://doi.org/10.1016/j.bbmt.2015.10.009.

52. Vos R, et al. A randomised controlled trial of azithromycin to prevent chronic rejection after

lung transplantation. Eur Respir J. 2011;37:164–72. https://doi.org/10.1183/09031936.00068310.

53. Bergeron A, et al. Effect of azithromycin on airflow decline-free survival after allogeneic hematopoietic stem cell transplant: the ALLOZITHRO randomized clinical trial. JAMA. 2017;318:557–66. https://doi.org/10.1001/jama.2017.9938.

54. Inamoto Y, et al. Incidence, risk factors, and outcomes of sclerosis in patients with chronic graft-versus-host disease. Blood. 2013;121:5098–103. https://doi.org/10.1182/blood-2012-10-464198.

55. Stevens AM, Sullivan KM, Nelson JL. Polymyositis as a manifestation of chronic graft-versus-host disease. Rheumatology (Oxford). 2003;42:34–9.

56. Ruutu T, et al. Prophylaxis and treatment of GVHD: EBMT-ELN working group recommendations for a standardized practice. Bone Marrow Transplant. 2014;49:168–73. https://doi.org/10.1038/bmt.2013. 107.

57. Bram RJ, Hung DT, Martin PK, Schreiber SL, Crabtree GR. Identification of the immunophilins capable of mediating inhibition of signal transduction by cyclosporin A and FK506: roles of calcineurin binding and cellular location. Mol Cell Biol. 1993;13:4760–9.

58. Gething MJ, Sambrook J. Protein folding in the cell. Nature. 1992;355:33–45. https://doi.org/10.1038/355033a0.

59. Petric R, Freeman D, Wallace C, McDonald J, Stiller C, Keown P. Effect of cyclosporine on urinary prostanoid excretion, renal blood flow, and glomerulotubular function. Transplantation. 1988;45:883–9.

60. Wong R, et al. Tacrolimus-associated posterior reversible encephalopathy syndrome after allogeneic haematopoietic stem cell transplantation. Br J Haematol. 2003;122:128–34.

61. Nevill TJ, et al. Influence of post-methotrexate folinic acid rescue on regimen-related toxicity and graft-versus-host disease after allogeneic bone marrow transplantation. Bone Marrow Transplant. 1992;9: 349–54.

62. Morris RE, Hoyt EG, Murphy MP, Eugui EM, Allison AC. Mycophenolic acid morpholinoethylester (RS-61443) is a new immunosuppressant that prevents and halts heart allograft rejection by selective inhibition of T- and B-cell purine synthesis. Transplant Proc. 1990;22:1659–62.

63. Storb R, et al. Stable mixed hematopoietic chimerism in DLA-identical littermate dogs given sublethal total body irradiation before and pharmacological immunosuppression after marrow transplantation. Blood. 1997;89:3048–54.

64. Hardinger KL, Koch MJ, Brennan DC. Current and future immunosuppressive strategies in renal transplantation. Pharmacotherapy. 2004;24:1159–76.

65. Cutler C, et al. Tacrolimus/sirolimus vs tacrolimus/methotrexate as GVHD prophylaxis after matched, related donor allogeneic HCT. Blood. 2014;124:

1372–7. https://doi.org/10.1182/blood-2014-04-567 164.

66. Cutler C, et al. Sirolimus is associated with veno-occlusive disease of the liver after myeloablative allogeneic stem cell transplantation. Blood. 2008;112:4425–31. https://doi.org/10.1182/blood-2008-07-169342.

67. Euvrard S, et al. Sirolimus and secondary skin-cancer prevention in kidney transplantation. N Engl J Med. 2012;367:329–39. https://doi.org/10.1056/NEJMoa 1204166.

68. Berenbaum MC, Brown IN. Prolongation of homograft survival in mice with single doses of cyclophosphamide. Nature. 1963;200:84.

69. Brunstein CG, et al. Alternative donor transplantation: results of parallel phase II trials using HLA-mismatched related bone marrow or unrelated umbilical cord blood grafts. Blood. 2011;118:282. https://doi.org/10.1182/blood-2011-03-344853.

70. Arango M, Combariza JF. Fever after peripheral blood stem cell infusion in haploidentical transplantation with post-transplant cyclophosphamide. Hematol Oncol Stem Cell Ther. 2017;10:79–84. https://doi.org/10.1016/j.hemonc.2017.03.001.

71. Malik SW, Myers JL, DeRemee RA, Specks U. Lung toxicity associated with cyclophosphamide use. Two distinct patterns. Am J Respir Crit Care Med. 1996;154:1851–6. https://doi.org/10.1164/ajrccm. 154.6.8970380.

72. Braverman AC, Antin JH, Plappert MT, Cook EF, Lee RT. Cyclophosphamide cardiotoxicity in bone marrow transplantation: a prospective evaluation of new dosing regimens. J Clin Oncol. 1991;9:1215–23. https://doi.org/10.1200/JCO.1991.9.7.1215.

73. Koura DT, et al. In vivo T cell costimulation blockade with abatacept for acute graft-versus-host disease prevention: a first-in-disease trial. Biol Blood Marrow Transplant. 2013;19:1638–49. https://doi.org/10.1016/j.bbmt.2013.09.003.

74. Watkins B, et al. T cell costimulation blockade with abatacept nearly eliminates early severe acute graft versus host disease after HLA-mismatched (7/8 HLA matched) unrelated donor transplant, with a favorable impact on disease-free and overall survival. Paper presented at the 59th ASH annual meeting. 2017.

75. Champlin RE, et al. T-cell depletion of bone marrow transplants for leukemia from donors other than HLA-identical siblings: advantage of T-cell antibodies with narrow specificities. Blood. 2000;95: 3996–4003.

76. Keever CA, et al. Immune reconstitution following bone marrow transplantation: comparison of recipients of T-cell depleted marrow with recipients of conventional marrow grafts. Blood. 1989;73: 1340–50.

77. Marmont AM, et al. T-cell depletion of HLA-identical transplants in leukemia. Blood. 1991;78:2120–30.

78. Bayraktar UD, et al. Ex vivo T cell-depleted versus unmodified allografts in patients with acute myeloid

leukemia in first complete remission. Biol Blood Marrow Transplant. 2013;19:898–903. https://doi.org/10.1016/j.bbmt.2013.02.018.

79. Walker I, et al. Pretreatment with anti-thymocyte globulin versus no anti-thymocyte globulin in patients with haematological malignancies undergoing haemopoietic cell transplantation from unrelated donors: a randomised, controlled, open-label, phase 3, multicentre trial. Lancet Oncol. 2016;17:164–73. https://doi.org/10.1016/S1470-2045(15)00462-3.

80. Di Ianni M, et al. Tregs prevent GVHD and promote immune reconstitution in HLA-haploidentical transplantation. Blood. 2011;117:3921–8. https://doi.org/10.1182/blood-2010-10-311894.

81. Beelen DW, Elmaagacli A, Muller KD, Hirche H, Schaefer UW. Influence of intestinal bacterial decontamination using metronidazole and ciprofloxacin or ciprofloxacin alone on the development of acute graft-versus-host disease after marrow transplantation in patients with hematologic malignancies: final results and long-term follow-up of an open-label prospective randomized trial. Blood. 1999;93:3267–75.

82. Auphan N, DiDonato JA, Rosette C, Helmberg A, Karin M. Immunosuppression by glucocorticoids: inhibition of NF-kappa B activity through induction of I kappa B synthesis. Science. 1995;270:286–90.

83. Scheinman RI, Cogswell PC, Lofquist AK, Baldwin AS Jr. Role of transcriptional activation of I kappa B alpha in mediation of immunosuppression by glucocorticoids. Science. 1995;270:283–6.

84. Zhang G, Zhang L, Duff GW. A negative regulatory region containing a glucocorticosteroid response element (nGRE) in the human interleukin-1beta gene. DNA Cell Biol. 1997;16:145–52. https://doi.org/10.1089/dna.1997.16.145.

85. Chao NJ, et al. Equivalence of 2 effective graft-versus-host disease prophylaxis regimens: results of a prospective double-blind randomized trial. Biol Blood Marrow Transplant. 2000;6:254–61.

86. De Jong CN, Saes L, Klerk CPW, Van der Klift M, Cornelissen JJ, Broers AEC. Etanercept for steroid-refractory acute graft-versus-host disease: a single center experience. PLoS One. 2017;12:e0187184. https://doi.org/10.1371/journal.pone.0187184.

87. Korngold R, Marini JC, de Baca ME, Murphy GF, Giles-Komar J. Role of tumor necrosis factor-alpha in graft-versus-host disease and graft-versus-leukemia responses. Biol Blood Marrow Transplant. 2003;9:292–303.

88. Levine JE, et al. Etanercept plus methylprednisolone as initial therapy for acute graft-versus-host disease. Blood. 2008;111:2470–5. https://doi.org/10.1182/blood-2007-09-112987.

89. van Groningen LF, Liefferink AM, de Haan AF, Schaap NP, Donnelly JP, Blijlevens NM, van der Velden WJ. Combination therapy with Inolimomab and Etanercept for severe steroid-refractory acute graft-versus-host disease. Biol Blood Marrow Transplant. 2016;22:179–82. https://doi.org/10.1016/j.bbmt.2015.08.039.

90. Bolanos-Meade J, et al. Pentostatin in steroid-refractory acute graft-versus-host disease. J Clin Oncol. 2005;23:2661–8. https://doi.org/10.1200/JCO.2005.06.130.

91. Alousi AM, et al. Etanercept, mycophenolate, denileukin, or pentostatin plus corticosteroids for acute graft-versus-host disease: a randomized phase 2 trial from the Blood and Marrow Transplant Clinical Trials Network. Blood. 2009;114:511–7. https://doi.org/10.1182/blood-2009-03-212290.

92. Verstovsek S, et al. A double-blind, placebo-controlled trial of ruxolitinib for myelofibrosis. N Engl J Med. 2012;366:799–807. https://doi.org/10.1056/NEJMoa1110557.

93. Ma HH, et al. Sequential activation of inflammatory signaling pathways during graft-versus-host disease (GVHD): early role for STAT1 and STAT3. Cell Immunol. 2011;268:37–46. https://doi.org/10.1016/j.cellimm.2011.01.008.

94. Laurence A, et al. STAT3 transcription factor promotes instability of nTreg cells and limits generation of iTreg cells during acute murine graft-versus-host disease. Immunity. 2012;37:209–22. https://doi.org/10.1016/j.immuni.2012.05.027.

95. Zeiser R, et al. Ruxolitinib in corticosteroid-refractory graft-versus-host disease after allogeneic stem cell transplantation: a multicenter survey. Leukemia. 2015;29:2062–8. https://doi.org/10.1038/leu.2015. 212.

96. Tefferi A, Pardanani A. Serious adverse events during ruxolitinib treatment discontinuation in patients with myelofibrosis. Mayo Clin Proc. 2011;86:1188–91. https://doi.org/10.4065/mcp.2011.0518.

97. Byrd JC, et al. Targeting BTK with ibrutinib in relapsed chronic lymphocytic leukemia. N Engl J Med. 2013;369:32–42. https://doi.org/10.1056/NEJMoa1215637.

98. Miklos D, et al. Ibrutinib for chronic graft-versus-host disease after failure of prior therapy. Blood. 2017;130:2243–50. https://doi.org/10.1182/blood-2017-07-793786.

99. Mock J, et al. Risk of major bleeding with Ibrutinib. Clin Lymphoma Myeloma Leuk. 2018;18:755. https://doi.org/10.1016/j.clml.2018.07.287.

100. Brown JR, et al. Characterization of atrial fibrillation adverse events reported in ibrutinib randomized controlled registration trials. Haematologica. 2017;102:1796–805. https://doi.org/10.3324/haematol.2017.171041.

101. Gorgun G, Miller KB, Foss FM. Immunologic mechanisms of extracorporeal photochemotherapy in chronic graft-versus-host disease. Blood. 2002;100:941–7. https://doi.org/10.1182/blood-2002-01-0068.

102. Kapoor N, Pelligrini AE, Copelan EA, Cunningham I, Avalos BR, Klein JL, Tutschka PJ. Psoralen plus ultraviolet A (PUVA) in the treatment of chronic

graft versus host disease: preliminary experience in standard treatment resistant patients. Semin Hematol. 1992;29:108–12.

103. Fauci AS, Dale DC, Balow JE. Glucocorticosteroid therapy: mechanisms of action and clinical considerations. Ann Intern Med. 1976;84:304–15.

104. Butler WT, Rossen RD. Effects of corticosteroids on immunity in man. I. Decreased serum IgG concentration caused by 3 or 5 days of high doses of methylprednisolone. J Clin Invest. 1973;52:2629–40. https://doi.org/10.1172/JCI107455.

105. Ashwell JD, Lu FW, Vacchio MS. Glucocorticoids in T cell development and function. Annu Rev Immunol. 2000;18:309–45. https://doi.org/10.1146/annurev.immunol.18.1.309.

106. Lanza L, et al. Prednisone increases apoptosis in in vitro activated human peripheral blood T lymphocytes. Clin Exp Immunol. 1996;103:482–90.

107. Mathian A, et al. Regulatory T cell responses to high-dose methylprednisolone in active systemic lupus erythematosus. PLoS One. 2015;10:e0143689. https://doi.org/10.1371/journal.pone.0143689.

108. Paliogianni F, Ahuja SS, Balow JP, Balow JE, Boumpas DT. Novel mechanism for inhibition of human T cells by glucocorticoids. Glucocorticoids inhibit signal transduction through IL-2 receptor. J Immunol. 1993;151:4081–9.

109. Wallen N, Kita H, Weiler D, Gleich GJ. Glucocorticoids inhibit cytokine-mediated eosinophil survival. J Immunol. 1991;147:3490–5.

110. Jegasothy BV, Ackerman CD, Todo S, Fung JJ, Abu-Elmagd K, Starzl TE. Tacrolimus (FK 506)–a new therapeutic agent for severe recalcitrant psoriasis. Arch Dermatol. 1992;128:781–5.

111. Schreiber SL, Crabtree GR. The mechanism of action of cyclosporin A and FK506. Immunol Today. 1992;13:136–42. https://doi.org/10.1016/0167-5699(92)90111-J.

112. Hirsch HH, et al. Polyomavirus BK replication in de novo kidney transplant patients receiving tacrolimus or cyclosporine: a prospective, randomized, multicenter study. Am J Transplant. 2013;13:136–45. https://doi.org/10.1111/j.1600-6143.2012.04320.x.

113. Kizilbash SJ, Rheault MN, Bangdiwala A, Matas A, Chinnakotla S, Chavers BM. Infection rates in tacrolimus versus cyclosporine-treated pediatric kidney transplant recipients on a rapid discontinuation of prednisone protocol: 1-year analysis. Pediatr Transplant. 2017;21:e12919. https://doi.org/10.1111/petr.12919.

114. Schwarz A, et al. Factors influencing viral clearing and renal function during polyomavirus BK-associated nephropathy after renal transplantation. Transplantation. 2012;94:396–402. https://doi.org/10.1097/TP.0b013e31825a505d.

115. Ruggeri A, et al. Incidence and risk factors for hemorrhagic cystitis in unmanipulated haploidentical transplant recipients. Transpl Infect Dis. 2015;17:822–30. https://doi.org/10.1111/tid.12455.

116. Rorije NM, et al. BK virus disease after allogeneic stem cell transplantation: a cohort analysis. Biol Blood Marrow Transplant. 2014;20:564–70. https://doi.org/10.1016/j.bbmt.2014.01.014.

117. Oz HS, Hughes WT. Novel anti-Pneumocystis carinii effects of the immunosuppressant mycophenolate mofetil in contrast to provocative effects of tacrolimus, sirolimus, and dexamethasone. J Infect Dis. 1997;175:901–4.

118. Geissler EK. The influence of mTOR inhibitors on immunity and the relationship to post-transplant malignancy. Transplant Res. 2013;2:S2. https://doi.org/10.1186/2047-1440-2-S1-S2.

119. Rao RR, Li Q, Odunsi K, Shrikant PA. The mTOR kinase determines effector versus memory CD8+ T cell fate by regulating the expression of transcription factors T-bet and Eomesodermin. Immunity. 2010;32:67–78. https://doi.org/10.1016/j.immuni.2009.10.010.

120. Brennan DC, et al. Effect of maintenance immunosuppressive drugs on virus pathobiology: evidence and potential mechanisms. Rev Med Virol. 2013;23:97–125. https://doi.org/10.1002/rmv.1733.

121. Cervera C, et al. Effect of mammalian target of rapamycin inhibitors on cytomegalovirus infection in kidney transplant recipients receiving polyclonal antilymphocyte globulins: a propensity score-matching analysis. Transpl Int. 2016;29:1216–25. https://doi.org/10.1111/tri.12848.

122. de Paula MI, et al. Long-term follow-up of de novo use of mTOR and Calcineurin inhibitors after kidney transplantation. Ther Drug Monit. 2016;38:22–31. https://doi.org/10.1097/FTD.0000000000000227.

123. Hirsch HH, Yakhontova K, Lu M, Manzetti J. BK polyomavirus replication in renal tubular epithelial cells is inhibited by sirolimus, but activated by tacrolimus through a pathway involving FKBP-12. Am J Transplant. 2016;16:821–32. https://doi.org/10.1111/ajt.13541.

124. Koo S, Marty FM, Baden LR. Infectious complications associated with immunomodulating biologic agents. Infect Dis Clin N Am. 2010;24:285–306. https://doi.org/10.1016/j.idc.2010.01.006.

125. Giles JT, Bathon JM. Serious infections associated with anticytokine therapies in the rheumatic diseases. J Intensive Care Med. 2004;19:320–34. https://doi.org/10.1177/0885066604267854.

126. Ahn IE, Jerussi T, Farooqui M, Tian X, Wiestner A, Gea-Banacloche J. Atypical *Pneumocystis jirovecii* pneumonia in previously untreated patients with CLL on single-agent ibrutinib. Blood. 2016;128:1940–3. https://doi.org/10.1182/blood-2016-06-722991.

127. Ghez D, et al. Early-onset invasive aspergillosis and other fungal infections in patients treated with ibrutinib. Blood. 2018;131:1955–9. https://doi.org/10.1182/blood-2017-11-818286.

128. Bercusson A, Colley T, Shah A, Warris A, Armstrong-James D. Ibrutinib blocks Btk-dependent

NF-kB and NFAT responses in human macrophages during *Aspergillus fumigatus* phagocytosis. Blood. 2018;132:1985. https://doi.org/10.1182/blood-2017-12-823393.

129. Ullmann AJ, et al. Posaconazole or fluconazole for prophylaxis in severe graft-versus-host disease. N Engl J Med. 2007;356:335–47. https://doi.org/10.1056/NEJMoa061098.

130. Tomblyn M, et al. Guidelines for preventing infectious complications among hematopoietic cell transplantation recipients: a global perspective. Biol Blood Marrow Transplant. 2009;15:1143–238. https://doi.org/10.1016/j.bbmt.2009.06.019.

131. Boeckh M, et al. Valganciclovir for the prevention of complications of late cytomegalovirus infection after allogeneic hematopoietic cell transplantation: a randomized trial. Ann Intern Med. 2015;162:1–10. https://doi.org/10.7326/M13-2729.

132. Saillard C, et al. Critically ill allogenic HSCT patients in the intensive care unit: a systematic review and meta-analysis of prognostic factors of mortality. Bone Marrow Transplant. 2018;53:1233. https://doi.org/10.1038/s41409-018-0181-x.

Stevens–Johnson Syndrome (SJS) and Toxic Epidermal Necrolysis (TEN)

Immunologic Reactions

19

Danielle Zimmerman and Nam Hoang Dang

Contents

Introduction 268

Etiology 268
Medications 268
Infections 269
Malignancies 269
Other Causes 270

Epidemiology 270
Genetics 270

Pathophysiology 271

Clinical Features 272
Mucocutaneous Manifestations 272
Ophthalmologic Manifestations 273
Bronchial Manifestations 273
GI Manifestations 273
Renal Manifestations 273
Hematologic Manifestations 273
Endocrine Manifestations 273
Other Manifestations and Laboratory Markers 273
Histopathology 274

Diagnosis 274

Management 274
Nonpharmacologic Management/Supportive Care 274
Pharmacologic Management 275
Prevention 277

Prognosis 277

References 277

D. Zimmerman · N. H. Dang (✉)
University of Florida Health Cancer Center,
Gainesville, FL, USA
e-mail: danielle.zimmerman@medicine.ufl.edu;
nam.dang@medicine.ufl.edu

© Springer Nature Switzerland AG 2020
J. L. Nates, K. J. Price (eds.), *Oncologic Critical Care*,
https://doi.org/10.1007/978-3-319-74588-6_195

Abstract

Stevens–Johnson syndrome (SJS) and toxic epidermal necrolysis (TEN) are immunologic reactions to several stimuli, mostly medications, which present as a spectrum of primarily widespread mucocutaneous lesions, but also with other organ involvement. Pathology is characterized by full thickness necrosis of the epithelial layer of the involved organ due to immune-mediated apoptosis of the resident keratinocytes. High suspicion for early detection and quick withdrawal of the culprit medication are the most important steps in stopping this reaction. Aggressive supportive care is often necessary as the patient recovers. Steroids, other immunosuppressants, and plasmapheresis have all been studied as treatments, but high-quality evidence supporting their contributions, either together or separately, in decreasing length of hospital stay or prolonging survival have not been consistently demonstrated. Further studies of the mechanism of action and novel treatment modalities are still needed to improve outcomes in patients with this rare but often fatal condition.

Keywords

Bullous lesion · Mucocutaneous involvement · Steroids · Stevens–Johnson syndrome · Toxic epidermal necrolysis

Introduction

Toxic epidermal necrolysis (TEN) and Stevens–Johnson syndrome (SJS) are potentially life-threatening type IVc immune reactions with inflammation mediated by cytotoxic T lymphocytes, that present with mucocutaneous blistering reactions with epidermal detachment and extensive necrosis [62].

The skin reaction is termed SJS when less than 10% of the body surface area (BSA) is involved. The intermediate form is classified as SJS/TEN and has 10–30% skin involvement. TEN describes the skin reaction when greater than 30% of the BSA is involved. Greater than 90% of patients with SJS have mucous membrane involvement, and nearly all patients will have mucous membrane involvement in TEN [54]. The overall range of disease will henceforth be referred to as SJS and TEN in this discussion. The whole spectrum of this disorder can involve other organs, which can complicate treatment and convalescence [69].

Epidermal cell necrosis is caused by aberrant immune activation by a variety of stimuli but mostly medications. Cytotoxic T lymphocytes are induced with CD4+ cells and innate immune cells to secrete granulysin and other cytokines that puncture the cell membrane and cause sufficient damage to induce widespread apoptosis in a rapid fashion [12].

Etiology

While approximately 5–20% of cases remain idiopathic [66], SJS and TEN are thought to be due to a combination of immune predisposition and exogenous stimuli such as medication [43] or infection that results in apoptosis of epithelial cells [59]. Medication exposure is associated with 50–95% of cases, depending on the population examined [55].

People with certain HLA serotypes, TCR subtypes, or differences in their ability to absorb, distribute to tissues, metabolize, or excrete medications have a higher likelihood of developing SJS and TEN [59].

Medications

There are 100–200 medications associated with the development of SJS and TEN. Though this group of medications includes many antibiotics and sulfa-containing compounds, there is no existing test to determine definitively if a given medication was responsible for causing the skin reaction [66]. However, there is an algorithm of drug causality for epidermal necrolysis (ALDEN) that was constructed to improve the individual assessment of medication causality in SJS and TEN [66].

A small selection of these medications causes about half of all cases of SJS and TEN oxicam NSAIDs; phenylbutzone; sulfonamides such as sulfamethoxazole, sulfadiazine, sulfapyridine, sulfadoxine, sulfasalazine; allopurinol; lamotrigine; nevirapine; phenytoin; and carbamazepine [62]. Acetaminophen has been identified as a possible cause in children but not in adults [59]. A review of severe skin reactions from 1950 to 2013 associated with antineoplastic agents revealed that the following medications have been strongly correlated with SJS and TEN: bendamustine, procarbazine, fludarabine, busulfan, chlorambucil, and lomustine [54]. Other drugs that can cause SJS and TEN include vancomycin, valproate, levofloxacin, etravirine, isotretinoin, quinolones, diclofenac, fluconazole, sitagliptin, oseltamivir, penicillins, barbiturates, sulfonamides, azithromycin, oxcarbazepine, zonisamide, modafinil, pyrimethamine, ethosuximide, bupropion, telaprevir, nystatin, cefixime, and trimethoprim [59].

Some medications that have been investigated but not found to have a strong link to development of SJS and TEN include aspirin, sulfonylureas, vitamins, thiazide diuretics, furosemide, aldactone, calcium channel blockers, beta blockers, hormones, angiotensin-converting enzyme inhibitors, angiotensin II receptor antagonists, and statins.

Infections

Mycoplasma pneumoniae is the most common bacterial infection associated with the development of SJS and TEN. Infection with this microorganism is noted to be the cause of SJS and TEN more often in children than in adults, and treatment of the infection has led to improvement of skin symptoms in some cases [31]. Less common bacterial agents implicated in its development include Yersinia, tuberculosis, syphilis, chlamydia, Streptococci, Salmonella, Enterobacter, and Pneumococcus [59].

Coccidiomycosis and histoplasmosis are the potential fungal causes of SJS and TEN [59]. Strongyloides infection was also associated with SJS and TEN in a case report [7].

The incidence of SJS and TEN in patients with HIV is about one thousand times higher than the incidence in patients without HIV [29]. This is likely due in part to the increased likelihood of HIV patients being exposed to potential culprit medications such as sulfonamides, but other cases are attributable to the HIV infection itself. Other viruses that may play a role in the pathogenesis of SJS and TEN include enterovirus, adenovirus, measles, mumps, CMV [29], herpes simplex, HHV-6, and influenza [59]. HHV has been recognized as a causative agent for SJS and TEN for several cases in children in particular. Some viral infections have been shown to increase expression of Fas ligand or sensitivity to Fas ligand-mediated apoptosis [29], but the importance of Fas ligand expression may have been overestimated, both overall and in virally induced cases of SJS and TEN. Speculation exists that changes to immune cell activity in keratinocytes induced by infection contributes to development of SJS and TEN in these cases.

Malignancies

Patients with hematologic malignancies, and to a lesser extent nonhematologic malignancies, have a higher risk of developing SJS and TEN. It is not known if the malignancies themselves, disrupted immune function, or exposure to a higher variety of pharmacologic agents is the key variable responsible in this patient cohort [41]. The magnitude of this risk has been estimated to be between two [18] and as much as sixty [70] times that of the patient without any malignancy, but this variance may depend on the patient population examined. Diagnoses of hepatocellular carcinoma and colorectal cancer (but not hematologic malignancy, lung cancer, or urothelial carcinoma), abnormal labs, and recent or current chemotherapy administration were associated with higher risks of death in a recent review of patients in the UK [68]. A study of patients in the USA found that SJS and TEN were most associated with multiple myeloma, leukemia, non-Hodgkin's lymphoma, and CNS malignancies [25]. An earlier review of patients at a

Roman hospital indicated that CNS malignancy and NHL were the most common malignancies associated with SJS and TEN [23].

Other Causes

There are rare cases in which vaccinations have been thought to lead to SJS and TEN, including the smallpox vaccination, the diphtheria-pertussis-tetanus (DPT) vaccination, Bacillus Calmette-Guérin (BCG) vaccination, and the measles-mumps-rubella (MMR) vaccination [55].

Cases of SJS and TEN have been reported after allogenic bone marrow transplantation; however, these cases have been difficult to distinguish from severe graft versus host disease due to similarity of skin appearance on exam and histology. Radiation therapy, inflammatory bowel disease, administration of IV contrast, and toxic chemical exposure have rarely been implicated in cases of SJS and TEN [62]. The cases of SJS and TEN associated with inflammatory bowel disease may have been associated with anti-TNF alpha therapy rather than the disease itself.

Epidemiology

The incidence of SJS and TEN is about one or two cases per one million people. TEN and SJS have been known to occur in patients of all ages, but the highest incidence is in adults greater than 40 years old [59]. Incidence is about equal in men and women [30]. Most cases tend to occur in winter or early spring, which could correlate with antibiotic prescriptions [18].

An observational study of patients with SJS and TEN in the UK indicated patients of African or Asian ancestry had twice the chance of developing SJS and TEN compared with white patients; however, the general applicability of the study is limited by the low sample size. Higher incidence in patients with epilepsy, gout, and autoimmune diseases was thought to be largely attributable to associated medications rather than to the diseases themselves. No association was found between SJS and TEN and tobacco use, alcohol use, or obesity [18].

Genetics

There appears to be a predilection for developing SJS and TEN in reaction to particular medications depending on patients' ethnicity and MHC I. People of Han Chinese or Thai ancestry living in Taiwan who also expressed HLA-B*1502, as well as HLA-B*1511, were more likely to have carbamazepine or phenytoin-induced SJS and TEN [11], while those who expressed HLA-B*5801 were more likely to have the reaction after allopurinol exposure [26]. Other MHC allotypes have also been associated with development of SJS and TEN upon exposure of these medications:

- People of Han Chinese descent with HLA-A*2402 have an increased risk of developing SJS and TEN in response to lamotrigine, carbamazepine, and phenytoin [57].
- Some association was also found in people of Japanese [27] and European [35] descent with expression of HLA-B*5801 and allopurinol-induced SJS and TEN.

Other HLA subtypes are associated with multiple types of skin reactions in addition to SJS and TEN upon exposure to the more common culprit medications:

- Expression of HLA-A*3101 in patients who are of European, Japanese, and Indian origin is associated with both SJS and TEN as well as drug reaction with eosinophilia and systemic symptoms (DRESS) [38].
- Patients of Thai ancestry who have the HLA-B*1301 allele tend to have a variety of drug-induced hypersensitivity reactions, including SJS and TEN, because of dapsone [61].

Noting these relationships has led to clinical recommendations in a minority of cases: There are some recommendations that patients of Asian ancestry who express HLA-B*1502 or HLA-A*3101 should undergo screening prior to initiation of carbamazepine treatment [2]. The carbamazepine-mediated reaction was not seen in people of Japanese [27], Korean, or European descent [36].

While the HLA subtype is a more commonly recognized genetic risk factor for the development of SJS and TEN, expression of certain cytochrome P450 enzyme subtypes can also be a predisposing factor: CYP2C9 is drug-metabolizing cytochrome P450 that metabolizes phenytoin. The CYP2C9*3 variant metabolizes phenytoin at a reduced rate and patients with CYP2C9*3 have been shown to have higher blood levels of phenytoin at similar doses as well as an increased incidence of SJS and TEN [37].

Pathophysiology

T-cell activation in SJS and TEN can be precipitated by a variety of stimuli that lead to unintended immune activation, primarily medications and/or their metabolites, but also including infections or malignancies. A favored theory regarding T-cell activation is termed the prohapten concept. A medication or its metabolite can bind with host protein to form a novel antigen. This antigen is taken up by APCs, which process the protein and then display the resulting peptides on the HLA component of their MHC for presentation to TCRs on CD8+ or CD4+ T cells. Upon binding of the HLA-novel antigen on the APC to the TCR of the CD4 or CD8+ T cell, the T lymphocyte is induced to replicate and these T cells will target host tissues [31]. Another model is termed the pharmacologic interaction of drugs with the immune system (p-i) concept. In this model, medications or their metabolites noncovalently bond with the type I MHC and TCR, which sets off production of T cells only. This theory could explain the lack of significant B cell populations found in the skin of patients studied with SJS and TEN.

However, other studies focusing on the role of APCs showed that production of T cells was absent when pathways responsible for antigen presentation and processing were inhibited by stimulating isolated lymphocytes from patients with known hypersensitivity reactions to sulfamethoxazole. In this same study, when this group of lymphocytes was isolated again and incubated with the inhibitors of antigen presentation, glutaraldehyde and glutathione, sulfamethoxazole metabolites were not able to stimulate T-cell proliferation [9]. This study provided positive evidence to support the prohapten concept. In fact, both models could explain in part the disease pathophysiology, although a complete understanding, including a coherent synthesis of the two, has yet to be achieved [55].

In cases of immune activation by means other than medication reaction, the stimuli, whether it is infection or malignancy, can promote propagation of memory T cells that have activity against self-antigens [44]. The process by which responses to stimuli such as infection or malignancy produces memory T-cell production is termed heterologous immunity. However, in many of these cases, it can be challenging to determine if SJS and TEN is occurring in response to the infection or malignancy itself or in response to its treatment. Furthermore, because such a preponderance of cases are due to medications rather than other causes, it is difficult to develop evidence for the mechanistic model by which these other stimuli propagate T-cell proliferation. Studies that reported lack of representative symptoms in CD8+ T-cell-deficient animal models reinforce the central role of cytotoxic T cells but do not elucidate the mechanism of their activation [52].

Several cytokines mediate apoptosis in SJS and TEN, including granulysin, perforin, and granzyme B, as well as tumor necrosis factor [46], with related molecules in a supportive role. Cytotoxic T cells can secrete granules that contain granulysin, perforin, and granzyme B. These granules penetrate cell membranes and lead to mitochondrial damage, resulting subsequently in cell death. Analysis of blister fluid from patients with SJS and TEN compared with blister fluid from burn patients showed that the blister fluid from patients with SJS and TEN contained up to twenty times more granulysin, eight times more granzyme B, three times more perforin, and twice as much Fas ligand (Fas-L) [55].

The presence of NK cells and macrophages alongside cytotoxic CD8+ T lymphocytes, which are the predominant immune cell population found in skin and blister fluid samples, supports the hypothesis that these cells behave in a cooperative manner to mediate keratinocyte apoptosis. These cells can secrete or support secretion of members of the tumor necrosis superfamily: tumor necrosis factor (TNF) alpha, CD40L, and Fas-L [1], which promote antigen presentation and other pathways of apoptosis [32].

The exact pathway through which T cells and NK cells produce these mediators has not yet been elucidated, but a study suggests that degranulation is potentially triggered by an interaction between HLA-E, an MHC1b molecule, on keratinocytes and CD94/NKG2CR on T cells [43]. Apoptosis of keratinocytes is the hallmark pathophysiologic feature of SJS and TEN.

Clinical Features

SJS and TEN most commonly start 4–28 days after the culprit medication is first administered [5]. If a medication is withdrawn and rechallenged, then onset more often occurs within a few hours to a few days [66]. Therefore, newly added drugs should merit more thorough consideration as the causative agent than medications with which the patient has been chronically treated.

The initial symptoms typically experienced include high fevers (>39 °C), pharyngitis, headache, arthralgias, malaise, and conjunctivitis, in addition to the skin lesions [58]. Of note is that fever, malaise, and arthralgias may be present in the first few days prior to any cutaneous involvement [66].

The next phase consists of epidermal detachment, which typically evolves over 5–7 days [62]. Subsequently, the "plateau" phase is characterized by progressive re-epithelization and lasts for a range of several days to several weeks, depending on disease severity and extent of comorbidities. Given the heavy burden of post SJS and TEN sequelae, frequent follow-up is often necessary on recovery to manage all the complications [50].

Mucocutaneous Manifestations

Mucosal involvement is noted in about 90% of cases and at least two different sites are typically involved [62].

The lesions characteristic of this syndrome are blisters with mucosal and epidermal detachment that results from epidermal necrosis without significant dermal inflammation. The blisters will develop on top of target lesions or macular lesions with significant involvement of the mucosal layer. These skin lesions can sometimes be confused with erythema multiforme (EM) associated with herpes simplex virus infection or the mucositis and blistering lesions seen in mycoplasma infection in children; however, these other phenomena have a less diffuse distribution than SJS and TEN [58].

When these lesions occur, they first emerge as erythematous, dusky, or purpuric plaques, papules, or blisters, sometimes with formation of vesicles [59]. Sometimes the lesions appear as targetoid lesions with dark centers [69]. They tend to first appear on the face, proximal limbs, and upper trunk. The lesions will grow and become confluent over hours to days, covering the rest of the body [62].

The lesions will then develop into painful ulcerations, which leave eroded areas covered with pseudomembrane and necrosis. Many patients will have tender hemorrhagic erosions with gray-white pseudomembranes and crusts over the vermillion border of the lips on presentation [58].

Nikolsky's sign is specific for SJS and TEN at this stage, but it is not sensitive as it also occurs in Staphylococcal scalded skin syndrome, pemphigus vulgaris, and mucous membrane pemphigoid. Nikolsky's sign is a dermatologic finding in which there is detachment of the epidermis at application of pressure, which results in an erythematous erosion. Nails can be shed in TEN [62].

There is not a strong correlation between severity of cutaneous and mucosal involvement [3].

Following the resolution of SJS and TEN, skin may be hypopigmented, hyperpigmented, or scarred. Nail growth may be abnormal in approximately one-third of surviving patients, with such defects as nail bed pigmentation changes, nail ridging, dystrophic nails, and permanent paronychia [62]. A similar proportion of surviving patients will suffer from dry mouth, altered sense of taste, and dental changes [20].

Ophthalmologic Manifestations

Odynophagia and burning or stinging of the eyes can start early and will portend mucous membrane involvement [62].

Approximately 80% of cases with have ocular involvement which is characterized by erythema, discharge, lacrimation, tenderness, and photophobia [62]. Severity of initial symptoms correlate with the development of subsequent complications [56].

Ophthalmologic sequelae occur due to altered conjunctival epithelium with abnormal lacrimal film. The ocular complications can include hyperemia, pseudomembrane formation, Sjorgen-like sicca syndrome, purulent conjunctivitis, dry eyes, entropion, trichiasis, symblepharon, inverted or loss of eyelashes, and corneal metaplasia causing corneal erosions/ulcerations [24]. These developments can lead to loss of vision. Bulbar conjunctiva and synechiae between eyelids are subsequent manifestations [56].

Genital, bronchial, esophageal, and pharyngolaryngeal lesions are less frequently occurring characteristics but merit special attention [58]. The genital lesions most often present as dysuria. Synechiae may also form because of genital lesions, especially if overlooked [39].

Bronchial Manifestations

Although patients may have normal chest radiographical findings and limited or no respiratory symptoms on initial presentation, careful monitoring is needed due to the potential for the rapid development of pulmonary changes. Approximately 25% of patients with SJS and TEN will have pulmonary involvement, which tends to first be heralded by cough and tachypnea. Interstitial lesions may appear that can lead to acute respiratory distress syndrome (ARDS). Bronchoscopy may be useful to help distinguish between infectious complications of ARDS versus ARDS due to SJS and TEN itself [62].

GI Manifestations

Necrosis of the esophageal, small bowel, or colonic epithelium occurs rarely but presents as diarrhea with melena, signs of malabsorption [40], and at worst perforation [8].

Renal Manifestations

Prerenal azotemia is a common complication. Renal failure due to acute tubular necrosis may occur due to apoptosis of the epithelial cells lining the tubules. Other renal manifestations can include proteinuria and hematuria. Elevated blood urea nitrogen (BUN) can signal severity of renal involvement [6].

Hematologic Manifestations

Neutropenia can occur rarely and tends to involve cases with poor prognosis. Anemia is often present. Eosinophilia does not commonly occur. A common hematologic finding is transient CD4+ lymphopenia, which corresponds to poor T cell function [62].

Endocrine Manifestations

Because SJS and TEN represent an extremely catabolic state, insulin secretion is often decreased, and insulin resistance can occur. These changes typically result in hyperglycemia and the development of diabetes. Blood glucose level greater than 14 mM portends severe disease and poor prognosis [5].

Other Manifestations and Laboratory Markers

Mental status changes because of SJS or TEN on their own are rare. As a result, patients tend to be cognizant of the changes, and extreme distress from severe pain is common [66].

Mild transaminitis and amylase elevation are commonly seen but do not affect prognosis [62].

Histopathology

The pathologic specimen is typically obtained from skin or mucous membrane biopsy; however, similar changes are found in other tissue types involved as well [48]. In the early stages of SJS and TEN, there are sparse apoptotic keratinocytes in the epithelium, which then rapidly changes to a full thickness necrosis with subepidermal detachment. Sweat glands and hair follicles can be involved. The later stages of the disease also feature inflammatory infiltrate of the papillary dermis, made up predominantly of CD8+ T cells and macrophages. Eosinophilia is not commonly seen in TEN [64].

Diagnosis

While there is no test or list of criteria to prove definitively that a patient has SJS and TEN [62], a skin biopsy can help rule out other conditions with similar presentations. The specimen is best obtained via a shave biopsy or punch biopsy that contains dermis. When preparing the sample for submission, it needs to be collected in formalin, the suspected diagnosis of SJS and TEN should be listed on the accompanying paperwork, and rapid processing (a few hours or less) should be requested [59].

It is difficult to distinguish clinically SJS and TEN from erythema multiforme (EM) early in the clinical presentation, but EM will manifest less extensively and floridly than SJS and TEN, and EM will not have the extensive mucosal involvement that often accompanies SJS and TEN [65].

Limited involvement of mucous membranes should prompt evaluation of alternative diagnoses, such as Staphylococcal scalded skin syndrome in infants, purpura fulminans in younger people, and in adults acute generalized exanthematous pustuosis, phototoxicity, or pressure ulcers

[65]. Trauma-induced scalding or thermal burns merits consideration if loss of consciousness was the first symptom in the patient's presentation [62]. Slower progression of disease would be more typical of linear IgA dermatosis and paraneoplastic pemphigus.

Skin biopsy should allow for differentiation between SJS and TEN and DRESS, exfoliative erythroderma, Staphylococcal scalded skin syndrome, bullous pemphigoid, pemphigus vulgaris, linear IgA dermatosis, paraneoplastic pemphigus, and pemphigus foliaceus. Hematoxylin and eosin staining and direct immunofluorescence will be done to distinguish among these diagnoses [59].

Management

There is not currently a proven effective cure or treatment for SJS and TEN, so the best approach given current data includes high suspicion for this syndrome, early clinical diagnosis, immediate cessation of suspected culprit medication [19], supportive therapy, and close monitoring for and treatment of complications with high morbidity, such as infection and ophthalmologic sequelae. If a patient has a SCORTEN score of less than or equal to one, has limited skin involvement, and has slower progression of disease, then care can take place in a nonspecialized setting, but all other patients need to be in an ICU or burn unit [16], as patients who receive care in burn units often have better morbidity and mortality outcome [33]. A dermatologic specialist should be consulted in all suspected cases.

Nonpharmacologic Management/ Supportive Care

Assessment of vital signs is an important first step in the evaluation of patient with suspected SJS or TEN as tachypnea and hypoxia can signal respiratory alkalosis from respiratory involvement [62].

Massive fluid loss through the skin lesions should be treated with aggressive fluid resuscitation as fluid loss causes hypotension due to hypovolemia, hypoalbuminemia, electrolyte disturbances, and renal dysfunction. While large doses of intravenous fluids are administered, smaller volumes than what are typically used for burns can be given due to the lack of interstitial edema in SJS and TEN [62].

Other supportive therapies in these cases usually include hemodynamic monitoring and stabilization, prophylaxis against infection, nutrient supplementation and/or replacement, temperature management, analgesia, and thorough care of skin, eyes, and mucous membranes [62].

Infectious complications are the first sequelae to appear and since sepsis is the primary cause of mortality in SJS and TEN, aggressive treatment is indicated [42]. The infectious agents most commonly detected are *Staphylococcus aureus* and *Pseudomonas* spp. As one-third of positive blood cultures in these patients contain noncutaneous Enterobacteriae, bacterial translocation from the GI tract is thought to be a common means of infection. Besides frequent daily mouth rinse with antiseptic or antifungal solution, prophylactic antibiotics are not indicated. Instead, careful aseptic technique should be stressed. Frequent culture specimens should be obtained from skin, blood, and urine [13].

Surgical debridement of wounds is not recommended since it can worsen skin lesions; however, the best methods for addressing the cutaneous lesions and optimizing skin care have not yet been determined [14].

Ocular lesions should be assessed by an ophthalmologist daily. Treatment with preservative-free emollients, antiseptic or antibiotic eye drops, and vitamin A are the interventions recommended early in the disease course to limit subsequent development of complications. These treatments tend to be more effective if administered earlier [64]. A retrospective review of patients with ocular complications of SJS and TEN who were fitted with scleral lens noted reduction in photophobia and tenderness [49].

Suction to prevent aspiration pneumonitis may be indicated in cases with oropharyngeal involvement [5].

Pharmacologic Management

Among the additional treatments to consider are several immunosuppressants, but these therapies could be a hindrance to recovery in cases complicated by infection [10].

Steroids

The efficacy of steroids in treatment of SJS and TEN remains to be elucidated, but this class of drugs remains the standard of care as first-line therapy in TEN after or in addition to supportive care [54]. If steroids are given, high dose pulse therapy is favored over smaller doses administered over a longer time period. Prednisone 1–2 mg/kg daily might be helpful early in the disease process, but prolonged use has led to increased mortality [51]. No prospective studies examining use of steroids compared to supportive care alone have yet been performed, but a large cohort study did not show any meaningful difference in survival with the use of steroids versus best supportive care [53].

Cyclosporine

Administration of cyclosporine could be considered based on the theoretical plausibility of the putative mechanism of action and several case reports and series [10]. Cyclosporine-mediated cytokine activation, CD8+ cell inhibition, Fas-L inhibition, NFKB inhibition, and TNF-alpha inhibition have all been hypothesized to affect SJS and TEN. Early administration of cyclosporine A in a couple case series at 3 mg/kg daily [63] or twice daily [3] has been described as resulting in lower than expected mortality rates than could be anticipated with steroid treatment.

IVIg

Treating SJS and TEN with IVIg has been recommended in some cases, but the overall effectiveness of this approach is still controversial [47].

The proposed mechanism of action that led originally to the consideration of IVIg as treatment is as follows: IVIg can act as a blocking antibody, which would interfere with the

Fas ligand-induced keratinocyte apoptosis that underlies this cutaneous reaction. However, examination of blister fluid and cells from wounds of patients with SJS and TEN contained two to four times as much granulysin as compared with Fas-ligand. This finding has led to the reconsideration of the putative mechanism of action described above [55].

Some reviews and retrospective analyses with smaller enrollments including adults who had received IVIg for SJS and TEN demonstrated a mortality benefit when patients had received IVIg in doses >2 g/kg over the course of 3–4 days. However, other studies did not show any benefit [4].

The efficacy of IVIg is likely dependent on timing of administration (early or late in disease course), variability in each IVIg dose, dose of IVIg given, and patient's morbidity burden, particularly renal failure [10].

Plasmapheresis

Plasmapheresis is thought to work by filtering off the inciting agent (the autoantibody or medication and/or its metabolites) or its downstream mediators [54]. Case series have been examined in which TEN patients received plasmapheresis with [34] or without [15] IVIg daily or every other day. These studies demonstrated lower than expected mortality. Reviews of plasmapheresis used in conjunction with pulse dose steroids have concluded that this combination could result in lower mortality rates or improved time to recovery [70]. Some case series suggested beneficial responses for patients refractory to other therapies [60]. In other case series, patients failed to exhibit any benefit from the use of plasmapheresis [17]. Plasmapheresis has been covered by insurance in Japan since 2006 as a second-line therapy for TEN [69]. The American Society of Apheresis lists plasmapheresis as a category 3 grade 2B recommendation [54].

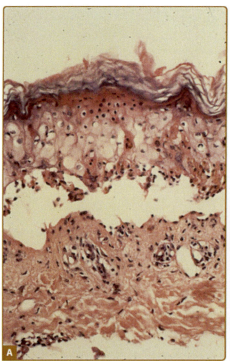
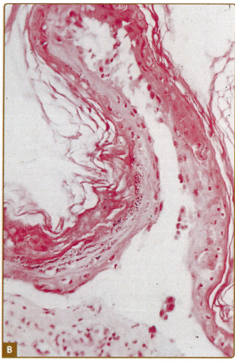

Fig. 1 Histologic appearance of toxic epidermal necrolysis. (**a**) Eosinophilic necrosis of the epidermis in the peak stage, with little inflammatory response in the dermis. Note cleavage in the junction zone. (**b**) The completely necrotic epidermis has detached from the dermis and folded like a sheet

Thalidomide

Thalidomide has been investigated for use in treatment of SJS and TEN, but its use cannot be recommended based on current evidence [36]. Because keratinocyte apoptosis in TEN is thought to be mediated by TNF alpha, it was hypothesized that the thalidomide-mediated TNF alpha inhibitor activity might grant it a role in the treatment of TEN. A prospective, randomized controlled study comparing the use of thalidomide to placebo in patients with TEN who had not received any therapy closed early after enrolling 22 of the planned 50 patients when 13 of the 22 patients died over the 16 months enrollment had been open. Upon unblinding of the results, it was found that 10 patients out of 12 had died in the thalidomide group, and 3 people out of 10 had died in the placebo group. The trial was then stopped at the recommendation of the group's safety board [29].

Prevention

Upon recovery, the patient should be alerted to the culprit medication and advised to never take that medication again. The patient should also be warned that other medications in the same class may cause the same reaction. The medication should be placed on the patient's allergy list and the patient may elect to wear a medical alert bracelet [5].

Prognosis

Prognosis correlates with extent of mucocutaneous necrosis, with SJS having a mortality rate of approximately 5–10% and TEN having a mortality rate of 30–40% [28]. Most deaths occur in elderly patients, with death being more likely in patients with greater comorbidity burden [67]. Sepsis is the primary cause of death in patients with SJS and TEN [33]. Pulmonary complications occur in approximately 15% of cases. Multisystem organ failure is noted in at least 30% of patients with SJS and TEN [45]. Purported cause does not play a role in risk of mortality. The SCORTEN scale allows for estimation of risk of death. Each of the following prognostic factors in the SCORTEN scoring system is worth one point: age greater than 40 years old, heart rate greater than 120 beats per minute, presence of malignancy, BSA greater than 10% involved, serum urea greater than 10 mM, serum bicarbonate less than 20 mM, and serum glucose greater than 14 mM. A score of 0–1 is associated with a mortality rate of 3.2%, 2 with 12.1%, 3 with 35.8%, 4 with 58.3%, and 5 or greater with 90% mortality [10]. Serum bicarbonate less than 20 mM indicates pulmonary involvement and also portends poor prognosis. GI involvement also indicates elevated morbidity and mortality should be anticipated [5].

Among patients who survive, complications are very common. Ninety percent of people in a cohort of European patients who remained alive after experiencing SJS and TEN had multiple persistent complications and a perception of worsened quality of life (Fig. 1).

References

1. Abe R, Shimizu T, Shibaki A, Nakamura H, Watanabe H, Shimizu H. Toxic epidermal necrolysis and Stevens-Johnson syndrome are induced by soluble Fas ligand. Am J Pathol. 2003;162(5):1515–20.
2. Amstutz U, Shear NH, Rieder MJ, Hwang S, Fung V, Nakamura H, Connolly MB, Ito S, Carleton BC, CPNDS clinical recommendation group. Recommendations for HLA-B*15:02 and HLA-A*31:01 genetic testing to reduce the risk of carbamazepine-induced hypersensitivity reactions. Epilepsia. 2014;55(4): 496–506.
3. Arevalo JM, Lorente JA, González-Herrada C, Jiménez-Reyes J. Treatment of toxic epidermal necrolysis with cyclosporine A. J Trauma. 2000;48(3): 473–8.
4. Bachot N, Revuz J, Roujeau JC. Intravenous immunoglobulin treatment for Stevens-Johnson and toxic epidermal necrolysis: a prospective noncomparative study showing no benefit on mortality or progression. Arch Dermatol. 2003;139(1):33–6.
5. Bastuji-Garin S, Fouchard N, Bertocchi M, Roujeau JC, Revuz J, Wolkenstein P. SCORTEN: a severity-of-illness score for toxic epidermal necrolysis. J Invest Dermatol. 2000;115(2):149–53.
6. Blum L, Chosidow O, Rostoker G, Philippon C, Revuz J, Roujeau JC. Renal involvement in toxic epidermal necrolysis. J Am Acad Dermatol. 1996; 34(6):1088–90.

7. Breslin ME, Garcia-Lloret M, Braskett M. A fatal case of drug reaction with eosinophilia and systemic symptoms (DRESS) – Stevens Johnson (SJS)/Toxic epidermal necrolysis (TEN) in the setting of strongyloides infection: treatment considerations. J Allergy Clin Immunol. 2015;135(2):AB124.

8. Carter FM, Mitchell CK. Toxic epidermal necrolysis – an unusual cause of colonic perforation. Report of a case. Dis Colon Rectum. 1993;36:773.

9. Castrejon JL, Berry N, El-Ghaiesh S, Gerber B, Pichler WJ, Naisbitt DJ. Stimulation of human T cells with sulfonamides and sulfonamide metabolites. J Allergy Clin Immunol. 2010;125(2):411–8.e4.

10. Chen ST, Velez NF, Saavedra AP. Adverse cutaneous drug reactions. In: McKean SC, Ross JJ, Dressler DD, Scheurer DB, editors. Principles and practice of hospital medicine, 2e. New York; 2017. Available via ACCESS MEDICINE. http://accessmedicine.mhmedical.com/content.aspx?bookid=1872&sectionid=146980847. Accessed 23 May 2018.

11. Chung WH, Hung SI, Hong HS, Hish MS, Yang LC, Ho HC, Wu JY, Chen YT. Medical genetics: a marker for Stevens Johnson syndrome. Nature. 2004;428(6982):486.

12. Chung WH, Hung SI, Yang JY, Su SC, Huang SP, Wei CY, Chin SW, Chiou CC, Chu SC, Ho HC, Yang CH, Lu CF, Wu JY, Liao YD, Chen YT. Granulysin is a key mediator for disseminated keratinocyte death in Stevens-Johnson syndrome and toxic epidermal necrolysis. Nat Med. 2008;14(12):1343–50.

13. de Prost N, Ingen-Housz-Oro S, Duong Ta, Valeyrie-Allanore L, Legrand P, Wolkenstein P, Brochard L, Brun-Buisson C, Roujeau JC. Bacteremia in Stevens-Johnson syndrome and toxic epidermal necrolysis: epidemiology, risk factors, and predictive value of skin cultures. Medicine (Baltimore). 2010;89(1):28–36.

14. Dorafshar AH, Dickie SR, Cohn AB, Aycock JK, O'Connor A, Tung A, Gottlieb LJ. Antishear therapy for toxic epidermal necrolysis: an alternative treatment approach. Plast Reconstr Surg. 2008;122(1):154–60.

15. Egan CA, Grant WJ, Morris SE, Saffle JR, Zone JJ. Plasmapheresis as an adjunct treatment in toxic epidermal necrolysis. J Am Acad Dermatol. 1999;40(3):458–61.

16. Ellis MW, Oster CN, Turiansky GW, Blanchard JR. A case report and a proposed algorithm for the transfer of patients with Stevens-Johnson syndrome and toxic epidermal necrolysis to a burn center. Mil Med. 2002;167(8):701–4.

17. Firoz BF, Henning JS, Zarzabal LA, Pollock BH. Toxic epidermal necrolysis: five years of treatment experience from a burn unit. J Am Acad Dermatol. 2012;67(4):630–5.

18. Frey N, Jossi J, Bodmer M, Bircher A, Jick SS, Meier CR, Spoendlin J. The epidemiology of Stevens-Johnson syndrome and toxic epidermal necrolysis in the UK. J Invest Dermatol. 2017;137(6):1240–7.

19. Garcia-Doval I, LeCleach L, Bocquet H, Otero XL, Roujeau JC. Toxic epidermal necrolysis and Stevens-Johnson syndrome. Does early withdrawal of causative drugs decrease the risk of death? Arch Dermatol. 2000;136(3):323–7.

20. Gaultier F, Rochefort J, Landru MM, Allanore L, Naveau A, Roujeau JC, Gogly B. Severe and unrecognized dental abnormalities after drug-induced epidermal necrolysis. Arch Dermatol. 2009;145(11):1332–3.

21. Goldsmith LA, Katz SI, Gilchrest BA, Paller AS, Leffell DJ, Wolff K (8th edition) Fitzpatrick's Dermatology in General Medicine. McGraw Hill, New York. 2012.

22. Gillis NK, Hicks JK, Bell GC, Daily AJ, Kanetsky PA, McLeod HL. Incidence and triggers of Stevens-Johnson syndrome and toxic epidermal necrolysis in a large cancer patient cohort. J Invest Dermatol. 2017;137(9):2021–3.

23. Gravante G, Delogu D, Marianetti M, Esposito G, Montone A. Toxic epidermal necrolysis and Steven-Johnson syndrome in oncologic patients. Eur Rev Med Pharmacol Sci. 2007;11(4):269–74.

24. Gueudry J, Roujeau JC, Binaghi M, Soubrane G, Muraine M. Risk factors for the development of ocular complications of Stevens-Johnson syndrome and toxic epidermal necrolysis. Arch Dermatol. 2009;145(2):157–62.

25. Hsu DY, Brieva J, Silverberg NB, Silverberg JI. Morbidity and mortality of Stevens-Johnson syndrome at toxic epidermal necrolysis in United States adults. J Invest Dermatol. 2016;136(7):1387–97.

26. Hung SI, Chung WH, Liou LB, Chu CC, Lin M, Huang HP, Lin YL, Lan JL, Yang LC, Hong HS, Chen MJ, Lai PC, Wu MS, Lai PC, Wu MS, Chu CY, Wang KH, Chen CH, Fann CS, Wu JY, Chen YT. HLA-B*5801 allele as a genetic marker for severe cutaneous adverse reactions caused by allopurinol. Proc Natl Acad Sci USA. 2005;102(11):4134–9.

27. Kaniwa N, Saito Y, Aihara M, Matsunaga K, Tohkin M, Kurose K, Sawada J, Furuya H, Takahashi Y, Muramatsu M, Kinoshita S, Abe M, Ikeda H, Kashiwagi M, Song Y, Ueta M, Sotozono C, Kkezawa Z, Hasegawa R, JSAR research group. HLA-B locus in Japanese patients with anti-epileptics and allopurinol-related Stevens-Johnson syndrome and toxic epidermal necrolysis. Pharmacogenomics. 2008;9(11):1617–22.

28. Kardaun SH, Jonkman MF. Dexamethasone pulse therapy for Stevens-Johnson syndrome/toxic epidermal necrolysis. Acta Derm Venereol. 2007;87(2):144–8.

29. Khalaf D, Toema B, Dabbour N, Jehani F. Toxic epidermal necrolysis associated with severe cytomegalovirus infection in a patient on regular hemodialysis. Mediterr J Hematol Infect Dis. 2011;3(1):e2011004.

30. Kinoshita Y, Saeiki H. A review of toxic epidermal necrolysis management in Japan. Allergol Int. 2017;66(1):36–41.

31. Koutlas IG. Diseases of the oral cavity. Clinical dermatology Eds. Carol Soutor, and Maria K. Hordinsky. New

York, NY: McGraw-Hill. 2013. http://accessmedicine. mhmedical.com.lp.hscl.ufl.edu/content.aspx?bookid= 2184&sectionid=165461482.

32. Le Cleach L, Delaire S, Boumsell L, Bagot M, Bourgault-Villada I, Bensussan A, Roujeau JC. Blister fluid T lymphocytes during toxic epidermal necrolysis are functional cytotoxic cells which express human natural killer inhibitory receptors. Clin Exp Immunol. 2000;119(1):225–30.

33. Lissia M, Mulas P, Bulla A, Rubino C. Toxic epidermal necrolysis (Lyell's disease). Burns. 2010;36(2): 152–63.

34. Lissia M, Figus A, Rubino C. Intravenous immuno-globulins and plasmapheresis combined treatment in patients with severe toxic epidermal necrolysis: pre-liminary report. Br J Plast Surg. 2005;58:504.

35. Lonjou C, Borot N, Sekula P, Ledger N, Thomas L, Halevy S, Naldi L, Bouwes-Bavinck JN, Sidoroff A, de Toma C, Schumacher M, Roujeau JC, Hovnanian A, Mockenhaupt M, RegiSCAR study group. A European study of HLA-B in Stevens-Johnson syndrome and toxic epidermal necrolysis related to five high-risk drugs. Pharmacogenet Genomics. 2008;18(2):99–107.

36. Lonjou C, Thomas L, Borot N, Ledger N, de Toma C, Lelouet H, Graf E, Schmacher M, Hovnanian A, Mockenhaupt M, Roujeau JC, RegiSCAR Group. A marker for Stevens-Johnson syndrome: ethnicity matters. Pharmacogenomics J. 2006;6(4):265–8.

37. Manuyakorn W, Siripool K, Kamchaisatian W, Pakakasama S, Visudtibhan A, Vilaiyuk S, Rujirawat T, Benjaponpitak S. Phenobarbital-induced severe cutaneous adverse drug reactions are associated with CYP2C19*2 in Thai children. Pediatr Allergy Immunol. 2014;24(3):299–303.

38. McCormack M, Alfirevic A, Bourgeois S, Farrell JJ, Kasperaviciute D, Carrington M, Sills GJ, Marson T, Jia X, de Bakker PI, Chinthapalli K, Molokhia M, Johnson MR, O'Conner GD, Chalia E, Alhusaini S, Shianna KV, Radtke RA, Keinzen EL, Walley N, Pandolfo M, Pichler V, Park BK, Depondt C, Sisodiya SM, Goldstein DB, Deloukas P, Delanty N, Cavalleri GL, Pirmohamed M. HLA-A*3101 and carbamazepine-induced hypersensitivity reactions in Europeans. N Engl J Med. 2011;364(12):1134–43.

39. Meneux E, Wolkenstein P, Haddad B, Roujeau JC, Revuz J, Paniel BJ. Vulvovaginal involvement in toxic epidermal necrolysis: a retrospective study of 40 cases. Obstet Gynecol. 1998;91(2):283–7.

40. Michel P, Joly P, Ducrotte P, Hemet J, Leblanc I, Lauret P, Lerebours E, Colin R. Ileal involvement in toxic epidermal necrolysis (Lyell syndrome). Dig Dis Sci. 1993;38(10):1938–41.

41. Mockenhaupt M, Viboud C, Dunant A, Naldi L, Halevy S, Bouwes Bavinck JN, Sidoroff A, Schneck J, Roujeau JC, Flahault A. Stevens-Johnson syndrome and toxic epidermal necrolysis: assessment of medication risks with emphasis on recently marketed drugs. The EuroSCAR-study. J Invest Dermatol. 2008;128(1):35–44.

42. Mockenhaupt M. Severe drug-induced skin reactions: clinical pattern, diagnostics and therapy. J Dtsch Dermatol Ges. 2009;7:142.

43. Morel E, Escamochero S, Cabanas R, Dias R, Fiandor A, Bellon T. CD94/NKG2R is a killer effector molecule in patients with Stevens-Johnson syndrome and toxic epidermal necrolysis. J Allergy Clin Immunol. 2010;125(3):703–10.

44. Okamoto-Uchida Y, Nakamura R, Sai K, Imatoh T, Matsunaga K, Aihara M, Saito Y. Effect of infectious disease on the pathogenesis of Stevens-Johnson syn-drome and toxic epidermal necrolysis. Biol Pharm Bull. 2017;40(9):1576–80.

45. Palmieri T, Greenhalgh DG, Saffle JR, Spence RJ, Peck MD, Jeng JC, Mozingo DW, Yowler CJ, Sheridan RL, Ahrenholz DH, Caruso DM, Foster KN, Kagan RJ, Voigt DW, Purdue GF, Hunt JL, Wolf S, Molitor F. A multicenter review of toxic epidermal necrolysis treated in U.S. burn centers at the end of the twentieth century. J Burn Care Rehabil. 2002; 23(2):87–96.

46. Paquet P, Nikkels A, Arrese JE, Vanderkelen A, Piérard GE. Macrophages and tumor necrosis factor alpha in toxic epidermal necrolysis. Arch Dermatol. 1994;130(5):605–8.

47. Prins C, Kerdel FA, Padilla RS, Hunziker T, Chimenti S, Viard I, Mauri DN, Flynn K, Trent J, Margolis DJ, Saurat JH, French LE, TEN-IVIG Study Group. Toxic epidermal necrolysis-intravenous immu-noglobulin. Treatment of toxic epidermal necrolysis with high-dose intravenous immunoglobulins. Arch Dermatol. 2003;139(1):26–32.

48. Quinn AM, Brown K, Bonish BK, Curry J, Gordon KB, Sinacore J, Gamelli R, Nickoloff BJ. Uncovering histologic criteria with prognostic signifi-cance in toxic epidermal necrolysis. Arch Dermatol. 2005;141(6):683–7.

49. Rosenthal P, Cotter J. The Boston Scleral Lens in the management of severe ocular surface disease. Ophthalmol Clin North Am. 2003;16(1):89–93.

50. Roujeau JC, Kelly JP, Naldi L, Rzany B, Stern RS, Anderson T, Auquier A, Bastuji-Garin S, Correia O, Locati F, et al. Medication use and the risk of Stevens-Johnson syndrome or toxic epidermal necrolysis. N Engl J Med. 1995;333(24):1600–7.

51. Rzany B, Hering O, Mockenhaupt M, Schröder W, Goerttler E, Ring J, Schöpf E. Histopathological and epidemiological characteristics of patients with ery-thema multiforme major, Stevens-Johnson syndrome and toxic epidermal necrolysis. Br J Dermatol. 2006; 135(1):6–11.

52. Saito N, Yoshioka N, Abe R, Qiao H, Fujita Y, Hoshina D, Suto A, Kase S, Kitaichi N, Ozaki M, Shimizu H. Stevens-Johnson syndrome/toxic epider-mal necrolysis mouse model generated by using PBMCs and the skin of patients. J Allergy Clin Immunol. 2013;131(2):434–41.

53. Schneck J, Fagot JP, Sekula P, Sassolas B, Roujeau JC, Mockenhaupt M. Effects of treatments on the mortality

of Stevens-Johnson syndrome and toxic epidermal necrolysis: a retrospective study on patients included in the prospective EuroSCAR Study. J Am Acad Dermatol. 2008;58(1):33–40.

54. Schwartz J, Padmanabhan A, Aqui N, Balogun RA, Connelly-Smith L, Delaney M, Dunbar M, Dunbar NM, Witt V, Wu Y, Shaz BH. Guidelines on the use of therapeutic apheresis in clinical practice – evidence based approach from the Writing Committee of the American Society for Apheresis: the seventh special issue. J Clin Apher. 2016;31(3):149–62.

55. Schwartz RA, McDonough PH, Lee BW. Toxic epidermal necrolysis: Part 1. Introduction, history, classification, clinical features, systemic manifestations, etiology, and immunopathogenesis. J Am Acad Dermatol. 2013;69(2):173.e1–13.

56. Shay E, Kheirkhah A, Liang L, Sheha H, Gregory DG, Tseng SC. Amniotic membrane transplantation as a new therapy for the acute ocular manifestations of Stevens-Johnson syndrome and toxic epidermal necrolysis. Surv Ophthalmol. 2009;54(6):686–96.

57. Shi YW, Min FL, Zhou D, Qin B, Wang J, Hu FY, Cheung YK, Zhou JH, Hu XS, Zhou JQ, Zhou LM, Zheng ZZ, Pan J, He N, Liu ZS, Hou YQ, Lim KS, Ou YM, Hui-Ping Khor A, Ng CC, Mao BJ, Liu XR, Li BM, Kuan YY, Yi YH, He XL, Deng XY, Su T, Kwan P, Laio WP. HLA-A*24:02 as a common risk factor for antiepileptic drug-induced cutaneous adverse reactions. Neurology. 2017;88(23):2183–91.

58. Shinkai K, Stern RS, Wintroub BU. Cutaneous drug reactions. In: Kasper D, Fauci A, Hauser S, Longo D, Jameson J, Loscalzo J, editors. Harrison's principles of internal medicine, 19e. New York; 2014. Available in ACCESS MEDICINE. http://accessmedicine.mhmedical.com/content.aspx?bookid=1130&sectionid=79727466. Accessed 23 May 2018.

59. Smith C. Erythema multiforme, Stevens–Johnson syndrome, toxic epidermal necrolysis, staphylococcal scalded skin syndrome. In: Soutor C, Hordinsky MK, editors. Clinical dermatology. New York; 2013. Available via ACCESS MEDICINE. http://accessmedicine.mhmedical.com.lp.hscl.ufl.edu/content.aspx?bookid=2184&sectionid=165460970. Accessed 28 May 2018.

60. Szczeklik W, Nowak I, Seczynska B, Sega A, Krolikowski W, Musial J. Beneficial therapeutic effect of plasmapheresis after unsuccessful treatment with corticosteroids in two patients with severe toxic epidermal necrolysis. Ther Apher Dial. 2010;14(3):354–7.

61. Tempark T, Satapornpong P, Rerknimitr P, Nakkam N, Saksit N, Wattanakrai P, Jantararoungtong T, Koomdee N, Mahakkanukrauh A, Tassaneeyakul W, Suttisai S, Pratoomwun J, Klaewsongkram J, Rerkpattanapipat T, Sukasem C. Dapsone-induced severe cutaneous adverse drug reactions are strongly linked with HLA-B*13: 01 allele in the Thai population. Pharmacogenet Genomics. 2017;27(12):429–37.

62. Valeyrie-Allanore LL, Roujeau J. Epidermal necrolysis (Stevens–Johnson syndrome and toxic epidermal necrolysis). In: Goldsmith LA, Katz SI, Gilchrest BA, Paller AS, Leffell DJ, Wolff K (8th edition). Fitzpatrick's dermatology in general medicine, McGraw Hill, New York; 2012. Available via ACCESS MEDICINE. http://accessmedicine.mhmedical.com/content.aspx?bookid=392&sectionid=41138737. Accessed 28 May 2018.

63. Valeyrie-Allanore L, Wolkenstein P, Brochard L, Ortonne N, Maître B, Revuz J, Bagot M, Roujeau JC. Open trial of ciclosporin treatment for Stevens–Johnson syndrome and toxic epidermal necrolysis. Br J Dermatol. 2010;163(4):847–53.

64. Williams GP, Mudhar HS, Leyland M. Early pathological features of the cornea in toxic epidermal necrolysis. Br J Ophthalmol. 2007;91(9):1129–32.

65. Williams R, Hodge J, Ingram W. Indications for intubation and early tracheostomy in patients with Stevens-Johnson Syndrome and Toxic Epidermal Necrolysis. Am J Surg. 2016;211(4):684–688e1.

66. Wolff K, Johnson R, Saavedra AP, Roh EK. The acutely ill and hospitalized patient. In: Fitzpatrick's color atlas and synopsis of clinical dermatology, 8e. New York; 2012. Available via ACCESS MEDICINE. http://accessmedicine.mhmedical.com/content.aspx?bookid=2043&sectionid=154897923. Accessed 23 May 2018.

67. Wolkenstein P, Latarjet J, Roujeau JC, Duguet C, Boudeau S, Vaillant L, Maignan M, Schuhmacher MH, Milpied B, Pilorget A, Bocquet H, Brun-Buisson C, Revuz J. Randomized comparison of thalidomide versus placebo in toxic epidermal necrolysis. Lancet. 1998;352(9140):1586–9.

68. Wu J, Lee YY, Su SC, Wu TS, Kao KC, Huang CC, Chang WC, Yang CH, Chung WH. Stevens-Johnson syndrome and toxic epidermal necrolysis in patients with malignancies. Br J Dermatol. 2015;173(5):1224–31.

69. Yamane Y, Matsukura S, Watanabe Y, Nakamura K, Kambara T, Ikezawa Z, Aihara M. Retrospective analysis of Stevens-Johnson syndrome and toxic epidermal necrolysis in 87 Japanese patients – treatment and outcome. Allergol Int. 2016;65(1):74–81.

70. Ye LP, Zhang C, Zhu QX. The effect of intravenous immunoglobulin combined with corticosteroid on the progression of Stevens-Johnson syndrome and toxic epidermal necrolysis: a meta-analysis. PLoS One. 2016;11(11):e0167120.

Mycosis Fungoides in Critically Ill Cancer Patients

20

Brian H. Ramnaraign and Nam Hoang Dang

Contents

Introduction 282

Epidemiology 282

Pathophysiology 282

Clinical Features 283

Diagnosis 284

Staging 284

Clinical Stages 285

Management Algorithm 285

Nonpharmacologic Treatment 286
Phototherapy (UVB or PUVA) 286
Local Radiation 286
Extracorporeal Photopheresis 287

Pharmacologic Treatment 287
Topical Corticosteroids 287
Topical Chemotherapy 287
Topical Retinoid 288
Imiquimod 288
Methotrexate 288
Systemic Chemotherapy 288
Systemic Retinoids 289
Interferon 289
Histone Deacetylase Inhibitors 289
Brentuximab Vedotin 290
Denileukin Diftitox 290

Infections 291

B. H. Ramnaraign · N. H. Dang (✉)
University of Florida Health Cancer Center,
Gainesville, FL, USA
e-mail: Brian.Ramnaraign@medicine.ufl.edu;
nam.dang@medicine.ufl.edu

© Springer Nature Switzerland AG 2020
J. L. Nates, K. J. Price (eds.), *Oncologic Critical Care*,
https://doi.org/10.1007/978-3-319-74588-6_196

Prognosis 292

Conclusion 292

References 292

Abstract

Mycosis fungoides is a rare disease that is part of a larger group of conditions known as cutaneous T-cell lymphomas and is likely caused by genetic and epigenetic changes in the DNA of affected individuals. For the critical care team, diagnosis of this condition can be confusing as mycosis fungoides-related skin lesions can appear very similar to other dermatologic conditions. The International Society of Cutaneous Lymphoma and the European Organization of Research and Treatment of Cancer have devised a diagnostic algorithm based on clinical, histopathologic, molecular biological, and immunopathogenic criteria. Staging is based on the extent of skin, lymph node, visceral organ, and blood involvement, with higher stage portending a worse prognosis. Patients with higher stage disease have low chance at cure, and these patients find themselves cycling through multiple lines of therapy with limited long-term efficacies. Such therapies include nonpharmacologic agents, such as UV light phototherapy or electron beam therapy, as well as pharmacologic agents, including topical and systemic agents such as steroids, retinoids, chemotherapy, imiquimod, methotrexate, histone deacetylase inhibitors, interferon, brentuximab vendotin, and denileukin diftitox. While the acute treatment of mycosis fungoides lies outside the realm of the intensive care unit, important issues facing the critical care team include disease manifestations and the potential side effects and complications of treatment including the risk of infections.

Keywords

Mycosis fungoides · Sezary syndrome · T-cell lymphoma · Methotrexate · Bexarotene · Romidepsin · Vorinostat · Brentuximab vedotin · Denileukin diftitox

Introduction

The term cutaneous T-cell lymphoma (CTCL) describes a group of diseases characterized by a clonal proliferation of malignant T cells in the skin [1]. Mycosis fungoides (MF) is the most common lymphoma in this group and was originally described in 1806 by French dermatologist Louis Alibert, who published observations of patients with skin lesions described as tumors with a mushroom-like appearance, thus coining the term [2].

This chapter will provide an overview of the epidemiology, pathophysiology, clinical features, diagnosis, staging, management, and prognosis of MF, for the critical care team. An emphasis here will be placed on clinical features encountered in the critical care setting including the side effects of the various treatment options.

Epidemiology

A rare disease, the incidence of MF in the USA is approximately 0.36 per 100,000 person-years [3]. African-Americans appear to be more affected with an age-adjusted incidence rate ratio of 1.7 compared to Whites whereas Asian-Americans appear to be less affected with an age-adjusted incidence rate ratio of 0.6 compared to Whites [3].

Rates of CTCL increase exponentially with age and seem to peak around age 80 with men appearing to be more effected than women with an overall incidence ratio of 1.7 [4].

Pathophysiology

MF can be best understood as a cancer of T cells which home to the skin and remain there in an activated state, thus accumulating in the skin, and in later stages, the lymph nodes and peripheral blood [1].

The etiology of MF is unclear. Environmental and occupational exposures have been suggested as a potential etiology but a large case-controlled trial found no consistent or biologically plausible differences between MF patients and the control group [5].

In addition, no infectious etiology has ever been confirmed as studies have failed to show a consistent association between CTCL and investigated microorganisms such as *Staphylococcus aureus*, retroviruses, or herpesviruses [6]. While human T-cell lymphotrophic virus type I (HTLV-1) is involved in the pathogenesis of adult T-cell leukemia-lymphoma, it has no established role in the pathogenesis of MF [7].

MF has been postulated to be caused by genetic and epigenetic changes. Investigators have implicated several genes in the pathogenesis of MF including promoter hypermethylation of tumor suppressor genes BCL7a, PTPRG, and p73 [8].

Clinical Features

MF patients commonly present with skins lesions that are either patches, plaques, or tumors that can be localized or widespread. Such lesions represent a diverse array of cutaneous manifestations and can be difficult to distinguish from other dermatologic disorders.

Patients often have a premycotic period, ranging from months to decades, where they complain of nonspecific scaly skin lesions with associated nondiagnostic skin biopsies [9]. These lesions wax and wane over several years and patients are often misdiagnosed with having other dermatoses such as parapsoriasis en plaque or nonspecific dermatitis. MF has been colloquially dubbed "the great imitator" [10].

The initial lesions in MF are usually scaly patches or plaques that vary in size, shape, and color and are often pruritic [11]. The majority of MF patients at this stage of disease never progress to more advanced stages (i.e., less than 10%), and these patients do not have an altered life expectancy [12]. In patients with darker skin,

hypopigmented lesions can be seen and can have an annular appearance [13].

For those whose disease does progress, patches grow to become plaques which then evolve to become more generalized and can eventually lead to ulcerations or exophytic tumors [11]. MF can continue to spread to involve the lymph nodes, internal organs, and peripheral blood. When there is significant involvement of the peripheral blood, the disease is renamed Sezary syndrome (SS).

Pruritus is the most common symptom experienced in patients with MF as up to 62% of patients with early stage disease and 83% of patients with late stage disease having this complaint [14].

Alopecia is observed in 2.5% of patients with MF/SS with one-third having patchy alopecia clinically similar to alopecia areata and two-thirds having hair loss within the discrete patch, plaque, or follicular lesions of MF or total body hair loss in those with generalized erythroderma and SS [15].

Patients with MF and SS are at significantly elevated risk for other non-Hodgkin lymphomas as well as Hodgkin lymphoma, melanoma, urinary, and biliary cancers [16].

Folliculotropic variant MF is a histologic and clinical variant of MF characterized by infiltration of follicles [17]. It has been associated with worse prognosis and having around twice the risk of disease progression but no difference in overall survival [18]. In advanced stages, folliculotropic variant was not seen as an adverse prognostic marker and this is most likely due to other prognostic factors that have more importance on survival outcomes such as age, LDH, extracutaneous involvement, and large cell transformation [19].

Large cell transformation includes a subgroup of patients with MF whose disease has transformed to a large T cell lymphoma, with histopathological studies showing the tumor cells to be at least four times greater in size than a small lymphocyte. This diagnosis is made when these cells occupy at least 25% of the infiltrate or if they form microscopic nodules [20]. Transformation is more likely to be seen in higher stages of MF and is clinically significant because median survival of transformed MF is 3 years while that for untransformed MF is 14 years [20].

Diagnosis

The International Society for Cutaneous Lymphoma (ISCL) and the cutaneous lymphoma task force of the European Organization of Research and Treatment of Cancer (EORTC) have created a diagnostic algorithm for MF. It includes clinical, histopathologic, molecular biological, and immunopathologic criteria. Points are assigned to each category and the diagnosis of MF is assigned when four or more points are attained from any combination of categories [11].

Clinical criteria: Two points for the basic criteria and two additional criteria; or 1 point for the basic criteria and one additional criterion.

Basic criteria: Persistent and/or progressive patches/thin plaques

Additional criteria:
1. Non-sun-exposed location
2. Size/shape variation
3. Poikiloderma

Histopathologic criteria: 2 points for the basic criteria and two additional criteria; or 1 point for the basic criteria and one additional criterion.

Basic criteria: Superficial lymphoid infiltrate

Additional criteria:
1. Epidermotropism without spongiosis
2. Lymphoid atypia

Molecular biological criteria: 1 point for clonal T cell receptor gene rearrangement

Immunopathologic criteria: 1 point for one or more of the following criteria
1. <50% CD2+, CD3+, and/or CD5+ T cells
2. <10% CD7+ T cells
3. Epidermal/dermal discordance in CD2, CD3, CD5, or CD7

The above algorithm seeks to increase the diagnostic accuracy of MF as the skin lesions of MF are easily confused with other disorders such as eczema, psoriasis, drug reactions, or even other CTCL such as cutaneous B cell lymphoma, cutaneous gamma/delta T cell lymphoma, primary cutaneous anaplastic large cell lymphoma, subcutaneous panniculitis-like T cell lymphoma, or adult T cell leukemia-lymphoma.

Another important distinction to make is that between MF and Sezary syndrome (SS). Patients who have MF may eventually evolve into SS [21]. SS is diagnosed when cutaneous erythroderma occupies more than 80% of the body surface area with circulating Sezary cells (atypical lymphocytes with cerebriform nuclei) in the peripheral blood accounting for more than 1000 cells/μL [22]. This is equivalent to the T4 and B2 designation in the TNMB staging system for MF [62]. SS should be considered an aggressive leukemic variant of CTCL.

Staging

Clinical staging of MF is based on the TNMB system where each letter represents the degree of involvement in the skin, lymph nodes, visceral organs, and blood, respectively. The following staging guidelines are taken from the ISCL/EORTC revision to the classification of MF and SS [62].

Skin (T)

T1 stage disease: Limited patches, papules, and/or plaques covering <10% of the skin surface. May further stratify into T1a (patch only) versus T1b (plaque ± patch)

T2 stage disease: Patches, papules, or plaques covering ≥10% of the skin surface. May further stratify into T2a (patch only) versus T2b (plaque ± patch)

T3 stage disease: One or more tumors (≥1 cm diameter)

T4 stage disease: Confluence of erythema covering ≥80% body surface area

Lymph Node (N)

N0 stage disease: No clinically abnormal peripheral lymph nodes; biopsy not required

N1 stage disease: Clinically abnormal peripheral lymph nodes; histopathology Dutch grade 1 or NCI LN0-2

N2 stage disease: Clinically abnormal peripheral lymph nodes; histopathology Dutch grade 2 or NCI LN3

N3 stage disease: Clinically abnormal peripheral lymph nodes; histopathology Dutch grades 3-4 or NCI LN4; clone positive or negative

Nx stage disease: Clinically abnormal peripheral lymph nodes; no histologic confirmation

Visceral (M)

M0 stage disease: No visceral organ involvement

M1 stage disease: Visceral involvement (must have pathology confirmation and organ involved should be specified)

Blood (B)

B0 stage disease: Absence of significant blood involvement: ≤5% of peripheral blood lymphocytes are atypical (Sézary) cell

B1 stage disease: Low blood tumor burden: >5% of peripheral blood lymphocytes are atypical (Sézary) cells but does not meet the criteria of B2

B2 stage disease: High blood tumor burden: ≥1000/μL Sézary cells with positive clone

Clinical Stages

Stage I

IA: T1 stage disease with no lymph node (N0) or visceral (M0) involvement with no or low blood tumor burden (B0-1)

IB: T2 stage disease with no lymph node (N0) or visceral (M0) involvement with no or low blood tumor burden (B0-1)

Stage II

IIA: T1 or T2 stage disease with lymph node involvement (N1-2) but no visceral involvement (M0) and no or low blood tumor burden (B0-1)

IIB: T3 stage disease with or without lymph node involvement (N0-2) but no visceral involvement (M0) and no or low blood tumor burden (B0-1)

Stage III

IIIA: T4 stage disease with or without lymph node involvement (N0-2) but no visceral involvement (M0) and no blood tumor burden (B0)

IIIB: T4 stage disease with or without lymph node involvement (N0-2) but no visceral involvement (M0) and with low blood tumor burden (B1)

Stage IV

IVA1: *Any* T stage disease (T1-4), with lymph node involvement (N0-2), no visceral involvement (M0) but with *high* blood involvement (B2)

IVA2: *Any* T stage disease (T1-4), *high* lymph node involvement (N3), no visceral involvement (M0) with any blood involvement (B0-2)

IVB: *Any* T stage disease (T1-4), *any* lymph node involvement (N0-3), *with* visceral involvement (M1) and any blood involvement (B0-2)

Management Algorithm

Treatment of MF depends on the clinical stage of the disease. Patients with early stage disease (stages IA to IIA) primarily present with skin manifestations only.

These patients are treated with skin-directed therapies, which include topical agents such as topical corticosteroids, topical chemotherapy, topical retinoids, topical imiquimod, or local radiation or phototherapy. These agents can be used alone or in combination. Systemic biologic therapies are reserved for patients with extensive or severe symptoms or those with a worse prognostic profile such as folliculotropic MF, large cell transformation, or early blood involvement. Total systemic electron beam therapy (TSEBT) is usually reserved for those patients with rapidly progressive and generalized plaques when a quick response is needed.

For patients with advanced disease (Stages IIB to IV), the course of the disease is often chronic, persistent, and with multiple relapses. There is no standard first-line therapy and the goal of treatment for this patient population is to provide disease control and symptom relief.

In these advanced patients, there is no advantage to early aggressive combination therapy with chemotherapy and radiation therapy compared to conservative management with sequential topical therapies in terms of overall survival [23]. Given the chronic nature of the disease, patients typically cycle through multiple treatment options, either as monotherapies or in combination with others, since the disease will eventually progress. For example, the median time to next treatment (TTNT) for interferon use is 8.7 months, while the median TTNT for histone deacetylase inhibitors (HDACi) is 4.5 months, versus 3.9 months for single or multi-agent chemotherapy [24].

Patients with clinically aggressive disease requiring an immediate response for symptomatic relief often need treatment with single or combination chemotherapy. Those with difficult to control aggressive disease should be referred for allogeneic stem cell transplantation to induce a graft-versus-lymphoma effect, which has been shown to produce an overall survival rate of 66% at 1 year and 54% at 3 years [25].

Nonpharmacologic Treatment

Phototherapy (UVB or PUVA)

Ultraviolet B (UVB) treatments are used to treat CTCL with the observation that UVB irradiation may serve an immunoregulatory role [26]. In a retrospective nonrandomized study of 37 non-consecutive patients with early stage CTCL, 83% of patients with disease limited to patches achieved a remission, and of these patients, 80% had no documented recurrence of their CTCL. Overall, the median duration of response was 22 months; however, none of the patients with plaque level disease achieved remission [26].

Treatment with UVB is usually administered in the dermatology office three to five times per week with improvement seen after 20–40 treatments. Once a complete response is obtained, treatments are tapered slowly and eventually

discontinued [27]. Adverse events are rare, but in a trial of 23 patients with MF treated with narrow band (NB) UVB treatments, two developed pruritis, two developed postinflammatory pigmentation, one developed severe erythema, and another developed burning of the skin [28].

Psoralen and ultraviolet A photochemotherapy (PUVA) treatments are more appropriate for patients with thicker patch/plaque lesions. Treatment consists of exposure to UVA light phototherapy for approximately 1.5–2 hours after oral psoralen is administered. Similar to UVB treatments, it is administered three times a week until a complete response is obtained and then slowly tapered until discontinuation. In a phase III trial of 93 patients with stage IB or IIA MF randomized to either PUVA with bexarotene or PUVA alone, patients in the PUVA alone arm had an overall response rate of 71% with a median duration of response of 9.7 months. Interestingly, there was no significant difference in the response rate or response duration between the two arms of this trial. Grade 3 or 4 toxicities were rare with the PUVA treatment arm with only two events, one patient developing renal toxicity and another developing pruritis, out of 41 patients [29].

As UV light exposure is a risk factor for skin cancers, the repetitive use of these therapies should be cautioned in all patients especially those with history of skin cancer.

Local Radiation

Total skin electron beam therapy (EBT) is usually reserved for patients with progressive or extensive disease or for those who are very symptomatic as the depth of penetration is further than UVB or PUVA treatments [30]. Treatment with EBT consists of delivering daily radiation over several weeks for a total dose between 12 Gy and 36 Gy. In a retrospective review of one center's experience delivering EBT to a total of 57 patients with T1 or T2 MF between 1975 and 2001, with radiation being delivered at 2 Gy/day, 4 days/week, for 4 weeks, for a mean total dose of 30 Gy, an overall response rate of 94.7% was achieved 3 months after completion of therapy. Fifty-four percent of these patients did experience a skin failure within 1 year and more than half of these patients received further reirradiation with EBT [31].

Complications from EBT are usually mild in nature and include erythema, desquamation, blisters, hyperpigmentation, and skin pain. Superinfection of skin lesions are seen in 32% of cases [32].

Extracorporeal Photopheresis

Extracorporeal photopheresis (ECP) is an apheresis procedure where the patient's leukocytes are removed, exposed to PUVA, and then reinfused back into the patient. This method is performed in order to provide systemic exposure to PUVA, rather than just topical, and is primarily used when there is peripheral blood involvement.

Response rates have been reported at 73% and were seen in patients with lymph node involvement, exfoliative erythroderma, and those patients resistant to standard chemotherapy [33]. The etiology of ECP benefit is unclear but is suspected to be related to an immune reaction to reinfused UV-damaged cells. Adverse effects seen with traditional chemotherapy including bone marrow suppression, gastrointestinal erosions, or hair loss were not seen.

ECP is a time-consuming procedure with treatment lasting several weeks to months, and it can only be provided at specialized centers.

Pharmacologic Treatment

Topical Corticosteroids

Topical corticosteroids are commonly used as the first-line agent in low-stage disease and are available as ointments, creams, solutions, foams, or gels and administered once or twice daily until the lesions are completely cleared. In a single institution retrospective review of 79 patients with early stage (predominantly patch) MF, treatment

with clobetasol produced an overall response rate of 94% in patients with T1 stage disease and 82% in patients with T2 stage disease. With a median follow-up period of 9 months, 80% of T1-stage patients were still in complete or partial response while 68% of T2-stage patients were still in complete or partial response. In this study, 10–20% of patients developed irritant dermatitis or purpura and skin atrophy or striae were seen in a small number of patients but were reversible [34]. Although systemic absorption is low with topical use, chronic use of high potency topical steroids applied over a large body surface area can cause adrenal suppression or Cushing's syndrome.

Topical Chemotherapy

Another commonly used first-line agent in low-stage disease is topical nitrogen mustards (i.e., mechlorethamine hydrochloride) which is available in a gel, ointment, or aqueous preparation, applied daily, and used until skin lesions are cleared.

In a single institution retrospective review of 117 patients with stage I, II, or III MF treated with mechlorethamine hydrochloride, response rates (defined as the probability of obtaining a complete remission within 2 years of treatment) of 75.8%, 44.6%, and 48.6% were seen, with a median time to complete remission of 6.5 months, 41.1 months, and 39.1 months, respectively. In this study, 58.1% of patients developed a delayed hypersensitivity reaction which was treated with dose alteration, with only one patient having to discontinue therapy [35]. Other adverse events are rare, and a 30-year population-based cohort study showed no increased risk of secondary cancers or any category of comorbidity including chronic pulmonary disease, congestive heart failure, diabetes, or dementia [36]. Approximately 20% of patients treated with mechlorethamine will achieve long-term complete responses lasting from 4 to 14 years [37].

Carmustine (BCNU) is another nitrogen mustard that has been used for MF and is applied topically to affected areas once daily. In a single institution retrospective study of 143 patients with CTCL treated with BCNU, a complete response rate of 86%, 48%, and 21% was observed in patients with stage T1, T2, and erythroderma stage disease, respectively. In this study, 7.4% of patients developed bone marrow suppression, 6.6% developed an irritant dermatitis, and skin erythema occurred in almost all patients, except those with dark skin, and was accompanied by skin tenderness and telangiectasias [38]. Given the fact that hematologic toxicities are common, BCNU is not widely used in practice.

Topical Retinoid

Bexarotene is a synthetic retinoid that is used in the treatment of MF and applied topically between 1 and 4 times daily in a 1% gel formulation. This agent was studied in an open-label phase III trial with 50 patients who had stage IA to IIA CTCL who were refractory or intolerant to at least two prior lines of therapy. Response rates to treatment with bexarotene were found to be 62% for stage IA disease and 50% for stage IB disease. These results were lower than the response rates for topical prednisone or topical nitrogen mustards; however, the patients in this study were all previously treated and thus had more aggressive disease. Bexarotene is generally well tolerated, with the most common side effects from use being irritant dermatitis, pruritis, burning pain at the skin application site, skin inflammation, excoriation, or new skin lesions [39].

Imiquimod

Imiquimod is an immune-response modifier with antitumor and antiviral properties via its stimulation of proinflammatory cytokines and its ability to induce apoptosis. Topical imiquimod has been used as an investigational agent in MF in the off-label setting, usually for patients with resistant or refractory skin-only disease. Imiquimod 5% cream is applied over the affected areas daily. In a case series report of 20 patients

from 5 individual studies, all with Stage IA to IIB MF treated with topical imiquimod, 16 (80%) achieved a complete or partial response. Imiquimod can cause a local inflammatory reaction producing erythema, edema, vesicles, and/or ulcerations or erosions. Systemic adverse events can occur and resemble flu-like symptoms with fevers, malaise, and myalgias [40].

Methotrexate

Methotrexate is a folate analog that competitively binds to and inhibits dihydrofolate reductase. It is used for a variety of medical indications, including as an immunosuppressive drug and as anti-neoplastic therapy. In MF, low-dose methotrexate is administered orally as a 5–50 mg dose per week or given intravenously as a 25–50 mg/m^2 dose weekly. In a single institution retrospective review of 29 patients with erythrodermic CTCL treated with methotrexate, a response rate of 58% was obtained, with a median freedom from treatment failure of 31 months being observed [41]. In a larger retrospective study with 69 patients, side effects seen included mucositis (17.4%), gastro-intestinal side effects (15.9%), myelosuppression (13%), minor neurologic symptoms (8.7%), elevated transaminase levels (6%), with one patient each developing pneumonitis and drug eruption [42]. It is also important to emphasize that methotrexate is a teratogen, similar to other chemotherapeutic agents described below.

Systemic Chemotherapy

Multiple systemic chemotherapy options exist for MF/SS. As of the writing of this chapter, the National Comprehensive Cancer Network (NCCN) guidelines have several chemotherapy options listed with no preference or category 1 indication. In general, chemotherapy does not offer long-term control of disease in MF. In a retrospective review of 198 patients with MF/SS from Australia, it was discovered that the median time to next treatment (TTNT) for single or multiagent chemotherapy was only

3.9 months [24]. This ranges from 1.8 months for single-agent anthracycline to 5.8 months for mitoxantrone-based therapy.

Gemcitabine has been studied as a single agent in MF/SS. In a single-arm phase II study, 44 patients with MF and PTCLU (peripheral T-cell lymphoma, unspecified), with relapsed or refractory disease, were given gemcitabine 1200 mg/m^2/day on days 1, 8, 15 on a 28-day cycle for 3–6 cycles. Overall response rate was 70.5% and the median duration of complete response and partial response was 15 months and 10 months, respectively [43].

Gemcitabine is generally well tolerated in these patients with neutropenia (38.5%), thrombocytopenia (46%), and transient increase in liver enzymes (36%) being the most common adverse effects with no patients reported to have alopecia, nausea, or emesis [44].

Liposomal doxorubicin has also been used in MF/SS patients. A prospective, open, multicenter single-arm study was conducted of 25 patients with stage II to stage IV CTCL, previously treated with at least two prior lines of therapy (or histologically transformed epidermotropic CTCL requiring chemotherapy), who were given pegylated liposomal doxorubicin hydrochloride 40 mg/m^2 once every 4 weeks.

The observed objective response rate here was 56%. Of the patients having a positive response to treatment, the median progression free survival at the end of treatment was 5 months [45].

In this study, the most common grade 3 or 4 toxicity was sepsis (12%) with two patients both developing *Staphylococcus aureus* septicemia. However, the most common adverse events considering all grades were anemia (36%), asthenia (20%), nausea/vomiting (20%), erythema (12%), palmoplantar erythrodysesthesia (12%), stomach pain (12%), and neutropenia (12%). No febrile neutropenia was observed.

Systemic Retinoids

The previously described bexarotene can also be given systemically as an oral treatment, dosed at 200–300 mg/m^2 per day or as a flat dose of 150 mg daily initially with subsequent upward titration based on response and tolerability. In a phase II/III trial of 94 patients with refractory advanced (Stage IIB-IV) MF treated with oral bexarotene, overall response rates between 45% and 55% were seen. With a dose of 300 mg/m^2/day, the median duration of response was 299 days. The most common adverse effects noted were hypertriglyceridemia (82%), hypercholesterolemia (30%), central hypothyroidism (29%), headache (20%), asthenia (16%), pruritis (13%), leukopenia (11%), skin disorder (11%), and rash (11%) while pneumonia (5%), fever (4%), and infection (3%) were also seen [46]. Dyslipidemia and hypothyroidism are common reasons for discontinuation of bexarotene; however, a strategy of early use of agents to lower lipids and elevate thyroid hormones with close monitoring may be effective [47].

Interferon

Interferon alfa 2a has been used for patients with all stages of relapsed or refractory MF. Administration is given as a subcutaneous injection of 3–5 million units three times a week, with a gradual increase in the dose depending on clinical response and side effects experienced. In one study of 22 patients with CTCL of any stage (the majority of whom had previous lines of therapy) who were treated with interferon, an objective antitumor response was seen in 64% of patients. Side effects were common and include fatigue (100%), fevers/chills (86%), myalgias (55%), anorexia (55%), weight loss (55%), as well as others [48].

Histone Deacetylase Inhibitors

Histone deacetylase inhibitors (HDACi) include both the intravenous drug romidepsin and the oral drug vorinostat. While romidepsin is approved by the FDA after one line of systemic therapy for persistent, progressive, or recurrent CTCL, vorinostat is approved for treatment after two previous lines of therapy.

Romidepsin was studied in an open-label phase II single-arm trial consisting of 96 patients with stage IB to IVA disease who received at least one prior systemic therapy. It was given as an IV infusion at 14 mg/m^2 on days 1, 8, and 15 every 28 days. It exhibited an overall response rate of 34% with a median duration of response of 15 months. Clinically improved pruritis was seen in 43% of patients including some who did not achieve a response. Grade 3 and 4 toxicities were rare but included asthenic conditions (asthenia, fatigue, lethargy, malaise, 6%), anemia (2%), and nausea (2%). Fifty-six percent of patients developed nausea of any grade. Two patients developed oral or oropharyngeal candidiasis, one developed sepsis, and one developed isolated pyrexia. Nonspecific EKG changes that were clinically insignificant were also seen in few patients [49]. The manufacturer of romidepsin recommends to consider cardiovascular monitoring in patients with congenital long QT syndrome, patients with a history of significant cardiovascular disease, or those on medications known to cause QT prolongation.

Vorinostat was evaluated in a single-arm, open-label phase IIb trial of 74 patients with stage IB-IV MF/SS who had received at least two prior lines of therapy including bexarotene. It was given as 400 mg PO daily until disease progression or intolerable toxicity. The overall response rate was 29.7%, with the median duration of response not reached (but estimated to be greater than or equal to 185 days) and with 32% of patients achieving relief of their pruritis. The most common grade 3 or 4 toxicities were fatigue (5%), thrombocytopenia (5%), nausea (4%), muscle spasms (3%), and anorexia (3%) [61]. EKG changes were seen in 15 patients, 10 of whom had a history of cardiovascular disease or baseline abnormal EKG; however, there were no grade 3 or higher EKG adverse events and no dose reduction or discontinuation was required.

Brentuximab Vedotin

An antibody-drug conjugate, brentuximab vedotin (BV) is an anti-CD30 antibody that is conjugated to monomethyl auristatin E (MMAE), which is a tubulin-disrupting agent. BV is an option for patients who have relapsed after at least one line of systemic therapy and have documented expression of CD30. It is given as an IV infusion once every 3 weeks for up to 16 cycles. In an open-label phase III trial of 131 patients with at least one previous systemic treatment for MF, patients were randomly assigned to one of two arms comparing BV to treatment of physician's choice (TPC, either bexarotene or methotrexate). 56.3% of patients in the BV arm achieved an objective global response of at least 4 months compared to 12.5% in the TPC arm. In this trial, there were no grade 4 toxicities with BV and grade 3 toxicities were rare with the most common being peripheral neuropathy and fatigue which were both seen at 5%. When considering all grades of toxicity, peripheral sensory neuropathy was seen in 45% of patients treated with BV, while only two patients (3%) treated with BV developed a skin infection, both of grade 3 severity [50].

Denileukin Diftitox

Denileukin diftitox (DD) is a recombinant fusion protein consisting of interleukin 2 (IL-2) linked to the enzymatically active and membrane translocation domains of diphtheria toxin. It inhibits protein synthesis in cells that express the IL-2 receptor (IL-2R), thereby resulting in cell death. It is administered 5 consecutive days every 3 weeks for up to 8 cycles.

The efficacy, safety, and pharmacokinetics of DD were studied in patients with CTCL that had stage IB-III disease that recurred or persisted after at least four previous treatments (not including topical or systemic steroids) or patients with stage IVA disease that failed at least one prior line of therapy. In this phase III trial of 71 patients randomly assigned to either 9 μg/kg/d or 18 μg/kg/d of DD, investigators found an objective response rate of 30% with a median duration of response of 6.9 months with no statistical difference between the two doses [51].

Adverse effects were similar between the two doses with the most common grade 3 or 4 toxicities being constitutional symptoms of chills, fevers, asthenia, arthralgia, myalgia, or headaches (37–47%), infection (33–43%, with systemic infection seen in 11% of patients), gastrointestinal symptoms of diarrhea, anorexia, nausea, or vomiting (20–36%), CNS side effects of headache, confusion, or dementia (17–25%), vascular leak syndrome with hypotension, edema, and/or hypoalbuminemia (17–25%), rash (19–23%), back pain (6–11%), hypotension (8–11%), and dyspnea (6–11%).

In a subsequent phase III placebo-controlled randomized trial involving patients with CTCL who had received up to three prior therapies, patients were randomly assigned to DD to be given at 9 μg/kg/d, or DD to be given at 18 μg/kg/d, or to placebo.

Overall response rate was 44% for patients randomly assigned to DD versus 15.9% to those randomly assigned to placebo. Progression free survival also favored DD with a median PFS of more than 2 years compared 124 days for the placebo arm [52].

The most common adverse events seen in this study with DD (both doses) included fatigue (12%), rigors (12%), pyrexia (11%), and nausea (10%). There was no apparent increase in the incidence of infections. One of the more concerning adverse events, capillary leak syndrome (CLS), was seen in about 10% of patients receiving DD – two of these patients had moderately severe CLS (these patients received the 9 μg/kg/d dose) and two others had severe (these patients received the 18 μg/kg/d dose).

CLS, or vascular leak syndrome as it is otherwise known, was first identified in 2001 [51]. It is defined by the presence of any two of the following adverse events that can occur individually any time during the course of treatment: hypotension, edema, or serum albumin less than 3.0 g/dL.

To prevent CLS, patients are medicated with corticosteroids prior to each infusion of DD. Patients are also educated to report any new or worsening edema, weight gain, or dyspnea, which can easily be treated with a mild diuretic for 3–7 days [53].

Infections

There is an increased risk of infections in MF patients due to decreased host humoral and cellular immunity [54]. This underlying risk of infection is magnified when these patients are treated with chemotherapy or immunosuppressive drugs.

Patients with MF/SS have higher rates of skin (63%) and nasal (54%) colonization with *Staphylococcus aureus* compared to the general population (10%) and treatment and eradication of staphylococcus is associated with clinical improvement [55].

Infections are commonly seen in MF/SS and can lead to significant morbidity. These include cutaneous bacterial infections (17.0 infections per 100 patients years), cutaneous herpes simplex virus and herpes zoster virus infection (3.8 infections per 100 patients-years), bacteremia (2.1 infections per 100 patient-years), bacterial pneumonia (1.7 infections per 100 patients-years), and urinary tract infection (1.4 infections per 100 patient-years) [56].

Disseminated cutaneous herpes simplex virus has been reported in a patient with MF [57]. Fungal superinfection with Coccidioides immitis of the skin has also been reported in the literature [58].

Nosocomial infections can have dire consequences and account for 19% of cutaneous bacterial infections, 59% of bacteremias, 62% of pneumonias, and 88% of infections that lead to death in these patients [56].

The major cause of death in erythrodermic and Sezary syndrome is line sepsis most often secondary to *Staphylococcus aureus* [59]. Given the underlying impaired host immunity and the high rates of skin colonization with *Staphylococcus aureus*, it is recommended that IV lines be avoided unless absolutely necessary.

Clinical risk factors for cutaneous infections include ulcerated lesions, hyperkeratotic lesions, scratched lesions, oozing lesions, severe pruritus, and plaque/patch or erythrodermic lesions [60].

Prognosis

The prognosis of MF is highly dependent on the TNMB staging of the disease with poorer prognosis associated with higher stage. The 5-year overall survival rate by clinical stage is as follows: IA: 94%, IB: 84%, IIA: 78%, IIB/IIIA: 47%, IIIB: 40%, IVA1:37%, and IVA2/IVB: 18% [18].

Prognostic variables affecting overall survival were evaluated prospectively in a cohort of 1263 patients at MD Anderson from 1982 to 2009, with study authors reporting that advanced age, plaque stage, lactate dehydrogenase (LDH) level, and tumor area, were all associated with risk of progression or death [59].

In this same study, there were 273 deaths, however, only 102 (37%) were directly attributable to MF or SS.

Conclusion

MF is an indolent non-Hodgkin lymphoma and is the most common of the cutaneous T-cell lymphomas. Life expectancy for low-stage disease is equivalent to those without the disease, while those patients with advanced disease or with high risk features can have a significantly reduced life expectancy. Treatment of patients with advanced disease involves a chronic and relapsing course of multiple lines of therapy which were described above with their associated adverse effects. Superinfection of skin lesions is a serious concern and can occur in patients with any stage of the disease.

The critical care team must be aware of the clinical features of this disease and of the adverse effects and potential complications associated with disease treatments which can complicate the care of this patient population.

References

1. Girardi M, Heald PW, Wilson LD. The pathogenesis of mycosis fungoides. N Engl J Med. 2004;350:1978–88.
2. Lessin SR. Alibert lymphoma: renaming mycosis fungoides. Arch Dermatol. 2009;145(2):209–10.
3. Weinstock MA, Gardstein B. Twenty-year trends in the reported incidence of mycosis fungoides and associated mortality. Am J Public Health. 1999;89:1240–4.
4. Bradford PT, Devesa SS, Anderson WF, Toro JR. Cutaneous lymphoma incidence patterns in the United States: a population-based study of 3884 cases. Blood. 2009;113:5064–73.
5. Whittemore AS, Holly EA, Lee IM, Abel EA, Adams RM, Nickoloff BJ, Bley L, Peters JM, Gibney C. Mycosis fungoides in relation to environmental exposures and immune response: a case-control study. J Natl Cancer Inst. 1989;81(20):1560–7.
6. Mirvish ED, Pomerantz RG, Geskin LJ. Infectious agents in cutaneous T-cell lymphoma. J Am Acad Dermatol. 2011;64(2):423–31.
7. Li G, Vowels BR, Benoit BM, Rook AH, Lessin SR. Failure to detect human T-lymphotropic virus type-I proviral DNA in cell lines and tissues from patients with cutaneous T-cell lymphoma. J Invest Dermatol. 1996;107(3):308–13.
8. van Doorn R, Zoutman WH, Dijkman R, de Menezes RX, Commandeur S, Mulder AA, van der Velden PA, Vermeer MH, Willemze R, Yan PS, Huang TH, Tensen CP. Epigenetic profiling of cutaneous T-cell lymphoma: promoter hypermethylation of multiple tumor suppressor genes including BCL7a, PTPRG, and p73. J Clin Oncol. 2005;23(17):3886–96.
9. Morales MM, Olsen J, Johansen P, Kaerlev L, Guénel P, Arveux P, Wingren G, Hardell L, Ahrens W, Stang A, Llopis A, Merletti F, Villanueva MA. Viral infection, atopy and mycosis fungoides: a European multicentre case-control study. Eur J Cancer. 2003;39(4):511–6.
10. Zackheim HS, McCalmont TH. Mycosis fungoides: the great imitator. J Am Acad Dermatol. 2002;47(6):914–8.
11. Pimpinelli N, Olsen EA, Santucci M, Vonderheid E, Haeffner AC, Stevens S, Burg G, Cerroni L, Dreno B, Glusac E, Guitart J, Heald PW, Kempf W, Knobler R, Lessin S, Sander C, Smoller BS, Telang G, Whittaker S, Iwatsuki K, Obitz E, Takigawa M, Turner ML, Wood GS, International Society for Cutaneous Lymphoma. Defining early mycosis fungoides. J Am Acad Dermatol. 2005;53(6):1053–63.
12. Kim YH, Jensen RA, Watanabe GL, Varghese A, Hoppe RT. Clinical stage IA (limited patch and plaque) mycosis fungoides. A long-term outcome analysis. Arch Dermatol. 1996;132(11):1309–13.
13. Uhlenhake EE, Mehregan DM. Annular hypopigmented mycosis fungoides: a novel ringed variant. J Cutan Pathol. 2012;39(5):535–9.

14. Vij A, Duvic M. Prevalence and severity of pruritus in cutaneous T cell lymphoma. Int J Dermatol. 2012;51(8):930–4.
15. Bi MY, Curry JL, Christiano AM, Hordinsky MK, Norris DA, Price VH, Duvic M. The spectrum of hair loss in patients with mycosis fungoides and Sézary syndrome. J Am Acad Dermatol. 2011;64(1):53–63.
16. Huang KP, Weinstock MA, Clarke CA, McMillan A, Hoppe RT, Kim YH. Second lymphomas and other malignant neoplasms in patients with mycosis fungoides and Sezary syndrome: evidence from population-based and clinical cohorts. Arch Dermatol. 2007;143(1):45–50.
17. Hodak E, Amitay-Laish I, Feinmesser M, Davidovici B, David M, Zvulunov A, Pavlotsky F, Yaniv I, Avrahami G, Ben-Amitai D. Juvenile mycosis fungoides: cutaneous T-cell lymphoma with frequent follicular involvement. J Am Acad Dermatol. 2014;70(6):993–1001.
18. Agar NS, Wedgeworth E, Crichton S, Mitchell TJ, Cox M, Ferreira S, Robson A, Calonje E, Stefanato CM, Wain EM, Wilkins B, Fields PA, Dean A, Webb K, Scarisbrick J, Morris S, Whittaker SJ. Survival outcomes and prognostic factors in mycosis fungoides/Sézary syndrome: validation of the revised International Society for Cutaneous Lymphomas/European Organisation for Research and Treatment of Cancer staging proposal. J Clin Oncol. 2010;28(31):4730–9.
19. Scarisbrick JJ, Prince HM, Vermeer MH, Quaglino P, Horwitz S, Porcu P, Stadler R, Wood GS, Beylot-Barry M, Pham-Ledard A, Foss F, Girardi M, Bagot M, Michel L, Battistella M, Guitart J, Kuzel TM, Martinez-Escala ME, Estrach T, Papadavid E, Antoniou C, Rigopoulos D, Nikolaou V, Sugaya M, Miyagaki T, Gniadecki R, Sanches JA, Cury-Martins J, Miyashiro D, Servitje O, Muniesa C, Berti E, Onida F, Corti L, Hodak E, Amitay-Laish I, Ortiz-Romero PL, Rodríguez-Peralto JL, Knobler R, Porkert S, Bauer W, Pimpinelli N, Grandi V, Cowan R, Rook A, Kim E, Pileri A, Patrizi A, Pujol RM, Wong H, Tyler K, Stranzenbach R, Querfeld C, Fava P, Maule M, Willemze R, Evison F, Morris S, Twigger R, Talpur R, Kim J, Ognibene G, Li S, Tavallaee M, Hoppe RT, Duvic M, Whittaker SJ, Kim YH. Cutaneous lymphoma international consortium study of outcome in advanced stages of mycosis Fungoides and Sézary syndrome: effect of specific prognostic markers on survival and development of a prognostic model. J Clin Oncol. 2015;33(32):3766–73.
20. Diamandidou E, Colome-Grimmer M, Fayad L, Duvic M, Kurzrock R. Transformation of mycosis fungoides/Sezary syndrome: clinical characteristics and prognosis. Blood. 1998;92(4):1150–9.
21. Hurabielle C, Michel L, Ram-Wolff C, Battistella M, Jean-Louis F, Beylot-Barry M, d'Incan M, Bensussan A, Bagot M. Expression of Sézary biomarkers in the blood of patients with erythrodermic mycosis fungoides. J Invest Dermatol. 2016;136 (1):317–20.
22. Olsen EA, Whittaker S, Kim YH, Duvic M, Prince HM, Lessin SR, Wood GS, Willemze R, Demierre MF, Pimpinelli N, Bernengo MG, Ortiz-Romero PL, Bagot M, Estrach T, Guitart J, Knobler R, Sanches JA, Iwatsuki K, Sugaya M, Dummer R, Pittelkow M, Hoppe R, Parker S, Geskin L, Pinter-Brown L, Girardi M, Burg G, Ranki A, Vermeer M, Horwitz S, Heald P, Rosen S, Cerroni L, Dreno B, Vonderheid EC, International Society for Cutaneous Lymphomas, United States Cutaneous Lymphoma Consortium, Cutaneous Lymphoma Task Force of the European Organisation for Research and Treatment of Cancer. Clinical end points and response criteria in mycosis fungoides and Sézary syndrome: a consensus statement of the International Society for Cutaneous Lymphomas, the United States Cutaneous Lymphoma Consortium, and the cutaneous lymphoma task force of the European Organisation for Research and Treatment of Cancer. J Clin Oncol. 2011;29 (18):2598–607.
23. Kaye FJ, Bunn PA Jr, Steinberg SM, Stocker JL, Ihde DC, Fischmann AB, Glatstein EJ, Schechter GP, Phelps RM, Foss FM. A randomized trial comparing combination electron-beam radiation and chemotherapy with topical therapy in the initial treatment of mycosis fungoides. N Engl J Med. 1989;321(26):1784.
24. Hughes CF, Khot A, McCormack C, Lade S, Westerman DA, Twigger R, Buelens O, Newland K, Tam C, Dickinson M, Ryan G, Ritchie D, Wood C, Prince HM. Lack of durable disease control with chemotherapy for mycosis fungoides and Sézary syndrome: a comparative study of systemic therapy. Blood. 2015;125(1):71–81.
25. Duarte RF, Canals C, Onida F, Gabriel IH, Arranz R, Arcese W, Ferrant A, Kobbe G, Narni F, Deliliers GL, Olavarría E, Schmitz N, Sureda A. Allogeneic hematopoietic cell transplantation for patients with mycosis fungoides and Sézary syndrome: a retrospective analysis of the Lymphoma Working Party of the European Group for Blood and Marrow Transplantation. J Clin Oncol. 2010;28(29):4492–9.
26. Ramsay DL, Lish KM, Yalowitz CB, Soter NA. Ultraviolet-B phototherapy for early-stage cutaneous T-cell lymphoma. Arch Dermatol. 1992;128(7):931–3.
27. Boztepe G, Sahin S, Ayhan M, Erkin G, Kilemen F. Narrowband ultraviolet B phototherapy to clear and maintain clearance in patients with mycosis fungoides. J Am Acad Dermatol. 2005;53(2):242–6.
28. Gökdemir G, Barutcuoglu B, Sakiz D, Köşlü A. Narrowband UVB phototherapy for early-stage mycosis fungoides: evaluation of clinical and histopathological changes. J Eur Acad Dermatol Venereol. 2006;20(7):804–9.
29. Whittaker S, Ortiz P, Dummer R, Ranki A, Hasan B, Meulemans B, Gellrich S, Knobler R, Stadler R, Karrasch M. Efficacy and safety of bexarotene combined with psoralen-ultraviolet A (PUVA) compared

with PUVA treatment alone in stage IB-IIA mycosis fungoides: final results from the EORTC cutaneous lymphoma task force phase III randomized clinical trial (NCT00056056). Br J Dermatol. 2012;167 (3):678–87.

30. Jones GW, Kacinski BM, Wilson LD, Willemze R, Spittle M, Hohenberg G, Handl-Zeller L, Trautinger F, Knobler R. Total skin electron radiation in the management of mycosis fungoides: consensus of the European Organization for Research and Treatment of Cancer (EORTC) Cutaneous Lymphoma Project Group. J Am Acad Dermatol. 2002;47 (3):364–70.

31. Ysebaert L, Truc G, Dalac S, Lambert D, Petrella T, Barillot I, Naudy S, Horiot JC, Maingon P. Ultimate results of radiation therapy for T1-T2 mycosis fungoides (including reirradiation). Int J Radiat Oncol Biol Phys. 2004;58(4):1128–34.

32. Lloyd S, Chen Z, Foss FM, Girardi M, Wilson LD. Acute toxicity and risk of infection during total skin electron beam therapy for mycosis fungoides. J Am Acad Dermatol. 2013;69(4):537–43.

33. Edelson R, Berger C, Gasparro F, Jegasothy B, Heald P, Wintroub B, Vonderheid E, Knobler R, Wolff K, Plewig G, et al. Treatment of cutaneous T-cell lymphoma by extracorporeal photo-chemotherapy. Preliminary results. N Engl J Med. 1987;316(6):297–303.

34. Zackheim HS. Treatment of patch-stage mycosis fungoides with topical corticosteroids. Dermatol Ther. 2003;16(4):283–7.

35. Ramsay DL, Halperin PS, Zeleniuch-Jacquotte A. Topical mechlorethamine therapy for early stage mycosis fungoides. J Am Acad Dermatol. 1988;19 (4):684–91.

36. Lindahl LM, Fenger-Grøn M, Iversen L. Secondary cancers, comorbidities and mortality associated with nitrogen mustard therapy in patients with mycosis fungoides: a 30-year population-based cohort study. Br J Dermatol. 2014;170(3):699–704.

37. Vonderheid EC, Tan ET, Kantor AF, Shrager L, Micaily B, Van Scott EJ. Long-term efficacy, curative potential, and carcinogenicity of topical mechlorethamine chemotherapy in cutaneous T cell lymphoma. J Am Acad Dermatol. 1989;20(3):416–28.

38. Zackheim HS, Epstein EH Jr, Crain WR. Topical carmustine (BCNU) for cutaneous T cell lymphoma: a 15-year experience in 143 patients. J Am Acad Dermatol. 1990;22(5 Pt 1):802–10.

39. Heald P, Mehlmauer M, Martin AG, Crowley CA, Yocum RC, Reich SD, Worldwide Bexarotene Study Group. Topical bexarotene therapy for patients with refractory or persistent early-stage cutaneous T-cell lymphoma: results of the phase III clinical trial. J Am Acad Dermatol. 2003;49(5):801–15.

40. Shipman AR, Scarisbrick J. New treatment options for mycosis fungoides. Indian J Dermatol. 2016;61:119.

41. Zackheim HS, Kashani-Sabet M, Hwang ST. Low-dose methotrexate to treat erythrodermic cutaneous T-cell lymphoma: results in twenty-nine patients. J Am Acad Dermatol. 1996;34(4):626–31.

42. Zackheim HS, Kashani-Sabet M, McMillan A. Low-dose methotrexate to treat mycosis fungoides: a retrospective study in 69 patients. J Am Acad Dermatol. 2003;49(5):873–8.

43. Zinzani PL, Baliva G, Magagnoli M, Bendandi M, Modugno G, Gherlinzoni F, Orcioni GF, Ascani S, Simoni R, Pileri SA, Tura S. Gemcitabine treatment in pretreated cutaneous T-cell lymphoma: experience in 44 patients. J Clin Oncol. 2000;18(13):2603–6.

44. Zinzani PL, Venturini F, Stefoni V, Fina M, Pellegrini C, Derenzini E, Gandolfi L, Broccoli A, Argnani L, Quirini F, Pileri S, Baccarani M. Gemcitabine as single agent in pretreated T-cell lymphoma patients: evaluation of the long-term outcome. Ann Oncol. 2010;21:860–3.

45. Quereux G, Marques S, Nguyen JM, Bedane C, D'incan M, Dereure O, Puzenat E, Claudy A, Martin L, Joly P, Delaunay M, Beylot-Barry M, Vabres P, Celerier P, Sasolas B, Grange F, Khammari A, Dreno B. Prospective multicenter study of pegylated liposomal doxorubicin treatment in patients with advanced or refractory mycosis fungoides or Sezary syndrome. Arch Dermatol. 2008;144(6):727–33.

46. Duvic M, Hymes K, Heald P, Breneman D, Martin AG, Myskowski P, Crowley C, Yocum RC, Bexarotene Worldwide Study Group. Bexarotene is effective and safe for treatment of refractory advanced-stage cutaneous T-cell lymphoma: multinational phase II-III trial results. J Clin Oncol. 2001;19(9):2456–71.

47. Assaf C, Bagot M, Dummer R, Duvic M, Gniadecki R, Knobler R, Ranki A, Schwandt P, Whittaker S. Minimizing adverse side-effects of oral bexarotene in cutaneous T-cell lymphoma: an expert opinion. Br J Dermatol. 2006;155(2):261–6.

48. Olsen EA, Rosen ST, Vollmer RT, Variakojis D, Roenigk HH Jr, Diab N, Zeffren J. Interferon alfa-2a in the treatment of cutaneous T cell lymphoma. J Am Acad Dermatol. 1989;20(3):395–407.

49. Whittaker SJ, Demierre MF, Kim EJ, Rook AH, Lerner A, Duvic M, Scarisbrick J, Reddy S, Robak T, Becker JC, Samtsov A, McCulloch W, Kim YH. Final results from a multicenter, international, pivotal study of romidepsin in refractory cutaneous T-cell lymphoma. J Clin Oncol. 2010;28(29):4485–91.

50. Prince HM, Kim YH, Horwitz SM, Dummer R, Scarisbrick J, Quaglino P, Zinzani PL, Wolter P, Sanches JA, Ortiz-Romero PL, Akilov OE, Geskin L, Trotman J, Taylor K, Dalle S, Weichenthal M, Walewski J, Fisher D, Dréno B, Stadler R, Feldman T, Kuzel TM, Wang Y, Palanca-Wessels MC, Zagadailov E, Trepicchio WL, Zhang W, Lin HM, Liu Y, Huebner D, Little M, Whittaker S, Duvic M, ALCANZA study group. Brentuximab vedotin or physician's choice in CD30-positive cutaneous T-cell lymphoma (ALCANZA): an international, open-label, randomised, phase 3, multicentre trial. Lancet. 2017;390(10094):555–66.

51. Olsen E, Duvic M, Frankel A, Kim Y, Martin A, Vonderheid E, Jegasothy B, Wood G, Gordon M, Heald P, Oseroff A, Pinter-Brown L, Bowen G, Kuzel T, Fivenson D, Foss F, Glode M, Molina A, Knobler E, Stewart S, Cooper K, Stevens S, Craig F, Reuben J, Bacha P, Nichols J. Pivotal phase III trial of two dose levels of denileukin diftitox for the treatment of cutaneous T-cell lymphoma. J Clin Oncol. 2001;19(2):376–88.

52. Prince HM, Duvic M, Martin A, Sterry W, Assaf C, Sun Y, Straus D, Acosta M, Negro-Vilar A. Phase III placebo-controlled trial of denileukin diftitox for patients with cutaneous T-cell lymphoma. J Clin Oncol. 2010;28:1870–7.

53. Walker PL, Dang NH. Denileukin diftitox as novel targeted therapy in non-Hodgkin's lymphoma. Clin J Oncol Nurs. 2004;8(2):169–74.

54. Krejsgaard T, Odum N, Geisler C, Wasik MA, Woetmann A. Regulatory T cells and immunodeficiency in mycosis fungoides and Sézary syndrome. Leukemia. 2012;26(3):424–32.

55. Talpur R, Bassett R, Duvic M. Prevalence and treatment of *Staphylococcus aureus* colonization in patients with mycosis fungoides and Sézary syndrome. Br J Dermatol. 2008;159(1):105–12.

56. Axelrod PI, Lorber B, Vonderheid EC. Infections complicating mycosis fungoides and Sézary syndrome. JAMA. 1992;267(10):1354–8.

57. Mallo-García S, Coto-Segura P, Suárez-Casado H, Caminal L, Sánchez-del-Río J, Santos-Juanes J. Fatal outcome due to bacterial superinfection of eczema herpeticum in a patient with mycosis fungoides. Dermatol Online J. 2008;14(6):21.

58. Poonawalla T, Diwan H, Duvic M. Mycosis fungoides with coccidioidomycosis. Clin Lymphoma Myeloma. 2006;7(2):148–50.

59. Talpur R, Singh L, Daulat S, Liu P, Seyfer S, Trynosky T, Wei W, Duvic M. Long-term outcomes of 1,263 patients with mycosis fungoides and Sézary syndrome from 1982 to 2009. Clin Cancer Res. 2012;18(18):5051–60.

60. Lebas E, Arrese JE, Nikkels AF. Risk factors for skin infections in mycosis fungoides. Dermatology. 2016;232(6):731–7.

61. Olsen EA, Kim YH, Kuzel TM, Pacheco TR, Foss FM, Parker S, Frankel SR, Chen C, Ricker JL, Arduino JM, Duvic M. Phase IIb multicenter trial of vorinostat in patients with persistent, progressive, or treatment refractory cutaneous T-cell lymphoma. J Clin Oncol. 2007a;25(21):3109–15.

62. Olsen EA, Vonderheid E, Pimpinelli N, Willemze R, Kim Y, Knobler R, Zackheim H, Duvic M, Estrach T, Lamberg S, Wood G, Dummer R, Ranki A, Burg G, Heald P, Pittelkow M, Bernengo MG, Sterry W, Laroche L, Trautinger F, Whittaker S, ISCL/EORTC. Revisions to the staging and classification of mycosis fungoides and Sezary syndrome: a proposal of the International Society for Cutaneous Lymphomas (ISCL) and the cutaneous lymphoma task force of the European Organization of Research and Treatment of Cancer (EORTC). Blood. 2007b;110 (6):1713–22.

Part IV

Neurologic Diseases

Delirium and Psychosis in Critically Ill Cancer Patients

21

Kimberly F. Rengel, Daniel A. Nahrwold, Pratik P. Pandharipande, and Christopher G. Hughes

Contents

Introduction	300
Definition	301
Diagnosis	301
Epidemiology	303
Prevalence	303
Risk Factors	303
Pathophysiology	305
Neuroinflammation	305
Neurotransmitters	306
Structural Changes	307
Neurological Aging	308
Prevention	308
Pain Management	308
Sedation Management	309

K. F. Rengel · C. G. Hughes (✉)
Department of Anesthesiology, Division of Anesthesiology Critical Care Medicine, Vanderbilt University Medical Center, Nashville, TN, USA
e-mail: kimberly.rengel@vumc.org; Christopher.hughes@vumc.org

D. A. Nahrwold
Department of Anesthesiology, Moffitt Cancer Center, Tampa, FL, USA

Department of Oncologic Sciences, University of South Florida, Morsani College of Medicine, Tampa, FL, USA
e-mail: daniel.nahrwold@moffitt.org

P. P. Pandharipande
Department of Anesthesiology and Surgery, Division of Anesthesiology Critical Care Medicine, Vanderbilt University Medical Center, Nashville, TN, USA
e-mail: pratik.pandharipande@vumc.org

© Springer Nature Switzerland AG 2020
J. L. Nates, K. J. Price (eds.), *Oncologic Critical Care*,
https://doi.org/10.1007/978-3-319-74588-6_33

Early Mobilization 309
Improving Sleep 309
Multicomponent Intervention 310
Pharmacologic Prophylaxis 311

Treatment 313

Conclusion 314

References 314

Abstract

Delirium is a common diagnosis within the critically ill cancer population. It is characterized by acute and rapid fluctuations in mental status and consciousness. The diagnosis of delirium can be difficult and is often accomplished with the use of a validated delirium assessment tool. The prevalence of delirium varies widely with higher rates in patients who are elderly, have severe critical illness including cancer, or are known to have preexisting cognitive impairment and dementia. The pathophysiology of delirium is highly complex and may be related to changes in the brain as a result of neuroinflammation, endothelial dysfunction, aberrant cerebral perfusion patterns, and deficiency or abnormal activity of neurotransmitters. The prevention of delirium in the critically ill involves multiple components including choice of pain and sedating medications, early physical and occupational therapy, improving sleep, and daily awakening and breathing trials. There are no FDA-approved pharmacologic treatments available for delirium, though some of the antipsychotics and dexmedetomidine have shown promise in various studies. Delirium can be a challenging and deleterious diagnosis for critically ill cancer patients, but with proper recognition, as well as validated preventative and management strategies, the negative consequences associated with delirium can be decreased.

Keywords

Delirium · Cancer · Coma · Agitation · Sedation · Antipsychotics · Dexmedetomidine · Neuroinflammation · Pain · Psychosis

Introduction

Delirium is a manifestation of acute brain dysfunction that is characterized by rapid fluctuations in mental status and consciousness. It is a syndrome that spans many healthcare domains but is particularly prevalent in the aging population, the critically ill, and patients with cancer. Understanding delirium and developing strategies for prevention and treatment are of utmost importance in the intensive care unit (ICU) as delirium is associated with significant short- and long-term consequences. In the acute period, delirium is associated with prolonged duration of hospitalization, family distress, increased mortality, higher risk of discharge to a facility other than home, and increased economic burden. Persistence of delirium is also independently associated with worse short-term prognosis in patients with advanced cancer. Survivors of critical illness who experience delirium while hospitalized face long-term consequences including higher mortality in the year following discharge, long-term cognitive impairment, and persistent physical disability. Unfortunately the diagnosis of delirium is frequently missed despite being common in the critically ill and oncology populations, and it is often considered a minor and expected complication of critical illness by clinicians regardless of its independent associations with worse outcomes. This chapter discusses the diagnosis of delirium, contributing factors for developing delirium, and strategies for prevention and management of delirium in critically ill patients with an emphasis on unique factors and considerations in the setting of cancer.

Definition

The term "delirium" has been generally applied to describe a variety of symptoms related to a state of altered mentation. *The Diagnostic and Statistical Manual of Mental Disorders, Fifth Edition (DSM-5)*, provides clear criteria for formal diagnosis, defining delirium as a disturbance in attention manifested by a reduced ability to direct, focus, sustain, or shift attention with concurrent disturbances in cognition such as memory deficit, disorientation, and visuospatial or perception deficit. Symptoms develop acutely and fluctuate throughout the day and must not be accounted for by a preexisting neurocognitive disorder. Patients may display differing psychomotor behavior profiles that are further classified into one of three

Table 1 Richmond Agitation-Sedation Scale (RASS)

Score	Term	Description
+4	Combative	Combative or violent behavior that poses danger to patient or care team
+3	Very agitated	Hyperactive agitation, attempting to remove lines, drains, and tubes with aggression towards caretakers
+2	Agitated	Restlessness with nonpurposeful movements or dyssynchrony with mechanical ventilation
+1	Restless	Uneasy and apprehensive behaviors without aggression toward caregivers
0	Alert and calm	Spontaneously and appropriately interactive and arousable
−1	Drowsy	Not fully alert but will awaken to voice and sustain at least 10 s of eye contact
−2	Lightly sedated	Awakening to voice with less than 10 s eye contact
−3	Moderately sedated	Spontaneous movement in response to vocal stimulus without eye contact
−4	Deep sedation	No response to verbal stimulation with movement to physical stimulation
−5	Unarousable	No response to verbal or physical stimulation

Adapted from Sessler et al. [49]

delirium subtypes: hyperactive, hypoactive, or mixed. Patients with hyperactive delirium often appear agitated, hypervigilant, and restless, whereas those with hypoactive delirium are lethargic with decreased movement and slowed mentation. If features of both types are present within 24 h, patients are considered to have a mixed delirium. This distinction is important as hypoactive delirium is much more common and, due to the subtlety of the symptom profile, is often missed by care providers.

Diagnosis

The gold standard for delirium diagnosis is a formal evaluation by a psychiatrist using *DSM-5* criteria. Recognizing that formal evaluation is not feasible in many hospital settings, a number of validated screening instruments have been developed for bedside assessment that can be administered by various members of the clinical care team. Rapid and reliable assessment tools are important, as a large percentage of delirium in the critically ill and cancer populations will go unrecognized, in particular the hypoactive subtype, without targeted screening. This has prompted the addition of routine delirium screening for all ICU patients to current practice guidelines [14]. To complete a delirium assessment, patients must be arousable to voice. Thus, an important first step in delirium assessment is the use of an arousal/sedation tool such as the Richmond Agitation-Sedation Scale (RASS) (Table 1) or the Sedation-Agitation Scale (SAS). While multiple validated delirium assessment tools are widely available, the Confusion Assessment Method for the Intensive Care Unit (CAM-ICU) and Intensive Care Delirium Screening Checklist (ICDSC) have been studied most frequently in the ICU, whereas the Memorial Delirium Assessment Scale (MDAS) is widely studied in cancer patients.

The CAM-ICU (Table 2) was adapted from the Confusion Assessment Method (CAM) for use in critically ill patients, including those that may be nonverbal or supported by mechanical ventilation.

Table 2 Confusion Assessment Method for the Intensive Care Unit (CAM-ICU)

Feature 1: Acute onset or fluctuating course
Acute change in mental status from baseline
Abnormal behavior fluctuating over the course of 24 h with increases or decreases in severity as evidenced by fluctuations in the Richmond Agitation Sedation Scale or Glasgow Coma Scale
Feature 2: Inattention
Difficulty focusing attention as evidenced by two or more errors on the Letters Attention Test
Feature 3: Altered level of consciousness
The patient is demonstrating an altered level of consciousness from alertness including vigilance, stupor, or coma:
Alert: spontaneously fully aware of the environment with appropriate interaction
Vigilant: hyperalert
Lethargic: drowsy but easily aroused, unaware of some elements in the environment or not spontaneously interacting with the interviewer; becomes fully aware and appropriately interactive when prodded minimally
Stupor: difficult to arouse, unaware of some or all elements in the environment or not spontaneously interacting with the interviewer; becomes in completely aware when prodded strongly; can be aroused only by vigorous and repeated stimuli and as soon as the stimulus ceases, stuporous subjects lapse back into an unresponsive state
Coma: unarousable, unaware of all elements in the environment with no spontaneous interaction or awareness of the interviewer so that the interview is impossible even with maximal prodding
Feature 4: Disorganized Thinking
Disorganized or incoherent thinking evidenced by incorrect answers to three or more of the following questions and inability to follow commands:
Questions
1. Will a stone float on water?
2. Are there fish in the sea?
3. Does 1 pound weight more than 2 pounds?
4. Can you use a hammer to pound a nail?
Commands
1. Are you having unclear thinking?
2. Hold up this many fingers. (Examiner holds two fingers in front of the patient.)
3. Now do the same thing with the other hand (without holding the two fingers in front of the patient)
CAM-ICU is positive if both Features 1 AND 2 are present WITH one of either Features 3 OR 4

Used with permission from Dr. Wes Ely

In addition, the assessment can be administered by non-physician care providers in 2–3 min at the bedside, allowing for easy adaptability into the daily care routine. The CAM-ICU tool evaluates four primary features of delirium: acute fluctuations in mental status, inattention, disorganized thinking, and altered levels of consciousness. Multiple validation studies have demonstrated >80% sensitivity and >95% specificity in critically ill patients. In a cohort of noncritically ill oncology patients, the CAM-ICU showed a lower sensitivity: specificity, however, remained >95%; thus in lower severity of illness patients, a brief assessment tool may miss some delirium, and a more detailed exam may be warranted. Importantly, assessments for delirium using the CAM-ICU have a very high positive predictive value across multiple patient populations and hospital settings. First introduced by Bergeron et al. in 2001, the ICDSC scores patients on eight features of delirium adapted from the DSM criteria: altered level of consciousness, inattention, disorientation, hallucination or delusion, psychomotor agitation or retardation, inappropriate mood or speech, sleep/wake cycle disturbance, and symptom fluctuation. Scores are collected over the course of a nursing shift without directly engaging patient participation. In validation studies, both sensitivity and specificity tend to be lower than with the CAM-ICU. Another scale designed to reflect diagnostic criteria of the DSM-IV, the MDAS (Table 3), was first introduced by Breitbart et al. to assess the presence and severity of delirium in medically ill patients. Clinicians grade patients on a four-point scale for ten items: awareness, disorientation, short-term memory impairment, impaired digit span, inattention, disorganized thinking, perceptual disturbance, delusions, change in psychomotor activity, and sleep-wake cycle disturbances. Initial assessment in a small group of inpatient cancer and acquired immuno-deficiency syndrome (AIDS) patients showed a sensitivity of 71% and specificity of 94%. The MDAS has subsequently been validated in the advanced cancer and critical illness populations. With growing interest in assessing severity of delirium and not only a positive/negative assessment value, the CAM-ICU was adapted to include a numbered scale (0–2) for each delirium feature. This severity scale, the CAM-ICU-7, has been validated in critically ill patients, and severe delirium scores have been found to correlate with

Table 3 Memorial Delirium Assessment Scale (MDAS). Patients are scored on a scale of 0–3 based on the severity of their symptoms in each category over the course of the previous several hours. A score of 0 indicates the absence of the behavior with 3 indicating severe symptomatology

Altered consciousness or reduced awareness of and interaction with the surrounding environment
A state of disorientation to self, surroundings, or time
Impaired short-term memory
Inability to repeat 3, 4, and 5 digits forward and backward
Impaired ability to focus attention or shift from one task to another when directed
Disorganization of thoughts, especially when addressing complex questions or tasks
Disturbances in perception including visual or auditory hallucinations
Delusional ideation or misinterpretations of surroundings/interactions with care team
Abnormal psychomotor activity including agitation or lethargy
Disruptions in normal sleep-wake cycles with decreased wakefulness

Adapted from Breitbart et al. [8]

an increase in mortality. Implementation of a validated delirium assessment tool promotes consistency and early identification of acute brain dysfunction. Current guidelines from the Society of Critical Care Medicine recommend utilizing the CAM-ICU or ICDSC for their strong psychometric properties and distinct design for use in critically ill patients who may require mechanical ventilation [14].

Epidemiology

Prevalence

The reported prevalence of delirium is highly variable with age, severity of illness, and assessment method. Delirium is estimated to occur in 19–30% of inpatient hospitalizations with a higher prevalence in the elderly population. In surgical patients, 45% will develop postoperative delirium in the acute recovery period, and of those admitted to the hospital postoperatively, rates range from 32% up to greater than 50% in high-risk surgical patients. The highest rates of

delirium have been found in the critically ill population where prevalence is generally reported at 30–50% overall. In patients requiring mechanical ventilation, however, up to 80% will experience delirium.

Delirium is also a common phenomenon in patients with cancer. In older cancer patients admitted to the hospital for symptom management, 50–60% meet criteria of delirium at admission or will develop delirium over the course of their hospital stay. Additionally, symptoms may persist for weeks after discharge. Similarly, 50% of patients in the palliative care setting have been found to meet criteria for delirium diagnosis. As the severity of illness progresses, delirium frequently accompanies, and up to 85% of terminally ill patients will demonstrate delirium in the final week of life.

Risk Factors

Multiple risk factors are associated with developing delirium. Risk factors can be stratified into two broad categories: predisposing and precipitating factors. Predisposing risk factors are those that the patient presents with versus precipitating factors, which are related to the course of critical illness and iatrogenic influences. While predisposing risk factors are important to understand, they are difficult to alter. However, precipitating factors provide targets for intervention for prevention of delirium. A summary of risk factors is provided in Table 4.

One of the most commonly cited predisposing risk factors for delirium is preexisting cognitive impairment and dementia. While it is intuitive that baseline cognitive dysfunction increases vulnerability to acute cerebral dysfunction in critical illness, studies have demonstrated that patients found to have baseline compromise in the microstructural integrity of white matter in the cerebellum, hippocampus, and thalamus were at increased risk of developing postoperative delirium, independent of clinical cognitive dysfunction. Increasing age has also been associated with increased risk of delirium development across a range of populations, including critical illness, oncology, and surgical patients.

Table 4 Risk factors for delirium

Predisposing	Precipitating	Cancer-related
Cognitive impairment	Mechanical ventilation	Primary brain tumors
Dementia	Increased severity of illness	Metastasis to brain
Compromised white matter integrity	Electrolyte abnormalities	Chemotherapeutics (immunomodulators, vinca alkaloids, and platinums)
Increasing age	Pain	Hypercalcemia
Frailty	Anticholinergics	Opioids
Comorbid diseases	Benzodiazepines	Dehydration
Depression	Steroids	
	Sepsis	
	Meperidine and morphine	
	Deep sedation	

Patients with higher comorbid disease burdens develop delirium at higher rates, especially hypertension and respiratory disease. Observation that patients with more cognitive and physical disease burden are more likely to develop delirium has increased interest in the relationship between frailty and delirium. Initial studies have focused on the surgical population and have demonstrated an increased risk of postoperative delirium in frail patients. In the palliative care setting, a lower score on the Palliative Performance Scale, indicative of worse physical function, has been associated with an increased risk of delirium during admission to a palliative care unit. Mental health also appears to play a role as baseline depression is associated with delirium development. This is particularly important in cancer patients where prevalence of depression is estimated to be 15–25%, more than twice the rate observed in the general population. A unique consideration in oncology patients is the presence of primary brain tumors or development of metastases to the brain or leptomeninges which may also contribute to acute cerebral dysfunction by reducing the brain's resiliency against insults such as acute illness. In addition, a number of chemotherapy agents are associated with neurologic toxicity and delirium including immunomodulators, vinca alkaloids, and platinums.

Identifying and understanding precipitating risk factors for delirium allow the care team an opportunity to apply increased attention, resources, and prevention strategies. Lawlor et al. [33] reported the presence of three or more precipitating factors per episode of delirium in oncology ward patients, which increased to more than ten risk factors per patient in the ICU in work by Ely and colleagues [17]. Worsening severity of illness and acute physiologic derangement as demonstrated by SOFA or APACHE II score has repeatedly been associated with delirium. Supporting this observation, the need for mechanical ventilation is also associated with an increased prevalence of delirium in the ICU and in critically ill cancer patients. Hypoxia, whether related to infection or tumor burden, has been associated with delirium, and progression to hypoxic encephalopathy has been associated with nonreversible delirium. Critically ill patients commonly present with or develop metabolic derangements that may provide a reversible target for intervention. Abnormalities associated with delirium include metabolic acidosis, elevated creatinine, sodium imbalance, and hepatic failure. Cancer and the therapies used for treatment frequently alter hematologic status. Evidence regarding anemia in delirium has been inconclusive, and lymphopenia has not been associated with delirium in critical illness.

Two precipitating factors fall most directly under control of the critical care team: (1) pain management and (2) medication selection with special attention to sedating and analgesic medications. Uncontrolled pain, particularly in the elderly population, may manifest as delirium and further preclude patients' ability to communicate their pain experience. In the surgical population, moderate to severe pain increases the risk of developing postoperative delirium. This has also been documented in case reports where severe pain from cancer caused agitated delirium that receded once the pain was managed. The sedating effects of traditional pain medications, predominantly opioids, present a challenge to providers in adequately managing pain without causing oversedation. Evidence regarding the relationship between opioids and delirium is currently inconclusive in the critically ill population. Opioid administration has been independently associated with delirium in some ICU populations. However, others have found no difference in delirium development in patients receiving opioids or that opioids reduced the incidence of delirium. The choice of opioid administered has been shown to impact outcomes. Patients given meperidine are more likely to develop delirium compared to other opioids. Morphine has also been associated with delirium in the critically ill population, and patients receiving morphine via patient-controlled analgesia (PCA) were more likely to develop delirium after surgery when compared to fentanyl PCA [51]. These effects may be related to the prolonged duration of action of these drugs, as well as active metabolite accumulation in the setting of renal or hepatic compromise. Evidence in the oncology population overwhelmingly identifies opioids as a modifiable risk factor for delirium development. In a cohort of severely medically ill cancer patients, 90% of those that developed delirium were on opioid therapy [7], and opioid administration appears to increase risk of delirium in a dose-dependent fashion [19]. Therefore, while pain management is a pillar of cancer therapy and symptom management, providers should exhibit caution in opioid choice and dose, seeking alternative means of pain control to minimize risk of delirium. Medication choice and dose are also important factors in providing sedation in the critical care setting. Benzodiazepines have been a common choice for sedation and anxiolysis but are now known to be strongly associated with delirium development in critical illness; these effects do not appear to be medication specific but rather an association with the entire class of benzodiazepines. Risk of developing delirium also increases with deeper levels of sedation.

Medications given for therapeutic intervention or symptom management in oncology patients may also increase risk of delirium. Many chemotherapy drugs have been associated with neurotoxicity and an increased risk of delirium. Steroids are often a component of therapy regimens and have been associated with an increased risk of delirium in advanced cancer and palliative care settings and promote transition to delirium in the ICU. Finally, many medications used for cancer symptom management, including promethazine, diphenhydramine, and cyclobenzaprine, have anticholinergic properties and may precipitate delirium development. Importantly, several medications associated with delirium are often started in the ICU and inappropriately continued upon transition out of the ICU or after discharge. As such, clinicians caring for the oncologic critically ill patient need to be vigilant about reducing medication exposure when appropriate.

Pathophysiology

The pathophysiology of delirium involves complex, multifactorial interactions that have not been clearly defined. The current prevailing hypotheses include neuroinflammation, endothelial dysfunction, changes in cerebral perfusion patterns, increased blood-brain barrier permeability, cholinergic deficiency, abnormal neurotransmitter activity, and structural changes to the brain including neuronal aging and cerebral atrophy (Fig. 1).

Neuroinflammation

It is well accepted that cancer induces a chronic state of inflammation, which is an established mediator of critical illness and acute brain

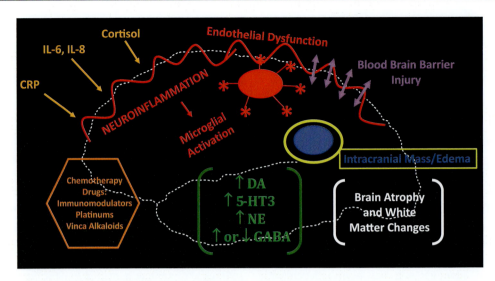

Fig. 1 Pathophysiology of delirium. The hypothesized mechanism of delirium during critical illness involves systemic inflammatory insults leading to neuroinflammation, neurotransmitter alterations, and structural changes. Chemotherapy drugs and intracranial lesions related to cancer also likely contribute to worse brain function

dysfunction. Elevated baseline C-reactive protein (CRP) levels have been associated with delirium in medical and surgical populations. In a cohort of patients awaiting noncardiac surgery, elevated CRP concentrations preoperatively and 2 days after surgical stress were associated with longer duration of delirium and increased severity of symptoms [60]. Plasma cytokines and inflammatory mediators including IL-6, IL-8, and cortisol have also been associated with delirium development.

Systemic inflammatory mediators communicate directly with the brain via peripheral primary afferent nerve activation. In addition, proinflammatory cytokines bind to the endothelium that comprises the blood-brain barrier (BBB), initiating an inflammatory signaling cascade, altering adhesion molecules, and promoting active cytokine transport across the BBB. Changes induced in the endothelium may lead to cell death and detachment, coagulation activation with microvascular thrombosis, and altered vascular permeability which subsequently result in ischemia and neuronal apoptosis. Hughes et al. found that elevated levels of biomarkers associated with endothelial dysfunction and BBB injury (S100B, E-selectin, plasminogen activator-1) were associated with increased duration of

delirium during critical illness [27]. A key mediator of inflammation in the brain are microglia, normally quiescent macrophages that are activated by inflammatory mediators to produce proinflammatory cytokines and reactive oxygen species that weaken astrocytic tight junctions and affect neuronal transmission. Once activated, microglia proliferate and further propagate the inflammatory insult by recruiting monocytes to the brain, resulting in neuronal apoptosis and brain edema. These acute insults likely lead to structural changes and subsequent long-term impairments in brain function.

Neurotransmitters

Early observations that patients frequently developed delirium after exposure to toxins and drugs known to impair cholinergic function led to an interest in the role of neurotransmitters in delirium development and the cholinergic deficiency hypothesis of delirium. Further investigation supporting this theory found increased serum anticholinergic activity was associated with delirium and that delirious patients had decreased levels of acetylcholine in cerebrospinal fluid (CSF) and plasma [35]. Proposed mechanisms of decreased cholinergic function include impaired synthesis pathways, decreased availability of precursor molecules such as Acetyl-CoA, and altered interaction at neural synapses in the presence of anesthetic drugs or anticholinergic medications. In addition, acetylcholine is depleted in high stress and inflammatory states, and further regeneration is impaired as synthesis is downregulated. Depletion of acetylcholine may contribute to an overall state of inflammation, as vagal stimulation and acetylcholine release have been found to attenuate the systemic inflammatory response and inhibit production of proinflammatory cytokines. Specific to the inflammatory response in the brain, microglia have acetylcholine receptors that, when activated, inhibit microglia activity. Loss of regulation of microglia activity promotes neuronal inflammation and further contributes to the development of delirium.

Acetylcholine is one component of a balanced network, and disruptions in normal levels and activity of other neurotransmitters, including dopamine, norepinephrine, and serotonin, have been associated with delirium. Excess dopamine levels have been associated with symptoms of psychosis and hyperactive delirium features. This is further supported in observations of drugs that interact with dopamine receptors. Dopamine agonists are known to potentially induce psychosis, and dopamine antagonists are used to treat psychotic episodes (and increasingly used to treat delirium). In a large observational study of critically ill patients, those receiving dopamine infusion for hemodynamic support were found to have higher odds of developing delirium [54]. Norepinephrine, normally involved in alertness and arousal pathways, has been found to be elevated in patients with delirium and associated with agitation, anxiety, impaired attention, psychosis, and hyperactive delirium [28]. The role of serotonin in delirium is less well characterized. Serotonin interacts with cholinergic pathways, and elevated levels, in the setting of deficient acetylcholine, have been associated with impairment in learning and memory in animal models. In critically ill patients, Pandharipande et al. [42] found elevated plasma levels of the serotonin precursor tryptophan were associated with

delirium. Gamma-aminobutyric acid (GABA) serves as the primary mediator of inhibitory pathways in the brain, and imbalance in GABA homeostasis has been associated with delirium. Administration of GABA agonists has been associated with increased risk of transition to delirium. Conversely, patients with postoperative delirium were found to have lower levels of GABA. Further, IL-6, which has been independently associated with delirium, appears to mediate central destruction of GABA neurons. Neurotransmitter pathway interactions are highly complex and overlapping, and likely each plays a role in the pathophysiology of delirium. Much ongoing work is dedicated to clarifying these pathways and selecting targeted interventions to restore balance in states of cerebral dysfunction.

Structural Changes

Neuroimaging studies have identified cerebral atrophy and disruption of white matter integrity as common features of patients with delirium. In addition, structural changes have been found to correlate with delirium severity and long-term cognitive outcomes. ICU patients who experienced delirium have an increased ventricle-to-brain ratio indicative of brain atrophy on imaging obtained at discharge and at 3-month follow-up. Atrophy of the superior frontal lobes and hippocampus was associated with longer duration of delirium, and brain atrophy at 3-month follow-up was associated with cognitive impairment up to 12 months after discharge [22]. White matter changes in the corpus callosum and anterior limb of the internal capsule have been observed in patients with prolonged duration of delirium. Failure of these changes to resolve within 3 months of discharge was associated with cognitive decline up to 12 months after discharge [38]. In elderly patients undergoing elective major noncardiac surgery, a postoperative decrease in integrity and increase in diffusion in periventricular, frontal, and temporal white matter, when compared to preoperative magnetic resonance imaging, were associated with postoperative delirium [11].

Neurological Aging

Cancer occurs at a disproportionately higher rate in the elderly population, who are also at a higher risk for developing delirium. The aging population often demonstrates a declining physiologic reserve when compared to a younger cohort. Exposure to systemic stressors, such as cancer and critical illness, increases their susceptibility to acute brain dysfunction. Many factors are proposed to contribute to this vulnerable state. Aging is associated with a decline in brain volume and the integrity of white matter. Neuronal tissue loss has also been observed to occur over time. Another well-defined phenomenon is a decrease in cerebral blood flow with increasing age. This has been demonstrated both in comparing older populations to a younger cohort and imaging the same cohort of individuals over time. Decreased blood flow provides less oxygen and may slow metabolism, altering activity and availability of neurotransmitters. One neurotransmitter demonstrated to change over time is acetylcholine with elderly populations expressing lower levels of acetylcholine. Many changes of normal aging mirror pathologic changes associated with delirium and highlight a possible mechanism of the increased prevalence of delirium in the elderly population.

Prevention

Pain Management

Pain is a common experience for patients with cancer and for those in the ICU. One meta-analysis estimated the prevalence of pain to be 59% for patients under ongoing anticancer treatment and 64% in those with metastatic or terminal disease, with 33% experiencing ongoing pain even after curative treatment [56]. In critical illness, up to 50% of patients report pain at rest or during a procedure. The first step in effective pain management is performing a pain assessment. Several pain assessment scales are available. Visual Analogue Scales (VAS), Verbal Rating Scales (VRS), and Numerical Rating Scales (NRS) have all been validated and found to be equivalent assessments in clinical oncology research and in palliative care. A visually enlarged version of the Numerical Rating Scale (NRS-V) demonstrated comparable validity and responsiveness to other scales in critically ill patients, but a superior negative predictive value, thus making it the scale of choice in the ICU. This scale is not always feasible in the setting of sedation and mechanical ventilation, leading to an increased risk of underassessment. The Critical-Care Pain Observation Tool (CPOT) and the Behavioral Pain Scale (BPS) meet this need by allowing providers to assess pain in intubated and nonverbal patients. Guidelines recommend the use of either CPOT or BPS due to their high inter-rater reliability and validity [14].

Opioids are generally the first-line therapy for pain in the ICU. Given their potential association with delirium development, it is important for critical care providers to consider a multimodal strategy including non-opioid medications and alternative interventions such as heat or ice, cutaneous stimulation (massage), and cognitive behavioral interventions (i.e., relaxation techniques). Cancer pain therapy is guided by the World Health Organization ladder that begins with non-opioids and escalates to short- and long-acting opioid medications and adjuncts, and patients may present with ongoing pain regimens at home. It is important to continue home regimens of scheduled chronic pain medications with as needed doses for breakthrough pain to prevent a pain crisis. In the setting of critical illness, home doses may need to be adjusted for renal or hepatic compromise to prevent overdose effects from prolonged activity or metabolite buildup. Opioid requirements may be decreased by adding adjuncts like acetaminophen and nonsteroidal anti-inflammatories (NSAIDs). If pain is neuropathic in nature, opioids have limited effect, whereas gabapentanoids and tricyclic antidepressants provide superior analgesia. Ongoing assessment of pain and evaluation of medication regimens will optimize patient care and address a significant risk factor for delirium.

Sedation Management

Sedation is nearly universal in patients requiring mechanical ventilation in the ICU. Two components of sedation have been shown to directly influence delirium development: choice of sedative and depth of sedation. A wide variety of sedation medications have been studied including benzodiazepines, dexmedetomidine, propofol, and morphine. Benzodiazepines were the first-line choice of sedative for many years; however, growing evidence indicates this regimen likely promotes delirium development. Dexmedetomidine has emerged as an alternative sedative with superior outcomes. When compared to continuous infusions of lorazepam or midazolam, patients receiving dexmedetomidine were less likely to develop delirium or coma and had more days alive and free of delirium or coma [43, 45]. Given the evidence supporting increased risk of delirium, current critical care guidelines recommend avoiding benzodiazepines for sedation. Propofol has become a common choice for ICU sedation due to its rapid onset (1–2 min) and short duration of action (2–8 min). In cardiac surgery patients, comparison of dexmedetomidine to propofol has shown reduced risk of delirium development and decreased duration of delirium [16] with dexmedetomidine. Large randomized controlled trials with robust delirium outcomes are needed to compare acute and long-term brain dysfunction between these two commonly used agents for ICU sedation. Another alternative strategy is analgesic-based sedation; current studies of this strategy, however, have not extensively evaluated delirium. In one trial of cardiac surgery patients, dexmedetomidine was associated with a decreased duration of delirium when compared to a morphine-based regimen [49].

Equally important as choice of sedative, monitoring and minimizing depth of sedation are associated with improved delirium outcomes. Contrary to the paradigm of deep sedation for all mechanically ventilated patients, Kress et al. [32] found that daily interruptions of sedative infusions decreased duration of mechanical ventilation and ICU stay. Girard et al. [20] then found that coordinated spontaneous awakening and breathing trials were associated with fewer days of coma, indicating an improvement in brain dysfunction. In addition to the spontaneous awakening and breathing trials, reducing the amount or level of sedation given is protective to the brain. Protocols that target lower levels of sedation and de-escalation of sedatives are associated with decreased duration of delirium.

Early Mobilization

In addition to early beliefs that mechanically ventilated patients required deep planes of sedation, ICU patients were conventionally thought to be unable to participate in mobility activities and physical therapy. Multiple studies have dispelled this notion, proving that early initiation of activity including passive and active range of motion, bed mobility, transferring, sitting, pre-gait exercise, and walking is safe and feasible in ICU patients and associated with improved outcomes. Early mobilization protocols engage participation from nursing, respiratory therapy, and physical and occupational therapy to provide daily activity sessions coordinated with periods of interrupted sedation. In randomized controlled trials across medical and surgical ICU populations, implementation of a coordinated mobility initiative has been associated with an increase in alertness and delirium-free days, reduced incidence of delirium, and decreased sedation requirements [46, 48].

Improving Sleep

It is well established that ICU patients do not sleep often and experience poor quality of sleep. When monitored with electrosomnography, patients were found to sleep as little as 2 h per 24-h period, though in some patients, no electrophysiologic identifiable sleep was detected [3]. Sleep patterns are characterized by severe fragmentation with a high arousal index and frequent disruptions [3]. Admission to the ICU is associated with disruption in normal circadian rhythm and sleep/wake cycles with up to 60% of sleep occurring during the day and only 40% overnight. Sleep deprivation causes similar symptomatology to delirium and is postulated to be a risk factor for delirium development.

Despite the lack of direct causality between sleep deprivation and delirium, efforts to improve sleep hygiene have shown improved delirium outcomes. Three primary areas for intervention include minimizing nighttime exposure to light, sound, and awakening for care, medication, or assessment. Simple interventions including providing ear plugs and eye masks to patients overnight have been associated with reduced incidence of delirium and an increase in delirium-/coma-free days. Multidisciplinary sleep bundles that focus on reducing light and noise, minimizing patient care interactions overnight, and promoting patient orientation during daytime hours have shown similar results. Though minimizing light exposure overnight has been beneficial, dynamic light application therapy has not been shown to reduce delirium.

Pharmacologic intervention with melatonin to improve sleep has gained interest based on observations that sedated and mechanically ventilated patients exhibit impaired or even abolished circadian rhythmic melatonin secretion and abnormally low levels of melatonin secretion have been detected in mechanically ventilated patients and postoperative critically ill patients who developed delirium. Trials of melatonin and melatonin agonists have produced mixed results with regard to delirium development. In a randomized controlled trial of elderly hospitalized internal medicine patients, melatonin administration was associated with a decreased risk of developing delirium [2]. However, postoperative administration of melatonin after hip fracture repair did not alter rates of delirium [12], and a Cochrane review did not find any reduction in delirium with melatonin [52]. Interestingly, Ramelteon, a melatonin agonist, has been associated with a lower risk of delirium in a mixed ICU and acute care population [23] and a tendency toward reduced delirium in patients after lung cancer surgery [37].

Multicomponent Intervention

As risk of delirium is multifactorial and ICU patients generally have multiple risk factors for delirium, implementation of evidence-based prevention bundles, which address multiple components of risk, has been highly effective. Bundled protocols were initially developed for medical ward patients and demonstrated efficacy in reducing delirium across medical and surgical inpatients. Included components targeted maintaining patient orientation through reminders of date and time, restoring vision and hearing aids, therapeutic activities with cognitive stimulation, and non-pharmacologic sleep hygiene. Early mobilization is also a key component, and early elimination of immobilizing equipment such as catheters and restraints is emphasized to facilitate in this goal. To meet the specific needs of ICU patients, a multicomponent intervention known as the Awakening and Breathing Coordination, Delirium monitoring/management, and Early exercise/mobility ("ABCDE") bundle was developed and demonstrated a reduction in delirium incidence and duration. Given the overall success of bundles in improving patient care, the Society of Critical Care Medicine initiated the ICU Liberation Collaborative with an expanded bundle now known as the ABCDEF bundle: Assess, prevent, and manage pain; Both spontaneous awakening trials (SAT) and spontaneous breathing trials (SBT) should be performed daily; Choice of sedation; Delirium – assess, prevent, and manage; Early mobilization; and Family engagement and empowerment [36]. In a large-scale implementation trial of seven community hospitals, as compliance with the ABCDEF bundle increased, significant increases in survival and days alive without delirium or coma were observed [5]. To incorporate factors specific to oncology patients, we have adapted the ABCDEF bundle to the CANCER bundle: Choice of sedation with daily sedation holidays, Assess and treat pain, Neuromonitoring with scheduled RASS and CAM assessments, Coordination of care with families and palliative medicine, Early mobility, and treat Reversible causes common to cancer including electrolyte imbalance, dehydration, and triggering medications used to for symptom management (Fig. 2).

Pharmacologic Prophylaxis

Multiple theories on the pathophysiology of delirium have led to the study of corresponding drug interventions for delirium prophylaxis, including antipsychotics to suppress excess dopamine and neurotransmitter imbalance, acetylcholinesterase inhibitors to increase cholinergic activity, and medications with anti-inflammatory properties including statins and ketamine.

Antipsychotics have been the most widely studied intervention and have produced conflicting results. In one study of critically ill patients evaluated to be at high risk for developing delirium, 1 mg of haloperidol administered intravenously every 8 h was beneficial in reducing delirium [57]. However, when applied to the general ICU population, two randomized controlled trials, the HOPE-ICU [41] and REDUCE [58] trials, found no difference in delirium outcomes with scheduled haloperidol. In the REDUCE trial, the most recent and largest study to date of prophylactic haloperidol in ICU patients, no

difference was found in delirium incidence, delirium-free days, length of stay, or survival overall or in pre-defined subgroups including type of ICU and severity of illness. Mixed results have also been observed in the surgical population. Atypical antipsychotics have demonstrated better results, though studies are primarily in surgical patients and may not extend to the general ICU population. In elderly patients undergoing joint replacement, perioperative administration of olanzapine significantly decreased the incidence of delirium. In cardiac surgery patients, risperidone given on arrival to the ICU has been associated with decreased postoperative delirium, and in post-cardiopulmonary bypass patients who develop subsyndromal delirium, initiation of scheduled risperidone was associated with decreased conversion to clinical delirium. This was further supported in a systematic review that found second-generation antipsychotics were more beneficial in preventing delirium when compared to placebo [25].

Despite the association between anticholinergic states and delirium, attempts to increase central cholinergic supply with acetylcholinesterase inhibitors have not improved delirium outcomes. Gamberini et al. [18] initiated scheduled rivastigmine to postoperative cardiac patients with no

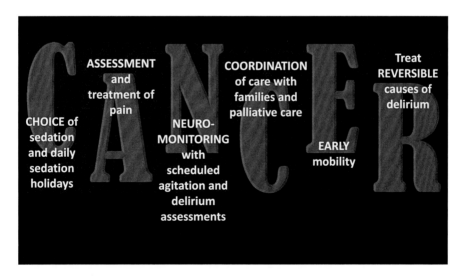

Fig. 2 Delirium prevention bundle. Multicomponent bundles, such as the one displayed, have been shown to reduce delirium and improve patient outcomes

effect on delirium development. Donepezil, an acetylcholinesterase inhibitor widely used for dementia, has also been studied in varied surgical populations with no difference in the incidence of delirium development.

Dexmedetomidine is a highly selective and potent alpha-2 agonist that is eight times more selective for the alpha-2 receptor than clonidine. It activates presynaptic alpha-2 receptors of sympathetic nerve endings, inhibiting the release of norepinephrine. Dexmedetomidine is thought to act at multiple points in the central nervous system (CNS) that are beneficial in preventing delirium. Central activity occurs at the locus ceruleus which modulates vigilance and nociceptive neurotransmission. In addition, direct action at the level of the spinal cord decreases transmission of pain signals. Importantly, the effects of dexmedetomidine on ventilation are minimal. Prophylactic dexmedetomidine for delirium prevention has been primarily studied in the surgical population. In one study of joint replacement surgery patients, a perioperative infusion of dexmedetomidine resulted in lower rates of delirium [34]. However, in a larger study of elderly noncardiac surgery patients, there was no difference in development of postoperative patients receiving a perioperative dexmedetomidine infusion with continuation for up to 2 h postoperatively when compared to usual care [13]. While results are mixed for patients receiving perioperative dexmedetomidine infusions, in a study of noncardiac patients admitted to the ICU postoperatively, dexmedetomidine infusion initiated at the time of admission and continued until 0800 the following morning was associated with a decreased incidence of delirium for up to 7 days, lower pain scores, and reduced duration of delirium [55]. In addition, a case report of intractable pain and delirium in a palliative care oncology patient was resolved with a continuous subcutaneous infusion of dexmedetomidine [24]. Prophylactic dexmedetomidine infusion has shown promise in critical care settings, though further studies are needed to confirm and characterize clinical utility.

The effects of systemic inflammation and proposed neuroinflammatory mechanism of delirium have prompted investigations into medications with known anti-inflammatory effects. Statins are known to exhibit complex pleiotropic anti-inflammatory effects including immunomodulation and enhancement of endothelial function. Similar to other pharmacologic interventions, statin use in the surgical population has demonstrated mixed results. In the ICU, continuing home statin therapy has been associated with decreased rates of delirium, and discontinuation of a home statin has been associated with an increased risk of developing delirium. Initiation of statin therapy in critically patients on mechanical ventilation, however, has not been associated any change in delirium development in randomized controlled trials. Therefore, it appears that continuing a home statin may be beneficial, but initiating new therapy in statin-naive patients is not likely to improve outcomes. Another drug of interest for its anti-inflammatory and pain control properties is ketamine. Infusion of ketamine, an N-methyl-D-aspartate (NMDA) receptor antagonist, after cardiac surgery was associated with attenuation of delirium in one randomized controlled trial [26]. However, in another trial of cardiac and noncardiac surgery patients, intraoperative administration of ketamine did not prevent postoperative delirium, and higher doses were associated with nightmares [4]. Further, in a retrospective study of patients undergoing hip and knee arthroplasty, intra- and postoperative ketamine administration was associated with increased risk of delirium [61]. Steroids are frequently a primary therapy in suppressing inflammatory states and have also been investigated for their ability to suppress inflammation and prevent delirium. In cardiac surgery, steroid administration has been trialed to reduce post-cardiopulmonary bypass inflammation and delirium; however no difference in postoperative delirium has been demonstrated in patients receiving perioperative steroids. Steroid use in the ICU has generated conflicting data regarding development of delirium. In a trial of mechanically ventilated patients in the ICU, steroid administration within the previous 24 h was associated with higher odds of developing delirium [47]. Conversely, in a cohort of ICU patients with severe sepsis, patients who received a 5-day course of hydrocortisone were less likely to develop delirium than those receiving a placebo [30]. Further work may characterize certain populations that would benefit from steroid administration. It is also important to remember that patients with metastatic or primary brain lesions may benefit from steroid administration for mass effect and edema.

Treatment

Delirium prevention should be the primary strategy for management as there are currently no FDA-approved pharmacologic treatments for delirium available, and evidence for pharmacologic options has demonstrated limited efficacy with myriad side effects. The first-line medication choice has traditionally been typical or atypical antipsychotics; large randomized controlled trials, however, are lacking, and current evidence regarding efficacy is conflicting. In a trial of critically ill patients randomized to haloperidol, ziprasidone, or placebo, there was no difference in delirium- or coma-free days between the groups [21]. This is one of the few trials currently that includes a placebo arm for comparison. Many trials have examined a difference in efficacy between different antipsychotic medications with variations in side-effect profile but no clear preferred treatment. While most of these trials demonstrate improvement in delirium symptoms over time, it is unclear as to whether the improvement results from the passing of time and resolution of underlying etiologies or medications administered, as there is often no placebo group for comparison. In a small study of palliative care patients, administration of haloperidol, risperidone, olanzapine, or aripiprazole showed equally effective reduction in delirium as measured by the MDAS over time. Patients receiving haloperidol were more likely to experience extrapyramidal symptoms, and those receiving olanzapine were more sedated [7]. Similarly, in an open trial of olanzapine for hospitalized cancer patients with delirium, symptoms resolved in 76% of patients, but 30% demonstrated sedation [9]. In a comparison between haloperidol and olanzapine in critically ill patients, delirium improved and benzodiazepine administration declined in both groups; however the haloperidol group developed extrapyramidal symptoms [53]. In a comparison

of risperidone and olanzapine in hospitalized patients (most with a primary diagnosis of cancer), both groups showed improvement over the 7-day trial without a superior treatment [31], indicating that risperidone may be used as alternative to haloperidol or olanzapine with fewer side effects. Quetiapine offers another alternative antipsychotic therapy that has been associated with improved delirium rating scores in elderly hospitalized patients with delirium. In addition, adding scheduled quetiapine (50 mg every 12 h) to as needed haloperidol in critically ill patients was associated with shorter time to resolution of delirium, decreased agitation, and increased likelihood of transfer to home instead of a rehabilitation facility [15]. A trial of multicomponent therapy targeted dopamine and acetylcholine pathways by adding rivastigmine, a centrally acting acetylcholinesterase inhibitor, to a haloperidol regimen. This study, however, was terminated due to increasing mortality trends and median duration of delirium in the rivastigmine group [59].

Antipsychotics have performed less favorably in patients with advanced cancer and terminal delirium. In one large study of palliative care patients with advanced cancer and agitated delirium, addition of risperidone or haloperidol to supportive care was associated with worse delirium symptom scores, more extrapyramidal symptoms, and worse survival in the haloperidol group when compared to placebo [1]. Another study of palliative care patients with advanced cancer, focused primarily on symptom management of agitated delirium, compared addition of lorazepam versus a placebo to haloperidol therapy and found less agitation as indicated by lower RASS scores in the group receiving haloperidol. This group also required fewer rescue neuroleptics, and caregivers and families perceived that patients receiving lorazepam were more comfortable [29]. It is important to note that patients in the group that received lorazepam were often over sedated with higher MDAS and thus reflective of agitated delirium being converted to a hypoactive form of delirium. In contrast, patients in the placebo group were more likely to remain alert and calm. While caregivers perceived that patients were more comfortable secondary to a reduction in agitation, sedation and hypoactive delirium can still be distressing to patients and reduce precious time patients may have with their loved ones at the end of their lives.

An alternative intervention that has shown promise in treating hyperactive delirium is dexmedetomidine. One trial randomized patients who were unable to be weaned from mechanical ventilation solely due to uncontrolled hyperactive delirium to a dexmedetomidine infusion versus placebo. Those receiving dexmedetomidine demonstrated more rapid resolution of delirium symptoms, shorter time to extubation, and an increase in ventilator-free hours [44]. Dexmedetomidine has also been used as a rescue therapy in non-intubated critically ill patients with agitated delirium refractory to haloperidol. In a non-randomized trial, patients found to respond to haloperidol were initiated on a haloperidol infusion, whereas non-responders received a dexmedetomidine infusion. The dexmedetomidine group demonstrated less agitation with higher quality of sedation, less oversedation, and a shorter time to ICU discharge [10]. While more randomized trials are needed, dexmedetomidine has shown promise as an intervention for delirium, particularly agitated delirium which is frequently seen in advanced cancer and distressing to patients and caregivers alike.

An important consideration for delirium management in advanced cancer patients is evaluation of opioid therapy and evaluation for opioid-related cognitive dysfunction. While the etiology is not well understood, the escalating doses of opioid often prescribed as cancer progresses are associated with a phenomenon known as opioid-induced neurotoxicity (OIN) which may manifest as delirium that is refractory to conventional therapy. Strategies for addressing OIN include opioid rotation and initiation of alternative therapies such as methadone or ketamine with the goal of adequately controlling pain, a precipitating factor for delirium, and reducing the dose of opioid administered to reduce the side-effect profile. Opioid rotation may allow for a reduction in dose, as well as removal of an opioid associated with delirium development, as illustrated in an open-label trial where patients transitioned from fentanyl to morphine demonstrated improved pain scores and improved delirium as evaluated by the MDAS

[39]. Another choice for opioid rotation is methadone, a long-acting mu-opioid agonist that also acts at NMDA receptors, is quick in onset (about 30 min), and has a half-life around 24 h. Rotation to methadone has been associated with improvement in uncontrolled pain and delirium [6, 40]. Non-opioid alternatives have also been used to treat OIN. In a case report of OIN in a hospice patient, adding a ketamine infusion allowed for rapid reduction of opioid dose with improved pain control and resolution of OIN symptoms including delirium [62].

Conclusion

Delirium is characterized by acute and rapid fluctuations in mental status and is a common diagnosis among the critically ill cancer population. The prevention of delirium in the critically ill involves multiple components including choice of pain and sedating medications, early physical and occupational therapy, improving sleep, and daily awakening and breathing trials. There are no FDA-approved pharmacologic prevention or treatment options available for delirium, though some of the antipsychotics and dexmedetomidine have shown promise in various studies. Delirium can be a challenging and deleterious diagnosis for critically ill cancer patients, but with proper recognition as well as validated preventative and management strategies, the negative consequences associated with delirium can be decreased.

References

1. Agar MR, et al. Efficacy of oral risperidone, haloperidol, or placebo for symptoms of delirium among patients in palliative care: a randomized clinical trial. JAMA Intern Med. 2017;177:34–42. https://doi.org/10.1001/jamainternmed.2016.7491.
2. Al-Aama T, Brymer C, Gutmanis I, Woolmore-Goodwin SM, Esbaugh J, Dasgupta M. Melatonin decreases delirium in elderly patients: a randomized, placebo-controlled trial. Int J Geriatr Psychiatry. 2011; 26:687–94. https://doi.org/10.1002/gps.2582.
3. Aurell J, Elmqvist D. Sleep in the surgical intensive care unit: continuous polygraphic recording of sleep in nine patients receiving postoperative care. Br Med J (Clin Res Ed). 1985;290:1029–32.

4. Avidan MS, et al. Intraoperative ketamine for prevention of postoperative delirium or pain after major surgery in older adults: an international, multicentre, double-blind, randomised clinical trial. Lancet. 2017;390:267–75. https://doi.org/10.1016/S0140-6736(17)31467-8.

5. Barnes-Daly MA, Phillips G, Ely EW. Improving hospital survival and reducing brain dysfunction at seven California community hospitals: implementing PAD guidelines Via the ABCDEF bundle in 6,064 patients. Crit Care Med. 2017;45:171–8. https://doi.org/10.1097/CCM.0000000000002149.

6. Benitez-Rosario MA, Feria M, Salinas-Martin A, Martinez-Castillo LP, Martin-Ortega JJ. Opioid switching from transdermal fentanyl to oral methadone in patients with cancer pain. Cancer. 2004;101:2866–73. https://doi.org/10.1002/cncr.20712.

7. Boettger S, Jenewein J, Breitbart W. Delirium and severe illness: etiologies, severity of delirium and phenomenological differences. Palliat Support Care. 2015;13:1087–92. https://doi.org/10.1017/S1478951514001060.

8. Breitbart W, Rosenfeld B, Roth A, Smith MJ, Cohen K, Passik S. The memorial delirium assessment scale. J Pain Symptom Manage 1997;13(3):128–37.

9. Breitbart W, Tremblay A, Gibson C. An open trial of olanzapine for the treatment of delirium in hospitalized cancer patients. Psychosomatics. 2002;43:175–82. https://doi.org/10.1176/appi.psy.43.3.175.

10. Carrasco G, Baeza N, Cabre L, Portillo E, Gimeno G, Manzanedo D, Calizaya M. Dexmedetomidine for the treatment of hyperactive delirium refractory to haloperidol in nonintubated ICU patients: a nonrandomized controlled trial. Crit Care Med. 2016;44:1295–306. https://doi.org/10.1097/CCM.0000000000001622.

11. Cavallari M, et al. Longitudinal diffusion changes following postoperative delirium in older people without dementia. Neurology. 2017;89:1020–7. https://doi.org/10.1212/WNL.0000000000004329.

12. de Jonghe A, et al. Effect of melatonin on incidence of delirium among patients with hip fracture: a multicentre, double-blind randomized controlled trial. CMAJ. 2014;186:E547–56. https://doi.org/10.1503/cmaj.140495.

13. Deiner S, et al. Intraoperative infusion of dexmedetomidine for prevention of postoperative delirium and cognitive dysfunction in elderly patients undergoing major elective noncardiac surgery: a randomized clinical trial. JAMA Surg. 2017;152:e171505. https://doi.org/10.1001/jamasurg.2017.1505.

14. Devlin JW, et al. Clinical practice guidelines for the prevention and management of pain, agitation/sedation, delirium, immobility, and sleep disruption in adult patients in the ICU. Crit Care Med. 2018;46:e825–73. https://doi.org/10.1097/CCM.0000000000003299.

15. Devlin JW, et al. Impact of quetiapine on resolution of individual delirium symptoms in critically ill patients with delirium: a post-hoc analysis of a double-blind, randomized, placebo-controlled study. Crit Care. 2011;15:R215. https://doi.org/10.1186/cc10450.

16. Djaiani G, Silverton N, Fedorko L, Carroll J, Styra R, Rao V, Katznelson R. Dexmedetomidine versus propofol sedation reduces delirium after cardiac surgery: a randomized controlled trial. Anesthesiology. 2016;124:362–8. https://doi.org/10.1097/ALN.0000000000000951.

17. Ely EW, Siegel MD, Inouye SK. Delirium in the intensive care unit: an under-recognized syndrome of organ dysfunction. Semin Respir Crit Care Med. 2001;22:115–26. https://doi.org/10.1055/s-2001-13826.

18. Gamberini M, et al. Rivastigmine for the prevention of postoperative delirium in elderly patients undergoing elective cardiac surgery – a randomized controlled trial. Crit Care Med. 2009;37:1762–8. https://doi.org/10.1097/CCM.0b013e31819da780.

19. Gaudreau JD, Gagnon P, Harel F, Roy MA, Tremblay A. Psychoactive medications and risk of delirium in hospitalized cancer patients. J Clin Oncol. 2005;23:6712–8. https://doi.org/10.1200/JCO.2005.05.140.

20. Girard TD, et al. Efficacy and safety of a paired sedation and ventilator weaning protocol for mechanically ventilated patients in intensive care (Awakening and Breathing Controlled trial): a randomised controlled trial. Lancet. 2008;371:126–34. https://doi.org/10.1016/S0140-6736(08)60105-1.

21. Girard TD, et al. Feasibility, efficacy, and safety of antipsychotics for intensive care unit delirium: the MIND randomized, placebo-controlled trial. Crit Care Med. 2010;38:428–37.

22. Gunther ML, et al. The association between brain volumes, delirium duration, and cognitive outcomes in intensive care unit survivors: the VISIONS cohort magnetic resonance imaging study*. Crit Care Med. 2012;40:2022–32. https://doi.org/10.1097/CCM.0b013e318250acc0.

23. Hatta K, et al. Preventive effects of Ramelteon on delirium: a randomized placebo-controlled trial. JAMA Psychiatry. 2014;71:397–403. https://doi.org/10.1001/jamapsychiatry.2013.3320.

24. Hilliard N, Brown S, Mitchinson S. A case report of dexmedetomidine used to treat intractable pain and delirium in a tertiary palliative care unit. Palliat Med. 2015;29:278–81. https://doi.org/10.1177/0269216314556923.

25. Hirota T, Kishi T. Prophylactic antipsychotic use for postoperative delirium: a systematic review and meta-analysis. J Clin Psychiatry. 2013;74:e1136–44. https://doi.org/10.4088/JCP.13r08512.

26. Hudetz JA, et al. Ketamine attenuates delirium after cardiac surgery with cardiopulmonary bypass. J Cardiothorac Vasc Anesth. 2009;23:651–7. https://doi.org/10.1053/j.jvca.2008.12.021.

27. Hughes CG, Pandharipande PP, Thompson JL, Chandrasekhar R, Ware LB, Ely EW, Girard TD. Endothelial activation and blood-brain barrier injury as risk factors for delirium in critically ill patients. Crit Care Med. 2016;44:e809–17. https://doi.org/10.1097/CCM.0000000000001739.

28. Hughes CG, Patel MB, Pandharipande PP. Pathophysiology of acute brain dysfunction: what's the cause of

all this confusion? Curr Opin Crit Care. 2012;18: 518–26. https://doi.org/10.1097/MCC.0b013e328357 effa.

29. Hui D, et al. Effect of lorazepam with haloperidol vs haloperidol alone on agitated delirium in patients with advanced cancer receiving palliative care: a randomized clinical trial. JAMA. 2017;318:1047–56. https://doi.org/10.1001/jama.2017.11468.

30. Keh D, et al. Effect of hydrocortisone on development of shock among patients with severe sepsis: the HYPRESS randomized clinical trial. JAMA. 2016;316:1775–85. https://doi.org/10.1001/jama.2016.14 799.

31. Kim SW, et al. Risperidone versus olanzapine for the treatment of delirium. Hum Psychopharmacol. 2010;25:298–302. https://doi.org/10.1002/hup.1117.

32. Kress JP, Pohlman AS, O'Connor MF, Hall JB. Daily interruption of sedative infusions in critically ill patients undergoing mechanical ventilation. N Engl J Med. 2000;342:1471–7. https://doi.org/10.1056/NEJM200005183422002.

33. Lawlor PG, Nekolaichuk C, Gagnon B, Mancini IL, Pereira JL, Bruera ED. Clinical utility, factor analysis, and further validation of the memorial delirium assessment scale in patients with advanced cancer: assessing delirium in advanced cancer. Cancer. 2000;88: 2859–67.

34. Liu Y, Ma L, Gao M, Guo W, Ma Y. Dexmedetomidine reduces postoperative delirium after joint replacement in elderly patients with mild cognitive impairment. Aging Clin Exp Res. 2016;28:729–36. https://doi.org/10.1007/s40520-015-0492-3.

35. Maldonado JR. Neuropathogenesis of delirium: review of current etiologic theories and common pathways. Am J Geriatr Psychiatry. 2013;21:1190–222. https://doi.org/10.1016/j.jagp.2013.09.005.

36. Marra A, Ely EW, Pandharipande PP, Patel MB. The ABCDEF bundle in critical care. Crit Care Clin. 2017;33:225–43. https://doi.org/10.1016/j.ccc.2016.1 2.005.

37. Miyata R, Omasa M, Fujimoto R, Ishikawa H, Aoki M. Efficacy of Ramelteon for delirium after lung cancer surgery. Interact Cardiovasc Thorac Surg. 2017;24:8–12. https://doi.org/10.1093/icvts/ivw297.

38. Morandi A, et al. The relationship between delirium duration, white matter integrity, and cognitive impairment in intensive care unit survivors as determined by diffusion tensor imaging: the VISIONS prospective cohort magnetic resonance imaging study*. Crit Care Med. 2012;40:2182–9. https://doi.org/10.1097/CCM.0b013e318250acdc.

39. Morita T, et al. Opioid rotation from morphine to fentanyl in delirious cancer patients: an open-label trial. J Pain Symptom Manage. 2005;30:96–103. https://doi.org/10.1016/j.jpainsymman.2004.12.010.

40. Moryl N, Kogan M, Comfort C, Obbens E. Methadone in the treatment of pain and terminal delirium in advanced cancer patients. Palliat Support Care. 2005; 3:311–7.

41. Page VJ, et al. Effect of intravenous haloperidol on the duration of delirium and coma in critically ill patients (Hope-ICU): a randomised, double-blind, placebo-controlled trial. Lancet Respir Med. 2013;1:515–23.

42. Pandharipande PP, Morandi A, Adams JR, Girard TD, Thompson JL, Shintani AK, Ely EW. Plasma tryptophan and tyrosine levels are independent risk factors for delirium in critically ill patients. Intensive Care Med. 2009;35:1886–92. https://doi.org/10.1007/s00134-009-1573-6.

43. Pandharipande PP, et al. Effect of sedation with dexmedetomidine vs lorazepam on acute brain dysfunction in mechanically ventilated patients: the MENDS randomized controlled trial. JAMA. 2007;298:2644–53. https://doi.org/10.1001/jama.298.22.2 644.

44. Reade MC, et al. Effect of dexmedetomidine added to standard care on ventilator-free time in patients with agitated delirium: a randomized clinical trial. JAMA. 2016;315:1460–8. https://doi.org/10.1001/jama.2016.2707.

45. Riker RR, et al. Dexmedetomidine vs midazolam for sedation of critically ill patients: a randomized trial. JAMA. 2009;301:489–99. https://doi.org/10.1001/jama.2009.56.

46. Schaller SJ, et al. Early, goal-directed mobilisation in the surgical intensive care unit: a randomised controlled trial. Lancet. 2016;388:1377–88. https://doi.org/10.1016/S0140-6736(16)31637-3.

47. Schreiber MP, et al. Corticosteroids and transition to delirium in patients with acute lung injury. Crit Care Med. 2014;42:1480–6. https://doi.org/10.1097/CCM.0000000000000247.

48. Schweickert WD, et al. Early physical and occupational therapy in mechanically ventilated, critically ill patients: a randomised controlled trial. Lancet. 2009;373:1874–82. https://doi.org/10.1016/S0140-6736(09)60658-9.

49. Sessler CN, Gosnell MS, Grap MJ, Brophy GM, O'Neal PV, Keane KA, Tesoro EP, Elswick RK. The richmond agitation-sedation scale: validity and reliability in adult intensive care unit patients. Am J Respir Crit Care Med. 2002;166(10):1338–1344.

50. Shehabi Y, Grant P, Wolfenden H, Hammond N, Bass F, Campbell M, Chen J. Prevalence of delirium with dexmedetomidine compared with morphine based therapy after cardiac surgery: a randomized controlled trial (DEXmedetomidine COmpared to Morphine-DEXCOM Study). Anesthesiology. 2009;111:1075–84. https://doi.org/10.1097/ALN.0b013e3181b6 a783.

51. Shiiba M, Takei M, Nakatsuru M, Bukawa H, Yokoe H, Uzawa K, Tanzawa H. Clinical observations of postoperative delirium after surgery for oral carcinoma. Int J Oral Maxillofac Surg. 2009;38:661–5. https://doi.org/10.1016/j.ijom.2009.01.011.

52. Siddiqi N, Harrison JK, Clegg A, Teale EA, Young J, Taylor J, Simpkins SA. Interventions for preventing delirium in hospitalised non-ICU patients. Cochrane Database Syst Rev. 2016;3:CD005563. https://doi.org/10.1002/14651858.CD005563.pub3.

53. Skrobik YK, Bergeron N, Dumont M, Gottfried SB. Olanzapine vs haloperidol: treating delirium in a

critical care setting. Intensive Care Med. 2004;30:444–9. https://doi.org/10.1007/s00134-003-2117-0.

54. Sommer BR, Wise LC, Kraemer HC. Is dopamine administration possibly a risk factor for delirium? Crit Care Med. 2002;30:1508–11.

55. Su X, et al. Dexmedetomidine for prevention of delirium in elderly patients after non-cardiac surgery: a randomised, double-blind, placebo-controlled trial. Lancet. 2016. https://doi.org/10.1016/S0140-6736 (16)30580-3.

56. van den Beuken-van Everdingen MH, de Rijke JM, Kessels AG, Schouten HC, van Kleef M, Patijn J. Prevalence of pain in patients with cancer: a systematic review of the past 40 years. Ann Oncol. 2007;18: 1437–49. https://doi.org/10.1093/annonc/mdm056.

57. van den Boogaard M, Schoonhoven L, van Achterberg T, van der Hoeven JG, Pickkers P. Haloperidol prophylaxis in critically ill patients with a high risk for delirium. Crit Care. 2013;17:R9. https://doi.org/10.1186/cc11933.

58. van den Boogaard M, et al. Effect of haloperidol on survival among critically ill adults with a high risk of delirium: the REDUCE randomized clinical trial. JAMA. 2018;319:680–90. https://doi.org/10.1001/jama.2018.0160.

59. van Eijk MM, et al. Effect of rivastigmine as an adjunct to usual care with haloperidol on duration of delirium and mortality in critically ill patients: a multicentre, double-blind, placebo-controlled randomised trial. Lancet. 2010;376:1829–37. https://doi.org/10.1016/S0140-6736(10)61855-7.

60. Vasunilashorn SM, et al. High C-reactive protein predicts delirium incidence, duration, and feature severity after major noncardiac surgery. J Am Geriatr Soc. 2017;65:e109–16. https://doi.org/10.1111/jgs.14913.

61. Weinstein SM, et al. Postoperative delirium in total knee and hip arthroplasty patients: a study of perioperative modifiable risk factors. Br J Anaesth. 2018;120: 999–1008. https://doi.org/10.1016/j.bja.2017.12.046.

62. Winegarden J, Carr DB, Bradshaw YS. Intravenous ketamine for rapid opioid dose reduction, reversal of opioid-induced neurotoxicity, and pain control in terminal care: case report and literature review. Pain Med. 2016;17:644–9. https://doi.org/10.1111/pme.12865.

Medication-Induced Neurotoxicity in Critically Ill Cancer Patients

Monica E. Loghin and Anne Kleiman

Contents

Chemotherapy-Induced Neurotoxicity 320
Introduction 320
Vinca Alkaloids 320
Taxanes 321
Platinum Analogues 321
Antimetabolites 322
Other Antimetabolites 323
Other 323
Management 323
Future Directions 324

Opiates-Induced Neurotoxicity 324
Introduction 324
Etiology 325
Epidemiology 325
Pathophysiology 325
Clinical Manifestations and Management 326
Sedation and Drowsiness 326
Delirium and Cognitive Impairment 326
Myoclonus 327
Opioid-Induced Hyperalgesia (OIH) 327
Future Directives 327

Antiepileptic Drugs-Induced Neurotoxicity 327
Introduction 327
Epidemiology 327
Pathophysiology 328
Clinical Manifestations 328
Management of AED Neurotoxicity 328
Future Directives 329

M. E. Loghin (✉) · A. Kleiman
Department of Neuro-Oncology, The University of Texas
MD Anderson Cancer Center, Houston, TX, USA
e-mail: mloghin@mdanderson.org;
AKleiman@mdanderson.org

© This is a U.S. government work and not under copyright protection in the U.S.;
foreign copyright protection may apply 2020
J. L. Nates, K. J. Price (eds.), *Oncologic Critical Care*,
https://doi.org/10.1007/978-3-319-74588-6_32

Immunosuppressants Neurotoxicity 329
  Introduction 329
  Epidemiology 329
  Pathophysiology 330
  Clinical Manifestations 330
  Neuroimaging 331
  Management 331
  Future Directions 331

References 332

Abstract

Neurotoxicity associated with cancer treatment and treatment for medical and surgical complications of cancer have been well recognized. Elderly patients, advanced cancer, concomitant polypharmacy, organ failure, and medical comorbidities are all confounders contributing to adverse events related to cancer therapy. Short-term and long-term neurotoxicities may lead to disabilities and poor quality of life in patients with cancer. As a result of early detection of cancer and advances in treatment, cancer survival rates have improved consistently over the last decades and thus long-term survivors may face physical and psychological challenges associated with cancer and cancer treatment. As such, understanding the pathogenic mechanisms, optimizing the strategies for clinical assessment and interventions for the management and prevention of medication-related neurotoxicity is of paramount importance in patient care.

This chapter will address the neurotoxicity induced by a number of drug classes commonly used in the treatment of cancer patients.

Keywords

Chemotherapy · Opiates · Antiepileptic drugs · Immunosuppressive drugs

Chemotherapy-Induced Neurotoxicity

Introduction

Neurotoxicity with chemotherapy is common and frequently the driving factor in limiting a course of treatment for malignancy. Although peripheral nervous system toxicity, led by peripheral neuropathy, is more common, central nervous system complications occur and more often require emergency management. Identifying toxicity early by optimizing clinical assessment and dose adjusting in a timely manner will decrease long-term sequelae of therapy. This becomes more critical and relevant as more people survive cancer and the sequelae of their treatments become more apparent.

Vinca Alkaloids

The vinca alkaloids cause their cellular effects through interacting with tubulin, the protein composing microtubules in cells and through their interaction preventing microtubule assembly. Their efficacy as an anticancer agent comes from disrupting microtubules necessary to form a mitotic spindle in cells that are actively dividing resulting in an arrest in the M phase of the cell cycle and specifically during metaphase. In rapidly proliferating cancer cells, this may result in desired cellular toxicity. The neurologic toxicity that results from binding tubulin requires microtubules for axonal transport, and this binding results in neuropathy. The toxicity is primarily peripheral, related in large part to these drugs not crossing the blood brain barrier, but central nervous system toxicity occurs as well.

Vincristine causes a peripheral neuropathy which is typically dose-dependent and cumulative. The onset is usually with sensory impairment and paresthesias in a glove and stocking distribution. But, mononeuropathy with wrist and foot drop or loss of deep tendon reflexes may occur. The sensory deficit is mostly reversible over months where the motor deficit is mostly irreversible. In clinical practice, many will continue vincristine in spite of loss of deep tendon reflexes and function. It is most typically when foot drop occurs both related to loss of position sense and motor strength that physicians will cease to administer additional vincristine in an attempt to avoid this becoming permanent.

With the first dose of vincristine, jaw pain is very typical and can be severe. It generally is refractory to traditional pain medications as it is neuropathic in origin. This symptom is usually related to damage to sensory nerves rather than true recovery. Occasionally, muscle cramps can herald the onset of the sensory symptoms. Sensory symptoms can also progress after drug is discontinued. Vincristine can affect cranial nerves causing facial palsy, diplopia, hoarseness, and pharyngeal or parotid pain. The aforementioned jaw pain is related to cranial nerve effects. Hearing and visual loss can occur as well. Vincristine can cause an autonomic neuropathy presenting with abdominal pain and cramping and constipation. In some instances, paralytic ileus or urinary retention may occur with single high doses in patients with hepatic impairment. More often this accumulates over time and some would view constipation as a relative contraindication for the administration of additional vincristine, at least until it has resolved as progression from constipation to ileus is well described. Other autonomic symptoms include orthostatic hypotension, arterial hypotension or hypertension [1].

Much less frequent central nervous system toxicity can present as confusion, agitation, hallucinations, seizures, parkinsonism, and hyponatremia from SIADH [2–8]. These usually improve after drug cessation.

Finally, intrathecal injection of vinca alkaloids, like vincristine, is lethal and well documented [9].

Other vinca alkaloids, such as vinblastine, vindesine, and vinorelbine, are overall less neurotoxic but have been reported to have similar side effects to vincristine with vinorelbine the least toxic.

Taxanes

Related to the vinca alkaloids, the taxanes similarly interfere with microtubule function but in this case, impacting microtubule disassembly rather than assembly. As this is the case, the impact of taxanes is slightly later in the M phase of the cell cycle. Their interaction with microtubules prevents anterograde axonal transport leading to its major toxicity of peripheral neuropathy. The incidence is affected by individual and total dose as well as rate of infusion and interaction with other cytotoxic chemotherapies. Examples of the taxanes include Paclitaxel and Docetaxel. Their neuropathy is mostly sensory, distal more than proximal and if severe will affect all sensory modalities and deep tendon reflexes. Symptoms can progress after the drug is discontinued. Uncommon are seizures, encephalopathy, Lhermitte sign, and stroke [10]. Rarely itching can be a manifestation of neuropathy as can joint or muscle pain [11]. Finally, separation of nail from nail beds can occur with use of these drugs. It is probably neurogenic in origin [12].

Platinum Analogues

Platinum therapies can cause both central and peripheral dysfunction. Cisplatin is the most commonly used platinum analogue. Its neurotoxicity is a close second to its renal toxicity. The mechanism of neurotoxicity might be related to cisplatin's disruption of normal cobalt metabolism – an important cofactor for vitamin B12 which is essential for nerve health. DNA is the cytotoxic target of cisplatin. Cisplatin directly forms a covalent bond linking DNA strands leading to mutations most of which will be deleterious and result in cell death. Cancer cells presumably have less time to repair DNA damage between cell cycles likely accounting for their relative sparing of normal cells compared to cancer cells. Since Schwann cells make myelin and are the only cells in peripheral nerve with DNA, then their loss could explain segmental demyelination seen in cisplatin-related peripheral neuropathy [13, 14]. Although peripheral neuropathy is the most common platinum-based neurotoxicity, hearing loss occurs frequently along with other less frequent toxicities such as visual impairment, including the rarer retrobulbar neuritis, papilledema, cortical blindness, and seizures.

The peripheral neuropathy presents in a classic glove and stocking in distribution, it is dose-dependent, related to both individual and cumulative dose. Sensory symptoms like numbness, tingling, and neuropathic pain predominate and strength is usually spared. Symptoms usually occur during treatment but may continue to progress afterwards and peak several months after therapy has been completed. This is a challenge when considering dose adjustment. There is gradual recovery for most over time but it is often partial with residual sensory, large fiber deficit. Infrequently patients may develop demyelination of the posterior columns which presents as a Lhermitte sign – electrical feelings down the back and into the extremities that is transient without permanent sequelae [10].

Hearing loss is usually in the high frequency range and related to the loss of outer hair cells on the cochlea. It is often heralded by tinnitus and is not reversible [15]. It can be compounded when given in conjunction with cranial radiation. It can also be exacerbated by concomitant administration of aminoglycosides. The hearing loss is almost invariable but predictably begins in high frequency and progresses from there.

Stroke syndromes have been reported when cisplatin has been given with other chemotherapy [16]. Carboplatin has much milder neurotoxicity. In high-dose regimens, peripheral neuropathy and ototoxicity may occur. Oxaliplatin can also cause a peripheral neuropathy, sometimes in an acute presentation with jaw tightening and paresthesias. It can cause painful muscle cramps as well.

Finally, other extremely rare platinum toxicities which have been reported are a myasthenic syndrome, autonomic neuropathy, and encephalopathy [17]. Considering these in an ICU setting may allow for better understanding of complex clinical pictures in the critically ill oncology patient.

Antimetabolites

Methotrexate is the prototypical antimetabolite that inhibits the synthesis of DNA and RNA, through its inhibition of dihydrofolate reducatase.

Dihydrofolate reducatase is an enzyme that produces a cofactor that is essential for thymidine production. Methotrexate also inhibits several enzymes in purine biosynthesis with a lower binding affinity. It can cause acute, subacute, and delayed neurotoxicity and varies with the dose and route of administration. Unlike the platinum-based and vinca-based therapies, its toxicity is limited to the central nervous system.

High dose intravenous methotrexate treatment may cause transient encephalopathy, including posterior reversible encephalopathy syndrome, chronic leukoencephalopathy, or stroke-like syndromes. The encephalopathy often presents after the second or third cycle of treatment and several days after the infusion. The symptoms usually resolve after a few days and do not preclude giving the drug again. The occurrence of this toxicity and its etiology are idiosyncratic and poorly understood.

It is understood, however, that leucovorin is used after methotrexate administration to reduce or prevent toxicity and is most effective when given in the first 24–48 h.

Chronic leukoencephalopathy can occur with repeated high dose exposure and presents with gradual progression of cognitive decline. It can stabilize or progress with devastating outcomes including dementia, weakness, or coma. Magnetic resonance imaging (MRI) can demonstrate abnormalities on the FLAIR sequences, typically diffuse bilateral periventricular white matter changes. Electroencephalogram (EEG) will demonstrate slowing. These impacts may be permanent. Cranial radiation can potentiate the leukoencephalopathy. Low-dose intravenous methotrexate can cause cognitive impairment, headaches, and/or dizziness which are usually transient. There has been a report of reversible posterior leukoencephalopathy syndrome with oral methotrexate [18].

Intrathecal methotrexate can also present with acute, subacute, or chronic sequelae. Acute intrathecal toxicity manifests as a chemical arachnoiditis with headache, vomiting, fever, and nuchal rigidity. Cerebrospinal fluid (CSF) analysis may demonstrate an inflammatory cell pleocytosis. A dose reduction or decrease in frequency may alleviate these symptoms. Sub-acute intrathecal toxicity may appear during the second or third week of treatment, often in patients with active meningeal leukemia, and present as cranial nerve deficits, seizures, or coma. Weakness of the extremities from lumbosacral radiculopathy occurs infrequently as well. Finally, chronic intrathecal toxicity may also present as a leukoencephalopathy.

Other Antimetabolites

Fludarabine, cytarabine, and nelarabine can cause also neurotoxicity. They are adenosine analogues which act to inhibit DNA synthesis. It is rare, but fludarabine can cause an irreversible syndrome of cortical blindness associated with encephalopathy, seizures, coma, or optic neuritis has been seen in patients receiving high doses. At lower doses, milder reversible symptoms can be seen. These include sedation and headache. Patients who receive high doses may become severely immunosuppressed putting them at risk for progressive multifocal leukoencephalopathy (PML) [19].

Cytarabine may cause an aseptic meningitis when given intrathecally. It is also infrequently responsible for a cerebellar and cerebral syndrome consisting of slurred speech, unsteady gait, dementia, and coma [20]. It is reversible over time unless there is permanent destruction to the Purkinje cells in the cerebellum. Peripheral nervous system toxicity is extremely rare but has been reported, including brachial plexopathy [21, 22].

Nelarabine can cause encephalopathy with a range of symptoms including somnolence, headache, memory loss, seizures, tremor, and weakness. Peripheral neuropathy can develop in a very small number of patients as well. Dose adjustment or cessation may be necessary and the only means to offset toxicity.

Mercaptopurine, thioguanine, and azathioprine are guanine analogs which directly are not neurotoxic. Mercaptopurine can rarely cause hepatotoxicity and therefore a related encephalopathy.

Other

Ifosfamide and cyclophosphamide are two of the more commonly used alkylating agents in the nitrogen mustard group. Ifosfamide may cause uncommon reversible encephalopathy. It is sometimes associated with seizures, hallucinations, extrapyramidal or cerebellar dysfunction. For unclear reasons, patients improve when treated with methylene blue. Cyclophosphamide has little neurotoxicity except in rare cases at high doses. In these instances, seizures and lethargy has been reported [23]. Oral cyclophosphamide can uncommonly cause confusion and blurry vision [24].

Temozolamide, another alkylator, acts by methylating nucleic acids rendering DNA abnormal and cytotoxic. It has very good penetration across the blood brain barrier. Rarely has it been associated with blurry vision, seizures, or confusion but this is difficult to separate from the underlying brain tumor for which it is being prescribed [25].

Hydroxyurea inhibits ribonucleotide reductase required for DNA synthesis. Neurotoxicity is rare and however has been associated with encephalopathy, headache, and dizziness.

The nitrosoureas including carmustine and lomustine do not have any significant neurotoxicity.

Bortezomib is a proteasome inhibitor used in multiple myeloma. Its primary adverse effect is peripheral neuropathy which is painful and dose-dependent. Predominantly large sensory fibers are affected but the symptoms are often reversible over time. Carfilzomib, a second generation proteasome inhibitor, has less toxicity. Central nervous system adverse effects are rare but include encephalopathy, language disturbance, and dizziness.

Management

Chemotherapy-induced neurotoxicity causes both central and peripheral nervous system dysfunction. Rapid identification and management of neurologic adverse effects most benefits each patient.

There is no known therapy which effectively and safely prevents peripheral neurotoxicity from chemotherapy. Active surveillance to identify toxicity and then begin dose reductions or drug cessation rapidly are necessary to limit toxicity. Patient reported outcomes usually reveal greater neurotoxicity than clinician assessment. When peripheral neuropathy is not well explained or appears out of proportion to an offending agent, then a neurology consult may be helpful. It is prudent to take a thorough history looking for comorbidity which might be augmenting chemotherapy-induced peripheral neuropathy. Check labs for the most common offenders, like B12 deficiency and diabetes mellitus. Obtain a thorough alcohol history, risk factors for HIV and hereditary neuropathy. Electromyography (EMG) can better characterize a neuropathy and add information supporting or refuting the suspected etiology or etiologies. A demyelinating neuropathy supported by EMG would prompt further evaluation for a possible immune-mediated process. Since neuroprotective agents have not been found to be effective, medical management is the best option for now.

Symptomatic relief with gabapentin, pregabalin, tricyclic antidepressants, and combination SSRI/SNRIs is possible.

More recently, Scrambler therapy has demonstrated promise as a nonpharmacological approach to treating pain and specifically chemotherapy-induced peripheral neuropathy. It treats pain by noninvasive cutaneous electrostimulation. The understanding is that transmission of pain signals will be blocked and allow the plasticity of the brain to not ascribe pain to the chronic pain area [26].

Early intervention with physical therapy to compensate for gait abnormalities or deficits related to mononeuropathies is helpful. Bracing may be necessary for foot drop induced by mononeuropathy, more frequent with vincristine.

Aggressive bowel regimens for chemotherapy-induced constipation, again common with vincristine, will help.

Oncologists routinely monitor audiograms while patients are treated with cisplatin and will cease treatment early if hearing loss encroaches on the range encompassed by normal speech as this will result in greater functional deficits including dysarthria. Some drugs have been tested in attempts to ameliorate the toxicity of cisplatin including amifostine [27]. These generally have not become standard of care as they are associated with other side effects such as emetogenicity and an unproven efficacy.

With the central nervous system (CNS) neurotoxicity including encephalopathy or seizures, other common contributing factors should be looked for, such as intraparenchymal or leptomeningeal metastatic disease or infection.

Future Directions

There are now millions of cancer survivors worldwide. The estimate of those with long-term adverse effects of therapies is expected to increase as we better identify disability. This can be achieved by adopting standardized clinician assessment as well as clinician-driven patient reporting of outcomes. Objective tools are available but not widely adopted yet for assessing peripheral neuropathy. These include the Total Neuropathy Score (TNS) for clinicians and the Patient Neurotoxicity Questionnaire (PNQ) for patients [28]. Long-term neurotoxicity is underappreciated and impacts on function and quality of life. Therefore, long-term follow-up is needed. Despite intensive research efforts to prevent chemotherapy-induced peripheral neuropathy, there lacks a suitable target for identifying neuroprotective pharmacological intervention. Improved understanding of the pathophysiology behind these adverse effects will drive the development of future neuroprotective strategies.

Opiates-Induced Neurotoxicity

Introduction

Most patients with cancer experience some degree of pain during their disease and up to 70–80% of patients with advanced stages of cancer experience significant pain. According to World Health

Organization guidelines for treatment of pain based on a "3-step analgesic ladder" algorithm, opioid analgesics constitute the cornerstone of analgesic therapy. Numerous factors, including patient characteristics, disease progression, opioid metabolites, and development of tolerance, may influence opioid responsiveness and occurrence of side effects.

Etiology

The opioids are metabolized by the liver and excreted via the kidney and thus renal or hepatic dysfunction may cause elevated concentrations of the drug which in turn may induce central nervous system toxicity. The neurotoxicity induced by opioid analgesics has been attributed to opioid metabolites such as morphine-3 glucuronide (M3G) or morphine-6-glucuronide (M6G) [29]. The overall analgesia and adverse events induced by opioids are variable and depend on the subtype of receptors stimulated by each opioid, individual opioid-receptor profile, and genetic expression of enzymes responsible for the metabolism of opioids [30]. Predisposition factors for opioid-induced neurotoxicity (OIN) have been studied and reported as long-term opioid use at high doses, rapid dose escalation, renal impairment, advanced age, dehydration, concurrent treatment with other drugs, and underlying brain disease or prior cognitive impairment [31].

Epidemiology

Data about tolerability of opioids and their adverse effects are scarce. A systematic review of prospective studies reporting adverse events (AE) of opioids for cancer-related pain reported variable rates of AE, as a result of large heterogeneity among the studies, and lack of methodical assessment of AE [32]. Drowsiness was reported from 18 studies with a rate ranging from 3% to 88%, while confusion, reported in only 5 studies, had an occurrence rate ranging from 7% to 80% [33, 34]. The incidence of delirium in cancer patients ranges between 25% and 40%

and increases up to 80% in terminally ill patients [35]. The reported incidence of myoclonus in cancer patients ranges from 3% to 87% and has been associated with opioids long-term use and high doses [36].

The effects of opioids on cognitive and psychomotor functions have not been well studied and the evidence is conflicting, as a result of multiple confounding variables in cancer population. In a consecutive admission series, the reported incidence of cognitive impairment in cancer patients ranged from 14% to 29% [37]. The opioid-induced hyperalgesia (OIH), defined as increased pain sensitivity, is associated with chronic opioid therapy. The true incidence of OIH is unknown as a result of paucity of literature. It can occur in patients who are receiving high doses of opioid intraoperatively or former opioid addicts who are on methadone maintenance [38]. Grand mal seizures have been reported in patients on parenteral high dose of morphine and may be related to preservatives in the solution.

Pathophysiology

Mechanisms of opioid-induced neurotoxicity are not fully understood. Neurotoxicity can occur with any opioid, but it is more commonly induced by opioids with active metabolites, such as meperidine, codeine, morphine, and to a lesser degree hydromorphone [39]. Meperidine-associated excitatory toxicities, such as seizures, myoclonus, and tremors, are believed to be induced by accumulation of active metabolite normeperidine [40]. All opioid analgesics work by binding to three major receptors, the mu, kappa, and delta receptors, located along the nociceptive pathways, including both peripheral and central nervous system. Most of the opioids act through mu receptors activation, causing both analgesic and euphoric effects. Morphine is metabolized into two active metabolites: morphine-3-glucuronide (M3G) and morphine-6-glucuronide (M6G). M6G binds to the mu receptor inducing analgesic effect, while M3G is not an agonist at opioid receptors and has been implicated in causing opioid-induced hyperalgesia and convulsions

[38]. Morphine metabolites are eliminated through the kidney and thus renal dysfunction induces accumulation of these metabolites, increasing the risk for neurotoxicity. Opioid analgesics antagonize other nonopioid receptors, such as N-methyl-D-aspartate (NMDA) receptors, and activate the serotonin and noradrenaline pathways in the brainstem, all of which induce analgesia by blocking the nociceptive transmission [41]. The overall analgesia and adverse events induced by opioids are variable and depend on the subtype of receptors stimulated by each opioid, individual opioid-receptor profile, genetic expression of enzymes responsible for the metabolism of opioids, as well as previous medical conditions, such as dehydration, nausea/vomiting, or renal impairment.

The central anticholinergic effect of morphine causing an imbalance in the dopaminergic/cholinergic system in the CNS has been considered a possible etiology for delirium in cancer patients [42]. Sedation and drowsiness is the result of opioid multiple inhibitory effects on cerebral activity, particularly on cholinergic pathways [43]. Myoclonus has been associated with chronic use of high doses opioids. It has been postulated that myoclonus could be mediated by an inhibition of glycine in dorsal horns neurons or perhaps through serotoninergic and GABA aminergic pathways in the brain stem. Another potential mechanism is indirect activation of the NMDA receptors [44]. The mechanisms responsible for OIH are complex and yet to be elucidated. The central glutaminergic system mediating the sensitization of spinal neurons via excitatory NMDA receptors is the most common explanation [45]. Other described mechanisms include spinal dynorphins and release of spinal excitatory neuropeptides, activation of facilitative descending pathways, decreased reuptake, and enhanced nociceptive response [46].

Clinical Manifestations and Management

Opioid-induced neurotoxicity is a syndrome of neuropsychiatry toxicity presenting with a variety of symptoms that can develop as a single feature or in any combination and order. Opiates can impair the level of consciousness (e.g., sedation, drowsiness), the mental process (e.g., cognitive and psychomotor impairment, delirium, hallucinations), or can cause a direct toxic effect on neurons.

Sedation and Drowsiness

Most commonly occur at initiation of opioid therapy or with rapid dose escalation. Comorbidities such as dementia, metabolic encephalopathy, or medications, (e.g., antidepressants, antihistamines, and anxiolytics) can contribute to sedation or reduce the opioid metabolism and thus increase or even prolong the opioid side effects for protracted periods. Management of persistent sedation is a stepwise approach including reducing the opioid dose minimizing polypharmacy, adding a psychostimulant such as methylphenidate or rotation to an alternate opioid [47]. For severe opioid-induced sedation, with respiratory depression, pinpoint pupils and hypotension, naloxone, an opioid antagonist, can be used in small doses with careful monitoring of the patient.

Delirium and Cognitive Impairment

Cognitive impairment and delirium occur frequently in terminally ill patients and has an underlying multifactorial etiology. Initiation of opioid analgesia or rapidly escalation doses of opioids are considered precipitation factors for delirium. Dehydration, organ failure, infection, disease process, previous cognitive deficits are often contributing factors, thus making difficult to determine the degree to which opioids contribute to delirium [48]. Management of delirium and cognitive impairment is a multistep strategy, first eliminating other causes, such as metabolic encephalopathy, reducing the dose of or rotating to an alternate opioid, and discontinuation of psychoactive medications. Pharmacological treatment of delirium involves the use of antipsychotics, of which haloperidol is considered first-line therapy especially for patients with agitated delirium. Atypical antipsychotics such as olanzapine, risperidone, and quetiapine have been used for delirium as well [42]. Cholinesterase inhibitors, e.g., donepezil or trazodone have been reported as potential treatment for delirium [43]. Benzodiazepines are not generally recommended, as a result of excessive sedation, and paradoxical exacerbation of delirium.

Myoclonus

Myoclonus or sudden, rapid involuntary jerking of a muscle or group of muscles is a symptom deriving from cortex, brainstem, or even spinal cord locations. The risk for myoclonus is increased with high doses of opioids, use of meperidine, and renal impairment. In mild to moderate cases, observation alone, dose reduction or opioid rotation maybe sufficient to alleviate symptoms. If severe, pharmacological therapy with benzodiazepines, muscle relaxants, or anticonvulsants has been recommended [44].

Opioid-Induced Hyperalgesia (OIH)

It is defined as increased sensitivity to pain, from painful or normal stimuli. OIH should be suspected when pain is escalating with an increase in opioid dose. Treatment of OIH is challenging and includes opioid rotation, use of nonopioid therapy, or use of NMDA antagonists.

Future Directives

Opioid-induced neurotoxicity occurs frequently in cancer population, commonly within the context of advanced disease and associated comorbidities. Methodical clinical assessment, management of concurrent acute or chronic medical conditions, opioid switch or dose reduction can achieve reversal of neurotoxicity in a significant number of cases. Further strategies and research initiatives are needed to develop

predictive models for neurotoxicity, as well as new approaches for prevention and treatment of drug-induced neurotoxicity in cancer patients. Prospective clinical trials incorporating pharmacogenetics and pharmacogenomics studies have the potential to tailor the best regimen for opioid-induced neurotoxicity.

Antiepileptic Drugs-Induced Neurotoxicity

Introduction

Antiepileptic drugs (AED) are commonly used in cancer patients, not only to manage seizures but also to treat other conditions, such as neuropathic pain, migraine headaches, and mood disturbances. Due to their complex pharmacokinetics, high potential for drug–drug interactions, and a narrow therapeutic window, AED are among the most common drug classes to induce neurotoxicity.

Epidemiology

The frequency of AED-related neurotoxicity in cancer population is overall similar to the general epilepsy population. Adverse events have been reported more frequently in patients on polytherapy and patients treated with older AED (e.g., phenytoin and phenobarbital) [49]. Dizziness and ataxia are among the most common side effects of AED. Data from several safety trials indicated that phenytoin, phenobarbital, and carbamazepine are more likely to cause dizziness or imbalance than newer AED (e.g., lamotrigine, gabapentin, or levetiracetam) [50]. Other susceptibility factors, such as individual pharmacokinetics, age, polytherapy, previous cerebellar atrophy, may contribute to the occurrence of neurotoxicity. AED-related cognitive side effects such as psychomotor slowing, executive problems, and memory impairment have been well documented in the literature [51]. In a retrospective study of nearly 1200 patients with focal seizures, the "intolerable cognitive" side effects reported by patients occurred more frequently with topiramate (21.5%) but also with carbamazepine (9.9%), gabapentine (7.3%), levetiracetam (10.4%), valproate (8.3%), and lamotrigine (8.9%) [52]. Dose-related tremor is a common side effect of valproic acid (VPA) and has been reported in 10–20% of cases [53]. Parkinsonism is a rare but potential severe adverse event of VPA treatment and is likely dose-dependent [54].

Pathophysiology

Experimental studies have documented Purkinje cell loss and swelling of Bergmann's glia with acute phenytoin toxicity [55]. Few reports indicated that cerebellar ataxia may occur with chronic therapeutic range-phenytoin therapy and suggested folate deficiency as a possible pathogenic mechanism [56]. Cerebellar atrophy with or without cerebellar symptoms has been identified by using computed tomography (CT) or MRI in several studies on patients with long-term phenytoin therapy [57]. Valproate-induced tremor may involve disturbances of dopamine and catecholamine neurotransmitters [58]. VPA-related parkinsonism may be induced by oxidative stress and mitochondrial dysfunction or through GABAergic mechanism in the basal ganglia [59].

Clinical Manifestations

Almost every single AED has a potential risk to induce CNS adverse events (Table 1). A variety of symptoms such as dizziness, somnolence, ataxia, imbalance, behavioral and mood changes, cognitive impairment have been frequently related to AED use. Phenobarbital and topiramate have the highest risk for causing cognitive adverse effects, including impairment of executive function and memory, word finding difficulties, and processing speed slowing [60, 61]. Dizziness and ataxia are common side effects of phenytoin, carbamazepine, and phenobarbital and they are often dose-dependent [56]. Current evidence shows a low incidence of dizziness and ataxia associated with the use of newer AED's such as lamotrigine, levetiracetam, or zonisamide. The tremor observed in patients receiving valproic acid treatment is often an action and postural tremor, although a resting tremor sometimes associated with extrapyramidal symptoms has been reported [62].

Management of AED Neurotoxicity

Management of AED adverse events in cancer patients is a complex and challenging process. Most AED should be started at a low dose and titrated up slowly. Screening for neurotoxicity symptoms should be considered shortly after initiation of AED as well as during the chronic

Table 1 CNS adverse events of commonly used AED in cancer patients

Drug	Dose frequency	Neurotoxic side effects
Phenobarbital	Once daily	Sedation, ataxia, behavioral changes
Phenytoin	Once daily	Confusion, slurred speech, ataxia, double vision
Lacosamide	BID	Dizziness
Lamotrigine	BID	Dizziness, ataxia, diplopia
Levetiracetam	BID	Irritability, mood and behavior changes
Gabapentine	TID	Dizziness, ataxia
Topiramate	BID	Cognitive impairment
Valproate	TID	Tremor, fatigue
Pregabaline	BID-TID	Sedation, dizziness, ataxia
Carbamazepine	BID	Drowsiness, dizziness, diplopia, ataxia
Zonisamaide	BID	Sedation, dizziness

Abbreviations: *BID* two times per day, *TID* three times per day

therapy, with special consideration for patients on polypharmacy and with medical comorbidities. When neurotoxic symptoms develop, the AED dose should be decreased or alternative AED with a lower toxicity profile should be considered. Beta blockers are the mainstay therapy for valproate tremor, with a 60 mg daily dose reported as effective in controlling the tremor. Other pharmacologic interventions include amantadine, diphenhydramine, benztropine, and cyproheptadine [53].

An important clinical implication is the drug–drug interactions between antiepileptic drugs and chemotherapy agents and other medications commonly prescribed in cancer patients. A number of studies reported that enzyme-inducing antiepileptics, such as carbamazepine, phenytoin and phenobarbital, can reduce the efficacy of several chemotherapy drug (e.g., methotrexate, cyclophosphamide, thiotepa, irinotecan, nitrosureas) through different mechanisms, including accelerated hepatic metabolism using the same pathways (e.g., cytochrome P450 or UGT glucuronidation system), faster digestion or decreased intestinal absorption [63]. When combined with enzyme inducing AED, tyrosine kinase inhibitors had a twofold increased clearance rate [64]. Similarly, chemotherapeutic drugs such as methotrexate, doxorubicin, cisplatin, fluorouracil, or tamoxifen can either decrease the efficacy of AED or increase the risk for toxicity [65]. Other interactions involve anticoagulants such as warfarin, corticosteroids, and antihypertensive medications with variable implications on drug metabolism and efficacy. Patients with cancer receiving AED's should be closely monitored for potential drug–drug interactions and serum drug concentrations should be closely followed to reduce the risk for toxicity and to ensure the efficacy of chemotherapy and seizure control.

Future Directives

Special attention should be focused on the unique setting of AED use in cancer patients. Multimodality treatment for active cancer, concomitant polypharmacy, organ dysfunction, and medical comorbidities carry a high risk for drug–drug interactions and neurotoxicity. A separate problem is the interaction of antiepileptics with chemotherapy agents that can result in ineffective antitumor therapy or in drug toxicity. Future research on seizure management may bring further guidance on use of antiepileptics in cancer patients, based on individual characteristics and the type of tumor.

Immunosuppressants Neurotoxicity

Introduction

Neurological complications of transplantation are common and can induce significant morbidity. Neurotoxicity associated with immunosuppressive therapy encompasses a broad spectrum of manifestations and can complicate the course of patients undergoing organ or stem cell transplantation. Recognition of heralding neurologic symptoms and early intervention may prevent permanent neurologic deficits and improve the survival rate.

Epidemiology

Calcineurin inhibitors (CI) such as cyclosporine and tacrolimus are considered the cornerstone therapy to prevent graft rejection. These agents have a narrow therapeutic index and thus therapeutic drug monitoring cannot predict the occurrence of neurotoxicity. The incidence of neurotoxicity in patients receiving immunosuppressants varies between 10% and 30% and can occur at any time after transplantation [66].

Tremor can develop in 40% of patients on cyclosporine or tacrolimus therapy and most often involves the upper extremities [67]. Other minor adverse events include headache, visual symptoms, paresthesia, and mood changes. Their incidence has been commonly underreported. Major central neurotoxicity includes akinetic mutism, acute confusional state, toxic encephalopathy, posterior reversible encephalopathy syndrome (PRES), and seizures. Up to 8% of patients after bone marrow transplantation may develop PRES [68]. Peripheral neurotoxicity can occur weeks to months after initiation of immunosuppressive therapy [69]. Some reports described CI-induced peripheral axonal and demyelinating neuropathy, sometime resembling chronic inflammatory demyelinating polyradiculopathy [70]. In a retrospective study describing the long outcome of allogeneic stem cell transplant recipients who developed CI-induced neurotoxicity, resolution of neurologic symptoms occurred in 70% of patients after either discontinuation or dose reduction of CI [71]. Approximately half of the patients who were rechallenged with the same or a different CI developed reoccurring symptoms that prompted discontinuation of the drug. Risk factors for CI-induced neurotoxicity include the use of corticosteroids, hypertension, hypocholesterolemia, posttransplant hypomagnesemia and hyponatremia, renal or hepatic dysfunction, and preexisting brain disease.

Pathophysiology

Calcineurin inhibitors are highly lipophilic drugs and are bounded to plasma cells, lipoproteins and low-density lipoprotein (LDL). Despite their lipophilic nature, cyclosporine and tacrolimus have to overcome the blood–brain barrier (BBB). The mechanism of injury to BBB is not fully understood. One proposed hypothesis is the vasogenic theory. Rapid increase in the blood pressure can surmount the cerebral autoregulation and lead to cerebral hyperperfusion, which may cause vasogenic edema. This occurs mainly in the posterior circulation, which has little sympathetic innervation [72]. The vasogenic theory does not explain the occurrence of PRES in patients with normal or slightly elevated blood pressure. The second theory is postulating endothelial dysfunction caused by circulating toxins that can trigger vascular leakage and brain edema. Endothelial activation can release vasoactive substances, mediating the cerebral vasospasm described frequently in cancer patients with PRES [73].

Numerous reports have linked calcineurin inhibitors with PRES development. The

pathogenic mechanism is unknown, but their neurotoxic properties may trigger the release of vasoactive substances and arterial hypertension. CI neurotoxicity may also be related to dysregulation of synaptic transmission and neuronal excitability [74]. The severity of neurotoxicity induced by CI does not correlate with the plasma levels of immunosuppressive agents. PRES has been reported in patients with plasma concentrations of immunosuppressants within therapeutic range. It has been observed that high dose of IV cyclosporine may cause endothelial damage, brain edema, and consequently PRES. Using oral formulations of cyclosporine or tacrolimus has reduced the incidence of neurotoxicity [75].

Clinical Manifestations

A high percentage of patients with CI neurotoxicity develop a fine, postural tremor in the upper extremities. Toxic encephalopathies with neurobehavioral abnormalities may develop, as a result of disruption of neural transmission in the white matter tracts. Clinical presentation varies from mild cases with inattention, forgetfulness, and changes in personality to severe cases with acute psychosis, akinetic mutism, and profound cognitive impairment [76]. Focal or generalized tonic-clonic seizures can occur with or without imaging or EEG abnormalities.

PRES is a neurotoxic encephalopathy well recognized in cancer patients receiving therapy. Typical clinical manifestations include confusion, headaches, seizures, and visual deficits. Patients may present with acute or subacute changes in mentation, blurred vision, visual hallucinations or cortical blindness, while focal weakness, aphasia or incoordination is rarely noted [77]. The majority of patients develop hypertension, although PRES has been reported in normotensive patients as well. Most of the patients will have a full recovery, although permanent neurologic deficits have been reported without prompt diagnosis and intervention. In a single institution retrospective study of PRES in cancer patients, thrombocytopenia, elevated blood pressure, electrographic seizures at the onset, atypical

MRI pattern, and delay in diagnostic imaging were reported risk factors associated with morbidity and mortality [78].

Neuroimaging

Typical brain MRI images demonstrate symmetric T2 signal abnormalities in the subcortical white matter in the parietal and occipital lobes. Additional radiographic abnormalities may involve frontal or temporal lobes, cerebellum or brainstem, as well as basal ganglia. Areas of diffusion-weighted-imaging (DWI) hypointensities or cortical gryriform enhancement may occur reflecting BBB disruption [79]. Atypical MRI pattern has been defined as petechial and intraparenchymal hemorrhages and has been noted in patients who had a bone marrow transplant and taking tacrolimus, patients with thrombocytopenia, and in patients with clotting abnormalities [78]. CT scans of the head that are commonly performed before the brain MRI may show subtle hypodensities. Correlation with clinical presentation should trigger MRI neuroimaging to confirm diagnosis. Prolonged vasoconstriction or hypoperfusion may induce intracellular cytotoxic edema and acute ischemia. Asymmetric lesions, acute ischemia, or parenchymal hemorrhage should be further investigated to eliminate other potential etiologies, such as cerebral aneurysm, stroke, cerebral venous thrombosis, encephalitis, or neoplasm.

Management

Early recognition of PRES and initiation of supportive therapy is of paramount importance in managing CI-induced neurotoxicity. Treatment should be focused to control blood pressure, in parallel with dose reduction or discontinuation of the offending agent. Acute hypertension should be managed in the intensive care unit with gradual lowering of the blood pressure with no more than 25% reduction within the first 6 h [80]. First-line intravenous antihypertensive agents include nicardipine and labetalol followed by hydralazine and enalaprilat. Oral medication including amlodipine, lisinopril, clonidine, losartan, and propranolol are commonly used in less severe cases.

Seizures are common and usually occur early in the course of disease. Oral anticonvulsants (e.g., levatiracetam, vimpat, valproate, or carbamazepine) should be promptly initiated and individualized based on associated medical comorbidities and metabolic abnormalities. Status epilepticus must be managed along with cardiorespiratory support in the intensive care setting. Management of status epilepticus should be in accordance with the guidelines for general populations: initial therapy with intravenous benzodiazepines (lorazepam or diazepam), followed by second-line therapy with fosphenytoin, valproate, or levatiracetam if status persists, and third-line therapy with anesthetic doses of either thiopental, midazolam, phenobarbital, or propofol for refractory status epilepticus, all with continuous EEG monitoring [81]. Long-term antiepileptic treatment is not commonly required. Correction of metabolic abnormalities, adjustments of concomitant medications, and platelet transfusion may decrease the incidence of complications associated with PRES and further improve the outcome.

Future Directions

Immunosuppressive therapy induced neurotoxicity, especially with calcineurin inhibitors, is a common complication after organ or stem cell transplantation and can be associated with high morbidity. Early clinical suspicion should prompt diagnostic workup, particularly brain MRI imaging, and immediate intervention to prevent irreversible neurologic deficits. Further research on the mechanism and pathophysiology of the CI neurotoxicity paired with large case-control studies can provide valid information about prevention and management of neurologic complications, resulting in prolonged survival rate for transplanted patients.

References

1. Magge RS, DeAngelis LM. The double-edged sword: neurotoxicity of chemotherapy. Blood Rev. 2015;29:93–100.
2. Robertson GL, Bhoopalam N, Zelkowitz LI. Vincristine neurotoxicity and abnormal secretion of antidiuretic hormone. Arch Intern Med. 1973;132:717–20.
3. Whittaker JA, Parry DH, Bunch C, Weatherall DJ. Coma associated with vincristine therapy. Br Med J. 1973;4:335–7.
4. Boranic M, Raci F. A Parkinson-like syndrome as side effect of chemotherapy with vincristine and adriamycin in a child with acute leukaemia. Biomedicine. 1979;31:124–5.
5. Byrd RL, Rohrbaugh TM, Raney RB Jr, Norris DG. Transient cortical blindness secondary to vincristine therapy in childhood malignancies. Cancer. 1981;47:37–40.
6. Dallera F, Gamoletti R, Costa P. Unilateral seizures following vincristine intravenous injection. Tumori. 1984;70:243–4.
7. Scheithauer W, Ludwig H, Maida E. Acute encephalopathy associated with continuous vincristine sulfate combination therapy: case report. Investig New Drugs. 1985;3:315–8.
8. Hurwitz RL, Mahoney DH, Armstrong DL, Browder TM. Reversible encephalopathy and seizures as a result of conventional vincristine administration. Med Pediatr Oncol. 1988;16:216–9.
9. Gaidys WG, Dickerman JD, Walters CL, Young PC. Report of a fatal case despite CNS washout. Cancer. 1983;52:799–801.
10. Walther PJ, Rossitch E, Bullard DE. The development of Lhermitte's sign during cisplatin chemotherapy. Possible drug-induced toxicity causing spinal cord demyelination. Cancer. 1987;60:2170–2.
11. DeAngelis LM, Posner JB. Neurologic complications of cancer. 2nd ed. Oxford: Oxford University Press; 2009.
12. Wasner G, Hilpert F, Schattschneider J, Binder A, Pfisterer J, Baron R. Docetaxel-induced nail changes – a neurogenic mechanism: a case report. J Neuro-Oncol. 2002;58:167–74.
13. Albers JW, Chaudhry V, Cavaletti G, Donehower RC. Interventions for preventing neuropathy caused by cisplatin and related compounds. Cochrane Database Syst Rev. 2001:CD005228. https://doi.org/10.1002/14651858.CD005228.pub3; 1–48
14. Chabner B, Longo DL. Cancer chemotherapy and biotherapy: principles and practice. 5th ed. Philadelphia: Wolters Kluwer Health/Lippincott Williams & Wilkins; 2011.
15. Rybak LP, Mukherjea D, Jajoo S, Ramkumar V. Cisplatin ototoxicity and protection: clinical and experimental studies. Tohoku J Exp Med. 2009;219:177–86.
16. Icli F, Karaoguz H, Dincol D, Demirkazik A, Gunel N, Karaoguz R, Oner A. Severe vascular toxicity associated with cisplatin-based chemotherapy. Cancer. 1993;72:587–93.
17. Lyass O, Lossos A, Hubert A, Gips M, Peretz T. Cisplatin-induced non-convulsive encephalopathy. Anti-Cancer Drugs. 1998;9:100–4.
18. Renard D, Westhovens R, Vandenbussche E, Vandenberghe R. Reversible posterior leucoencephalopathy during oral treatment with methotrexate. J Neurol. 2004;251:226–8.
19. Kiewe P, Seyfert S, Korper S, Rieger K, Thiel E, Knauf W. Progressive multifocal leukoencephalopathy with detection of JC virus in a patient with chronic lymphocytic leukemia parallel to onset of fludarabine therapy. Leuk Lymphoma. 2003;44:1815–8.
20. Benger A, Browman GP, Walker IR, Preisler HD. Clinical evidence of a cumulative effect of high-dose cytarabine on the cerebellum in patients with acute leukemia: a leukemiaintergroup report. Cancer Treat Rep. 1985;6:240–1.
21. Scherokman B, Filling-Katz MR, Tell D. Brachial plexus neuropathy following high-dose cytarabine in acute monoblastic leukemia. Cancer Treat Rep. 1985;69:1005–6.
22. Borgeat A, De Muralt B, Stalder M. Peripheral neuropathy associated with high-dose Ara-C therapy. Cancer. 1986;58:852–4.
23. Nagarajan R, Peters C, Orchard P, Rydholm N. Report of severe neurotoxicity with cyclophosphamide. J Pediatr Hematol Oncol. 2000;22:544–6.
24. Kende G, Sirkin SR, Thomas PR, Freeman AI. Blurring of vision: a previously undescribed complication of cyclophosphamide therapy. Cancer. 1979;44:69–71.
25. Cohen MH, Johnson JR, Pazdur R. Food and Drug Administration Drug approval summary: temozolomide plus radiation therapy for the treatment of newly diagnosed glioblastoma multiforme. Clin Cancer Res. 2005;11:6767–71.
26. Pachman DR, Weisbrod BL, Seisler DK, Barton DL, Fee-Schroeder KC, Smith TJ, Lachance DH, Liu H, Shelerud RA, Cheville AL, Loprinzi CL. Pilot evaluation of Scrambler therapy for the treatment of chemotherapy-induced peripheral neuropathy. Support Care Cancer. 2015;23:943–51.
27. Hu LY, Mi WL, Wu GC, Wang YQ, Mao-Ying QL. Prevention and treatment for chemotherapy-induced peripheral neuropathy: therapies based on CIPN mechanisms. Curr Neuropharmacol. 2017; https://doi.org/10.2174/1570159X15666170915143217.
28. Park SB, Goldstein D, Krishnan AV, Lin CS, Friedlander ML, Cassidy J, Koltzenburg M, Kiernan MC. Chemotherapy-induced peripheral neurotoxicity: a critical analysis. Cancer J Clin. 2013;63:419–37.
29. Quigley C, Joel S, Patel N, Baksh A, Slevin M. Plasma concentrations of morphine, morphine-6-glucuronide and morphine-3-glucuronide and their relationship with analgesia and side effects in patients with cancer-related pain. Palliat Med. 2003;17:185–90.

30. Ripamonti C, Dickerson ED. Strategies for the treatment of cancer pain in the new millennium. Drugs. 2001;61:955–77.
31. Grond S, Zech D, Diefenbach C, Bischoff A. Prevalence and pattern of symptoms in patients with cancer pain: a prospective evaluation of 1635 cancer patients referred to a pain clinic. J Pain Symptom Manag. 1994;9:372–82.
32. Oosten AW, Oldenmenger WH, Mathijssen RH, van der Rijt CC. A systematic review of prospective studies reporting adverse events of commonly used opioids for cancer-related pain: a call for the use of standardized outcome measures. J Pain. 2015;16:935–46.
33. De Conno F, Ripamonti C, Fagnoni E, Brunelli C, Luzzani M, Maltoni M, Arcuri E, Bertetto O. The MERITO Study: a multicentre trial of the analgesic effect and tolerability of normal-release oral morphine during 'titration phase' in patients with cancer pain. Palliat Med. 2008;22:214–21.
34. Mercadante S, Casuccio A, Agnello A, Serreta R, Calderone L, Baressi L. Morphine versus methadone in the pain treatment of advanced-cancer patients followed up at home. J Clin Oncol. 1998;16:3656–61.
35. Lawlor PG. The panorama of opioid-related cognitive dysfunction in patients with cancer: a critical literature appraisal. Cancer. 2002;94:1836–53.
36. Hagen N, Swanson R. Strychnine-like multifocal myoclonus and seizures in extremely high-dose opioid administration: treatment strategies. J Pain Symptom Manag. 1997;14:51–8.
37. Folstein MF, Fetting JH, Lobo A, Naiz U, Capozzoli KD. Cognitive assessment of cancer patients. Cancer. 1984;53:2250–7.
38. Compton P, Charuvastra VC, Ling W. Pain intolerance in opioid-maintained former opiate addicts: effect of long-acting maintenance agent. Drug Alcohol Depend. 2001;63:139–46.
39. Lotsch J. Opioid metabolites. J Pain Symptom Manag. 2005;29:S10–24.
40. Kaiko RF, Foley KM, Grabinski PY, Heidrich G, Rogers AG, Inturissi CE, Reidenberg MM. Central nervous system excitatory effects of meperidine in cancer patients. Ann Neurol. 1983;13:180–5.
41. Ripamonti C, Bianchi M. The use of methadone for cancer pain. Hematol Oncol Clin North Am. 2002;16:543–55.
42. Morita T, Tei Y, Tsunoda J, Inoue S, Chihara S. Underlying pathologies and their associations with clinical features in terminal delirium of cancer patients. J Pain Symptom Manag. 2001;22:997–1006.
43. Slatkin N, Rhiner M. Treatment of opioid-induced delirium with acetylcholinesterase inhibitors: a case report. J Pain Symptom Manag. 2004;27:268–73.
44. Mercadante S. Pathophysiology and treatment of opioid-related myoclonus in cancer patients. Pain. 1998;74:5–9.
45. Li X, Angst MS, Clark JD. A murine model of opioid-induced hyperalgesia. Brain Res Mol Brain Res. 2001;86:56–62.
46. Silverman SM. Opioid induced hyperalgesia: clinical implications for the pain practitioner. Pain Physician. 2009;12:679–84.
47. Ross JR, Riley J, Quigley C, Welsh KI. Clinical pharmacology and pharmacotherapy of opioid switching in cancer patients. Oncologist. 2006;11:765–73.
48. Cherny NI. The management of cancer pain. CA Cancer J Clin. 2000;50:70–116, quiz 117–20.
49. Bromfield EB. Epilepsy in patients with brain tumors and other cancers. Rev Neurol Dis. 2004;1(Suppl 1): S27–33.
50. Mattson RH, Cramer JA, Collins JF, Smith DB, Delgado-Escueta AV, Browne TR, Williamson PD, Treiman DM, McNamara JO, McCutchen CB. Comparison of carbamazepine, phenobarbital, phenytoin, and primidone in partial and secondarily generalized tonic-clonic seizures. N Engl J Med. 1985;313:145–51.
51. Taphoorn MJ, Klein M. Cognitive deficits in adult patients with brain tumours. Lancet Neurol. 2004;3:159–68.
52. Arif H, Buchsbaum R, Weintraub D, Pierro J, Resor SR Jr, Hirsch LJ. Patient-reported cognitive side effects of antiepileptic drugs: predictors and comparison of all commonly used antiepileptic drugs. Epilepsy Behav. 2009;14:202–9.
53. Karas BJ, Wilder BJ, Hammond EJ, Bauman AW. Valproate tremors. Neurology. 1982;32:428–32.
54. Jamora D, Lim SH, Pan A, Tan L, Tan EK. Valproate-induced Parkinsonism in epilepsy patients. Mov Disord. 2007;22:130–3.
55. Kokenge R, Kutt H, McDowell F. Neurological sequelae following Dilantin overdose in a patient and in experimental animals. Neurology. 1965;15:823–9.
56. Munoz-Garcia D, Del Ser T, Bermejo F, Portera A. Truncal ataxia in chronic anticonvulsant treatment. Association with drug-induced folate deficiency. J Neurol Sci. 1982;55:305–11.
57. De Marcos FA, Ghizoni E, Kobayashi E, Li LM, Cendes F. Cerebellar volume and long-term use of phenytoin. Seizure. 2003;12:312–5.
58. Hamed SA, Abdellah MM. The relationship between valproate induced tremors and circulating neurotransmitters: a preliminary study. Int J Neurosci. 2017;127:236–42.
59. Armon C, Shin C, Miller P, Carwile S, Brown E, Edinger JD, Paul RG. Reversible parkinsonism and cognitive impairment with chronic valproate use. Neurology. 1996;47:626–35.
60. Meador KJ, Loring DW, Moore EE, Thompson WO, Nichols ME, Oberzan RE, Durkin MW, Gallagher BB, King DW. Comparative cognitive effects of phenobarbital, phenytoin, and valproate in healthy adults. Neurology. 1995;45:1494–9.
61. Shorvon SD. Safety of topiramate: adverse events and relationships to dosing. Epilepsia. 1996;37(Suppl 2): S18–22.

62. Alonso-Juarez M, Torres-Russotto D, Crespo-Morfin P, Baizabal-Carvallo JF. The clinical features and functional impact of valproate-induced tremor. Parkinsonism Relat Disord. 2017;44:147–50.

63. Relling MV, Pui CH, Sandlund JT, Rivera GK, Hancock ML, Boyett JM, Schuetz EG, Evans WE. Adverse effect of anticonvulsants on efficacy of chemotherapy for acute lymphoblastic leukaemia. Lancet. 2000;356:285–90.

64. Reardon DA, Vredenburgh JJ, Desjardins A, Peters KB, Sathornsumetee S, Threatt S, Sampson JH, Herndon JE, Coan A, McSherry F, Rich JN, McLendon RE, Zhang S, Friedman HS. Phase 1 trial of dasatinib plus erlotinib in adults with recurrent malignant glioma. J Neuro-Oncol. 2012;108:499–506.

65. Avila EK, Graber J. Seizures and epilepsy in cancer patients. Curr Neurol Neurosci Rep. 2010;10:60–7.

66. Bartynski WS, Zeigler Z, Spearman MP, Lin L, Shadduck RK, Lister J. Etiology of cortical and white matter lesions in cyclosporin-A and FK-506 neurotoxicity. AJNR Am J Neuroradiol. 2001;22:1901–14.

67. Wijdicks EF, Wiesner RH, Dahlke LJ, Krom RA. FK506-induced neurotoxicity in liver transplantation. Ann Neurol. 1994;35:498–501.

68. Masetti R, Cordelli DM, Zama D, Vendemini F, Baigi C, Franzoni E, Pession A. PRES in children undergoing hematopoietic stem cell or solid organ transplantation. Pediatrics. 2015;135:890–901.

69. Wijdicks EF. Neurotoxicity of immunosuppressive drugs. Liver Transpl. 2001;7:937–42.

70. Ayres RC, Dousset B, Wixon S, Buckels JA, McMaster P, Mayer AD. Peripheral neurotoxicity with tacrolimus. Lancet. 1994;343:862–3.

71. Chohan R, Vij R, Adkins D, Blum W, Brown R, Tomasson M, Devine S, Graubert T, Goodnough LT, Dipersio JF, Khoury H. Long-term outcomes of allogeneic stem cell transplant recipients after calcineurin inhibitor-induced neurotoxicity. Br J Haematol. 2003;123:110–3.

72. Nishiguchi T, Mochizuki K, Shakudo M, Takeshita T, Hino M, Inoue Y. CNS complications of hematopoietic stem cell transplantation. AJR Am J Roentgenol. 2009;192:1003–11.

73. Marra A, Vargas M, Striano P, Del Guercio L, Buonanno P, Servillo G. Posterior reversible encephalopathy syndrome: the endothelial hypotheses. Med Hypotheses. 2014;82:619–22.

74. Baumgartel K, Mansuy IM. Neural functions of calcineurin in synaptic plasticity and memory. Learn Mem. 2012;19:375–84.

75. Wijdicks EF, Dahlke LJ, Wiesner RH. Oral cyclosporine decreases severity of neurotoxicity in liver transplant recipients. Neurology. 1999;52:1708–10.

76. Filley CM, Kleinschmidt-DeMasters BK. Toxic leukoencephalopathy. N Engl J Med. 2001;345:425–32.

77. Fugate JE, Claassen DO, Cloft HJ, Kallmes DF, Kozak OS, Rabinstein AA. Posterior reversible encephalopathy syndrome: associated clinical and radiologic findings. Mayo Clin Proc. 2010;85:427–32.

78. Kamiya-Matsuoka C, Paker AM, Chi L, Youssef A, Tummala S, Loghin ME. Posterior reversible encephalopathy syndrome in cancer patients: a single institution retrospective study. J Neuro-Oncol. 2016;128:75–84.

79. Lamy C, Oppenheim C, Meder JF, Mas JF. Neuroimaging in posterior reversible encephalopathy syndrome. J Neuroimaging. 2014;14:89–96.

80. Pinedo DM, Shah-Khan F, Shah PC. Reversible posterior leukoencephalopathy syndrome associated with oxaliplatin. J Clin Oncol. 2007;25:5320–1.

81. Glauser T, Shinnar S, Gloss D, Alldredge B, Arya R, Bainbridge J, Bare M, Bleck T, Dodson WE, Garrity L, Jagoda A, Lowenstein D, Pellock J, Riviello J, Sloan E, Treiman DM. Epilepsy based guideline: treatment of convulsive status epilepticus in children and adults: report of the guideline committee of the American Epilepsy Society. Epilepsy Curr. 2016;16:48–61.

Seizures and Status Epilepticus in Critically Ill Cancer Patients

23

Vishank A. Shah and Jose I. Suarez

Contents

Introduction 336

Epidemiology 336

Etiology 337
Brain Tumors 337
Systemic Malignancy 337

Pathophysiology 340

Clinical Features 341

Diagnosis 342

Management 344
Pharmacologic 344

Prognosis 349

Summary 349

References 350

Abstract

Seizures and status epilepticus (SE) occur more commonly in oncologic patients than the general population. Similarly, seizures are more common in critically ill patients, and thus critically ill oncologic patients are at high risk for having seizures and SE. There are several etiologic factors contributing to SE in critically ill oncologic patients including complications of existing brain tumors, brain metastasis, chemotherapy, radiation therapy, and paraneoplastic limbic encephalitides in addition to the etiologies that trigger seizures in non-tumor patients such as central nervous system (CNS) infections, electrolyte derangements, strokes, and hemorrhages. There is not much literature to guide the evaluation and management of

V. A. Shah
Stroke and Neurocritical Care, Department of Neurology, University of Arkansas for Medical Sciences College of Medicine, Little Rock, AR, USA
e-mail: VShah2@uams.edu

J. I. Suarez (✉)
Division of Neurosciences Critical Care, Departments of Anesthesiology and Critical Care Medicine, Neurology, and Neurosurgery, The Johns Hopkins University School of Medicine, Baltimore, MD, USA
e-mail: Jsuarez5@jhmi.edu

© Springer Nature Switzerland AG 2020
J. L. Nates, K. J. Price (eds.), *Oncologic Critical Care*,
https://doi.org/10.1007/978-3-319-74588-6_34

seizures and SE in this specific patient population. However, the principles of management of seizures and SE are identical to the management in non-cancer patients with the primary goal to achieve prompt seizure control. Long-term antiepileptic drug (AED) therapy should be tailored and taking into account the interactions with chemotherapeutic agents and adverse events specific to cancer patients. Non-pharmacologic treatment such as surgical resection and radiation therapy may also be indicated in long-term seizure control. The prognosis of patients with tumor-related SE is worse when compared to patients with non-tumor SE.

Keywords

Seizures · Status epilepticus · Antiepileptic drugs · Critically ill oncologic · Chemotherapy · Paraneoplastic · Prognosis

Introduction

Approximately 1.2% of the US population suffers from active epilepsy, which is 3.4 million persons [69]. Per the latest CDC report in 2015, there are approximately 480 new cases of cancer diagnosed per 100,000 persons each year. With the rising incidence of epilepsy and cancer, the overlap of these two seemingly distinct clinical entities is becoming more evident. In addition, with the advent of new immunological, radiological, and molecular technologies, it is becoming clearer that adult-onset "idiopathic" refractory epilepsy and status epilepticus (SE) may actually be linked to underlying undiagnosed neoplastic disease. In this chapter, we will review the epidemiology, etiology, clinical features, diagnosis, and management of seizures and SE in critically ill oncologic patients.

Epidemiology

It has been estimated that about 13% of patients with any type of cancer may have seizures during their lifetime, accounting for 5% of all the neurological problems that may occur in this patient pool [10]. On average, 30–40% of patients with any type of brain tumor develop seizures, and, of these, 30–50% may have seizures as a presenting symptom of the underlying tumor [63]. In addition, 4% of epilepsy patients have an underlying undiagnosed brain tumor [22]. Seizures in critically ill oncologic patients are poorly studied, but 3.3% of critically ill patients may have clinical seizures during their ICU stay with a higher prevalence of nonconvulsive seizures. Certainly, this number may be even higher in critically ill oncologic patients who have multiple risk factors for seizures.

SE is poorly studied in patients with neoplastic diseases. Per a study that derived data from the National Discharge Survey over 32 years, the incidence of SE in the USA increased to approximately 12.5/100,000 in 2010, and 2.29% of those patients with SE had associated brain neoplasms [15]. On the whole, 4–12% of patients with SE have underlying brain tumors. Contrary to isolated seizures, which occur more commonly in patients with low-grade gliomas, when SE was studied prospectively in glioma patients [29], a higher incidence was noted in patients with high-grade gliomas.

In contrast to convulsive SE, nonconvulsive SE (NCSE) is much more common in cancer patients. In one study evaluating patients with cancer and altered mental status, the incidence of NCSE was as high as 6% [11], although it is suspected that it may be even higher and remains underdiagnosed due to the lack of electroencephalographic (EEG) monitoring data in this patient population. When EEG monitoring was performed in any ICU patient with altered mentation, between 5% and 34% had underlying NCSE [62]. In addition, 4–12% of adults with NCSE have been shown to have an underlying undiagnosed intracranial tumor [40]. Needless to say, seizures and SE are frequent in patients with cancer and in critically ill patients and thus are likely to be even more common in critically ill cancer patients, contributing to increased mortality and morbidity.

Etiology

Etiology of seizures in patients with cancer can be divided into two broad categories:

Brain Tumors

Seizures occur most commonly in patients with slow-growing tumors which may be related to the longer median survival in these patients. Studies report that 100% patients with dysembryoplastic neuroepithelial tumors (DNETs) and 60–85% patients with low-grade gliomas have seizures. The incidence of epilepsy in patients with glioblastoma multiforme (GBM) ranges between 30% and 50% and in patients with meningiomas is approximately 25% [22, 33, 63, 65] (Table 1).

The location of the tumor also determines the risk of seizures. Frontal, temporal, and parietal lobe tumors are most likely to present with seizures when compared to occipital lobe, basal ganglia, and posterior fossa tumors. In fact, medulloblastomas and hemangioblastomas almost never present with seizures as they only occur in the posterior fossa.

Systemic Malignancy

Patients with systemic malignancy can have seizures due to several mechanisms:

Intracranial Metastasis

Patients with metastatic brain tumors are less likely to present with seizures, since often, there are multiple lesions, and they tend to involve the

Table 1 Frequency of seizures in patients with various intracranial neoplasms

Percentage (%)	Tumor
10–20	Leptomeningeal disease, primary CNS lymphoma
20–40	Metastasis, ependymoma
30–60	Meningioma, GBM
60–80	Astrocytoma, oligodendroglioma
80–90	Ganglioglioma
100	DNET

posterior fossa. Overall, 20–35% of patients with brain metastasis have seizures [22]. Lung cancer (both small cell and non-small cell) is the most common metastatic cancer that presents with seizures although seizures may also occur in patients with breast cancer, colon cancer, and melanoma [42]. In addition, 10–15% of patients with leptomeningeal carcinomatosis also present with seizures [47].

Chemotherapy-Induced Seizures

Most often, seizures occur within hours to days after exposure to the chemotherapeutic agents. Seizures and SE are most commonly seen after high doses of myelo-ablative chemotherapy (often administered prior to bone marrow transplant) or in the presence of hepatic and renal dysfunction which that which impair clearance of the drugs [56].

1. *Cisplatin*: This agent induces seizures 5–15 days after exposure by several mechanisms. Most commonly seizures occur in the setting of "posterior reversible encephalopathy syndrome" (PRES) which is characterized by confusion, cortical blindness, focal or generalized seizures, and nonconvulsive status epilepticus with imaging findings of T2-FLAIR hyperintensities in bilateral occipital lobes [58]. In addition cisplatin causes hypomagnesemia, hypocalcemia, and renal failure from renal tubular injury which may also provoke seizures.

2. *Busulfan*: Busulfan crosses the blood-brain barrier freely and causes excitotoxic neuronal injury. It reportedly causes generalized tonic-clonic seizures in a dose-dependent fashion most often when used in high doses for myelo-ablation prior to bone marrow transplants [30].

3. *Methotrexate*: Methotrexate is used to treat several malignancies including leukemias and lymphomas and is often given intrathecally for the treatment and prophylaxis against leptomeningeal disease. Seizures may occur within minutes after intrathecal administration and may be associated with focal neurological deficits due to associated inflammation. Imaging may be normal or may show diffusion

restricting lesions [34, 50]. Seizures may also occur several months after exposure, especially when methotrexate is administered concurrently with cranial irradiation. In this case it is usually associated with rapid cognitive decline and imaging often reveals a subcortical leukoencephalopathy.

4. *5-Fluorouracil*: This is a very commonly used chemotherapeutic agent in several cancers and has been anecdotally associated with seizures and a leukoencephalopathy syndrome, as seen with methotrexate, 15–20 weeks after exposure [56].

5. *Chlorambucil*: This is an alkylating agent used in the treatment of Hodgkin's lymphoma. Myoclonic or generalized tonic-clonic seizures are reported to occur when exposed to toxic doses [56].

6. *Cyclosporin-A*: Cyclosporin-A is an immunosuppressant most commonly used in leukemia patients after BMT to prevent graft rejection. It causes endothelial destruction in the intracranial blood vessels due to overexpression of endothelin-1 and reduction in nitric oxide levels [18]. Similar to cisplatin, cyclosporin-A also causes PRES and presents with acute-onset seizures and SE which resolve once the agent has been withdrawn [20].

7. *Immunomodulator therapy*: CD19-specific chimeric antigen receptor (CAR) T-cell therapy is a new therapy used in refractory ALL, but 62% of patients may develop neurotoxicity characterized by seizures, SE, and myoclonus [52].

8. *Other agents*: Interferon-alpha has been reported to cause seizures in 1–4% patients and may present as photosensitive seizures [5, 32]. Vincristine is also associated with PRES and can cause seizures and SE. Other agents that may rarely cause seizures include cyclophosphamide, ifosfamide, BCNU, etoposide, paclitaxel, and procarbazine, among others.

Cranial Irradiation

Cranial radiation therapy is used to treat metastatic brain lesions as well as primary brain tumors such as GBM. This has led to improved survival but in turn is associated with an increased incidence of radiation-related complications such as pseudoprogression and radiation necrosis. While the former occurs weeks to months after radiation exposure, the later can occur months to years after exposure. Both present with focal neurological deficits and seizures with enhancing lesions and surrounding mass effect on imaging [38]. Reports of refractory seizures related to postradiation sequelae exist. Rarely radiation therapy leads to formation of cavernous angiomas that also present with intractable epilepsy [56].

Paraneoplastic Syndromes

Paraneoplastic syndromes are autoimmune disorders involving sites distant from the primary cancer, triggered by an immune response to cancer epitopes. Any paraneoplastic syndrome involving the limbic lobes or cerebral cortex can present with seizures and SE. In a series of 50 cases, 12% of the patients with paraneoplastic limbic encephalitis presented with seizures and SE [21]. Patients may develop these syndromes several years prior to the detection of the underlying malignancy.

Seizures and SE in patients with limbic encephalitis are often refractory to medical therapy and may not resolve with tumor removal. Immunotherapy such as steroids, intravenous immunoglobulin (IVIG), or plasma exchange is often used, but response largely depends on the location of the epitopes. If epitopes are extracellular, the response to immunotherapy is excellent due to high volume of circulating antibodies that can be neutralized. However, if epitopes are intracellular, there is direct neuronal injury, and response is usually poor (Table 2) [12].

The common antibodies include:

(a) *Anti-Hu (ANNA) antibody*: This is the most common antibody associated with seizures and SE. It is most commonly seen with small cell lung cancer and is directed against intracellular epitopes causing a limbic encephalitis presenting with refractory seizures, epilepsia partialis continua (EPC), and focal SE with impairment of consciousness [25]. Often, this does not respond to immunotherapy.

Table 2 Most commons paraneoplastic disorders in patient with seizures

Paraneoplastic syndromes causing seizures					
Epitopes	Intracellular epitopes			Extracellular epitopes		
Antibodies	Hu	CRMP5	Ma2	NMDAR	VGKC	AMPAR
Malignancy commonly associated	Small cell lung cancer	Thymoma, small cell lung cancer	Germ cell tumor of the testis	Ovarian teratoma, testicular tumors	Thymoma, small cell lung cancer	Thymoma, small cell lung cancer, breast cancer
Clinical presentation	EPC, focal SE, limbic encephalitis	Limbic encephalitis, refractory seizures	Limbic, brain stem encephalitis, seizures, coma	Limbic encephalitis, seizures, psychosis, catatonia, dyskinesia, autonomic instability	Limbic encephalitis, Morvan's syndrome, seizures and SE	Limbic encephalitis, seizures, SE
Response to immune therapy	Poor	Poor	Moderate-30%	Good	Good	Good but has frequent relapses

Abbreviations: EPC, epilepsia partialis continua; SE, status epilepticus

(b) *Anti-CV2/CRMP5 antibody*: This is seen most commonly in patients with thymoma and small cell lung cancer and presents as a limbic encephalitis with refractory seizures. It is also directed against intracellular epitopes and thus has a poor response to immunotherapy [68].

(c) *Anti-Ma2 antibody*: Usually associated with germ cell tumors of the testes, this antibody is also directed against intracellular epitopes and causes a limbic encephalitis but often involves the diencephalon and brain stem as well. Patients with this syndrome present with seizures, SE, and coma. Unlike the prior, approximately 30% patients with these antibodies respond to immunotherapy and tumor removal [51].

(d) *Anti-NMDA receptor antibody*: This antibody is directed against extracellular NR-1 subunit of NMDA receptors and is typically seen young women. Patients present with behavioral changes and early-onset focal seizures, SE followed by altered sensorium, catatonia, orofacial dyskinesias, and autonomic instability. It has been found that about 60% of the female patients have underlying ovarian teratomas. In males, it may be associated with germ cell tumors of the testis. The condition responds very well to removal of the tumor

and immunotherapy, but recovery is slow [14].

(e) *Anti-VGKC antibody*: This antibody is directed against extracellular voltage-gated potassium channels and may be associated with thymoma or small cell lung cancer in 20% of the cases. Patients with these antibodies may either develop a limbic encephalitis or a more distinct syndrome known as Morvan's syndrome characterized by hallucinations, neuromyotonia, and insomnia, among other symptoms. In either case, patients may present with seizures and sometimes SE [60].

(f) *Anti-AMPA receptor antibody*: These antibodies are directed against extracellular AMPA receptors and are associated with thymoma and breast and lung cancer. Patients present with limbic encephalitis and have frequent seizures and SE. There is a good response to immunotherapy, but characteristically this disorder has frequent relapses and may need long-term immunosuppression [31].

Other Causes

Needless to say, oncologic patients may also have seizures due to all the usual causes of seizures seen in non-cancer patients [56]. These include:

(a) *Infections*:

Chemotherapy often causes immunosuppression which increases the risk of opportunistic infections. CNS infections, especially encephalitis, occur more commonly in this patient population and may present with seizures. Common infections include HSV, HHV-6, varicella zoster, toxoplasmosis, and aspergillosis, among others. In addition, patients with underlying brain tumors also have a higher propensity to have seizures in the setting of ongoing systemic infections.

(b) *Toxic-metabolic causes*:

These are the most common reversible causes of seizures. Chemotherapy often causes several metabolic derangements which can trigger seizures such as hyponatremia, hypomagnesemia, and hypocalcemia. Some tumors, such as insulinomas, may present as hypoglycemic seizures.

(c) *Postsurgical scarring*:

In certain cases, for example, after meningioma resection, seizures develop after surgical resection due to postsurgical inflammation, scarring, and gliosis. Often this requires lifelong antiepileptic drug therapy.

(d) *Cerebrovascular complications*:

Ischemic strokes, parenchymal hemorrhages, and venous sinus thrombosis are relatively common cerebrovascular complications in cancer patients and occur in approximately 15% of them [49]. These may often present with seizures and rarely SE.

Pathophysiology

Epileptogenesis in brain tumors has been postulated to occur due to several mechanisms. Tumor histology plays an important role in determining seizure risk. Slow-growing tumors are more epileptogenic. Although, in part, this might be due to the longer survival, slow-growing tumors (such as low-grade gliomas) and developmental tumors (DNETs or gangliogliomas) circumscribe and de-afferentate cortical and subcortical neural networks, impairing normal regulation [55]. Also, low-grade tumor cells are often well-differentiated and release excitatory neurotransmitters in an unsynchronized manner. Moreover, low-grade glial tumors infiltrate the surrounding parenchyma and may abnormally regulate the seemingly normal neuronal tissue. High-grade tumors on the other hand may be associated with seizures due to necrosis and hemosiderin deposition related to tumoral hemorrhage and rapid growth. Extrinsic tumors, such as meningiomas, cause seizures due to peritumoral edema and mass effect.

As previously mentioned, tumor location also plays an important role. Superficial and cortical tumors have a higher incidence of seizures when compared to deeper locations [26]. Seizures occur more commonly when lesions are closer to the Rolandic fissure [66]. Occipital lobe lesions are the least likely to cause seizures when compared to frontal, temporal, and parietal lobes.

Microscopically, peritumoral cells also have an uncharacteristic appearance with anomalous inefficient neuronal migration. Neurons may remain behind in the white matter with pyramidal neurons in the peritumoral tissue and excitatory synapses in abundance of inhibitory synapses, potentiating seizures [37]. In addition, peritumoral cortex is also shown to have significant differences in the form, size, and number of synaptic vesicles. There is also evidence that the interglial gap junctions in the peritumoral tissue are altered carrying higher amounts of CX43 membrane proteins [3, 9]. These altered gap junctions may be functionally adverse, propagating waves of calcium-mediated depolarization which propagates epileptic activity [55].

Metabolic dysfunction including changes in pH, ions, amino acid balance, receptors, and immunological milieu may also contribute to tumoral epileptogenicity. These changes have been studied by both pathological analysis as well as modern metabolic imaging including positron emission tomography (PET) scan and magnetic resonance spectroscopy (MRS). MRS demonstrates reduced N-acetylaspartate levels (a marker of neuronal viability) in the epileptogenic tumoral and peritumoral tissue [8].

Tumoral tissue, due to its rapid growth, is metabolically hyperactive and when the vascular supply cannot meet the regional metabolic needs, tumoral hypoxia ensues. This leads to impaired oxidative metabolism with lactate production and interstitial acidosis, known as the Warburg effect [54]. To add to this, high-grade gliomas have higher expression of glycolytic enzymes and decreased mediators of oxidative metabolism leading to further interstitial and cellular acidosis causing glial cell swelling and damage [48]. In addition, glioma cell membranes possess sodium channels that are activated by acidic pH leading to neuronal depolarization and triggering epileptogenicity. Moreover, it is postulated that the acidity of tumoral and peritumoral tissue may render AEDs inactive, contributing to the refractoriness of tumoral epilepsy [55]. In addition, glioma cells also have a high proportion of multidrug-resistant proteins which impair drug transport into the epileptogenic tissue further propagating refractoriness [6].

Peritumoral tissue has also been shown to have higher levels of calcium and sodium ions in the extracellular space which contribute to neuronal hyperexcitability. Peritumoral hemorrhage leads to higher levels of iron which also causes neuronal destabilization. Higher levels of glutamate and dysfunctional glutamate and GABA receptors have also been demonstrated in peritumoral tissue, further potentiating neuronal hyperexcitability contributing to tumoral epileptogenicity [55, 67].

In addition, as described in the previous section, seizures and SE can also occur in cancer patients without brain tumors by several pathophysiologic mechanisms including chemotherapeutic side effects, paraneoplastic syndromes, infections, and metabolic derangements. The underlying pathophysiology has already been discussed in the previous section.

Clinical Features

Age of onset of seizures in oncologic patients depends on the underlying etiology. In patients with brain tumors, the age of onset depends on the underlying tumor type. In general, patients with slow-growing brain neoplasms develop seizures at onset of the neoplastic disease and often lead to the diagnosis of the tumor. Average age of tumor diagnosis and thus seizure onset in patients with DNET and gangliogliomas is 15–19 years, whereas in patients with low-grade gliomas, it is 30–45 years. In patients with meningioma, the average age of onset is 50–60 years. The mean age for seizures in patients with glioblastoma and brain metastases is 60 and 70 years, respectively [17].

In patients with systemic malignancy, the temporal relation of new-onset seizures and SE to the phase of the disease course is more relevant than the specific age of onset. New-onset seizures or SE prior to diagnosis of the underlying systemic malignancy is usually common in patients with paraneoplastic limbic encephalitis, endocrine tumors, and brain metastases from malignancies with a high propensity to metastasize to the brain such as melanoma or lung cancer. Chemotherapy-induced seizures usually occur during the administration of the drugs, whereas seizures occurring weeks after chemotherapy may be related to CNS infections. Radiation necrosis-related seizures usually occur months after cranial irradiation and sometimes years after, if the patient develops a leukoencephalopathy syndrome or cavernous malformations [56].

Approximately 80% of patients with DNETs and GGs have focal seizures with loss of awareness, and about 50% of them will have secondary generalization [17]. Meningioma patients often present with headache and focal neurological deficits but may also present with seizures especially if the meningioma is supratentorial with peritumoral edema. About 20% of patients with meningioma may develop seizures after surgical resection [17].

Glioma patients classically present with focal-onset seizures with secondary generalization.

In a study analyzing 100 patients with primary brain tumors and seizures, 48% had tonic-clonic seizures. However, only half of these had a clear focal onset. Furthermore, 26% of them had focal motor, 10% had complex partial, and 8% had somatosensitive seizures.

SE is seen in 12% patients with brain tumors with a higher predilection for high-grade rather than low-grade gliomas [39]. About 48% of cases have focal-onset secondarily generalized SE, 26% have focal SE with impairment of consciousness, and 26% have focal SE without impairment of consciousness [29]. NCSE is found on continuous EEG monitoring in 2% of patients with brain tumors admitted to the hospital with altered sensorium. Moreover, 79% of patients have associated subclinical seizures, and only 42% patients will have visible motor manifestations such as twitching or automatisms [36].

In patients with systemic malignancy, generalized tonic-clonic seizures are usually seen in patients receiving chemotherapy or immunomodulators and patients with metabolic dysfunction, CNS infections, viral encephalitis, or vascular complications such as cerebral venous sinus thrombosis. Focal seizures with or without loss of awareness are more common in systemic cancer patients with intracranial metastases or paraneoplastic limbic encephalitis. Myoclonic seizures may be seen in busulfan-related neurotoxicity, whereas interferon-alpha may cause photosensitive seizures [56]. Generalized SE in systemic cancer patients is rare and is usually related to chemotherapeutic agents such as cyclosporin or ifosfamide and rarely due to intracranial metastasis. NCSE is seen in 6% of patients with systemic cancer presenting with altered mentation [11]. Paraneoplastic limbic encephalitis is the most common causes of focal NCSE or EPC in cancer patients without intracranial metastasis.

Critically ill oncologic patients presenting with seizures often have other neurological syndromes that can help provide clues to the diagnosis. Headaches and focal neurological deficits, such as motor weakness, are often suggestive of intraparenchymal tumors or metastasis. Headaches and altered sensorium with cranial nerve deficits may indicate leptomeningeal carcinomatosis. Severe encephalopathy, behavioral changes, psychosis, and refractory seizures suggest a diagnosis of paraneoplastic limbic encephalitis. Oral dyskinesias are classically seen in patients with NMDA receptor encephalitis in addition to above symptoms. Myoclonus may be seen in neurotoxicity due to CAR T-cell therapy or busulfan. Progressive dementia, behavioral changes, and gait disturbance may be seen in a leukoencephalopathy syndrome related to cranial radiation or methotrexate.

Diagnosis

The workup for critically ill oncologic patients presenting with seizures and status epilepticus is largely similar to patients without an underlying neoplasm (Algorithm 1). Diagnostic evaluation begins with evaluation for metabolic disturbances and infections. Complete blood count with differential count may reveal leukocytosis with neutrophilic predominance and pandemia suggesting an underlying infection, although seizures also cause neutrophilic demargination.

A comprehensive metabolic panel can help establish a rapidly reversible etiology for seizures in oncologic patients including hyponatremia, hypernatremia, hypomagnesemia, hypocalcemia, and hypoglycemia. Hyponatremia is very common in patients with underlying malignancy. Intracranial mass lesions as well as systemic malignancies such as small cell lung cancer lead to SIADH, triggering hyponatremia, which can lead to seizures. Severe intracranial hypertension from large tumors or pituitary neoplasms can lead to central diabetes insipidus which can cause hypernatremia and trigger seizures. Hypomagnesemia can trigger seizures and is commonly seen in patients receiving chemotherapeutic agents such as cisplatin. Hypocalcemia may also occur in cancer patients, due to osteoblastic-stimulating factors and side effects of chemotherapeutic drugs such as cisplatin, triggering seizures [16]. Severe hypoglycemia in tumor patients is rare but may be seen in patients with insulinomas, non-islet cell tumors producing insulin-like growth factor, massive tumor burden, and extensive tumor invasion of the liver [24]. Obtaining AED levels may aid with assessing non-compliance which remains the leading cause of recurrent seizures and SE in patients with epilepsy.

Next step in evaluating seizures and SE in critically ill oncologic patients includes neuroimaging. This should commence with an urgent non-contrast head computed tomography (CT) scan. Large intracranial metastatic lesions or primary brain tumors can be visualized as

New-onset seizures or SE in critically ill cancer patients

Clinical evaluation: history and clinical examination and seizure semiology

Basic workup: CBC with differential, Metabolic panel including sodium, magnesium, calcium and glucose, AED levels

CT head- to look for tumor hemorrhage, mass effect, shift

Continuous EEG monitoring if with patient altered sensorium

MRI Brain with Gadolinium - to evaluate tumor or non-neoplastic etiologies; consider MR Spectroscopy

Lumbar Puncture - if EEG and MRI are unrevealing or clinical suspicion high for infectious or paraneoplastic disease- send infectious, viral, cytology and paraneoplastic panel

Algorithm 1 Diagnostic workup of oncologic patients with seizures

hypodensities. Head CT can also evaluate peritumoral tissue for edema, midline shift, herniation, and tumoral hemorrhage in patients with known brain lesions, all of which can present with new-onset seizures or SE and can help guide emergent therapies.

Gadolinium-enhanced magnetic resonance imaging (MRI) of the brain is the most critical imaging modality in oncologic patients with seizures. The T2-weighted-fluid-attenuated inversion recovery (T2-FLAIR) and T1-post-contrast sequences are most useful when evaluating mass lesions. The pattern of contrast enhancement, tumor location, number of lesions, and surrounding tissue can indicate the underlying tumor type. In patients with known brain lesions presenting with SE, presence of a new or progression of an existing lesion has been shown to be associated with poor 2-month survival [36]. Leptomeningeal enhancement may indicate leptomeningeal carcinomatosis or infectious meningitis. Hippocampal T2-FLAIR hyperintensities may be seen with paraneoplastic limbic encephalitis [27]. Posterior white matter hyperintensities on T2-FLAIR in patients receiving chemotherapeutic drugs may indicate PRES. Diffusion restriction may be seen within hypercellular lesions such as GBM, CNS lymphoma, or brain abscesses or may indicate cerebrovascular complications such as arterial or venous infarcts. Cortical ribbon hyperintensity on diffusion-weighted imaging (DWI) and T2-FLAIR, not following a vascular distribution and without mass effect, is often a consequence of NCSE and is reversible [23].

Although, contrast-enhanced MRI provides abundant clinical information, advanced MR imaging may be necessary to resolve certain clinical dilemmas. In patients with new-onset seizures due to a ring-enhancing lesion of undetermined etiology, MRI alone may not be able to differentiate between a tumor, an abscess, and a demyelinating lesion. Patients with known brain tumors may present with seizures after initiation of radiation therapy and a new lesion or progression of an old lesion on MRI could either be related to radiation necrosis or tumor progression. MR spectroscopy in conjunction with MR perfusion imaging may help differentiate tumors from nonneoplastic lesions with a specificity of 92%. Elevated total choline (tCho) and reduced N-acetylaspartate (tNAA) are classic for brain tumors, whereas elevated lipids, lactate, and amino acids are more suggestive of nonneoplastic lesions. MR spectroscopy may also assist with differentiating infiltrative and high-grade lesions from low-grade lesions and in neurosurgical treatment planning such as identifying biopsy sites [44].

As previously mentioned, 6% of cancer patients presenting with altered sensorium may have ongoing NCSE on EEG even in the absence of CNS involvement. Thus, continuous EEG monitoring in critically ill oncologic patients presenting with altered sensorium, recurrent seizures, or SE is strongly recommended. It is important to note that 20-minute routine EEGs may not be able to detect intermittent subclinical seizures or NCSE in patients with persistent altered sensorium and should be reserved for patients who have returned to clinical baseline. We suspect that the incidence of NCSE is much higher but is underreported due to lack of EEG monitoring data in cancer and brain tumor patients. In a study of 1101 brain tumor patients, only 24% had EEG recordings [36]. The common EEG patterns described in tumor patients with altered sensorium due to NCSE included frequent focal nonconvulsive seizures (focal onset with clear electrographic evolution; seen in 50%), ictal-interictal continuum (ictal patterns without evolution; seen in 41%), epilepsia partialis continua (EPC) (unremitting motor seizures involving one side of the body; seen in 29%), and generalized nonconvulsive status epilepticus (generalized periodic discharges with 3 Hz or greater frequency; seen in 12%) [36].

If MRI and EEG monitoring do not reveal the etiology for new-onset refractory seizures or status epilepticus, then further evaluation with a large-volume lumbar puncture and cerebrospinal fluid (CSF) analysis may be warranted. Elevated opening pressure may be seen in leptomeningeal carcinomatosis and bacterial or fungal infections. CSF evaluation for protein, glucose, and cell count with differential count may be very revealing. Markedly elevated protein, low glucose, and elevated cell count may be seen in leptomeningeal carcinomatosis and bacterial or fungal meningitis, all of which may occur in cancer patients. CSF gram stain, acid-fast stain, cryptococcal antigen,

and bacterial and fungal cultures may help identify common CNS infections in immuno-suppressed cancer patients. Viral PCRs and antibody titers for HSV, VZV, CMV, EBV, HHV-6, enterovirus, and West Nile virus may also be helpful in identifying common viral encephalitides causing seizures in cancer patients. CSF cytology and flow cytometry can aid in diagnosing common cancers causing leptomeningeal carcinomatosis such as leukemias, lymphomas, and breast cancer. CSF paraneoplastic panel including anti-Hu, anti-CRMP5, anti-VGKC, anti-NMDAR, and anti-AMPA antibodies, among others, should also be sent if above workup is unrevealing or clinical suspicion for a paraneoplastic syndrome is high [41].

Management

Pharmacologic

Pharmacologic treatment is the mainstay when managing seizures and SE in critically ill oncologic patients. It includes emergent management of seizures and SE, management of the underlying etiology, and long-term antiepileptic drug therapy including seizure prophylaxis.

Management of SE

SE is a neuro-oncologic emergency, and management in patients with cancer is largely identical to the management in non-oncologic patients with the primary focus on prompt seizure control. For treatment purposes, the Neurocritical Care Society (NCS) guideline defines SE as continuous clinical and/or electrographic activity for 5 min or more or recurrent seizure activity without recovery between seizures [4]. In general, it is recommended to achieve definitive control of SE within 60 min (Algorithm 2). After ensuring adequate airway, oxygenation, and perfusion, the first line of treatment is benzodiazepines. Intravenous lorazepam (0.1 mg/kg; 4 mg per dose) and intramuscular midazolam (0.2 mg/kg up to a maximum of 10 mg) are the most effective in aborting SE [4]. While there may be concern for respiratory depression and need for intubation, a

Generalized seizure in a critically ill oncologic patient

-Elevate head of bed; continuous vital monitoring

-Airway: clear secretions/blood; supplemental oxygen, intubate if indicated

-Ensure MAP > 70 mm Hg (fluids and vasopressors)

-Establish peripheral IV access

-check glucose- give dextrose/thiamine if low

-send laboratory studies

1st line AED: Lorazepam 0.1 mg/kg (4 mg at a time) IV or Midazolam 0.2 mg/kg IM (max. 10 mg)

repeat dose if needed

2nd line IV AED: (regardless of whether seizure stopped):

- Fosphenytoin (20 mg/kg) OR

-valproate sodium 20-40 mg/kg OR

-levetiracetam (20-40 mg/kg) OR

-lacosamide 200-400 mg IV

Patient back to baseline?

NO

Intubate and initiate mechanical ventilation (only for generalized SE; not applicable for stable NCSE or EPC)

Continuous AED infusion

- Midazolam 0.2 mg/kg IV followed by 0.05-0.2 mg/kg/hr OR

-Propofol 1-2 mg/kg IV bolus followed by 20-200 mcg/kg/min OR

-Pentobarbital 5-15 mg/kg IV bolus followed by 0.5-5 mg/kg/hr infusion

(If EPC or stable NCSE- try another AED from above list; may need up to 3 AEDs)

Initiate continuous EEG monitoring for all SE types: GCSE, EPC and NCSE

titrate AEDs to achieve electrographic seizure control or burst suppression (in case of infusions) for 24-48 hours

-correct electrolyte abnormalities

-discontinue offending chemotherapeutic agents

-obtain neuroimaging- Head CT and MRI if possible

-consider Lumbar Puncture

-consider antibiotics and immune therapy if indicated

Algorithm 2   Management of the oncologic patient with seizure or SE

study showed that patients receiving benzodiazepines were less likely to be intubated compared to placebo in patients with GCSE (Table 3) [1].

Benzodiazepines should be followed by an urgent loading dose of a longer-acting AED regardless of whether SE was aborted. The latter serves two purposes: to abort SE if not aborted already or to prevent recurrence since benzodiazepines are short acting.

The choice of the best initial agent is a topic of contention. The VA Cooperative trial compared phenytoin, phenobarbital, lorazepam, and diazepam and found no difference between agents, but the newer agents have not been compared [1]. The 2012 NCS guidelines recommend either IV

fosphenytoin/phenytoin, IV valproate sodium, or IV levetiracetam. If a patient has been on an AED before, it is reasonable to give a loading dose of the same agent. Recently, IV lacosamide has also been shown to be effective in controlling SE [59]. In oncologic patients it might be preferable to use levetiracetam or lacosamide due to low risk of interactions with chemotherapeutic agents. Phenytoin and sodium valproate affect levels of steroids and chemotherapeutic agents. Regardless, aborting SE should be the first priority over the less imminent risk of drug interactions in the acute setting.

Refractory SE is defined as persistent clinical or electrographic seizures despite initial

Table 3 Medications available for oncologic patients presenting with seizures or SE

Status epilepticus pharmacologic therapy			
Drug name	Loading dose	Infusion rate	Adverse events
Lorazepam	0.1 mg/kg IV, may repeat in 5–10 mins	4 mg IV push per dose	Hypotension Respiratory depression
Midazolam IM	0.2 mg/kg IM up to maximum of 10 mg	NA	Hypotension Respiratory depression
Fosphenytoin/phenytoin	20 mg PE/kg IV, may give additional 5–10 mg/kg after 10 mins	Fosphenytoin: 150 mg/min Phenytoin: 50 mg/min	Hypotension Arrhythmias Bradycardia Drug interactions
Valproate sodium	20–40 mg/kg IV; repeat 20 mg/kg if needed	3–6 mg/kg/min	Hepatotoxicity Hyperammonemia Pancreatitis Thrombocytopenia Drug interactions
Levetiracetam	20–60 mg/kg IV	2–5 mg/kg/min	Drowsiness, agitation, no interactions
Lacosamide	200–400 mg IV	Over 15 min	PR prolongation No interactions
Midazolam infusion	0.2 mg/kg IV; repeat 0.1–0.2 mg/kg IV as needed for breakthrough seizures	0.05–2 mg/kg/hr., and then increase by 0.05–0.1 mg/kg/hr. as needed	Hypotension Tachyphylaxis Accumulation of active metabolite in renally impaired patients
Propofol infusion	1–2 mg/kg	20–200 mcg/kg/min as needed (avoid prolonged infusion >48 h)	Hypotension Bradycardia Cardiac depression Propofol infusion syndrome – rhabdomyolysis, lactic acidosis, heart failure, and death
Pentobarbital infusion	5–15 mg/kg, and repeat 5 mg/kg boluses as needed for breakthrough seizures	0.5–5 mg/kg/h	Hypotension Cardiac depression Infections/sepsis Paralytic ileus Prolonged duration of action – loss of neurologic function for days

benzodiazepine dose and a second control AED [4]. If a patient has not returned back to baseline after above therapy or continues to have subtle seizures, the patient should be monitored with continuous video EEG to determine the persistence of nonconvulsive SE which is fairly common following generalized SE.

In general, if patients have refractory generalized convulsive SE, they should be placed on mechanical ventilation, continuous EEG monitoring, and a continuous AED infusion such as midazolam or propofol. No evidence exists to support one over the other, although midazolam is less likely to cause hypotension and prolonged high-dose infusion of propofol carries an increased risk of propofol infusion syndrome. While pentobarbital infusion may be more effective than the other agents, it has a higher risk of adverse events and a very long duration of action. AED infusions should be titrated to achieve electrographic seizure control and/or burst suppression. Usually, this is continued for 24–48 h, and then the infusion is gradually weaned. If seizures recur, the infusions will have to be titrated back up, and another agent may need to be added [4].

In patients with NCSE or EPC who are hemodynamically stable and protecting their airway, emergent intubation and prolonged AED infusions are not recommended. It may be reasonable to add additional AEDs (levetiracetam, phenytoin, valproate, lacosamide, clobazam, phenobarbital, topiramate) till clinical and/or electrographic seizures have been aborted. Typically, EPC and NCSE are very refractory and may be difficult to achieve complete seizure control, although, these seizures are not associated with higher risk of permanent neurologic impairment.

Pharmacologic Management of Underlying Etiology of Seizures and SE

While SE management is ongoing, workup for the trigger of seizures/SE should be performed simultaneously, and reversible triggers should be addressed, as delineated above. If SE occurred due to electrolyte abnormalities (such as hypoglycemia, hypocalcemia, hypomagnesemia, or acute hyponatremia), these must be corrected rapidly. If CNS infections are suspected, then cultures

and lumbar puncture should be performed, and broad-spectrum antibiotics should be initiated as soon as possible. Attention should be given to the fact that these patients are immunosuppressed and may need IV ampicillin, antifungal agents, and acyclovir in addition to vancomycin and a third-generation cephalosporin until the specific pathogen is identified.

Patients may be receiving chemotherapeutic agents that trigger neurotoxicity and seizures, such as vinca alkaloids, cisplatin, busulfan, interferon-alpha, immunosuppressants, or CAR T-cell therapy. These agents should be held until SE is controlled, and alternative agents should be considered. If radiation necrosis is suspected, then steroids should be initiated, or dosage should be increased.

A special mention must be made regarding the management of paraneoplastic limbic encephalitis. Immunotherapy has been used with variable efficacy, and recommendations for immunotherapy are largely based on retrospective case series and expert opinions. A combination of intravenous immune globulin and/or plasma exchange with high-dose corticosteroids is considered the first line of immunotherapy. If there is no clinical improvement, rituximab or cyclophosphamide may be used. Rituximab has been reported to reduce relapses [13].

The use of chemotherapeutic agents in controlling seizures in brain tumor patients has been evaluated as one of the outcome measures in several clinical trials. Temozolomide has been shown to be efficacious in patients with high-grade gliomas in several studies. A few studies have also evaluated the use of temozolomide, for the purpose of seizure control, in patients with low-grade gliomas, with modest efficacy [45].

Long-Term Therapy for Prevention of Seizures in Oncologic Patients

While choosing long-term AED therapy in oncologic patients, care must be taken to evaluate drug interactions. While there is no direct comparison in the literature, in general, levetiracetam, lacosamide, gabapentin, and pregabalin are the preferred AEDs in oncologic patients due to their minimal side effects and drug interactions. If these are not effective, then oxcarbazepine, lamotrigine, topiramate, and zonisamide may be considered due to lesser degree of interactions [64].

Enzyme-inducing drugs such as phenytoin, phenobarbital, and carbamazepine reduce the efficacy of chemotherapeutic drugs such as nitrosoureas, etoposide, topotecan, doxorubicin, and methotrexate, among others. They also reduce the efficacy of corticosteroids. This has been shown to reduce survival and increase risk of tumor recurrence in glioma patients [43] and in children with acute lymphoblastic leukemia [46]. Similarly, chemotherapeutic agents are enzyme inducers and reduce plasma concentrations of AEDs. Cisplatin and doxorubicin lower levels of phenytoin, carbamazepine, and valproic acid. Valproic acid, a hepatic enzyme inhibitor, can lead to toxic levels of nitrosoureas, cisplatin, and etoposide and may increase occurrence of pancytopenia, which is already very common in cancer patients [64]. In a retrospective study, Kerkhoff et al. showed that use of valproic acid and levetiracetam in patients with glioblastoma may contribute to higher seizure control and when used in combination with temozolomide resulted in longer survival [28]. However, a pooled analysis of prospective trials was unable to show a benefit of valproic acid in GBM patients [28].

Long-term prophylaxis against seizures in patients with brain tumors is a common practice nationwide. There is a higher incidence of adverse effects from AED therapy in patients with brain tumors when compared to the general population. Brain tumor patients also have higher incidence of cognitive impairment when receiving AED therapy. No randomized-controlled trial has shown improved outcomes, survival, or reduced seizure occurrence with long-term AED prophylaxis. Thus, the American Academy of Neurology recommends against long-term seizure prophylaxis in brain tumor patients [57, 19]. Perioperatively, approximately 20% of patients may develop seizures and SE, and, in this setting, it may be prudent to initiate seizure prophylaxis for up to 1 week postoperatively. Levetiracetam is commonly used in clinical practice for perioperative seizure prophylaxis in brain tumor patients.

- **Non-pharmacologic**

While the mainstay of management of seizures and SE in critically ill oncologic patients is pharmacologic, there are a few points worth mentioning in the non-pharmacologic management of these patients.

In patients with SE, even prior to initiation of pharmacologic therapy, proper positioning, establishing a safe airway, and ensuring adequate oxygenation, ventilation, and hemodynamics are priority. Continuous vital sign monitoring should be initiated within 2 min of seizure onset. The patient should be positioned with head of bed at 30° or higher, to prevent aspiration of oral contents and to reduce intracranial pressure. Jaw thrust should be provided; airway should be cleared of secretions, foreign bodies, and blood; and noninvasive oxygenation such as nasal cannula or non-rebreather mask should be initiated. The patient should be emergently intubated if there is concern that the patient is not protecting his or her airway due to a low Glasgow Coma Scale (< 8), ongoing generalized convulsive SE despite two AEDs, excessive oral secretions coupled with poor cough, airway hemorrhage from tongue bite, poor ventilation characterized by elevated carbon dioxide levels, persistent hypoxemia, and concerns for raised intracranial pressure. Simultaneously adequate intravenous (IV) access, i.e., two large bore peripheral intravenous catheters, should be placed within the first 2 min. Benzodiazepines cause hypotension, and thus free-flowing IV crystalloids and/or vasopressors should be available to ensure adequate mean arterial pressure >70 mm Hg [4]. Finger-stick blood glucose should be checked, and if low, dextrose should be administered preceded by intravenous thiamine to prevent Wernicke's encephalopathy. A urinary catheter should also be placed. As previously mentioned, while the status epilepticus management algorithm is being performed, simultaneously, the evaluation for triggers should be ongoing as well. Comprehensive metabolic panel, antiepileptic drug levels, urine toxicology, and complete blood count should be sent. Chemotherapeutic agents that may have triggered the seizures should be held. Medication lists should be thoroughly reviewed, and any medications lowering the seizure threshold should be discontinued.

Surgical management for refractory epilepsy or SE in cancer patients may be considered. This is most relevant in two scenarios: (i) patients with brain tumors and (ii) patients with paraneoplastic syndromes. The purpose of surgical treatment is to ensure seizure control by removal of the tumor and the surrounding epileptogenic area. This requires thorough preoperative evaluation to delineate the epileptogenic focus and to ensure that the tumor is the sole epileptogenic focus and that its removal will result in minimal disability. In patients with benign and developmental brain tumors, 82% patients have been reported to have complete seizure control after surgery, provided there is a single focus on EEG, there are no other associated lesions, the duration of epilepsy is short, treatment is initiated early, and the tumor is completely resected [35]. Seizure freedom after resection of GBM occurs in around 77% patients. Seizure recurrence, in GBM patients, usually indicates tumor progression [17]. Similarly, early tumor removal in patients with paraneoplastic limbic encephalitis results in seizure freedom and improved clinical outcomes [13].

Radiotherapy for seizure control in patients with brain tumors has not been adequately studied, and the only available literature includes a short case series evaluating seven patients with low-grade astrocytoma who were found 75% seizure reduction after radiotherapy. However, more literature needs to be available before making recommendations on the use of radiotherapy to manage seizures in oncologic patients [64].

Prognosis

SE and seizures in critically ill oncologic patients are associated with worse prognosis when compared to non-tumor associated SE and seizures.

A meta-analysis and systematic review, involving 14 studies, demonstrated a higher mortality in brain tumor-related SE when compared to non-tumor-related SE (17.2% vs. 6.6%) with a relative risk of 2.78 [2]. Several other studies have also demonstrated a higher mortality in patients with SE secondary to a tumor (ranging 30–40%) when compared to other causes. In a study evaluating SE in 35 patients with a tumor, the average 30-day mortality was 23%, and patients with systemic cancer and older age correlated with a shorter survival [7]. Surprisingly, a diagnosis of epilepsy and seizures at presentation were associated with improved survival in a study that specifically evaluated GBM patients. This might be related to earlier detection and more complete resection of the tumors [61]. With regard to morbidity, a study demonstrated increased morbidity in tumor-related SE when compared to SE from other causes (33.3% vs. 15.2%) [53]. Overall, it is likely that mortality in critically ill oncologic patients presenting with seizures and SE is driven largely by the prognosis of the underlying malignancy, the stage of the neoplastic disease, and the functional status of the patient rather than the seizures themselves.

Summary

SE is a neurological emergency requiring prompt evaluation and management. It is becoming clearer that adult-onset "idiopathic" refractory epilepsy and SE may actually be linked to underlying undiagnosed neoplastic disease. Pharmacologic treatment is the mainstay when managing seizures and SE in critically ill oncologic patients. Such management includes emergent management of seizures and SE, management of the underlying etiology and long-term antiepileptic drug therapy including seizure prophylaxis. SE has been defined as continuous clinical and/or electrographic activity for 5 min or more or recurrent seizure activity without recovery between seizures. In general, it is recommended to achieve definitive control of SE within 60 min. After ensuring adequate airway, oxygenation, and perfusion, the first line of treatment is benzodiazepines. Intravenous loraze-pam and intramuscular midazolam are the most effective in aborting SE. Benzodiazepines should be followed by an urgent loading dose of a longer-acting AED regardless of whether SE was aborted. The sooner the treatment is initiated, the greater the chances of success and the better the outcome. Overall, SE and seizures in critically ill oncologic patients are associated with worse prognosis when compared to non-tumor associated SE and seizures. Prognosis is likely tied to the underlying malignancy and functional status of the patient.

References

1. Alldredge BK, Gelb AM, Isaacs SM, Corry MD, Allen F, Ulrich S, Gottwald MD, O'Neil N, Neuhaus JM, Segal MR, Lowenstein DH. A comparison of lorazepam, diazepam, and placebo for the treatment of out-of-hospital status epilepticus. N Engl J Med. 2001;345(9):631–7.

2. Arik Y, Leijten FS, Seute T, Robe PA, Snijders TJ. Prognosis and therapy of tumor-related versus non-tumor-related status epilepticus: a systematic review and meta-analysis. BMC Neurol. 2014;14:152–2377.

3. Aronica E, Gorter JA, Jansen GH, Leenstra S, Yankaya B, Troost D. Expression of connexin 43 and connexin 32 gap-junction proteins in epilepsy-associated brain tumors and in the perilesional epileptic cortex. Acta Neuropathol. 2001;101(5):449–59.

4. Brophy GM, Bell R, Claassen J, Alldredge B, Bleck TP, Glauser T, Laroche SM, Riviello JJ, Shutter L, Sperling MR, Treiman DM, Vespa PM, Neurocritical Care Society Status Epilepticus Guideline Writing Committee. Guidelines for the evaluation and management of status epilepticus. Neurocrit Care. 2012;17(1):3–23.

5. Brouwers PJ, Bosker RJ, Schaafsma MR, Wilts G, Neef C. Photosensitive seizures associated with interferon alfa-2a. Ann Pharmacother. 1999;33(1):113–4.

6. Calatozzolo C, Gelati M, Ciusani E, Sciacca FL, Pollo B, Cajola L, Marras C, Silvani A, Vitellaro-Zuccarello L, Croci D, Boiardi A, Salmaggi A. Expression of drug resistance proteins Pgp, MRP1, MRP3, MRP5 and GST-pi in human glioma. J Neuro-Oncol. 2005;74(2):113–21.

7. Cavaliere R, Farace E, Schiff D. Clinical implications of status epilepticus in patients with neoplasms. Arch Neurol. 2006;63(12):1746–9.

8. Chernov MF, Kubo O, Hayashi M, Izawa M, Maruyama T, Usukura M, Ono Y, Hori T, Takakura K. Proton MRS of the peritumoral brain. J Neurol Sci. 2005;228(2):137–42.

9. Chubinidze AI, Gobechiia ZV, Abramishvili VV, Samodurova GV, Chubinidze MA. Morphologic characteristics of cortical synapses in patients with epilepsy. Zhurnal nevropatologii i psikhiatrii imeni S.S. Korsakova (Moscow, Russia: 1952). 1989;89(6):23–6.

10. Clouston PD, DeAngelis LM, Posner JB. The spectrum of neurological disease in patients with systemic cancer. Ann Neurol. 1992;31(3):268–73.

11. Cocito L, Audenino D, Primavera A. Altered mental state and nonconvulsive status epilepticus in patients with cancer. Arch Neurol. 2001;58(8):1310.

12. Dalmau J. Status epilepticus due to paraneoplastic and nonparaneoplastic encephalitides. Epilepsia. 2009;50 Suppl 12:58–60.

13. Dalmau J, Graus F. Antibody-mediated encephalitis. N Engl J Med. 2018;378(9):840–51.

14. Dalmau J, Gleichman AJ, Hughes EG, Rossi JE, Peng X, Lai M, Dessain SK, Rosenfeld MR, Balice-Gordon R, Lynch DR. Anti-NMDA-receptor encephalitis: case series and analysis of the effects of antibodies. Lancet Neurol. 2008;7(12):1091–8.

15. Dham BS, Hunter K, Rincon F. The epidemiology of status epilepticus in the United States. Neurocrit Care. 2014;20(3):476–83.

16. Diniotis B, Sternberg E, Shakuntala S, Chiha M, Khosla P. Hypocalcemia in malignancy – unexpected but common. Cureus. 2015;7(12):e442.

17. Erturk Cetin O, Isler C, Uzan M, Ozkara C. Epilepsy-related brain tumors. Seizure. 2017;44:93–7.

18. Gijtenbeek JM, van den Bent MJ, Vecht CJ. Cyclosporine neurotoxicity: a review. J Neurol. 1999;246(5):339–46.

19. Glantz MJ, Cole BF, Forsyth PA, Recht LD, Wen PY, Chamberlain MC, Grossman SA, Cairncross JG. Practice parameter: anticonvulsant prophylaxis in patients with newly diagnosed brain tumors. Report of the Quality Standards Subcommittee of the American Academy of Neurology. Neurology. 2000;54(10):1886–93.

20. Gleeson JG, duPlessis AJ, Barnes PD, Riviello JJ. Cyclosporin A acute encephalopathy and seizure syndrome in childhood: clinical features and risk of seizure recurrence. J Child Neurol. 1998;13(7):336–44.

21. Gultekin SH, Rosenfeld MR, Voltz R, Eichen J, Posner JB, Dalmau J. Paraneoplastic limbic encephalitis: neurological symptoms, immunological findings and tumour association in 50 patients. Brain J Neurol. 2000;123(Pt 7):1481–94.

22. Herman ST. Epilepsy after brain insult: targeting epileptogenesis. Neurology. 2002;59(9 Suppl 5):S21–6.

23. Hormigo A, Liberato B, Lis E, DeAngelis LM. Nonconvulsive status epilepticus in patients with cancer: imaging abnormalities. Arch Neurol. 2004;61(3):362–5.

24. Iglesias P, Diez JJ. Management of endocrine disease: a clinical update on tumor-induced hypoglycemia. Eur J Endocrinol. 2014;170(4):R147–57.

25. Jacobs DA, Fung KM, Cook NM, Schalepfer WW, Goldberg HI, Stecker MM. Complex partial status epilepticus associated with anti-Hu paraneoplastic syndrome. J Neurol Sci. 2003;213(1–2):77–82.

26. Kargiotis O, Markoula S, Kyritsis AP. Epilepsy in the cancer patient. Cancer Chemother Pharmacol. 2011;67(3):489–501.

27. Kelley BP, Patel SC, Marin HL, Corrigan JJ, Mitsias PD, Griffith B. Autoimmune encephalitis: pathophysiology and imaging review of an overlooked diagnosis. AJNR Am J Neuroradiol. 2017;38(6):1070–8.

28. Kerkhof M, Dielemans JC, van Breemen MS, Zwinkels H, Walchenbach R, Taphoorn MJ, Vecht CJ. Effect of valproic acid on seizure control and on survival in patients with glioblastoma multiforme. Neuro-Oncology. 2013;15(7):961–7.

29. Knudsen-Baas KM, Power KN, Engelsen BA, Hegrestad SE, Gilhus NE, Storstein AM. Status epilepticus secondary to glioma. Seizure. 2016;40:76–80.

30. La Morgia C, Mondini S, Guarino M, Bonifazi F, Cirignotta F. Busulfan neurotoxicity and EEG abnormalities: a case report. Neurol Sci. 2004;25(2):95–7.

31. Lai M, Hughes EG, Peng X, Zhou L, Gleichman AJ, Shu H, Mata S, Kremens D, Vitaliani R, Geschwind MD, Bataller L, Kalb RG, Davis R, Graus F, Lynch DR, Balice-Gordon R, Dalmau J. AMPA receptor antibodies in limbic encephalitis alter synaptic receptor location. Ann Neurol. 2009;65(4):424–34.

32. Legroux-Crespel E, Lafaye S, Mahe E, Picard-Dahan C, Crickx B, Sassolas B, Descamps V. Seizures during interferon alpha therapy: three cases in dermatology. Ann Dermatol Venereol. 2003;130(2. Pt 1):202–4.

33. Lieu AS, Howng SL. Intracranial meningiomas and epilepsy: incidence, prognosis and influencing factors. Epilepsy Res. 2000;38(1):45–52.

34. Lovblad K, Kelkar P, Ozdoba C, Ramelli G, Remonda L, Schroth G. Pure methotrexate encephalopathy presenting with seizures: CT and MRI features. Pediatr Radiol. 1998;28(2):86–91.

35. Luyken C, Blumcke I, Fimmers R, Urbach H, Elger CE, Wiestler OD, Schramm J. The spectrum of long-term epilepsy-associated tumors: long-term seizure and tumor outcome and neurosurgical aspects. Epilepsia. 2003;44(6):822–30.

36. Marcuse LV, Lancman G, Demopoulos A, Fields M. Nonconvulsive status epilepticus in patients with brain tumors. Seizure. 2014;23(7):542–7.

37. McNamara JO. Emerging insights into the genesis of epilepsy. Nature. 1999;399(6738 Suppl):A15–22.

38. Mehta S, Shah A, Jung H. Diagnosis and treatment options for sequelae following radiation treatment of brain tumors. Clin Neurol Neurosurg. 2017;163:1–8.

39. Michelucci R, Pasini E, Meletti S, Fallica E, Rizzi R, Florindo I, Chiari A, Monetti C, Cremonini AM, Forlivesi S, Albani F, Baruzzi A, PERNO Study Group. Epilepsy in primary cerebral tumors: the characteristics of epilepsy at the onset (results from the PERNO study–Project of Emilia Romagna Region on Neuro-Oncology). Epilepsia. 2013;54(Suppl 7):86–91.

40. Neligan A, Shorvon SD. Frequency and prognosis of convulsive status epilepticus of different causes: a systematic review. Arch Neurol. 2010;67(8):931–40.

41. Niehusmann P, Dalmau J, Rudlowski C, Vincent A, Elger CE, Rossi JE, Bien CG. Diagnostic value of N-methyl-D-aspartate receptor antibodies in women with new-onset epilepsy. Arch Neurol. 2009;66(4):458–64.

42. Nussbaum ES, Djalilian HR, Cho KH, Hall WA. Brain metastases. Histology, multiplicity, surgery, and survival. Cancer. 1996;78(8):1781–8.

43. Oberndorfer S, Piribauer M, Marosi C, Lahrmann H, Hitzenberger P, Grisold W. P450 enzyme inducing and non-enzyme inducing antiepileptics in glioblastoma patients treated with standard chemotherapy. J Neuro-Oncol. 2005;72(3):255–60.

44. Oz G, Alger JR, Barker PB, Bartha R, Bizzi A, Boesch C, Bolan PJ, Brindle KM, Cudalbu C, Dincer A, Dydak U, Emir UE, Frahm J, Gonzalez RG, Gruber S, Gruetter R, Gupta RK, Heerschap A, Henning A, Hetherington HP, Howe FA, Huppi PS, Hurd RE, Kantarci K, Klomp DW, Kreis R, Kruiskamp MJ, Leach MO, Lin AP, Luijten PR, Marjanska M, Maudsley AA, Meyerhoff DJ, Mountford CE, Nelson SJ, Pamir MN, Pan JW, Peet AC, Poptani H, Posse S, Pouwels PJ, Ratai EM, Ross BD, Scheenen TW, Schuster C, Smith IC, Soher BJ, Tkac I, Vigneron DB, Kauppinen RA, MRS Consensus Group. Clinical proton MR spectroscopy in central nervous system disorders. Radiology. 2014;270(3):658–79.

45. Pace A, Vidiri A, Galie E, Carosi M, Telera S, Cianciulli AM, Canalini P, Giannarelli D, Jandolo B, Carapella CM. Temozolomide chemotherapy for progressive low-grade glioma: clinical benefits and radiological response. Ann Oncol. 2003;14(12):1722–6.

46. Relling MV, Pui CH, Sandlund JT, Rivera GK, Hancock ML, Boyett JM, Schuetz EG, Evans WE. Adverse effect of anticonvulsants on efficacy of chemotherapy for acute lymphoblastic leukaemia. Lancet (London, England). 2000;356(9226):285–90.

47. Riva M. Brain tumoral epilepsy: a review. Neurol Sci. 2005;26(Suppl 1):S40–2.

48. Rodriguez-Enriquez S, Moreno-Sanchez R. Intermediary metabolism of fast-growth tumor cells. Arch Med Res. 1998;29(1):1–12.

49. Rogers LR. Cerebrovascular complications in patients with cancer. Semin Neurol. 2010;30(3):311–9.

50. Rollins N, Winick N, Bash R, Booth T. Acute methotrexate neurotoxicity: findings on diffusion-weighted imaging and correlation with clinical outcome. AJNR Am J Neuroradiol. 2004;25(10):1688–95.

51. Rosenfeld MR, Eichen JG, Wade DF, Posner JB, Dalmau J. Molecular and clinical diversity in paraneoplastic immunity to Ma proteins. Ann Neurol. 2001;50(3):339–48.

52. Santomasso BD, Park JH, Salloum D, Riviere I, Flynn J, Mead E, Halton E, Wang X, Senechal B, Purdon T, Cross JR, Liu H, Vachha B, Chen X, DeAngelis LM, Li D, Bernal Y, Gonen M, Wendel HG, Sadelain M, Brentjens RJ. Clinical and biological correlates of neurotoxicity associated with CAR T-cell therapy in patients with B-cell acute lymphoblastic leukemia. Cancer Discov. 2018;8(8):958–71.

53. Scholtes FB, Renier WO, Meinardi H. Generalized convulsive status epilepticus: causes, therapy, and outcome in 346 patients. Epilepsia. 1994;35(5):1104–12.

54. Schwartz L, Supuran CT, Alfarouk KO. The Warburg effect and the hallmarks of cancer. Anti Cancer Agents Med Chem. 2017;17(2):164–70.

55. Shamji MF, Fric-Shamji EC, Benoit BG. Brain tumors and epilepsy: pathophysiology of peritumoral changes. Neurosurg Rev. 2009;32(3):275–84; discussion 284

56. Singh G, Rees JH, Sander JW. Seizures and epilepsy in oncological practice: causes, course, mechanisms and treatment. J Neurol Neurosurg Psychiatry. 2007;78 (4):342–9.

57. Sirven JI, Wingerchuk DM, Drazkowski JF, Lyons MK, Zimmerman RS. Seizure prophylaxis in patients with brain tumors: a meta-analysis. Mayo Clin Proc. 2004;79(12):1489–94.

58. Steeghs N, de Jongh FE, Sillevis Smitt PA, van den Bent MJ. Cisplatin-induced encephalopathy and seizures. Anti-Cancer Drugs. 2003;14(6):443–6.

59. Strzelczyk A, Zollner JP, Willems LM, Jost J, Paule E, Schubert-Bast S, Rosenow F, Bauer S. Lacosamide in status epilepticus: systematic review of current evidence. Epilepsia. 2017;58(6):933–50.

60. Thieben MJ, Lennon VA, Boeve BF, Aksamit AJ, Keegan M, Vernino S. Potentially reversible autoimmune limbic encephalitis with neuronal potassium channel antibody. Neurology. 2004;62(7):1177–82.

61. Toledo M, Sarria-Estrada S, Quintana M, Maldonado X, Martinez-Ricarte F, Rodon J, Auger C, Salas-Puig J, Santamarina E, Martinez-Saez E. Prognostic implications of epilepsy in glioblastomas. Clin Neurol Neurosurg. 2015;139:166–71.

62. Towne AR, Waterhouse EJ, Boggs JG, Garnett LK, Brown AJ, Smith JR, DeLorenzo RJ. Prevalence of nonconvulsive status epilepticus in comatose patients. Neurology. 2000;54(2):340–5.

63. van Breemen MS, Wilms EB, Vecht CJ. Epilepsy in patients with brain tumours: epidemiology, mechanisms, and management. Lancet Neurol. 2007;6(5): 421–30.

64. Villanueva V, Codina M, Elices E. Management of epilepsy in oncological patients. Neurologist. 2008;14(6 Suppl 1):S44–54.

65. Villemure JG, de Tribolet N. Epilepsy in patients with central nervous system tumors. Curr Opin Neurol. 1996;9(6):424–8.

66. White JC, Liu CT, Mixter WJ. Focal epilepsy; a statistical study of its causes and the results of surgical treatment; epilepsy secondary to intracranial tumors. N Engl J Med. 1948;238(26):891–9.

67. Wolf HK, Roos D, Blumcke I, Pietsch T, Wiestler OD. Perilesional neurochemical changes in focal epilepsies. Acta Neuropathol. 1996;91(4):376–84.

68. Yu Z, Kryzer TJ, Griesmann GE, Kim K, Benarroch EE, Lennon VA. CRMP-5 neuronal autoantibody: marker of lung cancer and thymoma-related autoimmunity. Ann Neurol. 2001;49(2):146–54.

69. Zack MM, Kobau R. National and state estimates of the numbers of adults and children with active epilepsy – United States, 2015. MMWR Morb Mortal Wkly Rep. 2017;66(31):821–5.

Posterior Reversible Encephalopathy Syndrome (PRES) in Cancer Patients

24

Bryan Bonder and Marcos de Lima

Contents

Introduction 354

Etiology 354

Epidemiology 355

Pathophysiology 356

Clinical Features 356

Diagnosis 357
Imaging 357
Cerebrospinal Fluid Examination 359
Laboratory Work 359
Electroencephalogram 359

Management 359
Pharmacologic Management 359
Nonpharmacologic Management 360

Prognosis 362

Conclusion 362

References 362

B. Bonder
Division of Hematology and Oncology, University Hospitals Cleveland Medical Center, Cleveland, OH, USA
e-mail: Bryan.Bonder@UHhospitals.org

M. de Lima (✉)
Stem Cell Transplant Program, Seidman Cancer Center, University Hospitals Cleveland Medical Center, and Case Western Reserve University, Cleveland, OH, USA
e-mail: Marcos.deLima@UHhospitals.org

Abstract

Posterior reversible encephalopathy syndrome (PRES) is a frequently dramatic clinical disorder characterized by a constellation of symptoms with imaging correlates. Typically, patients present with changes in mental status, visual disturbances, headaches, seizures, or focal neurological deficits. Imaging findings are classically in a posterior vascular distribution; however, PRES has been now recognized to involve other areas of the central nervous system. Once thought to be highly

© Springer Nature Switzerland AG 2020
J. L. Nates, K. J. Price (eds.), *Oncologic Critical Care*,
https://doi.org/10.1007/978-3-319-74588-6_37

associated with systemic hypertension, PRES has been identified to be secondary to a growing list of conditions and therapies. With the introduction of newer oncological drugs and more frequent usage of magnetic resonance imaging, PRES has been increasingly identified in cancer patients. Rapid recognition and intervention is critical to preventing morbidity or mortality.

Keywords

PRES · Posterior reversible encephalopathy syndrome · RPLS · Reversible posterior leukoencephalopathy syndrome · Neurological emergency · Seizure

Introduction

Posterior reversible encephalopathy syndrome (PRES) is a clinical syndrome involving the acute onset of neurological symptoms with vasogenic edema classically in a bilateral symmetric parieto-occipital distribution. PRES is also known as reversible posterior leukoencephalopathy syndrome, although it does not always present in a posterior distribution and may result in permanent disability or even death. PRES was first well characterized in 1996 by Hinchey et al. in 15 patients, the majority of whom were either receiving immunosuppressive therapy or were hypertensive [30]. Since then it has been described in a wide variety of clinical scenarios and with numerous etiologies. Patients can present with an assortment of symptoms including altered mental status, visual symptoms, headache, seizures, or focal neurological signs. PRES is commonly seen in cancer patients, especially those receiving chemotherapeutics, immunosuppressants, and undergoing stem cell transplantation. These patients may present without hypertension which was commonly thought to be the precipitant of PRES, leading to the formulation of numerous alternative theories of the underlying pathogenesis. Regardless of the causative physiological process, PRES is a neurological emergency and prompt recognition and management is necessary to prevent morbidity and mortality.

Etiology

A variety of conditions and treatments have been associated with the syndrome, including drugs, hypertension, electrolyte disturbances, renal failure, and autoimmune disorders among others (Table 1). Cancer patients are frequently exposed to therapies which are known to cause PRES (Table 2). Onset after exposure to a causative agent may be as short as 25 min [10] or may occur up to 3 months after exposure [30]. Multiagent chemotherapy regimens are frequently linked to PRES [41], but it does not appear that there is a dose-intensity relationship. Calcineurin inhibitors are often implicated (especially tacrolimus). Interestingly, plasma levels of immunosuppressants do not appear to correlate with the severity of imaging changes or symptoms. Other causative

Table 1 Etiologies and clinical conditions associated with PRES

Acute intermittent porphyria
Alcohol withdrawal
Autoimmune diseases (systemic lupus erythematosus, polyarteritis nodosa, and others)
Blood transfusion
Bone marrow transplantation
Cerebral spinal fluid leak
Contrast media exposure
Cryoglobulinemia
Diabetic ketoacidosis
Drugs (see Table 2)
Eclampsia or preeclampsia
Guillain-Barre syndrome
HELLP syndrome (hemolysis, elevated liver enzymes, low platelets)
Hypertension
Hypocalcemia
Hypomagnesemia
Infections
Intravenous immunoglobulins
Liver failure/cirrhosis
Neurosurgical procedures
Recent initiation of highly active antiretroviral therapy
Renal disease
Sickle cell anemia
Solid organ transplantation
Thrombotic microangiopathies (hemolytic uremic syndrome, thrombotic thrombocytopenic purpura)
Uremia

Table 2 Selected drugs and regimens associated with PRES

5-FU [51]
Adriamycin
All-trans retinoid acid and arsenic trioxide [15]
Apatinib [45]
Aurora kinase inhibitors [37]
Antithymocyte globulin
Bevacizumab [51]
Cabozantinib [12]
Carboplatin [68]
Cediranib [37]
Cetuximab [37]
Cisplatin [41]
Corticosteroids [56]
Cyclophosphamide [64]
Cyclosporine [30]
Cytarabine [59]
Dasatinib [37]
Daunorubicin [54]
Dexamethasone [33]
Docetaxel [65]
Enzalutamide [16]
EPOCH (etoposide, prednisone, vincristine, cyclophosphamide, doxorubicin) [24]
Eribulin mesylate [63]
Fludarabine
Gemcitabine [41]
Gemtuzumab [37]
Granulocyte colony-stimulating factor
Interferon
Ipilimumab and nivolumab [70]
Irinotecan [65]
L-asparaginase [53]
Lenvatinib [28]
Methotrexate (systemic and intrathecal) (21)
Mycophenolate mofetil [71]
Mitomycin-C [48]
Nivolumab [49]
Oxaliplatin [34]
Paclitaxel [65]
Pazopanib [19]
Pembrolizumab [42]
Pemetrexed [66]
R-CHOP (rituximab, cyclophosphamide, hydroxydaunorubicin, vincristine, prednisone) [31]
Rituximab [37]
Sorafenib [26]

(*continued*)

Table 2 (continued)

Sunitinib [13]
Tacrolimus (FK506) [30]
Trastuzumab [1]
Vincristine [32]
Ipilimumab [52]
Pembrolizumab [42]
Venlafaxine

agents include drugs that target vascular endothelial growth factor (VEGF) such as bevacizumab, sorafenib, and sunitinib [29, 65, 67].

PRES may also be triggered by infection, sepsis, and shock and may be an underlying etiology of approximately 20–25% of patients. The most common causative bacteria are gram-positive organisms [6].

Interestingly, radiation therapy including whole body and irradiation of the central nervous system does not appear to be associated with an increased risk [65]. Furthermore, the presence of brain metastases does not appear to dramatically increase risk of PRES [65].

Epidemiology

The overall incidence is unknown. PRES occurs in both adult and pediatric populations, and it has been described in patients from ages 2 to 90 years. In two large single center retrospective reviews, most cancer patients with PRES were between the ages of 19 to 78 years with a median age of 52–58 years [37, 65]. There appears to be a female predominance likely secondary to its association with pregnancy and autoimmune diseases [30, 65]. However, the possibility of hormonal influences cannot be excluded. PRES also is frequently seen in stem cell transplant patients at an incidence of up to 6–7% [5, 64] and may be the most common central nervous system complication associated with allogeneic hematopoietic stem cell transplantation [7]. Its high incidence in this population likely corresponds to frequent usage of chemotherapeutics and calcineurin inhibitors.

Pathophysiology

There are currently multiple theories to the underlying mechanism of this often dramatic syndrome, with the major theories being the vasogenic theory, immunogenic theory, and direct toxic effects of drugs on the endothelium.

The vasogenic theory is thought to involve dysfunction of cerebral vascular autoregulation and endothelial damage. The cerebral circulation maintains a steady blood flow in a range of 50–150 mm Hg through flow autoregulation. Regulation is dependent on the pressure supplied by cerebral arterioles, the back pressure from the venous system which is approximately equal to the intracranial pressure, and the resistance secondary to the diameter of small cerebral vessels [20]. The major site of regulation of the cerebral blood flow occurs through changes in cerebral arteriolar wall diameter which in turn is influenced by responses of smooth muscle to transmural pressure, carbon dioxide tension, and the autonomic nervous system. When systemic blood pressure decreases, cerebral arterioles dilate in an attempt to maintain blood flow to neural tissues. When blood pressure increases, cerebral arterioles constrict to prevent cerebral hypertension. This process is partially controlled by signaling from neurons, astrocytes, and vascular endothelial cells. Endothelial cells release relaxing agents such as nitric oxide or vasoconstrictors such as thromboxane A-2 and endothelin.

In PRES, it is thought that rapidly developing hypertension leads to hyperperfusion and subsequently decompensation of normal blood vessel regulatory mechanisms. This causes extravasation of plasma and macromolecules through the tight junctions into the brain parenchyma and interstitial space, with vasogenic edema. The posterior circulation has less sympathetic innervation as compared to the anterior circulation and therefore has less ability to autoregulate [21]. This difference innervation may explain the propensity of PRES to present in a posterior (parieto-occipital) distribution. However, approximately 15–20% of patients are not hypertensive when diagnosed, suggesting that multiple or alternative mechanisms may be involved [57].

Immune dysregulation and cytokines may also play a role in endothelial dysfunction and activation [50]. PRES is frequently seen in diseases with systemic activation of the immune system such as in autoimmune conditions, sepsis, transplantation, and post-cytotoxic chemotherapy. Tumor necrosis factor (TNF) alpha and interleukin 1, which are frequently elevated in the above conditions, induce expression of adhesion molecules such as intracellular adhesion molecule 1, vascular cell adhesion molecule 1, and E-selectin. These adhesion molecules recruit leukocytes which then release cytotoxic compounds such as reactive oxygen species and proteases which cause endothelial damage thus increasing vascular permeability. Also, TNF alpha increases VEGF expression and ultimately causes increased vascular permeability.

The cytotoxic drug theory proposes a direct effect of chemotherapy, immunosuppressive, or immunomodulatory drugs on endothelial cells. Endothelial injury is mediated by release of chemokines such as endothelin-1, leading to immune activation. This process also results in extravasation of plasma and macromolecules into the brain parenchyma causing cerebral edema. As listed in Table 2, PRES has been noted in an increasing number of patients receiving chemotherapeutic agents. These patients often present without hypertension suggesting that the cytotoxic and immunogenic hypotheses may play more of a role in the oncologic setting than the classic vasogenic theory.

Clinical Features

Acute and subacute presentations have been described. Symptoms in oncologic patients may include focal neurological deficits (~15%), headache (~48%), vomiting, seizures (~58%), altered mental status (~71%), and visual disturbances (~26%) [9, 65].

Hypertension may be secondary to treatment such as caused by steroids or cyclosporine, low magnesium levels or response to compression of renal vasculature causing activation of the renin-angiotensin-aldosterone system. Altered mental status can be as mild as personality changes or somnolence but can occasionally progress to stupor or coma.

Seizures are the one of the most common presentations of PRES occurring in up to two-thirds of cancer patients [37]. The etiology is likely cortical irritation induced by vasogenic edema. They may be self-limited but typically are recurrent and may require intensive therapy for status epilepticus. Seizures may be focal in onset but often progress to generalized tonic-clonic [3]. When focal EEG abnormalities are present, they frequently correspond to the location seen on imaging. Status epilepticus may be the presenting symptom and may occur in approximately 3–13% of patients [40, 43]. Status epilepticus should be managed with both treatments directed toward the seizures and the underlying etiology [40].

More focal neurological disturbances depend on the affected area location. Due to the predilection of PRES to involve structures in the posterior circulation, visual disturbances, tinnitus, and vertigo are commonly seen. Visual disturbances may include hemianopia, diplopia, blurred vision, visual hallucinations, and frank cortical blindness. Headaches and vomiting may represent signs of elevated intracranial pressure which may progress to cerebral herniation if left untreated. Headaches are frequently described as holocephalic.

Diagnosis

PRES should be suspected in the setting of acute onset neurological symptoms in patients with an inciting cause such as hypertension, renal failure, autoimmune disorders, or drugs known to be associated with the condition. Often the presenting symptoms are nonspecific therefore the diagnosis relies on a high index of suspicion and on magnetic resonance imaging (MRI). Clinical and radiological improvement with appropriate treatment often secures the diagnosis in uncertain cases. A partial list of etiologies which can mimic PRES is presented in Table 3.

Imaging

The classic imaging finding is subcortical and cortical edema in a parieto-occipital distribution. The

Table 3 Differential diagnosis

Acute disseminated encephalomyelitis
Cerebral metastases
Cerebral venous sinus thrombosis
Complex migraine
Hypertensive encephalopathy
Infectious encephalitis
Intracerebral hemorrhage
Ischemic stroke (particularly of the posterior circulation)
Leptomeningeal disease
Paraneoplastic or autoimmune encephalitis
Progressive multifocal leukoencephalopathy
Radiation necrosis
Reversible cerebral vasoconstriction syndrome
Seizures with or without postictal state
Toxic-metabolic encephalopathy
Vasculitis

gold standard method of detection is brain MRI with intensities best seen on T2 fluid-attenuated-inversion-recovery (FLAIR) sequences. This modified T2-weighted sequence nullifies the signal from the cerebral spinal fluid. If severe enough, changes related to vasogenic edema may be seen on computed tomography (CT) imaging. These will appear as areas of hypodensity. CT imaging is more sensitive for cerebral hemorrhage which may be associated with PRES. Overall, CT is less sensitive than MRI with only 50% of cases of PRES demonstrating lesions visible on CT [4].

PRES may involve other regions of the brain including the frontal and temporal lobes, cerebellum, brainstem, deep brain structures, and even spinal cord [8, 22]. Of note, frontal lobe involvement may be present in 50–79%, cerebellar involvement in 34–53%, brainstem in 13–21%, thalamic in 20–30%, and basal ganglia in 12–34% of cases [4, 39, 53]. Rarely, the spinal cord may be affected either in isolation or in additional to the cerebrum [58]. An example of typical imaging findings involving the parietal-occipital regions is shown in Fig. 1. Table 4 depicts a commonly used grading system for PRES-associated vasogenic edema. More severe grades portend poorer prognosis [38].

PRES may cause intraparenchymal and/or subarachnoid hemorrhage. Hemorrhages typically occur proximal to the area of vasogenic

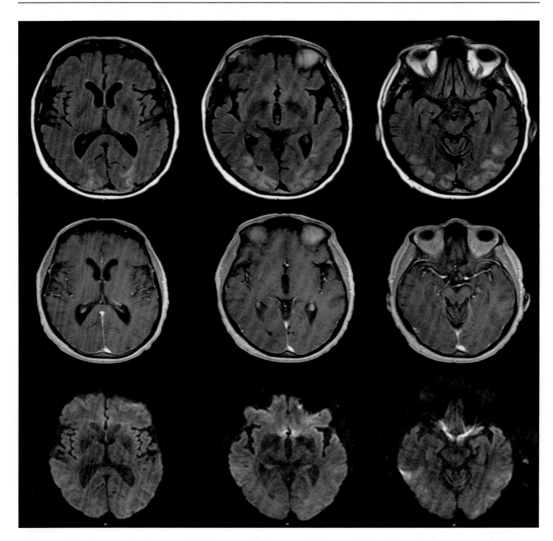

Fig. 1 MRI of a 65-year-old man who received an allo-geneic stem cell transplant and was on tacrolimus for GVHD prophylaxis who developed acute onset visual disturbance, headache, and hypertension. Hyperintensities in a watershed pattern in the posterior circulation on T2/FLAIR imaging (upper panels) without changes on T1 imaging with contrast (middle panels) is characteristic of PRES. Subtle changes on DWI (bottom panels) were without ADC correlate and likely represent T2 shine through

Table 4 Grading system for the severity of edema associated with PRES [53]

Grade	Extent of vasogenic edema	Structure involvement	Parenchymal hemorrhage	Mass effect
Mild	Cortical or subcortical white matter edema	None or one of the following: cerebellum, brainstem, or basal ganglia	Absent	Absent
Moderate	Confluent edema without involvement of periventricular white matter	Two of the following: cerebellum, brainstem, or basal ganglia	Present or absent	Mild – without midline shift or herniation
Severe	Confluent edema with extension to periventricular white matter	All three of the following: cerebellum, brainstem, and basal ganglia	Present or absent	Present with midline shift or herniation

edema. These may best be appreciated by the use of MRI gradient echo (GE) sequences or CT, while MRI diffusion-weighted imaging (DWI) can differentiate PRES from infarction. Hyperintensity on DWI with associated hypointensity on apparent diffusion coefficient (ADC) maps correspond to an area of infarction and cytotoxic edema. Stroke occurs in approximately 6% of cases [65]. It is important to distinguish this from vasogenic edema which will appear hypo- or isointense on DWI and hyperintense on ADC. Diffusion restriction may be seen in up to 11–26% of cases and is associated with a poorer outcome [62]. Similarly, increased intensity of signal on DWI is associated with a poor prognosis likely representing increased cytotoxic edema [14]. Gadolinium contrast enhancement is not typically needed but its presence represents disruption of the blood brain barrier and it may be seen in more than 40% of patients [38]. The presence of gadolinium enhancement, however, does not appear to be associated with a worse prognosis [53]. A small subset of patients may have clinical features consistent with PRES but no changes on brain MRI.

Angiography, if performed, will typically demonstrate vasoconstriction with focal vasospasm or a "string of beads" sign that indicates diffuse vasospasm. Distal branches of the cerebral arteries, particularly posterior cerebral artery, may be reduced in length which is described as "pruning" [61]. Note that these changes may also be seen in reversible cerebral vasoconstriction syndrome, and the two diagnoses may coexist in the same patient.

Cerebrospinal Fluid Examination

Examination of the cerebrospinal fluid (CSF) is not routinely done, however, if sampled may be normal or demonstrate albuminocytologic dissociation (elevated protein with normal white blood cell counts) [18]. This may indicate disruption of the blood brain barrier. Mild CSF pleocytosis may be present but it is uncommon, and consideration should be made for further diagnostic testing including ruling out CNS infection.

Laboratory Work

Laboratory investigation should be directed towards treatable electrolyte disturbances as well as the underlying cause as clinically appropriate. Correction of hypomagnesemia is particularly important [55]. Elevated serum uric acid, lactate dehydrogenase, and creatine may be predictors of poor outcome [23, 47]. High uric acid and creatine usually indicates underlying renal dysfunction and high lactate dehydrogenase (LDH) may represent microvascular hemolysis and/or endothelial dysfunction [27, 35]. Therefore, when elevated LDH levels are present, additional workup should be done to rule out thrombotic microangiopathy (TMA). This is especially important if the patient has been exposed to an agent such as gemcitabine, mitomycin C, or other chemotherapeutic which is known to cause TMA [2].

Electroencephalogram

Seizures are a common complication of PRES. Electroencephalography should be performed to assess for seizures due to the high incidence. They may occur in up to 92% of cases [43]. The most common findings on EEG according to a single center review of patients with PRES and cancer were diffuse theta or delta range slowing (36%), diffuse slowing with focal dysfunction (24%), focal dysfunction with epileptiform discharges (12%), and nonconvulsive status epilepticus (12%) [36].

Management

Rapid diagnosis and proper management of the underlying cause is key. Patients will often require admission to the intensive care unit.

Pharmacologic Management

A careful review of recent drugs the patient has been exposed to should be performed for agents which are known to cause PRES. Alternative agents should be used when feasible. Calcineurin inhibitors are frequently a precipitating cause and should be held whenever possible. Allogeneic transplant recipients frequently develop PRES in the context of GVHD, a scenario that requires careful transition of immunosuppressants. Although cross reactions among calcineurin inhibitors may happen, potential strategies include replacing a calcineurin inhibitor agent with another in the same class, or employing different pharmacologic classes. Steroids are often used to "bridge" the transition [37, 60, 65].

Nonpharmacologic Management

Blood Pressure Control

Blood pressure should be gradually lowered as per guidelines with a lowering of mean arterial blood pressure of up to 25% in the first hour then to 160/110 over the next 2–6 h, then to normal over the next 24–48 h [69]. Note that excessive reduction of blood pressure may result in end organ damage and ischemia and should be avoided. Parenteral antihypertensives are frequently required.

Seizures

Electroencephalogram monitoring and anti-epileptic drugs (AEDs) should be instituted as soon as seizures are suspected. Consideration should be given to using these agents prophylactically or empirically. Intubation may be necessary to protect the airway and may be required in approximately 40% of patients with a typical duration of 7 days [9]. Once control of seizures has been achieved, AEDs may be gradually tapered off over 1–6 months. Long-term risk of seizures after recovery from PRES is low [17]. AED choice should be governed by the patient's comorbidities and potential drug interactions.

Electrolytes

Prompt correction of electrolyte disturbances particularly hypercalcemia and hypomagnesemia should be pursued when clinically appropriate. Hypomagnesemia may especially be seen in patients taking calcineurin inhibitors,

proton pump inhibitors, loss due to gastrointestinal pathology, or excessive alcohol consumption [55].

Cerebral Edema

Posterior fossa edema or hemorrhage may cause brainstem compression or obstructive hydrocephalus. In these acute settings, prompt management of the edema and neurosurgical consultation is recommended. Hypertonic saline and/or mannitol may be needed to control intracranial pressure and temporize the edema until more definitive neurosurgical intervention can be performed. Corticosteroid therapy, unless directed at the underlying cause, does not appear to be helpful in management of vasogenic edema [56].

Thrombocytopenia

Thrombocytopenia should be aggressively managed due to the association of PRES with intracerebral hemorrhage. Transfusion should be performed in accordance with accepted guidelines with a goal of greater than $10 \times 10^3/mm^3$ in nonbleeding patients or greater than $100 \times 10^3/mm^3$ in patients with CNS bleeding or as the clinical scenario dictates. PRES has been associated with thrombotic microangiopathies such as hemolytic uremic syndrome and thrombotic thrombocytopenic purpura [48] and further investigations should be performed if these are suspected. Risk factors for the overlap of diagnoses include GVHD, sepsis, viral infections or reactivations such as EBV or CMV, and use of calcineurin inhibitors.

Cerebral Hemorrhage

Cerebral hemorrhage may occur in up to a third of patients. Minute hemorrhages are the most common followed by parenchymal and sulcal subarachnoid hemorrhage [46]. As would be expected, this is most frequently seen in patients with altered coagulation and worsened edema but not necessarily with elevated blood pressure [46]. When intracerebral hemorrhage is detected, prompt correction of hypertension to a goal systolic blood pressure of less than 140 is required to prevent expansion of the hemorrhage. Neurosurgical consultation is recommended as well. A proposed algorithm for diagnosis and management of PRES is presented in Fig. 2.

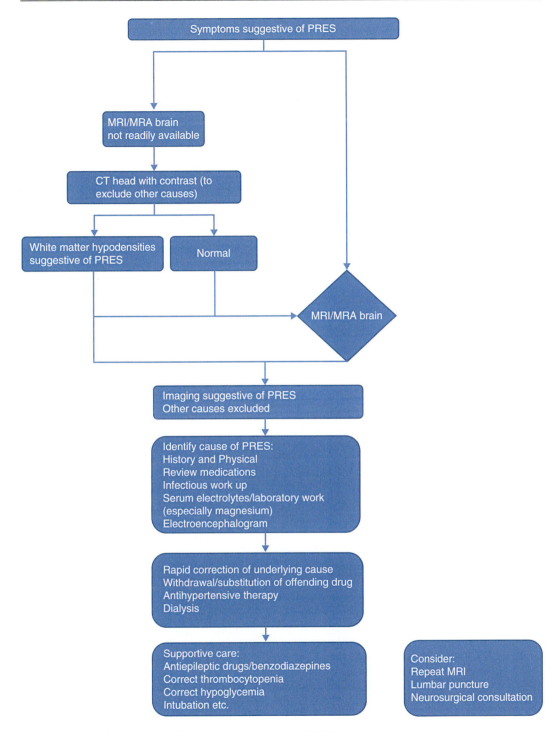

Fig. 2 Proposed algorithm for the diagnosis and management of PRES

Prognosis

The prognosis of PRES is generally favorable, and the syndrome typically resolves without permanent neurological damage. Some patients may have irreversible neurological injury with occasional fatalities. PRES often leads to prolonged hospital stays with a mean length of 20 days [9], but total recovery will occur in approximately 70% of patients [46]. Residual lesions may be seen on follow-up imaging in 35–45% of patients with focal gliosis, infarction, posthemorrhagic products, atrophy, and laminar necrosis being equally commonly seen [46]. Recurrent PRES is rare, however, can occur in approximately 6–8% of cases [25]. Mortality has been reported in the range of 10–20% of cases [44]. Risk factors for a worse outcome include advanced age, prior brain radiation, or sepsis [62]. Radiographic characteristics associated with poor outcomes include presence of hemorrhage, diffusion restriction, or meeting criteria for advanced radiologic PRES [11, 62]. Of note, active cancer does not appear to be associated with the clinical outcome suggesting alternative features like those mentioned above are more important drivers than the underlying malignancy [62].

Conclusion

Diagnosing PRES is sometimes difficult, and it is important to keep this condition high in the differential diagnoses list, especially in some of the clinical contexts discussed here. Early recognition is key, and a multidisciplinary approach is recommended given the complexities of management. Discontinuation of the triggering medication is usually helpful, but it has to be balanced with the needs of the underlying condition, as exemplified by calcineurin inhibitors in allogeneic transplant. Most patients recover well, but morbidity and mortality are high, and more research is needed to understand and prevent this rare but serious complication of oncologic therapy.

References

1. Abughanimeh O, Abu Ghanimeh M, Qasrawi A, Al Momani LA, Madhusudhana S. Trastuzumab-associated posterior reversible encephalopathy syndrome. Cureus. 2018;10:e2686. https://doi.org/10.7759/cureus.2686.
2. Aruch DB, Renteria A. Simultaneous PRES and TMA secondary to tacrolimus after allogeneic bone marrow transplant. Blood. 2015;125:3963.
3. Bakshi R, Bates VE, Mechtler LL, Kinkel PR, Kinkel WR. Occipital lobe seizures as the major clinical manifestation of reversible posterior leukoencephalopathy syndrome: magnetic resonance imaging findings. Epilepsia. 1998;39:295–9.
4. Bartynski WS, Boardman JF. Distinct imaging patterns and lesion distribution in posterior reversible encephalopathy syndrome. AJNR Am J Neuroradiol. 2007;28:1320–7. https://doi.org/10.3174/ajnr.A0549.
5. Bartynski WS, Zeigler ZR, Shadduck RK, Lister J. Variable incidence of cyclosporine and FK-506 neurotoxicity in hematopoeitic malignancies and marrow conditions after allogeneic bone marrow transplantation. Neurocrit Care. 2005;3:33–45. https://doi.org/10.1385/ncc:3:1:033.
6. Bartynski WS, Boardman JF, Zeigler ZR, Shadduck RK, Lister J. Posterior reversible encephalopathy syndrome in infection, sepsis, and shock. AJNR Am J Neuroradiol. 2006;27:2179–90.
7. Bhatt VR, et al. Central nervous system complications and outcomes after allogeneic hematopoietic stem cell transplantation. Clin Lymphoma Myeloma Leuk. 2015;15:606–11. https://doi.org/10.1016/j.clml.2015.06.004.
8. Brady E, Parikh NS, Navi BB, Gupta A, Schweitzer AD. The imaging spectrum of posterior reversible encephalopathy syndrome: a pictorial review. Clin Imaging. 2018;47:80–9. https://doi.org/10.1016/j.clinimag.2017.08.008.
9. Burnett MM, Hess CP, Roberts JP, Bass NM, Douglas VC, Josephson SA. Presentation of reversible posterior leukoencephalopathy syndrome in patients on calcineurin inhibitors. Clin Neurol Neurosurg. 2010;112:886–91. https://doi.org/10.1016/j.clineuro.2010.07.023.
10. Chen YH, Huang CH. Reversible posterior leukoencephalopathy syndrome induced by vinorelbine. Clin Breast Cancer. 2012;12:222–5. https://doi.org/10.1016/j.clbc.2012.01.006.
11. Chen Z, Zhang G, Lerner A, Wang AH, Gao B, Liu J. Risk factors for poor outcome in posterior reversible encephalopathy syndrome: systematic review and meta-analysis. Quant Imaging Med Surg. 2018;8:421–32. https://doi.org/10.21037/qims.2018. 05.07.
12. Chuk MK, et al. A phase 1 study of cabozantinib in children and adolescents with recurrent or refractory solid tumors, including CNS tumors: trial ADVL1211, a report from the Children's Oncology Group. Pediatr Blood Cancer. 2018;65:e27077. https://doi.org/10.1002/pbc.27077.

13. Costa R, Costa R, Costa R, Junior GM, Cartaxo HQ, de Barros AC. Reversible posterior encephalopathy syndrome secondary to sunitinib. Case Rep Oncol Med. 2014;2014:952624. https://doi.org/10.1155/2014/952624.

14. Covarrubias DJ, Luetmer PH, Campeau NG. Posterior reversible encephalopathy syndrome: prognostic utility of quantitative diffusion-weighted MR images. AJNR Am J Neuroradiol. 2002;23:1038–48.

15. Creutzig U, et al. First experience of the AML-Berlin-Frankfurt-Munster group in pediatric patients with standard-risk acute promyelocytic leukemia treated with arsenic trioxide and all-trans retinoid acid. Pediatr Blood Cancer. 2017;64. https://doi.org/10.1002/pbc.26461.

16. Crona DJ, Whang YE. Posterior reversible encephalopathy syndrome induced by enzalutamide in a patient with castration-resistant prostate cancer. Investig New Drugs. 2015;33:751–4. https://doi.org/10.1007/s10637-014-0193-3.

17. Datar S, Singh T, Rabinstein AA, Fugate JE, Hocker S. Long-term risk of seizures and epilepsy in patients with posterior reversible encephalopathy syndrome. Epilepsia. 2015a;56:564–8. https://doi.org/10.1111/epi.12933.

18. Datar S, Singh TD, Fugate JE, Mandrekar J, Rabinstein AA, Hocker S. Albuminocytologic dissociation in posterior reversible encephalopathy syndrome. Mayo Clin Proc. 2015b;90:1366–71. https://doi.org/10.1016/j.mayocp.2015.07.018.

19. Deguchi S, et al. Posterior reversible encephalopathy syndrome (PRES) induced by pazopanib, a multi-targeting tyrosine kinase inhibitor, in a patient with soft-tissue sarcoma: case report and review of the literature. Investig New Drugs. 2018;36:346–9. https://doi.org/10.1007/s10637-017-0521-5.

20. Donnelly J, Budohoski KP, Smielewski P, Czosnyka M. Regulation of the cerebral circulation: bedside assessment and clinical implications. Crit Care. 2016;20:129. https://doi.org/10.1186/s13054-016-1293-6.

21. Edvinsson L, Owman C, Sjoberg NO. Autonomic nerves, mast cells, and amine receptors in human brain vessels. A histochemical and pharmacological study. Brain Res. 1976;115:377–93.

22. Ferrara M, et al. Isolated pons involvement in posterior reversible encephalopathy syndrome: case report and review of the literature. eNeurologicalSci. 2017;6:51–4. https://doi.org/10.1016/j.ensci.2016.11.008.

23. Fitzgerald RT, et al. Elevation of serum lactate dehydrogenase at posterior reversible encephalopathy syndrome onset in chemotherapy-treated cancer patients. J Clin Neurosci. 2014;21:1575–8. https://doi.org/10.1016/j.jocn.2014.03.004.

24. Floeter AE, Patel A, Tran M, Chamberlain MC, Hendrie PC, Gopal AK, Cassaday RD. Posterior reversible encephalopathy syndrome associated with dose-adjusted EPOCH (etoposide, prednisone, vincristine, cyclophosphamide, doxorubicin) chemotherapy. Clin Lymphoma Myeloma Leuk. 2017;17:225–30. https://doi.org/10.1016/j.clml.2016.12.004.

25. Fugate JE, Claassen DO, Cloft HJ, Kallmes DF, Kozak OS, Rabinstein AA. Posterior reversible encephalopathy syndrome: associated clinical and radiologic findings. Mayo Clin Proc. 2010;85:427–32. https://doi.org/10.4065/mcp.2009.0590.

26. Furubayashi N, Negishi T, Iwai H, Nagase K, Nakamura M. Sorafenib-induced reversible posterior leukoencephalopathy in patients with renal cell carcinoma: a report of two cases. Mol Clin Oncol. 2017;7:281–4. https://doi.org/10.3892/mco.2017.1291.

27. Gao B, Liu FL, Zhao B. Association of degree and type of edema in posterior reversible encephalopathy syndrome with serum lactate dehydrogenase level: initial experience. Eur J Radiol. 2012;81:2844–7. https://doi.org/10.1016/j.ejrad.2011.12.010.

28. Ghidini M, Petrelli F, Ghidini A, Tomasello G, Hahne JC, Passalacqua R, Barni S. Clinical development of mTor inhibitors for renal cancer. Expert Opin Investig Drugs. 2017;26:1229–37. https://doi.org/10.1080/13543784.2017.1384813.

29. Hammerstrom AE, Howell J, Gulbis A, Rondon G, Champlin RE, Popat U. Tacrolimus-associated posterior reversible encephalopathy syndrome in hematopoietic allogeneic stem cell transplantation. Am J Hematol. 2013;88:301–5. https://doi.org/10.1002/ajh.23402.

30. Hinchey J, et al. A reversible posterior leukoencephalopathy syndrome. N Engl J Med. 1996;334:494–500. https://doi.org/10.1056/nejm199602223340803.

31. How J, Blattner M, Fowler S, Wang-Gillam A, Schindler SE. Chemotherapy-associated posterior reversible encephalopathy syndrome: a case report and review of the literature. Neurologist. 2016;21:112–7. https://doi.org/10.1097/nrl.0000000000000105.

32. Hualde Olascoaga J, Molins Castiella T, Souto Hernandez S, Becerril Moreno F, Yoldi Petri ME, Sagaseta de Ilurdoz M, Molina Garicano J. Reversible posterior leukoencephalopathy: report of two cases after vincristine treatment. Anales de pediatria. 2008;68:282–5. (Barcelona, Spain: 2003)

33. Irvin W, MacDonald G, Smith JK, Kim WY. Dexamethasone-induced posterior reversible encephalopathy syndrome. J Clin Oncol Off J Am Soc Clin Oncol. 2007;25:2484–6. https://doi.org/10.1200/jco.2007.10.9991.

34. Janjua TK, Hassan M, Afridi HK, Zahid NA. Oxaliplatin-induced posterior reversible encephalopathy syndrome (PRES). BMJ Case Rep. 2017;2017 https://doi.org/10.1136/bcr-2017-221571.

35. Junewar V, et al. Neuroimaging features and predictors of outcome in eclamptic encephalopathy: a prospective

observational study. AJNR Am J Neuroradiol. 2014;35:1728–34. https://doi.org/10.3174/ajnr.A3923.

36. Kamiya-Matsuoka C, Tummala S. Electrographic patterns in patients with posterior reversible encephalopathy syndrome and seizures. J Neurol Sci. 2017;375:294–8. https://doi.org/10.1016/j.jns.2017.02.017.

37. Kamiya-Matsuoka C, Paker AM, Chi L, Youssef A, Tummala S, Loghin ME. Posterior reversible encephalopathy syndrome in cancer patients: a single institution retrospective study. J Neuro-Oncol. 2016;128:75–84. https://doi.org/10.1007/s11060-016-2078-0.

38. Karia SJ, Rykken JB, McKinney ZJ, Zhang L, McKinney AM. Utility and significance of gadolinium-based contrast enhancement in posterior reversible encephalopathy syndrome. AJNR Am J Neuroradiol. 2016;37:415–22. https://doi.org/10.3174/ajnr.A4563.

39. Kastrup O, Schlamann M, Moenninghoff C, Forsting M, Goericke S. Posterior reversible encephalopathy syndrome: the spectrum of MR imaging patterns. Clin Neuroradiol. 2015;25:161–71. https://doi.org/10.1007/s00062-014-0293-7.

40. Kozak OS, Wijdicks EF, Manno EM, Miley JT, Rabinstein AA. Status epilepticus as initial manifestation of posterior reversible encephalopathy syndrome. Neurology. 2007;69:894–7. https://doi.org/10.1212/01.wnl.0000269780.45472.16.

41. Kwon EJ, Kim SW, Kim KK, Seo HS, Kim DY. A case of gemcitabine and cisplatin associated posterior reversible encephalopathy syndrome. Cancer Res Treat. 2009;41:53–5. https://doi.org/10.4143/crt.2009.41.1.53.

42. LaPorte J, Solh M, Ouanounou S. Posterior reversible encephalopathy syndrome following pembrolizumab therapy for relapsed Hodgkin's lymphoma. J Oncol Pharm Pract. 2017;23:71–4. https://doi.org/10.1177/1078155215620922.

43. Lee VH, Wijdicks EF, Manno EM, Rabinstein AA. Clinical spectrum of reversible posterior leukoencephalopathy syndrome. Arch Neurol. 2008;65:205–10. https://doi.org/10.1001/archneurol.2007.46.

44. Legriel S, et al. Determinants of recovery from severe posterior reversible encephalopathy syndrome. PLoS One. 2012;7:e44534. https://doi.org/10.1371/journal.pone.0044534.

45. Li X, Chai J, Wang Z, Lu L, Zhao Q, Zhou J, Ju F. Reversible posterior leukoencephalopathy syndrome induced by apatinib: a case report and literature review. Onco Targets Ther. 2018;11:4407–11. https://doi.org/10.2147/ott.S166605.

46. Liman TG, Bohner G, Heuschmann PU, Endres M, Siebert E. The clinical and radiological spectrum of posterior reversible encephalopathy syndrome: the retrospective Berlin PRES study. J Neurol. 2012;259:155–64. https://doi.org/10.1007/s00415-011-6152-4.

47. Lv C, Gao B. Serum lactate dehydrogenase as a predictor of outcome in posterior reversible encephalopathy syndrome: imperative to unify.

AJNR Am J Neuroradiol. 2015;36:E29–30. https://doi.org/10.3174/ajnr.A4243.

48. Makranz C, Khutsurauli S, Kalish Y, Eliahou R, Kadouri L, Gomori JM, Lossos A. Neurological variability in chemotherapy-induced posterior reversible encephalopathy syndrome associated with thrombotic microangiopathy: case reports and literature review. Mol Clin Oncol. 2018;8:178–82. https://doi.org/10.3892/mco.2017.1476.

49. Mancone S, Lycan T, Ahmed T, Topaloglu U, Dothard A, Petty WJ, Strowd RE. Severe neurologic complications of immune checkpoint inhibitors: a single-center review. J Neurol. 2018;265:1636. https://doi.org/10.1007/s00415-018-8890-z.

50. Marra A, Vargas M, Striano P, Del Guercio L, Buonanno P, Servillo G. Posterior reversible encephalopathy syndrome: the endothelial hypotheses. Med Hypotheses. 2014;82:619–22. https://doi.org/10.1016/j.mehy.2014.02.022.

51. Massey J. Posterior reversible encephalopathy syndrome (PRES) with sub-arachnoid haemorrhage after bevacizumab and 5-FU. J Clin Neurosci. 2017;40:57–9. https://doi.org/10.1016/j.jocn.2017.01.005.

52. Maur M, Tomasello C, Frassoldati A, Dieci MV, Barbieri E, Conte P. Posterior reversible encephalopathy syndrome during ipilimumab therapy for malignant melanoma. J Clin Oncol Off J Am Soc Clin Oncol. 2012;30:e76–8. https://doi.org/10.1200/jco.2011.38.7886.

53. McKinney AM, Short J, Truwit CL, McKinney ZJ, Kozak OS, SantaCruz KS, Teksam M. Posterior reversible encephalopathy syndrome: incidence of atypical regions of involvement and imaging findings. AJR Am J Roentgenol. 2007;189:904–12. https://doi.org/10.2214/ajr.07.2024.

54. Musiol K, Waz S, Boron M, Kwiatek M, Machnikowska-Sokolowska M, Gruszczynska K, Sobol-Milejska G. PRES in the course of hemato-oncological treatment in children. Childs Nerv Syst. 2018;34:691–9. https://doi.org/10.1007/s00381-017-3664-y.

55. Pandita A, Lehmann DF. Magnesium sulfate treatment correlates with improved neurological function in posterior reversible encephalopathy syndrome (PRES): report of a case. Neurologist. 2018;23:65–6. https://doi.org/10.1097/nrl.0000000000000174.

56. Parikh NS, et al. Corticosteroid therapy and severity of vasogenic edema in posterior reversible encephalopathy syndrome. J Neurol Sci. 2017;380:11–5. https://doi.org/10.1016/j.jns.2017.06.044.

57. Rabinstein AA, Mandrekar J, Merrell R, Kozak OS, Durosaro O, Fugate JE. Blood pressure fluctuations in posterior reversible encephalopathy syndrome. J Stroke Cerebrovasc Dis. 2012;21:254–8. https://doi.org/10.1016/j.jstrokecerebrovasdis.2011.03.011.

58. Ract I, Poujade A, Carsin-Nicol B, Mouriaux F, Ferre JC. Spinal cord involvement in posterior reversible encephalopathy syndrome (PRES). J Neuroradiol. 2016;43:56–8. https://doi.org/10.1016/j.neurad.2015.09.004.

59. Saito B, Nakamaki T, Nakashima H, Usui T, Hattori N, Kawakami K, Tomoyasu S. Reversible posterior leukoencephalopathy syndrome after repeat intermediate-dose cytarabine chemotherapy in a patient with acute myeloid leukemia. Am J Hematol. 2007;82:304–6. https://doi.org/10.1002/ajh.20772.

60. Schmidt V, Prell T, Treschl A, Klink A, Hochhaus A, Sayer HG. Clinical management of posterior reversible encephalopathy syndrome after allogeneic hematopoietic stem cell transplantation: a case series and review of the literature. Acta Haematol. 2016;135:1–10. https://doi.org/10.1159/000430489.

61. Schwartz R, Mulkern R, Vajapeyam S, Kacher DF. Catheter angiography, MR angiography, and MR perfusion in posterior reversible encephalopathy syndrome. AJNR Am J Neuroradiol. 2009;30: E19; author reply E20. https://doi.org/10.3174/ajnr. A1285.

62. Schweitzer AD, et al. Imaging characteristics associated with clinical outcomes in posterior reversible encephalopathy syndrome. Neuroradiology. 2017;59:379–86. https://doi.org/10.1007/s00234-017-1815-1.

63. Seol YM, Kim DY, Kim HJ, Choi YJ. Reversible posterior leukoencephalopathy syndrome after Eribulin mesylate chemotherapy for breast cancer. Breast J. 2017;23:487–8. https://doi.org/10.1111/tbj.12776.

64. Siegal D, et al. Central nervous system complications after allogeneic hematopoietic stem cell transplantation: incidence, manifestations, and clinical significance. Biol Blood Marrow Transplant. 2007;13:1369–79. https://doi.org/10.1016/j.bbmt.20 07.07.013.

65. Singer S, Grommes C, Reiner AS, Rosenblum MK, DeAngelis LM. Posterior reversible encephalopathy syndrome in patients with cancer. Oncologist. 2015;20:806–11. https://doi.org/10.1634/theoncologi st.2014-0149.

66. Smets GJ, Loyson T, Van Paesschen W, Demaerel P, Nackaerts K. Posterior reversible encephalopathy syndrome possibly induced by pemetrexed maintenance therapy for lung cancer: a case report and literature review. Acta Clin Belg. 2017;1–7. https://doi.org/ 10.1080/17843286.2017.1403103.

67. Tlemsani C, et al. Posterior reversible encephalopathy syndrome induced by anti-VEGF agents. Target Oncol. 2011;6:253–8. https://doi.org/10.1007/s11523- 011-0201-x.

68. Vieillot S, Pouessel D, de Champfleur NM, Becht C, Culine S. Reversible posterior leukoencephalopathy syndrome after carboplatin therapy. Ann Oncol. 2007;18:608–9. https://doi.org/10.1093/annonc/mdl4 36.

69. Whelton PK, et al. 2017 ACC/AHA/AAPA/ABC/ ACPM/AGS/APhA/ASH/ASPC/NMA/PCNA guideline for the prevention, detection, evaluation, and management of high blood pressure in adults: a report of the American College of Cardiology/American Heart Association Task Force on Clinical Practice Guidelines. J Am Coll Cardiol. 2018;71:e127–248. https://doi.org/10.1016/j.jacc.2017.11.006.

70. Win MA, Thein KZ, Yeung SJ. Cancer immunotherapy-induced posterior reversible encephalopathy syndrome in an ED. Am J Emerg Med. 2017;35:663.e661–2. https://doi.org/10.1016/j.ajem.2016.10.069.

71. Zhang L, Xu J. Posterior reversible encephalopathy syndrome (PRES) attributed to mycophenolate mofetil during the management of SLE: a case report and review. Am J Clin Exp Immunol. 2018;7:1–7.

Stroke in Critically Ill Cancer Patients

25

Ritvij Bowry and James C. Grotta

Contents

Introduction 368

Epidemiology 368

Etiology 368

Pathophysiology 368

Clinical Features 370

Diagnosis 370

Management 373
Pharmacologic 373

Non-pharmacologic 376

Prognosis 376

Conclusion 377

References 377

Abstract

Stroke and cancer have significant morbidity and mortality with heterogeneous risk factors. While conventional risk factors such as atherosclerosis and cardiac disease are important mechanisms in the occurrence of stroke, cancer is an unconventional risk factor that leads to both ischemic and hemorrhagic stroke in a myriad of ways. Although cancer-associated strokes have unique underlying mechanisms, the clinical features, diagnosis, and management scheme are similar for non-cancer-associated strokes. Prognosis is complex and is dependent on the stage and type of cancer, expected treatment course, and stroke burden.

R. Bowry
Department of Neurosurgery, Division of Neurocritical care, McGovern Medical School, University of Texas Health Science Center, Houston, TX, USA
e-mail: Ritvij.Bowry@uth.tmc.edu

J. C. Grotta (✉)
Clinical Innovation and Research Institute, Memorial Hermann Hospital, Houston, TX, USA
e-mail: james.c.grotta@uth.tmc.edu

Keywords

Cancer · Stroke · Tissue plasminogen activator · Ischemic stroke · Intracerebral hemorrhage · Hypercoagulability · Arterial embolism · Venous thromboembolism

Introduction

Compromised blood flow in arteries or veins can lead to impaired oxygen delivery to the central nervous system and result in irreversible tissue injury causing a stroke. Such injury can occur as a result of blood clots (ischemic strokes) or due to rupture of blood vessels leading to hemorrhage and secondary tissue injury (hemorrhagic strokes). Overall, stroke is the fifth leading cause of death in the United States, with an incidence of about 800,000 new cases annually and a high societal cost burden [27, 40].

Despite being a distinct clinical entity in itself, stroke is frequently the initial presenting "symptom" of cancer and thus the first expression of an underlying but unknown cancer state [39]. Ischemic strokes occur in a large number of cancer patients and can be both symptomatic and asymptomatic (silent infarctions). Hemorrhagic strokes have a higher association with hematological malignancies and lung cancer. In patients with leukemia and lymphoma, 72% and 36% of strokes, respectively, have found to be hemorrhagic. Other associated hematological abnormalities like chemotherapy-induced thrombocytopenia, disseminated intravascular coagulopathy (DIC), and other coagulation disorders also contribute to the risk of hemorrhagic strokes [46].

Epidemiology

Compared to the general population, patients with cancer have a higher prevalence of stroke, with an annual incidence up to 7% for ischemic strokes and a lifetime probability of occurrence of 50% [16]. 0.5–4.5% of all patients with ischemic strokes and up to 5% of those with strokes of undermined causes (cryptogenic strokes) are diagnosed of an unknown malignancy during hospitalization [39].

Stroke can be the initial clinical manifestation of an occult cancer state, with a majority being diagnosed during the first 6 months of follow-up after stroke [7, 16]. Ischemic strokes in cancer and non-cancer patients are mediated by similar risk factors such as older age, smoking, obesity, physical inactivity, hypertension, diabetes, hypercholesterolemia, and certain cardiac conditions like atrial fibrillation. Although the prevalence of various ischemic stroke mechanisms (mainly thromboembolism due to atherosclerosis, cardioembolism, and small vessel disease) is similar between patients with and without cancer, the traditional stroke mechanisms attributable to these specific risk factors are absent in up to 40% of patients with cancer [5].

Etiology

First described by Trousseau in 1865, hypercoagulability has been proposed as a central mechanism of ischemic strokes in patients with cancer. The risk of thrombosis in patients with cancer is an aggregate of individual vascular risk factors as described above, the type of cancer itself and the secondary effects of the cancer (non-bacterial thrombotic endocarditis leading to cardiac embolism, local compressive effects) and its treatment. Adenocarcinomas have been shown to have the greatest thrombotic risk overall [39] with high prevalence of prothrombotic states being associated with lung, prostate, colorectal, breast, gynecological cancers and lymphoma [41].

Patients with cancer-associated strokes have also been found to have lower body mass index and lower levels of hemoglobin, albumin, and triglycerides compared to non-cancer strokes, with higher levels of coagulation parameters such as prothrombin time (PT), international normalized ratio (INR), and D-dimer and fibrinogen levels [25, 47].

Pathophysiology

Cancer-associated ischemic strokes have several mechanisms that lead to hypercoagulability. These include derangements of the coagulation cascade, tumor mucin secretion, paraneoplastic effects, and a prothrombotic, inflammatory, vascular endothelium as a result of necrotizing factor and interleukins leading to the formation of fibrin- and platelet-rich thrombi in the vasculature or along normal heart valves that can embolize (non-bacterial, marantic endocarditis) [7, 15, 16, 33].

Solid and nonsolid tumors and the consequences of treatment also affect the mechanisms by which strokes occur. These effects occur as a result of (1) direct tumor effects, such as occlusive disease leading to thrombo-emboli, local compression of blood vessels, or meningeal extension of tumors, (2) consequences of medical complications of cancer such as coagulopathy and underlying infections (especially fungal), or (3) treatment related, such as chemotherapy-related thrombocytopenia, hypercoagulability, or radiation-induced accelerated atherosclerosis, leading to hemorrhagic strokes [11, 33]. Common chemotherapeutic agents that are associated with high incidence of strokes include newer anti-angiogenic agents such as bevacuzimab, along with cisplatin-based chemotherapy, cyclophosphamide, 5-flurouracil Taxol paclitaxel, L-asparaginase, and tamoxifen [45, 46] due to both systemic effects of the chemotherapy and direct effects on the coagulation cascade causing changes in platelet aggregation, increased levels of von Willebrand factor (cisplatin), and lower levels of anti-thrombin III and possibly protein C (tamoxifen). Complications of bone marrow transplantation can also cause thrombocytopenia and increased risk for hemorrhagic strokes.

Chemotherapeutic agents can also lead to posterior reversible encephalopathy syndrome (PRES), which consists of stroke-like symptoms, headache, disturbance of consciousness, seizures, and visual symptoms. Although associated with other etiologies such as malignant hypertension, eclampsia, renal failure, autoimmune conditions, and general anesthesia, there is a significant association of PRES and immunosuppressive therapies. The time interval between the last chemotherapy and first symptoms varies from a few hours after treatment to 5 weeks posttreatment and can occur within the first three cycles of chemotherapy. Proposed mechanisms by which immunosuppressive and cytotoxic agents cause PRES include endothelial injury and altered cerebral autoregulation that leads to breakdown of the blood–brain barrier and subsequent brain edema [6]. Specific antineoplastic agents like pemetrexed, methotrexate, vincristine, ifosfamide, cyclosporine, fludarabine, cytarabine, 5-fluorouracil, gemcitabine, and cisplatin have been associated with this condition, along with high-dose, multidrug chemotherapy, erythropoietin, and autologous stem cell transplants [43, 44]. Although PRES is a potentially reversible condition with supportive care and medical management that includes treatment of seizures, gradual reduction of blood pressure and removal of the offending agent(s), recurrences have been reported in 6% of cases and death in up to 15% of patients [22].

Cancer can also result in a vasculopathy involving the veins or arteries in various ways. Solid tumors can often cause venous infarctions by either exerting local mass effect or compression of venous sinuses or can proliferate along venous structures adjacent to the dura invading the sinuses leading to compromised venous drainage resulting in congestion and swelling causing hemorrhagic venous infarctions. Tumors can also spread into the leptomeningeal or Virchow Robin spaces and encompass the penetrating arteries, leading to vascular congestion and inflammation leading to vasculitis and compromise of cerebral blood flow (cerebral vasospasm). Commonly associated tumors with this process include lymphomas and primary lung cancer with lung metastases, where a tumor enters the pulmonary circulation and is distributed by arterial blood flow. Alternatively, intracardiac metastases or primary tumors such as myxomas can directly embolize to the cerebral circulation [33].

Cancer patients have up to a sevenfold increased risk of developing venous thromboembolism compared with those without cancer [8, 13]. This underlying hypercoagulability state predisposes cancer patients to developing deep venous thrombi in the pelvic and/or lower extremity venous system that can lead to arterial strokes by the migration of the these thrombi to the heart that can paradoxically embolize to the arterial system via a right-to-left shunt as a result of a patent foramen ovale [14, 48]. While there are no studies to-date directly linking immunotherapy to stroke, it can be associated with a higher risk of venous thromboembolism.

Tumor cells can also invade the walls of the intracranial vasculature, leading to aneurysm formation that are typically located in the distal vasculature and can result in parenchymal or sub-arachnoid hemorrhage [28]. The diagnosis is typically challenging and is made at autopsy or by observing growth of metastases at sites of previous infarction on neuroimaging scans. Patients with certain types of leukemia such as acute myelogenous leukemia and elevated leukocyte counts ($>100,000/mm^3$) can develop intravascular leukostasis leading to infarction that is usually hemorrhagic [33].

Surgical procedures and radiotherapy related to cancer treatments also confer an increased stroke risk, with up to 60% of ischemic strokes occurring in the post-operative period after resection of an intracranial neoplasm. Patients undergoing radical neck dissection for head and neck malignancies are at operative risk for infarction after ligation of the common carotid artery. There is also a delayed risk of stroke (twofold risk at about 5 years after a median radiation dose of 64 Gy) subsequent to irradiation of the head or neck, which can induce accelerated atherosclerosis [18] and an increased rate of carotid stenosis of greater than 70% in patients receiving an equivalent dose of radiotherapy (up to 66 Gy) to the neck [10, 33].

Clinical Features

The initial priority in the care of a stroke patient is similar to that of any potentially critically ill patient: stabilization of the airway, breathing, circulation (ABCs), followed by an assessment of neurological symptoms and medical comorbidities. The overall goal is not only to identify patients with possible strokes but also to exclude conditions that often present with stroke-like symptoms, such as hypoglycemia and migraines.

Common symptoms attributable to strokes include focal neurologic deficits such as sudden impairment in speech production or quality, vision, strength or sensation (variably affecting the face, arm, and leg), gait, and/or coordination. Subtle manifestations include cognitive dysfunction, reduced comprehension of language, and loss of fine motor skills [21]. Brain tumors or metastases can also have a stroke-like presentation as a consequence of lesion-induced seizures or acute hemorrhage into the tumor itself [33].

Diagnosis

The most crucial element in the history is the time of symptom onset or the last time the patient was at "normal" baseline state of health. A time window of 0–4.5 h from symptom onset/last seen normal is one of the main inclusion criteria for ischemic stroke patients to be able to receive fibrinolytic treatment. Other relevant history includes the time course and nature of symptoms, evaluation of risk factors for arteriosclerosis and cardiac disease, history of central nervous system cancer, anticoagulation or chemotherapy use, thrombocytopenia, drug abuse, migraine, seizure, infection, trauma, or pregnancy. Since the benefits of treatment with fibrinolytic therapy are time dependent, with faster treatment times resulting in better outcomes, the initial neurological examination consists of a standardized neurological assessment known at the National Institutes of Health Stroke Scale (Table 1) to ensure that the major components of a neurological examination are performed in a timely and uniform manner. Other tests that are emergently performed include a non-contrast head computed tomography (CT) scan to exclude any intracranial hemorrhage, blood glucose check, complete blood count with platelet count and PT, INR, and activated partial thromboplastin time (aPTT) if thrombocytopenia or coagulopathy is suspected, especially for patients on chemotherapy. Fibrinolytic therapy is not delayed however while awaiting the results of the PT, aPTT, or platelet count unless a bleeding abnormality or thrombocytopenia is suspected, the patient has been taking warfarin and heparin

Table 1 National Institutes of Health Stroke Scale (NIHSS)

Item	Title	Response/score
1A	Level of consciousness	0 – Alert 1 – Drowsy 2 – Obtunded 3 – Coma/unresponsive
1B	Orientation questions (2)	0 – Answers both correctly 1 – Answers 1 correctly 2 – Answers neither correctly
1C	Response to commands (2)	0 – Performs both tasks correctly 1 – Performs 1 task correctly 2 – Performs neither
2	Gaze	0 – Normal horizontal movements 1 – Partial gaze palsy 2 – Complete gaze palsy
3	Visual fields	0 – No visual field defect 1 – Partial hemianopia 2 – Complete hemianopia 3 – Bilateral hemianopia
4	Facial movement	0 – Normal 1 – Minor facial weakness 2 – Partial facial weakness 3 – Complete unilateral palsy
5	Motor function (arm) a. Left b. Right	0 – No drift 1 – Drift before 10 s 2 – Falls before 10 s 3 – No effort against gravity 4 – No movement
6	Motor function (leg) a. Left b. Right	0 – No drift 1 – Drift before 5 s 2 – Falls before 5 s 3 – No effort against gravity 4 – No movement
7	Limb ataxia	0 – No ataxia 1 – Ataxia in 1 limb 2 – Ataxia in 2 limbs
8	Sensory	0 – No sensory loss 1 – Mild sensory loss 2 – Severe sensory loss
9	Language	0 – Normal 1 – Mild aphasia 2 – Severe aphasia 3 – Mute or global aphasia
10	Articulation	0 – Normal 1 – Mild dysarthria 2 – Severe dysarthria
11	Extinction or inattention	0 – Absent 1 – Mild loss (1 sensory modality lost) 2 – Severe loss (2 modalities lost)

Source: National Institute of Neurological Disorders and Stroke. Available for download at: https://www.ninds.nih.gov/sites/default/files/NIH_Stroke_Scale.pdf

and is on chemotherapy, or anticoagulation use is uncertain. All acute stroke patients undergo cardiovascular evaluation with an admission electrocardiogram and telemetry monitoring after admission to the hospital, both for determination of the cause of the stroke and to optimize immediate and long-term management. Although atrial fibrillation may be evident on an admission electrocardiogram, its absence does not exclude its etiology as the cause of the event and thus warrants telemetry monitoring during the hospitalization and/or long-term monitoring after discharge.

Acute neuroimaging in stroke generally involves an initial non-iodinated contrast head CT scan to identify any acute intracranial hemorrhage and should be obtained within 25 min of the patient's arrival to the emergency department (ED) [21]. Other signs of early ischemia on a CT scan such as a hyperdense artery, loss of gray-white matter differentiation, sulcal effacement suggestive of early edema, and loss of the architecture of the deep gray nuclei corroborate the diagnosis of stroke but do not preclude treatment with fibrinolytic therapy [35]. For patients who have malignancies that have a high predilection for brain metastasis, a contrast-enhanced CT or magnetic resonance imaging (MRI) scan can be considered prior to tPA administration to ensure lack of parenchymal brain disease that could increase the risk of hemorrhage. Helical CT angiography (CTA) provides a means to rapidly and noninvasively evaluate the intracranial and extracranial vasculature in acute, subacute, and chronic stroke settings and provides important information about the presence of significant arterial vessel occlusions or stenosis that can be used in the acute stroke scenario to determine further endovascular treatment options in selected patients with large artery occlusions within 6 h of symptom onset [21]. Brain perfusion imaging using CT or MRI provides information about brain tissue undergoing ischemia but is not irreversibly infarcted, providing quantification of the ischemic penumbra. Combined with parenchymal (non-contrast CT or MRI) and vascular imaging (CTA or MR angiography), perfusion CT or MRI can be used to select certain stroke patients with large vessel occlusions in the intracranial internal or middle cerebral arteries for mechanical thrombectomy and clot extraction using cerebral angiography within 6–24 h from symptom onset/last seen normal time [1, 34].

Standard MRI sequences used to diagnose acute ischemic stroke include diffusion-weighted imaging (DWI) and apparent diffusion coefficient (ADC) sequences that are the most sensitive and specific imaging technique for acute infarction, with DWI having a high sensitivity (88–100%) and specificity (95–100%) for detecting infarcted within minutes of symptom onset. DWI/ADC sequences also allow for identification of the lesion size, site, and age, along with detection of relatively small cortical lesions and small deep or subcortical lesions (especially those in the brain stem or cerebellum) that can be poorly identifiable on a non-contrast head CT scan. Other MRI sequences such as T1-weighted, T2-weighted, fluid attenuated inversion recovery (FLAIR) are relatively insensitive to the changes of acute ischemia within the first hours, although they can be useful in identifying areas of infarcted that are more than 4.5 h [49] and provide estimates of the age of hemorrhage in relation to the initial occurrence [9, 21]. Patients with ischemic strokes and associated cancer have a higher prevalence of diffuse strokes that are generally multifocal, spanning different brain areas and cerebrovascular territories [5, 25, 39, 47].

An acutely hemorrhagic brain tumor lesion can be challenging to distinguish from a hemorrhagic stroke due to other more conventional causes, such as small vessel hypertensive lipohyalinosis or amyloid angiopathy. However, brain tumor hemorrhage is generally lobar (which is unusual for hypertension-associated hemorrhage) or located in an atypical location such as the corpus callosum, usually associated with marked edema surrounding the clot due to the underlying tumor, and can be associated with a ringlike, high-density area corresponding to the blood around a low-density center resulting from bleeding by tumor vessels at the junction of tumor and adjacent brain parenchyma [23]. Renal, thyroid, and germ cell carcinoma brain metastases, as well as melanoma, have the greatest tendency to be hemorrhagic, although brain metastases from lung cancer (bronchogenic carcinoma) are the most common cause [33]. The majority of underlying hemorrhagic primary brain tumors are malignant (i.e., high-grade gliomas), although meningiomas, oligodendrogliomas, and pituitary adenomas are also prone to hemorrhage. The most common primary brain neoplasms that bleed spontaneously are glioblastoma multiforme (GBM) and malignant astrocytoma. Less common tumors that cause parenchymal hemorrhage (but can cause primary intraventricular hemorrhage) are ependymoma, subependymoma, choroid plexus papilloma, intraventricular meningioma, neurocytoma, granular cell tumor, metastases, craniopharyngioma, and pituitary tumors that erode through the floor of the third ventricle [26].

Management

Pharmacologic

Administration of intravenous fibrinolytic therapy with tissue plasminogen activator (tPA) within 4.5 h of a suspected ischemic stroke is the standard of care and is associated with an increase in the odds of a favorable outcome [17, 50, 51]. The major risk of intravenous tPA treatment remains symptomatic intracranial hemorrhage with the initial evaluation focused toward screening patients with standard inclusion/exclusion criteria for tPA (Table 2). Since the benefit of therapy is time dependent, treatment should be initiated as soon as possible, targeting a door-to-bolus time of 60 min from hospital arrival. Standard dosing for tPA is 0.9 mg/kg (maximum dose 90 mg) with 10% of the dose given as a bolus over 1 min and the remainder as an infusion over an hour. Mechanical clot extraction via cerebral angiography can be performed at advanced stroke centers for a subgroup of stroke patients who are either ineligible for treatment with intravenous tPA or who receive tPA and have a concurrent large artery vessel occlusion in the internal or middle cerebral arteries and are within the first 6 h of symptom onset (Table 3). For other selected patients who present within 6–24 h from stroke-symptom onset, mechanical thrombectomy might also be considered, depending on specific clinical and neuroimaging (perfusion imaging) criteria [37, 38].

Besides coagulopathy and active hemorrhage, the most significant exclusion for intravenous tPA for cancer patients includes intracranial neoplasms, which can be divided into extra-axial and intra-axial tumors. Risks of intravenous tPA should thus be based on the anatomic and histological factors of a particular neoplasm if possible. Although data on intravenous tPA in the setting of intracranial neoplasms are confined to case reports, systemic thrombolysis appears safe in extra-axial, intracranial neoplasms, such as meningiomas. The same is not however applicable to intra-axial neoplasms such as intracranial metastases and primary brain neoplasms such as GBMs, and thus tPA should be avoided in cases where an intra-axial brain parenchymal tumor is suspected due to the risk of hemorrhage. Ultimately, the histology, location, and baseline bleeding risk of the tumor can inform reasonable intravenous tPA administration in these patients [12]. Such patients can alternatively be screened for potential mechanical thrombectomy based on current guidelines, especially if they are functionally independent and have a favorable prognosis and life expectancy given their underlying cancer and ongoing treatment course. A general history of cancer or active systemic malignancy (without brain or spinal cord metastases) should also not necessarily prevent stroke patients from receiving treatment with intravenous tPA (assuming other inclusion/exclusion criteria are met), although the risks and benefits must be carefully assessed, discussed with the patient/family, and considered with other medical providers involved in the oncologic care of the patient.

Subsequent care of the stroke patient after management in the ED largely depends on risk factor modification and investigation of the underlying etiology for the stroke. Oral administration of aspirin (initial dose 325 mg) within 24–48 h after stroke onset is recommended for treatment of most patients, depending on whether tPA is administered and consideration of the immediate bleeding risk. Patients who have elevated blood pressure on initial arrival and are otherwise eligible for treatment with intravenous tPA should have their blood pressure carefully lowered so that their systolic blood pressure is <185 mmHg

Table 2 Inclusion and exclusion criteria for treatment with intravenous tPA

Inclusions	Diagnosis of ischemic stroke causing measurable neurological deficits
	Aged ≥18 years
	Onset of symptoms/last known well 0–4.5[a] h before beginning treatment
Exclusions	CT brain with acute intracranial hemorrhage
	Severe head trauma or prior stroke in previous 3 months
	Arterial puncture at a non-compressible site in previous 7 days
	History of significant previous intracranial hemorrhage
	Intra-axial neoplasm, arteriovenous malformation, or aneurysm (safe if size <10 mm, unruptured and unsecured)
	Recent intracranial or intraspinal surgery within prior 3 months
	Persistently elevated blood pressure (systolic >185 mmHg or diastolic >110 mmHg) intractable to medical therapy
	Symptoms known or suspected to be associated with aortic arch dissection
	Active internal bleeding
	Platelet count <100,000/mm
	Heparin received within 48 h, resulting in abnormally elevated aPTT greater than the upper limit of normal
	Current use of direct thrombin inhibitors or direct factor Xa inhibitors with elevated sensitive laboratory tests (such as aPTT, INR, platelet count, and ECT; TT; or appropriate factor Xa activity assays)
	Treatment dose of LMWH within previous 24 h
	Symptoms consistent with infective endocarditis
	Current use of anticoagulant with INR >1.7, aPTT >40 s or PT >15 s
	Blood glucose concentration <50 mg/dL (2.7 mmol/L)
	CT demonstrates multi-lobar infarction (hypodensity >1/3 cerebral hemisphere)
Exclusions (relative)	Minor or rapidly improving stroke symptoms (potential disability of symptoms should be considered)
	Pregnancy (risks vs. benefits of tPA should be considered)
	Seizure at onset with postictal residual neurological impairments attributable to the seizure
	Major surgery or serious trauma within previous 14 days
	Significant gastrointestinal or urinary tract hemorrhage (within previous 21 days)
	Severe stroke (NIHSS>25)[a]
	Taking an oral anticoagulant regardless of INR[a]
	History of both diabetes and prior ischemic stroke[a]

Source: Refs. [21, 38]

aPTT activated partial thromboplastin time, *CT* computed tomography, *ECT* ecarin clotting time, *INR* international normalized ratio, *PT* partial thromboplastin time, *LMWH* low molecular weight heparin, *tPA* tissue plasminogen activator, *TT* thrombin time, *NIHSS* National Institutes of Health Stroke Scale

[a]Relative exclusions for treatment between 3 and 4.5 h from symptom onset/last known well time

and their diastolic blood pressure is <110 mmHg prior to tPA administration and <180/105 after tPA for the first 24 h. Beyond that, blood pressure goals and medications are initiated depending on the patient's neurologic and medical comorbidities based on optimizing cerebral perfusion in ischemic stroke or minimizing the risk of hematoma expansion in cases of hemorrhagic stroke. For patients with hemorrhagic strokes, systolic blood pressure is lowered to a goal of systolic of 140 for the first 24 h or beyond depending on the patient's clinical condition. Medications such as fresh frozen plasma, three- or four-factor prothrombin complex concentrate (PCC), or idarucizumab [36] can be used to acutely reverse the anticoagulation effects of warfarin or dabigatran, respectively, and are administered depending on the INR level and administration of last dose. Pharmacotherapy for management of diabetes and hypercholesterolemia is also initiated. Anticoagulation is generally initiated for prevention of venous thromboembolism within

Table 3 Evidence-based criteria for endovascular therapy with stent retrievers

(a) Pre-stroke mRS score 0–1
(b) Vascular occlusion of the ICA or proximal MCA (M1 segment) artery
(c) Age ≥18 years
(d) NIHSS score ≥6
(e) ASPECTS ≥6
(f) Treatment can be initiated (groin puncture) within 6 h of symptom onset/last known well time
(g) The use of endovascular therapy with stent retrievers can be considered on a case-by-case basis for causative occlusions of the M2 or M3 portion of the MCAs, anterior cerebral arteries, vertebral arteries, basilar artery, or posterior cerebral arteries
(h) Observation of patients after intravenous tPA to assess for clinical response before pursuing endovascular therapy is not required
Additional criteria for 6–24 h from symptom onset/last known well time
(a) In selected patients with acute ischemic stroke within 6–16 h of last known normal who have a LVO in the anterior circulation and meet DAWN[a] or DEFUSE 3[b] trials' inclusion/exclusion criteria, mechanical thrombectomy is recommended
(b) In selected patients with AIS within 6–24 h of last known normal who have LVO in the anterior circulation and meet other DAWN[a] trial inclusion/exclusion criteria, mechanical thrombectomy is reasonable

Source: Refs. [37, 38]

mRS modified Rankin scale, *tPA* tissue plasminogen activator, *ICA* internal carotid artery, *MCA* middle cerebral artery, *NIHSS* National Institutes of Health Stroke Scale, *ASPECTS* Alberta *stroke* program early CT *score*, *LVO* large vessel occlusion, *CT* computed tomography, *MRI* magnetic resonance imaging, *DWI* diffusion-weighted imaging

[a]*Inclusions* [34] = Pre-stroke mRS score 0–1; persistent occlusion >60 min after tPA administration; contraindications for tPA; NIHSS ≥10; clinical imaging mismatch [0–20 ml core infarct, NIHSS ≥10 if age ≥ 80; 0–30 ml core infarct, NIHSS ≥10 for age < 80; 31 ml to <50 ml core infarct, NIHSS ≥20 for age < 80]

[b]*Inclusions* [1] = Pre-stroke mRS score 0–2; Age 18–85; NIHSS ≥6; target mismatch profile on CT perfusion or MRI (ischemic core volume is <70 ml, mismatch ratio > 1.8, and mismatch volume > 15 ml or DWI lesion volume < 25 ml)

24–48 h, depending on clinical variables that might increase the risk of hemorrhage.

Atrial fibrillation is a well-known risk factor for ischemic stroke in cancer and non-cancer patients and generally warrants anticoagulation based on risk stratification scores and bleeding risks. Patients categorized as low risk are not routinely recommended anticoagulation prophylaxis. Cancer is known to increase the risk of ischemic stroke, but it is not clear to what extent cancer is a risk factor of ischemic stroke in patients with atrial fibrillation with a low stroke risk score. Cancer diagnosis within 1 year increases the risk of stroke in atrial fibrillation patients with low stroke risk score, particularly in patients greater than 65 years of age. These patients may thus benefit from anticoagulation treatment to lower the risk of ischemic stroke [3].

Patients with major ischemic infarctions are at high risk for brain edema and increased intracranial pressure, which are associated with major morbidity and mortality.

Medical management for cerebral edema includes hyperosmolar therapy and supportive care in a neuroscience intensive care unit with neuro-critical care and neurosurgical expertise in caring for such patients along with close monitoring for neurological deterioration. For selected patients based on age, medical comorbidities, and patient/family expectations for favorable outcomes, decompressive surgical evacuation of a space-occupying cerebellar infarction is effective in preventing and treating herniation and brain stem compression, as is decompressive surgery for malignant edema of the cerebral hemisphere in providing a life-saving benefit [52]. Placement of an external ventricular drain can be useful in patients with acute hydrocephalus secondary to ischemic stroke or intraventricular hemorrhage [19, 21]. For patients with occlusions of the major venous sinuses and associated venous infarctions, recanalization of a sinus is less likely to be achieved by conventional treatment with anticoagulation and can necessitate definitive therapy of the occluding tumor, usually with radiation [33]. Although there is no clear benefit of anticoagulation in the absence of a sinus thrombosis or venous thromboembolism, cancer patients with ischemic strokes attributable to cancer-related hypercoagulability are often anti-coagulated given the high risk of stroke recurrence (unless there is an excessive risk of systemic bleeding related to their cancer) [20, 32].

Non-pharmacologic

Cardiac monitoring is performed for at least the first 24 h to screen for atrial fibrillation and other potentially serious cardiac arrhythmias that can necessitate emergency cardiac interventions. Airway support is often needed for patients who have decreased consciousness or bulbar dysfunction. Supplemental oxygen should be provided to maintain oxygen saturation >94%. Sources of hyperthermia (temperature >38 °C) should be identified and treated, and antipyretic medications should be administered to lower temperature. In patients with elevated blood pressure who do not receive fibrinolysis, guidelines recommend permissive hypertension to promote cerebral perfusion and to only treat the blood pressure if the systolic blood pressure is >220 mmHg and diastolic blood pressure is >120 mmHg, unless there is concern for end-organ damage. Hypovolemia should be avoided, along with hypoglycemia (blood glucose <60 mg/dL) or hyperglycemia (>180 mg/dL). Appropriate antibiotics should be used for treatment of pneumonia, urinary tract infections, or other concurrent infections that can contribute to morbidity. Assessment of swallowing before the patient begins eating, drinking, or receiving oral medications is important, along with early mobilization with physical and occupational therapy for less severely affected stroke patients. The use of intermittent external compression devices is vital for treatment of patients who cannot receive anticoagulants for prevention of venous thromboembolism.

Prognosis

Cancer patients are at an increased risk of stroke, especially within 1 year of cancer diagnosis [33]. For ischemic stroke patients diagnosed with cancer within 6 months (~1.0%), it is likely that they already had an underlying, pre-existing malignancy at the time of stroke onset [41]. Patients newly diagnosed with common solid or hematologic cancers face a considerably increased short-term risk of arterial thromboembolism [31]. Advanced cancer stage, which is directly related to the overall tumor burden and extent of disease, is associated with increased stroke risk and carries a poor prognosis for survival, with a three-fold increased risk for death [31].

D-dimer is a marker for hypercoagulability, with increased D-dimer levels being associated with increased tumor burden and stage. Elevated D-dimer levels, however, have been associated with ischemic stroke in both cancer- and non-cancer-associated strokes. Some studies have found higher D-dimer levels to be associated with more widespread distribution of ischemic strokes across multiple vascular territories in cancer patients compared to non-cancer patients [5]. Along with high D-dimer levels, systemic metastases and diabetes are independent predictors of poor survival in cancer patients with cryptogenic strokes [4, 42, 45].

Patients with acute ischemic stroke in the setting of active cancer (especially adenocarcinoma) face a substantial short-term risk of recurrent ischemic stroke with cumulative rates of recurrent events being reported up to 7%, 13%, and 16% at 1, 3, and 6 months, respectively [29]. The stroke recurrence among cancer-related strokes was found to be associated with unconventional stroke etiologies, the absence of cancer treatment, extracranial stenosis, and cerebral microbleed numbers [25]. Other biomarkers such as erythrocyte sedimentation rate, high-sensitivity C-reactive protein, fibrinogen, and pro-b-type natriuretic peptide have also been shown to be higher in cancer patients with ischemic stroke compared with non-cancer patients and are associated with an increased frequency of large artery atherosclerosis as a potential etiology for ischemic strokes in cancer patients [24].

The increased risk of thrombosis in cancer patients also tends to correlate well with advanced stage of disease, increased tumor volume, and prolonged hospitalization [13]. The presence of venous thromboembolism (without any associated stroke) in patients with cancer is an independent predictor of poor survival in these patients [2].

Survival can be limited in patients with active systemic cancer who have a cryptogenic ischemic stroke independent of several potential confounders, such as age, functional status, presence of systemic metastases, and adenocarcinoma histology. The association of cryptogenic stroke with death is even stronger in patients with radiographic cardioembolic infarction patterns. In fact, only 17% of patients with cryptogenic stroke and 9% of those with radiographic cardioembolic infarction patterns survived to 1 year in one study. This is in contrast to the general stroke population, where cryptogenic strokes are typically associated with lower mortality and recurrence than strokes from known mechanisms [30].

Conclusion

The prognosis for patients with cancer and stroke is complex and is dependent on a multitude of variables related to a patient's conventional risk factors for stroke, type and stage of cancer, treatment course, and the nature and disability burden of the stroke. Although the outcome is poor for patients with systemic cancer, the survival rate is increasing with the development of more effective cancer treatments [11].

References

1. Albers GW, Marks MP, Kemp S, et al. Thrombectomy for stroke at 6 to 16 hours with selection by perfusion imaging. N Engl J Med. 2018;378:708–18. https://doi.org/10.1056/nejmoa1713973.
2. Amer M. Cancer-associated thrombosis: clinical presentation and survival. Cancer Manag Res. 2013;5:165. https://doi.org/10.2147/cmar.s47094.
3. Atterman A, Gigante B, Asplund K, et al. Cancer diagnosis as a risk factor of ischemic stroke in atrial fibrillation patients with low stroke risk score. Thromb Res. 2018;164:S209. https://doi.org/10.1016/j.thromres.2018.02.064.
4. Ay C, Dunkler D, Pirker R, et al. High D-dimer levels are associated with poor prognosis in cancer patients. Haematologica. 2012;97:1158–64. https://doi.org/10.3324/haematol.2011.054718.
5. Bang OY, Seok JM, Kim SG, et al. Ischemic stroke and cancer: stroke severely impacts cancer patients, while cancer increases the number of strokes. J Clin Neurol. 2011;7:53. https://doi.org/10.3988/jcn.2011.7.2.53.
6. Bartynski W. Posterior reversible encephalopathy syndrome, part 2: controversies surrounding pathophysiology of vasogenic edema. Am J Neuroradiol. 2008;29:1043–9. https://doi.org/10.3174/ajnr.a0929.
7. Bick RL. Cancer-associated thrombosis. N Engl J Med. 2003;349:109–11. https://doi.org/10.1056/nejmp030086.
8. Blom JW. Malignancies, prothrombotic mutations, and the risk of venous thrombosis. JAMA. 2005;293:715. https://doi.org/10.1001/jama.293.6.715.
9. Bradley WG. MR appearance of hemorrhage in the brain. Radiology. 1993;189:15–26. https://doi.org/10.1148/radiology.189.1.8372185.
10. Cheng SW, Wu LL, Ting AC, et al. Irradiation-induced extracranial carotid stenosis in patients with head and neck malignancies. Am J Surg. 1999;178:323–8. https://doi.org/10.1016/s0002-9610(99)00184-1.
11. Cocho D, Gendre J, Boltes A, et al. Predictors of occult cancer in acute ischemic stroke patients. J Stroke Cerebrovasc Dis. 2015;24:1324–8. https://doi.org/10.1016/j.jstrokecerebrovasdis.2015.02.006.
12. Demaerschalk BM, Kleindorfer DO, Adeoye OM, et al. Scientific rationale for the inclusion and exclusion criteria for intravenous alteplase in acute ischemic stroke. Stroke. 2015;47:581–641. https://doi.org/10.1161/str.0000000000000086.
13. Donati MB, Falanga A. Pathogenetic mechanisms of thrombosis in malignancy. Acta Haematol. 2001;106:18–24. https://doi.org/10.1159/000046585.
14. Gemmete JJ, Pandey AS, Chaudhary N, et al. Paradoxical embolus to the brain from embolization of a carotid body tumor. J Neurointerv Surg. 2011;4:e12.
15. Gonzalez-Quintela A, Candela M, Vidal C, et al. Non-bacterial thrombotic endocarditis in cancer patients. Acta Cardiol. 1991;46:1–9.
16. Graus F, Rogers LR, Posner JB. Cerebrovascular complications in patients with cancer. Medicine. 1985;64:16–35. https://doi.org/10.1097/00005792-198501000-00002.
17. Hacke W, Kaste M, Bluhmki E, et al. Thrombolysis with alteplase 3 to 4.5 hours after acute ischemic stroke. N Engl J Med. 2008;359:1317–29. https://doi.org/10.1056/nejmoa0804656.
18. Haynes JC, Machtay M, Weber RS, et al. Relative risk of stroke in head and neck carcinoma patients treated with external cervical irradiation. Laryngoscope. 2002;112:1883–7. https://doi.org/10.1097/00005537-200210000-00034.
19. Hemphill JC, Greenberg SM, Anderson CS, et al. Guidelines for the management of spontaneous intracerebral hemorrhage. Stroke. 2015;46:2032–60. https://doi.org/10.1161/str.0000000000000069.
20. Jang H, Lee JJ, Lee MJ, et al. Comparison of enoxaparin and warfarin for secondary prevention of cancer-associated stroke. J Oncol. 2015;2015:1–6. https://doi.org/10.1155/2015/502089.

21. Jauch EC, Saver JL, Adams HP, et al. Guidelines for the early management of patients with acute ischemic stroke: a guideline for healthcare professionals from the American Heart Association/American Stroke Association. Stroke. 2013;44:870–947. https://doi.org/10.1161/str.0b013e318284056a.

22. Kabre R, Kamble K. Gemcitabine and Cisplatin induced posterior reversible encephalopathy syndrome: a case report with review of literature. J Res Pharm Pract. 2016;5:297. https://doi.org/10.4103/2279-042x.192464.

23. Kase CS. Intracerebral hemorrhage: non-hypertensive causes. Stroke. 1986;17:590–5. https://doi.org/10.1161/01.str.17.4.590.

24. Kim K, Lee J-H. Risk factors and biomarkers of ischemic stroke in cancer patients. J Stroke. 2014;16:91. https://doi.org/10.5853/jos.2014.16.2.91.

25. Kim J-M, Jung K-H, Park KH, et al. Clinical manifestation of cancer related stroke: retrospective case–control study. J Neurooncol. 2013;111:295–301. https://doi.org/10.1007/s11060-012-1011-4.

26. Mohr JP. Stroke: pathophysiology, diagnosis, and management. Philadelphia: Elsevier/Saunders; 2011.

27. Mozaffarian D, Benjamin EJ, Go AS, et al. Heart disease and stroke statistics – 2016 update. Circulation. 2015;133:e38. https://doi.org/10.1161/cir.0000000000000350.

28. Murata J-I, Sawamura Y, Takahashi A, et al. Intracerebral hemorrhage caused by a neoplastic aneurysm from small-cell lung carcinoma. Neurosurgery. 1993;32:124–6. https://doi.org/10.1227/00006123-199301000-00019.

29. Navi BB, Singer S, Merkler AE, et al. Recurrent thromboembolic events after ischemic stroke in patients with cancer. Neurology. 2014a;83:26–33. https://doi.org/10.1212/wnl.0000000000000539.

30. Navi BB, Singer S, Merkler AE, et al. Cryptogenic subtype predicts reduced survival among cancer patients with ischemic stroke. Stroke. 2014b;45:2292–7. https://doi.org/10.1161/strokeaha.114.005784.

31. Navi BB, Reiner AS, Kamel H, et al. Risk of arterial thromboembolism in patients with cancer. J Am Coll Cardiol. 2017;70:926–38. https://doi.org/10.1016/j.jacc.2017.06.047.

32. Navi BB, Marshall RS, Bobrow D, et al. Enoxaparin vs aspirin in patients with cancer and ischemic stroke. JAMA Neurol. 2018;75:379. https://doi.org/10.1001/jamaneurol.2017.4211.

33. Nguyen T, DeAngelis LM. Stroke in cancer patients. Curr Neurol Neurosci Rep. 2006;6:187–92. https://doi.org/10.1007/s11910-006-0004-0.

34. Nogueira RG, Jadhav AP, Haussen DC, et al. Thrombectomy 6 to 24 hours after stroke with a mismatch between deficit and infarct. N Engl J Med. 2018;378:11–21. https://doi.org/10.1056/nejmoa1706442.

35. Patel SC, Levine SR, Tilley BC, et al. Lack of clinical significance of early ischemic changes on computed tomography in acute stroke. JAMA. 2001;286:2830–8. https://doi.org/10.1001/jama.286.22.2830.

36. Pollack CV, Reilly PA, Ryn JV, et al. Idarucizumab for dabigatran reversal – full cohort analysis. N Engl J Med. 2017;377:431–41. https://doi.org/10.1056/nejmoa1707278.

37. Powers WJ, Derdeyn CP, Biller J, et al. 2015 American Heart Association/American Stroke Association focused update of the 2013 guidelines for the early management of patients with acute ischemic stroke regarding endovascular treatment. Stroke. 2015;46:3020–35. https://doi.org/10.1161/str.0000000000000074.

38. Powers WJ, Rabinstein AA, Ackerson T, et al. 2018 Guidelines for the early management of patients with acute ischemic stroke: a guideline for healthcare professionals from the American Heart Association/American Stroke Association. Stroke. 2018;49:e46. https://doi.org/10.1161/str.0000000000000158.

39. Quintas S, Rogado J, Gullón P, et al. Predictors of unknown cancer in patients with ischemic stroke. J Neurooncol. 2018;137:551–7. https://doi.org/10.1007/s11060-017-2741-0.

40. Rha J-H, Saver JL. The impact of recanalization on ischemic stroke outcome: a meta-analysis. Stroke. 2007;38:967–73. https://doi.org/10.1161/01.str.0000258112.14918.24.

41. Selvik HA, Thomassen L, Bjerkreim AT, et al. Cancer-associated stroke: the Bergen NORSTROKE study. Cerebrovasc Dis Extra. 2015;5:107–13. https://doi.org/10.1159/000440730.

42. Shin Y-W, Lee S-T, Jung K-H, et al. Predictors of survival for patients with cancer after cryptogenic stroke. J Neurooncol. 2016;128:277–84. https://doi.org/10.1007/s11060-016-2106-0.

43. Sioka C, Kyritsis AP. Central and peripheral nervous system toxicity of common chemotherapeutic agents. Cancer Chemother Pharmacol. 2008;63:761–7.

44. Smets G-J, Loyson T, Paesschen WV, et al. Posterior reversible encephalopathy syndrome possibly induced by pemetrexed maintenance therapy for lung cancer: a case report and literature review. Acta Clin Belg. 2017;1–7. https://doi.org/10.1080/17843286.2017.1403103.

45. Sorgun MH, Kuzu M, Ozer IS, et al. Risk factors, biomarkers, etiology, outcome and prognosis of ischemic stroke in cancer patients. Asian Pac J Cancer Prev. 2018;19:649–53.

46. Stefan O, Vera N, Otto B, et al. Stroke in cancer patients: a risk factor analysis. J Neurooncol. 2009;94:221–6. https://doi.org/10.1007/s11060-009-9818-3.

47. Sun B, Fan S, Li Z, et al. Clinical and neuroimaging features of acute ischemic stroke in cancer patients. Eur Neurol. 2016;75:292–9. https://doi.org/10.1159/000447126.

48. Thaler DE, Saver JL. Cryptogenic stroke and patent foramen ovale. Curr Opin Cardiol. 2008;23:537–44. https://doi.org/10.1097/hco.0b013e32831311bd.

49. Thomalla G, Cheng B, Ebinger M, et al. DWI-FLAIR mismatch for the identification of patients with acute ischaemic stroke within 4·5 h of symptom onset (PRE-FLAIR): a multicentre observational

study. Lancet Neurol. 2011;10:978–86. https://doi.org/10.1016/s1474-4422(11)70192-2.

50. Wardlaw JM, Murray V, Berge E, et al. Recombinant tissue plasminogen activator for acute ischaemic stroke: an updated systematic review and meta-analysis. Lancet. 2012;379:2364–72. https://doi.org/10.1016/s0140-6736(12)60738-7.

51. Wardlaw JM, Murray V, Berge E, et al. Thrombolysis for acute ischaemic stroke. Cochrane Database Syst Rev. 2014. https://doi.org/10.1002/14651858.cd000213.pub3.

52. Wijdicks EFM, Sheth KN, Carter BS, et al. Recommendations for the management of cerebral and cerebellar infarction with swelling: a statement for healthcare professionals from the American Heart Association/American Stroke Association. Stroke. 2014;45:1222–38. https://doi.org/10.1161/01.str.0000441965.15164.d6.

Intracranial Hemorrhage Focused on Cancer and Hemato-oncologic Patients

26

Yasser Mohamad Khorchid and Marc Malkoff

Contents

Introduction 382

Etiology 382

Epidemiology 383

Pathophysiology 384

Clinical Features 385

Diagnosis 385

Management 388
Pharmacologic 388
Non-pharmacologic 390
Management Algorithm 391

Prognosis 391

Conclusion 392

References 392

Abstract

Intracranial hemorrhage (ICH) is the most fatal type of stroke and has the highest rate of disability. It is seen in less than 10% of cancer patients, including known intracranial neoplasms. Intratumoral hemorrhage and coagulopathy are the most common etiologies. ICH most commonly occurs supratentorially, in the cerebral parenchyma. The most common cancers associated with ICH are intracranial metastases, followed by glioblastoma multiforme and hematologic malignancies. Among hemorrhagic metastases, melanoma, lung, and breast cancers are the most common primary tumors. The exact mechanism of intratumoral hemorrhage is unknown, although vascular endothelial growth factor (VEGF) and matrix metalloproteinases (MMP) appear to play an important role. Most cancer patients with ICH are symptomatic. Change in mental status, hemiparesis, and headaches are the most common clinical presentations. A non-contrast head computed tomography (CT) scan is the

Y. M. Khorchid (✉) · M. Malkoff
Department of Neurology, University of Tennessee Health Science Center, Memphis, TN, USA
e-mail: ykhorchi@uthsc.edu; mmalkoff@uthsc.edu

© Springer Nature Switzerland AG 2020
J. L. Nates, K. J. Price (eds.), *Oncologic Critical Care*,
https://doi.org/10.1007/978-3-319-74588-6_40

initial diagnostic step if ICH is suspected. There are no specific guidelines for ICH management in cancer patients. Blood pressure needs to be controlled, and coagulopathy has to be corrected. Surgical interventions might be life-saving, especially in large hemorrhages in the posterior fossa. Overall, cancer patients have worse clinical outcomes than the general population when they develop ICH. Patients with coagulopathy have the poorest prognosis.

Keywords

Intracranial hemorrhage · Cancer · Brain tumor · Glioblastoma multiforme · Brain metastases · Intratumoral hemorrhage · Coagulopathy · Thrombocytopenia

Introduction

Intracranial hemorrhage (ICH) is the most fatal type of stroke and has the highest rate of disability among the survivors [64]. It can be defined as any bleeding that occur inside the cranial vault. This includes bleeding inside the brain tissue itself which is called intraparenchymal hemorrhage (IPH) and inside the brain ventricles known as intraventricular hemorrhage (IVH) and bleeding that occurs between the brain and its surrounding covers including subarachnoid hemorrhage (SAH), subdural hematoma (SDH), and epidural hematoma (EDH). Although the incidence of ICH in cancer patients is low [58], a good understanding of the relation between ICH and cancer is essential, as the pathophysiology, management, and clinical outcomes can be different from what is encountered in the community.

Etiology

Patients with cancer tend to have ICH from different pathologies comparing to the general population. Intratumoral hemorrhage and coagulopathy are the most common etiologies for ICH in cancer patients. Navi et al. retrospectively analyzed data of 208 cancer patients with IPH or SAH who presented to a single cancer center over a period of 7 years [48]. Sixty-one percent of cases were caused by intratumoral hemorrhage and 46% by coagulopathy. Thirty-three percent had multifactorial causes and 21% had both intratumoral hemorrhage and coagulopathy. Not surprisingly, solid tumors were more associated with intratumoral hemorrhage, whereas coagulopathy was more often found to be the cause of ICH in hematological malignancies. Interestingly, hypertension, which is the most common cause of spontaneous ICH in the community, only caused around 5% of ICH in cancer patients, which highlights the unique mechanisms of ICH in the setting of neoplasms [48, 53, 60, 69].

Other, but less frequent, etiologies were trauma (6%), hemorrhagic conversion of ischemic strokes (4%), cerebral venous thrombosis (2%) (which can be resulted either from hypercoagulability or neoplastic venous sinus compression) [48, 66], and aneurysmal rupture (2%).

Rare causes that are unique to patients with cancer include leukostasis which can occur in patients with leukemia when peripheral white blood cell counts rise above 100,000 cells/mm^3 and hyperviscosity [48, 66].

Besides intraparenchymal location, ICH in patients with cancer can involve other intracranial compartments [24, 34, 48, 68, 72]. SAH usually occurs in the setting of coagulopathy, trauma, or intratumoral hemorrhage that is adjacent to the cortex. Aneurysms and arteriovenous malformations are much less common etiologies of SAH in cancer patients comparing to the general population [48]. It is worth mentioning that when aneurysmal SAH occurs in patients with cancer, other atypical types of aneurysms, like mycotic and neoplastic (although the latter is extraordinarily rare), should be kept on the differential. Neoplastic and mycotic aneurysms are fusiform, typically develop in distal middle cerebral artery branches, and are most commonly associated with atrial myxoma, choriocarcinoma, and lung carcinoma [56, 66].

SDH is found frequently in patients with cancer and usually results from coagulopathy or from trauma [55]. A recent craniotomy can lead to SDH. Less frequently, the cause of SDH can be intratumoral hemorrhage from dura mater metastases [33, 46, 50]. In one report, 15–40% of patients with dural metastases have a coexistent SDH, mostly chronic [33].

Like SDH, EDH usually results from trauma or coagulopathy. In rare cases, it may occur from calvarial or dural neoplasms (primary or metastatic) [43, 66].

Epidemiology

Intracranial hemorrhage is responsible for about 50% of cerebrovascular events in patients with cancer and is more likely to be symptomatic than ischemic strokes [24]. Murphy et al. identified all patients diagnosed with spontaneous ICH from 2002 to 2011 in the Nationwide Inpatient Sample. Among 597,046 identified ICH patients, 22,394 (3.8%) had systemic cancer [47]. In patients who present as spontaneous ICH, brain neoplasm was found to be the underlying etiology in about 1–8% of cases [2, 32, 58, 59]. A prospective study of 692 patients who presented with ICH found intracranial tumor related to the ICH in 7.2% of the cases [58]. In another large autopsy series of ICH, an underlying and unsuspected cancer was discovered in only 4 of 430 (1%) cases [32, 58]. Similarly, a recent meta-analysis showed that an intracranial malignancy (including glioblastoma) as a cause of spontaneous ICH in young adults was rare, accounting for 2.3% of cases [28]. On the other hand, the incidence of ICH in known intracranial neoplasm patients was 2.4% according to a large prospective study that included 2041 patients with intracranial neoplasms [58].

ICH in cancer patients occur almost equally in both genders [68]. The median time from cancer diagnosis to ICH occurrence differs between patients based on the cancer type. In one study, the median time was 28 months for solid tumors, 22 months for hematologic tumors, and 6 months for primary brain tumors [48].

As far as ICH location goes, about three quarters of ICH in cancer patients are supratentorial. Infratentorial ICH sites are more common in the cerebellum than the brain stem.

Among intracranial compartments, bleeding occurs most frequently inside the brain parenchyma, followed by the subdural and then the subarachnoid spaces. Epidural location is less frequently encountered. In almost 25% of times, multiple hemorrhages can occur simultaneously, and in about 20% of cases, there are intraventricular hemorrhages [48, 58, 68].

Overall, any type of intracranial tumor can cause ICH, although the frequency varies widely among different neoplasms [58]. Usually, fast-growing and highly vascularized tumors with an irregular and fragile vascular architecture are most frequently associated with ICH [37]. Several tumors, particularly malignant ones, have an increased predilection for intratumoral hemorrhage [24, 31, 48, 58, 72]. The leading causes of tumor-related ICH were metastases of extracranial origin (36%), followed by glioblastoma multiforme (GBM) (30%) [38, 58]. In one retrospective study of ICH in patients with cancer, Navi et al. found that the cancer contributing to hemorrhage was a solid tumor in 68% of cases, a primary brain tumor in 16% of cases, and a hematologic tumor in 16% of cases.

Melanoma (15%), lung (14%), breast (7%), and renal cell (4%) cancers are the most common systemic solid tumors associated with ICH [48]. Their frequent association with ICH is partly explained by their ubiquity – these tumors have a high incidence in the population and account for most brain metastases – and their histological composition, which has elements of neoangiogenesis, tumor cell necrosis, and parenchymal blood vessel invasion [5, 35, 57]. On the other hand, thyroid cancer, hepatocellular carcinoma, and choriocarcinoma are rare causes of brain metastases but have an unusually high predisposition to hemorrhage, accounting for their overrepresentation of ICH in cancer series [11, 24, 35]. In addition, although prostate cancer rarely metastasizes to the brain, it accounted for a sizeable proportion (5%) of ICH in a recent clinical series of patients with cancer. This increased incidence compared to prior reports may be due to improvements in prostate cancer therapy, which may have altered the natural history of disease allowing for longer survival and increased risk of cerebrovascular complications [48].

Of primary brain tumors, glioblastoma multiforme (GBM) is most frequently associated with ICH, because it is the most common primary brain neoplasm and because its tumor cells are highly invasive and destructive [31, 34, 58, 72]. With their fragile retiform capillaries, oligodendrogliomas are also predisposed to hemorrhage even when low grade, despite the fact that they are much less frequent tumors than GBM [37]. Furthermore, benign neoplasms, including meningiomas, can also cause intratumoral hemorrhage. Benign neoplasms accounted for 23 of 110 (21%) and 9 of 50 (18%) cases of intratumoral hemorrhage [34, 58]; however, bleeding from meningioma is relatively rare. Wakai et al. found meningioma to cause only 4 of the 310 cases of intracranial neoplasm who presented with ICH [68]. Highly vascular meningotheliomatous and angioblastic meningiomas are most frequently the case. The majority of reported cases of meningioma associated with intracranial hemorrhage deal with SAH rather than IPH or hemorrhage within the substance of the tumor itself [36], probably due to their extra-axial location.

Hematological malignancies, particularly leukemia, are also frequently encountered in the setting of ICH in cancer patients. These tumors generally cause ICH through coagulopathy from severe thrombocytopenia or coagulation cascade dysfunction [24, 42, 48]. For instance, one study reported a mean platelet count of $13,500/mm^3$ in patients with leukemia (without intracranial invasion) and ICH. Despite the fact that lymphomas and leukemias can rarely metastasize to the brain parenchyma or arachnoid mater and cause brain hemorrhage, ICH still occur only in the setting of severe coagulopathy [24].

Pathophysiology

The mechanisms of ICH in cancer patients vary based on the cancer type. Solid tumors typically cause ICH from intratumoral hemorrhage. On the other hand, the vast majority of ICH in hematologic malignancies are related to coagulopathy and less frequently to leukostasis [24, 71]. In general, malignant and hypervascular neoplasms have the highest predilection for hemorrhage [31, 36, 48].

In 1889, Stephen Paget proposed the hypothesis of "seed and soil" which still, at least partially, explains the mechanism of metastases of systemic cancers to the central nervous system (CNS) [20]. In this hypothesis, tumor cells get their access to CNS capillary beds via hematogenous spread. Because 80% of the cerebral blood flow go to the anterior circulation, the majority of brain metastases and their related intratumoral hemorrhages are supratentorial as noted earlier. In addition, the "seed and soil" hypothesis can explain the propensity of certain tumors (e.g., melanoma) to establish brain metastases.

Although the exact mechanism that leads to intratumoral hemorrhage is still poorly understood, multiple factors that are possibly related to the pathophysiology have been identified. Several preclinical studies have suggested that new blood vessels induced by vascular endothelial growth factor (VEGF) have a propensity to lead to hemorrhage because of their fragility and permeability [10]. Immunohistochemical staining for VEGF was associated with intratumoral hemorrhage in surgical series [27]. Melanoma and renal cell carcinoma, two of the solid malignancies that their intracranial metastases have very high tendency to cause ICH, are highly vascularized tumors. Both of them are associated with angiogenesis and increased production of VEGF [40, 51].

In addition to VEGF, matrix metalloproteinases (MMP), which are substances that degrade extracellular matrix proteins and thereby allow for tumor invasion and metastasis [15], may also play a role in the pathogenesis of ICH secondary to malignancy. Jung et al. reported a study of 16 patients with brain metastases, 7 of whom had hemorrhagic complications and 9 did not. Patients in the hemorrhagic group had higher immunohistochemical expression of VEGF. In addition, they had evidence of increased basement membrane breakdown in the presence of immunohistochemical overexpression of matrix metalloproteinase-2 (MMP-2) and matrix metalloproteinase-9 (MMP-9) [29]. This suggests the possible contribution of increased MMP protein elaboration to the pathophysiology of ICH in the setting of underlying brain tumors.

Besides overexpression of VEGF and MMP in tumor cells, imbalances in the fibrinolytic cascade, rupture of thin-walled fistulous or friable large vessels, rapid tumor growth, aberrant neovascularization, tumor necrosis, and vascular invasion [35–37, 56, 66, 68] are all factors that might participate in the pathophysiology of intratumoral hemorrhage. ICH might arise from the rapidly growing peripheral portion of the tumor or from adjacent damaged brain tissue too [36, 39]. The inherent capacity of choriocarcinoma for vascular invasion appears to be a particularly important factor in the pathogenesis of ICH in this highly hemorrhagic neoplasm [36, 61, 65].

As mentioned above, coagulopathy play the key role in the pathogenesis of ICH in hematological cancers. Coagulopathy typically result from abnormalities of platelets, coagulation factors, or both. It can also be iatrogenic as many cancer patients have indications for anticoagulation agents (e.g., warfarin and direct oral anticoagulants). Thrombocytopenia often occurs from bone marrow suppression secondary to chemotherapy or radiation, tumor infiltration, or intrinsic failure (in hematological malignancies) [66]. Impairments of the coagulation cascade generally result from liver failure, vitamin K deficiency due to poor nutrition, or disseminated intravascular coagulation (DIC) [24, 66].

In hematological malignancies, hyperleukocytosis, defined as peripheral blast count for more than $100,000/mm^3$, stands as a unique but less frequent mechanism of ICH, especially in acute leukemias. One suggested mechanism is plugging of small cerebral vessels by blast cells, resulting in local hypoxia and vessel destruction. Another possibility is invasion of blood vessels by nodular growth of leukemia cells [55].

Clinical Features

Ninety-four percent of patients with cancer who develop ICH are symptomatic when the hemorrhage is diagnosed radiographically [48]. This is not the case when ICH is identified at surgery or autopsy [24, 68]. In a series of non-radiographically diagnosed ICH in brain tumor patients, Wakai et al. found about 42% of the patients with hemorrhage from brain tumors (other than pituitary adenoma) to be asymptomatic [68].

Clinical signs and symptoms of ICH in patients with cancer do not significantly differ from what is encountered in similar cases in the general population. Deterioration in the level of consciousness, hemiparesis, and headaches are the most common neurological findings following ICH [24, 36, 48, 58]. Nausea, vomiting, seizures, aphasia, hemisensory, and visual field disturbances are frequently seen [48], whereas unilateral dilated pupil and abducens cranial nerve (CN VI) palsy are present less often [58]. Coma can occur in 6–28% of cases [48, 58].

Diagnosis

As in all medical fields, clinical history and physical exam are the cornerstone in evaluating patients with cancer who might have ICH. History of trauma and coagulopathy (including taking anticoagulation medications) has a special importance. Acute onset of headaches, confusion, or focal neurological deficits such as aphasia, hemiparesis, hemisensory changes, and visual field disturbances are the main findings to look for. Asking about seizure-like activities is important as well.

When an intracranial central nervous system (CNS) process is suspected, a non-contrast head computed tomography (CT) scan is the first radiographic study to obtain because it can be done quickly, it is widely available, and it is pretty much sensitive for acute blood products detection [66]. As in other body parts, intracranial acute blood appears hyperdense on CT scan. If ICH is found, obtaining another CT study but this time with intravenous (IV) contrast along with CT angiography will add much more diagnostic value. Contraindications such as allergy to iodinated contrast and renal insufficiency need to be considered before proceeding with those studies. CT angiography of the head is particularly helpful in revealing underlying vascular malformations, an important etiology for ICH. Furthermore,

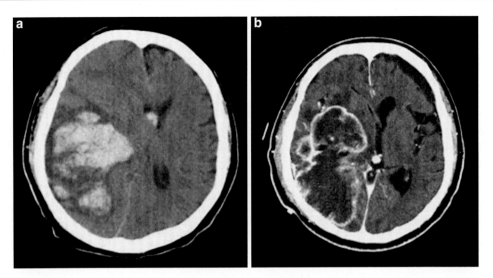

Fig. 1 (**a**) Axial CT head without contrast at admission of a 66-year-old male revealing a huge lobar acute hemorrhage in right temporoparietal region. (**b**) A follow-up CT head with contrast performed 2 months after the initial scan demonstrating giant mass with ringlike enhancement in the same region as the previous hemorrhage. (Photo is used with permission [Taniura S, Okamoto H, Tanabe M, Kurosaki M, Mizushima M, Watanabe T, Huge lobar intracerebral hemorrhage by glioblastoma multiforme. J Neurooncol (2007) 82:117–118. Fig. 1: page 118])

a "spot sign," which indicates active extravasation of blood products and fairly predicts hematoma expansion, might be found [67].

Cancer-related ICH shows distinct radiographic features, which should be carefully considered when interpreting ICH on CT scan [58] (Fig. 1). An atypical location of the hemorrhage can point at the possibility of the presence of a tumor. A bleeding in the cortical-subcortical junction or close to the dural membranes such as the falx or the tentorium or located close to major cerebral veins or sinuses can be related to tumor, comparing to deep basal ganglia and lobar locations which are more typical for hypertensive and cerebral amyloid angiopathy-related hemorrhages, respectively. Heterogeneous and irregular or ring-shaped appearance of the bleeding, the presence of calcification, and multifocal location are all clues that can suggest an underlying neoplasm. More importantly, contrast enhancement can reveal a tumor that would otherwise be concealed by the blood clot. Usually, peritumoral vascularization enhances, particularly, at its margins. Furthermore, excessive edema surrounding the hematoma on CT scan is often a very important clue to an underlying neoplasm because it is only rarely seen in the acute phase of spontaneous ICH [58]. One study reported a positive predictive value of 71% for underlying neoplasm if the vasogenic edema to mean hematoma diameter ratio was greater than 100% [63]. Additionally, persistent edema and delayed hematoma evolution are also suspicious for intratumoral hemorrhage [4].

Brain magnetic resonance imaging (MRI) with contrast offers better resolution than CT and shows all the findings that suggest tumor-related ICH noted earlier (Fig. 2). However, it takes much more time to be performed, in addition of being more costly. A special importance that favors MRI over CT scan is its ability to better evaluate for alternative etiologies of ICH. Ischemic stroke with hemorrhagic conversion (via diffusion-weighted imaging), venous sinus thrombosis (thrombosed veins demonstrate flow voids on pre-contrast images and restricted enhancement on post-contrast images), and amyloid angiopathy (lobar microhemorrhages on susceptibility-weighted sequences) are some examples [66].

Digital subtraction angiography (DSA) is an invasive diagnostic procedure that is still

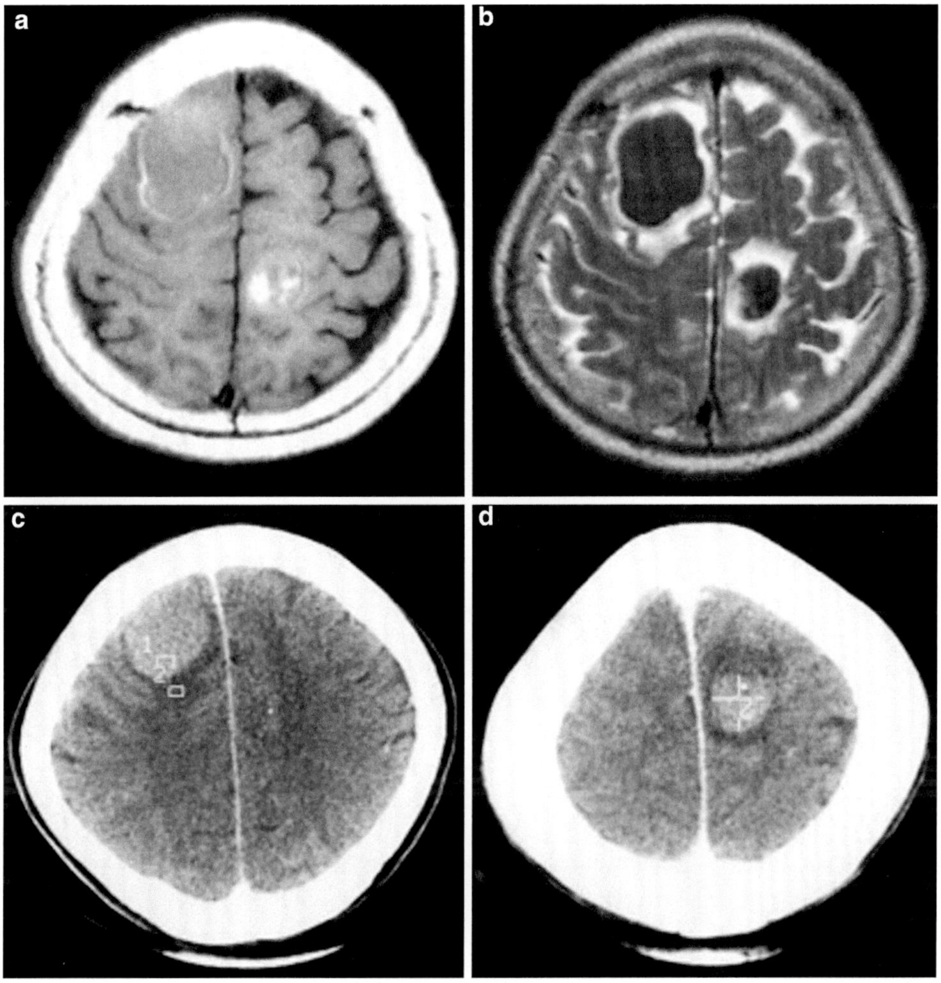

Fig. 2 This is a 69-year-old female with history of metastatic non-small cell lung cancer. She has left and right frontal hemorrhagic metastases. (**a**) MRI T1 and (**b**) MRI T2, both axial cuts, show acute to early subacute hemorrhages which appear isointense to hyperintense (bright) on T1 and hypointense (dark) on T2. Vasogenic edema surrounding the hemorrhages is easily identifiable on T2 (hyperintense). (**c**) and (**d**) CT head without contrast, axial cuts, show the same hemorrhagic metastases which appear as hyperdensities (bright). Vasogenic edema appears as hypodensity (dark) on CT. (Photo is used with permission from Ref. [29], p. 258)

sometimes used in the setting of ICH evaluation, mainly to rule out vascular malformations. In patients with cancer, abnormal tumor vessels and early venous filling were demonstrated in some cases, along with tumor mass effect [36].

Practically, a short-term neuroradiological follow-up is advisable in all cases in whom the clinico-radiological features do not correspond to the usual pattern of intracerebral hypertensive hemorrhage [47], although the timing and indication for contrast-enhanced brain MRI in the diagnostic evaluation of idiopathic IPH is more controversial [66]. In a study that included 148 patients with unexplained IPH evaluated with brain MRI, only 1 patient was found to have an underlying tumor [30]. In addition, acute IPH may obscure a tumor, leading to a false-negative study if MRI is performed too early [23]. With that being said, unless there is a high suspicion for cancer or another cause of IPH frequently detected on MRI (such as hemorrhagic conversion of an ischemic stroke or amyloid angiopathy), probably it is better idea to perform MRI 4–12 weeks after the ictus in order to enhance its diagnostic yield [66].

Besides diagnostic imagings, a focused laboratory evaluation should be performed as soon as possible in fairly all cases of ICH. Complete blood count (CBC), coagulation profile (e.g., PT, aPTT, and INR), and disseminated intravascular coagulation (DIC) panel (e.g., D-dimer and fibrinogen levels) are essential. A platelet function test can be checked if the patient is going to have an emergent surgical intervention. Moreover, if DIC is suspected, a peripheral blood smear should be obtained to evaluate for schistocytes [66].

Management

Since there are no specific protocols for management of ICH in cancer patients, existing guidelines for IPH, SDH, and SAH should be applied in those cases [13, 26, 66]. As in any serious and life-threatening medical illness, the management of cancer patients who present with ICH starts with a quick and focused evaluation of airways, breathing, and circulation (ABC). When the diagnosis of ICH is established, an urgent and, in case of rapidly declining mental status or ongoing clinical seizures, an emergent, neurological and neurosurgical consultation is mandatory. Admission to a dedicated intensive care unit with neurologic specialization is advised because that may decrease mortality in ICH patients according to a retrospective review of outcome data from the Project IMPACT database of intensive care units [18].

Pharmacologic

In patients with IPH, blood pressure should be controlled immediately after ictus similar to cases of spontaneous ICH. Intravenous antihypertensive agents, including nicardipine infusion, are usually used to rapidly control blood pressure. In a large prospective study of patients with spontaneous ICH, a systolic blood pressure (SBP) reduction to less than 140 within 1 h after randomization comparing to standard management (keeping SBP < 180) was safe. Although there was a statistically significant improvement in functional outcomes, the rates of severe disability and death were similar in both groups [3]. Moreover, a subsequent large prospective study compared SBP reduction to 110–139 versus 140–179 showed more renal adverse events in intensive blood pressure reduction group [54]. A recent meta-analysis that included 4360 patients from 5 randomized clinical trials (RCTs) showed that intensive blood pressure reduction was associated with a trend for lower risk of significant ICH expansion compared with standard treatment (OR, 0.82; 95% CI, 0.68 to 1.00, p = 0.056), especially in larger RCTs [6].

Besides blood pressure control, patients with intratumoral hemorrhage who have excessive vasogenic edema should be treated with steroids (e.g., dexamethasone) in order to reduce the mass effect [48]. Elevated intracranial pressure (ICP), which might be life-threatening, is not uncommon especially in large hemorrhages. Emergent therapy for increased ICP was administered to 13% of cancer patients with ICH in one study [48]. Raising the head of bed to 30–45° with maintaining midline head and neck position is the first step in high ICP management. Sedation and pain control (e.g., propofol or midazolam and fentanyl infusions) are essential. Osmotherapy with intravenous mannitol or hypertonic saline is frequently required. Neuromuscular paralysis, hyperventilation (which is a temporary measure), and even barbiturate coma are sometimes unavoidable in order to control ICP [22].

Seizures should be treated using antiepileptic medications [26]. Choosing among different agents depends on other comorbidities, particularly renal and hepatological functions. Status epilepticus is a neurocritical emergency that need to be managed according to current guidelines [7]. Any otherwise unexplained change in mental status has to trigger a continuous video electroencephalography (cvEEG) monitoring to evaluate for subclinical seizures, especially if repeated neuroimaging is stable and ICP is under control. If electrographic seizures are found, they have to be treated with anti-seizure drugs [26].

Patients with ICH should have intermittent pneumatic compression for prevention of venous thromboembolism (VTE) beginning the day of hospital admission. After documentation of cessation of bleeding, low-dose subcutaneous low-molecular-weight heparin or unfractionated heparin may be considered for prevention of VTE in patients with lack of mobility after 1–4 days from onset. Glucose should be monitored. Both hyperglycemia and hypoglycemia should be avoided. In all patients, a formal screening procedure for dysphagia should be performed before the initiation of oral intake to reduce the risk of pneumonia [26].

The management of acute SDH and EDH in patients with cancer is pretty much the same as in general population [66]. Small (less than 10 mm clot thickness) acute SDH without evidence of elevated intracranial pressure or severe neurological deficits can be managed conservatively without a surgical intervention [16]. Similarly, small and asymptomatic chronic SDH can be managed with observation [19]. On the other hand, surgery is required in large and/or symptomatic SDH, whether acute or chronic [16, 19].

Patients with cancer who develop acute SAH from saccular cerebral aneurysms should be treated according to current guidelines [13]. The ruptured aneurysm should be secured with endovascular coiling or surgical clipping (depending on its characteristics) as early as feasible to reduce the rate of rebleeding. Between the time of SAH symptom onset and aneurysm obliteration, blood pressure should be controlled with a titratable agent to balance the risk of stroke, hypertension-related rebleeding, and maintenance of cerebral perfusion pressure. For patients with an unavoidable delay in obliteration of aneurysm, a significant risk of rebleeding, and no compelling medical contraindications, short-term (72 h) therapy with tranexamic acid or aminocaproic acid is reasonable to reduce the risk of early aneurysm rebleeding [13]. Oral nimodipine should be administered to all patients with aneurysmal SAH as it has been shown to improve neurological outcomes.

Aneurysmal SAH is not a simple disease as many complications can come with it. When acute symptomatic hydrocephalus occurs, it should be managed by cerebrospinal fluid (CSF) diversion, either with external ventricular drain (EVD) or lumbar drainage, depending on the clinical scenario. Delayed cerebral ischemia (DCI) occurs in about 30% of patients with aneurysmal SAH, usually between 4 and 14 days after the onset of symptoms. DCI is defined as any neurologic deterioration (focal or global) presumed secondary to cerebral ischemia that persists for more than 1 h and cannot be explained by any other neurologic or systemic condition [62]. Maintenance of euvolemia and normal circulating blood volume is recommended to prevent DCI. In case it happens, induction of hypertension is recommended unless blood pressure is elevated at baseline or cardiac status precludes it. Cerebral angioplasty and/or selective intra-arterial vasodilator therapy is reasonable in patients with symptomatic cerebral vasospasm, particularly those who are not rapidly responding to hypertensive therapy [13]. Hyponatremia is seen often in patients with aneurysmal SAH. Fludrocortisone acetate and hypertonic saline solution are used for correcting sodium levels. Finally, heparin-induced thrombocytopenia (HIT) and deep venous thrombosis are relatively frequent complications after aneurysmal SAH. Early identification and targeted treatment are recommended, but further research is needed to identify the ideal screening paradigms [13].

It is worth mentioning that, in cancer patients, SAH might be related to mycotic, and in exceptional cases neoplastic, aneurysms [49, 66]. Those types of aneurysms are not easily amenable to surgery or endovascular coiling. Antibiotics are the mainstay of mycotic aneurysm-related SAH management, whereas radiation and chemotherapy are therapeutic options in case of neoplastic aneurysms [66].

As mentioned earlier in this chapter, bleeding diathesis is a major risk for ICH, and frequently it is the underlying etiology, especially in cancer patients. When ICH occurs in the setting of bleeding diathesis, treatment should be directed toward correcting the coagulopathy. If thrombocytopenia exists, platelet transfusions should be administered with a goal platelet value of more than $50,000–70,000/mm^3$ [48, 66]. On the other hand, the usefulness of platelet transfusions in ICH patients with a history of antiplatelet use is uncertain [26]. Patients with elevated prothrombin or partial thromboplastin times should be treated with intravenous vitamin K and fresh frozen plasma (FFP). In addition, an underlying etiology such as sepsis need to be treated in case of DIC [66].

Obviously, anticoagulation medications must be held in the setting of acute ICH. Patients who are receiving heparin should be given protamine sulfate as soon as possible. Antivitamin K agents (i.e., warfarin) need to be reversed. Intravenous vitamin K should be administered in all cases. Although FFP has been given frequently, prothrombin complex concentrate (PCC) may have fewer complications and correct the INR more rapidly than FFP. PCC might be considered over FFP according to the most recent ICH guidelines [26]. Importantly, the administration of rFVIIa is not recommended because it does not supply other vitamin K-dependent coagulation factors and does not improve survival or functional outcomes in patients with ICH [41].

As direct oral anticoagulants (DOAC) are being prescribed more, ICH in their presence is increasingly encountered. Specific reversal agents for management of serious hemorrhage in patients taking DOAC are being developed. Idarucizumab is a humanized monoclonal antibody fragment for dabigatran and is already approved by the FDA for the treatment of dabigatran-induced major hemorrhage [52]. Andexanet is a recombinant factor Xa protein without catalytic activity that captures circulating factor Xa inhibitors (e.g., rivaroxaban or apixaban). A multicenter, prospective, open-label, single-group study is ongoing to evaluate the safety and efficacy of andexanet, with promising preliminary results already published [14].

Non-pharmacologic

There is an important role for surgery in the management of ICH in cancer patients, depending on the location of the bleeding and the clinical status. Patients with cerebellar hemorrhage who are deteriorating neurologically or who have brainstem compression and/or hydrocephalus from ventricular obstruction should undergo surgical removal of the hemorrhage as soon as possible [17, 26].

In supratentorial hemorrhages, the underlying tumor should be considered for resection if surgically feasible [36, 58]. The presence of a brain neoplasm (whether primary or metastatic) was an exclusion criterion in the major clinical trials of surgical interventions in supratentorial ICH [44, 45], and subsequently their results cannot be applied in such cases. However, those trials can still be valid when ICH occurs in patients with systemic cancers who do not have known intracranial involvement. In STICH trial, surgical removal of supratentorial ICH did not improve functional outcomes [44]. Similar results were found in STICH II trial which included ICH patients with lobar locations only [44]. Of note, in both trials craniotomy was used in the vast majority of cases in order to remove the clot. On the other hand, MISTIE III is an ongoing large clinical trial aims to evaluate how a minimally invasive surgical approach of clot removal (using surgical aspiration followed by alteplase clot irrigation) can impact functional outcomes in supratentorial ICH [1].

Acute hydrocephalus can result from CSF outflow obstruction or intraventricular hemorrhage. An external ventricular drainage (EVD) should be placed in those situations, and it might be life-saving [36]. It is worth mentioning that administering intrathecal alteplase through EVD in cases of IVH that is obstructing third and/or fourth ventricles was evaluated in a large clinical trial (CLEAR III) [25]. Although it was safe, intrathecal alteplase did not improve functional outcomes.

Whole-brain radiation may be considered in patients with unresectable tumors or those with more than three metastatic lesions as a palliative measure [66]. In a retrospective study of cancer patients with ICH, 23% of them ultimately treated with cranial irradiation [48].

In patients with hyperleukocytosis (e.g., in acute myeloid leukemia), leukapheresis prior to chemotherapy initiation was suggested as a preventive measure in order to reduce the incidence of ICH [9, 70]. However, the data is conflicting. Furthermore, there is no evidence of any long-term survival benefit from this practice [9, 12].

Management Algorithm

ICH is suspected (acute onset of mental status change, headaches, or focal neurological deficit)
↓
Evaluate airway, breathing, and circulation (ABC)
↓
Obtain STAT CT head without contrast
↓ (If ICH is found)
Consult neurology and neurosurgery
Evaluate for coagulopathy (check CBC and coagulopathy panel, check for current anticoagulation medications use) → correct accordingly, reverse anticoagulation medication effect
Control blood pressure using intravenous agents (e.g., nicardipine infusion) for SBP goal of <140
If vasogenic edema is found → start steroids (e.g., dexamethasone)
↓
Admit to ICU (preferably NeuroICU)

Prognosis

Patients with cancer who suffer an intracranial hemorrhage have worse clinical outcomes than patients who develop ICH without a history of cancer [47]. From a large specimen of the Nationwide Inpatient Sample, Murphy et al. retrospectively compared outcomes in ICH patients with and without history of systemic cancer. In multivariate logistic regression analysis adjusted for demographics, comorbidities, and hospital-level characteristics, patients with cancer had higher odds of death (OR 1.62, 95% CI 1.56–1.69) and lower odds of favorable discharge (i.e., home or rehab) (OR 0.59, 95% CI 0.56–0.63) than patients without cancer. In this study, patients with cancer were more often diagnosed with coagulopathy than patients without cancer (14.1% vs. 5.4%, $P < 0.001$), a fact that

would, at least partially, explain the difference in outcomes as coagulopathy is well-known to be a predictor for hematoma expansion and poor prognosis in ICH patients [8, 21]. Moreover, cancer patients with ICH probably were managed less aggressively comparing to ICH patients without history of cancer, as the latter had more procedures done according to medical records in Murthy' study [47].

Cancer subtype may influence outcomes after ICH. Patients with nonmetastatic hematologic tumors and those with metastatic disease had worse outcomes than patients with nonmetastatic solid tumors. Interestingly, the rates of coagulopathy were higher in patients with nonmetastatic hematologic tumors (26.4%) and those with metastatic solid or hematologic tumors (16.5%) comparing to patients with nonmetastatic solid tumors (6.3%) [47]. In another study, Navi et al. found that patients with solid tumors had the best functional outcome at discharge, with 53% being completely or partially independent, compared with 44% of patients with primary brain tumors and 30% of patients with hematologic tumors [48].

Predictors of poor prognosis in patients with cancer and ICH include an underlying systemic malignancy (i.e., not a primary brain tumor), multiple hemorrhagic foci, hydrocephalus, treatment for increased intracranial pressure (likely reflects more severe disease), and the absence of ventriculostomy [48].

Mortality rates were the highest in patients with hematopoietic tumors (36% during hospitalization), whereas patients with primary brain tumors (8%) had the lowest. Thirty-day mortality was 31%, and 1-year mortality was 78% for the entire cohort. Median survival was 5.9 months for patients with primary brain tumors, 2.1 months for patients with solid tumors, and 1.5 months for patients with hematologic tumors [48].

In Navi' study, the multivariate models showed that impaired consciousness, not having a primary brain tumor, multiple foci of hemorrhage, hydrocephalus, increased ICP treatment, and not receiving ventriculostomy were significant predictors of 30-day mortality. All of these variables, except not having a primary brain tumor, were also independently predictive of 90-day mortality. Additionally, hemiparesis and current chemotherapy were significant predictors of mortality at 90 but not 30 days via multivariate analysis. Interestingly, neither anticoagulant nor antiplatelet use was a significant predictor of poor prognosis or mortality [48].

Conclusion

Intracranial hemorrhage is associated with high rates of morbidity and mortality, and it is encountered frequently in cancer patients. The most common etiologies in this population are intratumoral hemorrhage and coagulopathy. As the majority of patients are symptomatic, establishing the diagnosis with a CT scan as quickly as possible is vital. Most patients require an admission to a neurological intensive care unit and a neurosurgical consultation is almost always needed. Medical management is necessary, and, at times, surgical interventions might be life saving. Overall, clinical outcomes of intracranial hemorrhage remain poor, especially in cancer patients.

References

1. Minimally invasive surgery plus Rt-PA for ICH evacuation phase III (MISTIE III). Clinical Trials. gov Identifier: NCT 01827046
2. Abrahams NA, Prayson R. The role of histopathologic examination of intracranial blood clots removed for hemorrhage of unknown etiology: a clinical pathologic analysis of 31 cases. Ann Diagn Pathol. 2000;4:361–6.
3. Anderson CS, Heeley E, Huang Y, et al. Rapid blood-pressure lowering in patients with acute intracerebral hemorrhage. N Engl J Med. 2013;368:2355–65.
4. Atlas SW, Grossman RI, Gomori JM, et al. Hemorrhagic intracranial malignant neoplasms: spin-echo MR imaging. Radiology. 1987;164:71–7.
5. Barnholtz-Sloan JS, Sloan A, Davis FG, et al. Incidence proportions of brain metastases in patients diagnosed (1973 to 2001) in the Metropolitan Detroit Cancer Surveillance System. J Clin Oncol. 2004;22:2865–72.
6. Boulouis G, Morotti A, Goldstein JN, Charidimou A. Intensive blood pressure lowering in patients with acute intracerebral haemorrhage: clinical outcomes and haemorrhage expansion systematic review and meta-analysis of randomised trials. J Neurol Neurosurg Psychiatry. 2017;88:339–45.
7. Brophy GM, Bell R, Claassen J, Neurocritical Care Society Status Epilepticus Guideline Writing Committee, et al. Guidelines for the evaluation and management of status epilepticus. Neurocrit Care. 2012;17:3.
8. Brouwers HB, Chang Y, Falcone GJ, et al. Predicting hematoma expansion after primary intracerebral hemorrhage. JAMA Neurol. 2014;71:158–64.
9. Bug G, Anargyrou K, Tonn T, et al. Impact of leukapheresis on early death rate in adult acute myeloid leukemia presenting with hyperleukocytosis. Transfusion. 2007;47:1843–50.
10. Cao R, Eriksson A, Kubo H, Alitalo K, Cao Y, Thyberg J. Comparative evaluation of FGF-2-, VEGF-A-, and VEGF-C-induced angiogenesis, lymphangiogenesis, vascular fenestrations, and permeability. Circ Res. 2004;94:664–70.
11. Chang L, Chen Y-L, Kao M-CC. Intracranial metastasis of hepatocellular carcinoma: review of 45 cases. Surg Neurol. 2004;62:172–7.
12. Chang MC, Chen T, Tang JL, et al. Leukapheresis and cranial irradiation in patients with hyperleukocytic acute myeloid leukemia: no impact on early mortality and intracranial hemorrhage. Am J Hematol. 2007;82:976–80.
13. Connolly ES Jr, Rabinstein A, Carhuapoma JR, Derdeyn CP, Dion J, Higashida RT, Hoh BL, Kirkness CJ, Naidech AM, Ogilvy CS, Patel AB, Thompson BG, Vespa P, American Heart Association Stroke Council, Council on Cardiovascular Radiology and Intervention, Council on Cardiovascular Nursing, Council on Cardiovascular Surgery and Anesthesia, Council on Clinical Cardiology. Guidelines for the management of aneurysmal subarachnoid hemorrhage: a guideline for healthcare professionals from the American Heart Association/American Stroke Association. Stroke. 2012;43:1711–37.
14. Connolly SJ, Milling TJ, Eikelboom JW, ANNEXA-4 Investigators, et al. Andexanet alfa for acute major bleeding associated with factor Xa inhibitors. N Engl J Med. 2016;375:1131–41.
15. Coussens LM, Fingleton B, Matrisian LM. Matrix metalloproteinase inhibitors and cancer: trials and tribulations. Science. 2002;295:2387–92.
16. Croce MA, Dent D, Menke PG, Robertson JT, Hinson MS, Young BH, Donovan TB, Pritchard FE, Minard G, Kudsk KA, et al. Acute subdural hematoma: nonsurgical management of selected patients. J Trauma. 1994;36:820–6.
17. Dammann P, Asgari S, Bassiouni H, et al. Spontaneous cerebellar hemorrhage: experience with 57 surgically treated patients and review of the literature. Neurosurg Rev. 2011;34:77–86.
18. Diringer MN, Edwards D. Admission to a neurologic/neurosurgical intensive care unit is associated with reduced mortality rate after intracerebral hemorrhage. Crit Care Med. 2001;29:635–40.

19. Ducruet AF, Grobelny B, Zacharia BE, Hickman ZL, DeRosa PL, Anderson K, Sussman E, Carpenter A, Connolly ES Jr. The surgical management of chronic subdural hematoma. Neurosurg Rev. 2012;35:155–69.

20. Fidler IJ. The pathogenesis of cancer metastasis: the 'seed and soil' hypothesis revisited. Nat Rev Cancer. 2003;3:453–8.

21. Flibotte JJ, Hagan N, O'Donnell J, et al. Warfarin, hematoma expansion, and outcome of intracerebral hemorrhage. Neurology. 2004;63:1059–64.

22. Freeman WD. Management of intracranial pressure. Continuum (Minneap Minn). 2015;21:1299–323.

23. Golash A, Thorne J, West CG. Low grade pilocytic astrocytoma presenting as a spontaneous intracerebral haemorrhage in a child. Br J Neurosurg. 1998;12:59–62.

24. Graus F, Rogers L, Posner JB. Cerebrovascular complications in patients with cancer. Medicine (Baltimore). 1985;64:16–35.

25. Hanley DF, Lane K, McBee N, CLEAR III Investigators, et al. Thrombolytic removal of intraventricular haemorrhage in treatment of severe stroke: results of the randomised, multicentre, multiregion, placebo-controlled CLEAR III trial. Lancet. 2017;389:603–11.

26. Hemphill JC 3rd, Greenberg S, Anderson CS, Becker K, Bendok BR, Cushman M, Fung GL, Goldstein JN, Macdonald RL, Mitchell PH, Scott PA, Selim MH, Woo D, American Heart Association Stroke Council, Council on Cardiovascular and Stroke Nursing, Council on Clinical Cardiology. Guidelines for the management of spontaneous intracerebral hemorrhage: a guideline for healthcare professionals from the American Heart Association/American Stroke Association. Stroke. 2015;46:2032–60.

27. Jin Kim Y, Hyun Kim C, Hwan Cheong J, Min Kim J. Relationship between expression of vascular endothelial growth factor and intratumoral hemorrhage in human pituitary adenomas. Tumori. 2011;97:639–46.

28. Joseph DM, O'Neill A, Chandra RV, Lai LT. Glioblastoma presenting as spontaneous intracranial haemorrhage: case report and review of the literature. J Clin Neurosci. 2017;40:1–5.

29. Jung S, Moon K, Jung TY, Kim IY, Lee YH, Rhu HH, et al. Possible pathophysiological role of vascular endothelial growth factor (VEGF) and matrix metalloproteinases (MMPs) in metastatic brain tumor-associated intracerebral hemorrhage. J Neuro-Oncol. 2006;76:257–63.

30. Kamel H, Navi B, Hemphill JC. A rule to identify patients who require magnetic resonance imaging after intracerebral hemorrhage. Neurocrit Care. 2013;18:59–63.

31. Kondziolka D, Bernstein M, Resch L, et al. Significance of hemorrhage into brain tumors: clinico-pathological study. J Neurosurg. 1987;67:852–7.

32. Kothbauer P, Jellinger K, Falment H. Primary brain tumour presenting as spontaneous intracerebral haemorrhage. Acta Neurochir. 1979;49:35–45.

33. Laigle-Donadey F, Taillibert S, Mokhtari K, et al. Dural metastases. J Neuro-Oncol. 2005;75:57–61.

34. Licata B, Turazzi S. Bleeding cerebral neoplasms with symptomatic hematoma. J Neurosurg Sci. 2003;47:201–10.

35. Lieu AS, Hwang S, Howng SL, Chai CY. Brain tumors with hemorrhage. J Formos Med Assoc. 1999;98:365–7.

36. Little JR, Dial B, Bélanger G, Carpenter S. Brain hemorrhage from intracranial tumor. Stroke. 1979;10:283–8.

37. Liwnicz BH, Wu S, Tew JM Jr. The relationship between the capillary structure and haemorrhage in gliomas. J Neurosurg. 1987;66:536–41.

38. Maiuri F, D'Andrea F, Gallicchio B, Carandente M. Intracranial haemorrhages in metastatic brain tumours. J Neurosurg Sci. 1985;29:37–41.

39. Mandybur TI. Intracranial hemorrhage caused by metastatic tumors. Neurology (Minneap). 1977;27:650–5.

40. Marneros AG. Tumor angiogenesis in melanoma. Hematol Oncol Clin North Am. 2009;23:431–46.

41. Mayer SA, Brun N, Begtrup K, Broderick J, Davis S, Diringer MN, et al. Efficacy and safety of recombinant activated factor VII for acute intracerebral hemorrhage. N Engl J Med. 2008;358:2127–37.

42. McCormick WF, Rosenfield D. Massive brain hemorrhage: a review of 144 cases and an examination of their causes. Stroke. 1973;4:946–54.

43. McIver JI, Scheithauer B, Rydberg CH, et al. Metastatic hepatocellular carcinoma presenting as epidural hematoma: case report. Neurosurgery. 2001;49:447–9.

44. Mendelow AD, Gregson B, Fernandes HM, et al. Early surgery versus initial conservative treatment in patients with spontaneous supratentorial intracerebral haematomas in the international surgical trial in intracerebral Haemorrhage (STICH): a randomised trial. Lancet Neurol. 2005;365:387–97.

45. Mendelow AD, Gregson B, Fernandes HM, et al. Early surgery versus initial conservative treatment in patients with spontaneous supratentorial lobar intracerebral haematoma in the international surgical trial in intracerebral hemorrhage (STICH II): a randomised clinical trial. Lancet. 2013;382:397–408.

46. Minette SE, Kimmel D. Subdural hematoma in patients with systemic cancer. Mayo Clin Proc. 1989;64:637–42.

47. Murthy SB, Shastri A, Merkler AE, Hanley DF, Ziai WC, Fink ME, Iadecola C, Kamel H, Navi BB. Intracerebral hemorrhage outcomes in patients with systemic cancer. J Stroke Cerebrovasc Dis. 2016;25:2918–24.

48. Navi BB, Reichman J, Berlin D, Reiner AS, Panageas KS, Segal AZ, DeAngelis LM. Intracerebral and subarachnoid hemorrhage in patients with cancer. Neurology. 2010;74:494–501.

49. Omofoye OA, Barnett R., Lau W, Trembath D, Jordan JD, Sasaki-Adams DM. Neoplastic cerebral

aneurysm from metastatic non-small cell lung carcinoma: case report and literature review. Neurosurgery. 2018;83:E221–25.

50. Openshaw H, Ressler J, Snyder DS. Lumbar puncture and subdural hygroma and hematomas in hematopoietic cell transplant patients. Bone Marrow Transplant. 2008;41:791–5.

51. Pantuck AJ, Zeng G, Belldegrun AS, Figlin RA. Pathobiology, prognosis, and targeted therapy for renal cell carcinoma: exploiting the hypoxia-induced pathway. Clin Cancer Res. 2003;9:4641–52.

52. Pollack CV Jr, Reilly P, van Ryn J, et al. Idarucizumab for dabigatran reversal – full cohort analysis. N Engl J Med. 2017;377:431–41.

53. Qureshi AI, et al. Isolated and borderline isolated systolic hypertension relative to long-term risk and type of stroke: a 20-year follow-up of the national health and nutrition survey. Stroke. 2002;33:2781–8.

54. Qureshi AI, Palesch Y, Barsan WG, Hanley DF, Hsu CY, Martin RL, Moy CS, Silbergleit R, Steiner T, Suarez JI, Toyoda K, Wang Y, Yamamoto H, Yoon BW, ATACH-2 Trial Investigators and the Neurological Emergency Treatment Trials Network. Intensive blood-pressure lowering in patients with acute cerebral hemorrhage. N Engl J Med. 2016;375:1033–43.

55. Reichman J, Singer S, Navi B, Reiner A, Panageas K, Gutin PH, DeAngelis LM. Subdural hematoma in patients with cancer. Neurosurgery. 2012;71:74–9.

56. Rogers LR. Cerebrovascular complications in cancer patients. Neurol Clin. 2003;21:167–92.

57. Schouten LJ, Rutten J, Huveneers HA, Twijnstra A. Incidence of brain metastases in a cohort of patients with carcinoma of the breast, colon, kidney, and lung and melanoma. Cancer. 2002;94:2698–705.

58. Schrader B, Barth H, Lang EW, Buhl R, Hugo HH, Biederer J, Mehdorn HM. Spontaneous intracranial haematomas caused by neoplasms. Acta Neurochir (Wien). 2000;142:979–85.

59. Scott M. Spontaneous intracerebral hematoma caused by cerebral neoplasms. Report of eight verified cases. J Neurosurg. 1975;42:338–42.

60. Sessa M. Intracerebral hemorrhage and hypertension. Neurol Sci. 2008;29(Suppl 2):S258–9.

61. Shuangshoti S, Panyathanya R, Wichienkur P. Intracranial metastases from unsuspected choriocarcinoma. Neurology (Minneap). 1974;24:649–54.

62. Suarez JI. Diagnosis and management of subarachnoid hemorrhage. Continuum (Minneap Minn). 2015;21:1263–87.

63. Tung GA, Julius B, Rogg JM. MRI of intracerebral hematoma: value of vasogenic edema ratio for predicting the cause. Neuroradiology. 2003; 45:357–62.

64. van Asch CJ, Luitse M, Rinkel GJ, van der Tweel I, Algra A, Klijn CJ. Incidence, case fatality, and functional outcome of intracerebral haemorrhage over time, according to age, sex, and ethnic origin: a systematic review and meta-analysis. Lancet Neurol. 2010;9:167–76.

65. van den Doel EM, van Merriënboer F, Tulleken CA. Cerebral haemorrhage from unsuspected choriocarcinoma. Clin Neurol Neurosurg. 1985;87: 287–90.

66. Velander AJ, DeAngelis L, Navi BB. Intracranial hemorrhage in patients with Cancer. Curr Atheroscler Rep. 2012;14:373–81.

67. Wada R, Aviv R, Fox AJ, et al. CT angiography "spot sign" predicts hematoma expansion in acute intracerebral hemorrhage. Stroke. 2007;38:1257–62.

68. Wakai S, Yamakawa K, Manaka S, Takakura K. Spontaneous intracranial hemorrhage caused by brain tumor: its incidence and clinical significance. Neurosurgery. 1982;10:437–44.

69. Woo D, et al. Effect of untreated hypertension on hemorrhagic stroke. Stroke. 2004;35:1703–8.

70. Würthner JU, Köhler G, Behringer D, Lindemann A, Mertelsmann R, Lübbert M. Leukostasis followed by hemorrhage complicating the initiation of chemotherapy in patients with acute myeloid leukemia and hyperleukocytosis: a clinicopathologic report of four cases. Cancer. 1999;85:368–74.

71. Yamauchi K, Umeda Y. Symptomatic intracranial haemorrhage in acute non-lymphoblastic leukaemia: analysis of CT and autopsy findings. J Neurol. 1997;244:94–100.

72. Yuguang L, Meng L, Shugan Z, et al. Intracranial tumoural haemorrhage-a report of 58 cases. J Clin Neurosci. 2002;9:637–9.

Increased Intracranial Pressure in Critically Ill Cancer Patients

27

Abhi Pandhi, Rashi Krishnan, Nitin Goyal, and Marc Malkoff

Contents

Introduction 396
Monroe and Kellie Doctrine 396

Etiologies of Increased ICP [35] 397

Effect of Increased ICP 397

Intracranial Pressure Monitoring 398

Assessment of Intracranial Compliance and Elastance 398

Pressure Autoregulation (Fig. 3) 399

ICP and Outcome 400

Management of Increased ICP 400
Specific Therapy 401

Supportive Care 403

Role of Multimodality Monitoring 403

Upcoming Therapies 404

Conclusion 404

References 405

Abstract

Raised ICP can be seen with varied pathologies including traumatic brain injury (TBI), emergent large vessel occlusion stroke (ELVO), intracranial hemorrhage (ICH), primary versus metastatic neoplasms, diffuse brain processes such as cerebral edema, hepatic failure, inflammation and infection, hydrocephalus, and idiopathic.

ICP can be measured via an external ventricular drain (EVD) or a parenchymal bolt. Early clinical signs include headache, papilledema, nausea, stupor, and coma. Early recognition is helpful for early management to prevent cerebral hypoperfusion and brain death.

A. Pandhi (✉) · R. Krishnan · N. Goyal · M. Malkoff
Department of Neurology, University of Tennessee Health
Science Center, Memphis, TN, USA
e-mail: apandhi@uthsc.edu; rkrishn5@uthsc.edu;
ngoyal@uthsc.edu; mmalkoff@uthsc.edu

© Springer Nature Switzerland AG 2020
J. L. Nates, K. J. Price (eds.), *Oncologic Critical Care*,
https://doi.org/10.1007/978-3-319-74588-6_36

Management involves multiple tiers of therapies including head of bed up, sedation and analgesia, neuromuscular blockage, mild hyperventilation, and osmotherapy followed by barbiturate coma, therapeutic hypothermia, and aggressive hyperventilation. Last-ditch therapy involves decompressive hemicraniectomy. The use of multimodality monitoring helps in tailoring the appropriate therapy.

Keywords

Intracranial pressure · Cerebral herniation · Osmotherapy · Craniectomy · Indices indicated in green color

Introduction

The history behind ICP dates back to 1800s when Magendie discovered a small foramen in the floor of the fourth ventricle and pointed out the connection between the ventricular system and arachnoid spaces in the brain and spinal cord. In the later part of the century, Quincke discovered the use of lumbar puncture for diagnostic and therapeutic purposes which was later on used by many including. The use of lumbar puncture widely for measuring intracranial or CSF pressures fell out of favor due to the possibility of tonsillar herniation and death [26]. Intracranial pressure is defined as pressure within the intracranial vault and is measured in mm Hg.

Lundberg et al. did extensive research on approach to direct cannulation of the ventricular system especially lateral ventricle and connected to the fluid-filled transducer system [30]. He also described that spontaneous changes in ventricular fluid pressure (VFP) curve were of two types i.e., plateau waves and rhythmic oscillations [31]. These especially, the former could cause both transient and persistent damage to brain and therefore earlier diagnosis and prevention are of critical importance. Rhythmic fluctuations can be normal at a frequency of 1/min but the incidence increases with pathology and represent cerebral dysfunction.

The waves described by Lundberg include the following:

- A waves/plateau waves – high amplitude, i.e., 50–100 mm Hg, lasting 5–20 min. These waves are always pathological. Patients with these waveforms usually show early signs of herniation as well including bradycardia and hypertension. As the cerebral perfusion pressure (CPP) drops [CPP = MAP – ICP], cerebral vasodilation occurs which increases the cerebral blood volume. This leads to a vicious circle with eventual decrease in CPP.
- B waves – oscillating waves with frequency of 0.5–2/m and amplitude up to 50 mmHg likely while still in lower limits of pressure autoregulation.
- C waves – oscillating waves with frequency of 4–8/min and amplitude of up to 20 mmHg. These have been documented in healthy individuals as well.

Both A and B waves require intervention to reduce ICP and increase CPP, thus mandating the need for continuous monitoring of ICP.

Monroe and Kellie Doctrine

This doctrine stated by Professor Monroe and Kelly from Scotland (Monro et al.; [41, 69]) which states that in a closed system (i.e., when fontanelles and sutures are closed), the intracranial pressure-volume relationship can be represented as follows: VT = Vb+Vcsf+Vvasc (where Vt is the total intracranial volume, i.e., 1700 cc; Vb is brain volume, i.e., 1400 cc; Vcsf is 30 cc in ventricles; and Vvasc is circulatory volume, i.e., arteries and veins around 150 cc) [53]. When a central nervous system pathology occurs, a new volume Vx is added, such that now VT = Vb+Vcsf+Vvasc+Vx. To maintain the ICP constant, one of the other components must be displaced, which most commonly, CSF is the first one to egress from cerebral convexities through arachnoid granulations into the cerebral venous sinuses. With further increase in Vx, other reserves are exhausted and eventually leading to even rise in ICP and compression

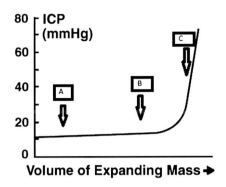

Fig. 1 Pressure volume curve

of intracranial structures including brain (Vb) or vasculature (Vvasc), causing brain ischemia and infarction.

Avezaat and Van Eijdhoven in the 1800s significantly contributed toward understanding of raised ICP which involves an interplay between intracranial volume and compliance of craniospinal axis. In Fig. 1, in the physiological range, i.e., near the origin of the x-axis on the graph (point a), intracranial pressure remains normal in spite of small additions of volume until a point of decompensation (point b), after which each subsequent increment in total volume results in an ever larger increment in intracranial pressure (point c) [53].

Etiologies of Increased ICP [35]

- Brain neoplasm: due to mass effect and vasogenic edema with symptoms of headache, blurred vision, decreased alertness, vomiting, and focal symptoms occasionally
- Traumatic brain injury (TBI): due to either diffuse axonal injury or focal cerebral edema, intracranial hemorrhage, or contusions with mass effect
- Large vessel ischemic stroke (could be internal carotid artery/middle cerebral artery occlusion) leading to large volume cytotoxic edema with mass effect causing secondary cerebral herniation and vascular occlusion of nearby arteries
- Intracranial hemorrhage (ICH): mass effect due to the space-occupying lesion within closed system, which could be either of

subdural hematoma or epidural hematoma or intracerebral hemorrhage, subarachnoid hemorrhage with or without hemorrhage
- Hydrocephalus: could be either non-communicating or communicating. Former a.k.a. obstructive hydrocephalus with mass effect/lesions obstructing the major CSF pathways or drainage. Latter a.k.a nonobstructive can be due to blockage of arachnoid granulations or microscopic CSF drainage from cells (e.g., meningitis, subarachnoid hemorrhage) or due to high proteins (such as Guillain-Barre syndrome)
- Diffuse edematous process such as acetaminophen overdose with hepatic failure and with or without hyperammonemia, acute on chronic live failure, encephalitis, vasogenic or other forms of cerebral edema
- Jugular venous obstruction or elevated right-sided cardiac venous pressure: could be due to central line insertion leading to jugular thrombosis or superior vena cava syndrome or severe congestive heart failure or chronic obstructive pulmonary disease (COPD) with clinically significant papilledema
- Idiopathic edema: pseudotumor cerebri (risk factors include female sex, obesity, and use of oral contraceptives)

Effect of Increased ICP

In a closed system (within the skull and split by dural membranes into anterior middle and posterior fossae), when an intracranial mass effect occurs (such as temporal lobe hematoma), it can encroach and extend into tentorium cerebelli causing displacement of adjacent intracranial structures, like third cranial nerve and subsequent ipsilateral pupil dilatation. If the mass effect extends across the brainstem to cause it to abut the contralateral tentorium, this can cause contralateral third nerve injury and pupillary dilatation (i.e., Kernohan's notch phenomenon) [13]. The initial mechanisms of reserve include CSF egress into ventricular system and compression of space between cortical sulci and CSF spaces. After that, brain tissue itself becomes compressed and shifts in path of least intracranial resistance, leading to mechanical movement of brain tissue, described as cerebral herniation. Examples include the following: (1) uncal herniation is defined as temporal lobe uncus shifting medially from middle cranial fossa into tentorium and medially downward toward lower posterior cranial fossa; (2) subfalcine herniation, when a part of frontal lobe moves under falx cerebri to the contralateral side which can cause compression of anterior cerebral artery and potential cerebral infarction from mechanical occlusion of these arteries (ipsilaterally and contralaterally if severe); (3) tonsillar herniation occurs when cerebellar tonsils herniate downward through foramen magnum; (4) diencephalic herniation, when diencephalon herniates downward through tentorium into posterior fossa, from bilateral cerebral edema or mass effect; and (5) external herniation occurs when part of calvarium is removed (surgically or by trauma) and brain herniates outside cranial vault [13].

Intracranial Pressure Monitoring

ICP can be measured at different sites in the brain – intraventricular and intraparenchymal measurements are more common, while extradural and subdural sensors are used occasionally. *Intraventricular catheters* are still the "gold standard" as they allow direct measurement by insertion of a catheter into one of the lateral ventricles, which is connected to an external pressure transducer [40, 63]. Benefits include that clinician can check for zero drift and sensitivity of the measurement system in vivo as well as excess CSF drainage when the pressure rises. Drawbacks include difficulty or failure to insert in patients with advanced brain swelling with slit ventricles. Another risk of infection is directly proportional to the amount of time catheter is in place, with rates up to 10% [3]. Antibiotic-coated tips (Codman Bactiseal® external ventricular drain catheter) that may reduce infection rates are available, but more studies are required before their use in clinical practice can be supported.

Intraparenchymal catheters are inserted through a support bolt or tunneled subcutaneously from a burr hole. These have a microminiature strain gauge pressure sensor side-mounted at the tip (Codman) or a fiber-optic catheter (Camino, InnerSpace). These have a low infection rate compared to intraventricular catheters [32]. Drawback includes small drift of the zero line and doesn't allow the in vivo pressure calibration. Some technical difficulties including kinking of the cable and dislocation of the sensor have been reported.

Subdural catheters are easily inserted following craniotomy, but measurements are unreliable because when ICP is elevated they are likely to underestimate the true ICP. They are liable to blockage as well. Extradural probes are even more unreliable compared to the former as the relationship between ICP and pressure in the extradural space is not certain. But both of these have lower risk of infection, epilepsy, and hemorrhage than ventricular catheters [15, 51].

Determination of cerebral perfusion pressure (CPP): ICP is an important determinant of CPP, i.e., $CPP = MAP - ICP$, which in turn affects CBF and CBV. Most of the studies recommend CPP in the range of 50–70 mm Hg with some variation through studies [11]. Treating ICP above the range of 20–25 is recommended as it is shown to decrease mortality and improve outcomes [25].

Measurement of intracranial pressure: ICP zero point is defined as center of the head or at the level of foramen of Monro, which is anatomically close to the tragus of the outer ear. When lying in lateral recumbent, the intrathecal pressure is equivalent to ICP, assuming craniocaudal axis is intact without any blockages [56, 64]. Performing a lumbar puncture in the sitting position makes measuring ICP problematic and may be inaccurate unless the tubing system is long enough to extend above the tragus. Normal ICP is usually less than 15–20 mm Hg. Conversion from Hg mm to cm H2O requires division by 1.35.

Assessment of Intracranial Compliance and Elastance

When ICP is normal, the shape of the ICP waveform has three distinct waves, sometimes called P1, P2, and P3. As additional intracranial volume is added, ICP increases precipitously, shown as P2 higher than P1 in Fig. 2.

Fig. 2 Intracranial pressure waveform

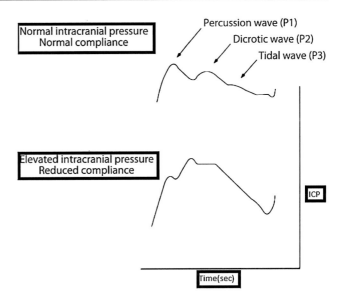

A simple bedside test to measure intracranial compliance is jugular venous compression (either unilateral or bilateral) while monitoring ICP. This is done by applying gentle pressure over each jugular while observing ICP under continuous monitoring. This is important for comatose patients who can't give a history or participate in Valsalva testing. Jugular pressure would raise the ICP similar to doing Valsalva, and after removal of pressure, it should decrease. The degree of ICP elevation in patients with high elastance/low compliance intracranial states can be striking and provide useful information to guide treatment.

A second test is by placing the head of the bed 0° (head flat test) from the common 30–40° elevation used in ICU. The ICP is first assessed at 30 or 40° position and then at head of bed flat (in case of EVD in place, EVD would need to be clamped and rezeroed after head position change). Increased ICP with the head of bed at 0° indicates poor intracranial compliance and demands caution, particularly when planning transportation outside of the intensive care unit or testing with the head in a flat position (e.g., radiology or procedures). This may be detrimental in case of patients with refractory intracranial hypertension, where being laid flat for the 20–30 min necessary can potentially lead to CPP crisis states (less than 60 mm Hg) and secondary brain injury [46, 47].

Another method is by injecting a small amount of saline into the ventricular catheter or lumbar drain followed by mathematical analysis of patient's elastance curve, which is still a topic of research.

Pressure Autoregulation (Fig. 3)

Cerebral blood flow (CBF) equation is important to know in the management of patients with increased ICP as the former is dependent on ICP values [56]:

$$CBF = CPP/CVR$$

where CVR is cerebrovascular resistance.

CBF is kept constant through a range of CPP values through mechanisms called cerebrovascular autoregulation. In normal states, as CPP increases, CVR increases as well and vice versa. Autoregulation is an energy-dependent process and starts to fail in case of an acute brain injury (i.e., stroke, TBI, or hemorrhage). When it fails, CBF becomes linearly proportional to CPP values. This presents as a challenge as low CPP may drop CBF below critical thresholds. Thus, these patients have two sets of problems: (1) compromised CPP from ICP elevation with or without preserved autoregulation and (2) loss

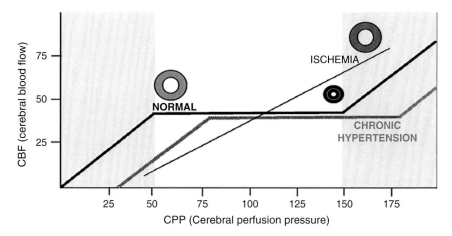

Fig. 3 CBF and CPP relationship

of autoregulation (leading to linear correlation between CBF and CPP), either or both leading to exacerbation of secondary injury. The ICP monitor can measure ICP, and multimodality monitoring helps in detection of failure or preservation of autoregulation [10, 71].

ICP and Outcome

ICP, as a simple numeric value, is not an independent outcome predictor, i.e., when used to predict outcome, the ICP data should be interpreted with clinical and demographic characteristics, CT findings, and other physiologic data. Recent studies suggest that individualized or patient-specific targets may provide a more robust relationship [27, 28, 68] retrospectively analyzed data from 327 TBI patients and defined individualized ICP thresholds and observed that individualized doses of intracranial hypertension were stronger predictors of death than doses derived from universal thresholds of 20 and 25 mm Hg [27]. Multiple modalities including physiologic monitors being used today, e.g., brain oxygen, microdialysis, and PET among others, demonstrate that brain energy dysfunction may occur even when ICP is normal or that the brain could be healthy despite an elevated ICP, thus advocating the concept of permissive intracranial hypertension, i.e., even if ICP is raised, other parameters such as the above should be looked at simultaneously [39].

Management of Increased ICP

The following are goals of therapy: (a) avoid sustained intracranial hypertension >20 mm Hg which predicts poor outcomes; (b) maintain CPP of 60 mm Hg (55–70) – higher CPP can predispose to acute respiratory distress syndrome (ARDS), and low CPP produces a fall in brain tissue PO2 [29].

General resuscitation involves appropriate cardiopulmonary support, ABCs, to maintain oxygenation [keep SaO2 >92–95% with ventilator settings with adjusting PEEP (no effect on ICP up to 15 cm H2O), FiO2 to improve hypoxia if any], adequate blood pressure (MAP >70, augmented with fluids or pressor support as well as blood transfusions as needed) and airway protection (rapid sequence intubation (RSI) for anyone with GCS <8), and fever treatment especially if >39 °C in first 24 h and immediate treatment of seizures if any [54].

Initial neurological exam should be undertaken along with history (signs of increased ICP including headache, stupor, nausea, vomiting, papilledema) early on to determine if patient is stable enough for further testing including neuroimaging. CT is preferred (alternatively MRI brain) in emergent setting to rule out life-threatening causes including TBI, ICH, brain herniation, malignant stroke, and hydrocephalus, and further as indicated, neurosurgical consultation is obtained for surgical decompression versus ICP monitor versus EVD placement [7, 16]. If cancer is suspected, then MRI brain with and without contrast is recommended.

Specific Therapy

First-Tier Therapies

This includes the first line of treatment for reducing raised ICP. Patient's head of bed should be raised up to 30° position and maximum of 45°, instead of keeping flat which can precipitate ICP crisis or higher than 45 which can drop the CPP [48]. Adequate sedation and pain control can reduce ICP somewhat by reducing Valsalva and jugular venous pressure elevation, but this comes at the cost of suppression of respiratory drive and clouding of sensorium and thus neurological examination. Subcutaneous route for analgesia is preferred at times if intractable vomiting [13]. Neuromuscular blockade is employed in these group of patients who are intubated to prevent coughing which can cause spikes of raised ICP. This approach is associated with clouding of neurological examination as well as increased risk of pneumonia and critical illness myopathy/polyneuropathy [49]. If EVD is in place, and ICP is raised, CSF can be drained as a temporizing measure [16]. Hyperventilation can be used temporarily or as a bridge therapy but avoided as a prolonged treatment modality. Latter can be associated with ischemia due to vasoconstriction. The suggested treatment plan includes mild hyperventilation (with PaCO2 of 32–34 mmHg) followed by a return to normocapnia (PaCO2 35–40 mmHg) [42].

Second-Tier Therapies: Osmotherapy

Mannitol: intravenous hyperosmolar agent which can be administered via peripheral line. It causes an increase in serum osmolality and an osmotic gradient between the serum and intracranial compartment with subsequent removal of brain water to reduce ICP. It has a reflection coefficient of 0.9, thus a theoretically increased risk of extravasating through blood-brain barrier into damaged brain tissue and exacerbating brain damage. The side effects associated with it include hypovolemia and secondary hypernatremia, thus mandating frequent electrolyte and serum osmolality monitoring. It can also precipitate hypokalemia and if sever enough can cause EKG changes as well. It can potentially worsen fluid status in patients with severe congestive heart failure or end-stage renal disease (contraindicated in latter as can't excrete mannitol out of body). It could be used a bolus therapy or even scheduled for patients with refractory ICP until the surgical therapy [61].

Hypertonic saline: comes in various concentrations including 1.5% vs. 3% vs. 10% vs. 14.6% vs. 23.4%. It requires a central venous access for administration to prevent peripheral thrombophlebitis. Similar to mannitol, it creates an osmotic gradient between serum and intracranial compartment to reduce ICP, but it doesn't have a diuretic effect and increases total body sodium and chloride concentrations and helps increase CPP. Patients who develop salt and volume overload due to the above can be given mannitol and hypertonic saline alternatively. It has a reflection coefficient of 1, thus lower theoretical risk of extravasation across blood-brain barrier and into damaged tissue. Caution exerted in using in patients with congestive heart failure. Frequent monitoring of electrolytes and osmolality is recommended to watch for signs of iatrogenic hypernatremia hyperchloremia and non-anion gap metabolic acidosis. Latter can be treated with enteral water pushes or infusions. Infusions of hypotonic solutions are generally avoided as they can increase the brain edema and ICP. Lastly, patients who develop high urine output and hypernatremia regardless of osmotherapy should be monitored for development of diabetes insipidus that can be a complication of the underlying severe brain injury. The clinical picture can be confused even with diuresis produced due to mannitol [14, 16, 28].

Third-Tier Therapy

Therapeutic hypothermia: hypothermia reduces brain metabolism and brain blood flow, thus reducing ICP. Mild to moderate hypothermia (32–34 °C) is effective in reducing ICP. NABIS II (National Acute Brain Injury Study:

Hypothermia II) study was a randomized controlled trial comparing normothermia with hypothermia and didn't demonstrate a difference in outcomes between two groups at 6 months [37]. A study by Jiang et al. demonstrated favorable outcomes with longer use of hypothermia up to 48–72 h [19]. Eurotherm 3235 trial provides evidence against therapeutic hypothermia to lower intracranial pressure but no clear guidance on its use for refractory intracranial hypertension [1].

The use of this modality has been associated with increased risk of infections and prolonged effects of sedatives and analgesics due to alteration in their metabolism. For patients who are febrile, normothermia is targeted as high temperatures are associated with worse outcomes. Controlled normothermia with cooling devices is being studied as well [34].

Barbiturate coma: includes pentobarbital and thiopental. The use of barbiturate in the setting of high ICP works in the following ways: (a) decreased cerebral metabolic rate (CMRO2), caused by decrease in synaptic transmission which is due to its effect on GABA transmission; (b) decrease in cerebral blood volume and flow and thus ICP due to increased cerebrovascular resistance because of vasoconstriction; (c) induction of hypothermia; (d) increase in intracranial glucose, glucagon, and phosphocreatine energy store; (e) decrease in nitrogen excretion following acute head injury; (f) anticonvulsant effect; (g) stabilization of lysosomal membranes; (h) decrease in excitatory neurotransmitters and intracellular calcium; and (i) free radical scavenging. Adverse effects of barbiturate therapy include (1) direct myocardial depressant, (2) impaired gastrointestinal motility, (3) direct CNS depressant, and (4) possible allergic reaction [20].

Aggressive hyperventilation: used as a last-ditch therapy. The details of hyperventilation are discussed above in first-tier therapy.

Role of steroids: use of steroids as temporizing measures for reducing vasogenic edema in primary and metastatic cancers. Patient is initially given dexamethasone 8 mg IV. If the patient responds and is stable and not vomiting, then continue with dexamethasone oral 4 mg four times daily. If the patient remains unwell or continues to vomit, then continue with IV dexamethasone; doses of up to 8 mg three to four hourly can be given IV for up to 2–3 days if needed. Consider prophylactic gastroprotection while the patient is on high-dose corticosteroids (omeprazole oral 20 mg daily or lansoprazole oral 30 mg daily). However, steroid use has been associated with worse outcomes in patients with high ICP and related brain edema [52, 55, 57, 59].

ICP and Malignancy

As stated above, steroids are sued for high ICP due to primary or metastatic malignancy. For intractable vomiting, cyclizine SC can be used. If the patient doesn't respond to the above regimen of steroids, then mannitol IV may be considered. Long-term mannitol is contraindicated.

Therefore, unless there is a rapidly acting therapeutic maneuver likely to provide longer-term stabilization of ICP (usually this requires surgery), mannitol should not be used. Mannitol total dose is 1 g/kg. First give 100 ml of a 20% solution (20 g mannitol) over 15 min. Then give the remainder over approximately 45 min. Repeat the following day if required but not long term [22].

Role of Surgery: Last Resort Therapy

Decompressive craniectomy (DC) involves removal of a part of the skull to let the swollen brain expand out. It is done to for cases of refractory intracranial hypertension [23] especially in operable cases such as posterior fossa hemorrhage with mass effect or large posterior fossa stroke (>3 cm) with effacement or midline shift or extra-axial hematomas [16, 24]. Replacement of original bone flap versus cranioplasty can be done typically within 6–12 weeks. If the follow-up surgery gets delayed beyond 12 weeks, then patients may develop severe headaches, tinnitus, dizziness, behavioral or emotional symptoms, sensorimotor or autonomic deficits, and cognitive impairments, which collectively can be referred to as syndrome of trephined, which gets reversed after the surgery [66].

DECRA (decompressive craniectomy) trial was conducted in Australia, New Zealand, and Saudi Arabia and included 155 adults randomized to medical management or medical management plus DC. After 6 months, the craniectomy group patients had worse outcomes with more complications than former [8]. In comparison, Randomized Evaluation of Surgery with Craniectomy for Uncontrollable Elevation of Intracranial Pressure (RESCUEicp) trial included 408 patients with severe TBI and refractory elevated intracranial pressure and found that even though 6-month mortality was lower in the DC group, the risk of vegetative state or severe disability was higher as compared to the medical management group [18].

The following recommendations regarding DC have been proposed:

- Brain Trauma Foundation (BTF) guidelines, 2017: Bifrontal DC is not recommended to improve outcomes in severe TBI patients with diffuse injury and with ICP elevations to >20 mm Hg for more than 15 min duration in an hour period that are refractory to first-tier therapies. But it does reduce ICP and days in the ICU [5].
- American College of Surgeons (ACS) 2015: Recommended as third-tier treatment after positioning, sedation, ventricular drainage, osmotherapies, and neuromuscular paralysis have been tried [9].
- Joint Trauma System Clinical Practice guidelines (JTS CPG), 2017: DC should be strongly considered following penetrating combat brain trauma [36].
- Recent systematic review and meta-analysis by Zhang et al. included multiple RCTs as well as several retrospective and observational studies and concluded that the mortality was reduced with DC compared to medical arm, but no significant difference found for the functional outcomes (except if DC was done within 36 h of the injury) [70]. Determination of whether an individual patient should undergo DC rests on clinical judgment and surrogate engagement.

Surgery has a role in elevated ICP and intracranial malignancy including removal or debulking of tumor to target symptom relief or management of focal resistant epilepsy, biopsy of the lesion especially if near or surrounding eloquent areas of the brain, as well as a definitive therapy for increased intracranial pressure [38].

Supportive Care

Mechanical DVT prophylaxis should be instituted right away, whereas chemical DVT prophylaxis should be started within 1–2 days of injury, sometimes at the discretion of the treating physician [16].

Nutrition: early feeding is important because of high metabolic requirement.

Supportive care also includes providing for anxiolysis, treatment of withdrawal syndromes, and seizure control [5].

Role of Multimodality Monitoring

No one method can provide complex information about the brain's functioning thus a combination of monitors or multimodality monitoring (MMM) has evolved in recent years.

Why do we need it?

- Detects damage caused by primary and secondary brain injury (SBI), before patient shows signs of clinical deterioration. SBI is seen sometimes hours to days after the injury and can be due to alteration in neurochemical mediators, glutamate-mediated influx of calcium/sodium leading to swelling and death, and alterations in glucose utilization such as mitochondrial dysfunction [39, 60, 67].
  - Evidence of microvascular injury and metabolic failure precedes an increase in ICP; thus detection of ICP (or CPP) may not always detect ingoing dysfunction/damage [12, 44].
  - Earlier detection can potentially lead to prompt intervention and better outcomes.

Indications

Clinical indications include (a) GCS < or = 8 + abnormal CT head and (b) GCS < or =8 +

normal CT head +2 of the following (hypotension or age >40 years or posturing)

Diagnostic indications – TBI, subarachnoid hemorrhage (SAH), ICH, anoxic injury, cerebral edema, and status epilepticus.

MMM tools include the following:

- ICP monitoring
- Brain tissue oxygen monitoring (PbtO2) or Licox monitoring
- Cerebral microdialysis (CMD)

MMM can help guide various therapies including hyperventilation, osmotherapy, glycemic control, transfusion, CPP augmentation, and therapeutic temperature modulation while making sure not to cause significant side effects from one type of therapy [21, 44]. It can also help differentiate between different pathologies causing similar clinic radiological picture as well as more accurate assessment of perfusion pressure compared to ICP/CPP monitoring alone [2] including those with diffuse brain damage. Some of the monitoring modalities including microdialysis and Licox monitoring, i.e., PbtO2, are associated with mortality and morbidity outcomes [33, 43, 65].

Monitoring by itself does not alter outcome. Instead, it is how the information is used that contributes to patient outcomes. RCT done by Chesnut et al. [6] revealed that patients undergoing MMM had 50% decrease in use of ICP lowering treatments but in fact ended up spending more days in ICU [6].

Study by Ponce et al. suggests that outcome is better when both PbtO2 and ICP/CPP therapy rather than ICP/CPP-only-based therapy are used in severe TBI [45]. BOOST 2 trial showed physiological efficacy and a trend toward improved outcomes in the population randomized to PbtO2 monitoring-based therapy [50]. The next phase, BOOST 3, is currently enrolling. The use of pressure reactivity (PRx) has been employed to determine an optimum CPP in a severe TBI group, but a study by Howell et al. found that CPP-targeted approach showed to be more successful in patients with preserved pressure reactivity and in contrast ICP-targeted approach was better when pressure reactivity was impaired [17].

Upcoming Therapies

Currently a trial is enrolling for possibility for use of hyperbaric oxygen for reducing brain injury in patients with severe TBIs. ProTeCT trial is currently underway as well studying the role of progesterone as a possible neuroprotective agent in moderate to severe TBI. The role of magnesium has been studied in TBI patients with variable results. Study by Temkin et al. [62] showed that serum concentration of 1.25–2.5 mmol/L was associated with increased mortality [62]. Review by Sen et al. suggested that a combination of magnesium and mannitol with dexanabinol and progesterone and interventions with hyperoxia or hypothermia could be a safe and clinically successful neuroprotective regimen for the treatment of TBI [58].

Specifically, for increased ICP and intracranial malignancies, various studies are underway in the field of regenerative medicine with the use of administration of healthy, functioning exogenous oligodendrocyte progenitor cells (OPCs) which maintain their normal function upon implantation into a previously irradiated brain migrating widely and generating oligodendrocytes and remyelinating lesioned area [4].

Conclusion

Increased ICP on critically ill patients can be multifactorial and can be monitored while in ICU with various modalities including external ventricular drain, intracranial bolt, multimodality monitoring. Various therapies available include positioning, sedation, analgesia, hypothermia, and medical management with steroids (specifically for increased intracranial pressure related to primary or secondary neoplasms) as well as osmotherapy. Surgical therapies as detailed above have been tried as a last resort to manage medically refractory ICP as well as for diagnostic purposes in case of suspicious lesions. The role of multimodality monitoring including PbtO2 or Licox monitoring, PRx, and CMD is being studied extensively in various studies as outlined above. Various neuroprotective agents including hyperbaric oxygen, magnesium, selenium, and progestin analogues have been studied as well as the use of OPCs for previously irradiated brain in the setting of a malignancy.

References

1. Andrews PJ, Sinclair HL, Rodriguez A, Harris BA, Battison CG, Rhodes JK, Murray GD, Eurotherm3235 Trial Collaborators. Hypothermia for intracranial hypertension after traumatic brain injury. N Engl J Med. 2015;373(25):2403–12. https://doi.org/10.1056/NEJMoa1507581.
2. Bouzat P, et al. Accuracy of brain multimodal monitoring to detect cerebral hypoperfusion after traumatic brain injury. Crit Care Med. 2014;43(2):445–52.
3. Bekar A, Goren S, Korfali E, Aksoy K, Boyaci S. Complications of brain tissue pressure monitoring with a fibreoptic device. Neurosurg Rev. 1998;21:254–9.
4. Burns TC, Awad AJ, Li MD, Grant GA. Radiation-induced brain injury: low-hanging fruit for neuroregeneration. Neurosurg Focus. 2016;40(5):E3. https://doi.org/10.3171/2016.2.FOCUS161.
5. Carney N, Totten AM, O'Reilly C, Ullman JS, Hawryluk GW, Bell MJ, Ghajar J. Guidelines for the management of severe traumatic brain injury, fourth edition. Neurosurgery. 2017;80(1):6–15. https://doi.org/10.1227/NEU.01432.
6. Chesnut RM, Temkin N, Carney N, et al. A trial of intracranial-pressure monitoring in traumatic brain injury. N Engl J Med. 2012;367(26):2471–81. https://doi.org/10.1056/NEJMoa1207363.
7. Connolly ES Jr, Rabinstein AA, Carhuapoma JR, et al. Guidelines for the management of aneurysmal subarachnoid hemorrhage: a guideline for healthcare professionals from the American Heart Association/American Stroke Association. Stroke. 2012;43(6):1711–37. https://doi.org/10.1161/STR.0b013e3182587839.
8. Cooper DJ, Rosenfeld JV, Murray L, Arabi YM, Davies AR, D'Urso P, New Zealand intensive care society clinical trials, G, et al. Decompressive craniectomy in diffuse traumatic brain injury. N Engl J Med. 2011;364(16):1493–502. https://doi.org/10.1056/NEJMoa1102077.
9. Cryer HG, Manley GT, Adelson PD, Alali AS, Calland JF, Cipolle M, Wright DW. ACS TQIP best practices in the management of traumatic brain injury. Chicago: American College of Surgeons; 2015.
10. Czosnyka M, Kirkpatrick PJ, Pickard JD. Multimodal monitoring and assessment of cerebral haemodynamic reserve after severe head injury. Cerebrovasc Brain Metab Rev. 1996;8(4):273–95.
11. Czosnyka M, Czosnyka Z, Pickard JD. Laboratory testing of the Spiegelberg brain pressure monitor: a technical report. J Neurol Neurosurg Psychiatry. 1997;63:732–5.
12. Eriksson EA, et al. Cerebral perfusion pressure and intracranial pressure are not surrogates for brain tissue oxygenation in traumatic brain injury. Clin Neurophysiol. 2012;123:1255–60.
13. Freeman WD. Management of intracranial pressure. Continuum (Minneap Minn). 2015;21(5 Neurocritical Care):1299–323. https://doi.org/10.1212/CON.0235.
14. Francony G, Fauvage B, Falcon D, et al. Equimolar doses of mannitol and hypertonic saline in the treatment of increased intracranial pressure. Crit Care Med. 2008;36(3):795–800. https://doi.org/10.1097/CCM.0B013E3181643B41.
15. Gaab MR, Heissler HE, Ehrhardt K. Physical characteristics of various methods for measuring ICP. In: Hoff JT, Betz AL, editors. Intracranial pressure VII. Berlin: Springer; 1989. p. 16–21.
16. Hemphill JC 3rd, Greenberg SM, Anderson CS, Becker K, Bendok BR, Cushman M, Fung GL, Goldstein JN, Macdonald RL, Mitchell PH, Scott PA, Selim MH, Woo D, American Heart Association Stroke Council, Council on Cardiovascular and Stroke Nursing, Council on Clinical Cardiology. Guidelines for the management of spontaneous intracerebral hemorrhage: a guideline for healthcare professionals from the American Heart Association/American Stroke Association. Stroke. 2015;46(7):2032–60. https://doi.org/10.1161/STR.0000000000000069.
17. Howells T, et al. Pressure reactivity as a guide in the treatment of cerebral perfusion pressure in patients with brain trauma. J Neurosurg. 2005;102(2):311–7.
18. Hutchinson PJ, Kolias AG, Timofeev IS, Corteen EA, Czosnyka M, Timothy J, Collaborators, R. E. T, et al. Trial of decompressive craniectomy for traumatic intracranial hypertension. N Engl J Med. 2016;375(12):1119–30. https://doi.org/10.1056/NEJMoa1605215.
19. Jiang JY, Xu W, Li WP, et al. Effect of long-term mild hypothermia or short-term mild hypothermia on outcome of patients with severe traumatic brain injury. J Cereb Blood Flow Metab. 2006;26(6):771–6. https://doi.org/10.1038/sj.jcbfm.9600253.
20. Greenberg J. Handbook of head and spine trauma. 1993. p. 230–3.
21. Johnston AJ, et al. Effect of cerebral perfusion pressure augmentation on regional oxygenation and metabolism after head injury. Crit Care Med. 2005;33(1):189–95.
22. Kaal EC, Vecht CJ. The management of brain edema in brain tumors. Curr Opin Oncol. 2004;16(6):593–600.
23. Kahraman S, et al. Heart rate and pulse pressure variability are associated with intractable intracranial hypertension after severe traumatic brain injury. J Neurosurg Anesthesiol. 2010;22(4):296–302.
24. Mostofi K. Neurosurgical management of massive cerebellar infarct outcome in 53 patients. Surg Neurol Int. 2013;4:28. https://doi.org/10.4103/2152-7806.107906.
25. Khormi YH, Gosadi I, Campbell S, Senthilselvan A, O'Kelly C, Zygun D. Adherence to brain trauma foundation guidelines for management of traumatic brain injury patients and its effect on outcomes: systematic

review. J Neurotrauma. 2018; https://doi.org/10.1089/neu.2017.5345.

26. Langfitt TW, Weinstein JD, Kassell NF, Simeone FA. Transmission of increased intracranial pressure I: within the craniospinal axis. J Neurosurg. 1964;21:989–97.

27. Lazaridis C, et al. Patient-specific thresholds of intracranial pressure in severe traumatic brain injury. J Neurosurg. 2014;120(4):893–900.

28. Lewandowski-Belfer JJ, Patel AV, Darracott RM, et al. Safety and efficacy of repeated doses of 14.6 or 23.4% hypertonic saline for refractory intracranial hypertension. Neurocrit Care. 2014;20(3):436–42. https://doi.org/10.1007/s12028Y013Y9907Y1.

29. Lou M, Xue F, Chen L, Xue Y, Wang K. Is high PEEP ventilation strategy safe for acute respiratory distress syndrome after severe traumatic brain injury? Brain Inj. 2012;26(6):887–90. https://doi.org/10.3109/02699052.2012.660514.

30. Lundberg N. Continuous recording and control of ventricular fluid pressure in neurosurgical practice. Acta Psychiat Neurol Scand. 1960;36(suppl):149.

31. Lundberg N, Troupp H, Lorin H. Continuous recording of the ventricular fluid pressure in patients with severe acute traumatic brain injury. J Neurosurg. 1965;22:581–90.

32. Mack WJ, King RG, Ducruet AF, Kreiter K, Mocco J, Maghoub A, Mayer S, Connolly ES Jr. Intracranial pressure following aneurysmal subarachnoid hemorrhage: monitoring practices and outcome data. Neurosurg Focus. 2003;14:1–5.

33. Maloney-Wilensky E, et al. Brain tissue oxygen and outcome after severe traumatic brain injury: a systematic review. Crit Care Med. 2009;37:2057–63.

34. Marion DW. Controlled normothermia in neurologic intensive care. Crit Care Med. 2004;32(2 suppl):S43–5. https://doi.org/10.1097/01.CCM.0000110731.69637.16.

35. May K. The pathophysiology and causes of raised intracranial pressure. Br J Nurs. 2009;18(15):911–4.

36. McCafferty R, et al. Joint trauma system clinical practice guideline: neurosurgery and severe head injury (CPG ID:30). 2017.

37. McCauley SR, Wilde EA, Moretti P, et al. Neurological outcome scale for traumatic brain injury: III. Criterion-related validity and sensitivity to change in the NABIS hypothermia-II clinical trial. J Neurotrauma. 2013;30 (17):1506–11. https://doi.org/10.1089/neu.2013.2925.

38. Macdonald DR, Cairncross JG. Surgery for single brain metastasis. N Engl J Med. 1990;323(2):132–3.

39. Menon DK, et al. Diffusion limited oxygen delivery following head injury. Crit Care Med. 2004;32:1384–90.

40. Miller JD. Measuring ICP in patients: its value now and in the future. In: Hoff JT, Betz AL, editors. Intracranial pressure VII. Berlin/Heidelberg/New York: Springer; 1989. p. 5–15.

41. Monro A. Observations on the structure and function of the nervous system. Edinburgh: Creech & Johnson; 1783.

42. Muizelaar JP, Marmarou A, Ward JD, et al. Adverse effects of prolonged hyperventilation in patients with severe head injury: a randomized clinical trial. J Neurosurg. 1991;75(5):731–9.

43. Oddo M, et al. Brain hypoxia is associated with short-term outcome after severe traumatic brain injury independently of intracranial hypertension and low cerebral perfusion pressure. Neurosurgery. 2011;69:1037–45.

44. Oddo M, et al. Anemia and brain oxygen after severe traumatic brain injury. Intensive Care Med. 2012;38:1497–504.

45. Okonkwo DO, Shutter LA, Moore C, Temkin NR, Puccio AM, Madden CJ, Andaluz N, Chesnut RM, Bullock MR, Grant GA, McGregor J, Weaver M, Jallo J, LeRoux PD, Moberg D, Barber J, Lazaridis C, Diaz-Arrastia RR. Brain oxygen optimization in severe traumatic brain injury phase-II: a phase II randomized trial. Crit Care Med. 2017;45 (11):1907–14. https://doi.org/10.1097/CCM.02619.

46. Peace K, Wilensky EM, Frangos S, et al. The use of a portable head CT scanner in the intensive care unit. J Neurosci Nurs. 2010;42(2):109–16. https://doi.org/10.1097/JNN.0b013e3181ce5c5b.

47. Peace K, Maloney-Wilensky E, Frangos S, et al. Portable head CT scan and its effect on intracranial pressure, cerebral perfusion pressure, and brain oxygen. J Neurosurg. 2011;114(5):1479–84. https://doi.org/10.3171/2010.11.JNS091148.

48. Pandhi A, Elijovich L. Postoperative positioning in the neurointensive care unit. In: Arthur A, Foley K, Hamm C, editors. Perioperative considerations and positioning for neurosurgical procedures. Cham: Springer; 2018. https://doi.org/10.1007/978-3-319-72679-3_19.

49. Pandit L, Agrawal A. Neuromuscular disorders in critical illness. Clin Neurol Neurosurg. 2006;108(7):621–7.

50. Ponce LL, et al. Position of probe determines prognostic information of brain tissue pO2 in severe traumatic brain injury. Neurosurgery. 2012;70(6):1492–502.

51. Raabe A, Totzauer R, Meyer O, Stockel R, Hohrein D, Schoeche J. Reliability of extradural pressure measurement in clinical practice: behaviour of three modern sensors during simultaneous ipsilateral intraventricular or intraparenchymal pressure measurement. Neurosurgery. 1998;43:306–11.

52. Rangel-Castilla L1, Gopinath S, Robertson CS. Management of intracranial hypertension. Neurol Clin. 2008;26(2):521–41. https://doi.org/10.1016/j.ncl.2008.02.003.

53. Rengachary SS, Ellenbogen RG, editors. Principles of neurosurgery. Edinburgh: Elsevier Mosby; 2005.

54. Reynolds SF, Heffner J. Airway management of the critically ill patient: rapid-sequence intubation. Chest. 2005;127(4):1397–412. https://doi.org/10.1378/chest.127.4.1397.

55. Roberts I, Yates D, Sandercock P, et al. Effect of intravenous corticosteroids on death within 14 days in 10008 adults with clinically significant head injury

(MRC CRASH trial): randomized placebo-controlled trial. Lancet. 2004;364(9442):1321–8. https://doi.org/10.1186/cc3813.

56. Rose JC, Mayer SA. Optimizing blood pressure in neurological emergencies. Neurocrit Care. 2004;1(3):287–99.

57. Ryken TC, McDermott M, Robinson PD, et al. The role of steroids in the management of brain metastases: a systematic review and evidence-based clinical practice guideline. J Neuro-Oncol. 2010;96(1):103–14. https://doi.org/10.1007/s11060Y009Y0057Y4.

58. Sen AP, Gulati A. Use of magnesium in traumatic brain injury. Neurotherapeutics. 2010;7(1):91–9. https://doi.org/10.1016/j.nurt.2009.10.014.

59. Shenkin HA. Steroids in treatment of high intracranial pressure. N Engl J Med. 1970;283(12):659.

60. Singh IN, et al. Time course of post-traumatic mitochondrial oxidative damage and dysfunction in a mouse model of focal traumatic brain injury: implications for neuroprotective therapy. J Cereb Blood Flow Metab. 2006;26:1407–18.

61. Stocchetti N, Picetti E, Berardino M, et al. Clinical applications of intracranial pressure monitoring in traumatic brain injury: report of the Milan consensus conference. Acta Neurochir. 2014;156(8):1615–22. https://doi.org/10.1007/s00701Y014Y2127Y4.

62. Temkin NR, Anderson GD, Winn HR, et al. Magnesium sulfate for neuroprotection after traumatic brain injury: a randomised controlled trial. Lancet Neurol. 2007;6:29–38.

63. The Brain Trauma Foundation, The American Association of Neurological Surgeons, The Joint Section on Neurotrauma and Critical Care. Recommendations for intracranial pressure monitoring technology. J Neurotrauma. 2000;17:497–506.

64. The Brain Trauma Foundation, American Association of Neurological Surgeons, Congress of Neurological Surgeons, Joint Section on Neurotrauma and Critical Care, AANS/CNS, Bratton SL, Chestnut RM, Ghajar J, et al. Guidelines for the management of severe traumatic brain injury. VII. Intracranial pressure monitoring technology. J Neurotrauma. 2007;24(suppl 1): S45–54.

65. Timofeev I, et al. Cerebral extracellular chemistry and outcome following traumatic brain injury: a microdialysis study of 223 patients. Brain. 2011;134: 484–94.

66. Vasung L, Hamard M, Soto MCA, Sommaruga S, Sveikata L, Leemann B, Vargas MI. Radiological signs of the syndrome of the trephined. Neuroradiology. 2016;58(6):557–68. https://doi.org/10.1007/s002 34-016-1651-8.

67. Vespa P, et al. Metabolic crisis without brain ischemia is common after traumatic brain injury: a combined microdialysis and positron emission tomography study. J Cereb Blood Flow Metab. 2005;25:763–74.

68. Vik A, et al. Relationship of "dose" of intracranial hypertension to outcome in severe traumatic brain injury. J Neurosurg. 2008;109(4):678–84.

69. Wu OC, Manjila S, Malakooti N, Cohen AR. The remarkable medical lineage of the Monro family: contributions of Alexander primus, secundus, and tertius. J Neurosurg. 2012;116(6):1337–46. https://doi.org/10. 3171/2012.2.JNS111366.

70. Zhang D, Xue Q, Chen J, Dong Y, Hou L, Jiang Y, Wang J. Decompressive craniectomy in the management of intracranial hypertension after traumatic brain injury: a systematic review and meta-analysis. Sci Rep. 2017;7(1):8800. https://doi.org/10.1038/s41598-017-08959-y.

71. Zweifel C, Dias C, Smielewski P, Czosnyka M. Continuous time-domain monitoring of cerebral autoregulation in neurocritical care. Med Eng Phys. 2014;36(5):638–45. https://doi.org/10.1016/j.medeng phy.2014.03.002.

Leptomeningeal Disease in Solid Cancers

28

Nazanin K. Majd and Monica E. Loghin

Contents

Introduction 410

Etiology 411

Epidemiology 411

Pathophysiology 412

Clinical Features 412

Diagnosis 412
Neuroimaging 412
CSF Studies 413
Neurological Assessment 414

Differential Diagnosis 414

Management 414

Pharmacological Treatments 415

Systemic Therapies 415
Breast Cancer 415
Non-Small Cell Lung Cancer 416
Melanoma 417
Intrathecal Chemotherapy 417

Non-pharmacological Treatments 418
Radiation 418
Surgery 418

Supportive Care 419

Prognosis 419

N. K. Majd · M. E. Loghin (✉)
Department of Neuro-Oncology, The University of Texas
MD Anderson Cancer Center, Houston, TX, USA
e-mail: NKMajd@mdanderson.org;
mloghin@mdanderson.org

Future Directions 419

Conclusion 421

References 421

Abstract

Leptomeningeal disease (LMD) is one of the most dreaded complications of solid and hematological malignancies and confers a poor prognosis. LMD occurs in about 5% of patients with solid cancers, most commonly in patients with breast cancer, lung cancer, and melanoma. Diagnosis of leptomeningeal disease is challenging and is dependent on the correlation of typical symptoms and signs, characteristic imaging findings, and evaluation of spinal fluid for malignant cells. The incidence of solid cancer LMD is rising due to improved survival of cancer patients and more frequent imaging. Treatment is dependent on patients' functional status, extent of systemic cancer, and availability of systemic treatment options. The landscape of treatment for solid cancer LMD is changing with the advent of novel blood-brain penetrant molecular targeted therapies and immunotherapy. More clinical trials are expected to include patients with solid tumors and LMD as novel treatment options have been developed. This chapter aims at reviewing the recent literature on LMD from solid cancers (focusing on breast cancer, lung cancer, and melanoma) and providing an algorithm that can be used to standardize our approach to management of this disease.

Keywords

Leptomeningeal disease · Malignant meningitis · Carcinomatous meningitis · Breast cancer · Lung cancer · Melanoma

Introduction

Leptomeningeal disease (LMD) also referred to as leptomeningeal metastasis or malignant meningitis describes metastasis to cerebrospinal fluid (CSF) and/or leptomeninges from solid and hematological cancers. The focus of this review is leptomeningeal disease from solid cancers, most commonly called carcinomatous or neoplastic meningitis. Breast cancer, lung cancer, and melanoma are the most common solid cancers to metastasize to leptomeninges [1]. LMD is one the most dreaded complications of solid cancers with a dismal prognosis and accounts for the third most common form of central nervous system (CNS) metastasis after brain and epidural metastasis. It is estimated that 5–8% of patients with solid cancers are diagnosed with LMD throughout the course of their illness accounting for 72,000 new cases per year [2]. The incidence of LMD is expected to steadily rise due to ongoing advances in systemic treatment of various solid cancers resulting in prolonged survival, frequent imaging as part of screening for clinical trials, and advanced imaging techniques.

LMD diagnosis is based on correlation of clinical symptoms, CSF analysis, and neuroimaging studies. Presentation of LMD may vary from incidental findings on imaging to isolated or multifocal neurological symptoms and signs. Presence of malignant cells in spinal fluid is the gold standard for diagnosis of LMD. Typical magnetic resonance imaging (MRI) findings include enhancement of the cranial nerves, linear enhancement of the leptomeninges, nodular enhancement within the spinal roots, and hydrocephalus, but normal MRI of the neuroaxis does not rule out LMD. In the setting of high clinical suspicion (new headaches, cranial neuropathies, cauda equina syndrome), diagnosis of probable and possible LMD can be made clinically with or without abnormal CNS MRI, respectively, even in the absence of positive CSF cytology [3].

Prognosis of LMD is very poor with a median overall survival (mOS) of 4–6 weeks if left untreated [4, 5] which can be improved to 3–6 months with a multimodality treatment approach. Survival rates vary by cancer type, with breast cancer having a better prognosis compared to lung or melanoma cancer with LMD [6, 7]. Prolonged survival of 12 months or longer has been reported in 15–20% of patients with breast cancer and LMD [8, 9].

Despite improved detection rates and recent advances in treatment of LMD, there is paucity of randomized clinical trials in patients with LMD since these patients are commonly excluded from clinical trials due to their poor functional status and survival. Therefore, no standard treatment algorithms exist. Here, we will discuss key concepts in pathophysiology, diagnosis, treatment, and prognosis of solid cancer LMD and will provide a management algorithm for use in common clinical practice.

Etiology

Breast cancer, lung cancer, and melanoma are the top three leading causes of solid cancer LMD accounting for 27–50%, 22–36%, and 12% of cases, respectively [10]. However, the prevalence of LMD is the highest in melanoma (30–75%) followed by lung cancer (9–25%) and breast cancer (5%) [11]. Other solid cancers that metastasize to leptomeninges less frequently include GI cancers, sarcoma, squamous cell carcinoma of the head and neck, genitourinary malignancies, and rarely unknown primaries. LMD from primary brain tumors is in general thought to be rare, but autopsy series report an incidence of 20–25% in cases of leptomeningeal gliomatosis from malignant glioma [12, 13]. Rare CNS tumors that are known to disseminate to leptomeninges include ependymoma, medulloblastoma, and germinoma [14].

Epidemiology

It is estimated that 5–8% of patients with solid cancers are diagnosed with LMD during their disease course [2]. The incidence of LMD is probably 30 in 100,000; however, this is likely an underestimate due to undiagnosed cases

[15]. In a large autopsy series, 8% of 2375 patients were diagnosed with LMD irrespective of clinical symptoms [16]. LMD is mostly diagnosed as a late complication of solid cancers in the setting of active systemic disease (70% of cases) [17, 18] but has also been described in the setting of stable systemic disease (20% of cases) or as the first manifestation of cancer in 5–10% of cases [5].

Brain metastasis occurs in 8–15% of all cancer patients, and 30% of patients with LMD have established diagnosis of brain metastasis [19]. Several studies have explored the risk factors of developing LMD in patients with brain metastasis in relation to the type of brain metastasis-directed therapies. There is a consensus in the literature regarding increased risk of LMD after surgical resection [20–22]. In two studies the increased risk of LMD was particularly associated with piecemeal rather than en block resection [20, 22]. With the widespread use of SRS in place of whole-brain radiation therapy (WBRT), several retrospective studies evaluated risk of LMD after SRS, but the results have been inconsistent [21, 23, 24].

In addition, cancer-specific molecular subtypes have been associated with varying risks of developing LMD. Hormone receptor (HR) and HER2 status have been shown to be associated with time to LMD diagnosis in breast cancer. Patients with triple negative breast cancer have a shorter time to LMD, and HR-positive patients have a longer time to LMD and better survival [25]. In addition, treatment with trastuzumab in HER2+ patients is associated with significantly longer time to LMD [26]. Epithelial growth factor receptor (EGFR) found in 10–35% of non-small cell lung cancer (NSCLC) patients confers an increased risk of LMD (9.4% vs. 1.7% in EGFR-mutated vs. wild-type NSCLC; $P < 0.001$) [27]. Incidence of LMD in anaplastic lymphoma kinase (ALK) mutated lung cancer (5% of NSCLC) is about 5%, similar to the incidence of 3.8% in molecularly unselected NSCLC patients [28].

Overall, the incidence of LMD is rising due to heightened awareness, increased detection rate, improved control of systemic disease leading to longer lifespan [5], and predilection for the CNS by the more resistant tumor cells.

Pathophysiology

Leptomeninges refer to the arachnoid and pia matter and the subarachnoid space where CSF resides. There are several leading theories regarding the involvement of leptomeninges by cancer cells: (1) hematogenous spread, (2) direct extension from metastatic tumor deposits through the venous plexus of Batson or arterial dissemination, and (3) tumoral spread along the perineural or perivascular spaces. Tumor cells in the CSF have predilection for areas of slow flow and gravity-dependent sites. This is in part the reason posterior fossa, basilar, and lumbar cisterns are locations of frequent involvement.

Clinical Features

Neurological manifestation of LMD is dependent on the CNS segments involved: cerebral hemispheres, cranial nerves, cerebellum, spinal cord, or roots. Symptoms are typically multifocal and subacute. Subacute neurological symptoms in patients with solid cancers otherwise unexplainable by frank intraparenchymal metastasis or neuropathy should raise concerns for LMD.

Clinical features depend on the type of LMD: (1) diffuse non-adherent free-floating cells in CSF typically cause headaches with or without communicative hydrocephalus, cranial neuropathies, and vision changes, and (2) nodular adherent cells located within spinal nerve roots usually present with pain, weakness, or cauda equina syndrome [15]. The most common presentations of LMD include headaches, cranial neuropathies (diplopia, hearing loss, perioral numbness), back/neck pain, extremity weakness, radicular pain, sensory loss, and gait impairment [29]. Seizures and altered mentation are usually later manifestations of LMD. LMD mostly presents late in the disease course in the setting of active systemic disease [17, 18], and up to 90% of patients can have concomitant brain metastasis [30] that may result in additional neurological symptoms and signs.

Diagnosis

Diagnosis of LMD is based on correlation of clinical findings suggestive of LMD, characteristic MRI brain and spine abnormalities, and CSF cytology in solid cancers – in addition to CSF flow cytometry in hematological malignancies.

Neuroimaging

Abnormalities on MRI brain that are suggestive of LMD can range from superficial intraparenchymal metastasis, cerebral gyri and cerebellar folia enhancement, or FLAIR hyperintensity to nodular enhancement in cauda equina (Fig. 1). Concurrent diagnosis of brain metastasis has been described in about 40–90% of patients with LMD from solid cancers [1, 30]. MRI of neuroaxis is more likely to be abnormal in LMD associated with solid cancers than LMD associated with hematological malignancies (72% vs. 50%) [31]. Overall 70–80% of suspected LMD cases have been reported to have abnormal MRI of neuroaxis [32]. MRI of the brain and spine with and without contrast should be done prior to lumbar puncture if not contraindicated to avoid false-positive leptomeningeal enhancement due to intracranial hypotension. If MRI is contraindicated, CT scan of the head is done prior to lumbar puncture to rule out large asymptomatic brain metastatic lesion that may alter the decision to drain large amounts of CSF due to risk of herniation and downward shift.

Because MRI findings characteristic of LMD are typically diffuse and small in volume (Fig. 1a, b, and e), using MRI changes as response assessment in LMD is challenging. The radiographic assessment in neuro-oncology (RANO) working group in leptomeningeal metastasis recommends to obtain contrast MRI of the entire neuroaxis at baseline as well as at pre-specified times thereafter and to focus on the presence or absence of nodules, leptomeningeal metastasis, cranial nerve, nerve root enhancement, hydrocephalus, and intraparenchymal, intramedullary, and epidural metastasis [33].

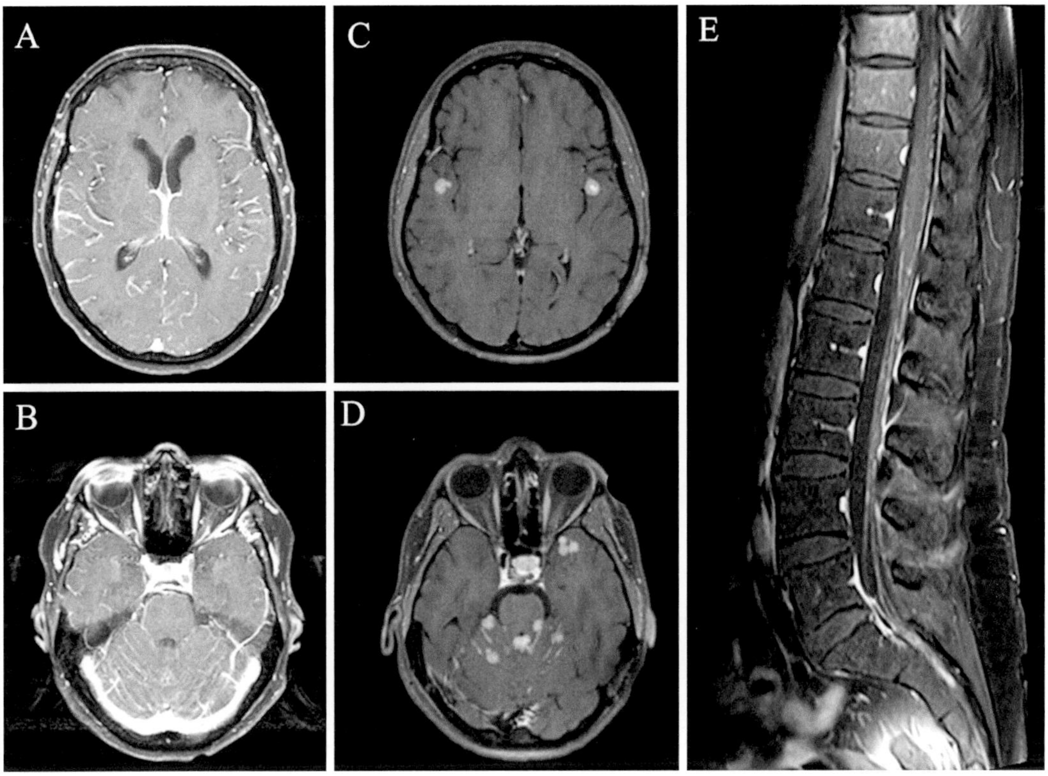

Fig. 1 Characteristic imaging findings in leptomeningeal disease. T1-postcontrast MRI images are from three different patients with breast cancer and LMD. Cerebral gyri (**a**) and cerebellar folia (**b**) enhancement. Superficial cortical (**c**) and cerebellar (**d**) enhancement. (**e**) Abnormal enhancement coating the nerve roots of the cauda equina

CSF Studies

Positive CSF cytology is the gold standard for diagnosis of LMD, and the yield increases with repeating the test. The false-negative rate for the first CSF analysis is as high as 50% and decreases to 20% with the third attempt [34]. CSF cytology is more likely to be positive in hematological than in solid malignancies (92% vs. 68%) [31]. It is a common practice to repeat the LP up to three times in order to increase the yield. The first LP is reported to be positive in 60–70% of cases of LMD suspected in solid cancers. The sensitivity increases by about 10–15% with the second attempt [30, 31] and only by 2% on subsequent LPs [15]. In addition to the number of sampling attempts, several other technical factors affect the yield of CSF cytology. CSF volume of ≥10.5 ml increases sensitivity, while delayed processing time and not obtaining CSF from a site of symptomatic or radiographically demonstrated disease decrease the sensitivity [35]. In addition, CSF cytology interpretation is subjective and typically reported as negative, atypical, suspicious, or positive in common clinical practice. Standardization of qualitative interpretation of CSF cytology has been recommended by RANO in leptomeningeal metastasis working group as positive versus negative [33] with a known caveat that the false-negative rate of CSF cytology may be as high as 50% [36]. The addition of CSF protein, glucose, and cell count is not recommended in assessing response to treatment in clinical trials [33] but can be used to screen for infection or for new pleocytosis or elevated CSF protein in cases of negative CSF cytology. Majority of patients with suspected LMD have non-specific abnormal CSF findings. These abnormalities include elevated cell count (25–64%) and protein (60–90%), decreased glucose (<50%), and elevated opening pressure (25%) [37].

CSF flow cytometry is more sensitive than CSF cytology in diagnosis of LMD from hematological malignancies [38]. However, the role of CSF flow cytometry in diagnosis of LMD from solid cancers is not well established. Subira et al. explored the role of CSF flow cytometry in diagnosis of solid cancer LMD and showed flow cytometry immunophenotyping using EpCAM antigen – an antigen highly expressed on malignant cells from colon, ovarian, stomach, pancreas, lung, and breast cancer – has higher sensitivity (75.5 vs. 65.3%) and similar specificity (96.1 vs. 100%) when compared with CSF cytology [39]. As the number of monoclonal antibodies directed against non-hematopoietic antigens is increasing, flow cytometry has the potential to serve as a novel tool to improve our diagnostic armamentarium in detection of malignant cells in CSF.

A radioisotope CSF study is recommended prior to consideration of intrathecal (IT) chemotherapy based on NCCN clinical practice guidelines in oncology in CNS cancers [40]. The purpose of the CSF flow study is to ensure that intrathecal chemotherapy will be evenly distributed within the subarachnoid space to reduce the risk of toxicity [41]. Impaired CSF flow over the cerebral convexities or in the spinal canal can be detected in up to 70% of patients with LMD [42] and may indicate an area of bulky disease even in the absence of radiographic findings [43]. Despite years of efforts in discovering CSF biomarkers that can improve CSF diagnostic yield, testing for CSF biomarkers is not established in common clinical practice.

Neurological Assessment

Diagnosis of probable and possible LMD can be made based on high clinical suspicion with or without abnormal CNS MRI, respectively, even in the absence of positive CSF cytology [3]. Neurological assessment should include surveying patients about typical symptoms of LMD (headaches, vision and hearing changes, facial numbness, and extremity pain or paresthesias) and a thorough neurological exam. RANO leptomeningeal metastases and neurological assessment working groups recommend assessing the following domains: gait, strength, sensation, vision, eye movement, facial strength, hearing, swallowing, level of consciousness, and behavior in order to generate a score card that can be used uniformly in clinical trials [33]. RANO leptomeningeal metastases assessment tools are the first step in standardizing response assessment in leptomeningeal clinical trials and are yet to be validated.

Differential Diagnosis

Other etiologies of subacute progressive neurological symptoms should be considered in differential diagnosis of leptomeningeal disease. The main categories include CNS infections and inflammatory and autoimmune neurological disorders which can have similar imaging findings of pachymeningitis (inflammation of the dura), cranial nerve enhancement, and nodular enhancement within the spine and the cauda equina. These conditions can also present with abnormal CSF findings of elevated WBC and protein and low glucose, similar to that of neoplastic LMD. CNS infections should be on top of the differential particularly since patients may be immunocompromised due to systemic chemotherapy.

Management

Treatment of LMD is challenging and difficult, with generally poor outcome. The primary treatment modalities may include a combination of radiation therapy and intrathecal and systemic chemotherapy, mainly aimed to improve symptoms and quality of life. The decision to initiate treatment for LMD is largely dependent on patients' functional status and the extent of the systemic disease. Ideal candidates for treatment of LMD would be patients with acceptable functional status and limited systemic disease or systemic disease with available treatment options. The next challenge would be to determine the role of radiation and the route of chemotherapy administration. The role of radiation therapy is mainly palliative in patients with LMD. Radiation is either delivered locally or as WBRT. The goal of local radiation is to treat bulky disease to allow for uniform CSF flow or to palliate symptoms such as in cases of cauda equina syndrome. The purpose of WBRT is to ameliorate symptoms of cranial neuropathies or to concomitantly treat brain metastatic lesions. The route of chemotherapy is dependent on availability of blood-brain penetrant systemic treatment options. Choices may include blood-brain penetrant chemotherapy, systemic chemotherapy that does not cross the blood-brain barrier (BBB), plus IT chemotherapy or IT chemotherapy alone in cases when systemic chemotherapy options are nonexistent and/or systemic disease is well controlled. Once the decision is made to use IT chemotherapy, route of administration needs to be determined, via lumbar puncture versus through surgically implanted subgaleal reservoir and intraventricular catheter (i.e., Ommaya reservoir) [44, 45].

Several intrathecal chemotherapeutic agents such as methotrexate, cytarabine, or topotecan have been tested in the context of clinical trials as single agent or combination for treatment of LMD and seem to have similar efficacies [46–49]. The limitations of these clinical trials include small number of patients, varying primary end points, lack of standardized response criteria, and inconsistent toxicity reporting. These limitations lead to RANO working group recommendations regarding assessing response in clinical trials for patients with LMD [33]. Chamberlain et al. recommended neurological exam, CSF analysis including cytology and flow cytometry (in case of hematological malignancies), and neuroimaging of the entire neuroaxis for all patients enrolled in LMD clinical trials. They prioritized neurological assessment over CSF analysis and neuroimaging given limitations of these diagnostic tests in LMD but allowed for "disease progression" based on progression on neuroimaging alone in the absence of progression in neurological exam and CSF studies. These assessment tools are yet to be validated in the context of clinical trials.

Pharmacological Treatments

Once the decision is made to treat LMD, the first step would be to determine the type of chemotherapy: systemic versus IT versus both. Seventy percent of patients present with LMD in the setting of active systemic disease [17, 18] and will need systemic therapies that cross the BBB or systemic and IT therapies simultaneously. However, the other 30% may have isolated LMD and warrant LMD-specific therapies in addition to continued surveillance of the systemic disease.

Systemic Therapies

Breast Cancer

Breast cancer is the most common solid cancer associated with LMD [37]. Determining hormone receptor (HR) and HER2 status in breast cancer is standard of care, and it derives the choices of systemic therapy, as these patients have varying prognosis and response to treatment. Anti-HER2 antibodies have improved the survival of patients with HER2-positive breast cancer, yet 4–19% of patients develop LMD, while their systemic tumor burden is well controlled [50]. This may be due to poor BBB penetration of first-generation anti-HER2 antibodies and or due to lack of HER2 positivity in CNS metastatic cells. Trastuzumab, the most commonly used and well-studied HER2 antibody, does not cross the BBB [51], and there have been no studies particularly addressing the effectiveness of systemic trastuzumab in treatment of LMD. Lapatinib, a HER2/EGFR dual tyrosine kinase inhibitor (TKI) thought to have improved BBB penetration, had a low CNS response rate of 6% in patients with brain metastasis [52]. Lapatinib in combination with capecitabine has shown CNS response rates of 66% in patients with brain metastatic HER2+ breast cancer [53]. This combination has not been tried in patients with LMD, but capecitabine monotherapy has demonstrated to have some activity against LMD in breast cancer patients in case reports [54, 55]. Ekenel and colleagues reported three patients with LMD from breast cancer whose symptoms improved on capecitabine therapy. Similarly, Giglio and colleagues reported response to treatment in three LMD patients (two with breast cancer and one with esophageal cancer). One paper reported an impressive long-term survival of 3.7 years in response to oral capecitabine in a breast cancer patient with positive CSF cytology [56]. Neratinib, an EGFR dual tyrosine kinase inhibitor with a small lipophilic molecule, is assumed to cross the blood-brain barrier. A randomized open-label trial of neratinib plus paclitaxel versus trastuzumab plus paclitaxel in previously untreated advanced meta-static HER2-positive breast cancer showed lower incidence of CNS recurrences and a longer time to CNS metastases in the neratinib arm [57].

The role of hormonal therapy for treatment of HR-positive breast cancer LMD has been described in several case reports with progression-free survival ranging from 6 months to more than 36 months [58, 59]. Given limited efficacy of IT chemotherapy in treatment of HR-positive breast cancer LMD and a more favorable side effect profile of hormonal therapies than IT chemotherapy, further research investigating the role of hormonal therapy in treatment of HR-positive breast cancer LMD is warranted.

Bevacizumab is an anti-VEGF monoclonal antibody that is thought to improve intratumoral penetration of cisplatin and etoposide in brain metastatic breast cancer [60, 61]. A pilot study of eight patients with breast cancer and LMD treated with bevacizumab combined with etoposide and cisplatin showed mOS of 4.7 months and neurologic progression-free survival of 4.7 months [61].

Aside from abovementioned isolated case reports and case series, there are overall no viable systemic chemotherapy options for treatment of breast cancer LMD patients at this time.

Non-Small Cell Lung Cancer

Lung cancer patients with LMD have worse outcome and response to IT chemotherapy than patients with LMD from breast cancer or lymphoma [32, 62]. However, recent therapeutic advances in targeted therapy in NSCLC with CNS metastasis have greatly improved survival [63] and have shown to be promising in treatment of a subgroup of patients with NSCLC LMD.

EGFR mutations account for 10–35% cases of NSCLC and provide an effective targeted therapy in EGFR mutant NSCLC patients. EGFR mutation confers an increased risk of LMD in NSCLC patients [27]. Gefitinib and erlotinib are first-generation EGFR TKIs with systemic response rates of 60–90% in EGFR mutant NSCLC [64, 65] and have been shown to delay the progression of CNS disease [66]. Jackman and colleagues performed a phase I study evaluating the safety, tolerance, and CSF penetration of high-dose gefitinib in seven NSCLC LMD patients with prior response to EGFR TKI and/or harboring EGFR mutation [67]. Four out of seven patients had improved in neurological symptoms, one patient's CSF cleared of malignant cells, and two patients had decreases in number of malignant cells in their CSF. However, a phase III study of gefitinib versus conventional chemotherapy (gemcitabine plus cisplatin) as first-line therapy for NSCLC patients resulted in similar cumulative incidence of LMD and time to LMD in the two treatment arms [68]. In a retrospective study, erlotinib was thought to be more effective than gefitinib in clearing CSF malignant cells [69], which may be due to its better BBB penetration and higher concentration in CSF in comparison with gefitinib [70]. The efficacy of erlotinib and gefitinib against LMD and their CSF concentration may be influenced by the dose and method of administration. High-dose erlotinib and pulsatile dosing erlotinib have shown improved response rates in patients with refractory CNS disease and improvement in neurological symptoms in one case report of EGFR mutant NSCLC patient with refractory LMD [71, 72]. Newer generations of TKIs such as osimertinib have demonstrated efficacy in NSCLC patients with CNS metastatic disease, who developed acquired resistance to first- or second-generation of TKI inhibitors [73–75].

Anaplastic lymphoma kinase (ALK) rearrangement is a therapeutically targetable oncogenic driver in 2–7% of patients with NSCLC [76]. Crizotinib, an ALK-specific tyrosine kinase inhibitor, has been effective in treatment of ALK-rearranged NSCLC [77, 78]. However, resistance typically occurs within 1 year with 41% of recurrent disease in the brain, likely as a result of poor BBB penetration of crizotinib [79]. One phase I trial tested the effect of ceritinib, a potent inhibitor of ALK that crosses the BBB, in 255 ALK-rearranged NSCLC patients and showed intracranial response rates of 79% in 19 ALK inhibitor-naïve patients and 69% in 75 ALK inhibitor pre-treated patients with retrospectively confirmed brain metastasis [80]. This has led to a phase II clinical trial testing the effectiveness of ceritinib in patients with ALK-rearranged NSCLC and brain or leptomeningeal metastasis (NCT02336451). Alectinib is another blood-brain penetrant ALK inhibitor with higher CNS response rates than crizotinib [81]. Qian and colleagues have reported five cases of improved clinical and radiographic LMD in patients with ALK-rearranged NSCLC treated with alectinib [82, 83]. Combination of first-generation TKIs with bevacizumab has shown promising results in isolated cases [84].

Overall, systemic targeted therapies have shown early promise for treatment of LMD in molecularly altered NSCLC. Effective treatment for LMD is limited, and blood-brain penetrant molecularly targeted therapies hold the promise to alter the outcome of LMD patients for the first time.

Melanoma

Targeted therapies (BRAF and MEK inhibitors) and immunotherapies such as checkpoint inhibitors (anti-CTLA4, anti-PD1, and anti-PDL1) have improved survival of patients with metastatic melanoma [85]. These treatments have also changed the life expectancy of patients with brain metastatic melanoma indicating that they are active against CNS disease.

Fifty percent of patients with melanoma harbor BRAF V600 mutations. The discovery of this targetable mutation has revolutionized the treatment of patients with metastatic melanoma [86–89]. BRAF inhibitors, dabrafenib and vemurafenib, have been shown to be active against brain metastatic melanoma [90, 91].

However, patients quickly develop resistance with duration response of a few months. Therefore, combination therapies using BRAF inhibitors and downstream targets of RAF, MEK, in the MAPK pathway have been tested and have demonstrated improved intracranial response rates [91, 92]. Trials of BRAF inhibitors in melanoma LMD are lacking, but isolated case reports have demonstrated activity of vemurafenib [93, 94] and dabrafenib [95] in melanoma patients with LMD.

Treatment with targeted therapy has been associated with a high- but short-lasting response rates in melanoma. In contrast, immune checkpoint blockade (anti-CTLA4, anti-PD1, and anti-PDL-1) has shown a lower- but longer-term responses in metastatic melanoma [96]. The data on immunotherapy in treating patients with CNS metastatic is scarce, mostly due to theoretical concerns with inducing an inflammatory response in CSF [97]. Scattered case reports in the literature demonstrated response to IT tumor-infiltrating lymphocytes or CD8+ cytotoxic T cells in patients with refractory melanoma LMD [98, 99]. Ipilimumab was shown to result in complete radiographic response in a patient with melanoma LMD who was alive 18 months after diagnosis of LMD [100]. There has also been an interest in combining immunotherapy with targeted therapy in metastatic melanoma, and several combinational trials are being conducted to determine the most effective timing and sequence of administration of these agents [96]. Whether or not targeted therapy, immunotherapy, or combination therapies are going to be effective in melanoma, patients with LMD remains to be tested in the context of clinical trials.

Intrathecal Chemotherapy

There are four FDA-approved intrathecal chemotherapies: methotrexate, cytosine arabinoside (Ara-C), liposomal cytarabine arabinoside (DepoCyt), and thiotepa [37]. These agents have been tested in the context of several randomized clinical trials for treatment of solid cancer LMD as single agents or in combination and seem to have overall similar efficacy [46–49]. The role of these FDA-approved agents for treatment of solid cancer LMD remains unclear and controversial [46, 101], but randomized trials are scarce and suffer from small heterogeneous patient populations and non-standardized response criteria and primary end points [33]. A growing number of retrospective studies and case reports suggest improved outcomes in patients receiving methotrexate [102–105], cytarabine [106, 107], and thiotepa [108].

Although not FDA approved, non-randomized trials and case series have shown that IT topotecan [107, 109, 110] and trastuzumab [106, 108, 111, 112] are well tolerated, have a low toxicity profile, and are not inferior to FDA-approved IT chemotherapies. In our practice, our therapy of choice for solid malignancies and LMD is IT topotecan except for cases of HER2+ breast cancer patients in whom our first choice is IT trastuzumab. The role of IT trastuzumab in treatment of LMD is being tested in two ongoing studies (NCT01325207, NCT01373710). In addition, an ongoing phase I trial (NCT00424242) is testing the safety and pharmacokinetics of CSF pemetrexed disodium in patients with LMD from different hematological and solid malignancies.

The route of administration of IT chemotherapy is largely institution dependent. One head-to-head trial comparing efficacy and complicate rates of lumbar puncture or intraventricular reservoir showed statistically significant improved progression-free survival favoring patients who received intraventricular over intralumbar methotrexate (19 vs. 42 days, $P = 0.048$), but the same was not true for sustained-release cytarabine. Authors concluded that the route of administration may be relevant with short half-life drugs such as methotrexate [44]. It is our common practice to use Ommaya reservoir for administration of IT chemotherapy as recommended by NCCN clinical practice guidelines in oncology on CNS cancers [40].

Concurrent radiation and chemotherapy is typically avoided in LMD patients as a result of potential increased toxicities related to combinational therapies. One relatively large study involving 59 patients with median Karnofsky Performance Status Scale (KPS) of 40 (range 20–70) with LMD from various solid cancers (42 lung cancer, 11 breast cancer, and 6 others) showed impressive response rates to concomitant weekly intrathecal methotrexate and involved field radiation, WBRT, and/or spinal canal radiation [113]. The overall response rate was 86.4%; the median overall survival was 6.5 months with 21.3% of patients alive in 1 year. However, 12 patients (20%) had grade III–IV toxic reactions including acute meningitis, chronic delayed encephalopathy, radiculitis, myelosuppression, and mucositis.

Non-pharmacological Treatments

Radiation

The role of radiation is mainly palliative in treatment of LMD. WBRT is commonly used prior to starting systemic or intrathecal chemotherapy as a palliative intent. However, in our practice we advocate for WBRT in cases where patients suffer from symptoms attributable to the cerebral cortex, cerebellum, or cranial nerves. In our opinion, WBRT in asymptomatic patients should be avoided as there is no proven survival benefit [114], and the palliative intent of WBRT is unclear. In a non-inferiority trial of 538 NSCLC patients with poor prognosis of brain metastasis, WBRT was not superior to optimal supportive care in overall survival and only showed marginal improvement in quality-adjusted life years (QALY) of 4.7 days [115]. Patients with symptomatic focal spine LMD can benefit from palliative radiation. Focal radiotherapy has been shown to improve symptoms of radiculopathies and bulky disease preventing CSF flow [41, 116]. Craniospinal radiation is usually avoided as bone marrow suppression may impede the patients' ability to receive other cytotoxic chemotherapies.

Surgery

The role of surgery in LMD is limited and includes biopsy, subgaleal intraventricular reservoir, and ventriculoperitoneal shunt placement. Biopsy may be indicated in cases of unknown primary cancer with equivocal CSF cytology or to rule out infectious etiologies mimicking neoplastic meningitis in the appropriate setting. Ventriculoperitoneal shunt with an on/off valve can be used to relieve the symptoms of increased intracranial pressure/hydrocephalus due to obstruction and to administer intrathecal chemotherapy, but it carries the theoretical risk of cancer cells seeding the peritoneum [6, 45]. Intraventricular subgaleal reservoir (i.e., Ommaya) placement is our preferred method of intrathecal chemotherapy administration due to ease of access and more reliable drug delivery [11, 15, 49]; however, use of these reservoirs to administer chemotherapy has not been shown to improve survival when compared with intrathecal chemotherapy administration through lumbar puncture [44].

Supportive Care

End of life and goals of care should be discussed with all patients and their families to delineate the course of palliative care. Education and emotional support for patients and their caregivers play an important role in the care provided for these patients and may be highly individualized as the disease progresses. Patients with poor functional status (KPS ≤ 50), major neurological deficits, and extensive systemic involvement with limited treatment options may be best suited for supportive care. Symptomatic care approaches include corticosteroids, analgesics, anticonvulsants, antidepressant, and/or anxiolytic. Radiation plays an important role in providing the best supportive care to patients as it may help relieve neurological symptoms [40]. Ventriculoperitoneal shunts can be used in cases of hydrocephalus to lower CSF pressure. In cases that a patient is not suited for a surgical procedure, implementation of a lumbar drain can transiently alleviate symptoms of hydrocephalus/somnolence.

Figure 2 provides a management algorithm for patients with solid cancer LMD.

Prognosis

LMD is the most feared CNS complication of solid cancers and carries a dismal prognosis of 4–6 months in general. Patients with breast cancer and LMD have the best prognosis with median

overall survival of 15 weeks when compared to 8.3 weeks for other solid cancers and 8.7 weeks for lung cancer in particular [117]. More recently efforts have been made to study the effect of breast cancer subtypes on prognosis. Hormone receptor (HR) and HER2 status in breast cancer have been shown to be associated with time to LMD diagnosis. Patients with triple negative breast cancer have a shorter time to LMD, and HR-positive patients have longer time to LMD and better survival [25]. In one study reviewing records of 190 patients diagnosed with LMD from breast cancer with available subtypes from 1997 to 2012, mOS from LMD diagnosis was 4.4 months for HER2+, 3.7 months for HR+/HER2-, and 2.2 months for triple negative breast cancer ($p = 0.0002$) [118]. The observed improved overall survival with combination of IT and systemic chemotherapy may be attributed to a selection bias of patients with good functional status and less severe systemic disease. Nevertheless, patients with HER2+ breast cancer had improved survival compared with HR+/HER2- and triple negative breast cancer patients after adjusting for age, IT and systemic chemotherapy, and extracranial disease burden.

The survival of patients with NSCLC and melanoma brain metastasis is improving [63, 85] owing, at least in part, to targeted therapies against EGFR and ALK abnormalities in NSCLC and against BRAF in melanoma as well as immunotherapy with checkpoint inhibitors [119]. The effect of these novel therapies in survival of patients with LMD remains to be identified.

The most important prognostic factor within a particular cancer type is the patients' functional status [120, 121]. Treatment decisions as well as goals of care should strongly take functional status into consideration.

Future Directions

Late diagnosis of LMD, rarity of molecularly driven randomized clinical trials, and lack of standardization in diagnosis and evaluation of treatment responses among the current available studies are roadblocks in improving the outcome of LMD patients.

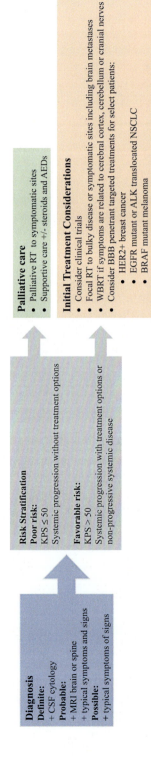

Diagnosis
Definite:
+ CSF cytology
Probable:
+ MRI brain or spine
+ typical symptoms and signs
Possible:
+ typical symptoms of signs

Risk Stratification
Poor risk:
KPS ≤ 50
Systemic progression without treatment options

Favorable risk:
KPS > 50
Systemic progression with treatment options or non-progressive systemic disease

Palliative care
• Palliative RT to symptomatic sites
• Supportive care +/- steroids and AEDs

Initial Treatment Considerations
• Consider clinical trials
• Focal RT to bulky disease or symptomatic sites including brain metastases
• WBRT if symptoms are related to cerebral cortex, cerebellum or cranial nerves
• Consider BBB penetrant targeted treatments for select patients:
  • HER2+ breast cancer
  • EGFR mutant or ALK translocated NSCLC
  • BRAF mutant melanoma
• Consider immunotherapy or combinational therapy for select patients
• Consider IT chemotherapy in the absence of above: got to next row

IT Chemotherapy: Induction Phase
• Consider Ommaya reservoir placement
• Consider VP shunt with on/off valve if symptoms of hydrocephalus exist
• Obtain CSF flow studies -> focal RT to areas of obstructive flow
• IT topotecan as first line for 4-6 weeks
• IT trastuzumab in HER2+ breast cancer for 4-6 weeks
• Continue systemic treatment if indicated

IT Chemotherapy: Maintenance Phase
• Assess response: Neurological exam, CSF studies, MRI brain and spine
• If improved or stable disease: continue IT chemotherapy and reduce interval of treatments
• If progressive disease:
  • IT methotrexate as second line
  • Add IT topotecan to IT trastuzumab in HER2+ breast cancer

Reassess response every 4-8 weeks and continue IT chemotherapy at reduced intervals till progression, in which case consider supportive care +/- palliative RT

Fig. 2 **Management algorithm of solid cancer leptomeningeal disease.** Below is a recommended management algorithm per MD Anderson Cancer Center Department of Neuro-oncology current clinical practice. Abbreviations: *CSF* cerebral spinal fluid, *KPS* Karofsky Performance Status Scale, *RT* radiation, *AED* anti-epileptic drug, *WBRT* whole brain radiation therapy, *BBB* blood brain barrier, *EGFR* endothelial growth factor receptor, *ALK* anaplastic lymphoma kinase, *NSCLC* non-small cell lung cancer, *IT* intrathecal chemotherapy, *VP* ventriculoperitoneal

CSF biomarkers aiding in early detection of LMD have the potential to significantly impact survival of patients with LMD. Poor prognosis of LMD patients may in part be due to delayed diagnosis using our current diagnostic armamentarium (MRI and CSF cytology). CSF biomarkers such as vascular endothelial growth factor (VEGF) levels and circulating tumor DNA (ctDNA) have shown promising results in early detection of LMD, but are not currently used in common clinical practice.

Solid cancer LMD has been historically studied as one entity without consideration of tumor types and varying molecular characteristics. However, LMD from different types of solid cancers has varying prognosis and response to therapy. For example, breast cancer patients with LMD seem to have better prognosis than other types of solid cancers, particularly those with HER2+ tumors. It is necessary to conduct cancer and molecular subtype-specific LMD treatment trials to better assess the effectiveness and specificity of particular treatments. In addition, the biology of the primary tumor and the tumor that has metastasized to leptomeninges may be different. Comprehensive genomic analysis of CSF tumor cells in comparison with primary cancer should be included in treatment trials to elucidate the mechanism by which cancer cells metastasize to the leptomeninges.

Finally, the evaluation of current available clinical trials in LMD is challenging due to heterogeneous inclusion criteria, diagnostic parameters, response assessment, and primary end points. The response assessment tools published in 2017 by Leptomeningeal Assessment in Neuro-oncology [3, 33, 122] and the European Association for Neuro-Oncology/European Society for Medical Oncology (EANO/ESMO) groups should be included in future clinical trials.

Conclusion

Leptomeningeal disease from solid tumors occurs in 5% of patients with solid cancer and confers a poor prognosis. The incidence of LMD is rising due to improved survival of cancer patients and more frequent imaging. Diagnosis and treatment of LMD is challenging and evolving with recent improvements in imaging techniques and advent of novel molecular targeted therapies and immunotherapy. Ultimately, diagnosis of LMD remains a clinical diagnosis supported by imaging findings and positive CSF cytology. Treatment decisions largely depend on patients' functional status and extent of systemic disease. Here, we have included a management algorithm to aid providers with diagnosis, risk stratification, and treatment of solid cancer LMD. Given lack of effective treatment that could significantly impact survival of patients with LMD, continuous efforts in refining tools for early diagnosis and designing standardized prospective clinical trials in LMD patients are warranted.

References

1. Chamberlain M, Soffietti R, Raizer J, Ruda R, Brandsma D, Boogerd W, Taillibert S, Groves MD, Le Rhun E, Junck L, van den Bent M, Wen PY, Jaeckle KA. Leptomeningeal metastasis: a Response Assessment in Neuro-Oncology critical review of endpoints and response criteria of published randomized clinical trials. Neuro-Oncology. 2014;16:1176–85.
2. Beauchesne P. Intrathecal chemotherapy for treatment of leptomeningeal dissemination of metastatic tumours. Lancet Oncol. 2010;11:871–9.
3. Le Rhun E, Weller M, Brandsma D, van den Bent M, de Azambuja E, Henriksson R, Boulanger T, Peters S, Watts C, Wick W, Wesseling P, Ruda R, Preusser M, EANO Executive Board and ESMO Guidelines Committee. EANO-ESMO Clinical Practice Guidelines for diagnosis, treatment and follow-up of patients with leptomeningeal metastasis from solid tumours. Ann Oncol. 2017;28:iv84–99.
4. Armstrong TS, Gilbert MR. The treatment of neoplastic meningitis. Expert Opin Pharmacother. 2004;5:1929–35.
5. Leal T, Chang JE, Mehta M, Robins HI. Leptomeningeal metastasis: challenges in diagnosis and treatment. Curr Cancer Ther Rev. 2011;7:319–27.
6. Le Rhun E, Taillibert S, Chamberlain MC. Carcinomatous meningitis: leptomeningeal metastases in solid tumors. Surg Neurol Int. 2013;4:S265–88.
7. Roth P, Weller M. Management of neoplastic meningitis. Chin Clin Oncol. 2015;4:26.
8. Clatot F, Philippin-Lauridant G, Ouvrier MJ, Nakry T, Laberge-LE-Couteulx S, Guillemet C, Veyret C, Blot E. Clinical improvement and survival

in breast cancer leptomeningeal metastasis correlate with the cytologic response to intrathecal chemotherapy. J Neuro-Oncol. 2009;95:421–6.

9. Rudnicka H, Niwinska A, Murawska M. Breast cancer leptomeningeal metastasis – the role of multimodality treatment. J Neuro-Oncol. 2007;84:57–62.

10. Chamberlain MC. Neoplastic meningitis. J Clin Oncol. 2005;23:3605–13.

11. Nayar G, Ejikeme T, Chongsathidkiet P, Elsamadicy AA, Blackwell KL, Clarke JM, Lad SP, Fecci PE. Leptomeningeal disease: current diagnostic and therapeutic strategies. Oncotarget. 2017;8:73312–28.

12. Erlich SS, Davis RL. Spinal subarachnoid metastasis from primary intracranial glioblastoma multiforme. Cancer. 1978;42:2854–64.

13. Yung WA, Horten BC, Shapiro WR. Meningeal gliomatosis: a review of 12 cases. Ann Neurol. 1980;8:605–8.

14. Louis DN, Perry A, Reifenberger G, von Deimling A, Figarella-Branger D, Cavenee WK, Ohgaki H, Wiestler OD, Kleihues P, Ellison DW. The 2016 World Health Organization classification of tumors of the central nervous system: a summary. Acta Neuropathol. 2016;131:803–20.

15. Mack F, Baumert BG, Schafer N, Hattingen E, Scheffler B, Herrlinger U, Glas M. Therapy of leptomeningeal metastasis in solid tumors. Cancer Treat Rev. 2016;43:83–91.

16. Posner JB, Chernik NL. Intracranial metastases from systemic cancer. Adv Neurol. 1978;19:579–92.

17. Chamberlain MC. Comprehensive neuraxis imaging in leptomeningeal metastasis: a retrospective case series. CNS Oncol. 2013;2:121–8.

18. Pauls S, Fischer AC, Brambs HJ, Fetscher S, Hoche W, Bommer M. Use of magnetic resonance imaging to detect neoplastic meningitis: limited use in leukemia and lymphoma but convincing results in solid tumors. Eur J Radiol. 2012;81:974–8.

19. Nayak L, Lee EQ, Wen PY. Epidemiology of brain metastases. Curr Oncol Rep. 2012;14:48–54.

20. Ahn JH, Lee SH, Kim S, Joo J, Yoo H, Lee SH, Shin SH, Gwak HS. Risk for leptomeningeal seeding after resection for brain metastases: implication of tumor location with mode of resection. J Neurosurg. 2012;116:984–93.

21. Ma R, Levy M, Gui B, Lu SE, Narra V, Goyal S, Danish S, Hanft S, Khan AJ, Malhotra J, Motwani S, Jabbour SK. Risk of leptomeningeal carcinomatosis in patients with brain metastases treated with stereotactic radiosurgery. J Neuro-Oncol. 2018;136:395–401.

22. Suki D, Hatiboglu MA, Patel AJ, Weinberg JS, Groves MD, Mahajan A, Sawaya R. Comparative risk of leptomeningeal dissemination of cancer after surgery or stereotactic radiosurgery for a single supratentorial solid tumor metastasis. Neurosurgery. 2009;64:664–74; discussion 674–6

23. Atalar B, Modlin LA, Choi CY, Adler JR, Gibbs IC, Chang SD, Harsh GRT, Li G, Nagpal S, Hanlon A, Soltys SG. Risk of leptomeningeal disease in patients treated with stereotactic radiosurgery targeting the postoperative resection cavity for brain metastases. Int J Radiat Oncol Biol Phys. 2013;87:713–8.

24. Ojerholm E, Lee JY, Kolker J, Lustig R, Dorsey JF, Alonso-Basanta M. Gamma Knife radiosurgery to four or more brain metastases in patients without prior intracranial radiation or surgery. Cancer Med. 2014;3:565–71.

25. Yust-Katz S, Garciarena P, Liu D, Yuan Y, Ibrahim N, Yerushalmi R, Penas-Prado M, Groves MD. Breast cancer and leptomeningeal disease (LMD): hormone receptor status influences time to development of LMD and survival from LMD diagnosis. J Neuro-Oncol. 2013;114:229–35.

26. Lee S, Ahn HK, Park YH, Nam DH, Lee JI, Park W, Choi DH, Huh SJ, Park KT, Ahn JS, Im YH. Leptomeningeal metastases from breast cancer: intrinsic subtypes may affect unique clinical manifestations. Breast Cancer Res Treat. 2011;129:809–17.

27. Yufen X, Binbin S, Wenyu C, Jialiang L, Xinmei Y. The role of EGFR-TKI for leptomeningeal metastases from non-small cell lung cancer. Springerplus. 2016;5:1244.

28. Cheng H, Perez-Soler R. Leptomeningeal metastases in non-small-cell lung cancer. Lancet Oncol. 2018;19: e43–55.

29. Pellerino A, Bertero L, Ruda R, Soffietti R. Neoplastic meningitis in solid tumors: from diagnosis to personalized treatments. Ther Adv Neurol Disord. 2018;11:1756286418759618.

30. Kaplan JG, Desouza TG, Farkash A, Shafran B, Pack D, Rehman F, Fuks J, Portenoy R. Leptomeningeal metastases: comparison of clinical features and laboratory data of solid tumors, lymphomas and leukemias. J Neuro-Oncol. 1990;9:225–9.

31. Prommel P, Pilgram-Pastor S, Sitter H, Buhk JH, Strik H. Neoplastic meningitis: how MRI and CSF cytology are influenced by CSF cell count and tumor type. ScientificWorldJournal. 2013;2013:248072.

32. Herrlinger U, Forschler H, Kuker W, Meyermann R, Bamberg M, Dichgans J, Weller M. Leptomeningeal metastasis: survival and prognostic factors in 155 patients. J Neurol Sci. 2004;223:167–78.

33. Chamberlain M, Junck L, Brandsma D, Soffietti R, Ruda R, Raizer J, Boogerd W, Taillibert S, Groves MD, Le Rhun E, Walker J, van den Bent M, Wen PY, Jaeckle KA. Leptomeningeal metastases: a RANO proposal for response criteria. Neuro-Oncology. 2017;19:484–92.

34. Glass JP, Melamed M, Chernik NL, Posner JB. Malignant cells in cerebrospinal fluid (CSF): the meaning of a positive CSF cytology. Neurology. 1979;29:1369–75.

35. Glantz MJ, Cole BF, Glantz LK, Cobb J, Mills P, Lekos A, Walters BC, Recht LD. Cerebrospinal fluid

cytology in patients with cancer: minimizing false-negative results. Cancer. 1998;82:733–9.

36. Jung H, Sinnarajah A, Enns B, Voroney JP, Murray A, Pelletier G, Wu JS. Managing brain metastases patients with and without radiotherapy: initial lessonsfrom a team-based consult service through a multidisciplinary integrated palliative oncology clinic. Support Care Cancer. 2013;21:3379–86.

37. Kak M, Nanda R, Ramsdale EE, Lukas RV. Treatment of leptomeningeal carcinomatosis: current challenges and future opportunities. J Clin Neurosci. 2015;22:632–7.

38. Ahluwalia SC, Chuang FL, Antonio AL, Malin JL, Lorenz KA, Walling AM. Documentation and discussion of preferences for care among patients with advanced cancer. J Oncol Pract. 2011;7:361–6.

39. Subira D, Serrano C, Castanon S, Gonzalo R, Illan J, Pardo J, Martinez-Garcia M, Millastre E, Aparisi F, Navarro M, Domine M, Gil-Bazo I, Perez Segura P, Gil M, Bruna J. Role of flow cytometry immunophenotyping in the diagnosis of leptomeningeal carcinomatosis. Neuro-Oncology. 2012;14:43–52.

40. Nabors LB, Pornow J, Baehring J, Brem H, Butowski N. Central Nervous System Cancers. NCCN Clinical Practice Guidelines in Oncology Version 1.2018. 2018.

41. Chamberlain MC. Radioisotope CSF flow studies in leptomeningeal metastases. J Neuro-Oncol. 1998b;38:135–40.

42. Grossman SA, Trump DL, Chen DC, Thompson G, Camargo EE. Cerebrospinal fluid flow abnormalities in patients with neoplastic meningitis. An evaluation using 111indium-DTPA ventriculography. Am J Med. 1982;73:641–7.

43. Glantz MJ, Hall WA, Cole BF, Chozick BS, Shannon CM, Wahlberg L, Akerley W, Marin L, Choy H. Diagnosis, management, and survival of patients with leptomeningeal cancer based on cerebrospinal fluid-flow status. Cancer. 1995;75:2919–31.

44. Glantz MJ, van Horn A, Fisher R, Chamberlain MC. Route of intracerebrospinal fluid chemotherapy administration and efficacy of therapy in neoplastic meningitis. Cancer. 2010;116:1947–52.

45. Lin N, Dunn IF, Glantz M, Allison DL, Jensen R, Johnson MD, Friedlander RM, Kesari S. Benefit of ventriculoperitoneal cerebrospinal fluid shunting and intrathecal chemotherapy in neoplastic meningitis: a retrospective, case-controlled study. J Neurosurg. 2011;115:730–6.

46. Boogerd W, van den Bent MJ, Koehler PJ, Heimans JJ, van der Sande JJ, Aaronson NK, Hart AA, Benraadt J, CHJ V. The relevance of intraventricular chemotherapy for leptomeningeal metastasis in breast cancer: a randomised study. Eur J Cancer. 2004;40:2726–33.

47. Glantz MJ, Jaeckle KA, Chamberlain MC, Phuphanich S, Recht L, Swinnen LJ, Maria B, Lafollette S, Schumann GB, Cole BF, Howell SB. A randomized controlled trial comparing intrathecal sustained-release cytarabine (DepoCyt) to intrathecal methotrexate in patients with neoplastic meningitis from solid tumors. Clin Cancer Res. 1999;5:3394–402.

48. Grossman SA, Finkelstein DM, Ruckdeschel JC, Trump DL, Moynihan T, Ettinger DS. Randomized prospective comparison of intraventricular methotrexate and thiotepa in patients with previously untreated neoplastic meningitis. Eastern Cooperative Oncology Group. J Clin Oncol. 1993;11:561–9.

49. Hitchins RN, Bell DR, Woods RL, Levi JA. A prospective randomized trial of single-agent versus combination chemotherapy in meningeal carcinomatosis. J Clin Oncol. 1987;5:1655–62.

50. Bendell JC, Domchek SM, Burstein HJ, Harris L, Younger J, Kuter I, Bunnell C, Rue M, Gelman R, Winer E. Central nervous system metastases in women who receive trastuzumab-based therapy for metastatic breast carcinoma. Cancer. 2003;97:2972–7.

51. Pestalozzi BC, Brignoli S. Trastuzumab in CSF. J Clin Oncol. 2000;18:2349–51.

52. Lin NU, Dieras V, Paul D, Lossignol D, Christodoulou C, Stemmler HJ, Roche H, Liu MC, Greil R, Ciruelos E, Loibl S, Gori S, Wardley A, Yardley D, Brufsky A, Blum JL, Rubin SD, Dharan B, Steplewski K, Zembryki D, Oliva C, Roychowdhury D, Paoletti P, Winer EP. Multicenter phase II study of lapatinib in patients with brain metastases from HER2-positive breast cancer. Clin Cancer Res. 2009;15:1452–9.

53. Bachelot T, Romieu G, Campone M, Dieras V, Cropet C, Dalenc F, Jimenez M, Le Rhun E, Pierga JY, Goncalves A, Leheurteur M, Domont J, Gutierrez M, Cure H, Ferrero JM, Labbe-Devilliers C. Lapatinib plus capecitabine in patients with previously untreated brain metastases from HER2-positive metastatic breast cancer (LANDSCAPE): a single-group phase 2 study. Lancet Oncol. 2013;14:64–71.

54. Ekenel M, Hormigo AM, Peak S, Deangelis LM, Abrey LE. Capecitabine therapy of central nervous system metastases from breast cancer. J Neuro-Oncol. 2007;85:223–7.

55. Giglio P, Tremont-Lukats IW, Groves MD. Response of neoplastic meningitis from solid tumors to oral capecitabine. J Neuro-Oncol. 2003;65:167–72.

56. Tham YL, Hinckley L, Teh BS, Elledge R. Long-term clinical response in leptomeningeal metastases from breast cancer treated with capecitabine monotherapy: a case report. Clin Breast Cancer. 2006;7:164–6.

57. Awada A, Colomer R, Inoue K, Bondarenko I, Badwe RA, Demetriou G, Lee SC, Mehta AO, Kim SB, Bachelot T, Goswami C, Deo S, Bose R, Wong A, Xu F, Yao B, Bryce R, Carey LA. Neratinib plus paclitaxel vs trastuzumab plus paclitaxel in previously untreated metastatic ERBB2-positive breast cancer: the NEfERT-T randomized clinical trial. JAMA Oncol. 2016;2:1557–64.

58. Boogerd W, Dorresteijn LD, van der Sande JJ, de Gast GC, Bruning PF. Response of leptomeningeal metastases from breast cancer to hormonal therapy. Neurology. 2000;55:117–9.

59. Zoghi B, Elledge R. Endocrine therapy for leptomeningeal metastases from ER-positive breast cancer: case report and a review of the literature. Breast J. 2016;22:218–23.

60. Chen IC, Lin CH, Jan IS, Cheng AL, Lu YS. Bevacizumab might potentiate the chemotherapeutic effect in breast cancer patients with leptomeningeal carcinomatosis. J Formos Med Assoc. 2016;115:243–8.

61. Wu PF, Lin CH, Kuo CH, Chen WW, Yeh DC, Liao HW, Huang SM, Cheng AL, Lu YS. A pilot study of bevacizumab combined with etoposide and cisplatin in breast cancer patients with leptomeningeal carcinomatosis. BMC Cancer. 2015;15:299.

62. Oechsle K, Lange-Brock V, Kruell A, Bokemeyer C, de Wit M. Prognostic factors and treatment options in patients with leptomeningeal metastases of different primary tumors: a retrospective analysis. J Cancer Res Clin Oncol. 2010;136:1729–35.

63. Sperduto PW, Yang TJ, Beal K, Pan H, Brown PD, Bangdiwala A, Shanley R, Yeh N, Gaspar LE, Braunstein S, Sneed P, Boyle J, Kirkpatrick JP, Mak KS, Shih HA, Engelman A, Roberge D, Arvold ND, Alexander B, Awad MM, Contessa J, Chiang V, Hardie J, Ma D, Lou E, Sperduto W, Mehta MP. The effect of gene alterations and tyrosine kinase inhibition on survival and cause of death in patients with adenocarcinoma of the lung and brain metastases. Int J Radiat Oncol Biol Phys. 2016;96:406–13.

64. Maemondo M, Inoue A, Kobayashi K, Sugawara S, Oizumi S, Isobe H, Gemma A, Harada M, Yoshizawa H, Kinoshita I, Fujita Y, Okinaga S, Hirano H, Yoshimori K, Harada T, Ogura T, Ando M, Miyazawa H, Tanaka T, Saijo Y, Hagiwara K, Morita S, Nukiwa T, North-East Japan Study Group. Gefitinib or chemotherapy for non-small-cell lung cancer with mutated EGFR. N Engl J Med. 2010;362:2380–8.

65. Mok TS, Wu YL, Thongprasert S, Yang CH, Chu DT, Saijo N, Sunpaweravong P, Han B, Margono B, Ichinose Y, Nishiwaki Y, Ohe Y, Yang JJ, Chewaskulyong B, Jiang H, Duffield EL, Watkins CL, Armour AA, Fukuoka M. Gefitinib or carboplatin-paclitaxel in pulmonary adenocarcinoma. N Engl J Med. 2009;361:947–57.

66. Di Lorenzo R, Ahluwalia MS. Targeted therapy of brain metastases: latest evidence and clinical implications. Ther Adv Med Oncol. 2017;9:781–96.

67. Jackman DM, Cioffredi LA, Jacobs L, Sharmeen F, Morse LK, Lucca J, Plotkin SR, Marcoux PJ, Rabin MS, Lynch TJ, Johnson BE, Kesari S. A phase I trial of high dose gefitinib for patients with leptomeningeal metastases from non-small cell lung cancer. Oncotarget. 2015;6:4527–36.

68. Lee Y, Han JY, Kim HT, Yun T, Lee GK, Kim HY, Lee JS. Impact of EGFR tyrosine kinase inhibitors versus chemotherapy on the development of leptomeningeal metastasis in never smokers with advanced adenocarcinoma of the lung. J Neuro-Oncol. 2013c;115:95–101.

69. Lee E, Keam B, Kim DW, Kim TM, Lee SH, Chung DH, Heo DS. Erlotinib versus gefitinib for control of leptomeningeal carcinomatosis in non-small-cell lung cancer. J Thorac Oncol. 2013a;8:1069–74.

70. Togashi Y, Masago K, Masuda S, Mizuno T, Fukudo M, Ikemi Y, Sakamori Y, Nagai H, Kim YH, Katsura T, Mishima M. Cerebrospinal fluid concentration of gefitinib and erlotinib in patients with non-small cell lung cancer. Cancer Chemother Pharmacol. 2012;70:399–405.

71. Kanemaru R, Morio Y, Takekawa H, Jo H, Kasuga F, Koyama R, Shiota S, Nagaoka T, Takahashi K. Successful treatment with weekly high-dose erlotinib against meningeal metastases from epidermal growth factor receptor (EGFR)-mutated lung adenocarcinoma. Respir Investig. 2016;54:372–5.

72. Kawamura T, Hata A, Takeshita J, Fujita S, Hayashi M, Tomii K, Katakami N. High-dose erlotinib for refractory leptomeningeal metastases after failure of standard-dose EGFR-TKIs. Cancer Chemother Pharmacol. 2015;75:1261–6.

73. Ballard P, Yates JW, Yang Z, Kim DW, Yang JC, Cantarini M, Pickup K, Jordan A, Hickey M, Grist M, Box M, Johnstrom P, Varnas K, Malmquist J, Thress KS, Janne PA, Cross D. Preclinical comparison of osimertinib with other EGFR-TKIs in EGFR-mutant NSCLC brain metastases models, and early evidence of clinical brain metastases activity. Clin Cancer Res. 2016;22:5130–40.

74. Mok TS, Wu YL, Ahn MJ, Garassino MC, Kim HR, Ramalingam SS, Shepherd FA, HE Y, Akamatsu H, Theelen WS, Lee CK, Sebastian M, Templeton A, Mann H, Marotti M, Ghiorghiu S, Papadimitrakopoulou VA, AURA3 Investigators. Osimertinib or platinum-pemetrexed in EGFR T790M-positive lung cancer. N Engl J Med. 2017;376:629–40.

75. Remon J, Le Rhun E, Besse B. Leptomeningeal carcinomatosis in non-small cell lung cancer patients: a continuing challenge in the personalized treatment era. Cancer Treat Rev. 2017;53:128–37.

76. Kwak EL, Bang YJ, Camidge DR, Shaw AT, Solomon B, Maki RG, Ou SH, Dezube BJ, Janne PA, Costa DB, Varella-Garcia M, Kim WH, Lynch TJ, Fidias P, Stubbs H, Engelman JA, Sequist LV, Tan W, Gandhi L, Mino-Kenudson M, Wei GC, Shreeve SM, Ratain MJ, Settleman J, Christensen JG, Haber DA, Wilner K, Salgia R, Shapiro GI, Clark JW, Iafrate AJ. Anaplastic lymphoma kinase inhibition in non-small-cell lung cancer. N Engl J Med. 2010;363:1693–703.

77. Shaw AT, Kim DW, Nakagawa K, Seto T, Crino L, Ahn MJ, de Pas T, Besse B, Solomon BJ, Blackhall F,

Wu YL, Thomas M, O'Byrne KJ, Moro-Sibilot D, Camidge DR, Mok T, Hirsh V, Riely GJ, Iyer S, Tassell V, Polli A, Wilner KD, Janne PA. Crizotinib versus chemotherapy in advanced ALK-positive lung cancer. N Engl J Med. 2013;368:2385–94.

78. Solomon BJ, Mok T, Kim DW, Wu YL, Nakagawa K, Mekhail T, Felip E, Cappuzzo F, Paolini J, Usari T, Iyer S, Reisman A, Wilner KD, Tursi J, Blackhall F, PROFILE 1014 Investigators. First-line crizotinib versus chemotherapy in ALK-positive lung cancer. N Engl J Med. 2014;371:2167–77.

79. Ou SH, Janne PA, Bartlett CH, Tang Y, Kim DW, Otterson GA, Crino L, Selaru P, Cohen DP, Clark JW, Riely GJ. Clinical benefit of continuing ALK inhibition with crizotinib beyond initial disease progression in patients with advanced ALK-positive NSCLC. Ann Oncol. 2014;25:415–22.

80. Kim DW, Mehra R, Tan DSW, Felip E, Chow LQM, Camidge DR, Vansteenkiste J, Sharma S, de Pas T, Riely GJ, Solomon BJ, Wolf J, Thomas M, Schuler M, Liu G, Santoro A, Sutradhar S, LI S, Szczudlo T, Yovine A, Shaw AT. Activity and safety of ceritinib in patients with ALK-rearranged non-small-cell lung cancer (ASCEND-1): updated results from the multicentre, open-label, phase 1 trial. Lancet Oncol. 2016;17:452–63.

81. Qian M, Zhu B, Wang X, Liebman M. Drug resistance in ALK-positiveNon-small cell lungcancer patients. Semin Cell Dev Biol. 2017;64:150–7.

82. Gainor JF, Chi AS, Logan J, Hu R, Oh KS, Brastianos PK, Shih HA, Shaw AT. Alectinib dose escalation reinduces central nervous system responses in patients with anaplastic lymphoma kinase-positive non-small cell lung cancer relapsing on standard dose alectinib. J Thorac Oncol. 2016;11:256–60.

83. Gainor JF, Sherman CA, Willoughby K, Logan J, Kennedy E, Brastianos PK, Chi AS, Shaw AT. Alectinib salvages CNS relapses in ALK-positive lung cancer patients previously treated with crizotinib and ceritinib. J Thorac Oncol. 2015;10:232–6.

84. Sakata Y, Kawamura K, Shingu N, Ichikado K. Erlotinib plus bevacizumab as an effective treatment for leptomeningeal metastases from EGFR mutation-positive non-small cell lung cancer. Lung Cancer. 2016;99:120–2.

85. Sloot S, Chen YA, Zhao X, Weber JL, Benedict JJ, Mule JJ, Smalley KS, Weber JS, Zager JS, Forsyth PA, Sondak VK, Gibney GT. Improved survival of patients with melanoma brain metastases in the era of targeted BRAF and immune checkpoint therapies. Cancer. 2018;124:297–305.

86. Bollag G, Hirth P, Tsai J, Zhang J, Ibrahim PN, Cho H, Spevak W, Zhang C, Zhang Y, Habets G, Burton EA, Wong B, Tsang G, West BL, Powell B, Shellooe R, Marimuthu A, Nguyen H, Zhang KY, Artis DR, Schlessinger J, Su F, Higgins B, Iyer R, D'Andrea K, Koehler A, Stumm M, Lin PS, Lee RJ, Grippo J, Puzanov I, Kim KB, Ribas A, Mcarthur GA, Sosman JA, Chapman PB, Flaherty KT, Xu X, Nathanson KL, Nolop K. Clinical efficacy of a RAF inhibitor needs broad target blockade in BRAF-mutant melanoma. Nature. 2010;467:596–9.

87. Flaherty KT, Puzanov I, Kim KB, Ribas A, Mcarthur GA, Sosman JA, O'Dwyer PJ, Lee RJ, Grippo JF, Nolop K, Chapman PB. Inhibition of mutated, activated BRAF in metastatic melanoma. N Engl J Med. 2010;363:809–19.

88. King AJ, Arnone MR, Bleam MR, Moss KG, Yang J, Fedorowicz KE, Smitheman KN, Erhardt JA, Hughes-Earle A, Kane-Carson LS, Sinnamon RH, Qi H, Rheault TR, Uehling DE, Laquerre SG. Dabrafenib; preclinical characterization, increased efficacy when combined with trametinib, while BRAF/MEK tool combination reduced skin lesions. PLoS One. 2013;8:e67583.

89. Tsai J, Lee JT, Wang W, Zhang J, Cho H, Mamo S, Bremer R, Gillette S, Kong J, Haass NK, Sproesser K, Li L, Smalley KS, Fong D, Zhu YL, Marimuthu A, Nguyen H, Lam B, Liu J, Cheung I, Rice J, Suzuki Y, Luu C, Settachatgul C, Shellooe R, Cantwell J, Kim SH, Schlessinger J, Zhang KY, West BL, Powell B, Habets G, Zhang C, Ibrahim PN, Hirth P, Artis DR, Herlyn M, Bollag G. Discovery of a selective inhibitor of oncogenic B-Raf kinase with potent antimelanoma activity. Proc Natl Acad Sci USA. 2008;105:3041–6.

90. Long GV, Trefzer U, Davies MA, Kefford RF, Ascierto PA, Chapman PB, Puzanov I, Hauschild A, Robert C, Algazi A, Mortier L, Tawbi H, Wilhelm T, Zimmer L, Switzky J, Swann S, Martin AM, Guckert M, Goodman V, Streit M, Kirkwood JM, Schadendorf D. Dabrafenib in patients with Val600Glu or Val600Lys BRAF-mutant melanoma metastatic to the brain (BREAK-MB): a multicentre, open-label, phase 2 trial. Lancet Oncol. 2012;13:1087–95.

91. Mcarthur GA, Maio M, Arance A, Nathan P, Blank C, Avril MF, Garbe C, Hauschild A, Schadendorf D, Hamid O, Fluck M, Thebeau M, Schachter J, Kefford R, Chamberlain M, Makrutzki M, Robson S, Gonzalez R, Margolin K. Vemurafenib in metastatic melanoma patients with brain metastases: an open-label, single-arm, phase 2, multicentre study. Ann Oncol. 2017;28:634–41.

92. Davies MA, Saiag P, Robert C, Grob JJ, Flaherty KT, Arance A, Chiarion-Sileni V, Thomas L, Lesimple T, Mortier L, Moschos SJ, Hogg D, Marquez-Rodas I, Del Vecchio M, Lebbe C, Meyer N, Zhang Y, Huang Y, Mookerjee B, Long GV. Dabrafenib plus trametinib in patients with BRAF(V600)-mutant melanoma brain metastases (COMBI-MB): a multicentre, multicohort, open-label, phase 2 trial. Lancet Oncol. 2017;18:863–73.

93. Lee JM, Mehta UN, Dsouza LH, Guadagnolo BA, Sanders DL, Kim KB. Long-term stabilization of leptomeningeal disease with whole-brain radiation therapy in a patient with metastatic melanoma treated with vemurafenib: a case report. Melanoma Res. 2013b;23:175–8.

94. Schafer N, Scheffler B, Stuplich M, Schaub C, Kebir S, Rehkamper C, Mack F, Niehusmann P, Simon M, Greschus S, Kuchelmeister K, Herrlinger U, Glas M. Vemurafenib for leptomeningeal melanomatosis. J Clin Oncol. 2013;31:e173–4.

95. Wilgenhof S, Neyns B. Complete cytologic remission of V600E BRAF-mutant melanoma-associated leptomeningeal carcinomatosis upon treatment with dabrafenib. J Clin Oncol. 2015;33:e109–11.

96. Kim T, Amaria RN, Spencer C, Reuben A, Cooper ZA, Wargo JA. Combining targeted therapy and immune checkpoint inhibitors in the treatment of metastatic melanoma. Cancer Biol Med. 2014;11:237–46.

97. Smalley KS, Fedorenko IV, Kenchappa RS, Sahebjam S, Forsyth PA. Managing leptomeningeal melanoma metastases in the era of immune and targeted therapy. Int J Cancer. 2016;139:1195–201.

98. Clemons-Miller AR, Chatta GS, Hutchins L, Angtuaco EJ, Ravaggi A, Santin AD, Cannon MJ. Intrathecal cytotoxic T-cell immunotherapy for metastatic leptomeningeal melanoma. Clin Cancer Res. 2001;7:917s–24s.

99. Glitza IC, Haymaker C, Bernatchez C, Vence L, Rohlfs M, Richard J, Lacey C, Mansaray R, Fulbright OJ, Ramachandran R, Toth C, Wardell S, Patel SP, Woodman SE, Hwu WJ, Radvanyi LG, Davies MA, Papadopoulos NE, Hwu P. Intrathecal administration of tumor-infiltrating lymphocytes is well tolerated in a patient with leptomeningeal disease from metastatic melanoma: a case report. Cancer Immunol Res. 2015;3:1201–6.

100. Bot I, Blank CU, Brandsma D. Clinical and radiological response of leptomeningeal melanoma after whole brain radiotherapy and ipilimumab. J Neurol. 2012;259:1976–8.

101. Orlando L, Curigliano G, Colleoni M, Fazio N, Nole F, Martinelli G, Cinieri S, Graffeo R, Peruzzotti G, Goldhirsch A. Intrathecal chemotherapy in carcinomatous meningitis from breast cancer. Anticancer Res. 2002;22:3057–9.

102. Boogerd W, Hart AA, van der Sande JJ, Engelsman E. Meningeal carcinomatosis in breast cancer. Prognostic factors and influence of treatment. Cancer. 1991;67:1685–95.

103. Fizazi K, Asselain B, Vincent-Salomon A, Jouve M, Dieras V, Palangie T, Beuzeboc P, Dorval T, Pouillart P. Meningeal carcinomatosis in patients with breast carcinoma. Clinical features, prognostic factors, and results of a high-dose intrathecal methotrexate regimen. Cancer. 1996;77:1315–23.

104. Gauthier H, Guilhaume MN, Bidard FC, Pierga JY, Girre V, Cottu PH, Laurence V, Livartowski A, Mignot L, Dieras V. Survival of breast cancer patients with meningeal carcinomatosis. Ann Oncol. 2010;21:2183–7.

105. Lara-Medina F, Crismatt A, Villarreal-Garza C, Alvarado-Miranda A, Flores-Hernandez L, Gonzalez-Pinedo M, Gamboa-Vignolle C, Ruiz-Gonzalez JD, Arrieta O. Clinical features and prognostic factors in patients with carcinomatous meningitis secondary to breast cancer. Breast J. 2012;18:233–41.

106. Mego M, Sycova-Mila Z, Obertova J, Rajec J, Liskova S, Palacka P, Porsok S, Mardiak J. Intrathecal administration of trastuzumab with cytarabine and methotrexate in breast cancer patients with leptomeningeal carcinomatosis. Breast. 2011;20:478–80.

107. Salgia S, Fleming GF, Lukas RV. Leptomeningeal carcinomatosis from breast cancer treated with intrathecal topotecan with concomitant intravenous eribulin. J Clin Neurosci. 2014;21:1250–1.

108. Ferrario C, Davidson A, Bouganim N, Aloyz R, Panasci LC. Intrathecal trastuzumab and thiotepa for leptomeningeal spread of breast cancer. Ann Oncol. 2009;20:792–5.

109. Groves MD, Glantz MJ, Chamberlain MC, Baumgartner KE, Conrad CA, Hsu S, Wefel JS, Gilbert MR, Ictech S, Hunter KU, Forman AD, Puduvalli VK, Colman H, Hess KR, Yung WK. A multicenter phase II trial of intrathecal topotecan in patients with meningeal malignancies. Neuro-Oncology. 2008;10:208–15.

110. Walker J, Schultz D, Grisdale K, Groves M. Intraventricular topotecan for the treatment of neoplastic meningitis: five case studies. J Adv Pract Oncol. 2012;3:237–41.

111. Mir O, Ropert S, Alexandre J, Lemare F, Goldwasser F. High-dose intrathecal trastuzumab for leptomeningeal metastases secondary to HER-2 overexpressing breast cancer. Ann Oncol. 2008;19:1978–80.

112. Oliveira M, Braga S, Passos-Coelho JL, Fonseca R, Oliveira J. Complete response in HER2+ leptomeningeal carcinomatosis from breast cancer with intrathecal trastuzumab. Breast Cancer Res Treat. 2011;127:841–4.

113. Pan Z, Yang G, He H, Zhao G, Yuan T, Li Y, Shi W, Gao P, Dong L, Li Y. Concurrent radiotherapy and intrathecal methotrexate for treating leptomeningeal metastasis from solid tumors with adverse prognostic factors: a prospective and single-arm study. Int J Cancer. 2016;139:1864–72.

114. Mix M, Elmarzouky R, O'Connor T, Plunkett R, Prasad D. Clinical outcomes in patients with brain metastases from breast cancer treated with single-session radiosurgery or whole brain radiotherapy. J Neurosurg. 2016;125:26–30.

115. Mulvenna P, Nankivell M, Barton R, Faivre-Finn C, Wilson P, Mccoll E, Moore B, Brisbane I, Ardron D, Holt T, Morgan S, Lee C, Waite K, Bayman N, Pugh C, Sydes B, Stephens R, Parmar MK, Langley RE. Dexamethasone and supportive care with or without whole brain radiotherapy in treating patients with non-small cell lung cancer with brain metastases unsuitable for resection or stereotactic radiotherapy (QUARTZ): results from a phase 3, non-inferiority, randomised trial. Lancet. 2016;388:2004–14.

116. Chamberlain MC. Leptomeningeal metastases: a review of evaluation and treatment. J Neuro-Oncol. 1998a;37:271–84.

117. Scott BJ, Oberheim-Bush NA, Kesari S. Leptomeningeal metastasis in breast cancer – a systematic review. Oncotarget. 2016;7:3740–7.

118. Abouharb S, Ensor J, Loghin ME, Katz R, Moulder SL, Esteva FJ, Smith B, Valero V, Hortobagyi GN, Melhem-Bertrandt A. Leptomeningeal disease and breast cancer: the importance of tumor subtype. Breast Cancer Res Treat. 2014;146:477–86.

119. Goldberg SB, Gettinger SN, Mahajan A, Chiang AC, Herbst RS, Sznol M, Tsiouris AJ, Cohen J, Vortmeyer A, Jilaveanu L, Yu J, Hegde U, Speaker S, Madura M, Ralabate A, Rivera A, Rowen E, Gerrish H, Yao X, Chiang V, Kluger HM. Pembrolizumab for patients with melanoma or non-small-cell lung cancer and untreated brain metastases: early analysis of a non-randomised, open-label, phase 2 trial. Lancet Oncol. 2016;17:976–83.

120. Niwinska A, Rudnicka H, Murawska M. Breast cancer leptomeningeal metastasis: propensity of breast cancer subtypes for leptomeninges and the analysis of factors influencing survival. Med Oncol. 2013;30:408.

121. Niwinska A, Rudnicka H, Murawska M. Breast cancer leptomeningeal metastasis: the results of combined treatment and the comparison of methotrexate and liposomal cytarabine as intra-cerebrospinal fluid chemotherapy. Clin Breast Cancer. 2015;15:66–72.

122. Olar A, Wani KM, Alfaro-Munoz KD, Heathcock LE, van Thuijl HF, Gilbert MR, Armstrong TS, Sulman EP, Cahill DP, Vera-Bolanos E, Yuan Y, Reijneveld JC, Ylstra B, Wesseling P, Aldape KD. IDH mutation status and role of WHO grade and mitotic index in overall survival in grade II-III diffuse gliomas. Acta Neuropathol. 2015;129:585–96.

Metastatic Spinal Cord Compression

29

John W. Crommett

Contents

Introduction 430

Epidemiology 430

Pathophysiology 430

Clinical Presentation 430

Diagnosis 431
History and Physical Examination 431
Imaging 431
Tissue Diagnosis 431

Management Options 432
Initial Care 432
Assessment of Spinal Stability 432
Pharmacological Treatments 432
Radiation Therapy 432
Surgical Management 433
Prognosis 433

References 433

Abstract

Metastatic spinal cord compression is a medical emergency characterized by its potential for rapid deterioration of neurological function, often leading to significant impairments in quality of life. The most common mechanism is growth of a vertebral metastatic lesion with invasion of the epidural space and compression of the spinal cord. Patients commonly present with progressive pain and may later develop motor and sensory weakness, and autonomic dysfunction. The preferred imaging study is an MRI of the entire spine, which should be performed urgently. In patients without known malignancy, tissue diagnosis through biopsy as well as evaluation for primary site of disease and other metastases is necessary. Initial management includes steroids and analgesics. Treatment options include radiation and surgical decompression, and considerations include tissue type, an assessment of spinal stability,

J. W. Crommett (✉)
Department of Critical Care Medicine, The University of Texas M.D. Anderson Cancer Center, Houston, TX, USA
e-mail: jwcrommett@mdanderson.org

and performance status. Patients with metastatic spinal cord compression should be managed at centers capable of providing specialized treatment including radiation oncology and neurosurgery.

Keywords

Metastatic spinal cord compression · Vertebral metastasis · Intramedullary · Corticosteroids · Dexamethasone · Magnetic resonance imaging · Surgical decompression · Stereotactic radiation · Cancer · Radiotherapy · Tetraplegia · Paraplegia

Introduction

Metastatic spinal cord compression is a medical emergency due to the strong potential for progression to tetraplegia or paraplegia if left untreated. This syndrome was described in detail by Dr. Charles Elsberg in a 1916 monograph, in which he stated that "more than 50% of all malignant tumors of the vertebrae are secondary to carcinomas of the breast" [9]. Spinal cord compression was also described in the medical literature by Dr. William Gibson Spiller 1925 as "rapidly progressive paralysis associated with carcinoma" [32]. Spinal cord compression is one of the most devastating complications of malignancies, leading to significant changes in quality of life and to associated comorbidities, including premature death. Early recognition, evaluation, and treatment may limit the extent of morbidity. Metastatic spinal cord compression is most commonly caused by compression of the dural sac and spinal cord from an extradural metastatic tumor, though direct extension by adjacent primary or metastatic disease, or extension from subdural or intramedullary metastases may occur [22].

Epidemiology

Approximately 60–70% of lesions associated with spinal cord compression occur in the thoracic vertebral bodies, with 20–30% occurring in the lumbar and sacral regions, and 10–15% occurring in the cervical spine ([3, 8]). Overall, approximately 5% of all cancer patients will develop cord compression,

with an additional 5% having undiagnosed cord compression at autopsy [3]. Between 45% and 61% of cases of metastatic spinal cord compression occur in patients with primary breast, lung, or prostate cancer; other malignancies commonly associated with this syndrome include renal cell carcinoma, multiple myeloma, colorectal carcinoma, sarcoma, lymphoma, and tumors of unknown primary [24, 25, 35]. It may occur in any malignancy, however. Spinal metastasis with cord compression may also occur as the initial manifestation of disease, though it is more commonly present in patients with disseminated disease [8].

Pathophysiology

There are two proposed mechanisms by which most metastatic tumors reach the epidural space. The most common mechanism involves hematogenous spread to the posterior portion of the vertebral body, where the metastasis grows in the bone, spreads to the epidural space, and leads to compression of the spinal cord [1]. The hematogenous spread has most recently been attributed to arterial tumor embolization rather than spread via Batson's venous plexus, but both theories are still prevalent in the literature [2, 4, 6]. The other, less common mechanism is direct extension of a paravertebral tumor into the spinal canal via an intervertebral foramen. This process is more common in lymphoma, Pancoast's tumor of the lung, and neuroblastoma [11]. Once the metastatic lesion has been established in the region, damage to the cord results from direct compression, leading to vascular compromise and axonal damage, which causes edema and stimulus of local inflammation, further inhibiting perfusion. Infarction of the cord with irreversible damage results from this process [18, 33].

Clinical Presentation

Back pain is the most common and earliest symptom in patients ultimately found to have metastatic spinal cord compression. It typically precedes the diagnosis by 2–5 months and affects 95% of patients [11, 16]. The back pain is commonly described as progressive and exacerbated by coughing, bending over, or sneezing, possibly awakening the patient from sleep. Radicular pain may also develop and is associated with nerve root involvement [16]. Vertebral body collapse may occur and is often associated with mechanical back pain, which is typically exacerbated by movement, and alleviated partially by lying still [5]. Intractable severe pain is often associated with lung metastasis [27].

Weakness is another common symptom at presentation, which may be described by patients more as "heaviness in legs," or "clumsiness," and the examiner discovers motor weakness. Approximately 60–85% of patients have weakness at the time of diagnosis, approximately two-thirds of whom are nonambulatory [13, 14].

Sensory deficits are also noted in a majority of patients at the time of diagnosis. These deficits typically start distally and ascend as the disease progresses. Autonomic dysfunction typically occurs later in the disease course and may be manifested by bladder or bowel dysfunction with urinary retention [7, 13].

Diagnosis

History and Physical Examination

When a cancer patient presents with back pain, clinicians should have a high index of suspicion for metastatic disease as a potential cause. A careful history and neurological examination will help elicit evidence of spinal cord compression, such as motor or sensory deficits. If these findings are present, an expedient workup is appropriate, as this is considered an acute oncologic emergency. The differential diagnosis, even in patients with cancer, includes degenerative spine disease, transverse myelitis, epidural hematoma, paraneoplastic syndromes, B_{12} deficiency, and radiation- or chemotherapy-induced myelopathies, and these potential etiologies must also be considered.

Imaging

Plain radiographs are often ordered, and have some clinical utility, but have limited overall clinical utility. Compression fractures may be noted,

and pedicle thinning, widening of the neural foramina, osteolytic or sclerotic lesions, and erosion of the margins of the spinal canal may be seen, providing evidence for metastatic disease that may be associated with cord compression [12, 26]. They are falsely negative in 10–17% of cases, however [3]. As a result, a large prospective study revealed that plain radiographs did not have enough predictive value to support the routine use [19]. Skeletal surveys with plain radiographs may still be quite useful, however, in patients with multiple myeloma.

Magnetic resonance imaging (MRI) is the first test usually ordered in a clinical scenario that is suggestive of spinal cord compression, and ideally, it should be performed within 24 hours. Studies have shown MRI to be superior to clinical examination plus plain radiographs [15]. The whole spine is usually evaluated, not just the symptomatic region, due to the high incidence of multiple spine metastases in these patients, and such findings would alter treatment plans for radiation or surgery [15]. Any indentation of the thecal sac in the region of symptoms is consistent with the diagnosis of spinal cord compression. MRI can be quite useful in ruling out cancer as the cause of a patient's symptoms due to the high specificity (97%) [21].

Computed tomography (CT), with or without myelography, is an appropriate test when MRI cannot be obtained, either due to lack of availability or due to a contraindication such as pacemaker, shrapnel, or patient size. It is also the preferred imaging modality for guided percutaneous biopsies [8].

Tissue Diagnosis

Obtaining tissue for diagnosis is crucial for patients without a known malignant diagnosis who present with cord compression from tumor. As above, CT-guided percutaneous biopsy of the spine lesion is usually recommended, though if early surgical decompression is planned, a histologic sample can be obtained as part of the procedure. Biopsy may also be indicated in patients with potentially more than one tumor type. Patients without a known malignant diagnosis at presentation will also require CT scans of the chest, abdomen, and pelvis in addition to routine blood counts and metabolic studies.

Management Options

Initial Care

Patients with suspected spinal cord compression should be initially managed as if they have spinal instability, and as such, the spine should be maintained in neutral alignment. They should be turned as a single unit (log-rolled) and the neck should not be flexed or extended in the event endotracheal intubation is required. These patients should also be transferred as soon as possible, in a safe, controlled manner, to a center that can provide specialized treatment, which includes having an available neurosurgeon and the capability to provide radiation therapy.

Assessment of Spinal Stability

Various algorithms have been developed for the management of epidural spinal cord compression, and the essential first step is to assess spinal stability. This assessment must be balanced by the patient's performance status, severity of other illnesses, and life expectancy. An MRI of the entire spine is the appropriate imaging study for assessing spinal stability. The classic definition of spinal instability was established by Panjabi and White: "the loss of the ability of the spine under physiologic loads to maintain relationships between the vertebrae in such a way that there is neither damage nor subsequent irritation to the spinal cord or nerve roots and, in addition, there is no development of incapacitating deformity or pain due to structural changes" [28]. If imaging reveals retropulsion of bone fragments into the spinal cord, then emergent surgical decompression and fixation is recommended. If unstable, but without retropulsed bony fragments, then consideration should be given to the radiosensitivity of the primary malignancy and previous radiation in the area. Typically radioresistant tumors

include renal cell, melanoma, sarcoma, non-small cell lung, and gastrointestinal malignancies. In these circumstances, or if previously irradiated, surgical decompression and fixation is also recommended, though stereotactic radiation may be an effective option. If the tumor is radiosensitive (myeloma, lymphoma, breast, ovary, prostate, small cell lung, germ cell tumors), then spine stabilization followed by external beam irradiation may be appropriate. In patients without spinal instability, the decision point considers radiosensitivity of the primary tumor and previous irradiation. If sensitive and no prior irradiation, then external beam irradiation is recommended, while stereotactic irradiation may be an option for radioresistant tumors and for those with prior external beam irradiation [23].

Pharmacological Treatments

Pain is often severe and usually requires narcotic analgesics. These should be used along with an effective bowel regimen, as constipation may be a consequence of the spinal cord dysfunction in addition to an opioid side effect. Corticosteroids are an important component of the treatment of metastatic spinal cord compression and may improve pain as well as spinal cord edema [33]. Dexamethasone is the preferred steroid, as it has been shown to increase the ambulatory period after diagnoses of metastatic spinal cord compression [31]. The dose of dexamethasone varies widely in the literature. Most agree that higher doses are associated with serious side effects of their use.

Radiation Therapy

Radiation therapy has long been the primary treatment for metastatic spinal cord compression. It can be effective in controlling both pain and neurological dysfunction [29]. The average time from initiation of radiotherapy to initial pain relief is about 2 weeks [17]. It is usually well-tolerated, though when the gastrointestinal tract is within the treatment field, mucositis may be an issue [30]. If the tumor is radiosensitive, then external beam irradiation is effective, though patients with multiple spinal metastases have shorter survival. Radioresistant tumors, such as sarcoma, renal cell, and melanoma may still benefit, with some palliation, but significant neurological improvement and long-lasting responses are unlikely. Stereotactic body radiotherapy is a newer option at specialized facilities and can achieve local control of disease without damage to the spinal cord, even in some patients with resistance to conventional radiation therapy [20, 30].

Surgical Management

The goals of surgical treatment of metastatic spinal cord compression are to provide prompt decompression of the spinal cord and to establish spinal stability, while avoiding further neurological deterioration. Many patients with spinal metastases have limited life expectancy, poor performance status, and other comorbidities, and this should be taken into consideration when planning surgical procedures [34]. In general terms, laminectomy alone should only be performed for isolated epidural metastases without spinal instability. In cases where metastases involve the vertebral body or otherwise affect stability, then posterior decompression with internal fixation should be performed.

For patients who undergo surgical decompression for metastatic spinal cord compression, postoperative radiotherapy should be considered as well. Patients who are ambulatory but with poor prognosis factors for successful radiotherapy and a reasonable survival expectancy may also be good candidates for decompressive surgery [10].

Prognosis

The prognosis for patients with metastatic spinal cord compression is overall poor. Many of these patients will have disseminated neoplastic disease, and the myelopathy represents a natural progression. The goals of care are usually palliative in nature, and steroids and opioid analgesics may provide short-

term relief. Despite the overall dismal outlook, early recognition and appropriate interventions may improve survival and almost certainly will improve a patient's quality of life. If the spine is unstable, surgical decompression and stabilization may be useful, though radiation therapy is the preferred treatment modality. Consideration should be given to stereotactic body radiation at experienced treatment centers, even for those patients with prior radiation, or radioresistant tumors.

References

1. Algra P, Heimans J, Valk J, Nauta J, Lachniet M, Van Kooten B. Do metastases in vertebrae begin in the body or pedicles? Imaging study in 45 patients. Am J Roentgenol. 1992;158(6):1275–9.
2. Arguello F, Duerst R, McQueen K, Frantz C, Baggs R, Johnstone L. Pathogenesis of vertebral metastases and epidural spinal cord compression. Cancer. 1990;65: 98–106.
3. Bach F, Larsen B, Rhode K, Borgesen S, Gjerris F, Boge-Rasmussen T, Agerlin N, Rasmusson B, Stjernholm P, Sorensen P. Metastatic spinal cord compression. Occurrence, symptoms, clinical presentations and prognosis in 398 patients with spinal cord compression. Acta Neurochir. 1990;107(1–2):37–43.
4. Batson O. The function of the vertebral veins and their role in the spread of metastases. Ann Surg. 1940;112(1):138–49.
5. Cole J, Patchell R. Metastatic epidural spinal cord compression. Lancet Neurol. 2008;7(5):459–66.
6. Coman D, Delong R. The role of the vertebral venous system in the metastasis of cancer to the spinal column. Experiments with tumor-cell suspensions in rats and rabbits. Cancer. 1951;4(3):610–8.
7. Constans J, de Divitiis E, Donzelli R, Spaziante R, Meder J, Haye C. Spinal metastases with neurological manifestations. J Neurosurg. 1983;59(1):111–8.
8. Desforges J, Byrne T. Spinal cord compression from epidural metastases. N Engl J Med. 1992;327(9): 614–9.
9. Elsberg C. Diseases of the spinal cord and membranes. Philadelphia: Saunders; 1916. p. 236–42.
10. George R, Jeba J, Ramkumar G, Chacko A, Tharyan P. Interventions for the treatment of metastatic extradural spinal cord compression in adults. Cochrane Database Syst Rev. 2015;4:1–30.
11. Gilbert R, Kim J, Posner J. Epidural spinal cord compression from metastatic tumor: diagnosis and treatment. Ann Neurol. 1978;3(1):40–51.
12. Graus F, Krol G, Foley K. Early diagnosis of spinal epidural metastases (SEM): correlation with clinical and radiographic findings. Proc Am Soc Clin Oncol. 1985;4(1):269.

13. Helweg-Larsen S, Sørensen P. Symptoms and signs in metastatic spinal cord compression: a study of progression from first symptom until diagnosis in 153 patients. Eur J Cancer. 1994;30(3):396–8.

14. Husband D. Malignant spinal cord compression: prospective study of delays in referral and treatment. BMJ. 1998;317(7150):18–21.

15. Husband D, Grant K, Romaniuk C. MRI in the diagnosis and treatment of suspected malignant spinal cord compression. Br J Radiol. 2001;74(877):15–23.

16. Jacobs W, Perrin R. Evaluation and treatment of spinal metastases: an overview. Neurosurg Focus. 2001;11(6):1–11.

17. Jennelle R, Vijayakumar V, Vijayakumar S. A systematic and evidence-based approach to the management of vertebral metastasis. ISRN Surg. 2011;2011:1–6.

18. Kato A, Ushio Y, Hayakawa T, Yamada K, Ikeda H, Mogami H. Circulatory disturbance of the spinal cord with epidural neoplasm in rats. J Neurosurg. 1985;63(2):260–5.

19. Kienstra G, Terwee C, Dekker F, Canta L, Borstlap A, Tijssen C, Bosch D, Tijssen J. Prediction of spinal epidural metastases. Arch Neurol. 2000;57(5):690.

20. Klimo P, Thompson C, Kestle J, Schmidt M. A meta-analysis of surgery versus conventional radiotherapy for the treatment of metastatic spinal epidural disease. Neuro-Oncology. 2005;7(1):64–76.

21. Li K, Poon P. Sensitivity and specificity of MRI in detecting malignant spinal cord compression and in distinguishing malignant from benign compression fractures of vertebrae. Magn Reson Imaging. 1988;6(5):547–56.

22. Lin A, Avila E. Neurologic emergencies in the patients with Cancer. J Intensive Care Med. 2016;32(2):99–115.

23. Lo S, Ryu S, Chang E, Galanopoulos N, Jones J, Kim E, Kubicky C, Lee C, Rose P, Sahgal A, Sloan A, Teh B, Traughber B, Van Poznak C, Vassil A. ACR appropriateness criteria® metastatic epidural spinal cord compression and recurrent spinal metastasis. J Palliat Med. 2015;18(7):573–84.

24. Loblaw D. A population-based study of malignant spinal cord compression in Ontario. Clin Oncol. 2003;15(4):211–7.

25. Maranzano E, Latini P, Checcaglini F, Ricci S, Panizza B, Aristei C, Perrucci E, Beneventi S, Corgna E, Tonato M. Radiation therapy in metastatic spinal cord compression. A prospective analysis of 105 consecutive patients. Cancer. 1991;67(5):1311–7.

26. Olcott E, Dillon W. Plain film clues to the diagnosis of spinal epidural neoplasm and infection. Neuroradiology. 1993;35(4):288–92.

27. Onimus M, Papin P, Gangloff S. Results of surgical treatment of spinal thoracic and lumbar metastases. Eur Spine J. 1996;5(6):407–11.

28. Panjabi M, White A. Basic biomechanics of the spine. Neurosurgery. 1980;7(1):76–93.

29. Rades D, Rudat V, Veninga T, Stalpers L, Basic H, Karstens J, Hoskin P, Schild S. A score predicting posttreatment ambulatory status in patients irradiated for metastatic spinal cord compression. Int J Radiat Oncol Biol Phys. 2008;72(3):905–8.

30. Sahgal A, Larson D, Chang E. Stereotactic body radiosurgery for spinal metastases: a critical review. Int J Radiat Oncol Biol Phys. 2008;71(3):652–5.

31. Sørensen P, Helweg-Larsen S, Mouridsen H, Hansen H. Effect of high-dose dexamethasone in carcinomatous metastatic spinal cord compression treated with radiotherapy: a randomized trial. Eur J Cancer. 1994;30(1):22–7.

32. Spiller W. Rapidly progressive paralysis associated with carcinoma. Arch Neurol Psychiatr. 1925;13(1):471–7.

33. Ushio Y, Posner R, Posner J, Shapiro W. Experimental spinal cord compression by epidural neoplasms. Neurology. 1977;27(5):422–9.

34. Van der Linden Y, Dijkstra S, Vonk E, Marijnen C, Leer J. Prediction of survival in patients with metastases in the spinal column. Cancer. 2005;103(2):320–8.

35. Wong D, Fornasier V, MacNab I. Spinal metastases: the obvious, the occult, and the impostors. Spine. 1990;15(1):1–4.

Frequent Central Nervous System (CNS) Infections in the Immunosuppressed Patient

30

Rafael Araos and Grecia Aldana

Contents

Introduction 436

Epidemiology 436

Classification 436

Clinical Presentation 437

Diagnosis 438

Treatment 440

References 441

Abstract

Infections of the central nervous system among immunocompromised patients are of major clinical relevance due to the high morbidity and mortality they convey.

The clinical approach to central nervous system (CNS) infections is based on keeping a low threshold of suspicion and recognizing the classic clinical syndromes together with the particularities that occur in immunocompromised patients: subacute onset, subtle and overlapped clinical presentation, and the presence of opportunistic agents in addition to traditional pathogens and sometimes the presence of more than one infectious agent.

The etiologic study should be oriented according to the clinical presentation syndrome and the underlying immunodepression model. Imaging studies should always be performed, and the cerebrospinal fluid should be analyzed. Finally, and particularly in the case of brain lesions with mass effect, early tissue collection should be considered.

The treatment has to be directed to agents related to the clinical syndrome and the underlying immune defect model identified. The timely initiation of empirical antimicrobials is warranted, and it should include broad-spectrum antimicrobials with adequate

R. Araos (✉)
Genomics and Resistant Microbes (GeRM) Lab, Facultad de Medicina Clínica Alemana Universidad del Desarrollo, Millennium Nucleus for Collaborative Research on Bacterial Resistance (MICROB-R), Santiago, Chile
e-mail: rafaelaraos@udd.cl

G. Aldana
Department of Pulmonary Medicine, The University of Texas MD Anderson Cancer Center, Houston, TX, USA
e-mail: glaldana@mdanderson.org

© Springer Nature Switzerland AG 2020
J. L. Nates, K. J. Price (eds.), *Oncologic Critical Care*,
https://doi.org/10.1007/978-3-319-74588-6_39

penetration to the central nervous system. Finally, the availability of adjunctive therapies to antimicrobials that may have additional utility in particular cases (e.g., corticoids in the case of pneumococcal meningitis) should be taken into account.

Keywords

Infection · Immunosuppression · CNS · Meningitis · Encephalitis

Introduction

Infections of the central nervous system (CNS) have unique characteristics that give them great clinical importance, especially in patients with some degree of immunocompromise. Although these are rare infections among the general population, in immunocompromised patients they occur more frequently, pose critical diagnostic challenges, and are associated with heightened morbidity and mortality. In particular, hematological neoplasms represent the most relevant group because they determine immunodeficiency states by itself, which are usually exacerbated and prolonged by their treatments. Patients with myelodysplastic syndromes and acute leukemias and those undergoing allogeneic hematopoietic stem cell transplants (HSCT) present models of immunocompromise that affect all compartments of innate and acquired immunity. This leaves these patients susceptible to a wide range of infectious agents, including both classic and opportunistic pathogens, either due to reactivation of latent infections or infections acquired de novo.

Epidemiology

There is a scarcity of data reporting the frequency of infectious complications of the CNS in immunocompromised patients. Although its general occurrence is uncommon, patients with hematological conditions have a notably higher burden of disease. In this patient group, the incidence of CNS infection can be as high as 15%, particularly during early stages after HSCT or during prolonged neutropenic episodes following chemotherapy [8]. A recent study from Japan showed that most CNS infection episodes occur within the first year after HSCT. In this study, the reported 1-year cumulative incidence of CNS infection among HSCT recipients was 4.1%, with a 5-year cumulative incidence of 5.5% [5]. In the absence of specific risk factors for bacterial infections such as invasive CNS procedures or devices, the epidemiology of bacterial infections of the CNS follows similar patterns when compared to the general population. Bacterial meningitis is the most common CNS syndrome among immunocompromised patients with differing incidences reaching up to 40 cases/100,000 patients per year among HSCT recipients [10]. Similar to other populations, *Streptococcus pneumoniae* is the most common etiologic agent of bacterial meningitis; less common agents such as *Listeria monocytogenes* and Gram-negative bacilli are also relevant among the immunocompromised host. Non-bacterial agents vary according to the type of underlying disease and the mechanism of associated immunosuppression, but in general infections caused by parasites such as *Toxoplasma gondii* and fungi such as *Cryptococcus* spp. and *Aspergillus* spp. explain most of the cases [8]. Finally, it is necessary to consider the geographic origin of each patient since the history of potential exposures influences the individual risk of presenting specific infections such as tuberculosis and endemic fungi (*Coccidioides* spp., *Paracoccidioides* spp., and *Histoplasma capsulatum*, among others) [14].

Classification

From a practical perspective, CNS infections in immunocompromised patients can be classified following the same factors that are usually considered among immunocompetent individuals. According to the predominantly compromised anatomical structure, it is possible to distinguish four syndromes that have different diagnostic and therapeutic approaches: (i) meningitis, (ii) meningoencephalitis, (iii) encephalitis, and (iv) focal lesions with or without mass effect.

Additionally, once the clinical syndrome has been identified, an effort must be made to identify the predominant underlying immunological defect, since this information allows the clinician to consider infectious agents associated with specific conditions. A simple but clinically useful categorization of immunological deficiencies should determine whether patients have, in isolation or combination, (a) disruption of anatomical and functional barriers, (b) granulocyte deficiencies, (c) alterations at the level of B lymphocytes/humoral immunity, and (d) T-lymphocyte/macrophage cell-mediated immune defect [3].

Clinical Presentation

Although CNS infections in cancer patients can occur following the classic clinical syndromes discussed above, they often manifest atypically. First, etiological agents can be multiple. Second, presenting symptoms and signs may be subtle and usually overlap with findings secondary to the underlying diseases and their treatments, in particular among patients with higher degrees of immunosuppression. For example, a brain abscess that is generating a mass effect in a patient with prolonged neutropenia may be manifested exclusively by fever and nonspecific alterations in consciousness [3]. Consequently, the threshold for triggering a diagnostic study to rule out a CNS infection in the immunocompromised host should be low, and the diagnostic strategy should include microbiological studies, imaging, and, in many cases, tissue procurement. Finally, and with the above considerations, it is still possible to distinguish specific clinical syndromes that are associated with particular etiological agents and should be approximated differentially.

Meningitis: The isolated presence of fever and meningeal signs (neck stiffness) are suggestive of the common etiologies of meningitis, with the classic bacterial agents being the most relevant [13]. Sudden onset of symptoms is associated with infections due to *Streptococcus pneumoniae,* *Haemophilus influenzae,* and *Neisseria meningitidis,* especially in patients with alterations in humoral immunity (e.g., functional or

anatomic splenectomy, multiple myeloma, and-anti-CD20 monoclonal antibody users). A subacute presentation suggests opportunistic agents such as *Listeria monocytogenes,* which can occasionally give isolated meningeal involvement, yeasts such as *Cryptococcus neoformans,* and dimorphic fungi including *Histoplasma capsulatum* or *Coccidioides* spp. (when there is a history of compatible environmental exposure). Isolated meningeal tuberculosis is a rare cause of meningitis but should also be included as an alternative to subacute meningitis. In this case, the finding of choroidal tubercles in the ophthalmological examination can support the diagnosis.

Meningoencephalitis, encephalitis, and mass lesions: In patients presenting with fever, with or without meningeal signs, associated with any type of mental status alteration or focal neurological signs, the differential diagnosis must be expanded and include agents according to the dominant clinical pattern. Encephalitis is defined by the presence of altered mental status in the absence of neck stiffness and is usually secondary to viral infections, with herpetic encephalitis caused by herpes simplex 1 being the most relevant due to the poor prognosis that it determines when it is not diagnosed and treated at an early stage [15]. Meningoencephalitis is characterized by the presence of neck stiffness together with encephalopathy, and the differential diagnosis should include *Listeria monocytogenes,* *Mycoplasma pneumoniae,* and *Mycobacterium tuberculosis.* Meningoencephalitis due to *Listeria monocytogenes* in immunocompetent patients often manifests as rhombencephalitis. However, in immunocompromised patients, the presentation is rather nonspecific, and therefore it should be suspected even in the absence of the classic manifestations [1]. Tuberculous meningoencephalitis, on the other hand, has a course that tends to be subacute or chronic and is characterized by neck stiffness and manifestations that suggest focal or diffuse encephalic compromise, such as cranial nerve palsies, altered mental status, and focal neurological signs, secondary to the mass effect determined by tuberculomas in the cerebral parenchyma [2]. Along with tuberculosis, the differential diagnosis of mass lesions should include toxoplasmosis and some fungal infections such as those caused by *Cryptococcus* spp., *Aspergillus* spp., and members of the order *Mucorales*.

Diagnosis

The diagnostic approach of a CNS infection in an immunocompromised patient should consider the clinical syndrome, its temporal course, and epidemiologically relevant exposures. Along with the above, noninfectious causes that simulate CNS infections must also be ruled out. In parallel, the clinician should estimate the degree of immune suppression and define, to the extent possible, the underlying immunodeficiency model to rationally direct the etiological study. Algorithm 1 summarizes the classical models of immunological defects and the agents that are associated with each of them. Notwithstanding the above, it is important to emphasize that in many situations it is not possible to identify the underlying immunological defect and it is a fact

that several alterations can coexist at the same time or sequentially [3]. The best example of this consists of the group of patients undergoing allogeneic HSCT. In this group of patients, the temporality of the transplant dictates the diagnostic possibilities. Thus, in the immediate post-HSCT period, infections associated with alteration of barriers and quantitative deficiencies in granulocytes predominate, which is why microorganisms such as *Staphylococcus* spp., Gram-negative bacilli (including non-fermenters such as *Pseudomonas* spp.), and *Candida* spp. must be considered. Subsequently, after the engraftment period, an intermediate period of profound immunodeficiency may occur, particularly in patients who develop graft-versus-host disease (GVHD) and those who receive immunosuppressive therapy for various indications. During this time, infections associated with defects in the function of T lymphocytes become relevant. Viral infections caused by agents such as cytomegalovirus and the varicella-zoster virus can cause encephalitis and meningoencephalitis and even simulate mass lesions, either due to

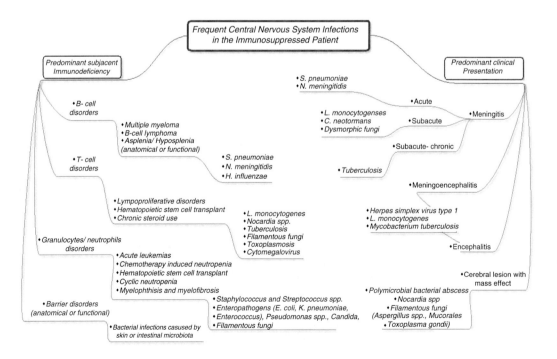

Algorithm 1

vasculitis, hemorrhagic complications, or nodular brain lesions. Among HSCT patients presenting with mass lesions, *Toxoplasma gondii* is a pathogen of high relevance. Toxoplasma lesions can be single or multiple, especially in patients with serological evidence of latent infection in the pretransplant study [8]. Similarly, infections caused by bacteria such as *Nocardia* spp. and *Listeria monocytogenes*, as well as those caused by molds including *Aspergillus* spp., *Fusarium* spp., and members of the order *Mucorales* should be considered. Finally, after the establishment of the immunological reconstitution, which depends mainly on the type of transplant and the occurrence of graft-versus-host disease, the etiologies to be considered tend to resemble infections in immunocompetent patients.

With the considerations presented above, the study of the immunosuppressed patient with suspected CNS infection should include images and laboratory techniques aimed at defining the etiological agent [8]. First, the images should evaluate the presence of mass lesions that are causing intracranial hypertension and that may preclude invasive CNS studies. Second, the images serve to rule out alternative non-infectious diagnoses and to determine or confirm the presenting clinical syndrome. Magnetic resonance is the ideal image; however, contrasted computed tomography can also be used as an initial approximation, is widely available, and is faster to obtain. Additional studies such as electroencephalogram should be indicated according to the particular context and can help to define the presence of encephalitis and even guide the etiology, as in the case of herpetic encephalitis. The primary laboratory study is the cerebrospinal fluid (CSF) analysis. The general characteristics of the CSF, such as its macroscopic aspect, its opening pressure, and its chemical and cytological analysis, are critical variables in the diagnosis process, and its interpretation does not differ to what has been classically described in immunocompetent patients. Findings such as hypercellularity at the expense of polymorphonuclear cells, hypoglycorrhachia, increased proteins, and elevated levels of lactic acid suggest a bacterial origin. On the other hand, viral infections determine less marked alterations of the CSF and are characterized by mononuclear pleocytosis. However, it should be considered that in the early stages, herpetic encephalitis can have a CSF similar to that of bacterial meningitis. Additionally, any CSF study must include a fundamental microbiological analysis oriented to the most probable causes. In the case of meningitis and meningoencephalitis, a Gram stain should always be included next to aerobic cultures. Depending on availability, the search for bacterial agents by standard culture techniques can be complemented using antigen-antibody detection techniques and molecular techniques that include polymerase chain reactions (PCR) primed against single or multiple microorganisms. Also, in subacute cases in which *Cryptococcus neoformans* is suspected, the India ink stain can detect capsulated yeast. Detection of the capsular polysaccharide antigen of *Cryptococcus neoformans* has excellent performance (sensitivity and specificity greater than 90%) and can be determined in both the CSF and blood [11]. Tuberculous meningoencephalitis is a significant cause to consider in patients with subacute or chronic conditions, especially when there is prior evidence of latent tuberculosis. Its diagnosis is challenging, and therapeutic decisions are often based on the presence of a compatible clinical picture together with suggestive findings in the CSF, including hypoglycorrhachia, increase in proteins, mononuclear pleocytosis, and elevated levels of adenosine deaminase (ADA). In all cases, an effort must be made to document the presence of *Mycobacterium tuberculosis* through the use of different techniques in combination, ideally in serial CSF samples, including Ziehl-Neelsen staining (smear microscopy), mycobacterial cultures, and molecular techniques. The latter has significantly increased the diagnostic performance (sensitivity 81% and specificity 98%), and some of them also allow the simultaneous detection of resistance to rifampin and isoniazid [4]. When viral meningitis or meningoencephalitis is suspected, relevant agents such as herpes simplex (mainly type 1), varicella-zoster virus, cytomegalovirus, and enterovirus should be tested by PCR in CSF.

Finally, the presence of focal brain lesions with mass effect usually requires invasive studies through brain biopsies, which can be obtained through stereotactic or open techniques. Tissue samples should be used for histopathological analyses and extensive microbiological studies, including stains (e.g., Gram stain, Kinyoun, Ziehl-Neelsen, and calcofluor-white), cultures (aerobic, anaerobic, mycobacteria, and fungal), and molecular techniques. In particular, *Toxoplasma gondii* can be detected by PCR in both CSF and tissues. Diagnosis of cerebral aspergillosis can be established by measuring the levels of galactomannan antigen and $(1, 3)$ β-D-glucan in CSF [7]. While PCR for *Aspergillus* spp. can play a role in the diagnosis, molecular techniques are not standardized. Therefore, its use in the usual practice is not currently recommended [9].

Treatment

CNS infections are severe conditions in any host, so their suspicion should trigger a rapid and efficient diagnostic workup that does not delay the start of empirical treatments aimed at covering the most likely agents according to each clinical situation. In this direction, the initial antimicrobial regimens must first consider the most common pathogens that cause particular syndromes in immunocompetent subjects. Secondly, consider the agents associated with the specific characteristics of each patient: the temporal course of the disease, the net state of immunosuppression, the predominant type of immunodeficiency, and the epidemiological exposures. In addition to favoring the early use of antimicrobials, the pharmacokinetics of each antimicrobial agent (CNS penetration) should be considered, and the indication of additional interventions should be evaluated. This includes the use of steroids when there is a suspicion of pneumococcal meningitis and immunoglobulin supplementation in hypogammaglobulinemic patients. The empirical therapeutic regimens recommended by clinical situation consist of the following:

Meningitis: *Streptococcus pneumoniae*, *Neisseria meningitidis*, *Haemophilus influenzae*, and *Listeria monocytogenes* should always be treated empirically. In this context, a first-line regimen should include a third-generation cephalosporin such as ceftriaxone in high doses (2 g every 12 h IV) together with ampicillin 12 g in 24 h IV. In patients with an allergy to beta-lactams or residents of geographical regions with a high prevalence of penicillin-resistant pneumococcus, vancomycin should also be included in the initial scheme in high doses, seeking baseline levels of 15–20 mcg/mL. In situations in which there is a risk of bacterial meningitis by less common agents, such as Gram-negative enteric bacilli including *Pseudomonas* spp. (as occurs in neutropenia), cefepime and meropenem are suitable alternatives to ceftriaxone. Although there is some controversy about the use of dexamethasone together with the first dose of antimicrobials, the data support that in the case of pneumococcal meningitis, the early use of dexamethasone is associated with a lower incidence of neurological sequelae and a reduction in mortality. Therefore, it should be considered when there is a high clinical suspicion of *Streptococcus pneumoniae* meningitis. It has been described that dexamethasone could hinder the penetration of vancomycin into the CNS, so in cases of confirmed pneumococcal meningitis (due to penicillin-resistant pneumococcus), some experts suggest adding rifampin to the baseline empirical regimen [12]. Staphylococcal meningitis is infrequent and usually related to alteration of anatomical barriers, particularly in neurosurgical patients. When suspected, it is essential to consider the local distribution of *Staphylococcus aureus* clones and their oxacillin resistance profiles. Suitable schemes to treat *Staphylococcus* spp. include nafcillin or vancomycin in high doses. At this point, it is important to mention that in many countries the treatment of choice for general infections caused by methicillin-susceptible *Staphylococcus aureus* is cefazolin, which has little or no penetration into the CNS, so it should not be part of schemes aimed at treating staphylococcal infections of the CNS. Alternatives then in countries without access to nafcillin are vancomycin, cotrimoxazole, linezolid, and daptomycin, usually together with rifampicin.

Meningoencephalitis and encephalitis: The initial empirical scheme should consider common bacterial agents such as those mentioned in the previous point, but it should also include intravenous acyclovir in doses of 10 mg/kg/8 h to treat herpes simplex type 1. In cases of suspicion of *Cryptococcus neoformans*, liposomal amphotericin B should be initiated together with flucytosine. In countries without access to flucytosine, an alternative regimen includes amphotericin with fluconazole in high doses (800 mg daily) [6].

Brain lesions with mass effect: Although in these cases the brain biopsy should be considered early, the initial empirical scheme should be active against polymicrobial bacterial abscesses (e.g., cefepime plus metronidazole or meropenem). Additionally, the use of therapy against *Toxoplasma gondii* (pyrimethamine plus sulfadiazine or cotrimoxazole) and molds, in particular, *Aspergillus* spp. should be considered initially. Voriconazole is the first-line agent in case of suspicion of cerebral aspergillosis, but agents with greater antifungal spectrum, such as lipid formulations of amphotericin and posaconazole, are alternatives to be considered in cases in which the presence of other non-aspergillus molds is suspected, either in association with voriconazole or as single agents. Finally, surgical drainage should be considered on a case-by-case basis in patients with confirmed cerebral aspergillosis [7, 9].

References

1. Armstrong R, Fung P. Brainstem encephalitis (Rhombencephalitis) due to *Listeria monocytogenes*: case report and review. Clin Infect Dis. 1993; 16:689–702. https://doi.org/10.1093/clind/16.5.689.

2. Balaguer Rosello A, Bataller L, Lorenzo L, et al. Infections of the central nervous system after unrelated donor umbilical cord blood transplantation or human leukocyte antigen–matched sibling transplantation. Biol Blood Marrow Transplant. 2017;23:134–9. https://doi.org/10.1016/j.bbmt.2016.10.005.

3. Cunha B. Central nervous system infections in the compromised host: a diagnostic approach. Infect Dis Clin N Am. 2001;15:567–90. https://doi.org/10.1016/s0891-5520(05)70160-4.

4. Denkinger C, Schumacher S, Boehme C, et al. Xpert MTB/RIF assay for the diagnosis of extrapulmonary tuberculosis: a systematic review and meta-analysis. Eur Respir J. 2014;44:435–46. https://doi.org/10.1183/09031936.00007814.

5. Hanajiri R, Kobayashi T, Yoshioka K, et al. Central nervous system infection following allogeneic hematopoietic stem cell transplantation. Hematol Oncol Stem Cell Ther. 2017;10:22–8. https://doi.org/10.1016/j.hemonc.2016.08.008.

6. Pappas P, Chetchotisakd P, Larsen R, et al. A phase II randomized trial of amphotericin B alone or combined with fluconazole in the treatment of HIV-associated cryptococcal meningitis. Clin Infect Dis. 2009;48:1775–83. https://doi.org/10.1086/599112.

7. Patterson T, Thompson G, Denning D, et al. Executive summary: practice guidelines for the diagnosis and management of aspergillosis: 2016 update by the Infectious Diseases Society of America. Clin Infect Dis. 2016;63:433–42. https://doi.org/10.1093/cid/ciw444.

8. Schmidt-Hieber M, Silling G, Schalk E, et al. CNS infections in patients with hematological disorders (including allogeneic stem-cell transplantation) – guidelines of the Infectious Diseases Working Party (AGIHO) of the German Society of Hematology and Medical Oncology (DGHO). Ann Oncol. 2016;27:1207–25. https://doi.org/10.1093/annonc/mdw155.

9. Schwartz S, Kontoyiannis D, Harrison T, Ruhnke M. Advances in the diagnosis and treatment of fungal infections of the CNS. Lancet Neurol. 2018;17:362–72. https://doi.org/10.1016/s1474-4422(18)30030-9.

10. Sonneville R, Magalhaes E, Meyfroidt G. Central nervous system infections in immunocompromised patients. Curr Opin Crit Care. 2017;23:128–33. https://doi.org/10.1097/mcc.0000000000000397.

11. Tanner D, Weinstein M, Fedorciw B, et al. Comparison of commercial kits for detection of cryptococcal antigen. J Clin Microbiol. 1994;32:1680–4.

12. Tunkel A, Hartman B, Kaplan S, et al. Practice guidelines for the management of bacterial meningitis. Clin Infect Dis. 2004;39:1267–84. https://doi.org/10.1086/425368.

13. van Veen K, Brouwer M, van der Ende A, van de Beek D. Bacterial meningitis in hematopoietic stem cell transplant recipients: a population-based prospective study. Bone Marrow Transplant. 2016;51: 1490–5. https://doi.org/10.1038/bmt.2016.181.

14. Wheat J, Myint T, Guo Y, et al. Central nervous system histoplasmosis: multicenter retrospective study on clinical features, diagnostic approach and outcome of treatment. Medicine. 2018;97:e0245. https://doi.org/10.1097/md.0000000000010245.

15. Wu M, Huang F, Jiang X, et al. Herpesvirus-associated central nervous system diseases after allogeneic hematopoietic stem cell transplantation. PLoS One. 2013;8: e77805. https://doi.org/10.1371/journal.pone.0077805.

Part V

Respiratory Diseases

Acute and Chronic Respiratory Failure in Cancer Patients

Steven P. Sears, Gordon Carr, and Christian Bime

Contents

Introduction 446

Epidemiology 447

Pathophysiology 447

Clinical Features 448

Etiology 449
Pulmonary Infections in the Cancer Patient 449
Opportunistic Infections 451
Fungal Pneumonia 452

Noninfectious Parenchymal Disorders 452
ARDS and ARDS Mimics 452
Radiation Injury and Fibrosis 453
Drug-Induced Lung Injury 453
Aspiration Pneumonitis and Pneumonia 455
Transfusion-Related Acute Lung Injury and Circulatory Overload
(TRALI/TACO) 455
Organizing Pneumonia 455
Parenchymal Disorders Common to HCT Patients 455
Vascular Disorders 456

S. P. Sears
Pulmonary and Critical Care Medicine,
University of Arizona, Tucson, AZ, USA
e-mail: ssears@deptofmed.arizona.edu

G. Carr
Banner-University Medical Center Tucson, Tucson, AZ,
USA
e-mail: Gordon.Carr@bannerhealth.com;
gcarr@deptofmed.arizona.edu

C. Bime (✉)
University of Arizona School of Medicine and Banner-
University Medical Center – Tucson,
Tucson, AZ, USA
e-mail: cbime@deptofmed.arizona.edu

© Springer Nature Switzerland AG 2020
J. L. Nates, K. J. Price (eds.), *Oncologic Critical Care*,
https://doi.org/10.1007/978-3-319-74588-6_43

Cardiac Causes of Acute Respiratory Failure 457
Other Causes of Acute Respiratory Failure 457

Diagnosis 457
Diagnostic Studies 458

Management 459
Noninvasive Positive Pressure Ventilation and High-Flow Nasal Oxygenation 460
Preparation for Mechanical Ventilation 462
Treatment Strategies for Hypercapnic Respiratory Failure 464
Ventilatory Therapies for Hypoxemic Respiratory Failure 464

Prognosis 465

References 466

Abstract

In 2016, there was an estimated 1.8 million new cases of cancer diagnosed in the United States. Remarkable advances have been made in cancer therapy and the 5-year survival has increased for most patients affected by malignancy. There are growing numbers of patients admitted to intensive care units (ICU) and up to 20% of all patients admitted to an ICU carry a diagnosis of malignancy. Respiratory failure remains the most common reason for ICU admission and remains the leading causes of death in oncology patients. There are many causes of respiratory failure in this population. Pneumonia is the most common cause of respiratory failure, yet there are many causes of respiratory insufficiency unique to the cancer patient. These causes are often a result of immunosuppression, chemotherapy, radiation treatment, or hematopoietic stem cell transplant (HCT). Treatment is focused on supportive care and specific therapy for the underlying cause of respiratory failure. Noninvasive modalities of respiratory support are available; however, careful patient selection is paramount as indiscriminate use of noninvasive positive pressure ventilation is associated with a higher mortality if mechanical ventilation is later required. Historically, respiratory failure in the cancer patient had a grim prognosis. Outcomes have improved over the past 20 years. Survivors are often left with significant disability.

Keywords

Respiratory failure · Noninvasive ventilation · Mechanical ventilation · Intensive Care Unit · Diffuse alveolar hemorrhage · Organizing pneumonia · Pulmonary embolism · High resolution computed tomography · Bronchoscopy

Introduction

In 2016, an estimated 1.8 million new cases of cancer were diagnosed and 595,690 cancer-related deaths in the United States [176]. In the United States, malignancy remains the second leading cause of death behind heart disease and has surpassed heart disease as the primary cause of death in those 45–79 years of age [155]. Worldwide there were 17.5 million new cancer diagnoses in 2015 [139]. With continued population growth, the number new cancer cases are expected to exceed 26 million by 2030 [174].

Despite the growing burden of cancer incidence, prevalence, and associated morbidity, remarkable advances have been made in cancer therapy. Until 1997, cancer deaths had been increasing for 70 years [155]. In 1969 the cumulative 5-year survival for patients with breast cancer was 64% [157]. Today with improvements in screening, precision medicine, anticancer agents, and treatment of side effects, 90% of patients with breast cancer will survive at least 5 years [155]. Likewise, over the last 50 years, 5-year survival in younger patients with acute leukemia has increased from 4% to 60% [142]. In essence, the paradigm of cancer has shifted from stigmatized terminal illness, to that of chronic disease.

Paralleling this, recent studies have documented progress in the care of critically ill cancer patients [11, 14, 26]. With an aging population and more patients surviving with cancer, there are growing numbers of patients admitted to intensive care units [127]. In fact, 20% of patients admitted to intensive care units (ICU) carry a diagnosis of malignancy [169]. Nearly 10% of cancer patients will at some point be afflicted with a life-threatening condition justifying ICU admission [14, 32]. The most common reason for transfer to a critical care ward is organ failure [134, 162]. Acute organ failure may be related to co-morbid illness, cancer treatment, or the malignancy itself. Any organ may be affected, yet respiratory failure is the most frequent and most feared indication for ICU admission [133, 162].

Historically, respiratory failure remains the leading cause of death of critically ill cancer patients, especially those requiring mechanical ventilation [11, 16, 159]. Twenty years ago, mechanical ventilation of the bone marrow transplant patient portended almost certain death [59]. Recent advances in both neoplastic therapies and intensive care medicine have improved outcomes in patients with solid tumors, hematologic malignancies, and those undergoing bone marrow transplant (HCT) [13].

This chapter reviews the numerous causes of acute and chronic respiratory failure that occur in patients with solid and hematologic malignancies. The importance of expeditious diagnostic precision is reviewed in the context of the outcomes of respiratory failure. The increased use of high resolution computer tomography (HRCT) has greatly aided in narrowing the differential diagnosis of respiratory failure in oncology patients which leads to more efficient use of invasive diagnostic modalities. We will review some classic patterns on HRCT that suggest specific diagnoses with a high sensitivity and specificity. In terms of management, we review the literature on the utility and risks of invasive

mechanical ventilation in immunocompromised cancer patients and further discuss the impact of current noninvasive ventilation strategies in this population. Finally, we will offer a general approach to diagnosis and management of respiratory failure in patients with active malignancy.

Epidemiology

Even in the absence of malignancy, acute and chronic respiratory failure have a high burden on patients, their families, and the health care system. In general the number of cases of acute respiratory failure is on the rise. In 2009 there were 1,917,910 cases of ARF in the United States resulting in 381,155 deaths and in inpatient cost of 54 billion dollars [166]. This translated into 784 cases of respiratory failure per 100,000 people, or an incidence of 0.7% [166]. Respiratory failure occurs in 5% of patients with solid tumors, 20% in those with hematologic malignancies, and in up to 50% of those undergoing bone marrow transplant [42]. For those cancer patients that survive respiratory-related critical illness, the estimated cost per year of life gained is nearly 83,000 dollars for patients with solid tumors and 189,000 dollars for patients with hematologic malignancy [151]. This figure is projected to increase with the use of novel antineoplastic treatments such as adoptive cell therapy with chimeric antigen receptor redirected T-cells (CAR-T) as such therapy itself is associated with a price tag of over 400,000 dollars [19]. Short-term survival of respiratory related critical illness in cancer patients has improved. However, the effects of chronic respiratory complications remain unclear.

Pathophysiology

Respiratory failure is insufficient gas exchange due to derangements in one more components of the respiratory system including the central nervous system, chest wall and diaphragm, airways, alveolar-capillary interface, or pulmonary circulation. Depending on the nature of the insult, failure of the respiratory system may be acute, subacute, or chronic. Respiratory failure may be further characterized by physiologic imbalance, each of which portends numerous differential diagnosis. Type I respiratory failure or hypoxemia is characterized by persistently low partial pressure of oxygen (PaO_2 less than 60 mmHg). Hypercapnic respiratory failure (type II) is characterized by an arterial partial pressure of carbon dioxide greater than 45 mmHg. Type III respiratory failure is that associated with perioperative complications, while type IV respiratory failure relates to mismatch of oxygen consumption and delivery related to shock states.

Respiratory failure mediated by arterial hypoxemia has numerous general causes including malperfusion, hypoventilation, mismatch of ventilation and perfusion, defect in gas transfer across the alveolar-capillary interface, and anatomic or physiologic shunt of blood flow from venous to arterial circulation. Any of these general derangements may precipitate hypoxemia and tissue hypoxia.

In the absence of significant anatomic shunt, the pulmonary capillary bed receives the entirety of the cardiac output. This large blood volume makes the lungs a target for metastatic and thromboembolic disease. The fragile lattice of the capillary bed as well as the pulmonary interstitium is also sensitive to the collateral damage of radiation and the cytokine storm associated with systemic chemotherapy. These cancer therapies are also frequently toxic to the cardiovascular system resulting in pericardial effusion or cardiogenic pulmonary edema. Local spread of disease may complicate the proximal airways leading to respiratory distress and postobstructive complications of endobronchial lesions. Procedural removal of such lesions or metastatic spread may also interfere with the neurologic pathways responsible for respiratory mechanics. In addition, cancer itself and many chemotherapy regimens ablate the immune systems leading to a multitude of infectious complications.

Patients with cancer often have multisystem comorbidities that may contribute to respiratory failure. For example, not only does smoking predispose to the development of lung cancer but is also fundamental to the pathophysiology of emphysema, pulmonary fibrosis, coronary artery disease, and more. Many of these preexisting comorbidities may themselves precipitate ARF.

Clinical Features

The clinical features of acute and chronic respiratory failure are nonspecific, evident in multiple systems, and are dependent on the underlying disease state. For example, patients with ventilatory failure and hypercapnia may be moribund, somnolent, or simply confused. They may be tachypnic with pursed lip breathing due to obstructive lung disease, or hypopnic with pinpoint pupils or other exam findings suspect of narcotic toxidromes. Myoclonus and asterixis may be observed with carbon dioxide narcosis. Respiratory acidosis may predispose to instability in the cardiac sarcolemma with resultant arrhythmias.

Evidence of hypoxemia may be gleaned in nearly every bodily system. Neurologic manifestations include restlessness, confusion, myoclonus, and seizures. Hypoxemia and global tissue hypoxia may create an acidotic intracellular milieu which may instigate tachy or bradyarrhythmias. Local pulmonary findings reflect the causal insult. For example, use of accessory muscles of respiration, diminished air movement, diffuse wheezing, and tripoding are evident in the asthmatic with impending respiratory collapse. Stridor may indicate proximal airway narrowing due to malignant disease within the trachea. Dullness to percussion and reduced tactile fremitus raise suspicion for a pleural effusion or consolidative process. Resonance on percussion and trachea shift suggest pneumothorax. Inspiratory "Velcro"-like crackles could suggest fibrotic lung disease, and with the appropriate historical context, might indicate radiation induced lung injury. Digital clubbing may indicate primary lung cancer [149]. In severe hypoxia, cyanosis can be found around the lips, nail beds, and mucous membranes.

Classic findings of pleuritic chest pain and productive cough may not be evident in the cancer patient. Rather, nonspecific symptoms of fever and malaise may herald the development of pneumonia in this population.

Adaptations to chronic hypoxia manifest as polycythemia, headaches, and potentially right heart failure from cor pulmonale.

Etiology

The causes of respiratory dysfunction requiring ICU admission are similar in those with and without cancer. However, cancer predisposes patients to etiologies of ARF not always common in the general populace. The numerous causes of respiratory failure in critically ill cancer patients are demonstrated in Table 1. Common causes include infections, exacerbation of underlying comorbid illness, aspiration pneumonia, thromboembolic disease, cardiogenic pulmonary edema, non-cardiogenic pulmonary edema from acute respiratory distress syndrome (ARDS), progression of malignancy, and complications of antineoplastic therapy. Numerous chemotherapeutic agents are associated with various forms of pulmonary toxicity. In addition, the use of stereotactic body radiation therapy has increased in the last two decades. This has translated to an increased incidence of radiation pneumonitis [188].

In general, the most common reason for respiratory failure in patients with cancer remains infection. However, there are also conditions that are unique to certain disease states. For example, patients with Acute Myeloid Leukemia (AML) are subject to leukostasis, while those who have undergone bone marrow transplant (BMT) are at risk for diffuse alveolar hemorrhage, idiopathic pneumonia syndrome, and more.

Pulmonary Infections in the Cancer Patient

Pneumonia is the most common infection in cancer patients [143]. Malignancy and chemotherapy both convey varying degrees of immunosuppression which in turn predispose to the development of infectious pneumonitis. The type of immune defect, humoral, cell-mediated, or qualitative granulocyte dysfunction, commonly influences microorganisms which breach host defenses. For example, defects in B-cell number or function as seen in acute leukemia and multiple myeloma predispose patients to infection with gram negative and encapsulated bacteria. Lymphoma or prolonged corticosteroid use may deplete T-cells leading to impairment in cell-mediated defense. Common infections in such patients include endemic mycosis and other fungal pathogens such as pneumocystis and Cryptococcus, mycobacteria, and viruses (especially CMV). Myeloproliferative disorders or the ablative effects of various chemotherapy may induce neutropenia leading one to be susceptible to virulent gram positive and negative bacteria, as well as opportunistic fungi including Aspergillus.

Bacterial Pneumonia

Bacterial pneumonia is the most common infection in the oncology patient predisposing to acute respiratory failure. In a cohort of 424 cancer patients with respiratory failure of determined etiology, bacterial pneumonia was diagnosed in 47%. Of these, the classic community acquired pathogens accounted for 25%. Streptococcus pneumonia was most frequently diagnosed. This followed by other streptococci, and more virulent and often resistant health care associated organisms such as *Staphylococcus aureus* (7.5%), *Pseudomonas aeruginosa* (16%), *Enterobacter cloacae* (10%), and *Klebsiella pneumonia* (4%). Ten percent culture positive pneumonia was documented due to intracellular organisms such as *Legionella pneumophilia* (5%), *Mycoplasma pneumonia* (2.5%), *Coxiella burnetii* (1%), and *Chlamydia pneumoniae* [153].

Viral Pneumonia

Seasonal respiratory viruses are often implicated as a cause of pneumonia in the immunocompromised host, more often in stem cell transplant patients and those with hematologic malignancy. Influenza is involved in one-third of such cases. Respiratory syncytial virus and parainfluenza are also commonly involved. With the advent

Table 1 Causes of acute respiratory failure in the cancer patient

Airway disorders	Parenchymal disorders	Cardiac disease	Vascular disorders	Chest wall and pleural disease	CNS disorders	Infections
Obstruction	ARDS and ARDS Mimics	Pericardial effusion	Thromboembolic disease	Obesity	Intracranial Malignancy	Viral
Bronchitis	Radiation injury	Congestive heart failure	Alveolar hemorrhage	Pleural effusion Malignant	Medications	Bacterial
COPD	Chemotherapy reactions	Coronary artery disease	Tumor emboli	Hemothorax	Metabolic encephalopathy	Fungal
Extrinsic compression	Pulmonary edema		Veno-occlusive disease	Pneumothorax	Iatrogenic injury	Opportunistic pathogens
Tumor invasion	TACO/TRALI		Pulmonary hypertension	Lung entrapment	Paraneoplastic syndrome	
	Aspiration			Chest wall invasion		
	Organizing pneumonia			Pathologic fractures		
	BOOP					
	Malignant infiltration					
	Lymphangitic spread					
	Leukostasis					
	Peri-engraftment syndrome					
	Idiopathic pneumonia syndrome					

of rapidly available viral PCR testing, human metapneumovirus has emerged as a common respiratory viral pathogen [154]. Immunocompromised oncology patients may present as symptoms of upper respiratory illness such as laryngitis, rhinorrhea, and congestion. In contrast to their immunocompetent counterparts, cancer patients may not rapidly improve over 3–5 days; rather they may progress to severe lower respiratory infection and manifest cough, wheezing, and hypoxia [88].

Opportunistic Infections

Opportunistic infections are common in these patients and may account for up to 30% of pulmonary infections [153]. Such infections include cytomegalovirus (CMV) pneumonia, invasive pulmonary aspergillosis, *Pneumocystis jirovecii*, tuberculosis, and atypical mycobacteria.

CMV Pneumonia

Largely characterized as an opportunistic infection, the incidence of CMV pneumonia in patients with hematologic malignancy is estimated near 40% of seropositive patients [110]. At least 60% of the US population has been exposed to CMV [189]. In patients with hematologic malignancy, steroid therapy, or bone marrow transplantation, latent CMV may reactivate and affect nearly any organ. Life threatening pneumonia may develop in this group. The radiographic presentation is variable and nonspecific including lobar consolidation mimicking bacterial processes, ground-glass opacities, or reticulonodular infiltrates. Serum CMV DNA polymerase chain reaction (PCR) has a high sensitivity but a low positive predictive value; thus, the diagnosis relies on culture or histopathology [63]. True infection warrants treatment with ganciclovir or foscarnet. Interestingly, increased incidence of co-infection with Nocardia and molds such as Aspergillus has been documented in patients with CMV pneumonia [44]. It is unclear if this is an epiphenomenon or what the mechanism is for such co-infection.

Pulmonary Aspergillosis

Invasive aspergillus is a major cause of death in patients following BMT. It commonly involves the lungs and sinuses of neutropenic patients and may present with fever, chest pain, and hemoptysis. Often, fever may be the only manifestation and the disease is suspected via lung imaging with CT scan. Specific patterns suggestive of various types of pulmonary aspergillosis are described in Table 2. Prompt diagnosis is imperative as the angioinvasive fungus may disseminate outside the respiratory tract to other organs. Such dissemination portends a mortality rate between 40% and 80% [20, 112]. Voriconazole is the drug of choice; however, combination therapy may be required.

Pneumocystis jirovecii Pneumonia

Infection with the opportunistic fungi *Pneumocystis jirovecii* is most common in individuals with T-cell deficiency. Classically described in patients with HIV/AIDS, this infection is also common and increasingly seen in those with hematologic malignancy or bone marrow transplant, as well as in those taking moderate doses of systemic corticosteroids. A Mayo Clinic series of 116 patients with PJP evaluated the epidemiology of the infection and noted hematologic malignancy as a risk factor in 30% of cases. Patients with solid tumors comprised 13% of infections [187]. Symptoms are often more severe in the non-HIV patient. Respiratory failure is common. Classic radiographic findings are listed in Table 2.

Nocardia

Often overlooked in the immunocompromised host is pulmonary infection with unusual pathogens such as Nocardia. Nocardia is a gram-positive infection in which two-thirds of patients demonstrate impaired cell medicated defense. Such deficiency is seen in lymphoma, bone marrow transplant, and with glucocorticoid use [178]. An inoculum is inhaled which leads to Nocardia pneumonia, the most common pulmonary manifestation. Pleural involvement and emphysema is common; as is disseminated CNS disease. Diagnosis if frequently delayed and is often radiographically confused with metastatic cancer [113].

Table 2 Computed tomography characteristics of select causes of acute respiratory failure in cancer patients

Disease	Radiographic correlates
ARDS	Diffuse, bilateral, and symmetric opacities which become more uniform in dependent areas. Often interlobular septal thickening and ground glass attenuation (crazy paving pattern) is present [79]
Acute interstitial pneumonia	Diffuse, bilateral, and symmetric ground glass opacities and parenchymal consolidation which may be most apparent in peripheral and lower lung regions. Later fibrotic phases may manifest with traction bronchiectasis and honeycombing [3]
Organizing pneumonia	Patchy areas of opacification which may be peripheral, subpleural or peribronchial. Centrilobular nodules may be present. Ground glass opacities may be surrounded by a rim of consolidation (Atoll or "reverse halo" sign) [70]
Diffuse alveolar hemorrhage	Ground glass attenuation with bilateral (often hilar) consolidation in a "butterfly" appearance. Typically spares the subpleural areas [140]
Lymphangitic spread of malignancy	Interlobular septal thickening which is nodular. Perilymphatic nodules present. Lung architecture is generally preserved. Mediastinal adenopathy may be present [93]
PJP pneumonia	Bilateral perihilar and central ground glass opacities often associated with smooth interlobular septal thickening (crazy paving pattern). Cysts may be found within the ground glass opacities. Cysts may have bizarre shapes [125]
Pulmonary aspergillosis	1. Angioinvasive disease: pulmonary nodules with a halo of ground glass surrounding the nodule (Halo sign). Ground glass represents hemorrhage. Wedge shaped infarct may be present. Necrosis and cavitation may occur 2. Allergic bronchopulmonary aspergillus: central or upper lobe bronchiectasis with mucoid impaction, often of high attenuation. Mucoid impaction may results in bronchocoele (finger-in-glove sign) 3. Aspergilloma: Thin or thick-walled cavity with soft tissue density within. Mass may be mobile with positioning [73]

Fungal Pneumonia

A useful way to categorize fungal pneumonia is based on the patient's pattern of immunodeficiency. For example, neutropenia predisposes to infection with angioinvasive molds such as Mucor and Aspergillus. On the other hand, patients with T-cell defects are subject to infections with Cryptococcus, PJP, and endemic mycosis such as *Coccidioides immitis, Blastomyces dermatitidis, and Histoplasma capsulatum.*

Isolated cryptococcal pneumonia is uncommon and pulmonary infection generally indicates widespread dissemination. In a review of 34 HIV-negative immunocompromised patients with cryptococcal pneumonia, 28 had evidence of extrapulmonary disease at time of diagnosis [98]. The clinical course may be quiescent with prolonged indolent infection, or the patient may present with fulminant respiratory failure and ARDS [132, 180]. CNS involvement should be sought out in all patients with pulmonary Cryptococcus. Mild cases may be treated with azole therapy, whereas severe respiratory failure and disseminated disease necessitate amphotericin B.

Noninfectious Parenchymal Disorders

ARDS and ARDS Mimics

The acute respiratory distress syndrome imparts a high mortality and is characterized by infiltration of the alveoli by protein-rich pulmonary edema with resultant severe mixed respiratory failure. Clinically it is defined as acute onset of respiratory symptoms within 1 week, bilateral radiographic airspace opacities, hypoxemia defined as arterial partial pressure of oxygen to fraction of inspired oxygen ratio less than 300 mmHg on at least 5 cmH$_2$O of PEEP, and exclusion of cardiogenic cause of the alveolar edema [9, 10]. Numerous conditions predispose to the syndrome, many of which are commonly found in the oncology patient. Sepsis, aspiration, massive transfusion and transfusion reactions, drugs, and even hematopoetic stem cell transplantation are associated with ARDS [99, 102, 136].

There is a selection of diffuse lung diseases that mimic ARDS both clinically and radiographically but have different etiologic and pathophysiologic characteristics. It is important to distinguish these from true ARDS as they typically respond well to systemic glucocorticoid therapy. These entities include: acute interstitial pneumonia (AIP), acute eosinophilic pneumonia, organizing pneumonia, diffuse alveolar hemorrhage, and acute hypersensitivity pneumonitis. Confusion is commonplace as malignancy, chemotherapy regimens, and bone marrow transplantation may predispose to either ARDS or respiratory failure from an ARDS mimic [4, 128, 163]. In practice, one often cannot distinguish between them without aid of bronchoscopy or surgical lung biopsy. Differentiation between true ARDS versus ARDS imitators is important as ARDS mimics may be more responsive to anti-inflammatory therapies.

Radiation Injury and Fibrosis

Radiation therapy (RT) is a mainstay of therapy for various stages of lung, neck, and breast cancer as well as lymphoma. The use of RT has increased, in part as it is tolerated well, generally with few side effects. The lung is radiosensitive and toxicity may occur as collateral damage with an incidence of up to 28%. The incidence is less frequent when radiation is used for treatment of breast cancer [115]. Clinically, the lung has two distinct pathologic responses to ionizing radiation. Radiation pneumonitis is an acute or subacute reaction which occurs within 6 months of thoracic radiotherapy. Risk for acute radiation pneumonitis depends on concomitant use of certain chemotherapy agents, prior radiation, total dose and field size, as well as host factors such as prior chronic lung disease [52]. Dyspnea, cough, and fever develop prior to radiographic changes. Pulmonary function tests demonstrate restrictive ventilatory defect. Reduction in the diffusion capacity (DLCO) is the most sensitive maker of acute and subacute radiation injury

[126]. Depending on the degree of lung tissue damaged, the course may be self-limited or progress to severe acute lung injury and fulminant hypoxic respiratory failure [82]. CT correlation can be used to assess the severity of disease. Oxygen and concomitant chemotherapy may worsen the lung injury [168]. The areas of RP tend to develop fibrosis over time [49]. Corticosteroids remain the mainstay of treatment.

Radiation fibrosis occurs 6 months to 1 year following completion of radiation therapy. The development of acute radiation pneumonitis is not a prerequisite for progression to fibrosis; patients may be asymptomatic until the late onset of breathlessness or in severe cases, respiratory failure and acute cor pulmonale. The diaphragm may also be affected resulting in hypoventilation [126]. Fibrosis tends to occur on the margins of the radiation field. Fibrosis may cause distortion of the interstitium or traction of the airways. Fibrosis may alter the function of the mucociliary elevator and predispose patients to infection [126]. Treatment is largely supportive and steroids have no role in therapy of radiation fibrosis. Radiation therapy may also lead to radiation-associated organizing pneumonia.

Drug-Induced Lung Injury

Pulmonary drug toxicity is a diagnosis of exclusion and can be difficult to diagnose owing to protean clinical and radiographic manifestations [147]. The presentation is often subacute or chronic and insidious as opposed to acute. It is estimated that up to 20% of patients treated with cytotoxic drugs may develop respiratory symptoms [158]. Numerous drugs are associated with various forms of pulmonary toxicity and the diagnosis should be considered in any cancer patient with new respiratory failure and pulmonary opacities on chest imaging. Drug-induced damage may be dose dependent or idiosyncratic [131]. Databases such as Pneumotox (https://www.pneumotox.com/drug/index/) have been established detailing the many histopathologic and radiologic findings associated with numerous agents. These resources are invaluable in formulating a differential diagnosis and it is often useful to correlate a specific radiographic pattern to a drug in question. In terms of pathophysiological mechanism, bleomycin toxicity is well understood and serves as an archetype for our understanding of drug-induced pulmonary toxicity. Bleomycin damages capillary endothelium and type I pneumocytes leading to free radical damage and exaggerated inflammatory response. Given the release of free radicals, oxygen therapy may worsen the lung injury. This is an unfortunate paradox as the very supportive care used in hypoxemia may be detrimental [46, 168, 171]. The clinical and/or radiographic pattern is variable and not specific to any drug. Common features include: organizing pneumonia, eosinophilic pneumonia, cardiac and noncardiac pulmonary edema, bronchoconstriction, diffuse alveolar hemorrhage, radiation recall, and more [92, 148, 150]. Table 3 lists radiographic manifestations of select commonly used antineoplastic drugs.

Newer antineoplastic agents now in circulation are also associated with various forms of pulmonary toxicity. These immunomodulating monoclonal antibody therapies targeting anticytotoxic T-lymphocyte antigen 4 (CTLA-4) and programed death 1 (PD-1) are being commonly used in non-small cell carcinoma as well as against melanoma. They have been associated with generalized dyspnea, pneumonitis, and even organizing pneumonia. Depending on the degree of severity, treatment may entail simply withdrawing the offending agent, or in severe cases, high dose glucocorticoids [22, 129].

Table 3 Pulmonary complications associated with common chemotherapeutic drugs. (Disease patterns referenced from Pneumotox)

Drug	Associated pulmonary complication
Bleomycin	ARDS, eosinophilic pneumonia, organizing pneumonia, pulmonary fibrosis, acute interstitial pneumonia, pneumothorax, pulmonary veno-occlusive disease, NSIP
5-FU	Pulmonary fibrosis, ARDS, pulmonary edema
Bevacizumab	ARDS, DAH, bronchospasm, pulmonary arterial hypertension
Bortezomib	Organizing pneumonia, ARDS, DAH, pulmonary arterial hypertension, infection
Carfilzomib	DAH, pulmonary arterial hypertension
Carmustine	Pulmonary fibrosis, ARDS, pleural effusion, pneumothorax, radiation recall pneumonitis, pleuroparenchymal fibroelastosis (PPFE)
Cyclophosphamide	Organizing pneumonia, pulmonary fibrosis, PPFE, ARDS, DAH, bronchospasm, pleural effusion, pulmonary veno-occlusive disease
Doxorubicin	Organizing pneumonia, pulmonary fibrosis, ARDS, radiation recall pneumonitis
Etoposide	ARDS, DAH, bronchospasm, angioedema
Fludarabine	Eosinophilic pneumonia (acute and chronic), organizing pneumonia, lung nodes, ARDS, DAH, pleuritic
Gemcitabine	Eosinophilic pneumonia, pulmonary fibrosis, radiation recall pneumonitis, AIP or ARDS, pulmonary edema, bronchospasm, pleural effusion, pleuritis
Ifosfamide	Pulmonary fibrosis, radiation recall pneumonitis, pulmonary edema, hypoxia
Melphalan	Pulmonary fibrosis, ARDS, bronchospasm, organizing pneumonia, NSIP, UIP
Methotrexate	Organizing pneumonia, pulmonary fibrosis, lung nodules, ARDS, AIP, DAH, bronchospasm, eosinophilic pleural effusion, pulmonary embolism, angioedema
Paclitaxel	ARDS and AIP, radiation recall pneumonitis
Pemetrexed	Organizing pneumonia, ARDS and AIP, DAH, pleuritis, capillary leak
Rituximab	Organizing pneumonia, pulmonary fibrosis, ARDS, pulmonary edema, hemoptysis, cough, asthma attack
Thalidomide	Eosinophilic pneumonia, organizing pneumonia, pulmonary embolism, pulmonary arterial hypertension
Vincristine	Cellular NSIP, laryngospasm
Nivolumab	Eosinophilic pneumonia, AIP, organizing pneumonia, shrinking lung, ARDS, pleural effusion

CAR-T therapy is associated with cytokine release syndrome, which affects multiple organs, including the lungs. Pulmonary side effects of this emerging therapy include pulmonary edema, pneumonitis, and subsequent respiratory failure, often severe enough to require mechanical ventilation [38].

Aspiration Pneumonitis and Pneumonia

Patients with head and neck cancer, gastrointestinal malignancy, or those who have undergone CNS or mediastinal radiation therapy are at risk for aspiration pneumonia. The use of opioid narcotics and sedatives further increases this risk. Only 20% of frank aspiration events result in clinical infection [111]. The majority of aspiration imparts a chemical pneumonitis. Yet the incidence of frank aspiration events is likely underreported, especially in the intensive care unit. Based on pepsin measurements in BAL, a multicenter study of 360 mechanically ventilated patients estimated that 89% of patients undergoing mechanical ventilation silently aspirate [118]. This is particularly detrimental in the cancer population with waning immune response and may lead to further catastrophic complications such as ARDS.

Transfusion-Related Acute Lung Injury and Circulatory Overload (TRALI/TACO)

Transfusion-related acute lung injury (TRALI) is an immune mediated inflammatory noncardiogenic pulmonary edema that occurs following transfusion of blood products, most frequently plasma [179]. It most often manifests within minutes to hours. Clinically it is defined as new hypoxia and diffuse bilateral infiltrates that occur within 6 h of transfusion [33, 156]. Fever is common as is hypotension. Oncology patients are especially at risk given their frequent need for transfusion. This diagnosis should be considered with any new respiratory failure following transfusion, even of allogenic stem cells. TRALI may be confused with transfusion related circulatory overload (TACO), though latter is more often associated with cardiac dysfunction, need for rapid infusion of fluids, and an overall positive fluid balance [51].

Organizing Pneumonia

Organizing pneumonia, often referred to as bronchiolitis obliterans organizing pneumonia or cryptogenic organizing pneumonia, is one of the idiopathic interstitial pneumonitis characterized by proliferation of granulation tissue with the alveoli and alveolar ducts [54]. Clinically its manifestations are nonspecific and often overlap with infectious pneumonia. When no precipitating cause can be identified, it is referred to as cryptogenic organizing pneumonia [56]. Characteristic radiographic findings are included in Table 2. There are many inciting causes including infection, autoimmune disease, vasculitis, immune deficiencies, and transplantation [43]. It has been reported after engraftment of in bone marrow recipients and is associated with acute and chronic graft versus host disease [4]. It may also occur in the context of lung cancer or hematologic malignancy including acute and chronic leukemias, myelodysplastic syndrome, t-cell leukemia, Evans syndrome, and Hodgkin disease [167]. It may also occur as a response to acute drug toxicity or even following radiation therapy [121, 170]. Diagnosis established definitively by lung or transbronchial biopsy but may be suggested on bronchoalveolar lavage. It is a particularly satisfying diagnosis to make as it demonstrates remarkable response to corticosteroid treatment. Relapses, however, are common following withdrawal of steroids [104].

Parenchymal Disorders Common to HCT Patients

Pulmonary complications of HCT are common as transplant conditioning and posttransplant immunosuppression predispose to numerous infections and noninfectious cause of respiratory failure.

Whereas some conditions occur in other cancer patients (organizing pneumonia, drug toxicity, infection, pulmonary edema, and diffuse alveolar hemorrhage and more), others are specific to the HCT patient. Such disease states include the engraftment syndrome and idiopathic pneumonia syndrome.

Peri-Engraftment Respiratory Distress Syndrome (PERDS)

Over 10% of patients undergoing HCT will develop PERDS. It presents during neutrophil recovery and is characterized by fever, rash, and hypoxia from noncardiogenic pulmonary edema. Respiratory failure requiring mechanical ventilation is common [2, 47]. The Spitzer criteria are used for diagnosis. Major criteria include fever, rash, and pulmonary edema. Minor criteria are weight gain, hepatic or renal injury, and encephalopathy. Diagnosis is established by incorporation of three major, or two major and one minor criteria [55].

Idiopathic Pneumonia Syndrome

The idiopathic pneumonia syndrome is a complication of allogenic stem cell transplant that may occur between weeks to months of transplantation. It has been defined as radiographic diffuse alveolar infiltrates with symptoms of pneumonia and objective hypoxia. To fulfil the criteria, infection must be ruled out by negative bronchoalveolar lavage or biopsy [48]. Disease progression is rapid and often requires mechanical ventilation. Tumor Necrosis Factor alpha inhibitors such as etanercept or corticosteroids may be of some benefit [47].

Diffuse Alveolar Hemorrhage (DAH)

Hemorrhage into the alveolar space with or without clinical hemoptysis defines DAH. Bleeding may be bland, or be due to pulmonary capillaritis or diffuse alveolar damage. Many disease states are associated with DAH, but in the cancer patient, DAH is most often linked to chemotherapy and HCT. Risk factors include advancing age, intensive ablative regimens, concomitant infection, and GVHD. Diagnosis is based on BAL with return of progressively bloodier aliquots of

fluid, or by demonstration of >20% hemosiderin laden macrophages [47].

Vascular Disorders

Pulmonary Embolism

Clinically significant deep venous thrombosis and pulmonary embolism may occur in 10% of patients with cancer as a result of a hypercoagulable state, tumor compression of blood vessels, and due to surgery and some chemotherapy agents [84, 175]. Risk also increases with advanced stage of cancer and tumor type. Of the solid tumors, brain, pancreatic, and stomach cancers are most associated with thromboembolic disease. Of the hematologic malignancies, AML is the most frequent culprit of thrombosis [186]. Most pulmonary emboli originate in the proximal veins of the lower extremities. Pulmonary embolism may be classified as acute or chronic, by size, or by hemodynamic characteristics [95, 96]. Low molecular weight heparin is the agent of choice for treatment [96, 105]. In cases of massive pulmonary embolism with hemodynamic compromise, the American College of Chest Physicians suggests use of thrombolytics or catheter directed thrombolysis (Grade 2B and 2C recommendations) [96]. Use of thrombolytics is contraindicated in the stable patient [96], though there is much debate if hemodynamically stable patients with high risk of deterioration (submassive PE) benefit from clot lysis [119]. Often patients with malignancy have contraindications to anticoagulation. These patients may benefit from placement of a filter within the inferior vena cava. However, recent evidence notes that in patients that can receive anticoagulation, the concomitant use of such filters may not prevent recurrence of pulmonary embolism [120].

Pulmonary Leukostasis

Pulmonary leukostasis occurs in patients with acute leukemia or chronic myeloid leukemia in blast crisis and is a result of symptomatic hyperleukocystosis [60, 62]. White blood cells are typically in excess of 50,000–100,000 per microliter of blood which greatly increases blood viscosity.

In addition to cellular occlusion of the microvasculature, metabolic activity of neutrophils results in hypoxemia and leads to cascade of cytokines and subsequent pulmonary injury [107]. Chest radiograph may or may not reveal infiltrates. Partial pressure of oxygen in an arterial blood gas may be spuriously low due to local metabolic activity of neutrophils. As such, pulse oximetry more accurately reflects oxygen balance in these patients. Prompt treatment with leukopheresis is necessary as left unchecked, mortality rates may exceed 40% [62].

Cardiac Causes of Acute Respiratory Failure

Congestive Heart Failure

Chemotherapy-induced cardiomyopathy may not become apparent until the development of a high-output challenge such as anemia or infection. Often it is discovered during fluid resuscitation or with subsequent chemotherapy [168]. Offending agents include anthracyclines, cyclophosphamide, and more. Monoclonal antibodies such as Trastuzumab are also associated with cardiac dysfunction [34]. Chemotherapy-induced heart failure may manifest as acute pulmonary edema and subsequent acute respiratory failure.

Pulmonary Veno-occlusive Disease

A particularly insidious cause of respiratory failure in the cancer patient (albeit rare) is pulmonary veno-occlusive disease. A unique form of postcapillary pulmonary hypertension, this disorder is rapidly fatal without lung transplant. Various chemotherapy regimens are associated with the development of this disorder including bleomycin and mitomycin. Bone marrow transplantation is also a risk factor [66, 77].

Other Causes of Acute Respiratory Failure

Pleural Effusions

Symptomatic pleural effusions may compress the lung with resultant ARF. These effusions represent sequela of a number of conditions common to the cancer patient including primary malignant effusion, infectious parapneumonic effusion and empyema, pulmonary embolism, heart failure, and more. Any new symptomatic effusion, especially in the context of infection, demands timely sampling [144]. Malignant pleural effusion typically represents an advanced stage of cancer and may be due to metastatic disease, lymphoma, or primary pleural malignancy such as mesothelioma. Treatment will be dictated by the underlying etiology. Depending on the rate of accumulation, malignant effusions may be dealt with by serial thoracentesis, indwelling pleural catheters, or pleurodesis [85].

Diagnosis

Respiratory failure is life threatening, and prompt diagnosis of the initiating cause may improve prognosis [14, 87]. The approach taken depends in part on the patient's clinical condition.

Subacute and chronic respiratory failure may afford more time to gather diagnostic data, whereas severe acute hypoxemia or impending cardiopulmonary collapse warrants empiric therapeutic action in concert with rapid diagnostic precision.

The history and pace of cardiopulmonary deterioration provide vital clues to the underlying etiology. Consideration of the nature of immunologic defect is paramount, as is adjunctive chemotherapy and radiation therapy, travel history, environmental exposures, recent hospitalizations, and procedures. A detailed review of prior chemotherapy regimens, past and current medications (prescription and over the counter) is obligatory. Careful attention to subtle clinical signs may reveal a diagnosis. Following a detailed history and physical examination, laboratory and radiographic investigations should selectively pursued to confirm or reject hypothesized differential diagnosis in a Bayesian approach.

Azoulay and colleagues outlined a diagnostic approach to ARF in cancer patients [12]. The utility of this strategy was found clinically useful

Table 4 DIRECT criteria for identifying causes of acute respiratory failure in cancer patients. (Adapted from Ref. [12])

DIRECT
Delay since malignancy onset or HSCT, since symptom onset and since implementation of antibiotics/prophylaxis
Nature of *immune* deficiency
Radiographic appearance
Experience and knowledge of the literature
Clinical picture
Findings by HR*CT*

in an original investigation published in the *European Respiratory Journal* [153]. This approach, easily remembered by the mnemonic DIRECT, is outlined in Table 4.

Diagnostic Studies

Historically, flexible bronchoscopy with bronchoalveolar lavage and biopsy has been the diagnostic modality of choice. Yet this procedure yields a diagnosis in approximately 50% of patients [39, 40, 114, 138, 177]. Some studies quote a higher diagnostic yield of nearly 90% in the bone marrow transplant population [165]. More recent data suggest that bronchoscopy changes the course of management in only 18% of cases [15]. The procedure is not without risk although the complication rates of bronchoscopy are generally low and occur in less than 1% of patients. However, in the hypoxemic cancer patient, the risk of complications increases tenfold. Open lung biopsy or video-assisted thoracoscopic surgery may provide a specific diagnosis more frequently than bronchoscopy. Yet the complication rates may be even higher with a surgical approach. Often the critically ill cancer patient is of poor protoplasm for undergoing surgery with general anesthesia [168]. In essence, the moderate diagnostic yield of bronchoscopy (or surgery) must be weighed against the risk of complications. The primary concern is worsening hypoxemia to the degree requiring invasive mechanical ventilation. This complication is a near death sentence as mechanical

ventilation in those with hematologic malignancy portends a mortality rate ranging from 44% to 100% [14]. Those with solid malignancy have improved outcomes undergoing mechanical ventilation compared to patients with hematologic disease. Given this risk, multiple simultaneous noninvasive modalities (echocardiography, computed tomography, etc.) should be considered prior to bronchoscopy. Noninvasive testing without bronchoscopy is noninferior to FO-BAL in identifying a cause of ARF in patients with cancer and may in fact identify the cause of ARF more quickly than FO-BAL [15].

Noninvasive testing such as bedside ultrasound and echocardiography is rapidly obtained and provides a wealth of information. Acute cardiogenic pulmonary edema is present in 10% of cancer patients with ARF. Given the wide prevalence of coronary artery disease and the use of cardiotoxic agents such as anthracyclines, pericardial effusions and cardiogenic pulmonary edema should be ruled out in all cancer patients with acute respiratory failure. History, exam, and review of medications may increase suspicion for acute heart failure. Interestingly, plasma brain natriuretic peptide may be spuriously elevated in patients with malignancy (sources). Therefore, caution is warranted in the use of BNP in cancer patients. Echocardiography is the diagnostic modality of choice to suggest the presence of cardiac dysfunction. Bedside ultrasound may reveal evidence of extra-vascular lung water or pleural effusions [137].

Infection leading to respiratory failure should be of chief concern. When suspecting infection, time course of the cancer patient's fundamental illness should be kept in mind, as should nature of the patient's immunosuppression. There has been an influx of biochemical assays that may reveal a culprit infection without the need for invasive diagnostics such as bronchoscopy or surgical lung biopsy. Nasopharyngeal viral PCR, immunofluorescence testing, and serum and urine antigen testing may provide valuable diagnostic data. Classic blood and sputum testing is a blunt instrument, yet exciting new tests are currently available, albeit costly. The Karius *Digital Culture*™ is a clinically validated test that can rapidly detect more than 1,250 bacteria, viruses, fungi, and parasites from a single blood draw. It has been demonstrated to have high diagnostic yield of fastidiously difficult to culture pathogens, as well in those patients who have already received broad spectrum antibiotics. A pilot study revealed probable infectious culprits (including Aspergillus fumigatus) in 18 patients with neutropenic fever, even in patients with no definitively positive blood cultures (need to add the source). This testing modality seems promising, but more research is needed before becoming mainstream, especially at the cost of 2,000 USD.

The radiographic pattern of illness is invaluable in the assessment of the hypoxemic cancer patient. However, keep in mind that the plain chest radiograph lacks sensitivity in this population due to muted inflammatory responses. In patients with febrile neutropenia, the plain chest radiograph has a sensitivity of only 36% when evaluating for suspected infection [78]. The sensitivity and specificity of thoracic computed tomography is greater in the evaluation of suspected infection. In addition it also provides detailed patterns such as nodules, infiltrates and consolidation, cysts, cavitation, and more, which can guide physicians in establishing a differential diagnosis and in planning invasive diagnostic procedures. For example, with the appropriate history of a patient with Hodgkin's disease or a patient on corticosteroids, a diffuse bilateral process with hilar ground glass opacities and interlobular septal thickening (crazy-paving) with cysts of varying size should be considered infection with *Pneumocystis jirovecii* pneumonia until proven otherwise. Often CT may itself be diagnostic. CT pulmonary angiography is now the gold standard for the diagnosis of acute pulmonary embolism [91]. Table 2 lists the radiographic characteristics of select causes of acute and chronic respiratory failure in patients with malignancy.

Simplicity is not the norm in the immunocompromised host and the principle of "Occam's razor" may not apply to this population. Often multiple simultaneous infections or conditions may coexist. Thus, a broad and thorough evaluation is warranted in any cancer patient with acute or chronic respiratory failure.

Management

Optimal care for the critical ill cancer patient with ARF requires not only a solid foundation in the principles of cardiopulmonary physiology and appropriate support, but also of the fundamental neoplastic disease-related and treatment-related complications that can occur in the cancer population. Staying abreast of the rapid development of novel chemotherapeutics and advances in ICU care is becoming increasingly difficult. Given this, and the complexity of the critically ill cancer patient, these patients should be cared for by a multidisciplinary team with expertise in pulmonary and critical care, oncology, and palliative care. Such combined efforts have been documented to improve patient outcomes in the ICU setting [141]. In addition, the collective experience of multiple specialists can hasten the diagnosis in the cancer patient with ARF. Given that the differential diagnosis for hypoxemia in the cancer patient is so large, it is important to approach the diagnosis through the lens of multiple looking glasses.

Although there are many causes of respiratory failure in those with malignancy, treatment principles are similar. Supportive care directed at the underlying root cause of a cancer patient's respiratory deterioration remains the goal of critical care admission. Treatment of type I respiratory failure should include oxygen therapy, whereas ventilatory support should be utilized in patients with hypercapnia. Often overlap of hypoxemia and hypercapnea may occur, further complicating therapy. The cause of ARF should be established as this has important prognostic and therapeutic implications. For example, the ventilatory strategy employed for the patient with head and neck cancer suffering from upper airway obstruction may differ from the method used to support a patient with hypoxemia from cardiogenic pulmonary edema. Likewise the tenets of treatment for a patient with diffuse lung disease and refractory hypoxemia will differ drastically compared to the therapy required for a patient with NSCLC and COPD exacerbation. Whatever the reason for respiratory failure in the cancer patient, establishing an

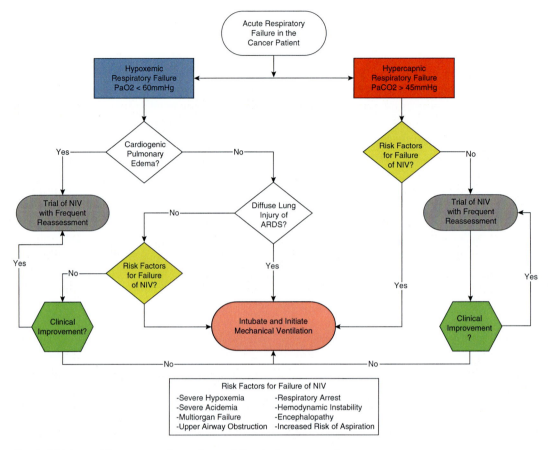

Fig. 1 Initial supportive treatment for respiratory failure in the cancer patient

airway, invasively or noninvasively takes precedence as in any other respiratory crisis. Figure 1 outlines an approach to supportive care for respiratory failure in the oncology patient.

Noninvasive Positive Pressure Ventilation and High-Flow Nasal Oxygenation

Twenty years ago, mechanical ventilation portended a near death sentence for the hematology and bone marrow transplant patient. With an already weakened immune system, these patients fell victim to virulent nosocomial infections and ventilator associated pneumonia [58]. The endotracheal cuff may also erode the trachea mucosa allowing the pooled nidus of bacteria infested secretions of the upper airway to translocate to

the blood stream or migrate to the lower respiratory tract [57]. Tracheal erosions also predispose to bleeding in the pancytopenic patient.

Given this, interest in treating hypoxic respiratory failure in this population with noninvasive modalities blossomed. In 2000, Antonelli et al. evaluated the use of NIV in postoperative solid organ transplant recipients. While cancer patients were not included, use of NIV in these immunocompromised patients following transplantation improved PaO_2 and reduced the rate of fatal complications. In addition, those treated with NIV less often required escalation to mechanical ventilation [8]. The following year, a single center, randomized controlled trail of 52 immunocompromised hypoxemic patients demonstrated that noninvasive positive pressure ventilation delivered by face mask reduced mortality and reduced complications when compared to oxygen therapy alone [89]. The population in this study was overwhelmingly comprised of patients with hematologic cancers. This study noted a 93% case mortality rate in those patients treated with oxygen alone. Over the subsequent decade, survival of cancer patients in the ICU improved, even among those undergoing mechanical ventilation. Along with this trend, fewer studies demonstrated benefit of NIV in hematology patients. Often the etiology of respiratory failure was not taken into account, nor was time on onset of ARF to trial of noninvasive ventilation controlled. Patients with cardiogenic pulmonary edema and hypercapnic respiratory failure were included, the presence of which may have further confounded the ability to parse out which patients truly benefited from an early trial of NIV [64].

In 2012 Wermke conducted a study evaluating early use of NIV in patients with hypoxic respiratory following allogenic hematopoietic stem cell transplant. Eighty-six patients with homogenous baseline characteristics were enrolled and randomized to oxygen therapy only versus treatment with NIV. This population of patients was studied within the wards rather than intensive care unit. There was no mortality difference between the two groups, nor was there a difference in escalation to ICU level care or implementation of invasive mechanical ventilation [184]. Studies in patients without cancer presenting with hypoxic respiratory failure due to community acquired pneumonia and without associated organ dysfunction have shown benefit with the use of NIV [36, 72, 97]. This is not borne out in the cancer patient. In fact, data indicate that cancer patients with documented respiratory infection may do worse when subjected to NIV as first line therapy for hypoxemia [71].

Presumably the same variables that plague outcomes of NIV in the noncancer patient with hypoxic respiratory failure also affect the outcomes in the cancer population. Hypoxic respiratory failure de novo is often prolonged and not immediately reversible. In contrast to hypercapnic respiratory failure or type I respiratory failure from cardiogenic pulmonary edema, NIV without substantial inspiratory support does not reduce the work of breathing in most cases of hypoxia [103]. The

inspiratory demand is increased in settings of hypoxia. This flow demand imparts more diaphragmatic inspiratory effort, ergo vast reductions in intrapleural pressure. Combining large negative pleural pressure with increased inspiratory pressures produces enormous swings in transpulmonary pressure and tidal volumes which may worsen diffuse lung injury [94]. In addition, many causes of type I respiratory failure are anatomically heterogeneous resulting in over distention of smaller, healthier sections of lung. Respiratory compliance is associated with the volume of this remaining functional lung. Recent data from a post hoc observational analysis of nine randomized trials have associated driving pressure (tidal volume divided by respiratory system compliance) as a surrogate marker of "adjusted lung size." In this study, the relative risk of death increased in a near linear fashion with increasing driving pressures, even when tidal volume is kept within a "lung protective" window of 6 ml/kg ideal body weight [7]. Higher driving pressures in NIV are associated with patient intolerance, leak around the mask, as well as gastric over distention with possible aspiration [103].

Specialized high-Flow nasal cannula (HFNC) is capable of delivering warmed and humidified oxygen at flow between 30 and 60 l/min and may circumvent some of the adverse physiology of NIV in hypoxemia. HFNC is also associated with improved patient tolerance, a modest degree of positive end-expiratory pressure, and reduced volume of dead space ventilation [23]. Benefits in patients with cancer have been demonstrated in the palliative arena [67, 83, 106]. Yet the place of this modality of support is not firmly established. A randomized controlled trial reported survival benefit in type I respiratory failure when HFNC was used in lieu NIV or standard oxygen therapy [74]. This was not borne out in a 2017 study specifically examining the use of HFNC in patients with hematologic malignancy and solid cancers. In this group, HFNC reduced the likelihood of intubation but had no significant effect on mortality [17]. Currently the HIGH study is enrolling patients to evaluate the survival benefit of HFNC in immunocompromised patients. This will be the largest multicenter, randomized controlled trial to date evaluating HFNC in cancer patients. The study completion date is estimated December 2018 [18].

Failure rates of NIV in the cancer patient vary widely from 25% up to 70% [14, 45, 161]. Unfortunately, data consistently indicate that outcomes are far worse following failure of NIV [41, 122, 181]. Whether this is due to delay of intubation, inappropriate utilization of NIV in a poorly monitored ward, impact of NiPPV on transpulmonary pressures with resultant volume and barotrauma, or other patient specific characteristics is not fully elucidated.

Previous studies have evaluated risk factors for failure of NIV in cancer patients. Such risks include high illness severity scores, presence of ARDS or multifocal lung involvement, prolonged duration of NIV, septic shock or concomitant use of vasoactive agents, male gender, high respiratory rate, and presence of documented pulmonary infection [11, 71] Within the last 2 years, predictive models have been created to assess a patient's risk for failing NIV. The HACOR score is one such model. This validated score ranging from 0 to 25 points takes into account the following variables of heart rate, acidosis, level of consciousness, oxygenation, and respiratory rate. Rate of failure of NIV in a patient scoring <5 is only 18%, whereas a score >5 predicts failure of NIV in 78% [65].

Truly this exemplifies the need for appropriate patient selection and to ascertain the cause of acute respiratory failure as indiscriminate application of NIV may be harmful. If used for hypoxemia, NIV should be restricted to areas of high monitoring (ICU level care) and performed early with a time sensitive trial and only in the absence of risk factors that portend high likelihood of failure. Such use is consistent with the use of NIV in the general population as outlined by the American Thoracic Society and European Respiratory Society. Otherwise NIV should be utilized in situations of established benefit such as hypercapnic respiratory failure, cardiogenic pulmonary edema, and in those patients with respiratory failure in the postoperative setting [146]. Many patients present advance directives that preclude the use of mechanical ventilation.

In these patients, it is reasonable to utilize NIV or even HFNC. Much as in ARDS, there is no place for non-invasive ventilation in cancer patients with hypoxemic respiratory failure and high risk of NIV failure. Such patients should simply be intubated and mechanically ventilated.

Preparation for Mechanical Ventilation

Patients with risk factors predicting failure of NIV, or in whom emergent airway management is needed, are candidates for invasive mechanical ventilation. The specifics of ventilator setup, different modes and indications, prolonged ventilator management and tracheostomy, postoperative considerations, weening, and ventilator specific strategies for treatment of refractory hypoxemia are beyond the scope of this chapter. These subjects require chapters (or books) dedicated to each topic. Rather, this section will cover the challenges and strategic evaluation of the cancer patient in preparation for transition to invasive positive pressure ventilation. For further reading, Walz et al. provide a comprehensive review of airway management in critical illness including preparation, drug selection, and algorithmic approach to the difficulty and failed airway [182].

Foremost the reason for ARF must be established and the appropriateness of noninvasive therapies must be weighed against the severity of illness and the potential risks of establishing an airway and proceeding with mechanical ventilation. Aside from physiologic challenges of respiratory failure, anatomic difficulties are frequent in the cancer population. This is exemplified in the case of a patient with head and neck squamous cell cancer and acute upper airway obstruction. Such anatomical distortion needs to be considered to minimize potential complications and avoid a situation in which one cannot oxygenate nor ventilate. The rate of complications of airway management differs by clinical setting. Failed intubation happens rarely (1 in 2000) in elective surgical cases in the controlled arena of the operating theatre. This number is far more frequent in the emergency department and ICU setting and failed intubation may occur in one of every 50 ICU patients [53]. In every patient requiring intubation and mechanical ventilation predictors of difficulty anatomy and physiology should be sought prior to initiating rapid sequence intubation (RSI). Indeed, RSI may be detrimental to securing the airway in selected patients with severe hypoxemia, right heart failure, hemodynamic instability, or profound obesity [123]. For initial evaluation of the difficult anatomic airway, the mnemonic LEMON is often used. This approach has the clinician evaluate for anatomical difficulties by Looking externally for unusual anatomy, body habitus, scars, etc., Evaluating incisor distance, the length from hyoid to mentum, and the thyroid to mouth, and assessing jaw mobility and mouth opening. Next the Mallampati score is determined on the classic I–IV scale. Class III and above predict a difficult intubation. Obstruction sought out next, especially in the patient with head and neck cancer. Finally, impairment in Neck mobility also presents an anatomic challenge to successful first pass endotracheal intubation. Neck mobility in cancer patients may occur due to prior surgery or as sequela of radiation therapy. If the difficulty anatomic airway is predicted and time allots, it is prudent to seek airway expertise or consider an awake, fiber optic intubation.

Physiologic challenges to establishing an airway are often overlooked, but of the utmost importance. Three physiologically difficult characteristics have been described including hypoxemia, hypotension, and right heart failure. Hypoxemic patients are at risk for rapid desaturation during intubation. Tissue hypoxia implies impaired oxygen delivery or grossly exaggerated oxygen consumption, often both. In a patient with central obesity, the oxygen reserve or functional residual capacity (FRC) is reduced, and when this patient is struck with hypoxia, the time to desaturation during RSI is rapid. It is suggested that if time permits, every patient undergo a period of preoxygenation prior to intubation [172], preferably with NIV [21]. Note that the indication for NIV in this instance is for preparation for mechanical ventilation. NIV has been shown to improve preoxygenation and end-tidal oxygen far better than standard oxygen alone [21, 164]. Once apneic, implementation of "diffusion respiration" or apneic oxygenation provides a buffer against hypoxia by providing a steady flow of oxygen though the upper airway which passively diffuses to the alveoli as oxygen is taken up into the blood stream [173]. HFNC is purportedly an ideal method of diffusion respiration [183]. While prolonged NIV and HFNC may not be appropriate therapy for hypoxemia, their place may be upheld in preparation for securing the airway for mechanical ventilation.

Many patients with malignancy present with both hypoxia and hypotension which presents challenges to establishing endotracheal intubation. This combination especially frequent and challenging in the cancer patient as hypotension is common. Side effects of chemotherapy predispose to volume loss by vomiting and dehydration [29]. Sequestration of intravascular fluid into the interstitium occurs later in disease as protein-calorie malnutrition becomes common. Sepsis, cytokine storm from novel therapy, pulmonary embolism, blood loss, and more may contribute to a state of poor perfusion which in turn imparts increased oxygen extraction and subsequent hypoxemia. Hypoxemia may contribute to tissue hypoxia and subsequent metabolic acidosis. This acidic milieu can impair the effect of native catecholamines and thereby worsen hypotension [30]. The negative intrathoracic pressure of spontaneous respiration acts to pull blood from the venous reservoir and increase venous return. Transition to positive pressure increases intrathoracic pressure and reduces this venous return. As such, a patient teetering on the brink may be subject to further hypotension as a result of commonly used induction agents or the implementation of positive pressure ventilation [75, 76]. As many as 30% of critically ill patients experience cardiovascular collapse following intubation [135]. This in turn contributes to longer runs of mechanical ventilation and increased ICU stay which can be detrimental to the immunocompromised cancer patient [75, 76, 86, 124]. Assessment of volume status and appropriate resuscitation and consideration of vasopressor infusion may be appropriate in the peri-intubation phase of the critically ill cancer patient requiring endotracheal intubation [123].

A brief note should be made regarding airway management with hypotension and hypoxia in the setting of right heart failure. Such physiology may develop as a result of pulmonary emboli, pulmonary hypertension, or cor pulmonale from any cause of hypoxemia in the cancer patient. Much like the pulmonary circulation, the right ventricle is a low-pressure, high-compliance pump. However, it has limited ability to adapt to acute insult. Hypotension due to right heart failure needs careful evaluation prior to initiation of positive pressure ventilation as increased intrathoracic pressure also increases right ventricular afterload. Hypoxia from ARF induces pulmonary vascular vasoconstriction which places further strain on an ailing RV. Measures normally thought of to restore perfusion pressures such as volume resuscitation or vasoactive agents may further impede RV function and perpetuate poor LV filling and hypotension. If RV dysfunction is suspected prior to intubation, bedside echocardiography should be performed to evaluate for signs of RV failure. In this situation, avoidance of hypoxemia with preoxygenation and apneic oxygenation are a must, and consider "blood pressure neutral" drugs for induction. Initial ventilator settings should target a lower mean airway pressure (if possible) until further stabilization. If available prior to intubation, one may consider application of inhaled nitric oxide or inhaled epoprostenol to improve V/Q mismatch and augment RV unloading and LV filling [123].

Treatment Strategies for Hypercapnic Respiratory Failure

Initial therapies for type II respiratory failure should be implemented at the bedside with attention to instigating causes. Many cancer patients take opioid narcotics for pain control. While a 2011 study identified that opioid related death is less common in cancer patients than in those taking narcotics for other reasons [31], the high doses of opioid often required to control malignant pain may subject one to hypoventilation and

subsequent respiratory failure. A trial of naloxone is reasonable and avoidance of sedatives is recommended. Care should be taken if attempting to reverse benzodiazepines as GABA antagonism may precipitate seizures in those patients with chronic use [5, 108].

Patients with hypercapnic respiratory failure may benefit from a trial of NIV. In cases of COPD exacerbation, therapy with NIV should be utilized early before the onset of acute respiratory acidosis. Suitable candidates for NIV in acute hypercapnia are those who are conscious and able to follow commands and have signs of respiratory distress, a pH <7.35 but greater than 7.20, and in whom close monitoring may occur. It should not be used as first line therapy in patients that are hemodynamically unstable, have multiorgan failure, severe hypoxemia or academia, encephalopathy, or are unable to follow commands, or in whom cardiac or respiratory arrest has occurred.

Optimal settings depend on the patient's body habitus and weight, degree of acidosis, and patient tolerance. Pressure controlled bilevel positive pressure is often used, though volume controlled NIV is also an option.

Frequent monitoring of the patient's clinical condition and arterial blood gas is a must as indiscriminate use of NIV can result in overcorrection and subsequent alkalemia. A time-limited trial should be performed, and if the patient worsens or develops contraindications to NIV, this therapy should be discontinued and mechanical ventilation initiated.

Extracorporeal carbon dioxide removal through a venovenous approach is available at some centers. Unfortunately many centers view active malignancy as a contraindication for extracorporeal membrane support of either oxygenation or CO_2 removal.

Ventilatory Therapies for Hypoxemic Respiratory Failure

Using the acute respiratory distress as a model for severe hypoxemia, there are basic principles of mechanical ventilation that afford a survival benefit. A "lung-protective" strategy should be

Table 5 Selection of PEEP based on required FiO_2. (Adapted from ARDSnet)

Lower PEEP and higher FiO_2									
FiO_2	0.3	0.4	0.4	0.5	0.5	0.6	0.7	0.7	0.7
PEEP	5	5	8	8	10	10	10	12	14
FiO_2	0.8	0.9	0.9	0.9	1.0				
PEEP	14	14	16	18	18–24				
Higher PEEP and lower FiO_2									
FiO_2	0.3	0.3	0.3	0.3	0.3	0.4	0.4	0.5	0.5
PEEP	5	8	10	12	14	14	16	16	18
FiO_2	0.5–0.8	0.8	0.9	1.0	1.0				
PEEP	20	22	22	22	24				

implemented with tidal volumes of 4–8 ml/kg ideal body weight, as well as selecting a modest level of positive end expiratory pressure (PEEP) and making best efforts to limit plateau pressures (in a volume targeted mode of ventilation) to less than 30 cmH$_2$0 [1]. Such remains the current standard of care despite studies over the last decade challenging this dogma. Once severe hypoxemia occurs, emphasis should be on providing adequate oxygenation while attempting to reduce or eliminate ventilator-induced lung injury. Whether pressure or volume targeted therapy is used, selection of appropriate PEEP may be especially important in the patient with suspected chemotherapy or radiation-induced lung injury as it may obviate the need for injurious levels of inspired oxygen [37, 80, 117]. While the three major studies in this area (ALVEOLI, LOV and EXPRESS) reported no survival benefit, they did demonstrate improvements in PaO$_2$/FiO$_2$. Many strategies to select PEEP area available, including incremental trial of PEEP, decremental selection of PEEP, and observation of the pressure-time curve during constant flow volume targeted ventilation (stress index) [80]. For simplicity, the ARDS Clinical Trial Network has created a table with suggested degrees of PEEP based on requirements for FiO$_2$ (Table 5).

Other modalities of ventilation may be utilized in cases of refractory hypoxemia. Such modalities, termed "rescue therapies," are associated with improvements in arterial oxygen tension, but not survival. These include such strategies as airway pressure release ventilation, recruitment maneuvers, and extracorporeal membrane oxygenation [68]. Some recent data are challenging

the belief that recruitment maneuvers are beneficial and even implicate them causing harm (Writing Group for the Alveolar Recruitment for Acute Respiratory Distress Syndrome Trial et al. [185]). In addition, most centers offering ECMO consider active or incurable malignancy as a contraindication to this service; thus, it is unfortunately unavailable for many cancer patients [109].

Prognosis

Whether or not to admit a patient with potentially severe illness to the ICU is a central dilemma faced by intensivists. Preconceived notions are difficult to abolish. Twenty years ago mechanical ventilation following bone marrow transplanted was associated with a mere 2–6% chance of survival. In this study from 1992, the authors elaborated that of 348 bone marrow transplant patients requiring mechanical ventilation, none survived if they required mechanical ventilation for more than 9 days [59]. Further studies in the early 1990s demonstrated high mortality rates of cancer patients in medical intensive care units [35, 151]. This perpetuated a mentality that admission of such patients to the ICU was futile care. Indeed attitudes toward the care of critically ill oncology patients vary by medical subspecialty [130]. Whereas intensivists may focus on organ failure and retain pessimistic notions of the outcomes of critically ill cancer patients [25], oncologists emphasize aspects of cancer therapy and tend to overestimate survival of oncologic patients with acute respiratory failure [50]. Therefore, a multidisciplinary approach with frequent communication between ICU teams, oncology, and palliative care is vital to minimize misconceptions and clarify viewpoints of patient care. Such comprehensive multidisciplinary care is associated with improved survival in this population [101].

In the last 25 years, the morality rates of cancer patients admitted to the ICU have improved and approached that of the general population (30–65%) [61, 159–161]. The notion of cancer as a chronic illness should be upheld when considering admission of the oncology patient to the ICU. Excluding individuals with hematopoietic stem cell transplant, oncology patients requiring mechanical ventilation for ARF have a 40% mortality rate. For perspective, a 2004 study identified a 38% mortality rate for chronic obstructive pulmonary disease patients undergoing mechanical ventilation for exacerbation of COPD [100]. Short term prognosis in critically ill adult oncology now depends on the nature of the acute illness rather than the stage of malignancy or by the complications of cancer therapy [27, 90, 116].

For patients with solid and hematologic malignancy, short term survival is best predicted by the type and number of organ failure [61, 152]. Highest rates of mortality is in those patients requiring mechanical ventilation [152]. When diagnosed with the acute respiratory distress syndrome, mortality rates may exceed 60% [16, 145]. Similarly, adult HCT recipients that require endotracheal intubation have mortality rates near 70% [6]. Variation between studies may be attributed to differences in indication for mechanical ventilation. However, several factors have been identified that portend an especially poor prognosis. These include respiratory failure from a poorly reversible cause [159], underlying chronic pulmonary illness [24], severe hypoxemia prior to intubation (PaO_2 <50 mmHg) [81], and prolonged need for mechanical ventilation [69]. In addition, a small study including patients undergoing chemotherapy while intubated in the ICU revealed an 87% mortality rate [61].

In those that survive ICU stay, 6-month outcomes are worse if mechanical ventilation was required. In a retrospective study of 37 patients with hematologic malignancy, only 36% of those surviving mechanical ventilation were alive 6 months post-ICU care [28].

References

1. Acute Respiratory Distress Syndrome Network, Brower RG, Matthay MA, Morris A, Schoenfeld D, Thompson BT, Wheeler A. Ventilation with lower tidal volumes as compared with traditional tidal volumes for acute lung injury and the acute respiratory distress syndrome. N Engl J Med. 2000;342:1301–8. https://doi.org/10.1056/NEJM200005043421801.
2. Afessa B, Abdulai RM, Kremers WK, Hogan WJ, Litzow MR, Peters SG. Risk factors and outcome of pulmonary complications after autologous hematopoietic stem cell transplant. Chest. 2012;141:442–50. https://doi.org/10.1378/chest.10-2889.
3. Akira M. Computed tomography and pathologic findings in fulminant forms of idiopathic interstitial pneumonia. J Thorac Imaging. 1999;14:76–84.
4. Alasaly K, Muller N, Ostrow DN, Champion P, FitzGerald JM. Cryptogenic organizing pneumonia. A report of 25 cases and a review of the literature. Medicine (Baltimore). 1995;74:201–11.
5. Albiero A, Brigo F, Faccini M, Casari R, Quaglio G, Storti M, Fiaschi A, Bongiovanni LG, Lugoboni F. Focal nonconvulsive seizures during detoxification for benzodiazepine abuse. Epilepsy Behav. 2012;23:168–70. https://doi.org/10.1016/j.yebeh.2011.11.005.
6. Allareddy V, Roy A, Rampa S, Lee MK, Nalliah RP, Allareddy V, Rotta AT. Outcomes of stem cell transplant patients with acute respiratory failure requiring mechanical ventilation in the United States. Bone Marrow Transplant. 2014;49:1278–86. https://doi.org/10.1038/bmt.2014.130.
7. Amato MB, Meade MO, Slutsky AS, Brochard L, Costa EL, Schoenfeld DA, Stewart TE, Briel M, Talmor D, Mercat A, Richard JC, Carvalho CR, Brower RG. Driving pressure and survival in the acute respiratory distress syndrome. N Engl J Med. 2015;372:747–55. https://doi.org/10.1056/NEJMsa1410639.
8. Antonelli M, Conti G, Bufi M, Costa MG, Lappa A, Rocco M, Gasparetto A, Meduri GU. Noninvasive ventilation for treatment of acute respiratory failure in patients undergoing solid organ transplantation: a randomized trial. JAMA. 2000;283:235–41.
9. Artigas A, Bernard GR, Carlet J, Dreyfuss D, Gattinoni L, Hudson L, Lamy M, Marini JJ, Matthay MA, Pinsky MR, Spragg R, Suter PM. The American-European Consensus Conference on ARDS, part 2: ventilatory, pharmacologic, supportive therapy, study design strategies, and issues related to recovery and remodeling. Acute respiratory distress syndrome. Am J Respir Crit Care Med.

1998a;157:1332–47. https://doi.org/10.1164/ajrccm. 157.4.ats2-98.

10. Artigas A, Bernard GR, Carlet J, Dreyfuss D, Gattinoni L, Hudson L, Lamy M, Marini JJ, Matthay MA, Pinsky MR, Spragg R, Suter PM. The American-European Consensus Conference on ARDS, part 2. Ventilatory, pharmacologic, supportive therapy, study design strategies and issues related to recovery and remodeling. Intensive Care Med. 1998b;24:378–98.

11. Azevedo LCP, Caruso P, Silva UVA, Torelly AP, Silva E, Rezende E, Netto JJ, Piras C, Lobo SMA, Knibel MF, Teles JM, Lima RA, Ferreira BS, Friedman G, Rea-Neto A, Dal-Pizzol F, Bozza FA, Salluh JIF, Soares M. Outcomes for patients with cancer admitted to the ICU requiring ventilatory support: results from a prospective multicenter study. Chest. 2014;146:257–66. https://doi.org/10.1378/chest.13-1870. S0012-3692(15)48814-2 [pii].

12. Azoulay E, Schlemmer B. Diagnostic strategy in cancer patients with acute respiratory failure. Intensive Care Med. 2006;32:808–22. https://doi.org/10.1007/s00134-006-0129-2.

13. Azoulay E, Alberti C, Bornstain C, Leleu G, Moreau D, Recher C, Chevret S, Le Gall JR, Brochard L, Schlemmer B. Improved survival in cancer patients requiring mechanical ventilatory support: impact of noninvasive mechanical ventilatory support. Crit Care Med. 2001;29:519–25.

14. Azoulay E, Thiery G, Chevret S, Moreau D, Darmon M, Bergeron A, Yang K, Meignin V, Ciroldi M, Le Gall JR, Tazi A, Schlemmer B. The prognosis of acute respiratory failure in critically ill cancer patients. Medicine (Baltimore). 2004;83:360–70. 00005792-200411000-00005 [pii].

15. Azoulay E, Mokart D, Lambert J, Lemiale V, Rabbat A, Kouatchet A, Vincent F, Gruson D, Bruneel F, Epinette-Branche G, Lafabrie A, Hamidfar-Roy R, Cracco C, Renard B, Tonnelier JM, Blot F, Chevret S, Schlemmer B. Diagnostic strategy for hematology and oncology patients with acute respiratory failure: randomized controlled trial. Am J Respir Crit Care Med. 2010;182:1038–46. https://doi.org/10.1164/rccm.20 1001-0018OC. 201001-0018OC [pii].

16. Azoulay E, Mokart D, Pene F, Lambert J, Kouatchet A, Mayaux J, Vincent F, Nyunga M, Bruneel F, Laisne LM, Rabbat A, Lebert C, Perez P, Chaize M, Renault A, Meert AP, Benoit D, Hamidfar R, Jourdain M, Darmon M, Schlemmer B, Chevret S, Lemiale V. Outcomes of critically ill patients with hematologic malignancies: prospective multicenter data from France and Belgium – a groupe de recherche respiratoire en reanimation onco-hematologique study. J Clin Oncol. 2013;31:2810–8. https://doi.org/10.1200/JCO.2012.47.2365. JCO.2012.47.2365 [pii].

17. Azoulay E, Pickkers P, Soares M, Perner A, Rello J, Bauer PR, van de Louw A, Hemelaar P, Lemiale V, Taccone FS, Martin Loeches I, Meyhoff TS, Salluh J, Schellongowski P, Rusinova K, Terzi N, Mehta S, Antonelli M, Kouatchet A, Barratt-Due A, Valkonen M, Landburg PP, Bruneel F, Bukan RB, Pene F, Metaxa V, Moreau AS, Souppart V, Burghi G, Girault C, Silva UVA, Montini L, Barbier F, Nielsen LB, Gaborit B, Mokart D, Chevret S, Efraim investigators and the Nine-I study group. Acute hypoxemic respiratory failure in immunocompromised patients: the Efraim multinational prospective cohort study. Intensive Care Med. 2017;43:1808–19. https://doi.org/10.1007/s00134-017-4947-1.

18. Azoulay E, Lemiale V, Mokart D, Nseir S, Argaud L, Pene F, Kontar L, Bruneel F, Klouche K, Barbier F, Reignier J, Stoclin A, Louis G, Constantin JM, Mayaux J, Wallet F, Kouatchet A, Peigne V, Perez P, Girault C, Jaber S, Oziel J, Nyunga M, Terzi N, Bouadma L, Lebert C, Lautrette A, Bige N, Raphalen JH, Papazian L, Rabbat A, Darmon M, Chevret S, Demoule A. High-flow nasal oxygen vs. standard oxygen therapy in immunocompromised patients with acute respiratory failure: study protocol for a randomized controlled trial. Trials. 2018;19:157. https://doi.org/10.1186/s13063-018-2492-z.

19. Bach PB, Giralt SA, Saltz LB. FDA approval of tisagenlecleucel: promise and complexities of a $475000 cancer drug. JAMA. 2017;318:1861–2. https://doi.org/10.1001/jama.2017.15218.

20. Baddley JW, Andes DR, Marr KA, Kontoyiannis DP, Alexander BD, Kauffman CA, Oster RA, Anaissie EJ, Walsh TJ, Schuster MG, Wingard JR, Patterson TF, Ito JI, Williams OD, Chiller T, Pappas PG. Factors associated with mortality in transplant patients with invasive aspergillosis. Clin Infect Dis. 2010;50:1559–67. https://doi.org/10.1086/652768.

21. Baillard C, Fosse JP, Sebbane M, Chanques G, Vincent F, Courouble P, Cohen Y, Eledjam JJ, Adnet F, Jaber S. Noninvasive ventilation improves preoxygenation before intubation of hypoxic patients. Am J Respir Crit Care Med. 2006;174:171–7. https://doi.org/10.1164/rccm.200509-1507OC.

22. Balaji A, Verde F, Suresh K, Naidoo J. Pneumonitis from anti-PD-1/PD-L1 therapy. Oncology (Williston Park). 2017;31:739–46, 754.

23. Barberi S, Ciprandi G, Verduci E, D'Auria E, Poli P, Pietra B, Incorvaia C, Buttafava S, Frati F, Riva E. Effect of high-dose sublingual immunotherapy on respiratory infections in children allergic to house dust mite. Asia Pac Allergy. 2015;5:163–9. https://doi.org/10.5415/apallergy.2015.5.3.163.

24. Bayraktar UD, Shpall EJ, Liu P, Ciurea SO, Rondon G, de Lima M, Cardenas-Turanzas M, Price KJ, Champlin RE, Nates JL. Hematopoietic cell transplantation-specific comorbidity index predicts inpatient mortality and survival in patients who received allogeneic transplantation admitted to the intensive care unit. J Clin Oncol. 2013;31:4207–14. https://doi.org/10.1200/JCO.2013.50.5867.

25. Benekli M. Challenging decision: ICU admission of critically ill elderly solid tumor patients. J Thorac Dis. 2017;9:3564–7. https://doi.org/10.21037/jtd.2017.09.25.

26. Benoit DD, Depuydt PO. Outcome in critically ill cancer patients: past and present. Rev Bras Ter Intensiva. 2008;20:82–7.

27. Benoit DD, Vandewoude KH, Decruyenaere JM, Hoste EA, Colardyn FA. Outcome and early prognostic indicators in patients with a hematologic malignancy admitted to the intensive care unit for a life-threatening complication. Crit Care Med. 2003;31:104–12. https://doi.org/10.1097/01.CCM.0000038213.27741.30.

28. Benoit DD, Depuydt PO, Vandewoude KH, Offner FC, Boterberg T, De Cock CA, Noens LA, Janssens AM, Decruyenaere JM. Outcome in severely ill patients with hematological malignancies who received intravenous chemotherapy in the intensive care unit. Intensive Care Med. 2006;32:93–9. https://doi.org/10.1007/s00134-005-2836-5.

29. Berk L, Rana S. Hypovolemia and dehydration in the oncology patient. J Support Oncol. 2006;4:447–54; discussion 455–7.

30. Biais M, Jouffroy R, Carillion A, Feldman S, Jobart-Malfait A, Riou B, Amour J. Interaction of metabolic and respiratory acidosis with alpha and beta-adrenoceptor stimulation in rat myocardium. Anesthesiology. 2012;117:1212–22. https://doi.org/10.1097/ALN.0b013e3182753264.

31. Bohnert AS, Valenstein M, Bair MJ, Ganoczy D, McCarthy JF, Ilgen MA, Blow FC. Association between opioid prescribing patterns and opioid overdose-related deaths. JAMA. 2011;305:1315–21. https://doi.org/10.1001/jama.2011.370.

32. Bos MM, Verburg IW, Dumaij I, Stouthard J, Nortier JW, Richel D, van der Zwan EP, de Keizer NF, de Jonge E. Intensive care admission of cancer patients: a comparative analysis. Cancer Med. 2015;4:966–76. https://doi.org/10.1002/cam4.430.

33. Boshkov LK. Transfusion-related acute lung injury and the ICU. Crit Care Clin. 2005;21:479–95. https://doi.org/10.1016/j.ccc.2005.05.005.

34. Bovelli D, Plataniotis G, Roila F, ESMO Guidelines Working Group. Cardiotoxicity of chemotherapeutic agents and radiotherapy-related heart disease: ESMO Clinical Practice Guidelines. Ann Oncol. 2010;21(Suppl 5):v277–82. https://doi.org/10.1093/annonc/mdq200.

35. Brenner H. Long-term survival rates of cancer patients achieved by the end of the 20th century: a period analysis. Lancet. 2002;360:1131–5. https://doi.org/10.1016/S0140-6736(02)11199-8.

36. Brochard L, Lefebvre JC, Cordioli RL, Akoumianaki E, Richard JC. Noninvasive ventilation for patients with hypoxemic acute respiratory failure. Semin Respir Crit Care Med. 2014;35:492–500. https://doi.org/10.1055/s-0034-1383863.

37. Brower RG, Lanken PN, MacIntyre N, Matthay MA, Morris A, Ancukiewicz M, Schoenfeld D, Thompson BT, National Heart, Lung, and Blood Institute ARDS Clinical Trials Network. Higher versus lower positive end-expiratory pressures in patients with the acute respiratory distress syndrome. N Engl J Med. 2004;351:327–36. https://doi.org/10.1056/NEJMoa032193.

38. Brudno JN, Kochenderfer JN. Toxicities of chimeric antigen receptor T cells: recognition and management. Blood. 2016;127:3321–30. https://doi.org/10.1182/blood-2016-04-703751.

39. Campbell JH, Raina V, Banham SW, Cunningham D, Soukop M. Pulmonary infiltrates – diagnostic problems in lymphoma. Postgrad Med J. 1989;65:881–4.

40. Cazzadori A, Di Perri G, Todeschini G, Luzzati R, Boschiero L, Perona G, Concia E. Transbronchial biopsy in the diagnosis of pulmonary infiltrates in immunocompromised patients. Chest. 1995;107:101–6.

41. Chandra D, Stamm JA, Taylor B, Ramos RM, Satterwhite L, Krishnan JA, Mannino D, Sciurba FC, Holguin F. Outcomes of noninvasive ventilation for acute exacerbations of chronic obstructive pulmonary disease in the United States, 1998–2008. Am J Respir Crit Care Med. 2012;185:152–9. https://doi.org/10.1164/rccm.201106-1094OC.

42. Chaoui D, Legrand O, Roche N, Cornet M, Lefebvre A, Peffault de Latour R, Sanhes L, Huchon G, Marie JP, Rabbat A. Incidence and prognostic value of respiratory events in acute leukemia. Leukemia. 2004;18:670–5. https://doi.org/10.1038/sj.leu.2403270.

43. Chaparro C, Chamberlain D, Maurer J, Winton T, Dehoyos A, Kesten S. Bronchiolitis obliterans organizing pneumonia (BOOP) in lung transplant recipients. Chest. 1996;110:1150–4.

44. Chemaly RF, Torres HA, Hachem RY, Nogueras GM, Aguilera EA, Younes A, Luna MA, Rodriguez G, Tarrand JJ, Raad II. Cytomegalovirus pneumonia in patients with lymphoma. Cancer. 2005;104:1213–20. https://doi.org/10.1002/cncr.21294.

45. Chen WC, Su VY, Yu WK, Chen YW, Yang KY. Prognostic factors of noninvasive mechanical ventilation in lung cancer patients with acute respiratory failure. PLoS One. 2018;13:e0191204. https://doi.org/10.1371/journal.pone.0191204.

46. Chi DC, Brogan F, Turenne I, Zelonis S, Schwartz L, Saif MW. Gemcitabine-induced pulmonary toxicity. Anticancer Res. 2012;32:4147–9.

47. Chi AK, Soubani AO, White AC, Miller KB. An update on pulmonary complications of hematopoietic stem cell transplantation. Chest. 2013;144:1913–22. https://doi.org/10.1378/chest.12-1708.

48. Clark JG, Hansen JA, Hertz MI, Parkman R, Jensen L, Peavy HH. NHLBI workshop summary. Idiopathic pneumonia syndrome after bone marrow transplantation. Am Rev Respir Dis. 1993;147:1601–6. https://doi.org/10.1164/ajrccm/147.6_Pt_1.1601.

49. Clarke M, Collins R, Darby S, Davies C, Elphinstone P, Evans V, Godwin J, Gray R, Hicks C, James S, MacKinnon E, McGale P, McHugh T, Peto R, Taylor C, Wang Y, Early Breast Cancer Trialists' Collaborative Group (EBCTCG). Effects of radiotherapy and of differences in the extent of surgery for early breast cancer on local recurrence and 15-year survival: an overview of the randomised trials. Lancet. 2005;366:2087–106. https://doi.org/10.1016/S0140-6736(05)67887-7.

50. Clement-Duchene C, Carnin C, Guillemin F, Martinet Y. How accurate are physicians in the prediction of patient survival in advanced lung cancer? Oncologist. 2010;15:782–9. https://doi.org/10.1634/theoncologist.2009-0149.

51. Clifford L, Jia Q, Subramanian A, Yadav H, Schroeder DR, Kor DJ. Risk factors and clinical outcomes associated with perioperative transfusion-associated circulatory overload. Anesthesiology. 2017;126:409–18. https://doi.org/10.1097/ALN.000 0000000001506.

52. Coggle JE, Lambert BE, Moores SR. Radiation effects in the lung. Environ Health Perspect. 1986;70:261–91.

53. Cook TM, MacDougall-Davis SR. Complications and failure of airway management. Br J Anaesth. 2012;109(Suppl 1):i68–85. https://doi.org/10.1093/bja/aes393.

54. Cordier JF. Cryptogenic organising pneumonia. Eur Respir J. 2006;28:422–46. https://doi.org/10.1183/09031936.06.00013505.

55. Cornell RF, Hari P, Drobyski WR. Engraftment syndrome after autologous stem cell transplantation: an update unifying the definition and management approach. Biol Blood Marrow Transplant. 2015;21:2061–8. https://doi.org/10.1016/j.bbmt.2015.08.030.

56. Cottin V, Cordier JF. Cryptogenic organizing pneumonia. Semin Respir Crit Care Med. 2012;33:462–75. https://doi.org/10.1055/s-0032-1325157.

57. Craven DE, Steger KA. Nosocomial pneumonia in the intubated patient. New concepts on pathogenesis and prevention. Infect Dis Clin North Am. 1989;3:843–66.

58. Craven DE, Kunches LM, Kilinsky V, Lichtenberg DA, Make BJ, McCabe WR. Risk factors for pneumonia and fatality in patients receiving continuous mechanical ventilation. Am Rev Respir Dis. 1986;133:792–6.

59. Crawford SW, Petersen FB. Long-term survival from respiratory failure after marrow transplantation for malignancy. Am Rev Respir Dis. 1992;145:510–4. https://doi.org/10.1164/ajrccm/145.3.510.

60. Cuttner J, Conjalka MS, Reilly M, Goldberg J, Reisman A, Meyer RJ, Holland JF. Association of monocytic leukemia in patients with extreme leukocytosis. Am J Med. 1980;69:555–8.

61. Darmon M, Thiery G, Ciroldi M, de Miranda S, Galicier L, Raffoux E, Le Gall JR, Schlemmer B, Azoulay E. Intensive care in patients with newly diagnosed malignancies and a need for cancer chemotherapy. Crit Care Med. 2005;33:2488–93. 00003246-200511000-00007 [pii].

62. Daver N, Kantarjian H, Marcucci G, Pierce S, Brandt M, Dinardo C, Pemmaraju N, Garcia-Manero G, O'Brien S, Ferrajoli A, Verstovsek S, Popat U, Hosing C, Anderlini P, Borthakur G, Kadia T, Cortes J, Ravandi F. Clinical characteristics and outcomes in patients with acute promyelocytic leukaemia and hyperleucocytosis. Br J Haematol. 2015;168:646–53. https://doi.org/10.1111/bjh.13189.

63. de la Hoz RE, Stephens G, Sherlock C. Diagnosis and treatment approaches of CMV infections in adult patients. J Clin Virol. 2002;25(Suppl 2):S1–12.

64. Depuydt PO, Benoit DD, Roosens CD, Offner FC, Noens LA, Decruyenaere JM. The impact of the initial ventilatory strategy on survival in hematological patients with acute hypoxemic respiratory failure. J Crit Care. 2010;25:30–6. https://doi.org/10.1016/j.jcrc.2009.02.016. S0883-9441(09)00131-2 [pii].

65. Duan J, Han X, Bai L, Zhou L, Huang S. Assessment of heart rate, acidosis, consciousness, oxygenation, and respiratory rate to predict noninvasive ventilation failure in hypoxemic patients. Intensive Care Med. 2017;43:192–9. https://doi.org/10.1007/s00134-016-4601-3.

66. Ellis DA, Capewell SJ. Pulmonary veno-occlusive disease after chemotherapy. Thorax. 1986;41:415–6.

67. Epstein AS, Hartridge-Lambert SK, Ramaker JS, Voigt LP, Portlock CS. Humidified high-flow nasal oxygen utilization in patients with cancer at Memorial Sloan-Kettering Cancer Center. J Palliat Med. 2011;14:835–9. https://doi.org/10.1089/jpm.2011. 0005.

68. Esan A, Hess DR, Raoof S, George L, Sessler CN. Severe hypoxemic respiratory failure: part 1 – ventilatory strategies. Chest. 2010;137:1203–16. https://doi.org/10.1378/chest.09-2415.

69. Ewer MS, Ali MK, Atta MS, Morice RC, Balakrishnan PV. Outcome of lung cancer patients requiring mechanical ventilation for pulmonary failure. JAMA. 1986;256:3364–6.

70. Faria IM, Zanetti G, Barreto MM, Rodrigues RS, Araujo-Neto CA, Silva JL, Escuissato DL, Souza AS Jr, Irion KL, Mancano AD, Nobre LF, Hochhegger B, Marchiori E. Organizing pneumonia: chest HRCT findings. J Bras Pneumol. 2015;41:231–7. https://doi.org/10.1590/S1806-37132015000 004544.

71. Ferreira JC, Medeiros P Jr, Rego FM, Caruso P. Risk factors for noninvasive ventilation failure in cancer patients in the intensive care unit: a retrospective cohort study. J Crit Care. 2015;30:1003–7. https://doi.org/10.1016/j.jcrc.2015.04.121.

72. Ferrer M, Esquinas A, Leon M, Gonzalez G, Alarcon A, Torres A. Noninvasive ventilation in severe hypoxemic respiratory failure: a randomized clinical trial. Am J Respir Crit Care Med. 2003;168:1438–44. https://doi.org/10.1164/rccm.200301-072OC.

73. Franquet T, Muller NL, Gimenez A, Guembe P, de La Torre J, Bague S. Spectrum of pulmonary aspergillosis: histologic, clinical, and radiologic findings. Radiographics. 2001;21:825–37. https://doi.org/10.1148/radiographics.21.4.g01jl03825.

74. Frat JP, Thille AW, Mercat A, Girault C, Ragot S, Perbet S, Prat G, Boulain T, Morawiec E, Cottereau A, Devaquet J, Nseir S, Razazi K, Mira JP, Argaud L, Chakarian JC, Ricard JD, Wittebole X, Chevalier S, Herbland A, Fartoukh M, Constantin JM, Tonnelier JM, Pierrot M, Mathonnet A, Beduneau G, Deletage-Metreau C, Richard JC, Brochard L, Robert R, FLORALI Study Group, REVA Network. High-flow oxygen through nasal cannula in acute hypoxemic respiratory failure. N Engl J Med. 2015;372:2185–96. https://doi.org/10.1056/NEJMoa1503326.

75. Funk DJ, Jacobsohn E, Kumar A. Role of the venous return in critical illness and shock: part II-shock and mechanical ventilation. Crit Care Med. 2013a;41:573–9. https://doi.org/10.1097/CCM.0b013e31827bfc25.

76. Funk DJ, Jacobsohn E, Kumar A. The role of venous return in critical illness and shock-part I: physiology. Crit Care Med. 2013b;41:255–62. https://doi.org/10.1097/CCM.0b013e3182772ab6.

77. Gagnadoux F, Capron F, Lebeau B. Pulmonary veno-occlusive disease after neoadjuvant mitomycin chemotherapy and surgery for lung carcinoma. Lung Cancer. 2002;36:213–5.

78. Gerritsen MG, Willemink MJ, Pompe E, van der Bruggen T, van Rhenen A, Lammers JW, Wessels F, Sprengers RW, de Jong PA, Minnema MC. Improving early diagnosis of pulmonary infections in patients with febrile neutropenia using low-dose chest computed tomography. PLoS One. 2017;12:e0172256. https://doi.org/10.1371/journal.pone.0172256.

79. Goodman LR, Fumagalli R, Tagliabue P, Tagliabue M, Ferrario M, Gattinoni L, Pesenti A. Adult respiratory distress syndrome due to pulmonary and extrapulmonary causes: CT, clinical, and functional correlations. Radiology. 1999;213:545–52. https://doi.org/10.1148/radiology.213.2.r99nv42545.

80. Grasso S, Stripoli T, De Michele M, Bruno F, Moschetta M, Angelelli G, Munno I, Ruggiero V, Anaclerio R, Cafarelli A, Driessen B, Fiore T. ARDSnet ventilatory protocol and alveolar hyperinflation: role of positive end-expiratory pressure. Am J Respir Crit Care Med. 2007;176:761–7. https://doi.org/10.1164/rccm.200702-193OC.

81. Hampshire PA, Welch CA, McCrossan LA, Francis K, Harrison DA. Admission factors associated with hospital mortality in patients with haematological malignancy admitted to UK adult, general critical care units: a secondary analysis of the ICNARC Case Mix Programme Database. Crit Care. 2009;13:R137. https://doi.org/10.1186/cc8016.

82. Hanna YM, Baglan KL, Stromberg JS, Vicini FA, Decker D. Acute and subacute toxicity associated with concurrent adjuvant radiation therapy and paclitaxel in primary breast cancer therapy. Breast J. 2002;8:149–53.

83. Harada K, Kurosawa S, Hino Y, Yamamoto K, Sakaguchi M, Ikegawa S, Hattori K, Igarashi A, Watakabe K, Senoo Y, Najima Y, Hagino T, Doki N, Kobayashi T, Kakihana K, Iino T, Sakamaki H, Ohashi K. Clinical utility of high-flow nasal cannula oxygen therapy for acute respiratory failure in patients with hematological disease. Springerplus. 2016;5:512. https://doi.org/10.1186/s40064-016-2161-1.

84. Hedderich GS, O'Connor RJ, Reid EC, Mulder DS. Caval tumor thrombus complicating renal cell carcinoma: a surgical challenge. Surgery. 1987;102:614–21.

85. Heffner JE, Klein JS. Recent advances in the diagnosis and management of malignant pleural effusions. Mayo Clin Proc. 2008;83:235–50. https://doi.org/10.4065/83.2.235.

86. Heffner AC, Swords DS, Neale MN, Jones AE. Incidence and factors associated with cardiac arrest complicating emergency airway management. Resuscitation. 2013;84:1500–4. https://doi.org/10.1016/j.resuscitation.2013.07.022.

87. Heussel CP, Kauczor HU, Ullmann AJ. Pneumonia in neutropenic patients. Eur Radiol. 2004;14:256–71. https://doi.org/10.1007/s00330-003-1985-6.

88. Hicks KL, Chemaly RF, Kontoyiannis DP. Common community respiratory viruses in patients with cancer: more than just "common colds". Cancer. 2003;97:2576–87. https://doi.org/10.1002/cncr.11353.

89. Hilbert G, Gruson D, Vargas F, Valentino R, Gbikpi-Benissan G, Dupon M, Reiffers J, Cardinaud JP. Noninvasive ventilation in immunosuppressed patients with pulmonary infiltrates, fever, and acute respiratory failure. N Engl J Med. 2001;344:481–7. https://doi.org/10.1056/NEJM200102153440703.

90. Hill QA, Kelly RJ, Patalappa C, Whittle AM, Scally AJ, Hughes A, Ashcroft AJ, Hill A. Survival of patients with hematological malignancy admitted to the intensive care unit: prognostic factors and outcome compared to unselected medical intensive care unit admissions, a parallel group study. Leuk Lymphoma. 2012;53:282–8. https://doi.org/10.3109/10428194.2011.614705.

91. Huisman MV, Klok FA. How I diagnose acute pulmonary embolism. Blood. 2013;121:4443–8. https://doi.org/10.1182/blood-2013-03-453050.

92. Jacobs C, Slade M, Lavery B. Doxorubicin and BOOP. A possible near fatal association. Clin Oncol (R Coll Radiol). 2002;14:262.

93. Johkoh T, Ikezoe J, Tomiyama N, Nagareda T, Kohno N, Takeuchi N, Yamagami H, Kido S, Takashima S, Arisawa J, et al. CT findings in lymphangitic carcinomatosis of the lung: correlation with histologic findings and pulmonary function tests. AJR Am J Roentgenol. 1992;158:1217–22. https://doi.org/10.2214/ajr.158.6.1590110.

94. Kallet RH, Diaz JV. The physiologic effects of noninvasive ventilation. Respir Care. 2009;54:102–15.

95. Kearon C, Akl EA, Comerota AJ, Prandoni P, Bounameaux H, Goldhaber SZ, Nelson ME, Wells PS, Gould MK, Dentali F, Crowther M, Kahn SR. Antithrombotic therapy for VTE disease: antithrombotic therapy and prevention of thrombosis, 9th ed: American College of Chest Physicians Evidence-Based Clinical Practice Guidelines. Chest. 2012;141:e419S–96S. https://doi.org/10.1378/chest.11-2301.

96. Kearon C, Akl EA, Ornelas J, Blaivas A, Jimenez D, Bounameaux H, Huisman M, King CS, Morris TA, Sood N, Stevens SM, Vintch JRE, Wells P, Woller SC, Moores L. Antithrombotic therapy for VTE disease: CHEST guideline and expert panel report. Chest. 2016;149:315–52. https://doi.org/10.1016/j.chest.2015.11.026.

97. Keenan SP, Sinuff T, Burns KE, Muscedere J, Kutsogiannis J, Mehta S, Cook DJ, Ayas N, Adhikari NK, Hand L, Scales DC, Pagnotta R, Lazosky L, Rocker G, Dial S, Laupland K, Sanders K, Dodek P, Canadian Critical Care Trials Group/Canadian Critical Care Society Noninvasive Ventilation Guidelines Group. Clinical practice guidelines for the use of noninvasive positive-pressure ventilation and noninvasive continuous positive airway pressure in the acute care setting. CMAJ. 2011;183:E195–214. https://doi.org/10.1503/cmaj.100071.

98. Kerkering TM, Duma RJ, Shadomy S. The evolution of pulmonary cryptococcosis: clinical implications from a study of 41 patients with and without compromising host factors. Ann Intern Med. 1981;94:611–6.

99. Khan H, Belsher J, Yilmaz M, Afessa B, Winters JL, Moore SB, Hubmayr RD, Gajic O. Fresh-frozen plasma and platelet transfusions are associated with development of acute lung injury in critically ill medical patients. Chest. 2007;131:1308–14. https://doi.org/10.1378/chest.06-3048.

100. Khilnani GC, Banga A, Sharma SK. Predictors of mortality of patients with acute respiratory failure secondary to chronic obstructive pulmonary disease admitted to an intensive care unit: a one year study. BMC Pulm Med. 2004;4:12. https://doi.org/10.1186/1471-2466-4-12.

101. Kim MM, Barnato AE, Angus DC, Fleisher LA, Kahn JM. The effect of multidisciplinary care teams on intensive care unit mortality. Arch Intern Med. 2010;170:369–76. https://doi.org/10.1001/archinternmed.2009.521.

102. Kotloff RM, Ahya VN, Crawford SW. Pulmonary complications of solid organ and hematopoietic stem cell transplantation. Am J Respir Crit Care Med. 2004;170:22–48. https://doi.org/10.1164/rccm.200309-1322SO.

103. L'Her E, Deye N, Lellouche F, Taille S, Demoule A, Fraticelli A, Mancebo J, Brochard L. Physiologic effects of noninvasive ventilation during acute lung injury. Am J Respir Crit Care Med. 2005;172:1112–8. https://doi.org/10.1164/rccm.200402-226OC.

104. Lazor R, Vandevenne A, Pelletier A, Leclerc P, Court-Fortune I, Cordier JF. Cryptogenic organizing pneumonia. Characteristics of relapses in a series of 48 patients. The Groupe d'Etudes et de Recherche sur les Malades "Orphelines" Pulmonaires (GERM"O"P). Am J Respir Crit Care Med. 2000;162:571–7. https://doi.org/10.1164/ajrccm.162.2.9909015.

105. Lee AY, Levine MN, Baker RI, Bowden C, Kakkar AK, Prins M, Rickles FR, Julian JA, Haley S, Kovacs MJ, Gent M, Randomized Comparison of Low-Molecular-Weight Heparin versus Oral Anticoagulant Therapy for the Prevention of Recurrent Venous Thromboembolism in Patients with Cancer (CLOT) Investigators. Low-molecular-weight heparin versus a coumarin for the prevention of recurrent venous thromboembolism in patients with cancer. N Engl J Med. 2003;349:146–53. https://doi.org/10.1056/NEJMoa025313.

106. Lee HY, Rhee CK, Lee JW. Feasibility of high-flow nasal cannula oxygen therapy for acute respiratory failure in patients with hematologic malignancies: a retrospective single-center study. J Crit Care. 2015;30:773–7. https://doi.org/10.1016/j.jcrc.2015.03.014.

107. Lichtman MA, Rowe JM. Hyperleukocytic leukemias: rheological, clinical, and therapeutic considerations. Blood. 1982;60:279–83.

108. Lugoboni F, Faccini M, Quaglio GL, Albiero A, Casari R, Pajusco B. Intravenous flumazenil infusion to treat benzodiazepine dependence should be performed in the inpatient clinical setting for high risk of seizure. J Psychopharmacol. 2011;25:848–9. https://doi.org/10.1177/0269881110393050.

109. Makdisi G, Wang IW. Extra Corporeal Membrane Oxygenation (ECMO) review of a lifesaving technology. J Thorac Dis. 2015;7:E166–76. https://doi.org/10.3978/j.issn.2072-1439.2015.07.17.

110. Marchesi F, Pimpinelli F, Ensoli F, Mengarelli A. Cytomegalovirus infection in hematologic malignancy settings other than the allogeneic transplant. Hematol Oncol. 2018;36:381–91. https://doi.org/10.1002/hon.2453.

111. Marik PE. Aspiration pneumonitis and aspiration pneumonia. N Engl J Med. 2001;344:665–71. https://doi.org/10.1056/NEJM200103013440908.

112. Marr KA, Carter RA, Boeckh M, Martin P, Corey L. Invasive aspergillosis in allogeneic stem cell transplant recipients: changes in epidemiology and risk factors. Blood. 2002;100:4358–66. https://doi.org/10.1182/blood-2002-05-1496.

113. Martinez R, Reyes S, Menendez R. Pulmonary nocardiosis: risk factors, clinical features, diagnosis and prognosis. Curr Opin Pulm Med. 2008;14:219–27. https://doi.org/10.1097/MCP.0b013e3282f85dd3.

114. Maschmeyer G, Link H, Hiddemann W, Meyer P, Helmerking M, Eisenmann E, Schmitt J, Adam D. Pulmonary infiltrations in febrile patients with neutropenia. Risk factors and outcome under empirical antimicrobial therapy in a randomized multicenter study. Cancer. 1994;73:2296–304.

115. McDonald S, Rubin P, Phillips TL, Marks LB. Injury to the lung from cancer therapy: clinical syndromes, measurable endpoints, and potential scoring systems. Int J Radiat Oncol Biol Phys. 1995;31:1187–203. https://doi.org/10.1016/0360-3016(94)00429-O.

116. McGrath S, Chatterjee F, Whiteley C, Ostermann M. ICU and 6-month outcome of oncology patients in the intensive care unit. QJM. 2010;103:397–403. https://doi.org/10.1093/qjmed/hcq032.

117. Mercat A, Richard JC, Vielle B, Jaber S, Osman D, Diehl JL, Lefrant JY, Prat G, Richecoeur J, Nieszkowska A, Gervais C, Baudot J, Bouadma L, Brochard L, Expiratory Pressure (Express) Study Group. Positive end-expiratory pressure setting in adults with acute lung injury and acute respiratory distress syndrome: a randomized controlled trial. JAMA. 2008;299:646–55. https://doi.org/10.1001/jama.299.6.646.

118. Metheny NA, Clouse RE, Chang YH, Stewart BJ, Oliver DA, Kollef MH. Tracheobronchial aspiration of gastric contents in critically ill tube-fed patients: frequency, outcomes, and risk factors. Crit Care Med. 2006;34:1007–15. https://doi.org/10.1097/01.CCM.0000206106.65220.59.

119. Meyer G, Vicaut E, Danays T, Agnelli G, Becattini C, Beyer-Westendorf J, Bluhmki E, Bouvaist H, Brenner B, Couturaud F, Dellas C, Empen K, Franca A, Galie N, Geibel A, Goldhaber SZ, Jimenez D, Kozak M, Kupatt C, Kucher N, Lang IM, Lankeit M, Meneveau N, Pacouret G, Palazzini M, Petris A, Pruszczyk P, Rugolotto M, Salvi A, Schellong S, Sebbane M, Sobkowicz B, Stefanovic BS, Thiele H, Torbicki A, Verschuren F, Konstantinides SV, PEITHO Investigators. Fibrinolysis for patients with intermediate-risk pulmonary embolism. N Engl J Med. 2014;370:1402–11. https://doi.org/10.1056/NEJMoa1302097.

120. Mismetti P, Laporte S, Pellerin O, Ennezat PV, Couturaud F, Elias A, Falvo N, Meneveau N, Quere I, Roy PM, Sanchez O, Schmidt J, Seinturier C, Sevestre MA, Beregi JP, Tardy B, Lacroix P, Presles E, Leizorovicz A, Decousus H, Barral FG, Meyer G, PREPIC2 Study Group. Effect of a retrievable inferior vena cava filter plus anticoagulation vs anticoagulation alone on risk of recurrent pulmonary embolism: a randomized clinical trial. JAMA. 2015;313:1627–35. https://doi.org/10.1001/jama.2015.3780.

121. Miwa S, Morita S, Suda T, Suzuki K, Hayakawa H, Chida K, Nakamura H. The incidence and clinical characteristics of bronchiolitis obliterans organizing pneumonia syndrome after radiation therapy for breast cancer. Sarcoidosis Vasc Diffuse Lung Dis. 2004;21:212–8.

122. Molina R, Bernal T, Borges M, Zaragoza R, Bonastre J, Granada RM, Rodriguez-Borregan JC, Nunez K, Seijas I, Ayestaran I, Albaiceta GM. Ventilatory support in critically ill hematology patients with respiratory failure. Crit Care. 2012;16:R133. https://doi.org/10.1186/cc11438. cc11438 [pii].

123. Mosier JM, Joshi R, Hypes C, Pacheco G, Valenzuela T, Sakles JC. The physiologically difficult airway. West J Emerg Med. 2015a;16:1109–17. https://doi.org/10.5811/westjem.2015.8.27467.

124. Mosier JM, Hypes C, Joshi R, Whitmore S, Parthasarathy S, Cairns CB. Ventilator strategies and rescue therapies for management of acute respiratory failure in the emergency department. Ann Emerg Med. 2015b;66:529–41. https://doi.org/10.1016/j.annemergmed.2015.04.030.

125. Moskovic E, Miller R, Pearson M. High resolution computed tomography of Pneumocystis carinii pneumonia in AIDS. Clin Radiol. 1990;42:239–43.

126. Movsas B, Raffin TA, Epstein AH, Link CJ Jr. Pulmonary radiation injury. Chest. 1997;111:1061–76.

127. Mullins PM, Goyal M, Pines JM. National growth in intensive care unit admissions from emergency departments in the United States from 2002 to 2009. Acad Emerg Med. 2013;20:479–86. https://doi.org/10.1111/acem.12134.

128. Muraoka M, Tagawa T, Akamine S, Oka T, Tsuchiya T, Araki M, Hayashi T, Nagayasu T. Acute interstitial pneumonia following surgery for primary lung cancer. Eur J Cardiothorac Surg. 2006;30:657–62. https://doi.org/10.1016/j.ejcts.2006.06.020.

129. Naidoo J, Wang X, Woo KM, Iyriboz T, Halpenny D, Cunningham J, Chaft JE, Segal NH, Callahan MK, Lesokhin AM, Rosenberg J, Voss MH, Rudin CM, Rizvi H, Hou X, Rodriguez K, Albano M, Gordon RA, Leduc C, Rekhtman N, Harris B, Menzies AM, Guminski AD, Carlino MS, Kong BY, Wolchok JD, Postow MA, Long GV, Hellmann MD. Pneumonitis in patients treated with anti-programmed death-1/programmed death ligand 1 therapy. J Clin Oncol. 2017;35:709–17. https://doi.org/10.1200/JCO.2016.68.2005.

130. Nassar AP Jr, Dettino ALA, Amendola CP, Dos Santos RA, Forte DN, Caruso P. Oncologists' and intensivists' attitudes toward the care of critically ill patients with cancer. J Intensive Care Med. 2017; 885066617716105. https://doi.org/10.1177/0885066617716105.

131. Ozkan M, Dweik RA, Ahmad M. Drug-induced lung disease. Cleve Clin J Med. 2001;68:782–5, 789–95.

132. Pappas PG, Perfect JR, Cloud GA, Larsen RA, Pankey GA, Lancaster DJ, Henderson H, Kauffman CA, Haas DW, Saccente M, Hamill RJ, Holloway MS, Warren RM, Dismukes WE. Cryptococcosis in human immunodeficiency virus-negative patients in the era of effective azole therapy. Clin Infect Dis. 2001;33:690–9. https://doi.org/10.1086/322597.

133. Pastores SM, Voigt LP. Acute respiratory failure in the patient with cancer: diagnostic and management strategies. Crit Care Clin. 2010;26:21–40. https://doi.org/10.1016/j.ccc.2009.10.001.

134. Paz HL, Crilley P, Weinar M, Brodsky I. Outcome of patients requiring medical ICU admission following

bone marrow transplantation. Chest. 1993;104: 527–31. S0012-3692(16)35370-3 [pii].

135. Perbet S, De Jong A, Delmas J, Futier E, Pereira B, Jaber S, Constantin JM. Incidence of and risk factors for severe cardiovascular collapse after endotracheal intubation in the ICU: a multicenter observational study. Crit Care. 2015;19:257. https://doi.org/10.1186/s13054-015-0975-9.

136. Pfeifer R, Heussen N, Michalewicz E, Hilgers RD, Pape HC. Incidence of adult respiratory distress syndrome in trauma patients: a systematic review and meta-analysis over a period of three decades. J Trauma Acute Care Surg. 2017;83:496–506. https://doi.org/10.1097/TA.0000000000001571.

137. Picano E, Pellikka PA. Ultrasound of extravascular lung water: a new standard for pulmonary congestion. Eur Heart J. 2016;37:2097–104. https://doi.org/10.1093/eurheartj/ehw164.

138. Pisani RJ, Wright AJ. Clinical utility of broncho-alveolar lavage in immunocompromised hosts. Mayo Clin Proc. 1992;67:221–7.

139. Pishgar F, Ebrahimi H, Saeedi Moghaddam S, Fitzmaurice C, Amini E. Global, regional and national burden of prostate cancer, 1990 to 2015: results from the Global Burden of Disease Study 2015. J Urol. 2018;199:1224–32. https://doi.org/10.1016/j.juro.2017.10.044.

140. Primack SL, Miller RR, Muller NL. Diffuse pulmonary hemorrhage: clinical, pathologic, and imaging features. AJR Am J Roentgenol. 1995;164:295–300. https://doi.org/10.2214/ajr.164.2.7839958.

141. Prin M, Wunsch H. International comparisons of intensive care: informing outcomes and improving standards. Curr Opin Crit Care. 2012;18:700–6. https://doi.org/10.1097/MCC.0b013e32835914d5.

142. Pulte D, Gondos A, Brenner H. Expected long-term survival of patients diagnosed with acute myeloblastic leukemia during 2006–2010. Ann Oncol. 2010;21:335–41. https://doi.org/10.1093/annonc/mdp309.

143. Rabello LS, Silva JR, Azevedo LC, Souza I, Torres VB, Rosolem MM, Lisboa T, Soares M, Salluh JI. Clinical outcomes and microbiological characteristics of severe pneumonia in cancer patients: a prospective cohort study. PLoS One. 2015;10:e0120544. https://doi.org/10.1371/journal.pone.0120544. PONE-D-14-35125 [pii].

144. Rahman NM, Chapman SJ, Davies RJ. Pleural effusion: a structured approach to care. Br Med Bull. 2004;72:31–47. https://doi.org/10.1093/bmb/ldh040.

145. Reichner CA, Thompson JA, O'Brien S, Kuru T, Anderson ED. Outcome and code status of lung cancer patients admitted to the medical ICU. Chest. 2006;130:719–23. https://doi.org/10.1378/chest.130.3.719.

146. Rochwerg B, Brochard L, Elliott MW, Hess D, Hill NS, Nava S, Navalesi P Members of the Steering Committee, Antonelli M, Brozek J, Conti G, Ferrer M, Guntupalli K, Jaber S, Keenan S, Mancebo J, Mehta S, Raoof S Members of the Task Force. Official ERS/ATS clinical practice guidelines: noninvasive ventilation for acute respiratory failure. Eur Respir J. 2017;50. https://doi.org/10.1183/13993003.02426-2016.

147. Rosenow EC 3rd, Limper AH. Drug-induced pulmonary disease. Semin Respir Infect. 1995;10:86–95.

148. Roychowdhury DF, Cassidy CA, Peterson P, Arning M. A report on serious pulmonary toxicity associated with gemcitabine-based therapy. Invest New Drugs. 2002;20:311–5.

149. Rutherford JD. Digital clubbing. Circulation. 2013;127:1997–9. https://doi.org/10.1161/CIRCULATIONAHA.112.000163.

150. Ryu JH. Chemotherapy-induced pulmonary toxicity in lung cancer patients. J Thorac Oncol. 2010;5:1313–4. https://doi.org/10.1097/JTO.0b013e3181e9dbb9.

151. Schapira DV, Studnicki J, Bradham DD, Wolff P, Jarrett A. Intensive care, survival, and expense of treating critically ill cancer patients. JAMA. 1993;269:783–6.

152. Schellongowski P, Sperr WR, Wohlfarth P, Knoebl P, Rabitsch W, Watzke HH, Staudinger T. Critically ill patients with cancer: chances and limitations of intensive care medicine-a narrative review. ESMO Open. 2016;1:e000018. https://doi.org/10.1136/esmoopen-2015-000018.

153. Schnell D, Mayaux J, Lambert J, Roux A, Moreau AS, Zafrani L, Canet E, Lemiale V, Darmon M, Azoulay E. Clinical assessment for identifying causes of acute respiratory failure in cancer patients. Eur Respir J. 2013;42:435–43. https://doi.org/10.1183/09031936.00122512.

154. Shah DP, Shah PK, Azzi JM, El Chaer F, Chemaly RF. Human metapneumovirus infections in hematopoietic cell transplant recipients and hematologic malignancy patients: a systematic review. Cancer Lett. 2016;379:100–6. https://doi.org/10.1016/j.canlet.2016.05.035.

155. Siegel RL, Miller KD, Jemal A. Cancer statistics, 2017. CA Cancer J Clin. 2017;67:7–30. https://doi.org/10.3322/caac.21387.

156. Silliman CC, Ambruso DR, Boshkov LK. Transfusion-related acute lung injury. Blood. 2005;105:2266–73. https://doi.org/10.1182/blood-2004-07-2929.

157. Silverberg E, Holleb AI. Major trends in cancer: 25 year survey. CA Cancer J Clin. 1975;25:2–8.

158. Snyder LS, Hertz MI. Cytotoxic drug-induced lung injury. Semin Respir Infect. 1988;3:217–28.

159. Soares M, Salluh JI, Spector N, Rocco JR. Characteristics and outcomes of cancer patients requiring mechanical ventilatory support for >24 hrs. Crit Care Med. 2005;33:520–6. 00003246-200503000-00008 [pii].

160. Soares M, Darmon M, Salluh JIF, Ferreira CG, Thiery G, Schlemmer B, Spector N, Azoulay E. Prognosis of lung cancer patients with life-threatening complications. Chest. 2007;131:840–6. https://doi.org/10.1378/chest.06-2244.

161. Soares M, Depuydt PO, Salluh JI. Mechanical ventilation in cancer patients: clinical characteristics and outcomes. Crit Care Clin. 2010a;26:41–58. https://doi.org/10.1016/j.ccc.2009.09.005. S0749-0704(09) 00078-5 [pii].

162. Soares M, Caruso P, Silva E, Teles JM, Lobo SM, Friedman G, Dal Pizzol F, Mello PV, Bozza FA, Silva UV, Torelly AP, Knibel MF, Rezende E, Netto JJ, Piras C, Castro A, Ferreira BS, Rea-Neto A, Olmedo PB, Salluh JI. Characteristics and outcomes of patients with cancer requiring admission to intensive care units: a prospective multicenter study. Crit Care Med. 2010b;38:9–15. https://doi.org/10.1097/CCM.0b013e3181c0349e.

163. Sohn JW. Acute eosinophilic pneumonia. Tuberc Respir Dis (Seoul). 2013;74:51–5. https://doi.org/10.4046/trd.2013.74.2.51.

164. Solis A, Baillard C. Effectiveness of preoxygenation using the head-up position and noninvasive ventilation to reduce hypoxaemia during intubation. Ann Fr Anesth Reanim. 2008;27:490–4. https://doi.org/10.1016/j.annfar.2008.04.006.

165. Springmeyer SC. The clinical use of bronchoalveolar lavage. Chest. 1987;92:771–2.

166. Stefan MS, Shieh MS, Pekow PS, Rothberg MB, Steingrub JS, Lagu T, Lindenauer PK. Epidemiology and outcomes of acute respiratory failure in the United States, 2001 to 2009: a national survey. J Hosp Med. 2013;8:76–82. https://doi.org/10.1002/jhm.2004.

167. Stemmelin GR, Bernaciak J, Casas JG. Bronchiolitis with leukemia. Ann Intern Med. 1991;114:912–3.

168. Stover DE, Kaner RJ. Pulmonary complications in cancer patients. CA Cancer J Clin. 1996;46:303–20.

169. Taccone FS, Artigas AA, Sprung CL, Moreno R, Sakr Y, Vincent JL. Characteristics and outcomes of cancer patients in European ICUs. Crit Care. 2009;13: R15. https://doi.org/10.1186/cc7713.

170. Takigawa N, Segawa Y, Saeki T, Kataoka M, Ida M, Kishino D, Fujiwara K, Ohsumi S, Eguchi K, Takashima S. Bronchiolitis obliterans organizing pneumonia syndrome in breast-conserving therapy for early breast cancer: radiation-induced lung toxicity. Int J Radiat Oncol Biol Phys. 2000;48:751–5.

171. Tamura M, Saraya T, Fujiwara M, Hiraoka S, Yokoyama T, Yano K, Ishii H, Furuse J, Goya T, Takizawa H, Goto H. High-resolution computed tomography findings for patients with drug-induced pulmonary toxicity, with special reference to hypersensitivity pneumonitis-like patterns in gemcitabine-induced cases. Oncologist. 2013;18:454–9. https://doi.org/10.1634/theoncologist.2012-0248.

172. Tanoubi I, Drolet P, Donati F. Optimizing preoxygenation in adults. Can J Anaesth. 2009;56: 449–66. https://doi.org/10.1007/s12630-009-9084-z.

173. Teller LE, Alexander CM, Frumin MJ, Gross JB. Pharyngeal insufflation of oxygen prevents arterial desaturation during apnea. Anesthesiology. 1988; 69:980–2.

174. Thun MJ, DeLancey JO, Center MM, Jemal A, Ward EM. The global burden of cancer: priorities for prevention. Carcinogenesis. 2010;31:100–10. https://doi.org/10.1093/carcin/bgp263.

175. Timp JF, Braekkan SK, Versteeg HH, Cannegieter SC. Epidemiology of cancer-associated venous thrombosis. Blood. 2013;122:1712–23. https://doi.org/10.1182/blood-2013-04-460121.

176. Torre LA, Siegel RL, Ward EM, Jemal A. Global cancer incidence and mortality rates and trends – an update. Cancer Epidemiol Biomarkers Prev. 2016;25:16–27. https://doi.org/10.1158/1055-9965. EPI-15-0578.

177. Torres A, Puig de la Bellacasa J, Xaubet A, Gonzalez J, Rodriguez-Roisin R, Jimenez de Anta MT, Agusti Vidal A. Diagnostic value of quantitative cultures of bronchoalveolar lavage and telescoping plugged catheters in mechanically ventilated patients with bacterial pneumonia. Am Rev Respir Dis. 1989;140:306–10. https://doi.org/10.1164/ajrccm/140.2.306.

178. Torres HA, Reddy BT, Raad II, Tarrand J, Bodey GP, Hanna H, Rolston KV, Kontoyiannis DP. Nocardiosis in cancer patients. Medicine (Baltimore). 2002;81:388–97.

179. Toy P, Popovsky MA, Abraham E, Ambruso DR, Holness LG, Kopko PM, McFarland JG, Nathens AB, Silliman CC, Stroncek D, National Heart, Lung and Blood Institute Working Group on TRALI. Transfusion-related acute lung injury: definition and review. Crit Care Med. 2005;33:721–6.

180. Vilchez RA, Linden P, Lacomis J, Costello P, Fung J, Kusne S. Acute respiratory failure associated with pulmonary cryptococcosis in non-aids patients. Chest. 2001;119:1865–9.

181. Walkey AJ, Wiener RS. Use of noninvasive ventilation in patients with acute respiratory failure, 2000–2009: a population-based study. Ann Am Thorac Soc. 2013;10:10–7. https://doi.org/10.1513/AnnalsATS.201206-034OC.

182. Walz JM, Zayaruzny M, Heard SO. Airway management in critical illness. Chest. 2007;131:608–20. https://doi.org/10.1378/chest.06-2120.

183. Weingart SD. Preoxygenation, reoxygenation, and delayed sequence intubation in the emergency department. J Emerg Med. 2011;40:661–7. https://doi.org/10.1016/j.jemermed.2010.02.014.

184. Wermke M, Schiemanck S, Hoffken G, Ehninger G, Bornhauser M, Illmer T. Respiratory failure in patients undergoing allogeneic hematopoietic SCT – a randomized trial on early non-invasive ventilation based on standard care hematology wards. Bone Marrow Transplant. 2012;47:574–80. https://doi.org/10.1038/bmt.2011.160.

185. Writing Group for the Alveolar Recruitment for Acute Respiratory Distress Syndrome Trial (ART) Investigators, Cavalcanti AB, Suzumura EA, Laranjeira LN, Paisani DM, Damiani LP, Guimaraes HP, Romano ER, Regenga MM, Taniguchi LNT,

Teixeira C, Pinheiro de Oliveira R, Machado FR, Diaz-Quijano FA, Filho MSA, Maia IS, Caser EB, Filho WO, Borges MC, Martins PA, Matsui M, Ospina-Tascon GA, Giancursi TS, Giraldo-Ramirez ND, Vieira SRR, Assef M, Hasan MS, Szczeklik W, Rios F, Amato MBP, Berwanger O, Ribeiro de Carvalho CR. Effect of lung recruitment and titrated positive end-expiratory pressure (PEEP) vs low PEEP on mortality in patients with acute respiratory distress syndrome: a randomized clinical trial. JAMA. 2017;318:1335–45. https://doi.org/10.1001/jama.2017.14171.

186. Wun T, White RH. Epidemiology of cancer-related venous thromboembolism. Best Pract Res Clin Haematol. 2009;22:9–23. https://doi.org/10.1016/j.beha.2008.12.001.

187. Yale SH, Limper AH. *Pneumocystis carinii* pneumonia in patients without acquired immunodeficiency syndrome: associated illness and prior corticosteroid therapy. Mayo Clin Proc. 1996;71:5–13.

188. Yamashita H, Nakagawa K, Nakamura N, Koyanagi H, Tago M, Igaki H, Shiraishi K, Sasano N, Ohtomo K. Exceptionally high incidence of symptomatic grade 2–5 radiation pneumonitis after stereotactic radiation therapy for lung tumors. Radiat Oncol. 2007;2:21. https://doi.org/10.1186/1748-717X-2-21.

189. Zhang LJ, Hanff P, Rutherford C, Churchill WH, Crumpacker CS. Detection of human cytomegalovirus DNA, RNA, and antibody in normal donor blood. J Infect Dis. 1995;171:1002–6.

Noninvasive Oxygen Therapies in Oncologic Patients

32

Michael C. Sklar, Bruno L. Ferreyro, and Laveena Munshi

Contents

Introduction 478

Spectrum of ARF in Oncologic Patients 478
What Is Unique About ARF in Oncologic Versus Nononcologic Patients 478

Noninvasive Oxygen Modalities 480
Continuous Oxygen Therapy 480
Noninvasive Ventilation 482
High-Flow Nasal Cannula 483

Evidence of NIV 484
General Population 484
Immunocompromised and Oncologic Patients 484

Evidence for HFNC 490
General Population 490
Immunocompromised and Oncologic Population 494

Conclusions 496

References 496

Abstract

Acute hypoxemic respiratory failure (ARF) is the most common cause of critical illness in oncologic patients. Despite significant advancements in survival of oncologic patients who develop critical illness, mortality rates in those requiring invasive mechanical ventilation have improved but remain high. Avoiding intubation is paramount to the management of oncologic patients with ARF. There are important differences between the oncologic patient with ARF compared to the general ICU population that likely underlie the increased mortality once intubated. Noninvasive oxygen modalities have been recognized as an important therapeutic approach to prevent intubation. Continuous low-flow oxygen therapy, noninvasive ventilation, and high-flow nasal cannula are the most commonly used noninvasive oxygen therapies in recent years. They have unique physiologic

M. C. Sklar · B. L. Ferreyro · L. Munshi (✉)
Interdepartmental Division of Critical Care Medicine, Mount Sinai Hospital, Sinai Health System, University of Toronto, Toronto, ON, Canada
e-mail: michaelcsklar@gmail.com;
bruno.ferreyro@uhn.ca;
Laveena.Munshi@sinaihealthsystem.ca

© Springer Nature Switzerland AG 2020
J. L. Nates, K. J. Price (eds.), *Oncologic Critical Care*,
https://doi.org/10.1007/978-3-319-74588-6_197

properties. The data surrounding their efficacy in the general ICU population and oncologic population has evolved over time reflecting the changes in the oncologic population. This chapter reviews the three different noninvasive oxygen modalities, their physiologic impact, and evidence surrounding their effectiveness.

Keywords

High-flow nasal cannula · High-flow oxygen therapy · Low-flow oxygen therapy · Continuous oxygen therapy · Noninvasive ventilation · Acute respiratory failure · Acute respiratory distress syndrome · Oncologic critical care · Immunocompromised

Introduction

Acute hypoxemic respiratory failure (ARF) is the most common cause of critical illness in oncologic patients [1–3]. Avoiding intubation is paramount to the management of oncologic patients with ARF. The risks associated with intubation are pronounced in the immunocompromised and oncologic population. These risks include numerous infectious, musculoskeletal, respiratory, and neurologic complications. Oncologic patients may present with a greater frequency of frailty at the time of critical illness, a higher likelihood of succumbing to aggressive or drug-resistant pathogens or they may experience a blunted or dysregulated host response [4–6]. As such, patients who progress to require invasive mechanical ventilation are subject to increased mortality compared to the general ICU population [7].

In hypoxemic oncologic patients, noninvasive oxygen therapy may be delivered via simple face mask (continuous oxygen therapy (COT)), noninvasive ventilation (NIV), or high-flow nasal cannula (HFNC). Earlier studies in immunocompromised patients receiving NIV compared to COT suggested a reduced need for intubation [6, 8]. This resulted in adoption of NIV as a noninvasive strategy to support oncologic patients in an attempt to prevent intubation. However, these results have been called into question in recent years [9]. Furthermore, we have recently

seen the development of HFNC with promising preliminary results across the general ICU population. It is unclear whether these promising results with HFNC translate to the oncologic population. With the goal to reserve intubation in those failing noninvasive oxygenation strategies, there remains a need to better understand these therapies in this unique population.

This chapter will focus on the rationale for preventing intubation in the oncologic population, the mechanisms of the various noninvasive oxygen modalities, evidence-to-date of these modalities across the general and oncologic patients, and future areas of consideration.

Spectrum of ARF in Oncologic Patients

The number of living patients with cancer has been increasing steadily over the last several years [10]. The spectrum of ARF in oncologic patients varies widely and may be induced by the underlying malignancy or be secondary to treatment-associated toxicities (Fig. 1).

What Is Unique About ARF in Oncologic Versus Nononcologic Patients

While mortality across critically ill oncologic patients has decreased significantly in recent decades with advancements in oncologic and critical care, mortality across ARF and acute respiratory distress syndrome (ARDS) remains high [11]. There are a series of factors that are theorized to be underlying this increased mortality. A thorough understanding of these factors is necessary when considering which noninvasive oxygen strategy one may choose.

Cause of ARF
ARF in the oncologic patient can broadly be categorized into disease-associated ARF and treatment-associated ARF. Disease associated causes of respiratory failure include tumor infiltration into the airway, pulmonary leukostasis, leukemic infiltrates, and malignant pleural effusions among others. Treatment-associated

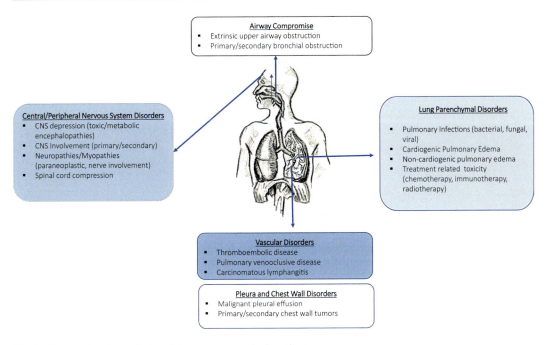

Fig. 1 Causes of acute respiratory failure across oncologic patients

toxicities may occur early during treatment (tumor lysis syndrome, cytokine release syndrome, all-transretinoic acid differentiation syndrome), at the height of treatment effect (neutropenic-associated infectious complications), during recovery (neutrophil reconstitution or engraftment syndrome associated with ARDS), or as a late toxicity (cardiomyopathy, pulmonary pneumonitis). These causes are unique to the oncologic population. While infectious etiologies remain the most common culprit, a higher proportion of non-infectious causes are noted in this population. Therefore, an accurate understanding of the differential is imperative to guide early recognition, anticipation of deterioration, and institution of appropriate supportive care and treatment. Recognizing and projecting the reversibility of the underlying cause is an important factor in deciding on the noninvasive or invasive modality one may choose as first line.

Diagnostic Challenge

Undiagnosed ARF is associated with a high mortality [12]. Given this, meticulous attention over previous decades has been dedicated to the optimal approach to diagnostic evaluation of

pulmonary infiltrates and ARF in the oncologic population. Diagnostic workup often includes, a series of noninvasive serum and sputum microbiologic tests (sputum cultures, induced sputum for pneumoncystic jirovecii pneumonia, cytomegalovirus serum evaluation, serum galactomannan, nasopharyngeal swab for viral polymerase chain reaction, etc.), imaging modalities (CT thorax, echocardiography if hydrostatic pulmonary edema is considered), and possible fiberoptic bronchoscopy for further microbiologic evaluation if no diagnosis has been yielded. This investigative workup is often more invasive and requires more imaging and transportation for the oncologic population compared to the general ICU population.

Frailty

Oncology patients represent a subgroup particularly susceptible to frailty. During intensive treatments, patients may be exposed to transient illnesses, hospitalizations, interruption in normal nutrition regimens, steroids, limited mobility due to toxic side effects, and recovery from surgery. All of these factors potentially put them at higher risk of developing frailty, particularly precritical illness. Frailty is increasingly being recognized as an important determinant of duration of mechanical ventilation, ICU survival and ICU functional recovery [13–15]. In this population, significant loss of muscle mass that may occur during treatment puts them at higher risk of frailty or prolonged mechanical ventilation due to the development of diaphragmatic dysfunction in the setting of ARF.

Increased Mortality

Over the last decade, there has been consistent evidence suggesting that oncologic patients with ARF who undergo invasive mechanical ventilation face a significantly increased risk of poor survival and functional outcomes [2, 16]. Although this association might be explained partially by indication bias, making it challenging to confirm a true causal effect, it is widely accepted that the initial oxygen delivery strategy is a key factor while approaching the management of ARF in this vulnerable population. Mortality across oncologic patients who require invasive mechanical ventilation can range from 40% to 50% and can reach as high as 80% in a certain subset of oncologic patients (i.e., allogenenic hematopoietic stem cell transplant patients, invasive fungal infections) [2, 17]. Risk factors for mortality are outlined in Table 2.

Long-Term Outcomes Trajectory

Despite evidence of a high mortality in the face of ARF, there is a paucity of data on the long-term outcomes of oncologic patients with ARF. What is unique about this population compared to the general population of ARDS survivors is that they have a potentially reversible underlying comorbid condition, and therefore their functional recovery and diseased trajectory could follow a different path. More data is needed to further delineate this dedicated to this population [11, 18].

Hematologic Malignancy Versus Solid Tumor

Outcomes of oncologic patients who develop critical illness have improved over the years with reports mirroring, in some studies, mortality rates across the general ICU populations. Critical illness is often associated with a higher severity of illness and, as a result, higher mortality [19, 20]. The more profound and prolonged nature of the immunocompromised state that is achieved, as a consequence of intensive curative therapies, render this vulnerable population to a greater risk of bacterial, viral, and invasive fungal infections. Noninfectious etiologies unique to the hematologic malignancy population include pulmonary leukostasis, pulmonary leukemic infiltrates, lung alveolar proteinosis in the setting of tumor lysis syndrome, alveolar hemorrhage, differentiation syndrome and capillary leak as a subset of treatment-associated toxicities, cytokine release syndrome-inducing ARDS, immune reconstitution-associated ARDS in the setting of neutrophil recovery, and radiation-associated pneumonitis [21]. In the allogeneic hematopoietic stem cell transplant, additional causes include engraftment syndrome, diffused alveolar hemorrhage, idiopathic pneumonia syndrome, and acute/chronic graft versus host disease [22, 23].

Noninvasive Oxygen Modalities

Noninvasive oxygenation strategies in the oncologic patient can be delivered by conventional face-mask oxygen therapy (COT), noninvasive ventilation (NIV), and high-flow nasal oxygen cannula therapy (HFNC). Each of these techniques have unique physiological considerations and important advantages and disadvantages that must be understood so that a clinician can deliver safe, effective, and personalized therapy to this high-risk patient population (Table 1). The following section will discuss the basic physiologic principles, advantages, and possible disadvantages of each.

Continuous Oxygen Therapy

Oxygen delivered to spontaneously breathing patients is most commonly delivered by masks. Broadly speaking, oxygen can be delivered by simple, partial rebreathing and non-rebreathing masks. Flow rates range from 6 L/min (simple) to 15 L/min (non-rebreather) with a fraction of

Table 1 Benefits and pitfalls of noninvasive oxygen modalities

	Benefits	Pitfalls
Continuous low-flow oxygen therapy	Comfortable Ease of application Amenable for transportation Does not impair cough/secretion management	In patients with high work of breathing, they may entrain a high volume of room air dissolving the delivered alveolar oxygen content Local toxic effects of high inspired FiO_2
Noninvasive ventilation	Continuous PEEP to facilitate recruitment Inspiratory positive pressure to support tidal volumes during poor compliance or fatigue Recruitment and decrease work of breathing may facilitate a decreased in FiO_2 requirements Decrease in preload/afterload in the setting of a cardiogenic pulmonary edema Amenable for transportation	Decrease in preload or increase in right ventricular afterload could precipitate or exacerbate shock Secretion clearance challenging with face mask interface Potential for injurious ventilation particularly in the setting of a high work of breathing May delay or impair administration of evidence-based ICU therapies or workup (nutrition, mobility, imaging, bronchoscopy) Facemask interface uncomfortable by some
High-flow nasal cannula	Comfortable Heated and humidified oxygen enhances mucociliary clearance Possible generation of PEEP to facilitate recruitment High flows help prevent entrainment of room air thus minimizing dilution of administered oxygen Deadspace washout may contribute to decreasing work of breathing Can facilitate fiberoptic bronchoscopy	Cannot transport Uncertainty surrounding levels of generated PEEP based upon patient features Highest flows may be considered uncomfortable by some

PEEP positive end expiratory pressure

inspired oxygen (FiO_2) of approximately 30–90% [24]. The advantages to COT is its noninvasive nature and its portability.

One of the major limitations of conventional face-mask oxygen delivery systems is the limited inspiratory flow rate it can deliver. In the setting of respiratory distress, the inspiratory flow rate of dyspneic patients often greatly exceeds the upper limit of flow rates delivered by these conventional systems and a significant entrainment of ambient air limits the delivery of the targeted FiO_2. As a result, oxygen delivery to the alveoli is the resultant fractions of high FiO_2 at a fixed delivered rate and ambient air (0.21) at a rate determined by any excessive inspiratory flow generated by a patient in respiratory distress. The greater the entrainment of ambient air, the greater dilution of the alveolar FiO_2. Furthermore, an additional shortcoming of COT is its lack of ability to provide any alveolar recruitment in the setting of a consolidated lung. Alveolar recruitment may result in a decreased need for excessive FiO_2 delivery through

recruitment of additional alveoli to participate in gas exchange. In the absence of this recruitment, a patient on COT may be exposed to unnecessarily high concentrations of inspired oxygen to maintain a sufficient saturation. The resultant negative effect of a prolonged exposure to high oxygen delivery is potentially oxygen toxicity which has been found to be associated with an increased mortality [25]. While we conceptualize oxygen toxicity as having the greatest harm in those with excessive dissolved oxygen content leading to excessive reactive oxygen species, the local toxic effect of the administration of high oxygen concentration of inspired O_2 has also been described leading to tracheal and bronchial irritation, impaired mucociliary clearance and surfactant impairment, alterations in microbial flora in the upper airways and alveolar nitrogen washout leading to absorptive atelectasis. Therefore, in critically ill patients, NIV and HFNC may be more attractive options to temporize or reverse acute respiratory failure given some mechanisms described below.

Noninvasive Ventilation

NIV refers to the delivery of positive pressure by devices other than an endotracheal tube [26]. In the critical care setting, NIV is most often delivered by application of a full oro-nasal facemask, but can be delivered through a nasal apparatus, or through use of a helmet [27]. When delivering NIV, clinicians will set an appropriate FiO_2, an inspiratory positive airway pressure (IPAP) and an expiratory positive airway pressure (EPAP).

The EPAP is synonymous with positive end-expiratory pressure, commonly referred to as PEEP. This is the positive pressure level (in cmH_2O) that is present at the end of expiration [26]. IPAP refers to the level of inspiratory pressure delivered. The difference between the delivered IPAP and EPAP will determine the amount of pressure support and amount of delivered tidal volume. Nomenclature for NIV settings is best demonstrated with an example: with an IPAP of 10 cmH_2O and an EPAP of 5 cmH_2O, a patient will receive a total inspiratory pressure of 10 cmH_2O with a PEEP of 5 cmH_2O. This patient will receive 5 cmH_2O of pressure support above their baseline pressure of 5 cmH_2O.

From a physiological perspective, the delivery of positive pressure has important implications. Positive pressure may improve arterial oxygenation through re-expansion of collapsed or atelectatic alveoli, redistribution of lung edema, and reducing areas of ventilation-perfusion mismatch [28]. Importantly, this oxygenation improvement is reliant on recruitable lung segments and avoidance of overdistension of normal pulmonary parenchyma [29]. In addition to changes in oxygenation, lung recruitment has important effects of respiratory mechanics. Lung compliance can improve when atelectatic alveoli are recruited or be reduced in situations of overdistension. These mechanisms may also result in the ability to decrease the FiO_2 delivered to the patient minimizing the potential risks associated with direct toxicity related to high inspired oxygen.

Heart–lung interactions must be considered when delivering positive pressure via NIV, and the clinician should appreciate and anticipate the potential hemodynamic alterations. Classically, positive pressure can affect hemodynamic performance through a variety of mechanisms. Positive pressure delivered may result in a decrease in right ventricular preload, a variable impact on right ventricular afterload, augment left ventricular preload through propelling blood volume from the pulmonary capillaries into the left atrium, and decrease left-ventricular afterload. It can both decrease right-ventricular afterload (through improving oxygenation and reversing hypoxic vasoconstriction/decreasing pulmonary vascular resistance) or increase right-ventricular afterload in the setting of alveolar overdistension if excessive PEEP were applied. This may result in a compression in pulmonary capillaries and increasing pulmonary vascular resistance [30].

One may anticipate the potential hemodynamic response to NIV by considering the patients underlying preload status and cardiac function. With normal cardiac function, the main hemodynamic response to an increase in intrathoracic pressure is a reduction in venous return and preload to the heart, which can manifest as a reduction in cardiac output and blood pressure [28]. This phenomenon underscores the need for adequate volume repletion in patients not in cardiogenic pulmonary edema. In contrast, those patients with reduced ventricular function and signs of cardiogenic induced hydrostatic pulmonary edema can greatly benefit from NIV. The physiologic impact of reducing right-ventricular preload and afterload reducing the left ventricle is ideal in the setting of congestive heart failure and an impaired left ventricle. This can result in the redistribution of extravascular lung water [30].

Finally, NIV has an important role in hypercapnic exacerbations of chronic obstructive pulmonary disease (COPD) by decreasing the work of breathing, off-loading the respiratory muscles, counteracting intrinsic PEEP, and preventing dynamic hyperinflation [31].

Despite the potential benefits of NIV, it is important to understand its limitations and relative contraindications. For safe delivery of NIV, patients must be awake and able to protect their airway. Therefore, caution must be employed when patients have a fluctuating level of consciousness, poor ability to clear secretions, nausea and vomiting, or have a full stomach at risk of pulmonary aspiration [26]. Contraindications may include, but are not limited to, cardiopulmonary arrest, head and neck surgery, upper airway obstruction, fresh esophageal anastomosis, bowel obstruction, hemoptysis, and untreated pneumothorax. Another important concern with NIV is that there is a challenge in measuring the delivered tidal volumes, which, when greater than 6–8 mL/kg of ideal body weight, may precipitate ventilator-associated lung injury [32, 33]. NIV is a modality that has the greatest evidence in rapidly reversible conditions (congestive heart failure, acute exacerbations of chronic obstructive pulmonary disease); however, in more protracted conditions (i.e., pneumonia, checkpoint-associated pulmonary toxicities), NIV may impair one's ability to proceed with other routine care-objectives, i.e., nutrition, mobility, bronchoscopy, calling into questions its role in longer term management of more complex patients. However, increasingly, evidence have demonstrated the safety of enteral nutrition, mobilization, and bronchoscopy mechanisms with various NIV interfaces [27, 34].

High-Flow Nasal Cannula

HFNC is a novel noninvasive oxygenation device that has rapidly gained popularity. HFNC is a heated, humidified oxygen delivery system that is capable of delivering flows of 40–60 L/min with an FiO_2 of up to a 100% through specialized nasal prongs [35]. One of the major benefits of this system is that the high flow rates can match those of severely dyspneic patients, thereby preventing entrainment of room air (with an FiO_2 of 21%). This mechanism prevents dilution of delivered oxygen [10]. Furthermore, the gas is heated and humidified to avoid mucosal injury and enhance patient comfort, overcoming the key problems of past use of high flow rates [36].

In addition to supplemental oxygen, high flow rates, and humidity, several other mechanisms are hypothesized to play an important role in the clinical benefits associated with HFNC. The use of HFNC is associated with a washout of carbon dioxide from the upper airways [36, 37]. This in turn reduces anatomic dead space fraction, rebreathing of expired, carbon dioxide rich gas, and ultimately making ventilation more efficient.

High inspiratory flow rates delivered by HFNC generate low amounts of PEEP [38]. Both human and benchwork studies have determined that at 60 L/min of flow, at least 2–4 cmH_2O (and perhaps even more) positive pressure can be generated. Through its flow-mediated generation of positive pressure, HFNC can improve oxygenation through recruitment of atelectatic lung regions in a mechanism comparable to NIV [36]. Given that the amount of PEEP is moderate, it may follow that the hemodynamic effects (both positive and negative) may be tempered compared to NIV.

Consistently, HFNC has been demonstrated to reduce respiratory rate, inspiratory effort, and improve oxygenation in patients with acute hypoxemic respiratory failure [35, 36, 39] and may play an important role in the mitigation of ventilation-associated lung and diaphragmatic injury [36]. The improved breathing pattern can limit expiratory diaphragm loading [36, 40] and therefore possibly constrain injurious eccentric diaphragm contractions. The above described mechanisms of HFNC ultimately reduce the metabolic cost of breathing and therefore reducing minute ventilation requirements, improve lung compliance, and ventilation-perfusion matching. Importantly, these processes may reduce lung stress and strain and repetitive opening and closing of alveoli (atelectrauma) [36, 41]. Cumulatively, the improved comfort and tolerance, improved oxygenation, and theoretical reduction in diaphragm and ventilation-induced lung injury lead to the improved clinical outcomes observed with HFNC [36].

HFNC has many promising advantages as a highly effective noninvasive oxygenation device. Firstly, it permits patients to be instrumented with nasal prongs and avoids the tight-fitting masks of conventional NIV. This allows patients to eat, sleep, and clear secretions more easily than with NIV. Especially in those patients who have not previously used full face mask NIV, the use of nasal prongs and HFNC may reduce claustrophobia and improve uptake, compliance, and allows for continuous use of the device. Perhaps as an extension of this, patients with acute hypoxemia have consistently rated HFNC to be more comfortable than NIV [35].

Although there are many benefits of HFNC, pathophysiological states such as cardiogenic pulmonary edema where increased amounts of PEEP are needed for redistribution of alveolar lung water, NIV may be a better option. Furthermore, more studies are needed to identify those patients who are at risk of HFNC failure requiring intubation and invasive mechanical ventilation. This is of paramount importance because these patients will have little to no oxygenation reserve and are at elevated risk of significant hypoxemia during airway instrumentation.

Evidence of NIV

General Population

The role of NIV for hydrostatic pulmonary edema or to support a patient with an exacerbation of chronic obstructive pulmonary disease is compelling which recent guidelines have made strong recommendations supporting its use [42]. Its role in ARF remains controversial [31, 42, 43]. However, as a result of its effectiveness for these isolated indications, we have seen a proliferation of use across the general and oncologic population for indications beyond hydrostatic pulmonary edema and chronic obstructive pulmonary disease [44, 45].

In one of the largest, multicenter, international, observational studies evaluating the diagnosis and management patients with ARDS, the Lung Safe Study, NIV was used as a first-line therapy in 15% of patients [46]. There was no major difference across severity of ARDS with reports of its use (mild = 14%, mod = 17%, severe = 13%). NIV failure occurred in a moderate proportion of these patients with failure rates of 22%, 42%, and 47% across mild, moderate, and severe ARDS, respectively. NIV failure was associated with a high mortality (45%) across all cohorts compared to NIV success (15% mortality). In a propensity matched analysis, NIV failure was associated with an increased ICU mortality and was found

to have a greater mortality rate than those who were managed with invasive mechanical ventilation as first line with moderate-severe ARDS (i.e., $PaO_2/FiO_2 < 150$).

Immunocompromised and Oncologic Patients

In the immunocompromised and oncologic population, the reported rates of NIV use for ARF has been increasing since 2000 [12, 46]. This increase in use overtime is likely attributable, in part to two seminal studies that hypothesized prevention of intubation would be associated with a decreased mortality.

Noninvasive Ventilation in Early ARF Versus Conventional Oxygen Therapy to Prevent Intubation

In a randomized controlled trial evaluating NIV versus COT for immunocompromised patients with early ARF, there was a significant reduction in invasive mechanical ventilation and mortality compared to patients who received COT [6]. Criteria for entry included patients who had evidence of early respiratory failure including pulmonary infiltrates, fever, dyspnea, and a PaO_2/FiO_2 less than 200 on a venturi mask. The majority of these patients were immunocompromised secondary to hematologic malignancies. NIV was applied for a median of 9 h per day in the first 24 h. Of note, the control arm had a very high mortality with an increased incidence of ventilator-associated pneumonia. These results were intriguing to many and led to an increased application of NIV for oncologic patients with ARF [3, 45]. Antonelli and colleagues conducted a randomized controlled trial evaluating a similar question in 40 solid organ transplantation and found a similar reduction in invasive mechanical ventilation and mortality [8]. However, this study was noted to have a high proportion of patients with hydrostatic pulmonary edema as the primary etiology of ARF – for which there is a strong, established evidence base. Squadrone and colleagues randomized 40 patients with hematologic malignancies with bilateral infiltrations, tachypnea, and mild hypoxia (saturation <90% on room air) to CPAP or COT as a means to prevent the development of acute lung injury and need for ICU admission [47]. Their study found a decreased need for admission to the ICU and need for invasive mechanical ventilation.

Given advancements oncology and hematologic malignancies, ventilator-associated pneumonia prevention, critical care management, and the small sample sizes of these seminal trials, the generalizability of these trials to current day management of oncologic patients with ARF was called into question, prompting a more recent study evaluating the role of NIV versus COT for early ARF. In the largest RCT to date of NIV versus COT for early ARF, Lemiale and colleagues randomized 374 critically ill immunocompromised patients (85% oncologic patients) to NIV versus COT [9]. ARF was defined the presence of $PaO_2 < 60$ mmHg on room air, tachypnea, or respiratory distress. After 28 days, noninvasive oxygen strategy had failed in 38% of the NIV and 45% of the COT ($p = 0.20$), and there was no difference in the 28-day mortality (24% in the NIV group vs. 27% in COT group $p = 0.47$). Study strengths include the large sample size included and the large proportion of oncologic patients allowing its generalizability to our population of interest with ARF. Limitations included the unblinded nature of the trial, low severity of illness across the population, inclusion criteria (although it does address this question in early ARF), and the use of HFNC in the COT group.

The data surrounding NIV compared to COT in the immunocompromised population was recently summarized [56]. Huang and colleagues found 5 RCTs including almost 600 patients. This group found that early NIV significantly reduced short-term mortality (RR 0.62, 95% CI 0.40 – 0.97, p = 0.04) and intubation rate (RR 0.52, 95% CI 0.32 – 0.85, p=0.01) when compared with COT; however, these results were associated with significant statistical heterogeneity. The controversy and inconsistencies in patient response might be addressed in the evidence summary that follows.

Noninvasive Ventilation in ARDS Versus Invasive Mechanical Ventilation (via Intubation)

Following the publications of trials by Hilbert and Antonelli and colleagues, adoption of noninvasive ventilation beyond early acute respiratory

failure was seen in the years that followed [16, 48, 65]. Given historic reports of increased mortality with invasive mechanical ventilation, centers theorized that perhaps a noninvasive approach to management may help mitigate the deleterious consequences associated with invasive mechanical ventilation in this population (ventilator-associated pneumonia/sedation/delirium). What followed were a series of studies that evaluated the impact of NIV versus invasive mechanical ventilation on mortality in oncologic patients with ARDS [56–58].

Reported rates of NIV use for ARDS in oncologic patients are much higher ranging from 32% to 49% [7, 16, 48]. In a post-hoc analysis of the Lung Safe study focusing on the immunocompromised population with ARDS, NIV was used in 21% of patients as the first ventilation modality of choice [65]. The application of NIV has been seen across all severities of ARDS in the setting of oncologic patients [2, 65]. While NIV is associated with a high incidence of failure noted in the Lung Safe study (48%) [65] across patients with ARDS, rates of failure in the oncologic population are even higher than the general ICU population ranging from 38% to 70% [2, 16]. NIV failure is associated with a higher in-hospital and ICU mortality (60–70%) compared to those who experience NIV success (28%) or invasive mechanical ventilation (50–60%) as first-line therapy [2, 16, 48] (Fig. 2). Pulmonary infection, increased severity of illness scores, hematologic malignancies, longer hospitalization prior to ICU admission, and severity of ARDS are consistent factors associated with NIV failure [16, 48] (Table 2). The remaining challenge is the identification of the subset who may benefit from NIV versus those in whom first-line intubation should be pursued. Table 3 outlines the evidence of NIV across oncologic patients across various severities of ARF/ARDS.

Theories of Harm Associated with NIV

1. *Injurious ventilation*

It is theorized that NIV could be associated with harm secondary to the pressure levels generated in NIV compared to pressure transmitted via low- or high-flow oxygen. During NIV, patients may generate tidal volumes that are above those considered lung protective (>8 mL/kg tidal volume based upon ideal body

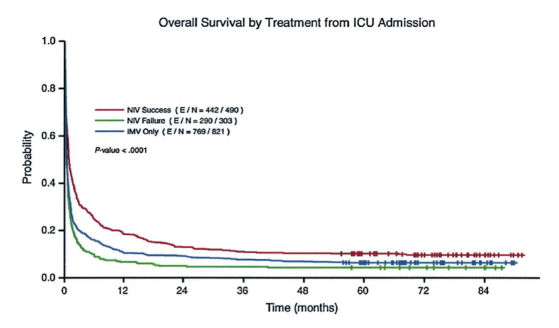

Fig. 2 Noninvasive ventilation mortality across successes and failures. Figure depicts overall survival difference in mortality across NIV success, NIV failure, and IMV. *NIV* noninvasive ventilation, *IMV* invasive ventilation

Table 2 Risk factors associated with an increased morality in oncologic patients with acute respiratory failure and noninvasive oxygen failure

Risk factors associated with an increased mortality in oncologic patients with ARF	Risk factors for noninvasive oxygen therapy failure
Demographic and clinical characteristics	
Hematologic malignancy, allogeneic hematopoietic stem cell transplantation	Hematologic malignancy
Cause of respiratory failure (infectious, PJP, invasive fungal infection, unclear etiology)	Pulmonary infection
Prolonged duration of hospitalization prior to admission to ICU	Prolonged duration of hospitalization prior to admission to ICU
Critical illness-associated features	
Greater severity of illness	Greater severity of illness
Worsened severity of ARDS	Worsened severity of ARDS
NIV failure as first line oxygen therapy	Lack of physiologic response to noninvasive ventilatory therapies (i.e., drop in respiratory rate, heart rate, improvement in oxygenation) evaluated early after initiation (1–4 h)
Vasopressors/renal failure	Vasopressors/renal failure
Tidal volume greater than 9 mL/kg 1 h after initiation of NIV	Tidal volume greater than 9 mL/kg 1 h after initiation of NIV

ARDS acute respiratory distress syndrome, *ICU* intensive care unit, *NIV* noninvasive ventilation, *PJP* pneumocystis jirovecii pneumonia

weight) [68]. Injurious tidal volumes could be exacerbated in the setting of spontaneous breathing facilitating further ventilator-induced lung injury [33, 50, 51]. This, in turn, could worsen

hypoxemia and generate conditions requiring invasive mechanical ventilation and multisystem organ failure. Immunocompromised patients typically present to ICU with higher illness

Table 3 Evidence across studies of noninvasive ventilation

NIV and other noninvasive oxygen modalities

Year	Design	N	Location	Population	Intervention	Control	Outcomes reported	Study outcomes	Limitations
Azoulay 2017	Prospective cohort study	(915) 859* analyzed	ICU	IC patients with ARF	HFNC	COT NIV	90-day mortality, in-hospital mortality, ICU mortality, IMV	After propensity score matching, HFNC but not NIV had an effect on IMV rate	Observational
Frat 2016	Post hoc analysis of randomized controlled trial	82	ICU	IC patients with ARF	HFNC	COT NIV	90-day mortality, ICU mortality	Odds ratios for intubation were higher in NIV versus HFNC or COT. NIV failure was associated with IMV and mortality	Post hoc analysis of RCT, exclusion of profound neutropenia
Coudroy 2016	Matched cohort study	115	ICU	IC patients with ARF	HFNC	NIV	28-day mortality, IMV	After PS score matching, NIV was associated with an increased mortality compared to HFNC	Observational
Mokart 2015	Retrospective cohort study; PS matching	178**	ICU	Oncologic patients with ARF	HFNC	COT or NIV	28-day mortality, IMV	Lower mortality at 28 days; however, HFNC group was exposed to intermittent NIV	Observational, cohorts contained a combination of modalities (i.e., HFNC with intermitted NIV)
Hui 2013	Randomized controlled trial	30	Acute care units	Advanced cancer and dyspnea	HFNC	NIV	Symptom resolution	Both modalities improved dyspnea compared but no significant difference existed between groups	End stage cancer, small sample size

(continued)

Table 3 (continued)

Year	Design	N	Location	Population	Intervention	Control	Outcomes reported	Study outcomes	Limitations
Noninvasive ventilation early acute respiratory failure									
Lemiale 2015	Randomized controlled trial	374	ICU	IC patients with ARF (85% oncology)	NIV	COT	28 day mortality and IMV	No difference in rates of IMV or mortality	COT arm included HFNC
Hilbert 2001	Randomized controlled trial	52	ICU	IC patients with ARF	NIV	COT	In-hospital mortality, ICU mortality, IMV	Lower in-hospital mortality (50% vs. 81%), lower ICU mortality (38% vs. 69%), lower IMV rates (46% vs. 77%) with NIV versus COT	Unblinded, small sample size, high mortality in control arm, possible outdated practices compared to recent years
Squadrone 2010	Randomized controlled trial	40	Ward	HM patients with early ARF	CPAP	COT	In-hospital mortality, CPAP	Lower in-hospital mortality in those admitted to ICU (15% vs. 75%) Lower IMV (20% vs. 80%)	Unblinded, small sample size
Noninvasive ventilation for acute respiratory distress syndrome									
Rathi 2017	Retrospective cohort study	1614	ICU	Hematologic malignancy and solid tumor	NIV success NIV failure	IMV	Overall survival (NIV vs. NIV failure vs. IMV)	38% NIV failure 80% hospital mortality in NIV failure group 28% hospital mortality in NIV success group 69% hospital mortality in IMV group	Observational

Neuschwander 2017	Post hoc analysis of prospective cohort study	1004	ICU	Hematologic malignancy and solid tumor	NIV success	NIV failure	Hospital mortality	71% NIV failure 63% hospital mortality in NIV failure group Risk factors for NIV failure see Table 2	Post hoc analysis, no comparator
Azevedo 2014	Prospective cohort study	717	ICU	Hematologic malignancy and solid tumor	NIV	IMV	Hospital mortality	53% NIV failure 69% hospital mortality in NIV failure group 40% hospital mortality in NIV success group 73% hospital mortality in IMV group	Observational
Adda 2008	Retrospective cohort study	99	ICU	Hematologic malignancy	NIV success	NIV failure	Factors predictive of NIV success or failure Hospital mortality	54% NIV failure 79% hospital mortality in NIV failures 41% hospital mortality in NIV success Risk factors for NIV failure see Table 2	Observational

ARF acute respiratory failure, *ARDS* acute respiratory distress syndrome, *COT* conventional oxygen therapy, *CPAP* continuous positive airway pressure, *HFNC* high-flow nasal cannula, *IC* immunocompromised, *ICU* intensive care unit, *IMV* invasive mechanical ventilation, *NIV* noninvasive ventilation

* - 915 included, only 859 analyzed

** - retrospective study that utilized propensity score matching

severity and multiple organ dysfunction [2] and are therefore at higher risk of ventilation-associated lung injury, potentially exacerbated by injurious tidal volumes during NIV.

2. *Delay in intubation*

It is further theorized that prolonged NIV without evidence of respiratory improvement may lead to a delay in intubation. In previous studies of patients with ARDS, there is a suggestion that a longer duration of NIV in those requiring intubation, the greater the mortality compared to those intubated sooner [51]; however, this was not found across a retrospective studies focused specifically on oncologic patients [16]. A delay in intubation or prolonged NIV prior to intubation potentially creates a setting of lower respiratory reserve, risk of aspiration pneumonitis, or potential greater instability around induction for intubation.

3. *ICU evidence-based care*

NIV may prevent ongoing evidence-based ICU care including mobilization, transport for imaging, enteral nutrition, and invasive diagnostic tests such as bronchoalveolar lavage. Sufficient recruitment to achieve adequate oxygenation may not be possible due to the facemask interface or discomfort by the patient.

Is There a Role for NIV in Oncologic Patients with ARDS?

The subset of those who experience NIV success consistently have been found to have the lowest mortality rate compared to those who undergo first-line invasive mechanical ventilation or fail NIV [16, 48]. Rates of NIV success have varied from reports across different institutions which may reflect important differences in patient selection and practice. Accurate identification of those who are at highest risk of NIV failure versus success is paramount to potentially defining any role for NIV in the setting of ARDS for oncologic patients. Data-to-date is limited by its retrospective nature subjecting it to selection bias – those who experience NIV failure are patients that the intensivist may not be keen to intubate given poor overall prognostic factors and therefore turned to NIV first line. Until further research clarifies its role in ARDS in oncologic patients, it should be reserved for those

patients in which one suspects underlying hydrostatic pulmonary edema as a plausible cause of ARF or contributor, or be applied for a time limited trial (1 or 4 h) in those with a low severity of illness with an early evaluation of physiologic improvement (decrease in respiratory rate, drop in FiO_2 requirements – Fig. 3). In the study by Rathi and colleagues, they evaluated improvement in respiratory rate, Glasgow coma score, oxygenation parameters, and acid-base status as markers of NIV success (and thus continuation) or NIV failure (potential indication to consider intubation) [16]. Frat and colleagues also evaluated factors associated with NIV failure. At 1 h following initiation, a persistent $PaO_2/FiO_2 < 200$ and tidal volumes greater than 9 mL/kg of predicted body weight were independently associated with the need for invasive mechanical ventilation and mortality [52]. It would be important that the intensivist considers (1) tidal volumes generated, (2) need for other invasive tests or imaging (CT/fiberoptic bronchoscopy), and (3) immediate response to its application with a projected rapid wean-off of NIV (i.e., drop in respiratory rate/oxygenation response). Furthermore, Patel and colleagues recently evaluated the interface of helmet versus face mask for NIV and found a decreased need for invasive mechanical ventilation and morality [27]. These findings are intriguing for which its role needs to be further elucidated in this population compared to alternative noninvasive oxygen strategies outlined below.

Evidence for HFNC

General Population

HFNC has recently emerged as a safe and comfortable device with a means to effectively administer high-flow oxygen to patients with ARF. Emerging data has demonstrated promising results compared to alternative noninvasive oxygen strategies (Table 4). In one of the largest RCTs to date, Frat and colleagues randomized 310 patients with ARF to HFNC versus COT versus NIV [32]. HFNC was associated with a lower incidence of 90-day mortality compared to the COT and NIV. In the subgroup of patients with a $PaO_2/FiO_2 < 200$,

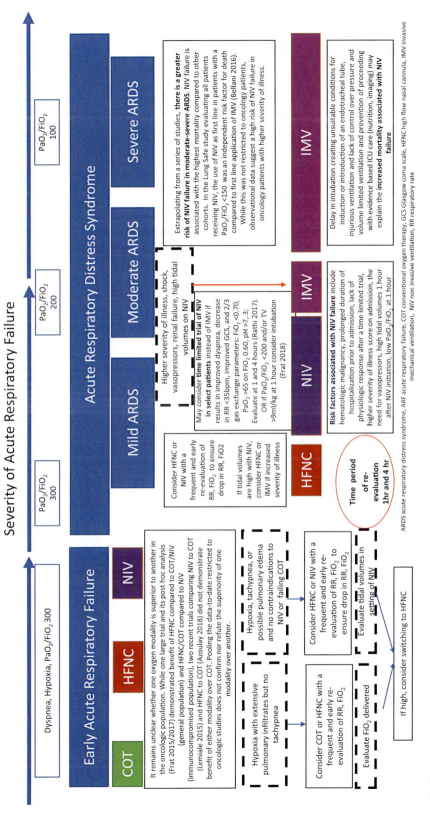

Fig. 3 Noninvasive oxygen strategy decision algorithm

Table 4 Summary of studies of high-flow nasal cannula in oncologic patients with acute respiratory failure

Year	Design	Sample size	Location	Population	Entry criteria	Intervention	Control	Outcomes	HFNC intubation rate	HFNC mortality[a]
Azoulay 2017	Prospective cohort study	859	ICU	IC patients with ARF	RR > 30/min or saturation <90% room air or $P_aO_2 \leq 60$ mmHg and requiring >6 L/min and respiratory symptoms less than 72 h	HFNC	COT NIV	90-day mortality, in-hospital mortality, ICU mortality, IMV	39%	42% (90-day)
Azoulay 2018	RCT	778	ICU	IC patients with ARF	RR > 30/min or saturation <90% room air or $P_aO_2 \leq 60$ mmHg and requiring >6 L/min	HFNC	COT	28-day mortality, IMV, P/F over 3 days, respiratory rate, ICU and hospital LOS, comfort, dyspnea	38.7%	35.6% (28-day)
Kim 2017	Retrospective cohort study	52	General ward, ICU	Non-HIV patients with PJP and ARF	Acute respiratory failure and PJP	HFNC	None	60-day mortality, IMV	56%	35% (60-day)
Lemiale 2017	Post hoc analysis of RCT; PS matching	353	ICU	IC patients with ARF	$PaO_2 < 60$ mmHg on room air or tachypnea >30/min or respiratory distress <72 h	HFNC	COT	28-day mortality, IMV	49%	24% (28-day)
Durey 2016	Retrospective cohort study	11	ER	Oncologic patients with solid malignancy	Any adult patient with solid malignancy	HFNC	None	Mortality, IMV	18%	36% (In-hospital)
Frat 2016	Post hoc analysis of RCT	82	ICU	IC patients with ARF	RR > 25 and $P_aO_2/FiO_2 < 300$ and $P_aCO_2 \leq 45$ mmHg	HFNC	COT NIV	90-day mortality, ICU mortality	46%	29% (90-day)

Study	Study type	N	Setting	Population / Inclusion criteria	Intervention	Comparator	Outcome	Result	Result
Coudroy 2016	Matched cohort study	115	ICU	IC patients with ARF / RR $\geq$ 25 breaths/min or clinical signs of respiratory distress $P_aO_2/FiO_2 < 300$	HFNC	NIV	28-day mortality, IMV	44%	30% (28-day)
Harada 2016	Retrospective cohort study	56	ICU	Hematologic malignancy with ARF / 4 L/min oxygen for $SpO_2 < 90\%$ RR > 25 Clinical signs of respiratory distress	HFNC	None	IMV	15% (64% palliated after HFNC failure)	
Lemiale 2015	RCT	100	ICU	IC patients with ARF / <72 h from admission 6 L/min oxygen for $SpO_2 > 95\%$ or RR > 30 and signs of respiratory distress	HFNC	COT	Invasive or Non-IMV	9% (evaluated on day 1 only)	
Mokart 2015	Retrospective cohort study; PS matching	178	ICU	Oncologic patients with ARF / $O_2 > 9$ L/min	HFNC[+]	COT or NIV	28-day mortality, IMV	50%	45% (28-day)
Lee 2015	Retrospective cohort study	45	ICU	Hematologic malignancy patients with ARF / Acute respiratory failure with hematological malignancy	HFNC	None	Mortality, IMV	58%	62% (In-hospital)
Hui 2013	RCT	30	Acute care units	Advanced cancer and dyspnea / Locally advanced cancer Dyspnea at least 3/10 (NRS) despite O_2 Life expectancy >1 week	HFNC	NIV	Symptom resolution	30%	

ABG arterial blood gas, *ARF* acute respiratory failure, *ARDS* acute respiratory distress syndrome, *BP* blood pressure, *CHF* congestive heart failure, *COT* conventional oxygen therapy, *ER* emergency department, *GVHD* graft versus host disease, *HIV* human immunodeficiency virus, *HR* heart rate, *ICU* intensive care unit, *IMV* invasive mechanical ventilation, *LOS* length of stay, *MOF* multiorgan failure, *NIV* noninvasive ventilation, *NRS* numeric rating scale, P_aCO_2 partial pressure of arterial carbon dioxide, P_aO_2/FiO_2 ratio of the partial pressure of arterial oxygen to the fraction of inspired oxygen, *PJP* pneumocystis jerovicii pneumonia, *PNA* pneumonia, *ROS* retrospective observational study, *RCT* randomized controlled trial, *RR* respiratory rate, SpO_2 oxygen saturation

[a]Mortality at longest follow-up

HFNC was associated with a lower incidence of invasive mechanical ventilation. However, the signal of benefit has not been consistent across all studies. A Cochrane review by Corley and colleagues evaluated the use of HFNC compared to COT or NIV for ARF or postextubation across 11 RCTs [53]. HFNC compared to COT was not associated with lower rates of invasive mechanical ventilation (reported in six studies) or mortality (reported in three studies). Confidence in the results using GRADE criteria [54] was downgraded to low given the risk of bias across these studies and different participant indications. Data comparing HFNC to NIV was not pooled given the low number of studies and their heterogeneity.

Immunocompromised and Oncologic Population

Given the important differences in the oncologic population and the general ICU population and evolving evidence of potential harm associated with NIV failure, HFNC has emerged as a promising modality in this population. High quality data evaluating use of HFNC compared to COT or NIV in this population is unfortunately limited. In a multinational, prospective observational study across 16 countries of immunocompromised patients with ARF (87% oncologic), noninvasive oxygen strategies were evaluated in 915 patients [12]. Fifty-three percent received COT, 17% received NIV, 20% received HFNC, and 9% received a combination of HFNC and NIV. After propensity score matching, HFNC had an impact on invasive mechanical ventilation but not NIV. HFNC was not independently associated with a lower mortality.

In a post hoc analysis of the RCT by Frat and colleagues evaluating HFNC versus COT and NIV, outcomes across the cohort of 82 immunocompromised patients (44% oncology) were evaluated [68]. NIV was associated with an increased need for invasive mechanical ventilation compared to HFNC or COT.

Finally, in a post hoc propensity score-matched analysis by Lemiale and colleagues of their prior RCT (NIV vs. COT) [9], they compared 90 patients who received HFNC in their control group matched to 90 patients who received COT

in their control group [55]. They found no difference in the rates of invasive mechanical ventilation or mortality.

Sklar and colleagues recently described the role of HFNC compared to any noninvasive oxygen control (COT or NIV) across immunocompromised patients (13 studies) [66]. Data from RCTs and observational studies that used matching techniques were meta-analyzed (8 studies). Mortality was found to be lower at the longest available follow-up with HFNC compared to the oxygen control groups (NIV or COT – 7 studies; 1429 patients, relative risk of 0.72, 95% CI 0.56–0.93, p=0.01). There was a lower rate of invasive mechanical ventilation with HFNC compared to the oxygen therapy controls across 8 studies (8 studies, 1529 patients, relative risk of 0.81, 95% CI 0.67–0.96, p=0.02). However, one of the limitations of this analysis was the pooling of the two control arm techniques and the inclusion of observational studies in the analysis.

Eleven studies have evaluated the use of HFNC specifically in oncologic patients (Table 4) reporting on 1,881 patients.

These studies included 6 retrospective, cohort studies [59, 60, 62–64], 1 prospective observational study [12], and 4 RCTs, 2 of which were post hoc analyses of previous RCTs outlined above [9, 55, 61, 68]. Eight studies compared HFNC to an oxygen therapy control (NIV or COT). Oncologic diagnosis or treatment associated effect was the leading cause of immunosuppression with a predominance of hematologic malignancy (9/11 studies). HFNC was initiated in the emergency department, acute care ward, or intensive care unit with the latter being the most common site of initiation. Various indications for the application of HFNC existed ranging from tachypnea or hypoxia on room air to more formalized PaO_2/FiO_2 thresholds. The median PaO_2/FiO_2 across the studies was 145 (IQR 115–175). The need for invasive mechanical ventilation, evaluated at 28-day intubation or hospital discharge, was 46% (IQR 25–67%). The longest follow-up mortality time points are reported in Table 3 with a median mortality of 36% (IQR 14–58%).

Mortality at longest available follow-up and the need for invasive mechanical ventilation was reported in 7 and 8 studies, respectively (Table 4).

Mortality at Longest Available Follow Up for HFNC compared to NIV

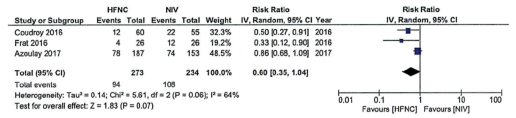

Mortality at Longest Available Follow Up for HFNC compared to COT

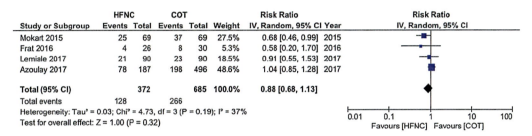

Need for Invasive Mechanical Ventilation for HFNC compared to NIV

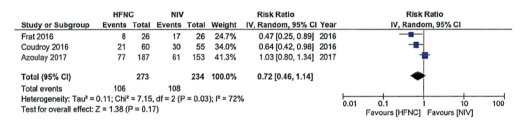

Need for Invasive Mechanical Ventilation for HFNC compared to COT

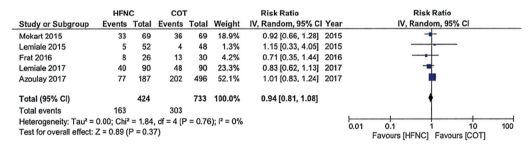

Fig. 4 Mortality and invasive mechanical ventilation across high-flow nasal cannula studies. This figure compares the effect of HFNC compared to NIV and COT on mortality at the longest available follow-up and need for invasive mechanical ventilation. Data are pooled using an inverse variance random effects model. Results are summarized as risk ratios. (Oncologic subgroup of studies extrapolated from a systematic review evaluating HFNC compared to other modalities-unpublished data)

Using a random effects model, HFNC compared to NIV or COT was not associated with a decreased mortality or need for invasive mechanical ventilation (Fig. 4) (unpublished work). These findings are primarily meant to be exploratory given the heterogeneous nature of the populations and low quality of evidence (observational studies, post hoc analyses of RCTs).

Most recently, Azoulay and colleagues performed the largest RCT to date of immunocompromised patients with ARF and randomized the approximately 800 patients to COT or HFNC [67]. These patients were mainly immunocompromised secondary to hematologic malignancy or its treatments. The primary outcome of 28-day survival was not different between the two groups (35.6% HFNC vs. 36.1% COT), nor were a number of secondary outcomes including intubation rates, ICU and hospital length of stay, or ICU-related complications. This trial therefore suggests that HFNC in all immunocompromised patients may not be better than COT and further subgroups of HFNC "responders" must be sought. Future directions would necessitate larger, randomized controlled trials specifically enrolling oncologic patients comparing COT, NIV, and HFNC head-to-head. In addition, there could exist a differential impact across varying severities and indications for ARF.

In deciding optimal noninvasive oxygen therapy, one needs to consider the etiology, timing of reversal, severity of illness, impact of the modality on tidal volumes, and immediate response of respiratory physiology variables and tidal volumes to the modality chosen [16, 52]. Figure 3 represents a proposed algorithm for consideration of noninvasive oxygen therapies and factors to consider in deciding upon first-line and second-line modalities. The figure attempts to capture some important factors that should be considered in deciding upon modality of choice.

Conclusions

COT, NIV, and HFNC are multimodal techniques to administer oxygen noninvasively in critically ill patients with ARF. Each has unique mechanisms, advantages, and disadvantages. Until further research is available, individual patient characteristics, severity of illness, and early response to each modality is imperative to guide selection of which strategy is most applicable. Most importantly, the physician needs to pay meticulous attention to the rapidity of reversibility of the underlying condition and reevaluate the impact of the strategy chosen at an early time

points (e.g., 1 and 4 h). An improved physiologic response to the modality of choice has been consistently found to be associated with success. While HFNC is a unique oxygen delivery modality that holds theoretical promise for the treatment of ARF in oncologic patients, the current body of literature demonstrates that there is a paucity of high-quality data in this specific population to guide evidence-based therapy. This chapter underscores the need for further research with clinical and physiological studies, including larger randomized controlled trials specifically of oncologic patients to more clearly elucidate the potential benefits of one modality over another.

References

1. Nava S, Cuomo AM. Acute respiratory failure in the cancer patient: the role of noninvasive mechanical ventilation. Crit Rev Oncol Hematol. 2004;51(2):91–103.
2. Azoulay E, Lemiale V, Mokart D, et al. Acute respiratory distress syndrome in patients with malignancies. Intensive Care Med. 2014;40(8):1106–15.
3. Cortegiani A, Madotto F, Gregoretti C, et al. Immunocompromised patients with acute respiratory distress syndrome: secondary analysis of the LUNG SAFE database. Crit Care. 2018;22:157–72.
4. Adda M, Coquet I, Darmon M, et al. Predictors of noninvasive ventilation failure in patients with hematologic malignancy and acute respiratory failure. Crit Care Med. 2008;36(10):2766–72.
5. Darmon MR, Bernal T, et al. Ventilatory support in critically ill hematology patients with respiratory failure. Crit Care. 2012;16(4):R133.
6. Hilbert G, Gruson D, Vargas F, et al. Noninvasive ventilation in immunosuppressed patients with pulmonary infiltrates. N Engl J Med. 2001;344:481–7.
7. Azevedo LCP, Caruso P, Silva UVA, et al. Outcomes for patients with cancer admitted to the ICU requiring ventilatory support: results from a prospective multicenter study. Chest. 2014;146(2):257–66.
8. Antonelli M, Conti G, Bufi M, et al. Noninvasive ventilation for treatment of acute respiratory failure in patients undergoing solid organ transplant: a randomized trial. JAMA. 2000;283:235–41.
9. Lemiale V, Mokart D, Resche-Rigon M, et al. Effect of noninvasive ventilation vs oxygen therapy on mortality among immunocompromised patients with acute respiratory failure: a randomized clinical trial. JAMA. 2015;314(16):1711–9.
10. Schellongowski P, Sperr W, Wohlfarth P, et al. Critically ill patients with cancer: chances and limitations of intensive care medicine – a narrative review. ESMO Open. 2016;1:e000018.

11. Azoulay E, Mokart D, Penne F, et al. Outcomes of critically ill patients with hematologic malignancies: prospective multicenter data From France and Belgium – a groupe de recherche respiratoire en réanimation onco-hématologique study. J Clin Oncol. 2013;31(22):2810–8.

12. Azoulay E, Pickkers P, Soares M, et al. Acute hypoxemic respiratory failure in immunocompromised patients: the Efraim multinational prospective cohort study. Intensive Care Med. 2017;43:1808–19.

13. Weijs PJM, Looijaard WGPM, Dekker IM, et al. Low skeletal muscle area is a risk factor for mortality in mechanically ventilated critically ill patients. Crit Care. 2014;18(2):R12.

14. Moisey LL, Mourtzakis M, Cotton BA, et al. Skeletal muscle predicts ventilator-free days, ICU-free days, and mortality in elderly ICU patients. Crit Care. 2013;17(5):R206.

15. Cesari M, Landi F, Vellas B, et al. Sarcopenia and physical frailty: two sides of the same coin. Front Aging Neurosci. 2014;6:192.

16. Rathi N, Haque S, Nates R. Non-invasive positive pressure ventilation vs invasive mechanical ventilation as first-line therapy for acute hypoxemic respiratory failure in cancer patients. J Crit Care. 2017;39:56–61.

17. Afessa B, Peters SG. Major complications following hematopoietic stem cell transplantation. Semin Respir Crit Care Med. 2006;27(3):297–309.

18. Herridge MS, Tansey CM, Matté A, et al. Functional disability 5 years after acute respiratory distress syndrome. N Engl J Med. 2011;364(14):1293–304.

19. Taccone F, Artigas A, Sprung C, et al. Characteristics and outcomes of cancer patients in European ICUs. Crit Care. 2009;13:R15.

20. Van Vliet M, Verburg I, Boogaard M. Trends in admission prevalence, illness severity and survival of hematological patients treated in Dutch intensive care units. Intensive Care Med. 2014;40:1275–84.

21. Squadrone V, Ferreyra G, Ranieri V. Non-invasive ventilation in patients with hematologic malignancy: a new prospective. Minerva Anestesiol. 2015;81(10):1118.

22. Kotloff RM, Ahya VN, Crawford F. Pulmonary complications of solid organ and hematopoietic stem cell transplantation. Am J Respir Crit Care Med. 2004;170:22–48.

23. Lucena CM, Torres A, Rovira M, et al. Pulmonary complications in hematopoietic SCT: a prospective study. Bone Marrow Transplant. 2014;49:1293–9.

24. Bateman NT, Leach RM. ABC of oxygen. Acute oxygen therapy. BMJ. 1998;317:798–801.

25. Chu D, Kim L, Young P, et al. Mortality and morbidity in acutely ill adults treated with liberal versus conservative oxygen therapy (IOTA): a systematic review and meta-analysis. Lancet. 2018;391:1693–705.

26. Mehta S, Hill NS. Non-invasive ventilation. Am J Respir Crit Care Med. 2001;163:540–77.

27. Patel BK, Wolfe KS, Pohlman AS, et al. Effect of noninvasive ventilation delivered by helmet vs face mask on the rate of endotracheal intubation in patients with acute respiratory distress syndrome: a randomized clinical trial. JAMA. 2016;315:2435–41.

28. Lenique F, Habis M, Lofaso F, et al. Ventilatory and hemodynamic effects of continuous positive airway pressure in left heart failure. Am J Respir Crit Care Med. 1997;155:500–5.

29. Mertens M, Tabuchi A, Meissner S, et al. Alveolar dynamics in acute lung injury: heterogeneous distension rather than cyclic opening and collapse. Crit Care Med. 2009;37:2604–11.

30. Chadda K, Annane D, Hart N, et al. Cardiac and respiratory effects of continuous positive airway pressure and noninvasive ventilation in acute cardiac pulmonary edema. Crit Care Med. 2002;30:2457–61.

31. Brochard L, Mancebo J, Wysocki M, et al. Noninvasive ventilation for acute exacerbations of chronic obstructive pulmonary disease. N Engl J Med. 1995;333:817–22.

32. Frat J-P, Thille AW, Mercat A, et al. High-flow oxygen through nasal cannula in acute hypoxemic respiratory failure. N Engl J Med. 2015;372:2185–96.

33. Brochard L, Slutsky A, Pesenti A. Mechanical ventilation to minimize progression of lung injury in acute respiratory failure. Am J Respir Crit Care Med. 2017;195:438–42.

34. Agarwal R, Khan A, Aggarwal AN, et al. Bronchoscopic lung biopsy using noninvasive ventilatory support: case series and review of literature of NIV-assisted bronchoscopy. Respir Care. 2012;57(11):1927–36.

35. Papazian L, Corley A, Hess D, et al. Use of high-flow nasal cannula oxygenation in ICU adults: a narrative review. Intensive Care Med. 2016;42:1336–49.

36. Goligher EC, Slutsky AS. Not just oxygen? Mechanisms of benefit from high-flow nasal cannula in hypoxemic respiratory failure. Am J Respir Crit Care Med. 2017;195:1128–31.

37. Möller W, Feng S, Domanski U, et al. Nasal high flow reduces dead space. J Appl Physiol. 2017;122:191–7.

38. Parke R, McGuinness S, Eccleston M. Nasal high-flow therapy delivers low level positive airway pressure. Br J Anaesth. 2009;103:886–90.

39. Rittayamai N, Tscheikuna J, Praphruetkit N, et al. Use of high-flow nasal cannula for acute dyspnea and hypoxemia in the emergency department. Respir Care. 2015;60:1377–82.

40. Pellegrini M, Hedenstierna G, Roneus A. The diaphragm acts as a brake during expiration to prevent lung collapse. Am J Respir Crit Care Med. 2016;195:1608–16.

41. Cressoni M, Chiumello D, Algieri I, et al. Opening pressures and atelectrauma in acute respiratory distress syndrome. Intensive Care Med. 2017;43:603–11.

42. Rochwerg B, Brochard L, Elliott M, et al. Official ERS/ATS clinical practice guidelines: noninvasive ventilation for acute respiratory failure. Eur Respir J. 2017;50:1602426.

43. Vital FM, Ladeira MT, Atallah AN. Non-invasive positive pressure ventilation (CPAP or bilevel NPPV) for cardiogenic pulmonary oedema. Cochrane Database Syst Rev. 2013;5:CD005351.

44. Mehta A, Douglas I, Walkey A. Evidence-based utilization of noninvasive ventilation and patient outcomes. Ann Am Thorac Soc. 2017;14(11):1667–73.

45. Bellani G, Laffey J, Pham T. Noninvasive ventilation of patients with acute respiratory distress syndrome: insights from the LUNG SAFE Study. Am J Respir Crit Care Med. 2017;195(1):67–77.

46. Bellani G, Laffey J, Pham T, et al. Epidemiology, patterns of care, and mortality for patients with acute respiratory distress syndrome in intensive care units in 50 countries. JAMA. 2016;315(8):788–800.

47. Squadrone V, Massaia M, Bruno B, et al. Early CPAP prevents evolution of acute lung injury in patients with hematologic malignancy. Intensive Care Med. 2010; 36(10):1666.

48. Neuschwander A, Lemiale V, Darmon M, et al. Noninvasive ventilation during acute respiratory distress syndrome in patients with cancer: trends in use and outcome. J Crit Care. 2017;38:295–9.

49. Brochard L. Ventilation-induced lung injury exists in spontaneously breathing patients with acute respiratory failure: yes. Intensive Care Med. 2017;43(2):250–2.

50. Amato MBP, Meade MO, Slutsky AS, et al. Driving pressure and survival in the acute respiratory distress syndrome. N Engl J Med. 2015;372(8):747–56.

51. Esteban A, Frutos-Vivar F, Ferguson ND, et al. Noninvasive positive-pressure ventilation for respiratory failure after extubation. N Engl J Med. 2004;350(24):245–54.

52. Frat JP, Ragot S, Coudroy R, et al. Predictors of intubation in patients with acute hypoxemic respiratory failure treated with a noninvasive oxygenation strategy. Crit Care Med. 2018;46(2):208–15.

53. Corley A, Rickard C, Aitken L, et al. High flow nasal cannulae for respiratory support in adult intensive care patients. Cochrane Database Syst Rev. 2017; 5:CD010172.

54. Higgins JPT, Green S. Cochrane handbook for systematic reviews of interventions. Hoboken: Wiley; 2011.

55. Lemiale V, Resche-Rigon M, Mokart D, et al. High-flow nasal cannula oxygenation in immunocompromised patients with acute hypoxemic respiratory failure: A Groupe de Recherche Respiratoire en Réanimation Onco-Hématologique Study. Crit Care Med. 2017;45(3):e274–81.

56. Liu J, Bell C, Campbell V, et al. Noninvasive ventilation in patients with hematologic malignancy. J Intensive Care Med. 2017. https://doi.org/10.1177/0885066617690725. Epub ahead of print.

57. Huang H-B, Xu B, Liu G-Y, et al. Use of noninvasive ventilation in immunocompromised patients with acute respiratory failure: a systematic review and meta-analysis. Crit Care. 2017;21(1):4–29.

58. Wang T, Zhang L, Luo K, et al. Noninvasive versus invasive mechanical ventilation for immunocompromised patients with acute respiratory failure: a systematic review and meta-analysis. BMC Pulm Med. 2016;16:129–43.

59. Lee HY, Rhee CK, Lee JW. Feasibility of high-flow nasal cannula oxygen therapy for acute respiratory failure in patients with hematologic malignancies: a retrospective single-center study. J Crit Care. 2015; 30(4):773–8.

60. Durey A, Kang S, Suh Y, et al. Application of high-flow nasal cannula to heterogeneous condition in the emergency department. Am J Emerg Med. 2017; 35(8):1199–201.

61. Hui D, Morgado M, Chisholm G, et al. High-flow oxygen and bilevel positive airway pressure for persistent dyspnea in patients with advanced cancer: a phase II randomized trial. J Pain Symptom Manage. 2013; 46(4):463–80.

62. Coudroy R, Jamet A, Petua P, et al. High-flow nasal cannula oxygen therapy versus noninvasive ventilation in immunocompromised patients with acute respiratory failure: an observational cohort study. Ann Intensive Care. 2016;6(1):45–56.

63. Mokart D, Geay C, Chow-Chine L, et al. High-flow oxygen therapy in cancer patients with acute respiratory failure. Intensive Care Med. 2015;41(11): 2008–10.

64. Kim WY, Sung H, Hong SB, et al. Predictors of high flow nasal cannula failure in immunocompromised patients with acute respiratory failure due to non-HIV pneumocystis pneumonia. J Thorac Dis. 2017;9(9): 3013–22.

65. Cortegiani A, Madotto F, Gregoretti C et al. Immunocompromised patients with acute respiratory distress syndrome: secondary analysis of the LUNG SAFE database. Critical Care. 2018;22:157–172.

66. Sklar MC, Mohammed A, Orchanian-Cheff A et al. The impact of high-flow nasal oxygen in the immunocompromised critically ill: A systematic review and meta-analysis, Respir Care. 2018;63 (12):1555–1566

67. Azoulay E, Lemiale V, Mokart D et al. Effect of high-flow nasal oxygen vs. standard oxygen on 28-day mortality in immunocompromised patients with acute respiratory failure. JAMA 2018; (Epub ahead of print) October 24, 2018.

68. Frat JP, Ragot S, Girault C, Perbet S, Prat G, Boulain T, Demoule A, Ricard JD, Coudroy R, Robert R, Mercat A. Effect of non-invasive oxygenation strategies in immunocompromised patients with severe acute respiratory failure: a post-hoc analysis of a randomised trial. The Lancet Respiratory Medicine. 2016 Aug 1;4 (8):646–52.

Respiratory Support Strategies and Nonconventional Ventilation Modes in Oncologic Critical Care

33

Yenny R. Cardenas and Joseph L. Nates

Contents

Introduction 500

Nonconventional Ventilation Modes 500
Biphasic Ventilation 501
High-Frequency Ventilation 503
Pressure-Regulated Volume Control (PRVC) 505
Neurally Adjusted Ventilatory Assist Ventilation (NAVA) 505

ECMO 505

Conclusion 505

References 506

Abstract

Nonconventional modes of ventilation have been around for decades. Starting in the 1970s, several modes of high-frequency ventilation (HFV) were introduced and have been used as experimental or rescue ventilation modes since then. More recently, close-loop dual modes of ventilation have been developed. Biphasic ventilation (BiPAP/APRV) and pressure-regulated volume control (PRVC) are among the most accepted and popular. Other less known include proportional assist ventilation (PAV) and neurally adjusted ventilatory assist (NAVA), among many others. To date, there is little to no evidence available for the use of these modes in cancer patients. We review some of the most important modes in current clinical practice and share our experience in the MD Anderson Cancer Center Intensive Care Units with the use of HFV, BiPAP, and APRV as well our respiratory support strategy to manage cancer patients in respiratory failure.

Y. R. Cardenas
Critical Care Department, Universidad del Rosario
Hospital Universitario Fundacion Santa Fe de Bogota,
Bogota, Colombia
e-mail: yennyrocio24@gmail.com

J. L. Nates (✉)
Department of Critical Care and Respiratory Care, The
University of Texas, MD Anderson Cancer Center,
Houston, TX, USA
e-mail: jlnates@mdanderson.org

Keywords

Ventilation strategies · Cancer · Critically ill ·
Oncology · Mechanical ventilation · Bi-level ·
Biphasic ventilation · BiPAP · APRV · HFV ·
VDR · HFOV · NAVA · ECMO · Recruitment
maneuvers · Prone positioning

© Springer Nature Switzerland AG 2020
J. L. Nates, K. J. Price (eds.), *Oncologic Critical Care*,
https://doi.org/10.1007/978-3-319-74588-6_54

Introduction

Respiratory failure remains the most frequent reason for admission to the intensive care unit (ICU). Recent large epidemiological studies indicate that over 50% of the ICU patients require ventilatory support [3]. However, not all the patients require ventilatory support on admission to the units. A prospective multicenter observational study in 40 European units showed that 32% of the patients were admitted for respiratory failure with moderate hypoxemia and need immediate ventilatory support, while 35% of the patients required support later for a total of 67% of the patients [35]. Oxygen therapy and ventilatory support are therefore at the center of the management of critically ill patients and a clear respiratory support strategy is essential in any environment that manages patients in respiratory distress.

Despite a myriad of additional diagnoses, the progression in the management of cancer patients with hypoxemic respiratory failure is similar to the management of patients in this condition without cancer. It usually starts with low-flow and transitions to high-flow oxygen therapy or noninvasive ventilation. If the patients fail to improve with the indicated medical care and these noninvasive strategies, additional respiratory support includes escalation to invasive mechanical ventilation using conventional modes of ventilation such as intermittent mandatory ventilation, assist control ventilation, and pressure control ventilation among others. In ARDS patients, these ventilation modes are accompanied by adjunctive treatments such as high-dose steroids, neuromuscular blockers (37.8%), recruitment maneuvers (32.7%), and prone positioning (16.3%) [2] (Fig. 1).

An epidemiological study of acute respiratory failure, describing causes and practices trends, showed that among the 1,364,624 medical patients that developed respiratory failure in 2009 in the USA, only 16% had a diagnosis of ARDS [33]. The initial intervention included noninvasive ventilation in 11.9%, while 38% were treated with invasive mechanical ventilation. In contrast, 552,971 surgical patients developed respiratory failure and ARDS accounted for 45.5% of them, consequently they required more invasive (52.9%) and less noninvasive (5.8%) ventilation. The overall hospital mortality for the medical patients was 22% and for the surgical patients 18.6%. The latter increased with age and underlying cause for failure. In a 50-countries ARDS study including 2377 patients diagnosed with ARDS, 30% had mild disease, 46% moderate disease, and 24.2% severe disease [2]. The overall unadjusted ICU mortality was reported to be 35.3% and the hospital mortality was 40%.

It is not clear what the actual use of nonconventional ventilation to treat respiratory failure patients is. However, based on the above epidemiological studies, it seems that most probably, these modes are used in less than 20% (less than 1 in 5) of all patients with ARDS. In addition, if this diagnosis is described in 16% of all patients with respiratory failure and 20% of them deteriorate to severe ARDS, the approximate percentage of patients with severe ARDS using requiring advanced modes of ventilation is 3.2%. This calculation is supported by a large prospective multicenter/multinational study, which found that ARDS was the cause of acute respiratory failure in 3% of the patients [40].

Nonconventional Ventilation Modes

The most common, well-known, and newer nonconventional modes include Biphasic Positive Airway Pressure ventilation or **BiPAP** [13] also known as Bi-Level positive airway pressure or Bi-vent (depending on what company's ventilator we use), Biphasic Airway Pressure Release Ventilation or **APRV**, and Pressure-Regulated Volume Control (PRVC) [40]. Other nonconventional modes such as neurally adjusted ventilatory assist (NAVA), proportional assist ventilation (PAV) [37], NeoGanesh, and mandatory minute ventilation (MMV), among others, are more recent and still less popular but their use varies among the units and there is no specific data about the real utilization rates of any of these modes [32]. The oldest nonconventional

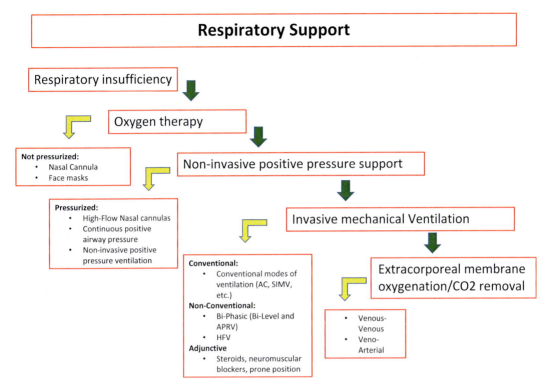

Fig. 1 AC – Assist Control; SIMV – Synchronized Intermittent Mechanical Ventilation; APRV – Airway Pressure Release ventilation; HFV – High-Frequency Ventilation

ventilation modes include the high-frequency modes developed in the 1970s [18]. These modes have been considered mostly experimental or rescue therapies in the adult population. No relevant studies using any of these modes have been published in the adult cancer patient population. However, a handful of retrospective studies have been published in pediatric cancer patients with ARDS [8, 26, 36].

The most comprehensive study describing the mortality of patients receiving mechanical ventilation over time was published in 2013 [40]. This study included three prospective cohorts of patients admitted to 927 intensive care units of 40 countries in the years 1998, 2004, and 2010. In the latter cohort including 8151 patients, the most frequent modes of invasive ventilation were conventional (82.5%), including: assist-control (33%), pressure support ventilation (23.7%), pressure control ventilation (13%), synchronized intermittent mandatory ventilation with pressure support (9.4%), and synchronized

intermittent mandatory ventilation alone (3.4%). Among the nonconventional (15.2%) modes, APRV or BiPAP were used 9.1% of the time, pressure release volume control 6.1%; other modes of ventilation were used only in 2.3% of the patients. In the 1998 cohort, conventional ventilation was used in 96.5% of the patients; nonconventional modes were reported among the other modes (3.5%). This study highlighted the development and progressive introduction of these modes in clinical practice over the past 20 years.

Biphasic Ventilation

BiPAP and APRV are a continuum of Biphasic ventilation. The main difference between them is that BiPAP has a normal inspiratory to expiratory (I:E) ratio, and in APRV the I:E ratio is inverted. Biphasic ventilation was developed and described as a combination of spontaneous breathing and pressure control in the 1980s [1].

Biphasic ventilation is a close-loop, partial support, time-cycled, pressure-controlled mode set at two levels of continuous positive airway pressure (CPAP), and unrestricted spontaneous breathing. Essentially, the mode integrates two levels of CPAP switching from high to low pressure in time-cycled periods, while allowing the patient to breath spontaneously at all times of the inspiratory or expiratory cycle. The tidal volume is determined by the difference between PEEP high, PEEP low, and lung compliance. PEEP low and PEEP high are set according to the low and high inflections points of the static pressure-volume curve respectively [20]. PEEP low can also be set identifying the optimal PEEP low level using different techniques (e.g., using esophageal pressure or best compliance) [11], and PEEP high according to the driving pressure needed to obtain the target tidal volume. The spontaneous breaths are supported with pressure support, which is set above the PEEP low to achieve the calculated tidal volume according to ideal body weight table or formula.

Some of the many benefits attributed to Biphasic ventilation may be a reduced biological impact seen in experimental animal models where we have seen a reduction in the markers of inflammation, apoptosis, fibrinogenesis, and epithelial/endothelial damage compared with pressure control or continuous mandatory ventilation (CMV) [7, 27]. When compared with CMV, APRV reduces endothelial permeability and preserved surfactant proteins A and B concentrations. In clinical practice, it has been associated with lower needs of sedatives and analgesics post cardiac surgery and trauma [22, 23] and an improvement in ventilation-perfusion matching, possibly secondary recruitment of previously non-ventilated areas [21]. Other potential benefits of this ventilatory approach are the improvement in glomerular filtration rate and sodium excretion seen in ARDS patients [12], a decreased intrathoracic pressure leading to reduced venous return, higher cardiac output, and increased oxygen delivery [21]. All these occur when maintaining spontaneous breathing during 10% to 40% of the minute ventilation; this is not necessarily a contraindication in patients with ventricular dysfunction [14].

No studies in adult cancer patients are available. However, an interesting retrospective study in immunosuppressed children transitioning patients that failed conventional ventilation to either APRV or HFOV showed that less than a 15% reduction in the oxygenation index or less than 90% improvement in PaO_2/FiO_2 ratio was a cutoff associated with no survival [36]. There was a significant difference between the two modes of ventilation with respect to CO_2 control and use of neuromuscular blockade (higher in HFOV); although the mortality was high and not different between the two groups (APRV 62% and HFOV 65%).

Two recent randomized studies of APRV versus low tidal volume (LTV) have been published [41, 39]. The first study in 63 trauma patients (31 APRV and 32 LTV) did not show any differences between these two groups in regards to ventilator days, ICU length of stay (LOS), pneumothorax, ventilator-associated pneumonia, need for tracheostomy, modality failure, or mortality (6.45% vs. 6.25% respectively). In the second study, differences were too remarkable to consider without additional confirming studies, and given the previous study showing no differences. In this 138 medical patients' study, APRV was associated with shorter LOS ($p = 0.003$), ventilator days ({19 [interquartile range (IQR) 8-22] vs. 2 (IQR 0-15); $P < 0.001$}), and the ICU mortality was 19.7% versus 34.3% ($p = 0.053$).

Although we have not published our experience at MD Anderson Cancer Center, we have been using Biphasic ventilation following a standardized protocol for over 15 years. In our ICUs, Biphasic ventilation became the standard mode of ventilation and integral part of the ventilatory support strategy to manage all patients requiring invasive mechanical ventilation. As highlighted in figure 1, our first line ventilatory support includes noninvasive ventilation, transition to invasive mechanical ventilation using Biphasic ventilation (BiPAP as first line) and, in addition to adjunctive measures, transition to APRV if progression of hypoxemia (Tables 1 and 2). If APRV fails, next level options include prone positioning, HFPV, and/or ECMO if not contraindicated. Our weaning process includes CPAP/PS and

Table 1 MD Anderson Cancer Center ICU ventilator initial general settings management protocol

1. Initial **biphasic (BiPAP or Bi-level or Bi-vent) ventilation** settings
a. Adjust the **fraction of inspired oxygen** (FiO$_2$) to achieve pulse saturation (SpO$_2$) >92% but <96%
b. Set **positive end-expiratory pressure** (PEEP) low to lower inflection point (or alternative method used)
c. Set **time high** to 1.5 s and rate at 10 breaths per minute
d. Set PEEP high to **achieve tidal volume** (Vt) calculated by IBW
e. Vt adjustments to a maximum of 7 cc/kg and a minimum of 4 mL/kg of the IBW
i. Males IBW (kg) = 50 + 2.3 [height (inches) − 60]
ii. Females IBW (kg) = 45.5 + 2.3 [height (inches) − 60]
f. Arterial blood gases (ABG) within the first hour of initiation of ventilation to adjust settings
2. If plateau pressure (P$_{plat}$) is greater than 30 cm H$_2$O: Decrease V$_T$ by 1 mL/kg
3. Adjust respiratory rate (f) to achieve desired minute ventilation based on ABG results or available clinical parameters
4. Adjust pressure support (PS) above PEEP low to match the set Vt during spontaneous breathing
5. Do not exceed a set rate of 35 breaths/min. Goal pH (if ABG results available)
a. Normal: 7.35–7.45
b. Chronic CO$_2$ retention or metabolic acidosis: 7.30–7.45
c. ALI/ARDS: 7.25–7.45
6. Consider use of incremental FiO$_2$/PEEP combinations to achieve PaO$_2$ ≥60 or SpO$_2$ ≥90% (refer to Table 2)
7. Notify ICU provider if set PEEP is greater than 15 cmH$_2$O
8. Heat moisture exchangers (HME) may be used for mechanical ventilation less than 48 h
9. All patients receiving continuous ventilation greater than 48 h shall be placed on active humidification not exceeding 98.6 °F or 37 °C
Transition to biphasic ventilation with inverse inspiratory/expiratory (I:E) ratio (APRV)
1. Convert plateau pressure to PEEP-high, it should not exceed 35 cm H$_2$O
2. Convert PEEP-low to 0 cmH$_2$O
3. Set time-high from 4 to 6 s
4. Set time-low from 0.5 to 1 s

Table 2 Modified ARDS Net PEEP table

FiO$_2$ (%)	[a]PEEP (cmH$_2$O)
30	5
40	5–8
50	8–10
60	10
70	10–14
80	14
90	14–18
100	18–24

NEJM 2000; 342: 1301–1308
[a]*PEEP* positive end expiratory pressure

protocolized interruption of sedation/analgesia with spontaneous breathing trials on a daily basis.

High-Frequency Ventilation

High-frequency ventilation (HFV) is a mode of ventilation that includes respiratory frequencies above 2 Hertz (1 Hertz is equal to 1 oscillation/breath per second) and tidal volumes equal or below the dead space (0.5 to 5 cc/kg). The Food and Drug Administration (FDA) considers a ventilator capable to provide HFV when it is able to deliver more than 150 breaths per minute. There are many proposed mechanisms of gas exchange in HFV, including convective ventilation, Taylor dispersion, the Pendelluft effect, cardiogenic mixing, molecular diffusion, and asymmetrical velocity profiles [16, 42]. Oxygenation is mainly determined by the inspiratory fraction of oxygen and the mean airway pressure. At the same time, ventilation is determined by gas transport coefficient (tidal volume to the square multiplied by frequency, Vt^2 X f). The most frequent high-frequency ventilator used in the USA is the 3100 (3100-A for children and 3100-B for adults).

There are many types of HFV including HF jet ventilation (HFJV), high frequency oscillation

(HFOV), percussive ventilation (HFPV) delivered by the volumetric diffusive respirator (VDR). These ventilation modes started to appear in the 1970s when Sjöstrand, in Sweden, described high frequency positive pressure ventilation (HFPPV) using a pneumatic valve interrupting the gas flow to the ventilator at a constant driving pressure. He used no entrainment, frequencies between 2 and 4 Hertz, and passive expiration. Lunkenheimer described another mode known as HFOV which delivers frequencies of 2 to 15 Hertz. A new feature of this type of HFV was that it included *active* expiration and used a piston or a speaker diaphragm [18]. A third mode described a few years later was high-frequency jet ventilation (HFJV), initially described by Klain and Smith in the USA [15]. This mode had gas entrapment, the pressure was modulated, expiration was passive, and used frequencies between 2 and 8 Hz. A fourth mode of HFV, the HFPV, was described by Forrest Bird in the early 1980s [17]. The VDR uses a high-frequency flow generator with an interphase called phasitron that allows air entrapment creating a Venturi effect. It also has a passive expiration.

Severe hypoxemic respiratory failure is an indication to use HFV. Studies have described early thresholds including severe or moderate (early use) ARDS requiring positive end expiratory pressures above 5 cmH$_2$O. The above HFV have different applications and have gained popularity according to specific patient populations and the different performing characteristics of each mode. HFJV has been used for multiple head and neck and thoracic surgery operations and in the pediatric ICU. HFOV has been used in the pediatric, adult trauma, and medical ICUs excluding COPD or neurological patients. The latter because of the limited to very poor ventilation and risks for elevated intracranial pressure with this type of HFV. HFPV has been very popular by the military in the field and trauma centers for many years to manage burn patients, neurological critically ill patients, and trauma, as well as medical and pediatric patients.

The controls of the HFOV and the settings are relatively simple in the 3100-A and 3100-B ventilators, basically requiring regulation of the start/ stop button, the inspiratory fraction of oxygen, the amplitude, the inspiratory time percentage, the frequency, and monitoring the mean airway pressure. However, the settings and controls of HFPV with the VDR are extremely complicated and require highly skilled and trained individuals to handle these ventilators. These include among others, the pulsatile flow rate, pulse frequency, oscillatory CPAP, demand CPAP, inspiratory and expiratory times, inspiratory fraction of oxygen, failsafe sensitivity, and convective pressure. The humidification in these systems is a key part of their management. Another significant challenge is the lack of the pressure–volume graphs and other standard monitoring features found in any conventional ventilator.

Two small retrospective studies have suggested that HFOV is useful in managing ARDS in immunosuppressed children. In 12 pediatric patients where the mode was tried in Jordan, the A-a gradient decreased from a median of 564 to 267 ($p = 0.001$) after 24 h on HFOV and the mortality was 42% (5 of 12 patients) [8]. In another retrospective study of 222 patients from 12 US pediatric centers, there was a trend toward improved survival with early HFOV (early HFOV 30%, conventional ventilation 24%, and late HFOV 9%) [26]. Among these patients, 85 were placed on HFOV and their ICU mortality was 76.5%.

The most recent randomized studies have led to a significant drop in the utilization of HFV, particularly because of a higher complication rate. These findings have led to suggest that HFOV is dead [19]. In the OSCAR study [38], 397 patients were randomized to HFOV versus usual ventilatory management. HFOV did not improve 30-day mortality; the hospital mortality for HFOV was 50.1% versus 48.4% in the conventional group. In another randomized study known as the OSCILLATE study [9], in-hospital mortality was higher in the HFOV versus conventional ventilation (47% vs. 35% respectively) showing a lower probability of survival among patients ventilated with HFOV ($p = 0.004$). The study was terminated earlier given the RR 1.33;95%CI 1.09–1.64; $p = 0.005$. Two meta-analysis have reaffirmed the lack of benefit of this modality in ARDS [43, 34].

At the University of Texas, we have been using HFOV and HFPV with VDRs for over two decades. Our experience with cancer patients at MD Anderson Cancer Center has not been encouraging. Preliminary analysis about 10 years ago demonstrated a very high mortality in cancer patients with severe ARDS ranging from 79% to 90%, and not significant difference between HFOV and HFPV. Following the OSCAR and OSCILLATE studies, and based on our own unpublished experience, we abandoned the use of HFOV, and only use HFPV in selected cases.

Pressure-Regulated Volume Control (PRVC)

Although this mode is available in several ventilators under various names, the literature is extremely scarce and there are no studies in cancer patients. This mode of ventilation basically delivers a set tidal volume under a predetermined pressure. This feature has the disadvantage of risking hypoventilation in cases where patients' demands increase during stressful conditions. Riverso et al. compared volume controlled with PRVC in a small number of ARDS patients with some improvement in oxygenation and decrease in the peak inspiratory pressure [25]. The mode has been compared to pressure control in patients with traumatic brain injury [28]. In this small randomized study, there were no differences in intracranial pressure (ICP) or CO_2 levels. In patients with COPD exacerbation in respiratory failure, PRVC was able to maintain a low peak inspiratory pressure while improving oxygenation when compared to SIMV [4]. The mode does not seem to confer any particular advantage that is not found in other modes.

Neurally Adjusted Ventilatory Assist Ventilation (NAVA)

NAVA is a close-loop mode of ventilation that uses the diaphragmatic electrical activity as a surrogate of the respiratory center to control ventilation. In this mode, the patients determine time and assist levels, regulating their tidal volumes. It

has evolved from the initial experimental works in animals [24] and humans to introduction in clinical practice [30, 31]. The only ventilator capable to deliver NAVA is the Servo-air mechanical ventilator using an esophageal catheter to monitor the diaphragmatic electrical activity (EAdi catheter; Maquet Critical Care) and are among the limitations to use this mode in clinical practice.

No ARDS or cancer adult patients' studies have been performed using this mode of ventilation. Its current clinical application in the adult population seems to have focused mostly in noninvasive NAVA or the weaning processes comparing it to pressure support ventilation (PSV). Most studies have been performed in the pediatric patient population; not the focus of this chapter.

Studies comparing NAVA to PSV have shown that NAVA reduces patient-ventilator asynchrony when compared during weaning [5, 10]. However, NAVA did not seem to shorten the ventilator days or mortality. A recent meta-analysis supports the use of NAVA when compared to PSV [29]. The authors found a significant reduction in the risk of having a higher severe asynchrony index when compared to PSV (RR 3.43;95%, CI 1.57–7.51). NAVA has also been associated with greater diaphragmatic efficiency after 48 h ventilation when compared to PSV [6].

ECMO

This intervention is currently the last resource to rescue patients in severe hypoxemic respiratory failure who do not respond to intensive conventional and nonconventional therapies. This approach, its indications, contraindications, and literature are extensively discussed in the ECMO chapter therefore we do not believe there is a need to address them again here.

Conclusion

In summary, nonconventional modes of ventilation are numerous; however, only a few seem to have been adopted more broadly. Among these,

Biphasic ventilation (BiPAP/APRV) seems to be the most popular and widely used worldwide. Our service adopted this mode as part of our routine ventilatory support in all patients mechanically ventilated with great acceptance among all practitioners, and we have used it for over 15 years and continue using it satisfactorily. It is too early to assess the potential impact of newer nonconventional modes such as NAVA; however, the fact that this mode increases the cost of management by requiring additional invasive equipment (esophageal catheter) and needs special ventilators suggest that newer nonconventional modes will not gain much acceptance. Older nonconventional ventilation modes such as HFV have suffered serious setbacks as a result of recent large randomized studies such as the OSCILLATE study and have been abandoned in many places including the University of Texas MD Anderson Cancer Center's intensive care units. Finally, there is little, if any, literature about the use of these new modes in cancer patients or other populations indicating the need for more research.

References

1. Baum M, Benzer H, Putensen C, Koller W, Putz G. Biphasic positive airway pressure (BiPAP) – a new form of augmented ventilation. Anaesthesist. 1989;38(9):452–8.
2. Bellani G, Laffey JG, Fan E, Brochard L, Esteban A, Gattinoni L, van Haren F, Larsson A, McAuley DF, Ranieri M, Rubenfeld G, Thompson BT, Wrigge H, Slutsky AS, Presenti A, for the LUNG SAFE Investigators and the ESICM Trials Group. Epidemiology, patters of care, and mortality for patients with acute respiratory distress syndrome in intensive care units in 50 countries. JAMA. 2016;315(8):788–800.
3. Carlucci A, Richard J-C, Wysocki M, Lepage E, Brochard L, SRLF Collaborative Group on Mechanical Ventilation. Noninvasive versus conventional mechanical ventilation: an epidemiologic survey. Am J Respir Crit Care Med. 2001;163:874–80.
4. Chang S, Shi J, Fu C, Wu X, Li S. A comparison of synchronized intermittent mandatory ventilation and pressure-regulated volume control ventilation in elderly patients with acute exacerbations of COPD and respiratory failure. Int J Chron Obstruct Pulmon Dis. 2016;17(11):1023–9.
5. Demoule A, Clavel M, Rolland-Debord C, Perbet S, Terzi N, Kouatchet A, Wallet F, Roze H, Vargas F, Guerin C, Dellamonia J, Jaber S, Brochjard L, Similowski T. Neurally adjusted ventilatory assist as an alternative to pressure support ventilation in adults: a French multicenter randomized trial. Intensive Care Med. 2016;42:1723–32.
6. Di Mussi R, Spadaro S, Mirabella L, Volta CA, Serio G, Staffieri F, Dambrosio M, Cinella G, Bruno F, Grasso S. Impact of prolonged assisted ventilation on diaphragmatic efficiency: NAVA versus PSV. Crit Care. 2016;20:1. https://doi.org/10.1186/s13054-015-1178-0.
7. Emr B, Gatto LA, Roy S, Satalin J, Ghosh A, Snyder K, Andrews P, Habashi N, Marx W, Ge L, Wang G, Dean DA, Vodovotz Y, Nieman G. Airway pressure release ventilation prevents ventilator induced lung injury in normal lungs. JAMA Surg. 2013;148(11):1005–12.
8. Faqih NA, Qanbba'h SH, Rihani RS, Ghonimat IM, Yamani YM, Sultan IY. The use of high frequency oscillatory ventilation in a pediatric oncology intensive care unit. Pediatr Blood Cancer. 2012;58(3):384–9.
9. Ferguson ND, Cook D, Guyatt GH, Mehta S, Hand L, Austin P, Zhou Q, Matte A, Walter SD, Lamontagne F, Granton JT, Arabi YM, Arroliga AC, Stewart TE, Slutsky AS, O'Meade MO, Oscillate Trial Investigators and the Canadian Critical Care Trials Group. High-frequency oscillation in early acute respiratory distress syndrome. NEJM. 2013;368(9):795–805.
10. Ferreira JC, Diniz-Silva F, Moriya HT, Alencar AM, Amato MBP, Carvalho CRR. Neurally adjusted ventilatory assist (NAVA) or pressure support ventilation (PSV) during spontaneous breathing trials in critically ill patients: a crossover trial. BMC Pulm Med. 2017;17(1):139.
11. Gattinoni L, Colino F, Maiolo G, Rapetti F, Romitti F, Tonetti T, Vasques F, Quintel M. Positive end-expiratory pressure: how to set it an individual level. Ann Transl Med. 2017;5(14):288.
12. Hering R, Peters D, Zinserling J, Wrigge H, von Spiegel T, Putensen C. Effects of spontaneous breathing during airway pressure release ventilation on renal perfusion and function in patients with acute lung injury. Intensive Care Med. 2002;28(10):1426–33.
13. Hörman C, Baum M, Putensen C, Mutz NJ, Benzer H. Biphasi positive airway pressure (BiPAP) – a new mode of ventilatory support. Eur J Anesthesiol. 1994;11(1):37–42.
14. Kaplan L, Bailey H, Formosa V. Airway pressure release ventilation increases cardiac performance in patients with acute ling injury/adult respiratory distress syndrome. Crit Care. 2001;5(4):221–6.
15. Klain M, Smith RB. High frequency percutaneous transtracheal jet ventilation. Crit Care Med. 1977;5:280–7.
16. Krishnan JA, Brower RG. High-frequency ventilation for acute lung injury and ARDS. Chest. 2000;118:795–807.
17. Lukangelo U, Fontanesi L, Antonaglia V, Pellis T, Berlot G, Liguori G, Bird FM, Gullo A. High frequency percussive ventilation (HFPV). Minerva Anestesiol. 2003;69:841–51.

18. Lunkenheimer PP, Rafflenbeul W, Keller H, Frank I, Dickhut HH, Fuhrmann C. Application of transtracheal pressure oscillations as a modification of "diffusion respiration". Br J Anaesth. 1972;44:627.

19. Nguyen AP, Schmidt UH, Macintyre NR. Should high-frequency in the adult be abandoned? Respir Care. 2016;61(6):791–800.

20. Putensen C, Wrigge H. Clinical review: biphasic positive airway pressure and airway pressure release ventilation. Crit Care. 2004;8:492–7. https://doi.org/10.1186/cc2919.

21. Putensen C, Mutz NJ, Putensen-Himmer G, Zinserling J. Spontaneous breathing during ventilatory support improves ventilation-perfusion distributions in patients with respiratory distress syndrome. Am J Respir Crit Care Med. 1999;159(4 Pt 1):1241–8.

22. Putensen C, Zech S, Wrigge H, Zinserling J, Stüber F, von Spiegel T, Mutz N. Long-term effects of spontaneous breathing during ventilatory support in patients with acute lung injury. Am J Respir Crit Care Med. 2001;164:43–9.

23. Rathgeber J, Schorn B, Falk V, Kazmaier S, Spiegel T. The influence of controlled mandatory ventilation (CMV), intermittent mandatory ventilation (IMV), and biphasic intermittent positive airway pressure (BiPAP) on duration of intubation and consumption of analgesics and sedatives. A prospective analysis in 596 patients following cardiac surgery. Eur J Anesthesiol. 1997;14:576–82.

24. Remmers JE, Gautier H. Servo respirator constructed from a positive pressure ventilator. J Appl Physiol. 1976;41:252–5.

25. Riverso P, Bernard PL, Corsa D, Morra MG, Pagannini G, Parigi F. A comparison of ventilation techniques in ARDS. Volume controlled vs pressure regulated volume control. Minerva Anesthesiol. 1998;64(7–8):339–43.

26. Rowan CM, Loomis A, McArthur J, Smith LS, Gertz SJ, Fitzgerald JC, Nitu ME, Moser EA, Hsing DD, Duncan CN, Mahadeo KM, Moffet J, Hall MW, Pinos EL, Tamburro RF, Cheifetz IM, Investigators of the Pediatric Acute Lung Injury and Sepsis Network. High-frequency oscillatory ventilation use and severe pediatric ARDS in the pediatric hematopoietic cell transplant recipient. Respir Care. 2018;63(4):404–11.

27. Saddy F, Moraes L, Santos CL, Pena G, Morales MM, Capelozzi VL, Game de Abreu M, Baez CS, Pelosi P, Rieken P. Biphasic positive airway pressure minimizes biological impact on lung tissue in mild acute lung injury independent of etiology. Crit Care. 2013;17:R228.

28. Schirmer-Mikalsen K, Vik A, Skogvoll E, Moen KG, Solheim O, Klepstad P. Intracranial pressure during pressure control and pressure-regulated volume control ventilation in patients with traumatic brain injury: a randomized crossover trial. Neurocrit Care. 2016;24(3):332–41.

29. Sehgal IS, Dhooria S, Aggarwal AN, Behera D, Agarwal R. Asynchrony index in pressure support ventilation (PSV) versus neurally adjust ventilator assist (NAVA) during non-invasive ventilation (NIV) for respiratory failure: a systematic review and meta-analysis. Intensive Care Med. 2016;42(11):1813–5.

30. Sinderby C, Beck J. Proportional assist ventilation and neurally adjusted ventilatory assist – better approaches to patient ventilator synchrony? Clin Chest Med. 2008;29(2):329–42.

31. Sinderby C, Navalesi P, Beck J, Skrobik Y, Comtois N, Friberg S, Gottfried SB, Lindström L. Neural control of mechanical ventilation in respiratory failure. Nature Med. 1999;5:1433–6.

32. Singh PM, Borle A, Trikha A. Newer nonconventional modes of mechanical ventilation. J Emerg Trauma Shock. 2014;7(3):222–7.

33. Stefan MS, Shieh MS, Pekow PS, Rothberg MB, Steingrub JS, Lagu T, Lindenauer PK. Epidemiology and outcomes of acute respiratory failure in the United States, 2001–2009: a national survey. J Hosp Med. 2013;8(2):76–82.

34. Sud S, Sud M, Friedrech JO, Wunsch H, Meade MO, Ferguson ND, Adhikari NK. High-frequency oscillatory ventilation versus conventional ventilation for acute respiratory distress syndrome. Cochrane Database Syst Rev 2016;4(4):CD004085.

35. Vincent JL, Akca S, De Mendonca A, Haji-Michael P, Sprung C, Moreno R, Antonelli M, Sutter PM, SOFA Working Group. The epidemiology of acute respiratory failure in critically ill patients. Chest. 2002;121(5):1602–9.

36. Yehya N, Topjian AA, Thomas NJ, Fricss SH. Improved oxygenation 24 hours after transition to airway pressure release ventilation of high-frequency oscillatory ventilation accurately discriminates survival in immunocompromised pediatric patients with acute respiratory distress syndrome. Pediatr Crit Care Med. 2014;15(4):e147–56.

37. Younes M. Proportional assist ventilation, a new approach to ventilatory support. Theory. Am Rev Respir Dis. 1992;145:114–20.

38. Young D, Lamb SE, Shah S, MacKenzie I, Tunnicliffe W, Lall R, Rowan K, Cuthbertson BH, OSCAR Study Group. High-frequency oscillation for acute respiratory distress. NEJM. 2013;368(9):806–13.

39. Zhou Y, Jin X, Lv Y, Wang P, Yang Y, Liang G, Wang B, Kang Y. Early application of airway pressure release ventilation may reduce the duration of mechanical ventilation in acute respiratory distress syndrome. Intensive Care Med. 2017;43:1648–59.

40. Esteban A, Frutos-Vivar F, Muriel A, Ferguson ND, Peñuelas O, Abraira V, Raymondos K, Rios F, Nin N, Apezteguía C, Violi DA, Thille AW, Brochard L, González M, Villagomez AJ, Hurtado J, Davies AR, Du B, Maggiore SM, Pelosi P, Soto L, Tomicic V, D'Empaire G, Matamis D, Abroug F, Moreno RP, Soares MA, Arabi Y, Sandi F, Jibaja M, Amin P, Koh Y, Kuiper MA, Bülow HH, Zeggwagh AA, Anzueto A.

Evolution of mortality over time in patients receiving mechanical ventilation. Am J Respir Crit Care Med 2013;188(2):220–230.

41. Maxwell RA, Green JM, Waldrop J, Dart BW, Smith PW, Brooks D, Lewis PL, Barker DE. A randomized prospective trial of airway pressure release ventilation and low tidal volume ventilation in adult trauma patients with acute respiratory failure. J Trauma 2010;69(3):501–510.

42. Pillow JJ. High-frequency oscillatory ventilation: mechanisms of gas exchange and lung mechanics. Crit Care med 2005;33(3):S135–141.

43. Gu XL, Wu GN, Yao YW, Shi DH, Song Y. Is high-frequency oscillatory ventilation more effective and safer than conventional protective ventilation in adult acute respiratory distress syndrome patients? A meta-analysis of randomized controlled trials. Crit Care 201418:R111

Prone Ventilatory Therapy in Critically Ill Cancer Patients

34

Alex Pearce and Rebecca E. Sell

Contents

Introduction 510

Etiology 510

Epidemiology 510

Pathophysiology 511

Clinical Features 512

Diagnosis 513

Management 513
Pharmacologic 513
Non-pharmacologic 513

Prognosis 514

References 514

Abstract

Mortality in critically ill cancer patients requiring mechanical ventilation approaches 60%. When mechanical ventilation is required for severe hypoxemia and acute respiratory distress syndrome, mortality ranges from 70% to 100%, with worse outcomes in patients with hematologic malignancy and stem cell transplant. While overall mortality has improved with the use of lung protective strategies like low tidal volume ventilation and conservative fluid management, prone positioning has been shown to improve gas exchange and decrease ventilator-associated lung injury. By recruiting collapsed lung units and redistributing transpulmonary pressures, prone positioning is associated with improved hemodynamics, decreased organ dysfunction, and improved mortality. Observational studies and retrospective case series suggest that prone positioning may improve mortality in patients with cancer and ARDS but in practice may be underutilized.

A. Pearce (✉)
Department of Internal Medicine, University of California San Diego, La Jolla, San Diego, CA, USA
e-mail: apearce@ucsd.edu

R. E. Sell
Department of Internal Medicine, University of California San Diego, La Jolla, San Diego, CA, USA

Division of Pulmonary and Critical Care, University of California San Diego, San Diego, CA, USA
e-mail: rsell@ucsd.edu

© Springer Nature Switzerland AG 2020
J. L. Nates, K. J. Price (eds.), *Oncologic Critical Care*,
https://doi.org/10.1007/978-3-319-74588-6_57

Keywords
Acute lung injury · Acute respiratory distress syndrome · Prone position · Critical care · Malignancy

Introduction

Mortality in critically ill cancer patients requiring mechanical ventilation approaches 60% [3]. When mechanical ventilation is required for severe hypoxemia (PaO2/fIO2 <150 on mechanical ventilation) and acute respiratory distress syndrome (ARDS), mortality ranges from 70% to 100% [28] with worse outcomes in patients with hematologic malignancy and stem cell transplant. ARDS is an inflammatory lung response to injury or infection leading to bilateral pulmonary infiltrates on chest imaging and hypoxic respiratory failure with a PaO2/FiO2 ratio of less than 300. For moderate to severe ARDS (PaO2/FiO2 ratio <150), mortality for all comers approaches 40%.

While there is no cure for ARDS, management includes treating the underlying condition and lung protective strategies such as low tidal volumes and higher positive end-expiratory pressure (PEEP) designed to mitigate damage caused by mechanical ventilation. Conservative fluid management is also associated with improved outcomes [37]. The original ARMA protocol comparing tidal volumes of 6 ml/kg (low) with 12 ml/kg (high) excluded patients with bone marrow transplant or malignancy with estimated 6-month mortality >50% [7]. Low tidal volume ventilation, however, was associated with lower mortality (OR 0.37) in a retrospective review of patients with ARDS and hematologic malignancy [32].

Early trials showed that prone positioning improved oxygenation and hemodynamics and likely decreased ventilator-induced lung injury (VILI) in mechanically ventilated patients [6, 9]. These observed benefits prompted additional studies translating these physiologic benefits into unique ventilatory strategies for the treatment of ARDS. Several early studies evaluating the use of prone positioning in ARDS failed to show a mortality benefit [11, 14, 35]. However, the PROSEVA (Proning Severe ARDS Patients) trial in 2013 specifically addressed only patients with severe ARDS (PaO2/FiO2 <150) and showed a 28-day and 90-day mortality benefit [15]. Early prone positioning has now been adopted in the treatment of severe ARDS in most major academic centers and is no longer considered solely a salvage therapy. This chapter will discuss the pathophysiology, practical applications, and management recommendations for prone positioning in the treatment of severe ARDS. It will also highlight elements of prone positioning to be considered specifically in the oncologic population.

Etiology

ARDS is an inflammatory response to injury or infection. Common triggers include sepsis, pneumonia, and aspiration. Azoulay et al. [2] report that in their cohort of over 1000 patients with malignancy and ARDS, 90% were infection related. Blood and blood product transfusions are also factors associated with the development of acute lung injury and ARDS, putting patients with cancer, especially those on chemotherapy or in the post stem cell transplant period at higher risk. Other noninfectious causes that may predispose stem cell transplant patients to the development of ARDS include the use of chemotherapy and radiation, diffuse alveolar hemorrhage, engraftment syndrome, and idiopathic pneumonia syndrome.

Epidemiology

ARDS occurs in approximately 190,000 patients per year in the United States, with an estimated 74,000 deaths [31]. A large observational study across ICUs in 50 different countries identified that ARDS patients make up approximately 10% of ICU admissions [5]. Of the 3022 patients with ARDS, 4.7% had hematologic disease. Similarly, 4.4% of patients enrolled in all ARDSNet clinical trials had cancer [34].

Respiratory failure is frequent in patients with solid and hematologic malignancies. Of patients with cancer transferred to the ICU, 16.5% will have ARDS [2]. Patients with leukemia and lymphoma are more likely to require ICU transfer, require mechanical ventilation, and have higher mortality [22]. A retrospective review of 280 patients with newly diagnosed AML (acute myeloid leukemia) identified 9% with ARDS, making it a relatively common complication [36]. Of patients with solid tumors and ARDS, lung cancer is most commonly identified [1, 22].

The use of prone positioning in the management of ARDS is not universal. In the Bellani et al. [5] observational study, prone positioning was used in only 7.9% of all patients with ARDS. It was more commonly used in patients with severe ARDS (16.3%). The landmark PROSEVA trial was pivotal in establishing a mortality benefit for prone positioning in severe ARDS [15]. Although this trial did not specifically focus on the effects of prone positioning in the oncologic population, 13% of the participants in the control group and 10% of the participants in the prone positioning group had cancer. It is likely that these positive results can be applied to oncologic patients in the ICU with severe ARDS.

Pathophysiology

ARDS has both local and systemic pathologic consequences. Local effects include profound hypoxemia driven by poor gas exchange due to non-compliant lungs and ventilation/perfusion (VQ) mismatch. Tissue hypoxia results, leading to organ damage. Inflammatory cytokines released by overdistended and stressed lung units, also known as ventilator-induced lung injury (VILI), are associated with multi-organ failure including acute renal failure and hypotension [17].

Prone positioning in ARDS is advantageous for many reasons. Prone positioning is unique in its ability to recruit additional alveoli for gas exchange. The ARDS lung is edematous and inflamed leading to loss of functionally aerated lung, primarily in the dependent lung regions [10]. As mechanically ventilated patients are traditionally positioned supine, these changes predominately result in loss of functional lung parenchyma dorsally. This has important implications as anatomically there is a greater lung volume located dorsally compared to ventrally. In addition to the increased stress on the dorsal lung units due to gravity-dependent edema and inflammation, the dorsal lung is also compressed by the heart and mediastinal structures when the patient is in the supine position. The prone position relieves this compression and recruits dorsal lung tissue [29]. Prone positioning also shifts the gravity-dependent edema to the ventral lung regions, thus affecting less of the overall lung volume. Overall, prone positioning adds additional functional pulmonary units from the previously compressed dorsal lung region. Increased recruitment of the dorsal alveoli allows for more of the total lung volume to be involved in functional gas exchange.

Prone positioning is also associated with improved VQ matching. While prone positioning improves ventilation to the dorsal lung parenchyma, it does not significantly impact perfusion [13]. Blood flow in the lung remains directed dorsally to alveoli that are now open resulting in improved ventilation perfusion matching, reducing shunting of blood past collapsed and atelectatic lung units.

Prone positioning also improves the transpulmonary pressure gradient between the dorsal and ventral lung regions creating more homogenous lung inflation [24]. Transpulmonary pressure is the pressure at airway opening minus pressure in the pleural space and is responsible for the distention of the lung. In the traditional supine position, the transpulmonary pressure of the ventral lung is greater than the dorsal lung leading to increased distention of ventral alveoli compared to those dorsally located [24]. This difference forces regional distribution of tidal volume and PEEP to the open ventral lung units, resulting in ventral alveoli overdistention and compression of the dorsal pulmonary units. Anatomically, prone positioning more evenly distributes transpulmonary pressure, leading to less dorsal alveolar collapse and decreased hyperinflation of the ventral alveoli [9]. Thus, alveolar distention and pressures are more evenly distributed across the lung.

The concept of a more homogenous lung produced by prone positioning has been proposed to be protective against ventilator-induced lung injury (VILI) as well. Damage from regional over distention of alveoli seen in the ventral portions of the lung in the supine position is mitigated by improved homogeneity and more uniformly distributed pleural pressure and mechanical strain [9]. PEEP is also more evenly distributed; thus once an alveolus is recruited it stays open and avoids the inflammatory consequences associated with cyclical opening and closing with each respiratory cycle [8]. Overall, by improving regional hyperdistention, facilitating more even distribution of pressure, and preventing atelectasis, prone positioning reduces VILI in the mechanically ventilated patient.

Prone positioning has a beneficial effect on systemic and organ hemodynamics [17]. There was no difference in the rates of hypotension between the prone and standard groups in the PROSEVA trial. More recently, a study of 18 patients with ARDS evaluated the effect of prone positioning on hemodynamics [19]. In this study, prone position resulted in a small increase in intra-abdominal pressure and in preload. There was a notable decreased in pulmonary vascular resistance which may be related to the effect of prone positioning on attenuating hypoxic-induced vasoconstriction of the pulmonary vasculature. In those patients with preload reserve, prone positioning resulted in an increase in cardiac index. Several studies have also evaluated the effect of prone positioning on distal organ hemodynamics [18, 26]. They found, using hepatic vein catheters to measure blood flow, oxygen delivery, and lactate production, that perfusion was unaffected in the prone position. Taken together, this suggests that using prone positioning in early ARDS may lead to improved hemodynamics and tissue perfusion.

Clinical Features

There are several features that are clinically important in the application of prone positioning in severe ARDS: integration with standard lung protective ventilator strategies, logistics of prone positioning, associated complications, contraindications, as well as the impact on other organ symptoms.

It is important that prone positioning be used in conjunction with other lung protective ventilatory strategies. Specifically, low tidal volume ventilation should be emphasized as this was a consistent feature of the studies showing a mortality benefit with prone positioning [15]. For example, the average tidal volume utilized by Guerin et al. [15] in the PROSEVA study was 6.1 ml/kg. While the use of low tidal volume strategies has been evaluated in conjunction with prone positioning, the optimal PEEP while prone is not yet defined, no studies have specifically evaluated high PEEP strategies and prone positioning. Animal models evaluating the effect of PEEP titration on lung mechanics, hemodynamics, and oxygenation in the supine and prone position demonstrated that both PEEP and prone positioning improved lung mechanics independent of one another [20]. Theoretically, there should be a synergistic effect of higher PEEP in recruiting and evenly distributing ventilation through the prone lung [4].

Experienced staff are required to implement safe and effective prone positioning. Patients should be positioned prone for a minimum of 16 h [33] and supine for the remainder of the day. While a "proning bed" may be utilized, placing the patient face down in the "swimmer's position" alternating the arms superiorly and turning the head from side to side is as effective. Possible complications in physically moving a patient to the prone position include displacement of the endotracheal tube and unintended extubation, loss of vascular access, and pressure sores [25].

There are several contraindications to prone positioning that should be considered. High likelihood of necessitating cardiopulmonary resuscitation, recent sternotomy, facial trauma, and pelvic and spinal instability are general contraindications to prone positioning [33]. One could extrapolate concerns related to facial trauma to patients with active head and neck cancer or recent facial surgery.

Hemoptysis is also a relative contraindication to prone positioning and of significance in patients with malignancy and ARDS. Cancer patients may have hemoptysis due to airway tumor or from invasive fungal infection and would be hard to manage in the prone position. Diffuse alveolar hemorrhage (DAH) as a cause of hemoptysis, however, may benefit from prone positioning. A case report of DAH from vasculitis reported improvement in oxygenation and hemodynamics when prone [16]. The author postulates that prone positioning resulted in improved V/Q matching and improved drainage of blood and edema from the dorsal lung.

Elevated intracranial pressure (ICP) is another contraindication that may be specifically relevant in oncologic patients. Due to the rotation of the head during prone positioning and indirect compression of the internal jugular vein, ICP may increase [30]. In patients with brain metastasis, this may be a significant contraindication.

Prone positioning also indirectly affects other organ systems and cardiovascular hemodynamics. Prone positioning increases venous return and decreases right ventricular afterload [19], improving cardiac output and blood pressure. Alternatively, some studies suggest that prone positioning increases intra-abdominal hypertension; however the exact significance of this is still debatable [21], and there are no reports of abdominal compartment syndrome due to prone positioning. It is also suggested that prone positioning allows for improved drainage of respiratory secretions and decreased risk of infectious complications [23].

Bronchoscopy, a procedure commonly required in ARDS patients in the ICU, is not routinely done while a patient is in the prone position. Ideally this procedure should be done during the 8 h when patient will be in the supine position.

Diagnosis

In general, consideration of prone positioning for a patient with severe ARDS should be undertaken early in the course of disease if the patient has a PaO2/FiO2 ratio <150. It should be noted that this PaO2/FIO2 ratio is slightly different than

standard definitions of severe ARDS which defines severe ARDS as a PaO2/FiO2 ratio <100. Trials evaluating prone positioning in patients with only mild to moderate ARDS did not show a mortality benefit [12, 14]. In addition to the criteria mentioned above, with the decision to pursue prone positioning as part of ventilatory management in a patient with malignancy and ARDS, the physician should take into account the entire clinical picture for each individual patient.

Management

Pharmacologic

Although there are no specific recommendations concerning prone positioning and sedation strategies, the majority (91%) of the patients in the PROSEVA test group received neuromuscular blockade, specifically cisatracurium besylate, which was strongly recommended in the first 48 h per the study protocol [15]. Early use of cisatracurium in patients with severe ARDS resulted in improved mortality at 90 days [27]. The combination of early prone positioning along with early paralytics is likely to be synergistic. All patients also received appropriate analgesia and sedation.

A conservative fluid management strategy with an even to slightly negative fluid balance during the first 7 days has also been associated with better oxygenation and fewer ventilator and ICU days than a liberal strategy [37]. There was also a trend toward improved mortality. Intravenous loop diuretics should be considered to assist in maintaining an appropriate fluid balance.

Prophylaxis against constipation, deep vein thrombosis, and gastrointestinal bleeding should be considered.

Non-pharmacologic

Prone positioning should be implemented early in patients meeting criteria for severe ARDS. The best results are seen when prone positioning is initiated within the first 48 h. Logistically, placing a patient in the prone position requires significant preparation and experienced staff. One staff member is dedicated to management and maintenance of the endotracheal tube which often require suctioning during the transition from supine to prone due to movement of secretions. Careful attention is paid to prevent dislodgement. Vascular access should be placed prior to prone positioning and must be carefully monitored during turning to prone position. The other staff members carefully turn the patient prone, positioning an arm above the head and the other arm down by the patient's side. The face is turned to one side to protect the airway.

Patients should be positioned prone for a minimum of 16 h [33] and supine for the remainder of the day. The decision to discontinue prone positioning is made on an individual basis. In general, sustained improvement in PaO2/FiO2 ratio (>150) with decreased needs for high FiO2 (≤60%) or PEEP ≤10 cm water) may indicate that prone positioning can be discontinued. However, it is recommended that patient have a clear improvement in both respiratory status and overall clinical picture before discontinuing prone positioning.

To prevent pressure ulcers, the patient's arms and head should be turned every 2 h. Pressure points should be examined routinely and adjusted to prevent ulcers. Prophylaxis against deep vein thrombosis is recommended.

Enteral nutrition should be considered; however, high gastric residuals may predispose to aspiration events and ventilator-associated pneumonia. The prone position may lead to higher gastric residuals if abdominal pressures increase.

Prognosis

ARDS mortality has improved with the implementation of low tidal volume ventilation and conservative fluid management but remains around 40%; this risk is increased in patients with solid and hematologic malignancy. The PROSEVA trial showed that patients with severe ARDS who were managed with early prone positioning had a 28-day mortality of 16% as opposed to the standard care group (HR for death 0.39). With early recognition, lung protective strategies and prone positioning appear to improve outcomes in patients with malignancy and ARDS.

References

1. Adam AK, Soubani AO. Outcome and prognostic factors of lung cancer patients admitted to the medical intensive care unit. Eur Respir J. 2008;31(1):47–53. https://doi.org/10.1183/09031936.00031607.
2. Azoulay E, Lemiale V, Mokart D, Pène F, Kouatchet A, Perez P, Vincent F, Mayaux J, Benoit D, Bruneel F, Meert AP, Nyunga M, Rabbat A, Darmon M. Acute respiratory distress syndrome in patients with malignancies. Intensive Care Med. 2014;40(8):1106–14. https://doi.org/10.1007/s00134-014-3354-0.
3. Azoulay E, Mokart D, Pène F, Lambert J, Kouatchet A, Mayaux J, Vincent F, Nyunga M, Bruneel F, Laisne LM, Rabbat A, Lebert C, Perez P, Chaize M, Renault A, Meert AP, Benoit D, Hamidfar R, Jourdain M, Darmon M, Schlemmer B, Chevret S, Lemiale V. Outcomes of critically ill patients with hematologic malignancies: prospective multicenter data from France and Belgium – a groupe de recherche respiratoire en réanimation onco-hématologique study. J Clin Oncol. 2013;31(22):2810–8. https://doi.org/10.1200/JCO.2012.47.2365.
4. Beitler JR, Guérin C, Ayzac L, Mancebo J, Bates DM, Malhotra A, Talmor D. PEEP titration during prone positioning for acute respiratory distress syndrome. Crit Care. 2015;19:436. https://doi.org/10.1186/s13054-015-1153-9.
5. Bellani G, Laffey JG, Pham T, Fan E, Brochard L, Esteban A, Gattinoni L, van Haren F, Larsson A, McAuley DF, Ranieri M, Rubenfeld G, Thompson BT, Wrigge H, Slutsky AS, Pesenti A, LUNG SAFE Investigators, ESICM Trials Group. Epidemiology, patterns of care, and mortality for patients with acute respiratory distress syndrome in intensive care units in 50 countries. JAMA. 2016;315(8):788–800. https://doi.org/10.1001/jama.2016.0291.
6. Broccard A, Shapiro RS, Schmitz LL, Adams AB, Nahum A, Marini JJ. Prone positioning attenuates and redistributes ventilator-induced lung injury in dogs. Crit Care Med. 2000;28(2):295–303.
7. Brower RG, Matthay MA, Morris A, Schoenfeld D, Thompson BT, Wheeler A, Network ARDS. Ventilation with lower tidal volumes as compared with traditional tidal volumes for acute lung injury and the acute respiratory distress syndrome. N Engl J Med. 2000;342(18):1301–8. https://doi.org/10.1056/NEJM200005043421801.
8. Cornejo RA, Díaz JC, Tobar EA, Bruhn AR, Ramos CA, González RA, Repetto CA, Romero CM,

Gálvez LR, Llanos O, Arellano DH, Neira WR, Díaz GA, Zamorano AJ, Pereira GL. Effects of prone positioning on lung protection in patients with acute respiratory distress syndrome. Am J Respir Crit Care Med. 2013;188(4):440–8. https://doi.org/10.1164/rccm.201207-1279OC.

9. Galiatsou E, Kostanti E, Svarna E, Kitsakos A, Koulouras V, Efremidis SC, Nakos G. Prone position augments recruitment and prevents alveolar overinflation in acute lung injury. Am J Respir Crit Care Med. 2006;174(2):187–97. https://doi.org/10.1164/rccm.200506-899OC.

10. Gattinoni L, Pesenti A. ARDS: the non-homogenous lung; facts and hypothesis. Intensive Crit Care Dig. 1987;6:1–4.

11. Gattinoni L, Tognoni G, Pesenti A, Taccone P, Mascheroni D, Labarta V, Malacrida R, Di Giulio P, Fumagalli R, Pelosi P, Brazzi L, Latini R, Prone-Supine Study Group. Effect of prone positioning on the survival of patients with acute respiratory failure. N Engl J Med. 2001;345(8):568–73. https://doi.org/10.1056/NEJMoa010043.

12. Gattinoni L, Carlesso E, Taccone P, Polli F, Guérin C, Mancebo J. Prone positioning improves survival in severe ARDS: a pathophysiologic review and individual patient meta-analysis. Minerva Anestesiol. 2010;76(6):448–54.

13. Glenny RW, Lamm WJ, Albert RK, Robertson HT. Gravity is a minor determinant of pulmonary blood flow distribution. J Appl Physiol (1985). 1991;71(2):620–9. https://doi.org/10.1152/jappl.1991.71.2.620.

14. Guerin C, Gaillard S, Lemasson S, Ayzac L, Girard R, Beuret P, Palmier B, Le QV, Sirodot M, Rosselli S, Cadiergue V, Sainty JM, Barbe P, Combourieu E, Debatty D, Rouffineau J, Ezingeard E, Millet O, Guelon D, Rodriguez L, Martin O, Renault A, Sibille JP, Kaidomar M. Effects of systematic prone positioning in hypoxemic acute respiratory failure: a randomized controlled trial. JAMA. 2004;292(19):2379–87. https://doi.org/10.1001/jama.292.19.2379.

15. Guérin C, Reignier J, Richard JC, Beuret P, Gacouin A, Boulain T, Mercier E, Badet M, Mercat A, Baudin O, Clavel M, Chatellier D, Jaber S, Rosselli S, Mancebo J, Sirodot M, Hilbert G, Bengler C, Richecoeur J, Gainnier M, Bayle F, Bourdin G, Leray V, Girard R, Baboi L, Ayzac L, PROSEVA Study Group. Prone positioning in severe acute respiratory distress syndrome. N Engl J Med. 2013;368(23):2159–68. https://doi.org/10.1056/NEJMoa1214103.

16. Hayes-Bradley C. Hypoxia from vasculitic pulmonary haemorrhage improved by prone position ventilation. Br J Anaesth. 2004;92(5):754–7. https://doi.org/10.1093/bja/aeh114.

17. Hepokoski ML, Malhotra A, Singh P, Crotty Alexander LE. Ventilator-induced kidney injury: are novel biomarkers the key to prevention? Nephron. 2018;1–4. https://doi.org/10.1159/000491557.

18. Hering R, Wrigge H, Vorwerk R, Brensing KA, Schröder S, Zinserling J, Hoeft A, Spiegel TV, Putensen C. The effects of prone positioning on intraabdominal pressure and cardiovascular and renal function in patients with acute lung injury. Anesth Analg. 2001;92(5):1226–31.

19. Jozwiak M, Teboul JL, Anguel N, Persichini R, Silva S, Chemla D, Richard C, Monnet X. Beneficial hemodynamic effects of prone positioning in patients with acute respiratory distress syndrome. Am J Respir Crit Care Med. 2013;188(12):1428–33. https://doi.org/10.1164/rccm.201303-0593OC.

20. Keenan JC, Cortes-Puentes GA, Zhang L, Adams AB, Dries DJ, Marini JJ. PEEP titration: the effect of prone position and abdominal pressure in an ARDS model. Intensive Care Med Exp. 2018;6(1):3. https://doi.org/10.1186/s40635-018-0170-9.

21. Kirkpatrick AW, Pelosi P, De Waele JJ, Malbrain ML, Ball CG, Meade MO, Stelfox HT, Laupland KB. Clinical review: Intra-abdominal hypertension: does it influence the physiology of prone ventilation? Crit Care. 2010;14(4):232. https://doi.org/10.1186/cc9099.

22. Kress JP, Christenson J, Pohlman AS, Linkin DR, Hall JB. Outcomes of critically ill cancer patients in a university hospital setting. Am J Respir Crit Care Med. 1999;160(6):1957–61. https://doi.org/10.1164/ajrccm.160.6.9812055.

23. Ladoire S, Pauchard LA, Barbar SD, Tissieres P, Croisier-Bertin D, Charles PE. Impact of the prone position in an animal model of unilateral bacterial pneumonia undergoing mechanical ventilation. Anesthesiology. 2013;118(5):1150–9. https://doi.org/10.1097/ALN.0b013e31828a7016.

24. Lai-Fook SJ, Rodarte JR. Pleural pressure distribution and its relationship to lung volume and interstitial pressure. J Appl Physiol (1985). 1991;70(3):967–78. https://doi.org/10.1152/jappl.1991.70.3.967.

25. Lee JM, Bae W, Lee YJ, Cho YJ. The efficacy and safety of prone positional ventilation in acute respiratory distress syndrome: updated study-level meta-analysis of 11 randomized controlled trials. Crit Care Med. 2014;42(5):1252–62. https://doi.org/10.1097/CCM.0000000000000122.

26. Matejovic M, Rokyta R, Radermacher P, Krouzecky A, Sramek V, Novak I. Effect of prone position on hepatosplanchnic hemodynamics in acute lung injury. Intensive Care Med. 2002;28(12):1750–5. https://doi.org/10.1007/s00134-002-1524-y.

27. Papazian L, Forel JM, Gacouin A, Penot-Ragon C, Perrin G, Loundou A, Jaber S, Arnal JM, Perez D, Seghboyan JM, Constantin JM, Courant P, Lefrant JY, Guérin C, Prat G, Morange S, Roch A, ACURASYS Study Investigators. Neuromuscular blockers in early acute respiratory distress syndrome. N Engl J Med. 2010;363(12):1107–16. https://doi.org/10.1056/NEJMoa1005372.

28. Poe RH, Wahl GW, Qazi R, Kallay MC, Utell MJ, Morrow GR. Predictors of mortality in the immunocompromised patient with pulmonary infiltrates. Arch Intern Med. 1986;146(7):1304–8.

29. Puybasset L, Cluzel P, Chao N, Slutsky AS, Coriat P, Rouby JJ. A computed tomography scan assessment of regional lung volume in acute lung injury. The CT Scan ARDS Study Group. Am J Respir Crit Care Med. 1998;158(5 Pt 1):1644–55. https://doi.org/10.1164/ajrccm.158.5.9802003.

30. Roth C, Ferbert A, Deinsberger W, Kleffmann J, Kästner S, Godau J, Schüler M, Tryba M, Gehling M. Does prone positioning increase intracranial pressure? A retrospective analysis of patients with acute brain injury and acute respiratory failure. Neurocrit Care. 2014;21(2):186–91. https://doi.org/10.1007/s12028-014-0004-x.

31. Rubenfeld GD, Herridge MS. Epidemiology and outcomes of acute lung injury. Chest. 2007;131(2):554–62. https://doi.org/10.1378/chest.06-1976.

32. Seong GM, Lee Y, Hong SB, Lim CM, Koh Y, Huh JW. Prognosis of acute respiratory distress syndrome in patients with hematological malignancies. J Intensive Care Med. 2018. https://doi.org/10.1177/0885066617753566.

33. Scholten EL, Beitler JR, Prisk GK, Malhotra A. Treatment of ARDS with prone positioning. Chest. 2017;151(1):215–24. https://doi.org/10.1016/j.chest.2016.06.032.

34. Soubani AO, Shehada E, Chen W, Smith D. The outcome of cancer patients with acute respiratory distress syndrome. J Crit Care. 2014;29(1):183.e187–12. https://doi.org/10.1016/j.jcrc.2013.10.011.

35. Taccone P, Pesenti A, Latini R, Polli F, Vagginelli F, Mietto C, Caspani L, Raimondi F, Bordone G, Iapichino G, Mancebo J, Guerin C, Ayzac L, Blanch L, Fumagalli R, Tognoni G, Gattinoni L, Prone-Supine II Study Group. Prone positioning in patients with moderate and severe acute respiratory distress syndrome: a randomized controlled trial. JAMA. 2009;302(18):1977–84. https://doi.org/10.1001/jama.2009.1614.

36. Van de Louw A, Desai RJ, Zhu J, Claxton DF. Characteristics of early acute respiratory distress syndrome in newly diagnosed acute myeloid leukemia. Leuk Lymphoma. 2018;1–8. https://doi.org/10.1080/10428194.2018.1435874

37. Wiedemann HP, Wheeler AP, Bernard GR, Thompson BT, Hayden D, deBoisblanc B, Connors AF, Hite RD, Harabin AL, National Heart Lung, and Blood Institute Acute Respiratory Distress Syndrome (ARDS) Clinical Trials Network. Comparison of two fluid-management strategies in acute lung injury. N Engl J Med. 2006;354(24):2564–75. https://doi.org/10.1056/NEJMoa062200.

Extracorporeal Membrane Oxygenation (ECMO) Critically Ill Cancer Patients

35

Thomas Staudinger, Peter Schellongowski, and Philipp Wohlfarth

Contents

Introduction 518

Principles of ECMO 519
Extracorporeal Gas Exchange 519
Circulatory Support 519

General Indications and Clinical Data 520

ECMO in Cancer Patients 521
Cancer Patients 521
Hematopoietic Stem Cell Transplantation 521
Indications for ECMO in Cancer Patients 522
Contraindications for ECMO in Cancer Patients 523

Special Considerations for the Management of Cancer Patients on ECMO 523
Bleeding and Anticoagulation 523
Ventilatory Management and Infection Control 524
Chemotherapy on ECMO 526
Ethical Considerations 526

Summary 526

References 526

Abstract

As prognosis of critically ill cancer patients has markedly improved during the last decades, a general reluctance to admit critically ill cancer patients to the ICU cannot be justified anymore.

T. Staudinger (✉) · P. Schellongowski · P. Wohlfarth
Department of Medicine I, Intensive Care Unit, Medical University of Vienna, Vienna General Hospital, Vienna, Austria
e-mail: thomas.staudinger@meduniwien.ac.at; peter.schellongowski@meduniwien.ac.at; philipp.wohlfarth@meduniwien.ac.at

This development leads to an increasing number of patients classified as prone to "full code management" which refers to the use of the whole armamentarium of intensive care medicine, comprising also respiratory or circulatory support by ECMO, if applicable. The term "ECMO" refers to either respiratory or circulatory support. As respiratory failure is the leading cause for ICU admission in cancer patients and is associated with high mortality, respiratory ECMO has been mainly used in selected patients suffering from severe pneumonia, ARDS, diffuse alveolar

© Springer Nature Switzerland AG 2020
J. L. Nates, K. J. Price (eds.), *Oncologic Critical Care*,
https://doi.org/10.1007/978-3-319-74588-6_60

hemorrhage, or involvement of the respiratory system by the underlying disease. General ECMO indication criteria also apply to cancer patients, provided that the status of the underlying malignancy allows for "full code" intensive care management. Outcome of critically ill cancer patients in need for ECMO is however worse compared to patients not suffering from malignancy. There are no defined criteria for predicting prognosis; it seems to be prudent, however, to prefer ECMO in patients in need for a therapeutic bridge to overcome a reversible acute and life-threatening complication. Patients undergoing hematopoietic stem cell transplantation are no good candidates for ECMO therapy during the peri-transplant period due to very poor outcome. Management of cancer patients during ECMO can be challenging due to immunosuppression leading to an increased risk for infectious complications as well as due to an increased risk for bleeding complications due to thrombocytopenia or derangements of plasmatic coagulation. An individually tailored anticoagulation concept should therefore be applied. If prerequisites for successful management cease to apply, withdrawal of care will be appropriate. In this situation, a clear communication strategy and adequate palliative care measures should be applied in a standardized way.

Keywords

ECMO · ARDS · Mechanical circulatory support · Cancer · Indications · Contraindications · Extracorporeal membrane oxygenation · Chemotherapy

Introduction

As survival for patients suffering from malignancy has markedly improved over the last decades due to advances in anticancer therapy as well as supportive measures, a rapidly increasing body of evidence has changed our attitude toward the admission these patients to an intensive care unit. A considerable proportion of adult ICU survivors regains a favorable quality of life and returns into a state in which the continuation of anticancer therapy is feasible. Their long-term survival is determined by the underlying disease and is not different from cancer patients who were never admitted to the ICU [1]. Thus, a general reluctance to admit critically ill cancer patients to the ICU cannot be justified anymore [2]. This development leads to an increasing number of patients classified as prone to "full code management" without restrictions, if well-established criteria like in newly diagnosed malignancies with favorable life expectation, and remission of the malignant disease, apply or when therapeutic options aiming for cure or at long-term survival are available. "Full code management" refers to the use of the whole armamentarium of intensive care medicine on principle comprising also respiratory or circulatory support by ECMO systems, if applicable [3]. A number of problems and unanswered questions however arise concerning the use of ECMO in patients suffering from hematological diseases and solid cancer: Most of the patients have to be regarded as immunosuppressed, many of them suffer from thrombocytopenia or derangements of plasmatic coagulation, and many are under treatment by chemotherapeutic or immunomodulatory therapies, all of which might interfere with extracorporeal circuits or per se represent relative contraindications to ECMO. Outcome of patients in need for ECMO has been shown to be associated with the number of patients treated per year ("volume dependency") as the management of technical issues and circuit-patient interactions is complex and warrants experience [4]. The same is true for the management of critically ill cancer patients [5, 6]. This leads to the conclusion that ideally centers treating critically ill cancer patients with ECMO should be highly specialized in both fields, which is rarely the case in most health-care systems. In the following, we shall shortly present the principles of extracorporeal gas exchange and circulatory support, as clinicians treating cancer patients are not always familiar with this kind of therapy, and then focus on indications and clinical data available for cancer patients on ECMO, followed by considerations on specific issues during the management of cancer patients undergoing ECMO therapy.

Principles of ECMO

The term "ECMO" (extracorporeal membrane oxygenation) implicates a focus on oxygenation. ECMO, however, dependent on the circuit's configuration, may enhance gas exchange, i.e., oxygenation and decarboxylation, as well as support circulation. The therapeutic intention to primarily enhance decarboxylation is referred to as $ECCO_2$-R (extracorporeal CO_2 removal), while more or less full respiratory support including decarboxylation and oxygenation is called "respiratory" ECMO (mostly as veno-venous configuration, VV-ECMO). Additional circulatory support by bypassing the pump function of the heart is usually called "circulatory" ECMO or "extracorporeal life support" (ECLS) and mandates a veno-arterial setting (VA-ECMO). In order to clarify terminology, efforts have been made to link the different settings to therapeutic intentions as part of extracorporeal organ support (ECOS), in a way that $ECCO_2$-R and respiratory ECMO are tools for partial or full lung replacement, while cardiac ECMO refers to circulatory support due to a failing heart [7].

The main determinants to achieve a therapeutic goal are the way of cannulation and the setup of the circuit, mainly consisting of a pump and a gas exchange membrane ("oxygenator").

Extracorporeal Gas Exchange

A modern gas exchange membrane consists of polymethylpentene hollow fibers allowing diffusion between the gas inside the hollow fibers and the surrounding blood. The flow of gas through the fibers (oxygen or an oxygen/air blend) is referred to as "sweep gas flow." As concentration of oxygen in the sweep gas usually exceeds blood-oxygen concentration, oxygen will shift to the blood and will be transported back into the patient's circulation. Due to the CO_2 gradient in the opposite direction, CO_2 will be eliminated from the blood and is washed out by the sweep gas. The amount of oxygen transported to the patient is therefore mainly dependent on the amount of blood pumped through the membrane. The amount of CO_2 elimination is dependent on both, blood flow and sweep gas flow. Much lower blood flows are needed for CO_2 elimination compared to oxygenation. In VV settings, a clinically relevant CO_2 elimination will commence at blood flows as low as 300–400 mL/min, while a maximum will be achieved at blood flows of 1500–2000 mL/min. From that point on, CO_2 elimination is more or less exclusively dependent of sweep gas flow [8]. The amount of oxygen delivered to the arterial circulation is dependent of the gas exchange capacity of the membrane and – mainly – on the proportion of the maximally oxygenated blood from the extracorporeal circuit on venous admixture, i.e., cardiac output. It has been shown that adequate oxygenation in ARDS patients on VV-ECMO by concomitantly setting mechanical ventilation to a protective level could be achieved if extracorporeal blood flow exceeded 60% of patients´ innate cardiac output [9].

Circulatory Support

In VA-ECMO settings, gas exchange at the membrane follows the same principles, but blood from the extracorporeal circuit directly enters the arterial circulation. ECMO blood flow therefore determines mean arterial pressure. An oxygen blender for sweep gas flow is used to regulate oxygenation toward the desired level and to avoid hyperoxia. Dependent on return cannula site, ECMO flow may not be uniformly distributed within the arterial system possibly leading to regional hypoxia. This is mostly true in femoro-femoral cannulation settings when left ventricular function is partly preserved leading to a phenomenon called ECMO watershed or differential hypoxia: Blood from the ECMO circuit will meet the blood pumped by the left ventricle leading to a neutralization of these opposite blood flows on a certain levels within the aorta, possibly leading to hypoxia of the aortic arch and its branches in case of concomitant lung failure [10].

General Indications and Clinical Data

Traditionally, ECMO has been reserved for patients suffering of acute cardiac or respiratory failure refractory to conservative therapy in case of a potentially reversible disease expected to have a good quality of life should recovery occur. There are no generally accepted criteria for initiation of ECMO therapy. Table 1 lists possible indications for respiratory and cardiac ECMO. Table 2 lists the current recommendations of the Extracorporeal Life Support Organization (ELSO) for initiation of respiratory and cardiac ECMO, respectively. For ARDS patients, a prospective randomized trial has evaluated modern ECMO therapy with respect to outcome [13]. The results of this trial suggest a benefit of ECMO therapy compared to conventional management; however, the design of this study has provoked severe criticism as it more or less proved favorable

outcome for patients treated in a specialized center only, irrespective of ECMO itself. A second, large randomized multicenter study in severe ARDS comparing ECMO versus conservative treatment has been published recently (EOLIA trial). Although there was a trend toward higher 60-day survival rate, the difference did not reach statistical significance. There was, however, a 28% rate of crossover to ECMO in the control group due to treatment failure (refractory hypoxia in most cases), resulting in a significant benefit in favor of ECMO for a combined endpoint of death and treatment failure [14]. Of note, cancer patients with a life expectancy of less than 5 years had been excluded from study entry.

Cardiac ECMO plays an increasing role in refractory cardiogenic shock as bridge to revascularization or recovery or as a bridge to a ventricular assist device or transplantation [15, 16]. In selected patients with prolonged or refractory cardiac arrest,

Table 1 Possible indications for respiratory and cardiac ECMO

Respiratory ECMO (VV)	Cardiac ECMO (VA)
Severe ARDS	Refractory cardiogenic shock due to, e.g.:
Hypercapnia with pronounced respiratory acidosis	Acute coronary syndrome
Refractory status asthmaticus	Acute myocarditis
	Acute cardiomyopathy
Diffuse alveolar hemorrhage	Massive pulmonary embolism
Potentially reversible pulmonary infiltration by neoplastic disease (e.g., leukemia)	Cardiac arrest ("ECPR")
Mediastinal bulky disease leading to airway compression	Mediastinal bulky disease leading to compression of the heart or large vessels

VV, Veno-venous; VA, veno-arterial; ECPR, extracorporeal cardiopulmonary resuscitation

Table 2 Recommendations of the Extracorporeal Life Support Organization (ELSO) for initiation of respiratory and cardiac ECMO [11, 12]

Respiratory ECMO (VV)	Cardiac ECMO (VA)
Acute hypoxic respiratory failure with 80% mortality risk (associated with a PaO_2/FiO_2 <100 on FiO_2 >90% and/or Murray score 3–4, AOI >80, APSS 8 despite optimal care for 6 h or less)	Cardiogenic shock with Inadequate tissue perfusion manifested as hypotension and low cardiac output despite adequate intravascular volume
CO_2 retention on mechanical ventilation despite high P_{plat} (>30 cm H_2O)	Shock persistence despite volume administration, inotropes and vasoconstrictors, and intra-aortic balloon counterpulsation if appropriate
Severe air leak syndromes	
Need for intubation in a patient on lung transplant list	
Immediate cardiac or respiratory collapse (PE, blocked airway, unresponsive to optimal care)	

AOI, age-adjusted oxygenation index; APSS, Age, PaO_2/FiO_2, and Plateau Pressure Score; P_{plat}, plateau pressure; PE, pulmonary embolism

ECMO is used with increasing enthusiasm as CPR device ("ECPR"). Hospital mortality, however, depends on patient selection criteria and ranges between 70% and 80% [17, 18].

ECMO in Cancer Patients

Cancer Patients

The body of literature on the use of ECMO in patients suffering from malignant neoplastic diseases is sparse. Gow and co-workers analyzed the ELSO registry from 1992 to 2008 for adults suffering from cancer undergoing ECMO therapy [19]. Seventy-two patients were identified (47 (65%) with solid tumors, 21 (30%) with hematologic malignancies, and 4 (6%) after HSCT). The low proportion of patients within the vast registry underlines the obvious reluctance to establish ECMO therapy in critically ill cancer patients. About 50% of patients underwent VV-ECMO and VA-ECMO, respectively. Indication for ECMO was not described in detail. Interestingly, survival to discharge was significantly better in cardiac support patients (70%) compared to respiratory support (26%). Overall survival was 32%. Of note, infections were more common in cancer patients, whereas bleeding events were not.

A Korean group reported on 15 patients suffering from hematological malignancy undergoing predominantly VV-ECMO for acute respiratory failure [20]. Seven patients of this retrospectively analyzed cohort were treated after allogeneic stem cell transplantation. Unfortunately, all of these patients died. Bleeding complications, however, were not the main reason for death (major bleeding in five patients, three patients died due to pulmonary hemorrhage). Of note, survival rate in an immunocompetent non-cancer control group was still as low as 24%.

In our institution, ECMO has been an established therapy for severe acute respiratory failure for years. As our ICU is affiliated to oncology and hematology departments, ECMO has been also an option for cancer patients.

We retrospectively analyzed 14 adult patients with hematological malignancy undergoing ECMO therapy between 2000 and 2013 [21]. Of note, 541 patients suffering from malignancy were treated during this time period. Thus, the proportion of ECMO patients represents 2.5% of these and, hence, must be regarded as a highly selected cohort. VV-ECMO was used for pulmonary ARDS due to pneumonia in most patients. Three patients required VA-ECMO due to septic cardiomyopathy or life-threatening circulatory and respiratory failure due to massive mediastinal bulky disease. Of note, five patients received rescue chemotherapy during ECMO. Overall survival was as high as 50%; all survivors reached hematological remission and were alive at a follow-up at 36 months.

The so far largest cohort of cancer patients undergoing ECMO was published as part of the IDEA study, a retrospective multicenter analysis on immunocompromised patients in need for respiratory ECMO [22]. Out of 225 immunocompromised patients treated at 10 ICUs between 2008 and 2014, 62 (30%) suffered from hematological malignancies and 39 (19%) from solid tumors. Malignancies were associated with significantly worse outcome compared to other causes of immunosuppression like steroid therapy, AIDS, solid organ transplantation, or autoimmune diseases. Higher age, longer duration of mechanical ventilation, hypercapnia, and higher driving pressure prior to ECMO were identified as independent predictors of adverse prognosis, while newly diagnosed immunocompromised status, higher platelet count, and solid organ transplantation were associated with better prognosis. Six-month mortality of patients with hematological malignancies and solid tumors was 76% and 80%, respectively.

Hematopoietic Stem Cell Transplantation

In the last decade, survival of patients receiving allogeneic or autologous hematopoietic stem cell transplantation (HSCT) has constantly improved [23–25]. Respiratory failure and septic shock represent the most common causes of admission to ICU with a mortality rate >70% when there has been no response to maximal conventional therapy [26]. Development of ARDS due to different causes occurs in up to 15% and is therefore not a rare complication of allogeneic stem cell transplantation and is associated with high mortality [27].

Considering these poor results, debate is ongoing about the proper use of ECMO in these patients in case of refractory severe respiratory and/or circulatory failure. Actually, in children, allogeneic HSCT is considered an absolute contraindication for ECMO because of its poor survival [28]. Autologous HSCT instead seems to have a prognosis like all other hematological patients. In adults, pooled data from European centers show a very poor outcome in patients after allogeneic HSCT going for ECMO [29]. Survival ranged between 10% and 20% and survivors were usually admitted long after their stay (>240 days) for HSCT. No patient admitted during the peri-transplant period up to 100 days after HSCT survived; only one patient survived admitted during the first 240 days after HSCT. In the light of these data, ECMO therapy after allogeneic HSCT should be restricted to very carefully selected patients, if at all, at least during the first year after transplantation.

Indications for ECMO in Cancer Patients

Most cases of ARDS in cancer patients successfully treated by ECMO are due to respiratory infections. If patients fulfill criteria for "full code" management, ECMO is an option in case of severe, refractory hypoxia or pronounced respiratory acidosis with concomitant unacceptably invasive ventilation settings. It is difficult to refer to absolute numbers with respect to hypoxia or hypercapnia; there are, however, recommendations for considering ECMO: The Extracorporeal Life Support Organization has lowered its threshold to a PaO_2/FiO_2 ratio below 100 plus a lung injury score of 3.0–4.0 [11], which comprises PEEP level, radiological findings, and compliance additionally to hypoxia [30]. A recently finished large randomized trial on

ECMO use in ARDS used more stringent criteria for inclusion (PaO_2/FiO_2 ratio <50 for >3 h or PaO_2/FiO_2 ratio <80 for >6 h) [14]. With respect to hypercapnia, ELSO does not define $PaCO_2$ or pH thresholds for ECMO indication, yet just mentions "CO_2 retention" despite a plateau pressure >30 cm H_2O [11], while the EOLIA trial specified an arterial blood pH of <7.25 with a $PaCO_2$ of ≥ 60 mmHg for >6 h with the respiratory rate increased to 35 breaths per minute and mechanical ventilation settings adjusted to keep a plateau pressure of ≤ 32 cm of water [14]. These indication criteria might also be used in cancer patients together with considerations on the risk-benefit ratio as well as assessment of antineoplastic treatment options and long-term prognosis.

Specific malignancy associated complications may rarely lead to severe refractory respiratory or circulatory failure. VV-ECMO has been successfully used in cases malignant lymphomas leading to mediastinal bulky disease to buy time for salvage chemotherapy [31, 32]. If bulky disease leads to additional circulatory failure due to compression of heart and/or large vessels, implementation of VA-ECMO may be necessary [21]. VA-ECMO has also been successfully used for refractory cardiogenic shock associated with malignant diseases as chemotherapy-associated heart failure [33] or in pheochromocytoma-induced cardiomyopathy as a bridge to surgery [34]. As malignant diseases predispose to thrombosis and pulmonary embolism (PE), VA-ECMO might be an option in massive PE leading to refractory cardiogenic shock or a cardiac peri-arrest situation. Use of ECMO for massive thrombotic PE [35] or tumor-associated pulmonary arterial obstruction [36] has however been described only as single cases. VA-ECMO may serve as short-term support in case of refractory acute septic cardiomyopathy [37], while during distributive shock with hyperdynamic circulatory pattern, VA-ECMO did not turn out to serve as successful therapeutic strategy [38, 39]

Hematological malignancies and antineoplastic chemotherapy may lead to severe thrombocytopenia as a risk factor for diffuse alveolar hemorrhage (DAH). Successful rescue VV-ECMO has been described in DAH cases, most of them associated with autoimmune pulmonary vasculitis [40], but also with anticoagulation in a patients with lung cancer [41]. We performed VV-ECMO in two patients with pulmonary infiltration of acute myelogenous leukemia and severe respiratory failure to enable rescue chemotherapy, which turned out to lead to remission and survival in one patient, while the other died due to severe pulmonary and cerebral bleeding.

Conclusively, indications for ECMO in cancer patients resemble the more or less acknowledged indications in the general population plus rare specific syndromes associated with distinct cancer entities. As ECMO always serves as a bridge to recovery in these patients, reversibility, i.e., the possibility of treating the underlying cause – which sometimes might be the malignant disease itself – has to be a precondition for initiating ECMO therapy. Time may play a pivotal role as it could be assumed that shorter time on ECMO will reduce the risk for complications. In our series of hematological patients on ECMO, a trend for shorter duration of ECMO could be observed in survivors [21].

Contraindications for ECMO in Cancer Patients

According to ELSO guidelines "there are no absolute contraindications to ECLS, as each patient is considered individually with respect to risks and benefits" [11]. The only absolute contraindication will therefore remain a patient's (or a legal representative's) declared unwillingness to undergo ECMO therapy. There are conditions, however, that are associated with a poor outcome despite ECLS and can be considered relative contraindications. Table 3 lists relative contraindications according to ELSO guidelines [11]. First of all, any invasive and aggressive therapeutic approach including ECMO has to be weighed against overall prognosis of the underlying disease, expected life span, and quality of life. In case of critically ill cancer patients, the term "full code management" refers to patients with favorable long-term prognosis and should be a precondition for initiating ECMO support. Immunosuppression is

Table 3 Relative contraindications to ECMO therapy in respiratory failure [11]

Mechanical ventilation at high settings (FiO$_2$ >0.90, P$_{plat}$ >30) for 7 days or more
Major pharmacologic immunosuppression or absolute neutrophil count < 400/mm^3
CNS hemorrhage that is recent or expanding
Nonrecoverable comorbidity such as major CNS damage or terminal malignancy
Age: no specific age contraindication but consider increasing risk with increasing age

CNS Central nervous system

commonly regarded as a relative contraindication, yet will usually be present in cancer patients and by itself must be regarded rather as an immanent factor of adverse prognosis within this specific group of patients than a contraindication. Thrombocytopenia and bleeding diathesis are a common problem in cancer patients, especially in patients suffering from hematological neoplasms. The need for anticoagulation in a patient at high risk for bleeding or ongoing bleeding leads to reluctance to initiate extracorporeal therapy in many ECMO centers. Individually targeted anticoagulation strategies, however, make successful operation of the extracorporeal circuit possible (see below).

Special Considerations for the Management of Cancer Patients on ECMO

Bleeding and Anticoagulation

Bleeding is one of the leading complications in the general ECMO population, occurs in 30–60% of patients, and is associated with increased mortality [42–45]. Bleeding occurred in 43% of a series of hematological patients on ECMO [21] and in 38% of patients undergoing ECMO after HSCT [29], thus seemingly not excessively more common than in the general ECMO population. Thrombocytopenia was commonly present in these patients, being more pronounced in the non-survivors. Low platelet count was independently associated with adverse prognosis in a large cohort of immunosuppressed patients on ECMO, while bleeding events were not different between survivors and non-survivors [22]. Management of anticoagulation is a challenge in patients at high risk for bleeding or active hemorrhage. Usually, unfractionated heparin to target an ACT of 180–220 s or an aPTT of 1.5–2.5 times baseline values is recommended for ECMO patients [46]. Newer data suggest that monitoring of anti-Xa levels may exert a better correlation with heparin dose than ACT and aPTT [47]. Moreover, reducing heparin dose to lower targets [48] or administering low molecular weight heparin in prophylactic doses only [49] were shown to reduce bleeding risk. Anticoagulation may be withheld in case of active bleeding, which has been successfully done in trauma patients [50] or during diffuse alveolar hemorrhage [41, 51]. Heparin-coated circuits (which is the standard in modern ECMO systems) allow for anticoagulation-free ECMO runs over several days, especially when high blood flow is maintained. The risk for circuit clotting with consecutive system exchange may be the better choice than major bleeding in patients at risk. Severe thrombocytopenia may even allow for anticoagulation-free management of ECMO over a longer period. We usually stop heparin when platelet count falls below 30 G/L in hematological patients or if patients exert active bleeding with a platelet count below 50 G/L. In seven patients with severe refractory thrombocytopenia treated at our center, anticoagulation-free ECMO was run for a median of 20 days (range 5–317 days) without occurrence of serious clotting events. We nevertheless aim at keeping platelet count above 50 G/L, as severe thrombocytopenia has been shown to be a risk factor for fatal intracranial bleeding on ECMO [52]. In a more recent analysis, independent risk factors for cerebral bleeding events were rather renal failure as well as a fast drop in $PaCO_2$ after initiating ECMO [53].

Bleeding, however, is not always associated with the underlying malignant disease or its therapy. In any case of a pronounced drop in platelet count, heparin-induced thrombocytopenia has to be ruled out. Hemorrhagic diathesis may be multifactorial, and thorough monitoring and in-depth diagnosis are warranted to identify risk factors. Table 4 suggests diagnostic workup and possible therapeutic approach in case of overt bleeding on ECMO.

Ventilatory Management and Infection Control

Setting of mechanical ventilation ARDS patients on ECMO has been subject to discussion for many years. More or less, a strict "put the lungs at rest" strategy rivals an "(ultra-)protective open lung" strategy using higher PEEP levels. Some recent, retrospective data rather support the open lung approach, using adequate PEEP levels to keep the lung "open" while reducing FiO_2 and tidal volume as far as possible [54, 55]. A tidal volume <6 mL/kg of predicted body weight thus reducing plateau pressure and – more importantly – driving pressure is referred to as "ultraprotective" ventilation.

Cancer patients have to be regarded as immunosuppressed due to several reasons, like anticancer drugs or the underlying disease itself. Infection is therefore not only a common cause for severe respiratory failure, but also a complication during treatment. Mechanical ventilation increases the risk for respiratory infections, as well as intravascular catheters and cannulas increase the risk for blood-stream infections. An analysis of adult cancer patients within the ELSO registry reported on a higher infection rate compared to a general ECMO population without cancer, whereas the rate of bleeding events was not increased [19]. Infection control should consist of broad-spectrum antibiotics and close microbiological surveillance. Due to an inadequate immune response, many cancer patients are prone for opportunistic infections, making extensive diagnostic measures inevitable. Reviewing the available data, there is, however, no signal toward beneficial effects of using ECMO as a tool to avoid mechanical ventilation. In a case series of six patients with ARDS, four of them being immunosuppressed, two due to leukemia, intubation and mechanical ventilation was avoided by initiating ECMO in first place [56]. Three patients had to be intubated, yet out of four survivors, three

Table 4 Assessment of coagulation disturbances associated with bleeding on ECMO and possible therapeutic approaches

Assessment of…	Routine tests	Additional tests	Management
Level of anticoagulation	ACT ↑ and/or APTT ↑ and/or Anti-Xa ↑	TEG/ROTEM® (for prolonged APTT exclude factor XII deficiency and lupus anticoagulant)	Stop heparin Restart after cessation of bleeding Adjust dose
Lack of coagulation factors II, V, VII, and X (liver failure, vitamin K antagonists)	Prothrombin time (INR) ↑	Factor activity	Prothrombin complex concentrates, plasma, and vitamin K
Thrombocytopenia	Platelets <50 G/L	Exclude DIC and HIT	Platelet transfusion
Disseminated intravascular coagulation (DIC)	Fibrinogen, D-Dimer ↑, Platelets ↓	Prothrombin fragment F_{1+2} ↑	Find and treat cause! Substitute platelets and fibrinogen if overt bleeding Search for clotting events Consider system change
Platelet dysfunction	No change	Multiplate, TEG/ROTEM®	Platelet transfusion Desmopressin
Hyperfibrinolysis	Fibrinogen ↓, D-Dimer ↑	TEG/ROTEM®	Substitute fibrinogen Consider antifibrinolytics Consider system change
Acquired von Willebrand syndrome	No change	vWF:RCo/vWF:Ag ratio <0,6	Desmopressin, plasma, and vWF concentrate Reduce shear stress (pump speed) if possible

ACT, activated clotting time; aPTT, activated partial thromboplastin time; TEG, thromboelastography; INR, international normalized ratio; DIC, disseminated intravascular coagulation; HIT, heparin-induced thrombocytopenia; vWF, von Willebrand factor; RCo, ristocetin co-factor; vWF:Ag, von Willebrand factor antigen

were managed without mechanical ventilation. In a series of 37 patients undergoing ECMO after HSCT, 24% remained without spontaneous ventilation, which did not turn out to be associated with survival [29]. Given the risk of ECMO and regarding the sparse evidence concerning avoidance of mechanical ventilation in cancer patients, this strategy has to be regarded as highly experimental and cannot be recommended to date.

Patients suffering from severe respiratory failure however bear a high risk for development of ICU-acquired weakness [57]. Patients undergoing ECMO therapy suffer from even more pronounced impairment of their physical and mental outcome [58]. Enabling spontaneous breathing, even as assisted breathing during ventilation,

(early) physiotherapy and mobilization has been proposed and investigated to overcome these long-term sequelae [59] and has been shown to be feasible and effective even in ventilated patients [60]. The concept can also be implemented in patients on ECMO [61] leading to a success rate of more than 30% with respect to active physiotherapy [62]. An impact on outcome has not been shown so far unless for patients during bridging to lung transplantation by avoiding immobilization and mechanical ventilation [63]. It can be assumed, however, that patients suffering from a high risk for infectious complications and from a per se consuming underlying disease might benefit from early spontaneous breathing and mobilization.

Chemotherapy on ECMO

Critical illness per se is no absolute contraindication to salvage chemotherapy, especially if the life-threatening problem is due to cancer progression. It has been shown that these patients benefit from early ICU admission [64, 65]. Need for ECMO should not be the reason for withholding lifesaving chemotherapy. It has been shown that chemotherapy obviously works [21], although the changes in pharmacokinetics on ECMO makes the relationship between dose and side effects hard to predict [66].

Ethical Considerations

In case patients do not fulfill criteria for "full code" management, the initiation of ECMO should be considered only for highly selected patients. However, each patient's case should be considered carefully before either offering or restricting ECLS from their therapeutic options. The known 5-year survival of a patient's underlying disease together with concomitant diseases and performance status should be taken into consideration when evaluating candidacy. Patients with malignancies and an expected 5-year survival of less than 50% irrespective of their acute critical illness should be considered less favorable candidates ECMO. This has been shown, for instance, for lung cancer patients, whose 6-month survival after admission to an ICU for respiratory failure leading to mechanical ventilation was as low as 15% [67].

If ECLS is offered as a support measure, a clear understanding of therapy goals as well as criteria for withdrawal of ECLS support is critical for both the caregivers and the family. If prerequisites for successful management cease to apply, withdrawal of care will be appropriate. In this situation, a clear communication strategy and adequate palliative care measures should be applied in a standardized way. Close collaboration between the critical care team, oncologists, as well as the family is then warranted.

Summary

The prognosis of critically ill cancer patients admitted to an ICU has substantially improved over the last decades. In patients admitted for "full code" treatment, ECMO may be a therapeutic option. As outcome has been shown to be significantly worse compared to non-cancer populations, careful selection of patients is mandatory. ECMO may be a valuable tool in patients in need for a short-term therapeutic bridge to overcome a reversible acute and life-threatening complication. Rescue chemotherapy during ECMO therapy has been done successfully, yet has to be regarded as highly experimental. Patients undergoing hematopoietic stem cell transplantation are no good candidates for ECMO therapy during the peri-transplant period due to very poor outcome. Management of cancer patients during ECMO can be challenging due to immunosuppression leading to an increased risk for infectious complications as well as due to an increased risk for bleeding complications due to thrombocytopenia or derangements of plasmatic coagulation. An individually tailored anticoagulation concept should therefore be applied. If prerequisites for successful management cease to apply, withdrawal of care will be appropriate. In this situation, a clear communication strategy and adequate palliative care measures should be applied in a standardized way.

References

1. Azoulay E, et al. Outcomes of critically ill patients with hematologic malignancies: prospective multicenter data from France and Belgium–a groupe de recherche respiratoire en reanimation onco-hematologique study. J Clin Oncol. 2013;31:2810–8. https://doi.org/10.1200/JCO.2012.47.2365.
2. Azoulay E, Afessa B. The intensive care support of patients with malignancy: do everything that can be done. Intensive Care Med. 2006;32:3–5. https://doi.org/10.1007/s00134-005-2835-6.
3. Lecuyer L, Chevret S, Thiery G, Darmon M, Schlemmer B, Azoulay E. The ICU trial: a new admission policy for cancer patients requiring mechanical ventilation. Crit Care Med. 2007;35:808–14. https://doi.org/10.1097/01.CCM.0000256846.27192.7A.
4. Barbaro RP, Odetola FO, Kidwell KM, Paden ML, Bartlett RH, Davis MM, Annich GM. Association of

hospital-level volume of extracorporeal membrane oxygenation cases and mortality. Analysis of the extracorporeal life support organization registry. Am J Respir Crit Care Med. 2015;191:894–901. https://doi.org/10.1164/rccm.201409-1634OC.

5. Lecuyer L, Chevret S, Guidet B, Aegerter P, Martel P, Schlemmer B, Azoulay E. Case volume and mortality in haematological patients with acute respiratory failure. Eur Respir J. 2008;32:748–54. https://doi.org/10.1183/09031936.00142907.

6. Zuber B, et al. Impact of case volume on survival of septic shock in patients with malignancies. Crit Care Med. 2012;40:55–62. https://doi.org/10.1097/CCM.0b013e31822d74ba.

7. Ranieri VM, Brodie D, Vincent JL. Extracorporeal organ support: from technological tool to clinical strategy supporting severe organ failure. JAMA. 2017;318:1105–6. https://doi.org/10.1001/jama.2017.10108.

8. Hermann A, et al. A novel pump-driven veno-venous gas exchange system during extracorporeal CO2-removal. Intensive Care Med. 2015;41:1773–80. https://doi.org/10.1007/s00134-015-3957-0.

9. Schmidt M, et al. Blood oxygenation and decarboxylation determinants during venovenous ECMO for respiratory failure in adults. Intensive Care Med. 2013;39:838–46. https://doi.org/10.1007/s00134-012-2785-8.

10. Hoeper MM, et al. Extracorporeal membrane oxygenation watershed. Circulation. 2014;130:864–5. https://doi.org/10.1161/CIRCULATIONAHA.114.011677.

11. ELSO. Adult respiratory failure guideline. 2017. https://www.elso.org/Portals/0/ELSO%20Guidelines%20For%20Adult%20Respiratory%20Failure%201_4.pdf

12. ELSO. Guidelines for adult cardiac failure. 2017. https://www.elso.org/Portals/0/IGD/Archive/FileManager/e76ef78eabcusersshyerdocumentselsoguidelinesforadultcardiacfailure13.pdf

13. Peek GJ, et al. Efficacy and economic assessment of conventional ventilatory support versus extracorporeal membrane oxygenation for severe adult respiratory failure (CESAR): a multicentre randomised controlled trial. Lancet. 2009;374:1351–63. https://doi.org/10.1016/S0140-6736(09)61069-2.

14. Combes A, et al. Extracorporeal membrane oxygenation for severe acute respiratory distress syndrome. N Engl J Med. 2018;378:1965–75. https://doi.org/10.1056/NEJMoa1800385.

15. Muller G, et al. The ENCOURAGE mortality risk score and analysis of long-term outcomes after VA-ECMO for acute myocardial infarction with cardiogenic shock. Intensive Care Med. 2016;42:370–8. https://doi.org/10.1007/s00134-016-4223-9.

16. Schmidt M, et al. Predicting survival after ECMO for refractory cardiogenic shock: the survival after veno-arterial-ECMO (SAVE)-score. Eur Heart J. 2015;36:2246–56. https://doi.org/10.1093/eurheartj/ehv194.

17. Fagnoul D, Combes A, De Backer D. Extracorporeal cardiopulmonary resuscitation. Curr Opin Crit Care. 2014;20:259–65. https://doi.org/10.1097/MCC.0000000000000098.

18. Lamhaut L, et al. A pre-hospital extracorporeal cardio pulmonary resuscitation (ECPR) strategy for treatment of refractory out hospital cardiac arrest: an observational study and propensity analysis. Resuscitation. 2017;117:109–17. https://doi.org/10.1016/j.resuscitation.2017.04.014.

19. Gow KW, Lao OB, Leong T, Fortenberry JD. Extracorporeal life support for adults with malignancy and respiratory or cardiac failure: The Extracorporeal Life Support experience. Am J Surg. 2010;199:669–75. https://doi.org/10.1016/j.amjsurg.2010.01.018.

20. Kang HS, Rhee CK, Lee HY, Kim YK, Kwon SS, Kim SC, Lee JW. Clinical outcomes of extracorporeal membrane oxygenation support in patients with hematologic malignancies. Korean J Intern Med. 2015;30:478–88. https://doi.org/10.3904/kjim.2015.30.4.478.

21. Wohlfarth P, et al. Extracorporeal membrane oxygenation in adult patients with hematologic malignancies and severe acute respiratory failure. Crit Care. 2014;18:R20. https://doi.org/10.1186/cc13701.

22. Schmidt M, et al. Six-month outcome of immunocompromised severe ARDS patients rescued by ECMO. An International Multicenter Retrospective Study. Am J Respir Crit Care Med. 2018; https://doi.org/10.1164/rccm.201708-1761OC.

23. Huynh TN, Weigt SS, Belperio JA, Territo M, Keane MP. Outcome and prognostic indicators of patients with hematopoietic stem cell transplants admitted to the intensive care unit. J Transp Secur. 2009;2009:917294. https://doi.org/10.1155/2009/917294.

24. Lengline E, et al. Changes in intensive care for allogeneic hematopoietic stem cell transplant recipients. Bone Marrow Transplant. 2015;50:840–5. https://doi.org/10.1038/bmt.2015.55.

25. Mokart D, et al. Allogeneic hematopoietic stem cell transplantation after reduced intensity conditioning regimen: Outcomes of patients admitted to intensive care unit. J Crit Care. 2015;30:1107–13. https://doi.org/10.1016/j.jcrc.2015.06.020.

26. Afessa B, Azoulay E. Critical care of the hematopoietic stem cell transplant recipient. Crit Care Clin. 2010;26:133–50. https://doi.org/10.1016/j.ccc.2009.09.001.

27. Yadav H, et al. Epidemiology of acute respiratory distress syndrome following hematopoietic stem cell transplantation. Crit Care Med. 2016;44:1082–90. https://doi.org/10.1097/CCM.0000000000001617.

28. Di Nardo M, et al. Extracorporeal membrane oxygenation in pediatric recipients of hematopoietic stem cell transplantation: an updated analysis of the Extracorporeal Life Support Organization experience. Intensive Care Med. 2014;40:754–6. https://doi.org/10.1007/s00134-014-3240-9.

29. Wohlfarth P, et al. Characteristics and outcome of patients after allogeneic hematopoietic stem cell transplantation treated with extracorporeal membrane oxygenation for acute respiratory distress syndrome. Crit Care Med. 2017;45:e500–7. https://doi.org/10.1097/CCM.0000000000002293.

30. Murray JF, Matthay MA, Luce JM, Flick MR. An expanded definition of the adult respiratory distress

syndrome. Am Rev Respir Dis. 1988;138:720–3. https://doi.org/10.1164/ajrccm/138.3.720.

31. Aboud A, Marx G, Sayer H, Gummert JF. Successful treatment of an aggressive non-Hodgkin's lymphoma associated with acute respiratory insufficiency using extracorporeal membrane oxygenation. Interact Cardiovasc Thorac Surg. 2008;7:173–4. https://doi.org/10.1510/icvts.2007.159921.

32. Oto M, Inadomi K, Chosa T, Uneda S, Uekihara S, Yoshida M. Successful use of extracorporeal membrane oxygenation for respiratory failure caused by mediastinal precursor T lymphoblastic lymphoma. Case Rep Med. 2014;2014:804917. https://doi.org/10.1155/2014/804917.

33. Rateesh S, Shekar K, Naidoo R, Mittal D, Bhaskar B. Use of extracorporeal membrane oxygenation for mechanical circulatory support in a patient with 5-fluorouracil induced acute heart failure. Circ Heart Fail. 2015;8:381–3. https://doi.org/10.1161/CIRCHEARTFAILURE.115.002080.

34. Kaese S, Schulke C, Fischer D, Lebiedz P. Pheochromocytoma-induced takotsubo-like cardiomyopathy and global heart failure with need for extracorporal life support. Intensive Care Med. 2013;39:1473–4. https://doi.org/10.1007/s00134-013-2942-8.

35. Kurakazu M, Ueda T, Matsuo K, Ishikura H, Kumagai N, Yoshizato T, Miyamoto S. Percutaneous cardiopulmonary support for pulmonary thromboembolism caused by large uterine leiomyomata. Taiwan J Obstet Gynecol. 2012;51:639–42. https://doi.org/10.1016/j.tjog.2012.09.023.

36. Chung JH, et al. Treatment of pulmonary tumor embolism from choriocarcinoma: extracorporeal membrane oxygenation as a bridge through chemotherapy. Cancer Res Treat. 2017;49:279–82. https://doi.org/10.4143/crt.2016.125.

37. Brechot N, et al. Venoarterial extracorporeal membrane oxygenation support for refractory cardiovascular dysfunction during severe bacterial septic shock. Crit Care Med. 2013;41:1616–26. https://doi.org/10.1097/CCM.0b013e31828a2370.

38. Huang CT, Tsai YJ, Tsai PR, Ko WJ. Extracorporeal membrane oxygenation resuscitation in adult patients with refractory septic shock. J Thorac Cardiovasc Surg. 2013;146:1041–6. https://doi.org/10.1016/j.jtcvs.2012.08.022.

39. Park TK, et al. Extracorporeal membrane oxygenation for refractory septic shock in adults. Eur J Cardiothorac Surg. 2015;47:e68–74. https://doi.org/10.1093/ejcts/ezu462.

40. Abrams D, Agerstrand CL, Biscotti M, Burkart KM, Bacchetta M, Brodie D. Extracorporeal membrane oxygenation in the management of diffuse alveolar hemorrhage. ASAIO J. 2015;61:216–8. https://doi.org/10.1097/MAT.0000000000000183.

41. Lee JH, Kim SW. Successful management of warfarin-exacerbated diffuse alveolar hemorrhage using an extracorporeal membrane oxygenation. Multidiscip Respir Med. 2013;8:16. https://doi.org/10.1186/2049-6958-8-16.

42. Aubron C, et al. Predictive factors of bleeding events in adults undergoing extracorporeal membrane oxygenation. Ann Intensive Care. 2016;6:97. https://doi.org/10.1186/s13613-016-0196-7.

43. Thiagarajan RR, et al. Extracorporeal life support organization registry international report 2016. ASAIO J. 2017;63:60–7. https://doi.org/10.1097/MAT.0000000000000475.

44. Vaquer S, de Haro C, Peruga P, Oliva JC, Artigas A. Systematic review and meta-analysis of complications and mortality of veno-venous extracorporeal membrane oxygenation for refractory acute respiratory distress syndrome. Ann Intensive Care. 2017;7:51. https://doi.org/10.1186/s13613-017-0275-4.

45. Zangrillo A, et al. A meta-analysis of complications and mortality of extracorporeal membrane oxygenation. Crit Care Resusc. 2013;15:172–8.

46. ELSO. ELSO anticoagulation guideline. 2014. https://www.elso.org/Portals/0/Files/elsoanticoagulationguideline8-2014-table-contents.pdf

47. Liveris A, et al. Anti-factor Xa assay is a superior correlate of heparin dose than activated partial thromboplastin time or activated clotting time in pediatric extracorporeal membrane oxygenation*. Pediatr Crit Care Med. 2014;15:e72–9. https://doi.org/10.1097/PCC.0000000000000028.

48. Yeo HJ, Kim DH, Jeon D, Kim YS, Cho WH. Low-dose heparin during extracorporeal membrane oxygenation treatment in adults. Intensive Care Med. 2015;41:2020–1. https://doi.org/10.1007/s00134-015-4015-7.

49. Krueger K, Schmutz A, Zieger B, Kalbhenn J. Venovenous extracorporeal membrane oxygenation with prophylactic subcutaneous anticoagulation only: an observational study in more than 60 patients. Artif Organs. 2017;41:186–92. https://doi.org/10.1111/aor.12737.

50. Muellenbach RM, et al. Prolonged heparin-free extracorporeal membrane oxygenation in multiple injured acute respiratory distress syndrome patients with traumatic brain injury. J Trauma Acute Care Surg. 2012;72:1444–7. https://doi.org/10.1097/TA.0b013e3 1824d68e3.

51. Herbert DG, Buscher H, Nair P. Prolonged venovenous extracorporeal membrane oxygenation without anticoagulation: a case of Goodpasture syndrome-related pulmonary haemorrhage. Crit Care Resusc. 2014;16:69–72.

52. Kasirajan V, Smedira NG, McCarthy JF, Casselman F, Boparai N, McCarthy PM. Risk factors for intracranial hemorrhage in adults on extracorporeal membrane oxygenation. Eur J Cardiothorac Surg. 1999;15:508–14.

53. Luyt CE, et al. Brain injury during venovenous extracorporeal membrane oxygenation. Intensive Care Med. 2016;42:897–907. https://doi.org/10.1007/s00134-016-4318-3.

54. Schmidt M, et al. Mechanical ventilation management during extracorporeal membrane oxygenation for acute respiratory distress syndrome: a retrospective international multicenter study. Crit Care Med. 2015;43:654–64. https://doi.org/10.1097/CCM.0000000000000753.

55. Serpa Neto A, et al. Associations between ventilator settings during extracorporeal membrane oxygenation for refractory hypoxemia and outcome in patients with

acute respiratory distress syndrome: a pooled individual patient data analysis: mechanical ventilation during ECMO. Intensive Care Med. 2016;42: 1672–84. https://doi.org/10.1007/s00134-016-4507-0.

56. Hoeper MM, et al. Extracorporeal membrane oxygenation instead of invasive mechanical ventilation in patients with acute respiratory distress syndrome. Intensive Care Med. 2013;39:2056–7. https://doi.org/10.1007/s00134-013-3052-3.

57. Herridge MS, et al. Functional disability 5 years after acute respiratory distress syndrome. N Engl J Med. 2011;364:1293–304. https://doi.org/10.1056/NEJMoa1011802.

58. Schmidt M, et al. The PRESERVE mortality risk score and analysis of long-term outcomes after extracorporeal membrane oxygenation for severe acute respiratory distress syndrome. Intensive Care Med. 2013;39: 1704–13. https://doi.org/10.1007/s00134-013-3037-2.

59. Schweickert WD, et al. Early physical and occupational therapy in mechanically ventilated, critically ill patients: a randomised controlled trial. Lancet. 2009;373:1874–82. https://doi.org/10.1016/S0140-6736(09)60658-9.

60. Schaller SJ, et al. Early, goal-directed mobilisation in the surgical intensive care unit: a randomised controlled trial. Lancet. 2016;388:1377–88. https://doi.org/10.1016/S0140-6736(16)31637-3.

61. Wells CL, Forrester J, Vogel J, Rector R, Tabatabai A, Herr D. Safety and feasibility of early physical therapy for patients on extracorporeal membrane oxygenator:

University of Maryland medical center experience. Crit Care Med. 2018;46:53–9. https://doi.org/10.1097/CCM.0000000000002770.

62. Abrams D, et al. Early mobilization of patients receiving extracorporeal membrane oxygenation: a retrospective cohort study. Crit Care. 2014;18:R38. https://doi.org/10.1186/cc13746.

63. Fuehner T, et al. Extracorporeal membrane oxygenation in awake patients as bridge to lung transplantation. Am J Respir Crit Care Med. 2012;185:763–8. https://doi.org/10.1164/rccm.201109-1599OC.

64. Benoit DD, et al. Outcome in severely ill patients with hematological malignancies who received intravenous chemotherapy in the intensive care unit. Intensive Care Med. 2006;32:93–9. https://doi.org/10.1007/s00134-005-2836-5.

65. Wohlfarth P, et al. Prognostic factors, long-term survival, and outcome of cancer patients receiving chemotherapy in the intensive care unit. Ann Hematol. 2014;93:1629–36. https://doi.org/10.1007/s00277-014-2141-x.

66. Shekar K, Fraser JF, Smith MT, Roberts JA. Pharmacokinetic changes in patients receiving extracorporeal membrane oxygenation. J Crit Care. 2012;27:741 e749–18. https://doi.org/10.1016/j.jcrc.2012.02.013.

67. Slatore CG, et al. Intensive care unit outcomes among patients with lung cancer in the surveillance, epidemiology, and end results-medicare registry. J Clin Oncol. 2012; 30:1686–91. https://doi.org/10.1200/JCO.2011.40.0846.

Cancer Treatment-Related Lung Injury

36

Vickie R. Shannon

Contents

Introduction 532

Chemotherapy-Induced Lung Injury 532
General Principals 532

Lung Injury Associated with Cancer Immunotherapies 547
Immune Checkpoint Blocking Agents 547
Genetically Engineered Immunotherapies 547

Radiation-Induced Lung Injury 549
Clinical Presentation 549
Radiation Recall Pneumonitis 550
Other Manifestations of Radiation-Induced Lung Injury 550
Management of Radiation-Induced Lung Injury 551

References 552

Abstract

Lung injury associated with cancer therapeutics is often the limiting factor that trumps otherwise successful cancer therapy. Thoracic radiation as well as cancer pharmacotherapeutics, including conventional chemotherapy, molecular targeted agents, and cancer immunotherapies, have been associated with a unique spectrum of histopathologic injury patterns that may involve the lung parenchyma, pleura, airways, and/or pulmonary vasculature. Injury patterns may be idiosyncratic, unpredictable, and highly variable from one agent class to the next. Variability in lung injury patterns within a specific therapeutic class of drugs also occurs, adding to the conundrum. Drug-induced toxicities to the thoracic cavity are infrequent, and early recognition of clinical clues portends a good outcome in most cases. Failure to recognize early clinical signs, however, may result in irreversible and potentially lethal consequences.

This chapter provides an overview of our current knowledge of thoracic complications associated with cancer pharmacotherapies.

Author Contributions: VS: conception and design, acquisition of radiological data, drafting the chapter, critical revision of intellectual content, and final approval of the version to be published

V. R. Shannon (✉)
Department of Pulmonary Medicine, Division of Internal Medicine, The University of Texas at MD Anderson Cancer Center, Houston, TX, USA
e-mail: vshannon@mdanderson.org

The review is not intended to be a treatise of all cancer agents that adversely affect the lungs, but rather a discussion of established risk factors and histopathologic patterns of lung injury associated with broad classes of cancer agents. Optimal management strategies, based on existing clinical experience, will also be discussed. Complications associated with thoracic radiation are also reviewed. It is hoped that these discussions will facilitate early recognition and management of treatment-related thoracic complications and, ultimately, better patient outcomes.

Keywords

Drug-induced lung disease · Lung injury · Toxicity · Chemotherapy · Immunotherapy · Targeted therapy · Radiation · Pneumonitis · Malignancy · Pulmonary · Interstitial pneumonitis · Pleural effusions · Respiratory · Cancer treatment

Introduction

Recent advancements in the understanding of cancer biology have fueled a new era in anticancer therapeutics that extends beyond the class of conventional cytotoxic chemotherapy and radiation therapy regimens. Strategies that exploit the cancer genome in the development of molecular-targeted therapies and schemes that harness the immune system to tilt immune equilibrium in favor of enhanced tumor killing have rapidly emerged as standard of care for patients with a variety of malignancies and have joined the ranks of cytotoxic drugs in the medical management of some cancers. Each class of cancer therapeutics has been limited by a unique spectrum of toxicities that may target the lung parenchyma, pleura, and/or pulmonary circulation. Although drug-related adverse events within the thoracic cavity are infrequent relative to other organ systems, they are an important source of severe and life-threatening toxicity. Therefore, failure to recognize early clinical clues may have catastrophic consequences. Respiratory distress is a frequent reason for ICU transfer in cancer patients and is attributable to infectious

causes associated with cytotoxin-related immune suppression in most cases. In addition, cytotoxic therapies as well as the molecular-targeted and immune therapies are reported to cause a unique spectrum of noninfectious complications that affect the lung parenchyma, pleura, and vascular structures. For example, interstitial pneumonitis is an important sequela of cancer therapy and frequent reason for drug withdrawal [1–9]. Inhibitors of antiangiogenetic pathways are a source of severe vascular side effects within the lungs, including thromboembolic events and pulmonary hemorrhage. The cardiotoxic effects of these agents as well as the Bcr-Abl inhibitors may result in pulmonary edema associated with congestive heart failure [10, 11]. The emergence of pleural and pericardial effusions owing to Bcr-Abl inhibition has also been described [12–16].

Familiarity with established common adverse lung events and management of potentially life-threatening complications relating to conventional and new anticancer agents are essential for treating clinicians, including the ICU staff, oncologists, and organ specialists. This chapter provides an update and review of the clinical and pathophysiologic findings associated with specific notorious cancer pharmacotherapies and presents evidence-based algorithms, where available, in the management of thoracic complications associated with chemotherapeutic agents and radiation therapy.

Chemotherapy-Induced Lung Injury

General Principals

Incidence and Risk Factors

Pneumotoxicity may be predictable and dose dependent with some agents (busulfan, bleomycin, nitrosoureas). Other reactions are idiosyncratic and dose independent, occurring as a result of immune-mediated processes, bioactivation, or toxic drug metabolites. The frequent use of complex multi-drug and multimodality regimens and overlapping clinical and radiographic manifestations of lung injury caused by drug toxicity, infection, and cancer relapse render precise estimates difficult. Predisposing factors, including patient age, tobacco use history, cumulative dose, renal dysfunction, oxygen therapy, and preexisting lung disease, may influence the incidence, severity, and latency period of lung toxicity following drug exposure. The significance of these risk factors varies with individual agents within a particular drug class and across drug classes. For example, preexisting fibrosis is a significant independent risk factor in the development of severe and accelerated pulmonary toxicity following therapies with conventional cytotoxic therapies such as gemcitabine, oxaliplatin, amrubicin, bleomycin, methotrexate, and the molecular targeted therapies everolimus, temsirolimus, erlotinib, gefitinib [17–21]. Whether prior lung fibrosis potentiates toxicities associated with the class of drugs known as immune checkpoint inhibitors has not been established. Cancer agents within one therapeutic class may produce histopathologic patterns of lung injury with widely varying frequencies. For instance, pulmonary hypertension is a well-established adverse event following the Bcr-Abl inhibitor, dasatinib, but extremely rare among other agents within this class of drugs. Thus, estimates of the incidence of lung injury caused by individual chemotherapeutic agents vary broadly. Reported estimates are included in discussions of individual agents.

Diagnosis

Pneumotoxicity associated with chemotherapeutic agents represents a diagnostic conundrum. Toxicity is typically assessed through clinical, radiographic, and histopathologic studies, although no single abnormality is pathognomonic. Biomarkers and laboratory studies are not sufficiently sensitive to distinguish drug-related lung injury from competing diagnoses. Histopathologic features of chemotherapy-induced lung injury are not specific for DILD and can be seen in a wide variety of clinical contexts and competing diagnoses, including pneumonia, congestive heart failure, and cancer progression. High-resolution CT (HRCT) scans may detect early abnormalities; however, imaging findings are nonspecific. Interstitial and mixed alveolar-interstitial abnormalities are frequent findings on computed tomography (CT). These abnormalities appear as bilateral (may be asymmetrical) reticular markings, septal thickening, and ground-glass opacities that typically localize to the subpleural and lower lung zones. Radiographic manifestations of pulmonary fibrosis, including traction bronchiectasis and honeycombing, herald the onset of end-stage lung disease. Other findings, including nodular lesions, pleural effusions, and lymphadenopathy, may be confused with cancer progression.

Bronchoalveolar lavage (BAL) with or without lung biopsies may be helpful in excluding competing diagnoses of infection or background disease. BAL findings of increased numbers of lymphocytes, eosinophils, fibroblasts, and dysplastic type II pneumocytes may aid in the diagnosis of chemotherapy-induced lung injury; however, none of these findings are diagnostic. Decreased CD4/CD8 ratios on BAL fluid are also supportive findings; however, ratios vary widely and cannot distinguish sufficiently between drug-induced and other causes of ILD [22–24]. The diagnosis of DAH is supported by findings of progressively bloody BAL samples on sequential aliquots and/or cytologic evidence of increased numbers of hemosiderin-laden macrophages on BAL fluid. Serum elevations of the WBC count, erythrocyte sedimentation rate, and C-reactive protein are also common but nonspecific findings. Toxicity to the lung parenchyma is usually signaled by a reduction in the diffusing capacity (DLCO). With disease progression, a restrictive ventilatory defect is seen [25–28]. Alteration in DLCO is generally accepted as the most sensitive parameter in assessing drug-related injury, although its predictive potential for the detection of early change has been variable. Irreversible changes in lung function are seen with end-stage lung disease. In earlier stages, normalization of pulmonary function may occur, typically within 2 years of toxin exposure [25, 27, 29, 30].

The diagnosis of DILD is, therefore, based on the exclusion of competing causes in the context of a compatible clinical presentation and temporal relationship between the administration of the suspected drug and onset of symptoms. Measureable improvements in clinical signs and symptoms following drug withdrawal and/or recrudescence of disease with drug rechallenge are supportive of the diagnosis. Delayed toxicities, occurring months to years after drug withdrawal (gentamycin, bleomycin, busulfan) and disease progression despite discontinuation of the offending agent (immune checkpoint inhibitors), are diagnostically challenging features of some agents. Drug rechallenge is justified only in a minority of patients, and its use as a diagnostic tool is discouraged.

Clinical Presentation

Manifestations of pneumotoxicity are nonspecific and protean. Most commonly, symptoms of cough (typically nonproductive), dyspnea, hypoxia, and low-grade fever develop insidiously over weeks to months after drug exposure. Fulminant disease, which may rapidly progress to respiratory failure and acute respiratory distress syndrome (ARDS), is also seen. Symptom onset varies with individual drugs and may be classified into acute (within hours to days of drug exposure), early (within the first 6 months of drug exposure), and late (6 months or more after exposure) time periods. Delayed pulmonary fibrosis, occurring months to years after exposure to bleomycin, busulfan, cyclophosphamide, gemcitabine, and the nitrosoureas as a late manifestation of DILD, has also been described [31–33].

Histopathologic Features of DILD

The response of the lungs to drug-related adverse events results in stereotyped histopathologic patterns of lung injury. Drug-induced interstitial lung diseases (DILD) (nonspecific interstitial lung disease, NSIP; pulmonary fibrosis, PF; hypersensitivity reactions, HP; sarcoid reactions) and alveolar processes (diffuse alveolar damage, DAD; diffuse alveolar hemorrhage, DAH; eosinophilic pneumonias, EP; noncardiogenic pulmonary edema, NCPE; alveolar proteinosis) are the most frequent histopathologic patterns of response to standard chemotherapeutic agents as well as molecular-targeted therapies and immunomodulating agents. Pleural diseases (pleural effusions, fibrosis), drug-induced vascular disorders (thrombosis, pulmonary hypertension, pulmonary veno-occlusive disease, PVOD),

airway disorders (bronchospasm, infusion reactions), and mediastinal diseases (lymphadenopathy, fibrosis) have also been described, particularly following molecular-targeted and immunomodulating therapies. Finally, immune suppression following conventional and targeted therapies as well as immune activation triggered by immunomodulating agents may incite a variety of opportunistic pneumonias. The often life-threatening pneumonias that may emerge in the setting of immune suppression are discussed elsewhere.

Specific Clinical and Histopathologic Patterns of DILD

Interstitial Lung Disease. Interstitial pneumonitis is one of the major patterns of lung injury following systemic cancer therapies. This pattern of lung injury may arise from direct cytotoxicity, oxidative stress, and immune-mediated mechanisms. Pneumonitis may be stratified into six major categories according to clinicoradiographic and histopathologic findings: (1) nonspecific interstitial pneumonitis, (2) organizing pneumonia, (3) hypersensitivity pneumonitis, (4) diffuse alveolar damage/acute respiratory distress syndrome, (5) diffuse alveolar hemorrhage, and (6) eosinophilic pneumonia. Characteristic imaging features and the cancer agents that have been implicated in the development of category of lung injury are listed in Tables 1 and 2. The diagnosis of drug-induced ILD requires a high index of suspicion. Individual agents may elicit multiple patterns of lung injury. Lung injury patterns within a single class of drugs may vary widely. Furthermore, there are pathognomonic imaging findings or histopathologic markers that distinguish drug-induced ILD from other causes. Drug interruption with or without the addition of systemic corticosteroids is the mainstay of treatment of drug-related IP. Optimal dose, timing, and duration of steroids in this setting have not been well established; however, 0.5–1 mg/kg/day of prednisone or its equivalent is generally given for 8–12 weeks. Although most patients present with mild disease, any of the ILD injury patterns may progress to pulmonary fibrosis, particularly with acute and fulminant presentations of ILD, such as that seen in the setting of ARDS/DAD.

Table 1 Drug-induced lung injury: Conventional chemotherapy

Radiographic pattern	Clinical findings	Imaging findings	Responsible agents: conventional chemotherapy						
			Alkylating agents	Antimetabolites	Cytotoxic antibiotics	Topoisomerase inhibitors	Podophyllotoxins	Taxanes/microtubule inhibitors	Others
Interstitial lung disease									
NSIP	Subacute onset of dry cough, dyspnea, low-grade fevers, evolving over weeks	GGOs, reticular opacities with predominant peripheral lung and lower lung distribution with subpleural sparing; traction bronchiectasis; volume loss over the lower lobes with advanced disease	Busulfan BCNU CCNU Cyclophosphamide Ifosfamide Temozolomide Oxaliplatin Melphalan	Methotrexate Cytarabine Fludarabine Azacitidine Gemcitabine Azathioprine 6-Mercaptopurine	Bleomycin Mitomycin C	Topotecan Irinotecan Amrubicin Daunorubicin Liposomal Doxorubicin	Etoposide Teniposide	Paclitaxel Docetaxel	ATRA Arsenic trioxide Procarbazine
OP	Subacute onset of dry cough, dyspnea, low-grade fevers, weight loss, evolving over weeks	Bilateral migratory, patchy areas of lung consolidation or GGOs in a predominant peripheral and lower lobe distribution; opacities tend to wax and wane (hallmark) nodular opacities; reverse halo sign	Busulfan Cyclophosphamide Ifosfamide Oxaliplatin	Methotrexate Azathioprine 6-Mercaptopurine	Bleomycin	Topotecan			L-asparaginase

(continued)

Table 1 (continued)

Radiographic pattern	Clinical findings	Imaging findings	Responsible agents: conventional chemotherapy						
			Alkylating agents	Antimetabolites	Cytotoxic antibiotics	Topoisomerase inhibitors	Podophyllotoxins	Taxanes/microtubule inhibitors	Others
HP	Acute, subacute and chronic forms of disease; dry cough, dyspnea,	Mosaic attenuation caused by air trapping; diffuse ground-glass opacification without interstitial thickening; poorly defined centrilobular ground-glass nodules		Methotrexate				Paclitaxel Docetaxel	
Eosinophilic pneumonia	Acute onset of dyspnea and dry cough, low-grade fever evolving over 1–3 weeks after initiation of the offending agent	Patchy, diffuse, ground-glass or reticular opacities randomly distributed throughout the bilateral lungs	Busulfan Cyclophosphamide Oxaliplatin BCNU Oxaliplatin	Methotrexate Cytarabine Fludarabine Gemcitabine Pentostatin	Bleomycin			Paclitaxel Docetaxel	Interleukin-2
AIP/ARDS/DAD	Dry cough and dyspnea, hypoxia may develop more rapidly (days – weeks) versus other forms of ILD	Diffuse bilateral septal thickening, GGOs and consolidations in the dependent areas of the lungs; volume loss	Busulfan, Cyclophosphamide, Ifosfamide, Temozolomide, Oxaliplatin Melphalan	Methotrexate Azathioprine Cytarabine Fludarabine Azacitidine Gemcitabine Pentostatin Pemetrexed Zinostatin	Bleomycin Mitomycin C	Topotecan	Etoposide Teniposide	Paclitaxel Docetaxel Vincristine Vinblastine Vindesine Vinorelbine Ixabepilone	ATRA Arsenic trioxide

	Clinical features	Radiographic/imaging features					
Vascular disease							
Thromboembolism	Dyspnea often accompanied by pleuritic chest pain or tightness. May be acute, subacute, or chronic; hemodynamic instability with right heart strain, shock if massive	Acute: complete or partial intraluminal filling defects on CTA	Cisplatin	5-Fluorouacil			Thalidomide
		Chronic: complete occlusive disease in vessels that are smaller than adjacent patent vessels; recanalization, webs, flaps, partial filling defects form obtuse angles with the vessel wall	Oxaliplatin				Lenalidomide L-asparaginase GM-CSF GCSF
Pulmonary hypertension	Progressive dyspnea, fatigue, chest pain, palpitations, LE edema, cyanosis	Abrupt narrowing/tapering of peripheral pulmonary vessels	Cyclophosphamide	Gemcitabine	Bleomycin		Interferon-α
		Right atrial/ventricular enlargement Dilatation of central pulmonary artery Mosaic attenuation due to variable lung perfusion	Procarbazine BCNU		Mitomycin		Interferon-β
Pleural disease							
Pleural effusions	Progressive dyspnea, pleuritic chest pain	CXR: Blunting of costophrenic angle, fluid within horizontal or oblique fissures, mediastinal shift as fluid progresses	Cyclophosphamide	Methotrexate	Mitomycin	Docetaxel	ATRA
		Echo-free space on ultrasound evaluation		Gemcitabine		Paclitaxel	Arsenic trioxide Procarbazine

(continued)

Table 1 (continued)

Radiographic pattern	Clinical findings	Imaging findings	Responsible agents: conventional chemotherapy						
			Alkylating agents	Antimetabolites	Cytotoxic antibiotics	Topoisomerase inhibitors	Podophyllotoxins	Taxanes/microtubule inhibitors	Others
Pleural fibrosis	Progressive dyspnea	Pleural thickening with/without calcification Associated volume loss of affected hemithorax	BCNU Bleomycin Cyclophosphamide						
Airway disease									
Infusion reaction/bronchospasm	Acute wheezing/bronchospasm; may be accompanied by hemodynamic instability, chest pain	Imaging studies of the chest may be normal	Cyclophosphamide Ifosfamide Carboplatin Cisplatin Oxaliplatin	Methotrexate Gemcitabine Pemetrexed	Bleomycin Mitomycin C	Amrubicin Daunorubicin Liposomal Doxorubicin	Etoposide Teniposide	Paclitaxel Docetaxel Vincristine Vinblastine Vindesine Vinorelbine	L-asparaginase
Other									
Methemoglobinemia	Shortness of breath, hypoxia headache, fatigue, exercise intolerance, cyanosis seizures, coma with higher levels of methemoglobin	CXR may be normal; discordant oxygen saturation via pulse oximetry versus arterial blood gas; Chocolate-brown color of blood	Cyclophosphamide Ifosfamide						
Acute chest pain syndrome	Acute chest pain, typically occurs during infusion	Chest imaging may be normal			Bleomycin				

Table 2 Drug-induced lung injury: Targeted agents and immunotherapies

Radiographic pattern	Clinical findings	CT findings	Molecular-targeted therapies		Rapamycin inhibitors	Proteosome inhibitors	ICIs	Other
			MoAB	TKIs				
NSIP	Subacute onset of dry cough, dyspnea, low-grade fevers, evolving over weeks	GGOs, reticular opacities with predominant peripheral lung and lower lung distribution with subpleural sparing; traction bronchiectasis; volume loss over the lower lobes with advanced disease	Cetuximab Panitumumab Alemtuzumab Rituximab Brentuximab	Gefitinib Erlotinib Imatinib Osimertinib Afatinib Dasatinib Sorafenib Sunitinib Vandetanib Idelalisib Trametinib Crizotinib Ceritinib Alectinib Brigatinib Ibrutinib	Everolimus Temsirolimus	Bortezomib Carfilzomib	Ipilimumab Nivolumab Pembrolizumab Atezolizumab Durvalumab Avelumab	Thalidomide IL-2
OP	Subacute onset of dry cough, dyspnea, low-grade fevers, weight loss, evolving over weeks	Bilateral migratory, patchy areas of lung consolidation or GGOs in a predominant peripheral and lower lobe distribution; opacities tend to wax and wane (hallmark) nodular opacities; reverse halo sign (nonspecific)	Rituximab Panitumumab	Imatinib	Everolimus Temsirolimus Sirolimus (rare)	Bortezomib Carfilzomib	Ipilimumab Nivolumab Pembrolizumab Atezolizumab Durvalumab Avelumab	
HP	Acute, subacute and chronic forms of disease; dry cough, dyspnea,	Mosaic attenuation caused by air trapping; diffuse ground-glass opacification without interstitial thickening; poorly defined					Ipilimumab Nivolumab Pembrolizumab Atezolizumab Durvalumab Avelumab	

(continued)

Table 2 (continued)

Radiographic pattern	Clinical findings	CT findings	Molecular-targeted therapies		Rapamycin inhibitors	Proteosome inhibitors	ICIs	Other
			MoAB	TKIs				
		centrilobular ground-glass nodules						
AIP/ARDS/ DAD	Dry cough and dyspnea, hypoxia may develop more rapidly (days – weeks) versus other forms of ILD	Diffuse bilateral septal thickening, GGOs and consolidations in the dependent areas of the lungs; volume loss	Cetuximab Panitumumab Alemtuzumab Rituximab Brentuximab Ofatumumab Ibritumomab Trastuzumab Pertuzumab Ado-trastuzumab Gemtuzumab	Gefitinib Erlotinib Imatinib Sorafenib Vandetanib Crizotinib Ruxolitinib	Everolimus Temsirolimus	Bortezomib	Ipilimumab Nivolumab Pembrolizumab Atezolizumab Durvalumab Avelumab	Thalidomide Lenalidomide CAR-T inhibitors Blinatumomab
Eosinophilic pneumonia	Homogeneous opacities, peripheral, and upper-lobe distribution (reverse batwing sign, also known as reverse pulmonary edema sign)	Peripheral opacities with upper-lobe predominant distribution					Ipilimumab Nivolumab Pembrolizumab	

Nonspecific Interstitial Pneumonitis (NSIP). Nonspecific interstitial pneumonitis and organizing pneumonia (OP) are the most common morphologic patterns of interstitial lung disease following systemic chemotherapy, including the molecular-targeted and immune checkpoint inhibitor therapies. Dry cough and progressive dyspnea, developing insidiously, over weeks to months following drug exposure are notable clinical features of both syndromes. Diffuse ground-glass and reticular opacities with peribronchovascular predominant fibrosis and sparing of the subpleural space help to distinguish NSIP from other forms of pulmonary fibrosis (Fig. 1). However ground-glass consolidations localizing to the lung periphery and bibasilar areas are also frequently seen, particularly in late forms of disease, rendering these diagnostic clues imperfect [34]. An extensive list of conventional cytotoxic chemotherapies has been linked to the development of NSIP. These most commonly include the cytotoxic antibiotics (bleomycin, mitomycin), the nitrosoureas (BCNU, CCNU), other alkylating agents (busulfan, cyclophosphamide), antimetabolites (methotrexate, gemcitabine, procarbazine, cytosine, arabinoside), the podophyllotoxins (etoposide), taxanes (paclitaxel), and the anti-angiogenesis inhibitors (thalidomide, pomalidomide, lenalidomide). Among the molecular-targeted

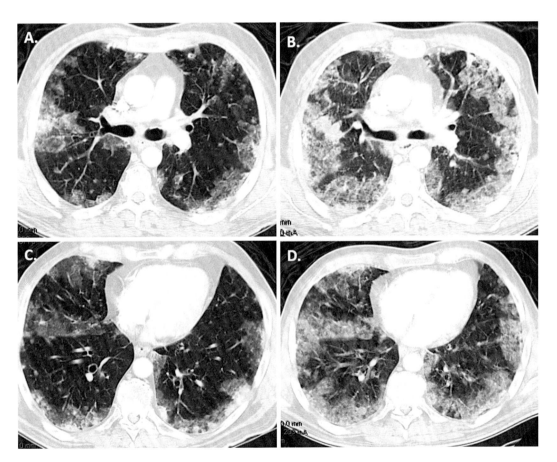

Fig. 1 Gemcitabine-induced lung injury. A 54-year-old man was hospitalized for progressive dyspnea, dry cough, and severe hypoxia 3 weeks after initiation of gemcitabine therapy for pancreatic cancer. The extensive nodular infiltrates with subpleural predominance seen on CT at baseline (**a, c**) were biopsy-proven to represent metastatic disease. The admitting CT of the chest (**b, d**) demonstrated relatively stable nodules with marked increase in the peripheral ground-glass and consolidative opacities bilaterally. Pathologic analysis of lung tissue obtained by transbronchial biopsies confirmed nonspecific interstitial pneumonitis (NSIP) superimposed on known metastatic disease, likely due to gemcitabine therapy

therapies, cetuximab, erlotinib, gefitinib, brentuximab, panitumumab, obinutuzumab, dasatinib, brigatinib, and m-tor inhibitors, everolimus and temsirolimus, are most frequently implicated. NSIP is also triggered by the programmed cell death-1/programmed cell death-ligand 1 (PD-1/PD-L1) inhibition and, to a lesser extent, the anti-cytotoxic T lymphocyte antigen (anti-CTLA-4) immune checkpoint inhibitors.

Organizing Pneumonia. The histologic hallmark of organizing pneumonia (OP) is fibrin plugs within the lumens of distal airways with associated chronic inflammation. This finding, coupled with patchy unilateral or bilateral areas of consolidation that migrate from one area of the lung to another on sequential chest imaging studies, should heighten the suspicion for OP. Other findings include tree-in-bud branching linear opacities, areas of nodular consolidation, and centrilobular nodules. A lymphocyte-predominant fluid is seen on bronchoscopically obtained sample analysis [35]. PFT abnormalities typically include a mixed obstructive-restrictive pattern in secondary OP. Chemotherapeutic agents that are most commonly implicated in the development of OP include conventional agents (cyclophosphamide, oxaliplatin, methotrexate, bleomycin, busulfan), targeted therapies (rituximab, cetuximab, adalimumab, alemtuzumab, everolimus), and immunomodulating agents (ipilimumab, pembrolizumab, nivolumab, atezolizumab, durvalumab). The prognosis of OP is generally favorable. Systemic steroids represent standard therapy, although the precise dose and duration of treatment have not been established. Most reports favor a slow steroid taper (4–6 weeks), to avoid disease relapse. Due to their anti-inflammatory properties, macrolides have also been used with occasional benefit [36].

Hypersensitivity Pneumonitis (HP). This immune-mediated ILD typically develops following repeated exposure to an offending agent. Imaging findings suggestive of HP include mosaic attenuation, reflective of air trapping and diffuse ground-glass opacification. A predilection for the upper lobes may be seen in chronic forms of the disease. Associated symptoms of fever, dyspnea, dry cough, and rash typically occur over the first 3–4 weeks following drug exposure and may wax and wane without adjustments in therapy. Poorly formed granulomas and BAL lymphocytic alveolitis are common histopathologic findings. Chemotherapeutic agents that most commonly provoke this type of reaction include bleomycin, busulfan, carmustine (BCNU), methotrexate, procarbazine, the taxanes (paclitaxel, docetaxel), and interferon-α. Methotrexate is the prototype agent associated with HP, which may develop regardless of route of methotrexate administration (oral, intrathecal, intramuscular, or intravenous). Hypersensitivity reactions have been reported following both Taxol and Taxotere administration, which may arise as a result of the drug or its diluent. Taxol is formulated in a highly allergenic polyoxyethylated castor oil (Cremophor EL) solvent. Up to 10% of patients develop HP following paclitaxel administration, which is marked by urticaria, bronchospasm, angioedema, and, in extreme cases, hypotension. Paclitaxel-induced HP has been attributed to its Cremophor EL suspension vehicle rather than the agent itself. A hypersensitivity reaction reported following interferon-α has been attributed to the immune-stimulating properties of interferon-α, rather than a reaction to the agent itself. Drug withdrawal and steroid therapy typically produce favorable outcomes, with complete resolution of clinical signs and symptoms in early-stage disease. Chronic HP may progress to pulmonary fibrosis with fatal outcomes.

Noncardiogenic Pulmonary Edema (NCPE), Diffuse Alveolar Damage (DAD), and Acute Respiratory Distress Syndrome (ARDS). Drug-induced injury to the alveolar-capillary membranes may result in capillary leak and a permeability (noncardiogenic) pulmonary edema. ARDS and its histologic hallmark, DAD, may ensue as the disease progresses. Early histopathologic findings include the accumulation of proteinaceous inflammatory debris, capillary congestion, atelectasis, alveolar edema, and intra-alveolar hemorrhage. This is followed days later by edema of the alveolar septa, thickened alveolar membranes, epithelial cell hyperplasia, and hyaline membrane deposition [37]. Corresponding imaging findings of DAD include septal thickening, atelectasis, and diffuse ground-glass and consolidative opacities, which are most pronounced in the dependent portions of the lungs. DAD may progress to irreversible pulmonary fibrosis. Drug-induced DAD/ARDS may be idiosyncratic, without any relationship to drug dosage or duration of therapy.

Compelling causal drug-related associations arise from nearly all classes of antineoplastic therapies, including cytotoxic antibiotics (bleomycin, mitomycin C); alkylating agents (busulfan, bis-chloroethyl nitrosourea (BCNU), chloroethyl cyclohexyl nitrosourea (CCNU), high-dose cyclophosphamide); antimetabolites (methotrexate, gemcitabine, azathioprine, cytosine-arabinoside, fludarabine); molecularly target agents (gefitinib, erlotinib, cetuximab); antilymphocyte monoclonal antibodies (rituximab, alemtuzumab, ofatumumab); and the rapamycin inhibitors (everolimus, temsirolimus) and the immunomodulating agents (immune checkpoint inhibitors, chimeric antigen receptor T cells [CAR-T], bispecific T cell engagers [BiTE], methotrexate). Chemotherapeutic agents such as bleomycin, mitomycin C, busulfan, gentamycin, everolimus, and the nitrosoureas may promote DAD by disrupting the alveolus via apoptosis. Others interfere with repair of the alveolar epithelial barrier (gefitinib, erlotinib, cetuximab) or immune mechanisms (immune checkpoint inhibitors, chimeric antigen receptor T cells [CAR-T], bispecific T cell engagers [BiTE], methotrexate). In many cases, specific mechanism of drug-induced DAD is unknown. Prompt discontinuation of the offending agent is vital, although disease progression may occur despite drug withdrawal.

NCPE leading to ARDS has been described following ruxolitinib, a novel Jakafi one-half inhibitor, as a result of a cytokine rebound reaction. This reaction is mitigated with the preemptive use of corticosteroids and supportive therapy [38, 39]. Cytokine storm has also been described following all-trans retinoic acid (ATRA) and arsenic trioxide therapies in the treatment of acute promyelocytic leukemia (APL). The differentiation syndrome is characterized by potentially fatal NCPE and ARDS and occurs in up to 25% of APL patients undergoing induction therapy. Unlike many of the lung injury processes, in patients with ATRA and arsenic-related differentiation syndrome, de-escalation of drug dose rather than drug withdrawal, along with systemic steroid

therapy, has been associated with successful resolution of toxicity in patients with mild to moderate forms of this syndrome [40, 41].

The onset of ARDS is heralded by acute dyspnea, hypoxia, and bilateral alveolar infiltrates. Reactions may be mild and self-limited, although progression to ARDS with fatal outcomes occasionally occurs. Drug withdrawal, supplemental oxygen, and the judicious use of diuretics usually effect a rapid recovery. With the exception of ATRA- and arsenic-induced NCPE (see above), drug rechallenge with the offending drug often results in recrudescence of symptoms and is not recommended. Aggravating factors that potentiate disease progression to ARDS include multi-agent protocols and the concomitant or sequential use of radiation or oxygen therapy, particularly following therapy with bleomycin or busulfan [42, 43]. Once established, the response of ARDS to drug withdrawal and corticosteroid therapy is variable. Progressive respiratory impairment, leading to respiratory failure and death, has been reported with some agents (busulfan, cyclophosphamide, bleomycin) despite drug withdrawal. Among molecular-targeted therapies, ARDS has been best described following agents that inhibit EGFR (gefitinib, erlotinib, cetuximab), the antilymphocyte monoclonal antibodies (rituximab, alemtuzumab, ofatumumab), and the rapamycin inhibitors (everolimus, temsirolimus). Acute withdrawal of the JAK1/2 inhibitor, ruxolitinib, has been associated with the development of ARDS as a result of a cytokine rebound reaction. Preemptive use of corticosteroids, along with supportive therapy and a slow taper off this agent, is recommended to mitigate this potential problem [38, 39].

Diffuse Alveolar Hemorrhage and Hemoptysis. DAH is typically seen as sequelae of alveolar-capillary membrane injury. Disruption of the alveolar and capillary basement membranes facilitates the entry of red blood cells into the alveoli and represents the histologic change that underlies DAD. Thus, any chemotherapeutic agent that prompts the development of DAD may cause DAH. However, DAH is an uncommon sequela of chemotherapeutic agents, with only a handful of drugs being implicated. Agents such as high-dose cyclophosphamide, cytarabine, gemcitabine, mitomycin, erlotinib, alemtuzumab, and rituximab are most frequently cited as causes of DAH, probably because of the propensity of these agents to trigger DAD. Occasionally, bland alveolar hemorrhage has been described in the absence of DAD following rituximab and alemtuzumab therapy [38, 44]. Affected patients may present with acute hypoxemic respiratory distress. Patients often present with abrupt dyspnea and cough which may progress to acute hypoxemic respiratory failure. Hemoptysis may be minimal or absent in approximately 25–30% of patients, despite massive bleeds [45, 46]. The diagnosis of DAH is confirmed by progressively bloody aliquots of bronchoalveolar lavage (BAL) fluid. Cytologic evidence of increased hemosiderin-laden macrophages (>20%) is also supportive. CT findings of diffuse, bilateral ground-glass opacities or consolidative changes are typical. Early recognition and discontinuation of the offending agent are crucial, as prompt diagnosis and treatment improve survival. Corticosteroids and immunosuppressive agents are often used, although their efficacy in this setting has not been formally evaluated.

Massive and sometimes fatal bleeding has been reported during bevacizumab therapy for treatment of central airway tumors [47]. The inhibition of VEGF is the putative mechanism, which may cause destruction of normal lung tissue and subsequent hemoptysis. Hemoptysis following VEGF inhibitor therapies has been reported more often in association with lung cancers of squamous cell histology, which is likely due to the central location of these tumors [48]. Treatment requires discontinuation of the drug and stabilization of the patient, preferably in an intensive care unit setting. Management of massive hemoptysis is beyond the scope of this chapter but typically includes early bronchoscopy performed with either rigid or flexible endoscope (or both), endovascular embolization, and, in selected cases, surgery, with goals of controlling the bleeding and prevention of aspiration.

Eosinophilic Pneumonia. Eosinophilic pneumonia is characterized by an inappropriate increase in the number of eosinophils and macrophages within alveoli, causing the alveolar septa to become engorged. Progressive dyspnea, dry cough, and occasionally fever are nonspecific clinical correlates. Elevated peripheral eosinophilia and elevated IgE levels and nonsegmental homogeneous opacities with peripheral and upper-lobe distribution (reverse batwing sign, also known as reverse pulmonary edema sign) are important clinical clues. Causative agents include the taxanes, methotrexate, gemcitabine, fludarabine, and interferon-α. Drug-related EP may resolve with cessation of therapy and initiation of systemic steroids.

Pleural Effusions. Drug-induced pleural effusions may occur as an isolated toxicity to the pleura (following methotrexate, dasatinib, bosutinib, docetaxel, ATRA, and granulocyte colony-stimulating factor (GCSF) administration) or as a manifestation of a generalized pleuroparenchymal abnormality [49, 50]. These small- to moderate-sized effusions are typically exudative and lymphocyte predominant and may be unilateral or bilateral. Withdrawal of the offending agent may result in spontaneous resolution in some cases.

Pulmonary Vascular Disorders (PVD). The development of thromboembolic disease, pulmonary hypertension, and pulmonary veno-occlusive disease has been described following conventional chemotherapeutic, molecularly targeted, and immunomodulating agents. Increased rates of venous thromboembolism (pulmonary embolism and deep venous thrombosis) have been reported with the ALK inhibitor crizotinib, Bcr-Abl inhibitor ponatinib, and VEGF inhibitors bevacizumab, sunitinib, sorafenib, and pazopanib [51, 52]. In addition, the angiogenesis inhibitors (thalidomide, revlimid, pomalidomide) in combination with steroids, doxorubicin, or BCNU are associated with 14–43% increased risk of thromboembolic events. Other agents, including hormonal therapies, growth factors, and erythropoietic agents, contribute to cancer-associated venous thromboembolism. The development of pulmonary arterial hypertension (PAH) has been associated with several drugs, including bleomycin, busulfan, BCNU, interferon, and dasatinib. Severe PAH following dasatinib, a multi-kinase Bcr-Abl tyrosine kinase inhibitor (TKI), is well described. Once dasatinib-associated

PAH develops, drug withdrawal without rechallenge is recommended. There are no reports of PAH following exposure to the more selective Bcr-Abl targeted TKIs (imatinib and nilotinib), which may be safely used in dasatinib-induced PAH [16, 53–55]. Bleomycin and BCNU have also been implicated in the development of PVOD, an irreversible and often fatal form of pulmonary hypertension that is characterized by fibrous obliteration of pulmonary venules.

Drug-Induced Airway Disease. Virtually all chemotherapeutic and targeted agents may trigger an infusion reaction (IR), a sometimes life-threatening acute reaction that may be associated with dry cough, dyspnea, wheezing, chest pain, and hypoxia. IRs may manifest as IgE-mediated, type 1 hypersensitivity reactions (carboplatin, oxaliplatin, and L-asparaginase) or as anaphylactoid reactions, mediated by cytokine release. The latter reaction is often seen following the administration of several monoclonal antibodies (mAbs). IRs may be triggered by the drug itself or in response to the vehicle in which the drug is formulated. This is particularly true of the taxane class of drugs. For example, paclitaxel is formulated in Cremophor EL, a highly allergenic poly-oxyethylated castor oil solvent. Docetaxel is formulated in polysorbate 80. Both vehicles may induce mast cell/basophil activation and subsequent hypersensitivity reaction. Other drugs that are formulated in Cremophor EL (cyclosporine, teniposide, ixabepilone) or polysorbate 80 (etoposide) may trigger similar reactions and should be avoided in patients with a history of IRs following taxane administration [56, 57]. Histamine receptor antagonists and steroids are recommended as standard prophylaxis prior to taxane administration, which has reduced the incidence of taxane-induced bronchospasm from 30% to 2% [58]. IRs may occur within minutes to several hours following drug exposure. Close monitoring during and immediately following drug infusion is critical, as breakthrough IRs may occur despite prophylaxis. Although vinca alkaloids are rarely associated with lung toxicity, severe bronchospasm has been described when these agents are given with concurrent or sequential administration of mitomycin therapy [59].

Infections. Lung infections are frequent sequelae of aggressive immunosuppressive regimens. The conventional chemotherapeutic agents as well as molecular-targeted therapies may promote recalcitrant and sometimes life-threatening opportunistic pneumonias [60–77]. Increased infection risk in this setting is primarily due to the development of drug-related neutropenia, lymphopenia, and/or impairment of T cell and B cell function. Reactivation of tuberculosis has been reported following anti-PD-1 therapies [78]. Agents that are more frequently linked to an increased infection risk are listed in Table 3.

Methemoglobinemia. Methemoglobinemia is a rare but potentially fatal blood disorder in which the iron of heme is oxidized in excess to the ferric ($Fe+++$) state. Ferric hemes of methemoglobin exhibit an impaired affinity for oxygen, while the remaining heme sites within the same tetrameric hemoglobin that are in ferrous state demonstrate an increased affinity for oxygen. This imbalance results in poor oxygen delivery, tissue hypoxia. As methemoglobin levels increase, clinical symptoms of shortness of breath, cyanosis, fatigue, exercise intolerance, dizziness, shock, neurologic disturbances (headache, mental status changes, seizures, coma), and death may ensue. Severe symptoms may occur at lower levels of methemoglobin in the setting of preexisting conditions, such as anemia, coexistent glucose-6-phosphate dehydrogenase (G6PD) deficiency, and chronic lung or heart disease. Exposure to dapsone, topical anesthetic agents, and other oxidant drugs are the most common precipitating agents associated with acquired methemoglobinemia. Two chemotherapeutic agents, cyclophosphamide, and a structurally similar compound, ifosfamide, are important causes of methemoglobinemia. This diagnosis should be considered in the differential of patients who develop acute shortness of breath, cyanosis, respiratory depression, or altered sensorium during treatment with one of these agents [79]. Hypoxia that is refractory to supplemental oxygen, abnormal chocolate coloration of the blood, and clinical cyanosis in the presence of normal PaO2 are important diagnostic clues. Drug withdrawal is the mainstay of therapy. Depending on the clinical presentation, blood

Table 3 Chemotherapeutic agents and infection risk

Agent class	Infection risk	Mechanism	Refs
Conventional chemotherapy			
Alkylating agents Chlorambucil Cyclophosphamide Bendamustine	Bacterial Fungal HBV reactivation (bendaustine, chlorambucil)	Neutropenia Lymphopenia (T cell dysfunction) Lymphopenia (B and T cell dysfunction, bendamustine, cladribine, pentostatin)	[113]
Purine/pyrimidine analogues Fludarabine Cladribine Pentostatin 6-Mercaptopurine Cytosine arabinoside Azathioprine	Listeria, PJP, nocardia Mycobacterial infections Opportunistic fungal infections Viral (CMV, VZV, HSV)	Lymphopenia (T cell dysfunction – fludarabine) Lymphopenia (B and T cell dysfunction – cladribine, pentostatin)	[114]
Targeted agents			
Bruton tyrosine kinase Inhibitors Ibrutinib Acalabrutinib	Opportunistic fungi (*Aspergillus*, *Cryptococcus*, PJP, *Fusarium*) HBV reactivation	Lymphopenia (B-cell dysfunction, ? T cell dysfunction)	[115]
Proteasome inhibitors Carfilzomib Bortezomib	Viruses (VZV)	T cell dysfunction	[116]
Anti-CD20-target Rituximab Obinutuzumab Ofatumumab	Viruses (herpesvirus-CMV, HSV, VZV, enterovirus, JC virus); HBV reactivation	Lymphopenia (B cell dysfunction) Neutropenia (obinutuzumab)	[64]
Anti-CD-52 target Alemtuzumab	Viruses (herpesviruses – CMV, HSV, VZV) Fungal (PJP, *Aspergillus*, *Zygomycetes*, *Candida*)	Lymphopenia (B, T and NK cell dysfunction)	[65]
mTOR inhibitors Temsirolimus Everolimus Sirolimus	Bacterial Fungal	B and T cell dysfunction	[66]
Pl3K inhibitors Idelalisib Brigatinib	Bacterial Fungal (PJP, *Aspergillus*)	Neutropenia Lymphopenia (B and T cell dysfunction)	[69]
BCL2 inhibitors Venetoclax	Bacteria Viruses (enterovirus)	Neutropenia Lymphopenia (B and T cell dysfunction)	[70]
Jak-1 inhibitors Ruxolitinib	Fungal (PJP, *Cryptococcus*) Mycobacteria (MTB); HBV reactivation	T cell dysfunction	[71–73]
Immunomodulators Thalidomide Lenalidomide	Viral Fungal	Neutropenia Lymphopenia (B and T cell dysfunction)	[75]
Anti-cytokines IFN-α TNF-α (infliximab)	Fungal (PJP, *Cryptococcus*) Mycobacteria (MTB) HBV reactivation	T cell dysfunction	[77]
Immune checkpoint inhibitors			
Anti-PD-1 therapies	TB reactivation	Anti-PD-1 activity	[78]

transfusions, methylene blue, and intensive care monitoring for stabilization of the airway and hemodynamics should be considered.

Lung Injury Associated with Cancer Immunotherapies

Immune Checkpoint Blocking Agents

A key responsibility of the host immune system is to target and destroy cancer cells. This process is mediated via a series of tightly regulated co-stimulatory and co-inhibitory immunomodulatory signals that result in a dynamic state of equilibrium between immune attack and immune tolerance. Immune-related adverse events (IrAEs) may involve virtually every major organ system, including the lungs. Lung involvement is infrequent; however, pneumonitis associated with immune checkpoint inhibitors (ICIs) represents one of the most severe and potentially fatal forms of IrAEs. The incidence of ICI-related pneumonitis ranges from 5% to 11%, with the most frequent and severe events occurring following combination strategies using concurrent or sequential anti-CTLA-4/PD-1 regimens [80–84]. Nonspecific symptoms of new or worsening dry cough, fatigue, and shortness of breath typically occur within the first 3–6 months of initiation of therapy. Fever and chest pain have also rarely been described. Tachycardia and hypoxia are ominous signs which may presage advance disease. Bronchoscopy and lung biopsy can be helpful in excluding competing diagnoses, such as lymphangitic carcinomatosis, pneumonia, pulmonary edema, alveolar hemorrhage, or preexisting lung disease. A lymphocyte-predominant bronchoalveolar lavage (BAL) fluid is common. Occasionally, peripheral and BAL eosinophilia, suggestive of eosinophilic pneumonia, may be seen. Histopathologic findings of a cellular interstitial pneumonitis, organizing pneumonia, or diffuse alveolar damage may progress to traction bronchiectasis with pulmonary fibrosis (Fig. 2). Ground-glass and reticular changes with subpleural and basilar predominance and patchy, consolidative changes on chest imaging studies are also nonspecific. These findings do not distinguish ICI-related IP from other causes. A concurrent or sequential history of extrapulmonary IrAEs involving the skin, gut, thyroid, or other organs may occur in more than 50% of patients and should raise the index of suspicion [82, 84–88]. Organizing pneumonia and cellular interstitial pneumonitis represent the most frequent histopathologic findings which may progress to traction bronchiectasis with pulmonary fibrosis with advanced stages of disease. Other ICI-mediated respiratory events include bronchitis, bronchiolitis, pleural disease, sarcoid-like reactions, pulmonary granulomatosis, and pseudoprogression of the underlying malignancy [89–93].

The Common Terminology Criteria for Adverse Events (CTCAE) has been widely utilized to establish guidelines for the management of IrAEs. This scoring system uses organ-specific parameters to stratify the severity of therapy-related organ toxicities. Accordingly, symptom scoring ranges from asymptomatic (grade 1) to severe (grade 4) pneumonitis (Table 4). For grade 1 pneumonitis, withholding the drug with close outpatient monitoring is recommended. Drug rechallenge among this group of patients may be considered on a case-by-case basis, if repeat imaging studies, performed 2–4 weeks after withholding the drug, demonstrate resolution of infiltrates. Current consensus favors inpatient management with initiation of systemic corticosteroid therapy among patients with grade 3–4 pneumonitis and patients with grade 2 pneumonitis who demonstrate progression of toxicity despite drug cessation [7, 87, 94–96]. Early grade (1–2) pneumonitis may rapidly progress to respiratory failure and death in 1–2% of patients. Thus, close monitoring of patients with all grades of pneumonitis is recommended.

Genetically Engineered Immunotherapies

Recent success in the use of genetically engineered T cells in the treatment of hematologic malignancies has inspired tremendous interest in this area. This process involves ex vivo modification of the naïve T cell to express a unique high-affinity T cell receptor (TCR) or a chimeric

Baseline   **Ipilimumab, (course 1, day 5)**

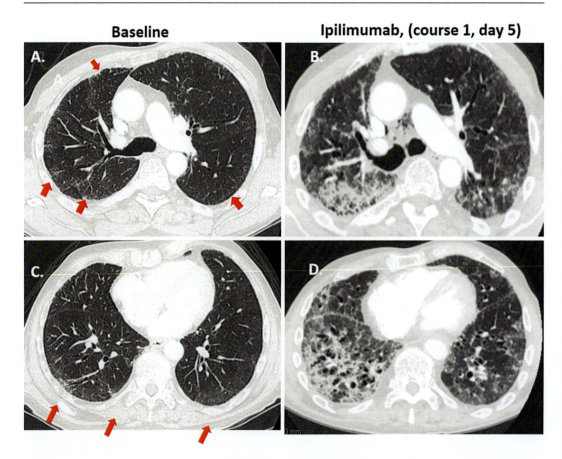

Fig. 2 Ipilimumab-induced lung injury. A 78-year-old man treated with combined ipilimumab monotherapy for melanoma presented 5 days after cycle 1 of therapy with dyspnea and dry cough. Asymptomatic idiopathic pulmonary fibrosis was coincidentally found on CT imaging studies 5 years prior to the cancer diagnosis. Subtle, subpleural reticular changes at baseline (arrows, **a**, **c**) are consistent with the patient's known history of pulmonary fibrosis. Extensive superimposed areas of bilateral ground-glass densities are seen on the admitting CT (**b**, **d**), which corresponded to organizing pneumonia on lung biopsies, felt to be related to ipilimumab

antigen receptor (CAR). The modified T cells are expanded and infused into the recipient through a process called adoptive cell transfer. The two major classes of engineered T cell therapies, known as chimeric antigen receptor T cells (CAR-T) and bispecific T cell engagers (BiTEs), have advantages over conventional therapies in their ability to target unique antigens on tumor cells with a precision that standard chemotherapy and radiation cannot, resulting in cytologic killing of specific antigen-positive tumor targets. In addition, these agents have the capacity to promote large-scale T cell expansion [96–101]. BiTEs are antibody-derived molecules with dual antigen specificity, allowing them to simultaneously bind unique antigens on the T cell and the tumor cell, thereby facilitating cytotoxic cell-to-cell interactions and tumor cell killing.

Engineered T cells are "living drugs" which may induce organ toxicity well after discontinuation of the agent. The most prominent toxicity of both CAR-T and BiTE therapies is cytokine release syndrome (CRS), a systemic inflammatory response that is thought to be caused by rapid T cell proliferation with the toxic release of pro-inflammatory cytokines, such as IFN-g, TNF-a, and IL-6 following therapy. These cytokines may promote damage to the endothelium and other organs, resulting in microvascular leakage, and potentially fatal organ system damage to the heart, liver, lung, and kidneys [102]. Patients may present with rapid onset of

Table 4 CTCAE scoring system and consensus guidelines in the management of lung injury associated with immune checkpoint inhibitor therapies

Pneumonitis grade	Clinical symptoms	Treatment recommendations
1	Asymptomatic	Withhold therapy; close clinical and diagnostic follow-up to determine timing and feasibility of resumption of therapy; if evidence of disease progression, treat as higher-grade pneumonitis
2	Mild symptoms of dyspnea with moderate exertion; minimal interference with activities of daily living	Withhold therapy; initiate corticosteroid therapy in select cases; close clinical and diagnostic follow-up to determine timing and feasibility of resumption of therapy; if evidence of disease progression, treat as higher-grade pneumonitis
3	Dyspnea at rest; dyspnea limits activities of daily living and self-care	Discontinue therapy; hospitalize and initiate corticosteroid therapy; if evidence of disease progression, treat as higher-grade pneumonitis
4	Severe, life-threatening symptoms, respiratory compromise	Permanent discontinuation of therapy; hospitalize with higher-level (ICU) care; initiate corticosteroid therapy

high fever, rigors, chills, myalgias, dyspnea, hypoxia, and hemodynamic instability 4–16 h following drug infusion (Fig. 3). Supportive care, including fluid resuscitation, vasopressor support, supplemental oxygen, and intubation, may be required for patients with severe symptoms. Systemic corticosteroids and treatment with IL-6 receptor-directed therapy with tocilizumab are also used to suppress the intense inflammatory response [96, 103, 104].

Radiation-Induced Lung Injury

Clinically significant radiation-induced lung injury (RILI) is the most common dose-limiting complication of thoracic radiation therapy (RT), occurring in 5–20% of patients. Recent advances in radiation techniques and delivery systems, such as proton therapy, three-dimensional conformal RT (CRT), intensity-modulated RT (IMRT), and stereotactic body RT (SBRT), purport lower lung injury rates while delivering higher target doses of radiation to the lung. Factors associated with radiation delivery (total radiation dose, dose per fraction, volume of irradiated lung, and beam characteristics and arrangements) and clinical factors (preexisting lung disease, underlying poor pulmonary reserve, prior radiotherapy, multimodality regiments, rapid steroid withdrawal) all potentiate the appearance and severity of radiation pneumotoxicity.

Radiographically apparent lung injury is common with total doses of radiation that exceed 40 Gy and is rare at doses below 20 Gy [105, 106]. Hyperfractionated radiation doses delivered to the smallest lung volume are recommended.

Clinical Presentation

Acute clinical radiation pneumonitis, heralded by dyspnea, low-grade fever, and dry cough, develops insidiously over 1–3 months after completion of radiation. Radiographic changes typically precede clinical symptoms, appearing 3–4 weeks following RT. Discrete ground-glass opacities, ill-defined patchy nodules, or consolidation with air bronchograms and volume loss within the irradiated field are common early findings which evolve over the ensuing 6–23 months, leaving a linear scar. Regional fibrosis is seen in nearly all patients, including those without clinical symptoms, and is characterized by the appearance of a well-demarcated area of volume loss, linear densities, bronchiectasis, retraction of the lung parenchyma, tenting and elevation of the hemidiaphragm, and ipsilateral pleural thickening within the irradiated field (Fig. 4). Post-radiation volume loss, bronchiectasis, and consolidation may occur following the newer modes of RT delivery but typically are less extensive than injury patterns following conventional radiation [107].

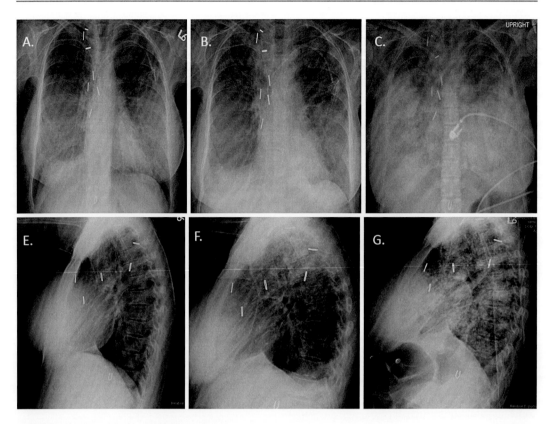

Fig. 3 Cytokine release syndrome associated with blinatumomab therapy. A 47-year-old woman developed acute, severe dyspnea, dry cough, and low-grade fever 7 h following infusion of blinatumomab for refractory ALL. Over the ensuing 24 h, the patient required vasopressor support and was intubated and placed on mechanical ventilation for hypoxemic respiratory failure. Bronchoscopically obtained distal airway samples were culture negative and without evidence of malignant cells. The patient was started on high-dose steroids and tocilizumab but succumbed to refractory hypoxemia and hypotension, felt to be due to cytokine release syndrome

Radiation Recall Pneumonitis

Radiation recall pneumonitis (RRP) is a rare inflammatory reaction that develops within a previously irradiated field following certain chemotherapy and molecularly targeted therapies. This reaction has been most often observed following taxane- and anthracycline-based therapies. Gemcitabine, etoposide, vinorelbine, trastuzumab, and erlotinib may also trigger this disease [108, 109]. Clinically, RRP is signaled by dry cough, fever, and dyspnea and accompanied by ground-glass opacities and areas of consolidation that conform to the prior radiation treatment portal. RRP may develop during the first or subsequent course of therapy with the inciting agent, which may be weeks to years following completion of RT. Drug withdrawal and corticosteroid therapy may mitigate symptoms of radiation pneumonitis but have not been shown to be of benefit in the treatment of radiation fibrosis. Drug reintroduction has been successful in some cases [110].

Other Manifestations of Radiation-Induced Lung Injury

Pleural effusions may develop as early (within 6 months) and late (1–5 years) sequelae of RT. Effusions are typically small, ipsilateral, or bilateral. Reactive mesothelial cells with

Baseline   **9 weeks post XRT**

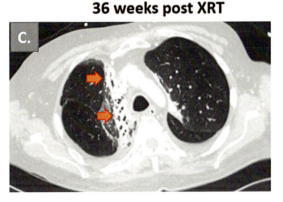

36 weeks post XRT

Fig. 4 Evolution of radiation-induced lung injury. A 56-year-old man underwent radiation therapy to the right upper and middle lobes and paramediastinal areas for primary bronchogenic carcinoma. At baseline, (**a**) a large central mass involving the right upper and middle lobes (*) along with a moderate-sized right pleural effusion (arrow) is seen. Nine weeks after completion of radiation therapy (**b**), there are dense consolidative opacities in the right lung (arrow), consistent with evolving radiation changes. The large mass-like consolidation has resolved. Nine months following completion of radiation therapy (**c**), linear densities outlining a well-demarcated area of volume loss (arrows), bronchiectasis, retraction of the lung parenchyma, and ipsilateral pleural thickening within the irradiated field are seen

negative pleural fluid cytology are common. Most radiation-induced pleural effusions are asymptomatic, although pleuritic chest pain and dyspnea are occasionally presenting symptoms. Radiation-related organizing pneumonia (OP) and eosinophilic pneumonia (EP) have been described in patients with breast cancer and may involve nonirradiated areas of the lung [107, 111]. These lung injury patterns are characterized by migratory pulmonary opacities that develop 1–3 months after completing RT. A prior history of asthma or atopy, coupled with blood or tissue eosinophilia, supports the diagnosis of radiation-induced EP. Both lung injury patterns are typically steroid-responsive.

Management of Radiation-Induced Lung Injury

Treatment recommendations for DILI in the cancer setting are generally provided by collective clinical experience and expert opinion. Pneumonitis grading schemes, based on the National Cancer Institute common terminology criteria for adverse events (NCI CTCAE) [112], offer limited guidelines for drug withdrawal and initiation of immunosuppressive therapies based on symptom severity. Permanent drug cessation is recommended for most DILI events associated with cytotoxic drugs; however, indications for drug interruption and resumption may vary with the specific class of agents in question. Resolution of pulmonary toxicity may occur following drug simple interruption in some patients. Thus, close follow-up while withholding corticosteroid therapy in asymptomatic patients with stable and mild disease is reasonable. Initiation of systemic corticosteroids is generally based on the acuity, severity, and rapidity of worsening of pulmonary impairment as well as the histopathologic patterns of disease. The benefits of corticosteroids in this setting are largely observational and gleaned from anecdotal reports and small case series. Evidence-based guidelines informing the optimal timing, dose, and duration of corticosteroid therapy do not exist. Prednisolone or its equivalent, dosed at 0.5–1 mg/kg/day, is typical, with dosing and tapering schedules guided by the radiologic and clinical symptoms and response to therapy. Additional therapies, such as cyclophosphamide, macrolides, cyclosporine, rituximab, and infliximab, may be indicated in steroid-refractory patients. Evidence favoring a benefit in these cases is also anecdotal and limited to small case series.

References

1. Bennett WM, Pastore L, Houghton DC. Fatal pulmonary bleomycin toxicity in cisplatin-induced acute renal failure. Cancer Treat Rep. 1980;64:921–4.
2. Azambuja E, Fleck JF, Batista RG, Menna SSB. Bleomycin lung toxicity: who are the patients with increased risk? Pulm Pharmacol Ther. 2005;18:363–6.
3. Massin F. Busulfan-induced pneumopathy. Rev Mal Respir. 1987;3:3–10.
4. Barlesi F, Villani P, Doddoli C, Gimenez C, Kleisbauer JP. Gemcitabine-induced severe pulmonary toxicity. Fundam Clin Pharmacol. 2004;18:85–91.
5. Steijfer S. Bleomycin-induced pneumonitis. Chest. 2001;120:617–24.
6. Vulsteke C, Dierickx D, Verbeken E, Wolter P, Thomas J, Schoffski P. Rituximab-induced fatal interstitial pneumonitis: case report. Leuk Lymphoma. 2010;51:546–8.
7. Naidoo J, Wang X, Woo KM, Iyriboz T, Halpenny D, Cunningham J, Chaft JE, Segal NH, Callahan MK, Lesokhin AM, Rosenberg J, Voss MH, Rudin CM, Rizvi H, Hou X, Rodriguez K, Albano M, Gordon RA, Leduc C, Rekhtman N, Harris B, Menzies AM, Guminski AD, Carlino MS, Kong BY, Wolchok JD, Postow MA, Long GV, Hellmann MD. Pneumonitis in patients treated with anti-programmed death-1/programmed death ligand 1 therapy. J Clin Oncol. 2017;35:709–17.
8. Nishino M, Ramaiya NH, Hatabu H, Hodi FS, Armand PF. PD-1 inhibitor-related pneumonitis in lymphoma patients treated with single-agent pembrolizumab therapy. Br J Haematol. 2016;180:752–5.
9. Mileshkin L, Prince HM, Rischin D, Zimet A. Severe interstitial pneumonitis following high-dose cyclophosphamide, thiotepa and docetaxel: two case reports and a review of the literature. Bone Marrow Transplant. 2001;27:559–63.
10. Herrmann J, Yang EH, Iliescu CA, Cilingiroglu M, Charitakis K, Hakeem A, Toutouzas K, Leesar MA, Grines CL, Marmagkiolis K. Vascular toxicities of cancer therapies: the old and the new – an evolving avenue. Circulation. 2016;133:1272–89.
11. Hedhli N, Russell KS. Cardiotoxicity of molecularly targeted agents. Curr Cardiol Rev. 2011;7:221–33.
12. Wattal S, Rao MS, Chandra GN, Razak UK, Shetty KR. Dasatinib induced cardiac tamponade-a rare association. J Clin Diagn Res. 2017;11:FD03–4.
13. Krauth MT, Herndlhofer S, Schmook MT, Mitterbauer-Hohendanner G, Schlogl E, Valent P. Extensive pleural and pericardial effusion in chronic myeloid leukemia during treatment with dasatinib at 100 mg or 50 mg daily. Haematologica. 2011;96:163–6.
14. Eskazan AE, Soysal T, Ongoren S, Gulturk E, Ferhanoglu B, Aydin Y. Pleural and pericardial effusions in chronic myeloid leukemia patients receiving low-dose dasatinib therapy. Haematologica. 2011;96:e15; author reply e16–17
15. Bergeron A, Rea D, Levy V, Picard C, Meignin V, Tamburini J, Bruzzoni-Giovanelli H, Calvo F, Tazi A, Rousselot P. Lung abnormalities after dasatinib treatment for chronic myeloid leukemia: a case series. Am J Respir Crit Care Med. 2007;176:814–8.
16. Montani D, Bergot E, Gunther S, Savale L, Bergeron A, Bourdin A, Bouvaist H, Canuet M, Pison C, Macro M, Poubeau P, Girerd B, Natali D, Guignabert C, Perros F, O'Callaghan DS, Jais X, Tubert-Bitter P, Zalcman G, Sitbon O, Simonneau G, Humbert M. Pulmonary arterial hypertension in patients treated by dasatinib. Circulation. 2012;125:2128–37.
17. Wilcox BE, Ryu JH, Kalra S. Exacerbation of pre-existing interstitial lung disease after oxaliplatin therapy: a report of three cases. Respir Med. 2008;102:273–9.
18. Niho S, Kubota K, Goto K, Yoh K, Ohmatsu H, Kakinuma R, Saijo N, Nishiwaki Y. First-line single agent treatment with gefitinib in patients with advanced non-small-cell lung cancer: a phase II study. J Clin Oncol. 2006;24:64–9.
19. Liu V, White DA, Zakowski MF, Travis W, Kris MG, Ginsberg MS, Miller VA, Azzoli CG. Pulmonary toxicity associated with erlotinib. Chest. 2007;132:1042–4.
20. Saravanan V, Kelly CA. Reducing the risk of methotrexate pneumonitis in rheumatoid arthritis. Rheumatology (Oxford). 2004;43:143–7.
21. Vahid B, Marik PE. Pulmonary complications of novel antineoplastic agents for solid tumors. Chest. 2008;133:528–38.

22. Akoun G, Cadranel JL, Milleron BJ, D'Ortho MP, Mayaud CM. Bronchoalveolar lavage cell data in 19 patients with drug-associated pneumonitis (except amiodarone). Chest. 1991;99:98–104.

23. Stover DE, Zaman MB, Hajdu SI, Lange M, Gold J, Armstrong D. Bronchoalveolar lavage in the diagnosis of diffuse pulmonary infiltrates in the immunosuppressed host. Ann Intern Med. 1984;101:1–7.

24. White DA, Kris MG, Stover DE. Bronchoalveolar lavage cell populations in bleomycin lung toxicity. Thorax. 1987;42:551–2.

25. Beinert T, Düll T, Wolf K, Holler E, Vogelmeier C, Behr J, Kolb H. Late pulmonary impairment following allogeneic bone marrow transplantation. J Med Res. 1996;1:343–8.

26. van Barneveld P, Veenstra G, Sleijfer D, van der Mark T, Mulder N, Schraffordt Koops H, Sluiter H, Peset R. Changes in pulmonary function during and after bleomycin treatment in patients with testicular carcinoma. Cancer Chemother Pharmacol. 1985;14:168–71.

27. Gore EM, Lawton CA, Ash RC, Lipchik RJ. Pulmonary function changes in long-term survivors of bone marrow transplantation. Int J Radiat Oncol Biol Phys. 1996;36:67–75.

28. Theuws JC, Muller SH, Seppenwoolde Y, Kwa SL, Boersma LJ, Hart GA, Baas P, Lebesque JV. Effect of radiotherapy and chemotherapy on pulmonary function after treatment for breast cancer and lymphoma: a follow-up study. J Clin Oncol. 1999;17:3091–100.

29. Hirsch A, Vander Els N, Straus DJ, Gomez EG, Leung D, Portlock CS, Yahalom J. Effect of ABVD chemotherapy with and without mantle or mediastinal irradiation on pulmonary function and symptoms in early-stage Hodgkin's disease. J Clin Oncol. 1996;14:1297–305.

30. Bruno B, Souillet G, Bertrand Y, Werck-Gallois MC, So Satta A, Bellon G. Effects of allogeneic bone marrow transplantation on pulmonary function in 80 children in a single paediatric centre. Bone Marrow Transplant. 2004;34:143–7.

31. Hasleton PS, O'Driscoll BR, Lynch P, Webster A, Kalra SJ, Gattamaneini HR, Woodcock AA, Poulter LW. Late BCNU lung: a light and ultrastructural study on the delayed effect of BCNU on the lung parenchyma. J Pathol. 1991;164:31–6.

32. O'Driscoll BR, Hasleton PS, Taylor PM, Poulter LW, Gattameneni HR, Woodcock AA. Active lung fibrosis up to 17 years after chemotherapy with carmustine (BCNU) in childhood. N Engl J Med. 1990;323:378–82.

33. Beynat-Mouterde C, Beltramo G, Lezmi G, Pernet D, Camus C, Fanton A, Foucher P, Cottin V, Bonniaud P. Pleuroparenchymal fibroelastosis as a late complication of chemotherapy agents. Eur Respir J. 2014;44:523–7.

34. Akira M, Inoue Y, Kitaichi M, Yamamoto S, Arai T, Toyokawa K. Usual interstitial pneumonia and nonspecific interstitial pneumonia with and without concurrent emphysema: thin-section CT findings. Radiology. 2009;251:271–9.

35. Cordier JF. Organising pneumonia. Thorax. 2000;55:318–28.

36. Drakopanagiotakis F, Paschalaki K, Abu-Hijleh M, Aswad B, Karagianidis N, Kastanakis E, Braman SS, Polychronopoulos V. Cryptogenic and secondary organizing pneumonia: clinical presentation, radiographic findings, treatment response, and prognosis. Chest. 2011;139:893–900.

37. Raanani P, Segal E, Levi I, Bercowicz M, Berkenstat H, Avigdor A, Perel A, Ben-Bassat I. Diffuse alveolar hemorrhage in acute promyelocytic leukemia patients treated with ATRA – a manifestation of the basic disease or the treatment. Leuk Lymphoma. 2000;37:605–10.

38. Tefferi A, Litzow MR, Pardanani A. Long-term outcome of treatment with ruxolitinib in myelofibrosis. N Engl J Med. 2011;365:1455–7.

39. Beauverd Y, Samii K. Acute respiratory distress syndrome in a patient with primary myelofibrosis after ruxolitinib treatment discontinuation. Int J Hematol. 2014;100:498–501.

40. Rogers JE, Yang D. Differentiation syndrome in patients with acute promyelocytic leukemia. J Oncol Pharm Pract. 2012;18:109–14.

41. Luesink M, Jansen JH. Advances in understanding the pulmonary infiltration in acute promyelocytic leukaemia. Br J Haematol. 2010;151:209–20.

42. Cooper J. Drug-induced lung disease. Adv Intern Med. 1997;42:231–68.

43. Shannon V, Price K. Pulmonary complications of cancer therapy. Anesthesiol Clin North Am. 1998;16:563–85.

44. Sachdeva A, Matuschak GM. Diffuse alveolar hemorrhage following alemtuzumab. Chest. 2008; 133:1476–8.

45. Hildebrand F, Rosenow EI, Haberman T. Pulmonary complications of leukemia. Chest. 1990;98 (5):1233–9.

46. Afessa B, Tefferi A, Litzow MR, Krowka MJ, Wylam ME, Peters SG. Diffuse alveolar hemorrhage in hematopoietic stem cell transplant recipients. Am J Respir Crit Care Med. 2002;166:641–5.

47. Sandler A. Bevacizumab in non small cell lung cancer. Clin Cancer Res. 2007;13:s4613–6.

48. Johnson DH, Fehrenbacher L, Novotny WF, Herbst RS, Nemunaitis JJ, Jablons DM, Langer CJ, DeVore RF 3rd, Gaudreault J, Damico LA, Holmgren E, Kabbinavar F. Randomized phase II trial comparing bevacizumab plus carboplatin and paclitaxel with carboplatin and paclitaxel alone in previously untreated locally advanced or metastatic non-small-cell lung cancer. J Clin Oncol. 2004;22:2184–91.

49. Huggins JT, Sahn SA. Drug-induced pleural disease. Clin Chest Med. 2004;25:141–53.

50. Wohlrab J, Liu M, Anderson E, Kia Noury D. Docetaxel induced pleural effusions [abstract]. Chest. 2002;122:94S–5S.

51. Procopio G, Verzoni E, Gevorgyan A, Mancin M, Pusceddu S, Catena L, Platania M, Guadalupi V, Martinetti A, Bajetta E. Safety and activity of

sorafenib in different histotypes of advanced renal cell carcinoma. Oncology. 2007;73:204–9.

52. Nalluri SR, Chu D, Keresztes R, Zhu X, Wu S. Risk of venous thromboembolism with the angiogenesis inhibitor bevacizumab in cancer patients: a meta-analysis. JAMA. 2008;300:2277–85.

53. Godinas L, Guignabert C, Seferian A, Perros F, Bergot E, Sibille Y, Humbert M, Montani D. Tyrosine kinase inhibitors in pulmonary arterial hypertension: a double-edge sword? Semin Respir Crit Care Med. 2013;34:714–24.

54. Abratt RP, Morgan GW. Lung toxicity following chest irradiation in patients with lung cancer. Lung Cancer. 2002;35:103–9.

55. Soultati A, Mountzios G, Avgerinou C, Papaxoinis G, Pectasides D, Dimopoulos MA, Papadimitriou C. Endothelial vascular toxicity from chemotherapeutic agents: preclinical evidence and clinical implications. Cancer Treat Rev. 2012;38:473–83.

56. Szebeni J, Alving CR, Savay S, Barenholz Y, Priev A, Danino D, Talmon Y. Complement activation-related pseudoallergy caused by liposomes, micellar carriers of intravenous drugs, and radiocontrast agents. Formation of complement-activating particles in aqueous solutions of Taxol: possible role in hypersensitivity reactions. Crit Rev Ther Drug Carrier Syst. 2001;18:567–606.

57. Lv Y, Tang B, Liu X, Xue C, Liu Y, Kang P, Zhang LA. Comparative study of scientific publications in health care sciences and services from Mainland China, Taiwan, Japan, and India (2007–2014). Int J Environ Res Public Health. 2016;13:79.

58. Markman M. Managing taxane toxicities. Support Care Cancer. 2003;11:144–7.

59. Rivera NP, Kris MG, Gralla RJ. Syndrome of acute dyspnea related to combined mitomycin plus vinca alkaloid chemotherapy. Am J Clin Oncol. 1995;18:245–50.

60. Hwang SD, Chung BH, Oh EJ, Choi BS, Park CW, Kim YS, Yang CW. Effect of pretransplant rituximab use on posttransplant clinical outcomes in patients with high panel reactive antibody scores. Nephron. 2015;130:239–44.

61. Voog E, Morschhauser F, Solal-Celigny P. Neutropenia in patients treated with rituximab. N Engl J Med. 2003;348:2691–4; discussion 2691–2694

62. Byrd JC, Peterson BL, Morrison VA, Park K, Jacobson R, Hoke E, Vardiman JW, Rai K, Schiffer CA, Larson RA. Randomized phase 2 study of fludarabine with concurrent versus sequential treatment with rituximab in symptomatic, untreated patients with B-cell chronic lymphocytic leukemia: results from Cancer and Leukemia Group B 9712 (CALGB 9712). Blood. 2003;101:6–14.

63. Hillmen P, Robak T, Janssens A, Babu KG, Kloczko J, Grosicki S, Doubek M, Panagiotidis P, Kimby E, Schuh A, Pettitt AR, Boyd T, Montillo M, Gupta IV, Wright O, Dixon I, Carey JL, Chang CN, Lisby S, McKeown A, Offner F, Investigators

CS. Chlorambucil plus ofatumumab versus chlorambucil alone in previously untreated patients with chronic lymphocytic leukaemia (COMPLE-MENT 1): a randomised, multicentre, open-label phase 3 trial. Lancet. 2015;385:1873–83.

64. Keating MJ, O'Brien S, Albitar M, Lerner S, Plunkett W, Giles F, Andreeff M, Cortes J, Faderl S, Thomas D, Koller C, Wierda W, Detry MA, Lynn A, Kantarjian H. Early results of a chemoimmunotherapy regimen of fludarabine, cyclophosphamide, and rituximab as initial therapy for chronic lymphocytic leukemia. J Clin Oncol. 2005;23:4079–88.

65. Martin SI, Marty FM, Fiumara K, Treon SP, Gribben JG, Baden LR. Infectious complications associated with alemtuzumab use for lymphoproliferative disorders. Clin Infect Dis. 2006;43:16–24.

66. Garcia CA, Wu S. Attributable risk of infection to mTOR inhibitors everolimus and temsirolimus in the treatment of cancer. Cancer Investig. 2016;34:521–30.

67. Zelenetz AD, Barrientos JC, Brown JR, Coiffier B, Delgado J, Egyed M, Ghia P, Illes A, Jurczak W, Marlton P, Montillo M, Morschhauser F, Pristupa AS, Robak T, Sharman JP, Simpson D, Smolej L, Tausch E, Adewoye AH, Dreiling LK, Kim Y, Stilgenbauer S, Hillmen P. Idelalisib or placebo in combination with bendamustine and rituximab in patients with relapsed or refractory chronic lymphocytic leukaemia: interim results from a phase 3, randomised, double-blind, placebo-controlled trial. Lancet Oncol. 2017;18:297–311.

68. O'Brien SM, Lamanna N, Kipps TJ, Flinn I, Zelenetz AD, Burger JA, Keating M, Mitra S, Holes L, Yu AS, Johnson DM, Miller LL, Kim Y, Dansey RD, Dubowy RL, Coutre SE. A phase 2 study of idelalisib plus rituximab in treatment-naive older patients with chronic lymphocytic leukemia. Blood. 2015;126:2686–94.

69. Jones JA, Robak T, Brown JR, Awan FT, Badoux X, Coutre S, Loscertales J, Taylor K, Vandenberghe E, Wach M, Wagner-Johnston N, Ysebaert L, Dreiling L, Dubowy R, Xing G, Flinn IW, Owen C. Efficacy and safety of idelalisib in combination with ofatumumab for previously treated chronic lymphocytic leukaemia: an open-label, randomised phase 3 trial. Lancet Haematol. 2017;4:e114–26.

70. Stilgenbauer S, Eichhorst B, Schetelig J, Coutre S, Seymour JF, Munir T, Puvvada SD, Wendtner CM, Roberts AW, Jurczak W, Mulligan SP, Bottcher S, Mobasher M, Zhu M, Desai M, Chyla B, Verdugo M, Enschede SH, Cerri E, Humerickhouse R, Gordon G, Hallek M, Wierda WG. Venetoclax in relapsed or refractory chronic lymphocytic leukaemia with 17p deletion: a multicentre, open-label, phase 2 study. Lancet Oncol. 2016;17:768–78.

71. Wysham NG, Sullivan DR, Allada G. An opportunistic infection associated with ruxolitinib, a novel janus kinase 1,2 inhibitor. Chest. 2013;143:1478–9.

72. Palandri F, Polverelli N, Breccia M, Nicolino B, Vitolo U, Alimena G, Cavo M, Vianelli N, Benevolo G. Safety and efficacy of ruxolitinib in myelofibrosis

patients without splenomegaly. Br J Haematol. 2016;174:160–2.

73. Heine A, Brossart P, Wolf D. Ruxolitinib is a potent immunosuppressive compound: is it time for anti-infective prophylaxis? Blood. 2013;122:3843–4.

74. Offidani M, Corvatta L, Polloni C, Gentili S, Brioni A, Visani G, Galieni P, Brunori M, Alesiani F, Catarini M, Centurioni R, Samori A, Blasi N, Ferranti M, Fraticelli P, Mele A, Rizzi R, Larocca F, Leoni P. Infectious complications in patients with multiple myeloma treated with new drug combinations containing thalidomide. Leuk Lymphoma. 2011;52:776–85.

75. Teh BW, Harrison SJ, Worth LJ, Thursky KA, Slavin MA. Infection risk with immunomodulatory and proteasome inhibitor-based therapies across treatment phases for multiple myeloma: a systematic review and meta-analysis. Eur J Cancer. 2016;67:21–37.

76. Jouanguy E, Altare F, Lamhamedi S, Revy P, Emile JF, Newport M, Levin M, Blanche S, Seboun E, Fischer A, Casanova JL. Interferon-gamma-receptor deficiency in an infant with fatal bacille Calmette-Guerin infection. N Engl J Med. 1996;335:1956–61.

77. Keane J, Gershon S, Wise RP, Mirabile-Levens E, Kasznica J, Schwieterman WD, Siegel JN, Braun MM. Tuberculosis associated with infliximab, a tumor necrosis factor alpha-neutralizing agent. N Engl J Med. 2001;345:1098–104.

78. Sakai S, Kauffman KD, Sallin MA, Sharpe AH, Young HA, Ganusov VV, Barber DL. CD4 T cell-derived IFN-gamma plays a minimal role in control of pulmonary *Mycobacterium tuberculosis* infection and must be actively repressed by PD-1 to prevent lethal disease. PLoS Pathog. 2016;12:e1005667.

79. Hadjiliadis D, Govert JA. Methemoglobinemia after infusion of ifosfamide chemotherapy: first report of a potentially serious adverse reaction related to ifosfamide. Chest. 2000;118:1208–10.

80. Abdel-Rahman O, Fouad M. Risk of pneumonitis in cancer patients treated with immune checkpoint inhibitors: a meta-analysis. Ther Adv Respir Dis. 2016;10:183–93.

81. Zimmer L, Goldinger SM, Hofmann L, Loquai C, Ugurel S, Thomas I, Schmidgen MI, Gutzmer R, Utikal JS, Goppner D, Hassel JC, Meier F, Tietze JK, Forschner A, Weishaupt C, Leverkus M, Wahl R, Dietrich U, Garbe C, Kirchberger MC, Eigentler T, Berking C, Gesierich A, Krackhardt AM, Schadendorf D, Schuler G, Dummer R, Heinzerling LM. Neurological, respiratory, musculoskeletal, cardiac and ocular side-effects of anti-PD-1 therapy. Eur J Cancer. 2016;60:210–25.

82. Nishino M, Giobbie-Hurder A, Hatabu H, Ramaiya NH, Hodi FS. Incidence of programmed cell death 1 inhibitor-related pneumonitis in patients with advanced cancer: a systematic review and meta-analysis. JAMA Oncol. 2016;2:1607–16.

83. Eigentler TK, Hassel JC, Berking C, Aberle J, Bachmann O, Grunwald V, Kahler KC, Loquai C,

Reinmuth N, Steins M, Zimmer L, Sendl A, Gutzmer R. Diagnosis, monitoring and management of immune-related adverse drug reactions of anti-PD-1 antibody therapy. Cancer Treat Rev. 2016;45:7–18.

84. Nishino M, Brais LK, Brooks NV, Hatabu H, Kulke MH, Ramaiya NH. Drug-related pneumonitis during mammalian target of rapamycin inhibitor therapy in patients with neuroendocrine tumors: a radiographic pattern-based approach. Eur J Cancer. 2016;53:163–70.

85. Nishino M, Chambers ES, Chong CR, Ramaiya NH, Gray SW, Marcoux JP, Hatabu H, Janne PA, Hodi FS, Awad MM. Anti-PD-1 inhibitor-related pneumonitis in non-small cell lung cancer. Cancer Immunol Res. 2016;4:289–93.

86. Nishino M, Ramaiya NH, Awad MM, Sholl LM, Maattala JA, Taibi M, Hatabu H, Ott PA, Armand PF, Hodi FS. PD-1 inhibitor-related pneumonitis in advanced cancer patients: radiographic patterns and clinical course. Clin Cancer Res. 2016;22:6051–60.

87. Balaji A, Verde F, Suresh K, Naidoo J. Pneumonitis from anti-PD-1/PD-L1 therapy. Oncology (Williston Park). 2017;31:739–46, 754

88. Nishino M, Hatabu H. Programmed death-1/programmed death ligand-1 inhibitor-related pneumonitis and radiographic patterns. J Clin Oncol. 2017;35:1628–9.

89. Lomax AJ, McGuire HM, McNeil C, Choi CJ, Hersey P, Karikios D, Shannon K, van Hal S, Carr U, Crotty A, Gupta SK, Hollingsworth J, Kim H, Fazekas de St Groth B, McGill N. Immunotherapy-induced sarcoidosis in patients with melanoma treated with PD-1 checkpoint inhibitors: case series and immunophenotypic analysis. Int J Rheum Dis. 2017;20:1277–85.

90. Berthod G, Lazor R, Letovanec I, Romano E, Noirez L, Mazza Stalder J, Speiser DE, Peters S, Michielin O. Pulmonary sarcoid-like granulomatosis induced by ipilimumab. J Clin Oncol. 2012;30: e156–9.

91. Gounant V, Brosseau S, Naltet C, Opsomer MA, Antoine M, Danel C, Khalil A, Cadranel J, Zalcman G. Nivolumab-induced organizing pneumonitis in a patient with lung sarcomatoid carcinoma. Lung Cancer. 2016;99:162–5.

92. Kolla BC, Patel MR. Recurrent pleural effusions and cardiac tamponade as possible manifestations of pseudoprogression associated with nivolumab therapy- a report of two cases. J Immunother Cancer. 2016;4:80.

93. Chiou VL, Burotto M. Pseudoprogression and immune-related response in solid tumors. J Clin Oncol. 2015;33:3541–3.

94. Champiat S, Lambotte O, Barreau E, Belkhir R, Berdelou A, Carbonnel F, Cauquil C, Chanson P, Collins M, Durrbach A, Ederhy S, Feuillet S, Francois H, Lazarovici J, Le Pavec J, De Martin E, Mateus C, Michot JM, Samuel D, Soria JC, Robert C, Eggermont A, Marabelle A. Management of immune

checkpoint blockade dysimmune toxicities: a collaborative position paper. Ann Oncol. 2016;27:559–74.

95. Kluetz PG, Chingos DT, Basch EM, Mitchell SA. Patient-reported outcomes in cancer clinical trials: measuring symptomatic adverse events with the National Cancer Institute's patient-reported outcomes version of the common terminology criteria for adverse events (PRO-CTCAE). Am Soc Clin Oncol Educ Book. 2016;35:67–73.

96. Barrett DM, Teachey DT, Grupp SA. Toxicity management for patients receiving novel T-cell engaging therapies. Curr Opin Pediatr. 2014;26:43–9.

97. Grupp SA, Kalos M, Barrett D, Aplenc R, Porter DL, Rheingold SR, Teachey DT, Chew A, Hauck B, Wright JF, Milone MC, Levine BL, June CH. Chimeric antigen receptor-modified T cells for acute lymphoid leukemia. N Engl J Med. 2013;368:1509–18.

98. Barrett DM, Singh N, Porter DL, Grupp SA, June CH. Chimeric antigen receptor therapy for cancer. Annu Rev Med. 2014;65:333–47.

99. Maude SL, Frey N, Shaw PA, Aplenc R, Barrett DM, Bunin NJ, Chew A, Gonzalez VE, Zheng Z, Lacey SF, Mahnke YD, Melenhorst JJ, Rheingold SR, Shen A, Teachey DT, Levine BL, June CH, Porter DL, Grupp SA. Chimeric antigen receptor T cells for sustained remissions in leukemia. N Engl J Med. 2014;371:1507–17.

100. Maude SL, Teachey DT, Porter DL, Grupp SA. CD19-targeted chimeric antigen receptor T-cell therapy for acute lymphoblastic leukemia. Blood. 2015;125:4017–23.

101. Porter DL, Levine BL, Kalos M, Bagg A, June CH. Chimeric antigen receptor-modified T cells in chronic lymphoid leukemia. N Engl J Med. 2011;365:725–33.

102. Brentjens RJ, Riviere I, Park JH, Davila ML, Wang X, Stefanski J, Taylor C, Yeh R, Bartido S, Borquez-Ojeda O, Olszewska M, Bernal Y, Pegram H, Przybylowski M, Hollyman D, Usachenko Y, Pirraglia D, Hosey J, Santos E, Halton E, Maslak P, Scheinberg D, Jurcic J, Heaney M, Heller G, Frattini M, Sadelain M. Safety and persistence of adoptively transferred autologous CD19-targeted T cells in patients with relapsed or chemotherapy refractory B-cell leukemias. Blood. 2011;118:4817–28.

103. Fitzgerald JC, Weiss SL, Maude SL, Barrett DM, Lacey SF, Melenhorst JJ, Shaw P, Berg RA, June CH, Porter DL, Frey NV, Grupp SA, Teachey DT. Cytokine release syndrome after chimeric antigen receptor T cell therapy for acute lymphoblastic leukemia. Crit Care Med. 2017;45:e124–31.

104. Teachey DT, Rheingold SR, Maude SL, Zugmaier G, Barrett DM, Seif AE, Nichols KE, Suppa EK, Kalos M, Berg RA, Fitzgerald JC, Aplenc R, Gore L, Grupp SA. Cytokine release syndrome after blinatumomab treatment related to abnormal macrophage activation and ameliorated with cytokine-directed therapy. Blood. 2013;121:5154–7.

105. Marks LB, Yu X, Vujaskovic Z, Small W Jr, Folz R, Anscher MS. Radiation-induced lung injury. Semin Radiat Oncol. 2003;13:333–45.

106. Movsas B, Raffin TA, Epstein AH, Link CJ Jr. Pulmonary radiation injury. Chest. 1997;111:1061–76.

107. Cornelissen R, Senan S, Antonisse IE, Liem H, Tan YK, Rudolphus A, Aerts JG. Bronchiolitis obliterans organizing pneumonia (BOOP) after thoracic radiotherapy for breast carcinoma. Radiat Oncol. 2007;2:1–5.

108. Schweitzer V, Juillard G, Bajada C. Radiation recall dermatitis and pneumonitis in a patient treated with paclitaxel. Cancer. 1995;76:1069–72.

109. Schwarte S, Wagner K, Karstens JH, Bremer M. Radiation recall pneumonitis induced by gemcitabine. Strahlenther Onkol. 2007;183:215–7.

110. Ding X, Ji W, Li J, Zhang X, Wang L. Radiation recall pneumonitis induced by chemotherapy after thoracic radiotherapy for lung cancer. Radiat Oncol. 2011;6:1–6.

111. Cottin V, Frognier R, Monnot H, Levy A, DeVuyst P, Cordier JF, Pulmonaires. GdEedRslMO. Chronic eosinophilic pneumonia after radiation therapy for breast cancer. Eur Respir J. 2004;23:9–13.

112. Hagelstein V, Ortland I, Wilmer A, Mitchell SA, Jaehde U. Validation of the German patient-reported outcomes version of the common terminology criteria for adverse events (PRO-CTCAE). Ann Oncol. 2016;27:2294–9.

113. Gafter-Gvili A, Gurion R, Raanani P, Shpilberg O, Vidal L. Bendamustine-associated infections-systematic review and meta-analysis of randomized controlled trials. Hematol Oncol. 2017;35(4):424–431. https://www.ncbi.nlm.nih.gov/pubmed/27734524.

114. Ravandi F, O'Brien S. Infections associated with purine analogs and monoclonal antibodies.Blood Rev. 2005;19(5):253–73. https://www.ncbi.nlm.nih.gov/pubmed/15963834.

115. Dias AL, Jain D. Ibrutinib: a new frontier in the treatment of chronic lymphocytic leukemia by Bruton's tyrosine kinase inhibition. Cardiovasc Hematol Agents Med Chem. 2013;11(4):265–71. https://www.ncbi.nlm.nih.gov/pubmed/24433470.

116. Teh BW, Harrison SJ, Worth LJ, Thursky KA, Slavin MA. Infection risk with immunomodulatory and proteasome inhibitor-based therapies across treatment phases for multiple myeloma: A systematic review and meta-analysis. Eur J Cancer. 2016;67:21–37. https://doi.org/10.1016/j.ejca.2016.07.025. https://www.ncbi.nlm.nih.gov/pubmed/27592069.

Acute Respiratory Distress Syndrome in Cancer Patients

37

Alisha Y. Young and Vickie R. Shannon

Contents

Introduction 558

Definition and Pathogenesis of ALI and ARDS 558

Pathophysiology and Pathogenesis of ALI/ARDS 559

Etiology and Predisposing Factors of ARDS in the Cancer Patient 562

Primary and Secondary Triggers of ALI/ARDS in the Cancer Patient 565
Pneumonia/Opportunistic Infections 565
Drug-Induced Acute Lung Injury (ALI)/ARDS 566
Postoperative ARDS 567
ALI/ARDS Post Hematopoietic Stem Cell Transplant 568
ALI/ARDS Due to Pulmonary Spread of Tumor: Lymphangitic Carcinomatosis
and Pulmonary Leukostasis 570

Clinical Presentation and Diagnostic Workup of ALI/ARDS 571

Cancer-Related ALI/ARDS: Outcomes and Treatment 572

Treatment 573
Pharmacologic Therapies 573
Noninvasive and Invasive Ventilation 574
Sedation and Neuromuscular Blockade 576

Conclusion 576

References 577

A. Y. Young
Department of Pulmonary Medicine, University of Texas at McGovern Medical School, Houston, TX, USA

V. R. Shannon (✉)
Department of Pulmonary Medicine, Division of Internal Medicine, The University of Texas at MD Anderson Cancer Center, Houston, TX, USA
e-mail: vshannon@mdanderson.org

Abstract

Acute respiratory distress syndrome (ARDS) is a heterogeneous form of acute, diffuse lung injury that is characterized by dysregulated inflammation, increased alveolar-capillary interface permeability, and non-cardiogenic pulmonary edema. In the general population, the incidence and mortality associated with ARDS over the last two decades have steadily declined in parallel with optimized approaches

© Springer Nature Switzerland AG 2020
J. L. Nates, K. J. Price (eds.), *Oncologic Critical Care*,
https://doi.org/10.1007/978-3-319-74588-6_48

to pneumonia and other underlying causes of ARDS as well as increased utilization of multimodal treatment strategies that include lung-protective ventilation. In the cancer settings, significant declines in the incidence and mortality of ARDS over the past two decades have also been reported, although these rates remain significantly higher than those in the general population. Epidemiologic studies identify infection, including disseminated fungal pneumonias, as a major underlying cause of ARDS in the cancer setting. More than half of cancer patients who develop ARDS will not survive to hospital discharge. Those who do survive often face a protracted and often incomplete recovery, resulting in significant long-term physical, psychological, and cognitive sequelae. The residual organ dysfunction and poor functional status after ARDS may delay or preclude subsequent cancer treatments. As such, close collaboration between the critical care physicians and oncology team is essential in identifying and reversing the underlying causes and optimizing treatments for cancer patients with ARDS. This chapter reviews the diagnosis and common causes of ARDS in cancer and gives an update on the general management principles for cancer patients with ARDS in the ICU.

Keywords
Acute respiratory distress syndrome · Malignancy · Pulmonary · Lung injury · Pneumonia · Mechanic ventilation · Intensive care unit

Introduction

Acute respiratory distress syndrome (ARDS) is a heterogeneous form of acute, diffuse lung injury that is characterized by dysregulated inflammation, increased alveolar-capillary interface permeability, and non-cardiogenic pulmonary edema. In the general population, the incidence and mortality associated with ARDS over the last two decades have steadily declined in parallel with optimized approaches to pneumonia and other underlying

causes of ARDS as well as increased utilization of multimodal treatment strategies that include lung-protective ventilation. In the cancer setting, significant declines in the incidence and mortality of ARDS have also been reported, although these rates remain significantly higher than those in the general population. Epidemiologic studies identify infection, including disseminated fungal pneumonias as a major underlying cause if ARDS in the cancer setting. More than half of cancer patients who develop ARDS will not survive to hospital discharge. Those who do survive often face a protracted and frequently incomplete recovery, resulting in significant long-term physical, psychological, and cognitive sequelae. The residual organ dysfunction and poor functional status after ARDS may delay or preclude subsequent cancer treatments. As such, close collaboration between the critical care physicians and oncology team is essential in identifying and reversing the underlying causes and optimizing treatments for cancer patients with ARDS.

Definition and Pathogenesis of ALI and ARDS

In 1965, Asbaugh and colleagues described 12 adult patients who developed diffuse pulmonary opacities, refractory hypoxemia, tachypnea, and tachycardia following acute medical illness or surgical trauma. At autopsy, prominent hyaline membranes lining the alveoli were seen. This syndrome was initially coined as adult respiratory distress syndrome and later renamed acute respiratory distress syndrome (ARDS) to emphasize the acuity of the syndrome and to include pediatric-aged patients with similar clinical and histopathologic findings [1].

In its original definition, the diagnosis of ARDS was established based on findings of a rapidly progressive respiratory failure that evolves over a 2-day period and results in respiratory distress, severe arterial hypoxemia, and the need for mechanical ventilation. Multiple definitions of ARDS have been proposed since the original description by Asbaugh. In 1994, the American-European Consensus Conference

(AECC) expanded the definition to include an arterial partial pressure of oxygen to fraction of inspired oxygen [PaO_2/FIO_2] of ≤ 200 mm Hg) with bilateral infiltrates on frontal chest radiograph, and no evidence of left atrial hypertension. The AECC also recognized a less severe form ARDS, referred to as acute lung injury (ALI), which used similar ARDS criteria but with milder hypoxemia ($PaO_2/FIO_2 < 300$ mm Hg) [2]. Although this definition of ARDS was widely adopted, criteria lacked explicit definitions for "acute." Furthermore, interobserver interpretations of chest radiographs were highly variable, and ventilator settings such as PEEP and/or FIO_2 render PaO_2/FIO_2 ratios inconsistent. Spurred by issues regarding the lack of a clear definition of ARDS, experts from the European Society of Intensive Care Medicine (ESICM), joined by the American Thoracic Society (ATS) and the Society of Critical Care Medicine (SCCM), were empaneled to create an ARDS definition task force [3]. Out of these meetings emerged the 2012 Berlin definition of ARDS. This definition defines "acute" as the at-risk period for the development of ARDS, which was designated as within 7 days of the original insult. The experts also proposed three mutually exclusive categories of ARDS, based on the degree of hypoxemia: mild (200 mmHg$>PaO_2/FIO_2 < 300$ mmHg), moderate (100 mmHg-$PaO_2/FIO_2 < 200$ mmHg), and severe ($PaO_2/FIO_2 < 100$ mmHg). The panel retained the requirements of bilateral pulmonary infiltrates consistent with pulmonary edema as defining criteria for ARDS and added chest computed tomography (CT) as a potential imaging tool. Comparisons of ARDS definitions based on AECC and Berlin criteria are shown in Table 1. An expanded definition of ARDS, proposed by Murray, classifies patients according to the severity of lung injury, associated clinical disorder(s), and the presence of nonpulmonary organ dysfunction. In this definition, lung injury severity is stratified according to the extent of abnormalities on chest radiographs, degree of hypoxemia, respiratory system compliance, and PEEP requirements, using the lung injury scoring system [4].

Pathophysiology and Pathogenesis of ALI/ARDS

ALI/ARDS is marked by three sequential phases, each characterized by different clinical, histopathologic, and radiographic manifestations. In the acute exudative phase, damage to the pulmonary epithelial and endothelial surfaces triggers a cascade of events in the evolution of ALI/ARDS. The loss of integrity of the epithelial and endothelial barriers that ensues results in extravasation of a protein-rich edema fluid into the alveolar space. This form of increased permeability pulmonary edema is commonly referred to as primary or non-cardiogenic pulmonary edema and has as its histopathologic hallmark the accumulation of a proteinaceous fluid in the interstitium as a result of breach of the integrity of the alveolar and microvascular barriers within the lungs. Inflammatory cells, including neutrophils, red blood cells, platelets, and fibrin, are also prominent features of the edema fluid which flood alveoli, creating large areas of ventilation-perfusion inequality or shunt formation. Widespread but patchy areas of destruction to alveolar type I epithelial cells, which are exquisitely sensitive to this type of lung injury, are a common early histologic finding. Type II pneumocytes are also injured, which results in disruption of normal epithelial ion transport activity, reduced surfactant turnover, and, consequently, reduced clearance of edema fluid from the airway. Loss of normal surfactant activity by activated polymorphonuclear neutrophils and plasma proteins also contributes to microatelectasis and shunt formation. Impaired epithelial cell ion transport further compounds efficient clearance of edema fluid from the distal airways. The precipitated plasma proteins, fibrin, and necrotic debris form hyaline membranes. Hyaline membranes along with marked hyperplasia of cytologically bizarre and pleomorphic type II pneumocytes are key components of diffuse alveolar damage (DAD), the histopathologic hallmark of ARDS [2, 5–8]. These physiologic changes promote decreased lung compliance and subsequent respiratory failure, characterized physiologically by severe ventilation/perfusion (V/Q) mismatching and marked refractory hypoxemia. The

Table 1 Evolution of ALI/DADS definition

	Ashbaugh	American-European Consensus Conference (AECC)	Berlin
Year	1967	1994	2012
ARDS description	Rapidly progressive respiratory failure associated with noncardiogenic pulmonary edema (permeability pulmonary edema) and severe hypoxemia; PCW < 18 mm Hg or no clinical evidence of left atrial hypertension	Rapidly progressive respiratory failure associated with noncardiogenic pulmonary edema (permeability pulmonary edema) and severe hypoxemia; PCW measurements not required; hydrostatic edema excluded via other clinical clues	Rapidly progressive respiratory failure not explained by cardiac failure or volume overload and occurring within 1 week of the triggering event
Definition of "Acute"	"Acute" without further definition	"Acute" without further definition	Onset within 1 week of a known clinical insult or new or worsening respiratory symptoms
ARDS stratification	None specified	Any patient with PaO_2/FIO_2 <200	Three mutually exclusive subgroups identified based on PaO_2/FIO_2 and PEEP >5 mm Hg
			Mild: 200 mmHg>PaO_2/FIO_2<300 mmHg
			Moderate: 100 mmHgPaO_2/FIO_2<200 mmHg
			Severe: PaO_2/FIO_2<100 mmHg
Oxygen/ PEEP specifications	None specified, other than hypoxemia requiring oxygenation	Arterial partial pressure of oxygen to fraction of inspired oxygen PaO_2/FIO_2 <200 mm Hg), regardless of PEEP	Stratified according to PEEP or CPAP requirements: mild, PEEP or CPAP <5 mmHg; moderate or severe, PEEP >5 cm H_2O
Risk factors	None specified	None specified	Pneumonia, sepsis, trauma pancreatitis; echocardiography recommended to exclude hydrostatic edema if no risk factor identified
ALI designation	ALI not recognized	Same as ARDS except PaO_2/FIO_2<300 mm Hg	ALI category removed from definition

ALI acute lung injury, *PaO₂* partial pressure of oxygen, *FIO₂* fraction of inspired oxygen, *PEEP* positive end-expiratory pressure

inhomogeneous lung injury pattern is marked by perfused alveoli which are not adequately ventilated (physiologic shunt), while others are ventilated but not adequately perfused (dead space).

Increased permeability pulmonary edema may also occur in the absence of DAD and is referred to as capillary leak syndrome. In the cancer setting, this type of pulmonary edema typically occurs following the administration of cytokines such as IL_2 and TNF, which disrupt the capillary endothelial cell integrity [9]. Both of these drugs may also

cause direct toxicity to the myocardium, resulting in mixed or overlap edema associated with normal and increased permeability etiologies. Neurogenic and re-expansion pulmonary edema represent two other causes of mixed edema, which are frequently observed in the cancer setting.

Lung injury may resolve after the exudative stage or progress through the proliferative phase to the final stage of fibrosing alveolitis. The proliferative phase of ARDS typically occurs 7–14 days after the triggering insult. During this phase, exuberant proliferation of type II cells, fibroblasts, and inflammatory cells and regeneration of epithelial cells occur in an attempt to reestablish alveolar barrier function and repair the damaged alveolar structures. Therapeutic measures, such as oxygen toxicity, may promote further lung injury during this phase of ARDS. The proliferative phase is marked by minimal edema fluid and abnormalities of coagulation, which may give rise to extensive microvascular microthrombi and disruption of the pulmonary-capillary bed. Subsequent elevations in pulmonary vascular resistance may be significant enough to induce cor pulmonale in some patients. An extensive neutrophil-predominant alveolitis on BAL fluid and histopathologic findings of bizarre-shaped cuboidal type II alveolar cells are common findings [10]. Fever, leukocytosis, diminished systemic vascular resistance, and diffuse areas of alveolar and interstitial consolidation on chest radiographs may mimic clinical infection/sepsis during this phase, although an infectious cause is rarely found.

The final fibrotic phase is heralded by extensive collagen deposition into the alveolar, vascular, and interstitial beds, which irreversibly obliterate the airspace and small vessels, and further promotes dead space ventilation, shunt formation, and pulmonary hypertension refractory hypoxemia [2, 11].

Activation of the innate immune response, including neutrophils, complement and humoral inflammatory mediators, is thought to play a key role in the development of DAD in ARDS. This leads to a cascade of events, including the production of the Toll-like receptors on lung epithelial cells and activation of neutrophils and alveolar macrophages. The activated alveolar macrophages trigger additional immune responses, including cytokine production, which damage the alveolar-capillary interface and cause leakage of proteinaceous fluid into the alveoli, leading to the clinical manifestations of ARDS. Earlier studies suggested that neutrophilic inflammation was central to the development of ARDS. However, ARDS may develop in patients with profound neutropenia. Furthermore, stimulation of neutrophil production with granulocyte colony-stimulating factor does not appear to trigger or worsen ARDS in most patients. These observations imply that neutrophilic inflammation occurs as a consequence rather than a cause of ARDS and suggest that additional mechanisms of acute lung injury may be important. A role for pro-inflammatory cytokines in the initiation and/or amplification of the inflammatory response in ARDS is suggested by increased levels of macrophage inhibitory factor, tumor necrosis factor (TNF-α), and interleukin-8 (IL-8) in the airways of patients with lung injury. Anti-inflammatory activities of tumor necrosis factor receptor (TNFr), interleukin-1 receptor antagonist (IL-1r), interleukin-10 (IL-10), and interleukin-11 (IL-11) have been shown to modulate the development of ALI/ARDS. Alterations in the delicate balance between pro- and anti-inflammatory cytokines in the airway likely play a critical role in ALI/ARDS development and offer therapeutic strategies in the management of this disorder [4, 10, 12]. Accumulating evidence increasingly implicates platelet activation in ARDS pathogenesis and suggests that these cells are pivotal in a host of inflammatory effects that contribute to ARDS development, including increased endothelial barrier permeability and augmented neutrophil recruitment into the airways [13]. These observations have laid the groundwork for ongoing studies to investigate the role of antiplatelet therapy in ARDS [14–16].

The majority of patients with clinical risk factors for ARDS do not develop ARDS. Thus, genetic susceptibility is thought to play a key role in the pathogenesis of this disorder. More than 40 candidate genes have been linked to ARDS risk, including the genes encoding angiotensin-converting enzyme (ACE), IL-10, tumor necrosis factor (TNF), vascular endothelial growth factor (VEGF), and LRRCI6A [17, 18]. Several molecular and immune biomarkers are being developed to identify distinct ARDS phenotypes. Although many of these biomarkers are currently in experimental stages of development, they hold promise in their potential for risk stratification of patients for ARDS and also in their ability to predict clinical outcomes [19–21]. For example, higher plasma levels of inflammatory biomarkers have been demonstrated in patients with a hyperinflammatory ARDS phenotype. This subgroup of patients may have a higher prevalence of sepsis and vasopressor use and require longer periods on the ventilator than their non-hyperinflammatory counterparts [22]. Elevated levels of specific inflammatory cytokines, such as TNF-α, IL-1B, IL-6, and IL-8, have been shown to correlate with lung injury severity and may predict unfavorable outcomes, particularly among patients in which elevated biomarkers occur early and persist throughout the course of ARDS [22, 23].

Etiology and Predisposing Factors of ARDS in the Cancer Patient

Cancer patients are susceptible to a variety of overlapping ARDS risk factors including primary lung insults (pneumonia, aspiration, surgical and nonsurgical chest and/or lung trauma) and secondary sources of injury (drug toxicity, polytrauma, pancreatitis, hypertransfusion, sepsis, or septic shock that originates from extrapulmonary infections or noninfectious etiologies) (Table 2). For example, cancer-related primary insults, such as increased susceptibility to pneumonia or the propensity to aspirate, may be compounded by a variety of malignancy-related secondary issues, including toxicity from pneumotoxic drugs, blood/blood product transfusions, or sepsis. Major categories of risk factors that account for most of the reported cases of ALI/ARDS include infection, sepsis, chemotherapeutic agents (including molecular targeted therapies and immune-modulating agents), trauma, and aspiration of gastric contents. Radiation toxicity, tumor lysis syndrome, and leukoagglutinin reactions have also been linked to ARDS in patients with cancer. These conditions may act synergistically to increase the risk of ALI/ARDS. In a study by Pepe and colleagues, ARDS risk increased by 3.2-fold among patients with three or more risk factors versus a single risk factor (85% versus 25%) [24]. Traditional widely held beliefs purported that specific lung injury triggers have no bearing on clinical expression of ARDS or disease progression, which are primarily dictated by the severity of the lung insult and efficacy of the therapeutic intervention. Recent studies have questioned the validity of support for concepts that suggest that the clinical and histopathologic features of ARDS are identical, regardless of etiology. These investigations have identified a differential effect of ARDS on lung compliance and responsiveness to positive end-expiratory pressures (PEEP), with more severe reductions in compliance and decreased responsiveness to PEEP, ventilatory recruitment maneuvers, prone positioning, and other adjunctive therapies among patients with primary causes of ARDS versus extrapulmonary (secondary) etiologies [25, 26]. Reduced respiratory compliance and response to positive end-expiratory pressure (PEEP) may correlate with a higher prevalence of lung consolidation in patients with primary ARDS as opposed to prevalent edema and alveolar collapse associated with secondary forms of the disease [27]. This distinction may be clinically important. The concept of ARDS as a heterogeneous disorder may offer more precise clinical management. However, frequent overlapping pathogenetic mechanisms and morphologic alterations often render distinctions between primary and secondary forms of ARDS imprecise, and the concept of treatment approaches based on etiology of ARDS remains controversial.

Severe ARDS represents a classic example of lung failure whereby associated ventilation/perfusion abnormalities, shunts, or alterations of alveolar-capillary diffusion lead to pure hypoxia, at least in its early stages. By contrast, primary failure of alveolar ventilation, or pump failure, leads to severe hypercapnia and acidosis with only mild hypoxemia (Fig. 1). Impairments to any component of the ventilatory pump, including the respiratory muscles, central nervous system, and peripheral nervous systems, may lead to pump failure. Cancer and its treatment may adversely affect all components of the respiratory pump. For example, increased resistance loads due to tumors within the lung may cause intrinsic or extrinsic obstruction of the large airways, bronchospasm associated with certain chemotherapeutic agents, or concomitant COPD, and obstructive sleep apnea associated with head and neck tumors are

Table 2 Common triggers of ALI/ARDS in cancer

	Clinical clues/risk factors	Clinical features and imaging findings	Diagnostic testing	Treatment
Infection/ pneumonia	Productive cough, pleuritic pain, fever, chills, shortness of breath	Pulmonary infiltrates may be lobar, multi-lobar, diffuse, or bilateral areas of consolidation and/or ground-glass change. Air bronchograms may be seen	Gram stain/cultures obtained on sputum or bronchoscopically; blood cultures; WBC may be elevated, normal, or decreased	Antibiotics, supportive care, ventilatory support, as indicated
Aspiration	Witnessed aspiration or high risk for aspiration; bronchial erythema, food, lipid-laden macrophages seen on bronchoscopy; low-grade fever	Infiltrates on chest imaging usually involving dependent pulmonary segments	Presumptive diagnosis with negative cultures	Supportive, ventilatory support; supplemental oxygen, antibiotics
Pancreatitis	Presence of risk factors – gallstones, drugs/alcohol, viral infection. Persistent abdominal pain, nausea/vomiting; elevated amylase and lipase, with or without abnormal imaging	Dyspnea due to diaphragmatic inflammation/ARDS; unexplained hypotension (5–10%); small pleural effusions	Elevated lipase, amylase	Supportive; IV fluid resuscitation, antibiotics, ventilatory support, oxygen, vasopressor support, dietary modifications, remove offending drugs
TRALI	History of transfused blood products within 6 h of clinical signs/symptoms: dyspnea, hypoxemia, fever, hypotension, cyanosis	Bilateral pulmonary infiltrates with normal cardiac silhouette	Diagnosis of exclusion; infiltrates, hypoxemia occurring within 6 h of blood/blood product transfusion that meets criteria for ARDS is designated transfusion-related ARDS; exclude hemolytic transfusion reactions	Supportive: oxygen supplementation, noninvasive respiratory support with continuous positive airway pressure (CPAP) or bi-level positive airway pressure (BiPAP) may be sufficient in less severe cases, endotracheal intubation with invasive mechanical ventilation if severe
Sepsis/ shock	Fever, hypotension, lactic acidosis, DIC; infectious source not identified in all cases; CRP >2 SD above normal; plasma prolactin >2 SD above normal; thrombocytopenia; CBC may demonstrate leukocytosis, leukopenia, or normal WBC with bandemia	Signs/symptoms of organ damage: nephritis, transaminitis, adrenal insufficiency, altered mental status	Appropriate clinical context and positive cultures	Supportive; IV fluid resuscitation, antibiotics, ventilatory support, oxygen, vasopressor support
HSCT	History of HSCT	Variable, diffuse infiltrates, nodules, consolidation; evidence of graft-versus-host disease (allogeneic transplants)	Diagnosis of exclusion	Supportive; antibiotics ventilatory support, oxygen, vasopressor support

(*continued*)

Table 2 (continued)

	Clinical clues/risk factors	Clinical features and imaging findings	Diagnostic testing	Treatment
Drug toxicity	History of exposure to offending agent or radiation; BAL may demonstrate nonspecific findings of predominant lymphocytosis, eosinophils, or foamy macrophages, depending on the suspected culprit	Bilateral subpleural reticulation; ground-glass changes or consolidation	Diagnosis of exclusion, lung biopsy occasionally helpful	Discontinue offending agent; supportive care, antibiotics, ventilatory support, oxygen, vasopressor support
Thoracic surgery	History of surgery, intraoperative ventilation, intraoperative transfusion	Elevated hemidiaphragm due to postoperative diaphragmatic dysfunction; partial/complete opacification of the ipsilateral thorax depending on the extent of resection and time interval postsurgery. Bronchopleural fistula formation with persistent air leak, depending on the type of surgery	Diagnosis of exclusion	Supportive; antibiotics, ventilatory support, oxygen, vasopressor support

ESR erythrocyte sedimentation rate, *CRP* C-reactive protein, *SD* standard deviation

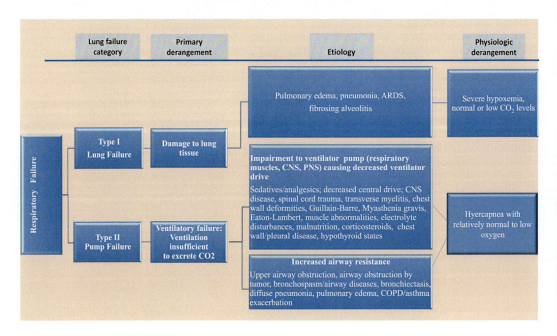

Fig. 1 Lung versus pump failure

common causes of respiratory compromise in patients with cancer. Peripheral muscle impairment owing to electrolyte disturbances, malnutrition, systemic corticosteroids, Eaton-Lambert syndrome, or chest wall disease may also occur. Neurologic and myopathic changes caused by chemo- and immunotherapeutic agents such as the taxanes, carboplatin, ipilimumab, and nivolumab are well described [28–31]. Finally, hypothyroidism, brain-stem lesions, and analgesic and sedating medications may cause profound suppression of the central nervous system and pump failure. In the cancer setting, overlapping causes of lung failure and pump failure often coexist, resulting in intractable hypoxemic, hypercarbic respiratory failure.

Primary and Secondary Triggers of ALI/ARDS in the Cancer Patient

Pneumonia/Opportunistic Infections

Infections are responsible for approximately 90% of all primary and secondary causes of ARDS in the cancer setting (Table 3) [32]. Pneumonia is the most common and potentially lethal form of infection in patients with cancer, complicating nearly 10% of all cancer-related hospital admissions. In patients with hematologic malignancies (HM), rates of pneumonia may exceed 80% and is a leading cause of death, particularly in the setting of hematopoietic stem cell transplantation (HSCT) and acute leukemias [33]. Studies by Azoulay and others have implicated pneumonia as the underlying trigger for ARDS in 66–80% of patients with either solid or hematological malignancies. This compares to an incidence of pneumonia-related ARDS of <60% among patients without cancer [32, 34, 35]. Opportunistic organisms, including invasive *Aspergillus*, pneumocystis pneumonia, and candidemia, are prominent causes of primary and secondary ARDS in cancer, accounting for up to 1/3 of cases [36]. Cancer-related and cancer treatment-related impairments in immune defense largely contribute to the increased vulnerability of these patients to infections and accounts for the disproportionately high incidence of ARDS in cancer. Cytopenias, treatment toxicities, and other immune derangements are frequent causes of recalcitrant pneumonias, particularly among patients with hematologic malignancies and following HSCT [37–39]. Bacterial pneumonia is the leading cause of ARDS in this setting [33]. Opportunistic fungal diseases, including invasive aspergillosis, *Pneumocystis* pneumonia, and systemic candidemia, are increasingly common and account for a disproportionate percentage (31–36%) of pneumonia-related ARDS in immunocompromised patients compared to the 5–10% incidence in immunocompetent patients with ARDS [40, 41]. In addition, profound impairments in cell mediated and humoral immunity are risk factors for pneumonias caused by reactivation of latent viral infections, such as cytomegalovirus, varicella zoster virus, and herpes simplex virus. These infections may lead to ARDS as a sequela of primary pneumonia or disseminated disease, particularly among the immune-suppressed HM/HSCT patients and the subgroup of HSCT patients with graft-versus-host disease. Progression of upper respiratory tract infections, including respiratory syncytial virus, influenza, and parainfluenza virus, leading to ARDS may also occur [42, 43]. Other causes of increased vulnerability to pneumonia in the cancer setting include derangements in lung architecture caused by surgery, radiation or cancer itself, prolonged mechanical ventilation, and swallowing difficulties associated with thoracic tumors, pain, and sedating medications. Finally, repeated exposures to antibiotics and frequent encounters with the healthcare system may promote the development of pneumonias caused by multidrug-resistant pathogens. Once established, these infections may exact an inexorable course, with high associated mortality. Early etiological assessment and initiation of appropriate antimicrobial therapy, along with prompt initiation of critical care, are vital steps in improving outcomes.

In the general patient population, ARDS is thought to complicate 6–7% of all cases of sepsis [44]. Rates of sepsis causing ALI/ARDS in the cancer setting is thought to be much higher, although the true incidence is unknown. Older age, shock, pneumonia, pancreatitis, Acute Physiology and Chronic Health Evaluation II (APACHE II) scores, and volume of fluid resuscitation over the first 6 h of presentation are significant risk factors for among septic patients with ARDS [45]. Rates of sepsis and septic shock caused by Gram-negative organisms, as well as other bacterial, fungal, and viral pneumonias, vary

Table 3 Infectious causes of ARDS

Bacteria	Fungi	Viruses	Parasites
Gram-positive bacteria			
Staphylococcus aureus	*Aspergillus*	Adenovirus	*Giardia lamblia*
Streptococcus pneumoniae	*Pneumocystis jirovecii*	Rhinovirus	*Babesia* spp.
Streptococcus pyogenes	*Candida* spp.	RSV	*Plasmodium* spp.
Nocardia spp.	*Rhizopus* spp.	Influenza A, B	*Strongyloides stercoralis*
Rhodococcus equi	*P. boydii*	Parainfluenza	*Toxoplasma gondii*
Gram-negative bacteria		Cytomegalovirus	
Escherichia coli		Herpes simplex virus	
Nontypeable *Haemophilus influenzae*		Herpes varicella zoster	
Enterobacteriaceae		Coronavirus	
Stenotrophomonas maltophilia		Metapneumovirus	
Serratia marcescens		Echoviruses	
Klebsiella pneumoniae			
Nocardia spp.			
Acinetobacter baumannii complex			
Alcaligenes/Achromobacter spp.			
Neisseria meningitidis			
Proteus spp.			
Pseudomonas spp.			
Chlamydia pneumoniae enterovirus			
Moraxella catarrhalis			
Burkholderia spp.			
Citrobacter spp.			
Enterobacter cloacae			
Listeria sp.			
Atypical bacteria			
Legionella spp.			
Mycoplasma pneumoniae			
Chlamydophila pneumoniae			
Mycobacteria spp.			

broadly in the cancer setting and roughly correlate with the degree of immune suppression.

Drug-Induced Acute Lung Injury (ALI)/ARDS

Estimates regarding the incidence of ARDS attributed to chemotherapy agents are imprecise, as the results depend heavily on individual case reports and competing diagnoses, such as infection, may occur concomitantly with drug-induced ARDS. In addition, many antineoplastic agents are prescribed as components of complex multidrug and multimodality regimens, which renders identification of individual drugs as specific culprits difficult. Although nonspecific pneumonitis and organizing pneumonia are the most frequent histopathologic findings in drug-induced lung injury, acute lung injury with DAD/ARDS has been reported in a small percentage of patients across the spectrum of antineoplastic therapies, including the conventional cytotoxic therapies, molecular targeted therapies, and the immune-modulating agents [46–50]. High supplemental oxygen, given concurrently or sequentially, and concurrent granulocyte-colony-stimulating factor or granulocyte macrophage-colony-stimulating factor (G-CSF, GM-CSF) may potentiate chemotherapy-related ARDS [51, 52]. Hyperoxia and increased ARDS risk has been most frequently reported in bleomycin-exposed patients [51, 53].

Postoperative ARDS

ALI/ARDS is a leading cause of postoperative respiratory failure, with mortality rates approaching 40% in the general population. Mortality rates in the cancer population vary broadly (6–76%), depending on the type of cancer surgery. Thoracic surgeries, in particular intrapericardial or extrapleural pneumonectomy and esophagectomy, confer the highest operative risk for lung injury (Fig. 2). Postoperative acute lung injury in these settings is most often due to pneumonia, pulmonary edema, atelectasis, persistent air leak, bronchopleural fistula, and prolonged mechanical dependence. Nosocomial pneumonias with related acute respiratory failure complicate approximately 20% of thoracic and upper abdominal cancer surgeries with an associated 50% mortality rate [54, 55]. Contributions to postoperative ARDS in cancer are similar to the general population and include aspiration pneumonitis, massive transfusion, shock (septic, hemorrhagic, or anaphylactic), and excessive perioperative fluids. Thoracic surgical resections that involve pneumonectomy, extended surgical manipulation, and single lung ventilation with inherent hyperoxia and volutrauma also confer an increased risk of postoperative ARDS [56]. Few data exist regarding the prevalence of lung injury following lung resection. Most recent series suggest that around 5% of patients develop some degree of lung injury. Those that develop frank ARDS have a poor prognosis compared to those who suffer lesser degrees of damage. The pathogenesis of ALI/ARDS following intrathoracic resection remains unknown. Perioperative fluid overload, increased blood flow through the remaining lung postoperatively, reoxygenation injury, and activation of

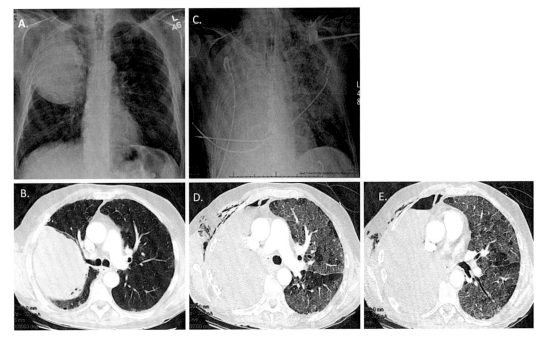

Fig. 2 A 48-year-old man developed severe hypoxemia 48 h after right pneumonectomy with chest wall resection for primary bronchogenic carcinoma. A large right upper lobe mass abutting the chest wall is seen on baseline chest radiograph and CT (**a, b**). Two days later, diffuse ground-glass opacities are noted throughout the left lung (**c–e**). Postoperative changes related to right pneumonectomy and partial right lateral chest wall resection, including a large amount of subcutaneous emphysema, are also seen. A large amount of subcutaneous emphysema is noted on the right. The patient remained ventilator dependent and succumbed to progressive respiratory failure

inflammatory mediators have been postulated as possible causes. Conventional parameters for preoperative assessment do not predict those patients most predisposed to develop lung injury following lung resection. Hypoxia and diffuse interstitial pulmonary edema may occur as early as 24–72 h following pneumonectomy or lobectomy and quickly progress to respiratory failure. Rales on lung examination may become clinically apparent within hours of presentation. Mimickers of ARDS, including pneumonia, pulmonary embolism, cardiogenic pulmonary edema, pulmonary embolism, and bronchopleural fistula formation, should be excluded. Positive pressure ventilation, supplemental oxygen, fluid restriction, and diuretics represent standard of care in this setting, although postpneumonectomy/lobectomy ARDS is inherently refractory to treatment, and 50% of patients will succumb to their illness [54] (Fig. 3).

The increased risk of ARDS following cardiothoracic surgeries has traditionally been associated with the use of cardiopulmonary bypass (CPB), the need for blood product transfusions, large volume shifts, mechanical ventilation, and direct surgical insult. The impact of ARDS in the cardiac population is substantial, affecting not only survival but also in-hospital length of stay and long-term physical and psychological morbidity. Early identification of high ARDS risk groups are crucial in improving postsurgical outcomes.

ALI/ARDS Post Hematopoietic Stem Cell Transplant

Lung injury following hematopoietic stem cell transplantation (HSCT) occurs in 30–60% HSCT recipients, with progression to ARDS in approximately 5% [57]. Risk factors for ARDS in this setting include pneumonia, shock, sepsis, and aspiration. ARDS is more frequent (61% versus 3%), more severe, and occurs at a later time point (median 55 days compared 14 days) among recipients of allogeneic transplants versus autologous HSCT. This likely reflects increased vulnerability to infection owing to more intense immune suppression among allogeneic recipients. Not surprisingly, posttransplant outcomes among this group of patients with ARDS are poor, with increased ICU days (9 days vs. 6.8 days among autologous recipients) and higher ICU mortality [58].

Transfusion-related acute lung injury (TRALI)/transfusion-related ARDS is a distinct clinical condition, characterized by acute lung injury with hypoxemia (PaO_2/FiO_2 <300 mm Hg), fever, hypotension, cyanosis, and bilateral pulmonary infiltrates. The diagnosis of TRALI requires a temporal relationship between transfusion of blood products and the development of acute lung injury and the exclusion of other competing risk factors for ARDS, such as pneumonia, sepsis, pancreatic, drug toxicity, or trauma. A growing consensus supports a "two-hit model" in the development of TRALI, in which an inflammatory condition, such as infection or trauma in the lungs, leads to sequestration and priming of lung neutrophils. With subsequent blood/blood product transfusion, antibodies and endotoxins in stored blood promote endothelial damage by inducing the release of oxidases and proteases from the primed neutrophils. This sequence of events results in capillary leak and acute lung injury [59, 60]. Although the precise incidence of TRALI in the general population is unknown, historical estimates suggest that TRALI develops in approximately 1 in 5000 transfused blood components, or 0.1% of transfused patients [61]. TRALI may be more frequent in the cancer setting and the ICU, where susceptible patients are some of the highest consumers of blood and blood product support.

Symptoms of TRALI typically occur early (within minutes of initiation a transfusion) but may be delayed up to 6 h following blood product administration. Chest imaging studies demonstrate patchy infiltrates unrelated to cardiogenic pulmonary edema. Virtually all blood products, including fresh frozen plasma, packed red blood cells (PRBCs), platelets, granulocytes, cryoprecipitate, intravenous immune globulin, and allogeneic stem cells, have all been implicated in the development of this syndrome [60, 62, 63]. Specific risk factors for TRALI may be stratified according to recipient factors and blood

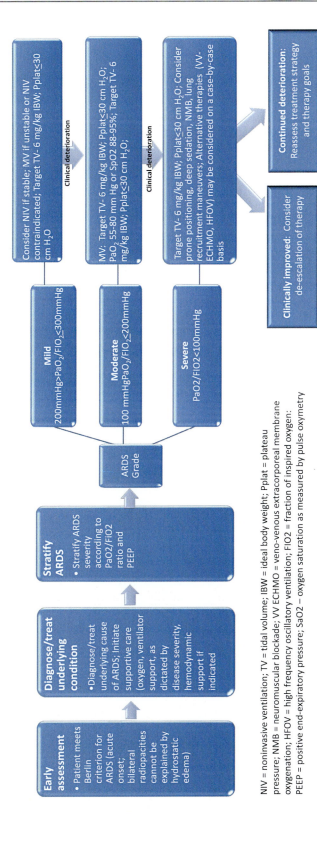

NIV = noninvasive ventilation; TV = tidal volume; IBW = ideal body weight; Pplat = plateau pressure; NMB = neuromuscular blockade; VV ECHMO = veno-venous extracorporeal membrane oxygenation; HFOV = high frequency oscillatory ventilation; FIO2 = fraction of inspired oxygen: PEEP = positive end-expiratory pressure; SaO2 – oxygen saturation as measured by pulse oxymetry

Fig. 3 Proposed Algorithm for Management of ARDS. NIV = noninvasive ventilation; TV = tidal volume; IBW = ideal body weight; Pplat = plateau pressure; NMB = neuromuscular blockade; VV ECHMO = veno-venous extracorporeal membrane oxygenation; HFOV = high frequency oscillatory ventilation; FIO$_2$ = fraction of inspired oxygen; PEEP = positive end-expiratory pressure; SaO$_2$ = oxygen saturation as measured by pulse oxymetry

product factors. Recipient factors include hematologic malignancy, critical illness, emergency cardiac surgery, massive transfusion, sepsis, mechanical ventilation, and a high APACHE II scores [64]. General surgery, cytokine infusion, and active infection have also been linked to TRALI, although these associations have not been confirmed. Blood product factors have included transfusions of whole blood and donor gender, with increased rates associated with increased plasma or whole blood from female donors [65–67]. Numerous studies have explored the influence of RBS storage time on transfusion-related adverse events, including TRALI and posttransfusion infections, with mixed results [68–70]. More recent studies suggest that transfusion of fresh (1–10 days old) RBCs does not confer superior transfusion outcomes to the standard practice of transfusing blood stored for up to 3 weeks [71]. Supportive measures, including initiation of supplemental oxygen and hemodynamic support, are the cornerstones of TRALI therapy. Noninvasive respiratory support with continuous positive airway pressure (CPAP) is indicated in patients with mild disease. However, approximately 70–80% of patients will require invasive mechanical ventilation [61, 72, 73]. High-dose intravenous steroids have been reported to have success in individual case reports, although no prospective trials exist and existing anecdotal evidence favoring the use of steroids in the management of TRALI is limited [74]. Upon suspicion of TRALI, the transfusion should be immediately discontinued and the blood bank alerted of a possible transfusion reaction. With the recognition that alloimmunization during pregnancy renders multiparous women as high-risk donors in the development of TRALI, national and international risk-reduction strategies have been implemented over the past decade that exclude multiparous women as donors with the preferential utilization of males and nulligravida donors in whole blood and high plasma volume components transfusions [75–78]. These mitigation strategies do not currently apply to platelet or red blood cell products, due to concerns that broader applications may result in donor shortages of platelets and red blood cell products. Other risk-reduction strategies, including use of solvent-detergent-treated plasma, and more stringent screening of blood and blood product donors have also been implemented. These efforts have resulted in a significant reduction in both TRALI-related incidence and mortality rates. The prognosis is substantially more favorable compared to other causes of acute lung injury, with many survivors exhibiting full recovery [74].

ALI/ARDS Due to Pulmonary Spread of Tumor: Lymphangitic Carcinomatosis and Pulmonary Leukostasis

Tumoral involvement of the pulmonary vascular bed may present as occlusion of small airways by tumor microemboli or macrovascular occlusion of central pulmonary vessels caused by large tumor emboli. Choriocarcinomas and tumors of mucinous origin from the breast, lung, gastrointestinal tract, and kidneys are associated with the highest rates of tumor embolization. Lymphangitic spread of tumor frequently accompanies tumor microembolization. However, either entity may exist in isolation. Hyperleukocytosis, variably defined as a WBC greater than $50 \times 10^9/L$ (50,000/microL) or $100 \times 10^9/L$ (100,000/microL) with leukostasis, may result in leukemic sequestration and leukocyte thrombus formation within the pulmonary microvasculature. This disorder is most often seen among patients with acute or chronic myeloid leukemias in blast crisis and is considered an oncologic emergency. The markedly elevated and poorly deformable blast cells are thought to plug the microcirculation, leading increased blood viscosity, leukostasis, and tissue hypoperfusion. Cytokine production by the dividing blast compound the problem by damaging the endothelial lining cells, resulting in alveolar hemorrhage [79, 80]. Patients with microvascular thrombosis typically present with an insidious dry cough, progressive dyspnea, and hypoxemia in association with echocardiographic evidence of pulmonary hypertension and cor pulmonale. Interstitial infiltrates suggestive of lymphangitic spread of disease may also be seen. The prognosis is conditioned by the type of malignancy (patients with acute myeloid leukemias in blast crisis tend to do worse) and evidence of end-organ damage (renal, neurologic, respiratory) [81]. Treatment of leukostasis with hyperleukocytosis includes stabilization with urgent efforts to reduce the WBC count with cytoreduction, hydroxyurea, and/or leukapheresis. Avoidance of whole blood transfusions may also help to mitigate blood hyperviscosity and symptomatic hyerleukostasis. Intravenous hydration, correction of coagulation abnormalities including disseminated intravascular coagulopathy, and aggressive platelet support are the mainstays of treatment.

Initiation of chemotherapy for treatment of acute nonlymphocytic leukemia has been reported to precipitate acute hypoxemic respiratory failure and is thought to be caused by chemotherapy-induced pulmonary leukostasis and perivascular hemorrhage. This syndrome, known as leukemic cell lysis pneumopathy, has been reported following chemotherapy for acute myelomonocytic leukemia. Patients typically present within the initial 48 h of treatment for leukemia with severe hypoxemia associated with new or worsening pulmonary infiltration on chest radiography. Lysis of leukemic cells, with subsequent release of their enzyme contents, leading to diffuse alveolar damage and ARDS is the postulated mechanism of lung injury [82]. Measured PaO_2 may be artificially low in patients with hyperleukocytic leukemias in the absence of lung involvement, owing to leukocyte metabolism of oxygen within the arterial blood gas syringe. In this setting oxygen saturations obtained by pulse oximetry are normal. Rapid analysis of the arterial blood gas specimen kept on ice or the addition of cyanide to the blood gas syringe effectively eliminates this problem.

Patients with macrovascular tumor emboli may present with acute onset dyspnea and hypoxemia with pleuritic chest pain. Symptoms and signs closely resemble acute pulmonary thromboembolic disease, and premortem distinctions between the two entities are often difficult to discern. Microvascular tumor embolization, however, typically presents with insidious symptoms of dyspnea, nonproductive cough, hypoxemia, and severe pulmonary artery pressure elevations.

Cor pulmonale and diffuse interstitial infiltrates, suggestive of lymphangitic spread of disease, are common findings and heighten the already poor prognosis.

Clinical Presentation and Diagnostic Workup of ALI/ARDS

The clinical, histopathologic, and radiographic manifestations of ALI/ARDS are highly varied. Acute respiratory failure with refractory hypoxemia is typical during the exudative stage of ALI/ARDS. Patients commonly develop clinical manifestations of lung injury early, usually within 24 h of exposure to the injurious agent. Progression to respiratory failure and the need for noninvasive and/or invasive ventilation also occurs early (within the first 72 h of onset) in 90% of patients [34, 83]. Imaging findings vary with the severity of ARDS. Bilateral areas of patchy airspace consolidation within the lung periphery with normal cardiac silhouette and absence of Kerley B lines are classic findings on chest radiographs. On computed tomography (CT), alveolar filling and consolidation within dependent areas of the lungs are also characteristic. These findings may appear as subtle ground-glass opacities during early stages of ALI/ARDS but evolve to dense consolidative changes as the disease progresses. Imaging abnormalities may closely mimic cardiogenic edema, which should be excluded. Clinical manifestations, including progressive dyspnea, tachypnea, tachycardia, cough, and diffuse rales, are notoriously nonspecific findings. With disease progression, respiratory distress, cyanosis, altered mental status, and chest pain (owing to pneumothorax in some cases) may occur. Acute hypoxemia and a compensatory respiratory alkalosis are common early derangements on arterial blood gases. The development of hypercapnic respiratory acidosis signals severe disease with impending respiratory failure and portends a poor prognosis.

The goal of the diagnostic evaluation of ARDS is to identify the underlying cause(s) and provide guidance for immediate empirical treatment. Early identification and treatment of the cause(s) of ARDS has been shown to favorably impact outcomes [36, 84–89]. Thus, the evaluation and relevant testing should be performed as early as possible, starting with a thorough history and clinical examination and chest imaging. Chest radiographs and CT imaging may provide critical clues to the diagnosis and help to exclude competing entities, such as pneumonia (lobar consolidation, air bronchograms, cavitation) and cardiogenic pulmonary edema (presence of Kerley B lines, cardiomegaly, pulmonary venous congestion, pleural effusions). Diagnostic yields of bronchoscopically obtained lavage (BAL) fluid in the cancer setting vary widely (30–89%) but may be helpful in evaluating infectious etiologies [28, 90]. Common underlying infectious triggers for ARDS in the cancer setting may be identified on BAL fluid, including bacteria, invasive mycotic infections, tuberculosis, pneumocystis, and viral pathogens. In addition, elevated eosinophils, bloody fluid with increased hemosiderin-laden macrophages, and malignant cells on BAL fluid are helpful clues in the diagnosis of acute eosinophilic pneumonia conditions, diffuse alveolar hemorrhage, or lymphangitis carcinomatosis, respectively. The utility of lung biopsies in this setting has been debated. The underlying trigger(s) for ARDS are typically identified using less invasive strategies, and the likelihood of obtaining additional information has to be carefully weighed against the overall risk of the surgical procedure. Nonetheless, surgical biopsies may be reasonable when a specific pathology and/or reversible etiology (such as lymphangitic spread of disease, vasculitis, or cryptogenic organizing pneumonia) is suspected but not obvious from less invasive studies or when surgically obtained biopsies may inform critical therapeutic and prognostic decision-making.

Complete blood count (CBC), coagulation studies, chemistries, liver function tests, and arterial blood gas (ABG) analysis should be included in the initial blood work. Brain natriuretic peptide (BNP) or pro-N terminal BNP (pro-NT BNP) and troponin levels may help to exclude cardiogenic causes of pulmonary edema. Serum lipase and amylase levels to evaluate for pancreatitis should be investigated in patients with abdominal symptoms and no other obvious triggers for ARDS. Laboratory evidence of organ injury associated with hypoxemia (transaminitis, acute renal insufficiency) are frequent findings with advanced disease. Metabolic acidosis may reflect major organ sites of involvement (liver, kidneys) or sepsis. Depending on the clinical suspicion, other components of the ARDS evaluation may include nasopharyngeal aspiration for respiratory viral panel, urinary antigens and cultures for legionella or *Streptococcus pneumoniae*, and PCR for *Pneumocystis jirovecii* and herpes simplex virus. Depending on the underlying trigger, the white cell count may be elevated, depressed, or normal. ARDS should be considered in any patient who develops progressive dyspnea, hypoxia, and bilateral pulmonary infiltrates on chest imaging within 6 h to 1 week of an inciting event. Unfortunately, the inciting event is frequently unknown, and early signs and symptoms are often missed. Recovery or death may occur at any stage of ARDS. Prognosis is primarily dependent on the severity, chronicity, and treatment of ARDS rather than the etiology of lung injury. Survivorship among those patients that progress to the fibrotic phase of ARDS is marked by long-term oxygen dependence and a decreased quality of life.

Cancer-Related ALI/ARDS: Outcomes and Treatment

Conditions common to ARDS, such as infection, respiratory failure, hemodynamic instability, disseminated intravascular coagulation, sepsis, and gastrointestinal (GI) bleed, are independent predictive variables that presage poor outcomes. Assessments of illness severity at the time of ICU admission, using SOFA (sequential organ failure assessment) scores, are also helpful in identifying the high-risk patients with predicted poor outcomes [91]. Although the treatment of ARDS in patients with cancer is similar to that in the non-cancer setting, unique manifestations of cancer and its treatment, including increased rates of neutropenia, infection, thrombocytopenia, mucositis, and thrombosis, represent decisive challenges that highlight the added complexity

Table 4 Prognosis of ARDS in cancer

Type of malignancy	# Patients	Mortality (%)			Reference
		28 day	In-hospital	6 months	
Leukemia patients post HSCT	2635			66.90%	Yadav et al. [58]
Hematologic	68	77%			Türkoğlu [134]
Hematologic	70	63%			Mokart (2012)
Mixed solid/hematologic	116	55.20%			Soubani et al. [25]
Mixed solid/hematologic	1004		64%		Azoulay et al. [32]
Hematologic			55.70%		Seong (2018)
Mixed cancers (13%), all others no cancer history	3022	34%	39.6		Bellani et al. [34]

of managing ARDS in cancer patients. Mortality rates in excess of 90% have been reported among cancer patients requiring mechanical ventilation for ARDS in the past, with the highest vulnerability among patients with hematologic malignancies and recipients of hematopoietic transplants [92, 93]. Recent investigations suggest significant declines in mortality rates (30–63%) and offer a more favorable perspective [25, 85, 90] Table 4. These survival gains have been attributed to early identification and management of precipitating condition(s) coupled with improvements in prophylaxis measures for infection and aspiration over the past decade [94]. In addition, improved HSCT techniques, including more aggressive use of hematopoietic growth factor support and the increasing use of donor stem cells from a peripheral rather than bone marrow source, have also had salutary effects on ARDS mortality. Convincing evidence has also shown earlier ICU transfer within 48 h of onset of respiratory symptoms is also associated with improved survival [85, 95]. Finally, the expanded use of NIV and lung protective strategies that attenuate ventilator-associated lung injury have been central to improved ventilator outcomes [90, 94, 96].

Pulmonary function usually may return to normal within 6–12 months following mild to moderate ARDS. Patients with severe disease and those requiring prolonged ventilatory support may develop persistent abnormalities in pulmonary function, disabling muscle weakness and neuropsychiatric deficiencies. Studies have shown the beneficial impact of daily interruption of sedation and spontaneous breathing trials

(wake up and breathe protocol) and of early mobilization of mechanically ventilated patients, as part of a comprehensive multifaceted strategy to curtail long-term complications from ARDS.

Treatment

Pharmacologic Therapies

Despite extensive investigations, evidence supporting the utility of most pharmacologic therapies in adult ARDS management are limited. Randomized controlled trials and cohort studies suggest that high-dose glucocorticoids may offer some mortality benefit, particularly if given early, during the fibroproliferative phase of ARDS; however a consistent mortality advantage has not been shown [97–99]. Furthermore, an optimal steroid dose (range 1 mg/kg/day to 120 mg/kg/day in various studies) has not been established. Exogenous surfactant therapy may be beneficial in the management of childhood ARDS, but has not been found to be of therapeutic utility in adults. Results of other pharmacologic investigations including anti-TNF-α, anti-interleukin-1, ketoconazole, prostaglandin E1, prostacyclin, and inhaled nitric oxide in attenuating ARDS risk and/or improving ARDS outcomes have been equally disappointing [100, 101].

Respiratory and hemodynamic support along with diuretics, vasopressors, and antibiotics, where indicated, are standard supportive care measures in ALI/ARDS. Intravenous fluids should be given judiciously, with careful attention to fluid homeostasis, as persistent positive fluid balance has been associated with increased days on the ventilator and poor clinical outcomes [102, 103]. Thus, conservative intravenous fluid hydration titrated to lower central pressures is recommended [104, 105]. Unless contraindicated prophylaxis against venous thromboembolism using low-molecular-weight heparin (40 mg of enoxaparin) or 5000 units of subcutaneous dalteparin per day) or low-dose, unfractionated subcutaneous heparin (5000 units twice daily) is recommended. Nonpharmacologic measures to reduce thrombus risk, such as intermittent pneumatic compression (IPC), should be considered when anticoagulant therapy is contraindicated. IPC therapy has proven benefit in reducing DVT in the postoperative setting, although rigorous investigations of this device as a stand-alone intervention in the nonsurgical setting are not available. Patients should also receive daily stress ulcer prophylaxis with sucralfate, ranitidine, or omeprazole, unless contraindicated. Nutritional support should be initiated within 24–48 h of ICU transfer and preferably by enteral route, in accordance with ADA guidelines [106]. Successful management of ARDS also requires an expeditious evaluation and treatment of nosocomial and community-acquired pneumonias and other secondary infections. Meticulous glycemic control, prevention of aspiration events, and careful management of gastrointestinal (GI) bleeding are also frequent issues among cancer patients with ARDS that mandate careful monitoring and coordination with other therapies.

Noninvasive and Invasive Ventilation

Noninvasive ventilation (NIV) has gained broad acceptance in the management of cancer patients with respiratory failure, based on pivotal randomized, controlled studies that have demonstrated unequivocal efficacy of NIV in the management of patients with pump failure [107, 108] as well as selected cases of lung failure [107]. In a recent retrospective study of the outcome of cancer patients following ICU transfer for ARF, the use of NIV was associated with marked improvements in patient survival [90]. In addition, significant reductions in both ICU and post ICU hospital mortality have been linked to the use of intermittent NIV during the early stages of hypoxemic ARF (PaO_2/FiO_2 ratio <250) [84, 108, 109]. The use of NIV has also been associated with significant declines in the need for conventional mechanical ventilation. However, these favorable results may apply only to a subset of patients in the early stages of ARDS and should be interpreted with caution. The application of NIV in the LUNG-SAFE study was associated with worse mortality [109]. Very few investigations have demonstrated improved survival among cancer patients with ARDS treated with NIV. In one small randomized controlled study of immunocompromised patients with hypoxemic acute lung injury, initiation of NIV resulted improved oxygenation and a reduced need for endotracheal intubation. However, intubation was associated with mortality rates of up to 94% in the control group, suggesting that survival gains in cancer patients with ARDS may be overestimated. Other studies have demonstrated equally high mortality rates among cancer patients who failed NIV and subsequently required mechanical ventilation. NIV may be sufficient in cancer patients with mild or incipient ARDS, with mechanical ventilation reserved for patients with more advanced disease. Increasing NIV duration, steroid therapy, other organ failure (including renal failure), the need for vasopressor support, and lack of definite etiological triggers for ARDS are reported predictors of NIV failure in the cancer setting. Knowledge of determinants of increased risk for NIV failure may help to better triage patients for NIV versus early intubation and mechanical ventilation as first-line ventilator support. Patients treated with NIV should undergo close surveillance for early signs of NIV failure. Persistent hypoxemia, advanced ARDS, end-organ dysfunction, and altered mental status signal a poor NIV outcome and the need for intubation and mechanical ventilation [87, 109, 110].

Mechanical ventilation, the cornerstone of ARDS treatment, poses a critical conundrum. This intervention is potentially lifesaving and, at the same time, potentially deadly [5]. The ability of this therapeutic intervention to potentiate lung injury and contribute to nonpulmonary organ failure is well established [96, 111]. Increased respiratory drive and excessive pulmonary dead space are key features of ARDS. As ARDS progresses, these physiologic derangements drive minute ventilation to unsustainable levels, resulting in progressive hypercapnia. The goals of mechanical ventilation – to improve oxygenation and eliminate CO_2 – are met through adjustments in tidal volumes, driving pressures, gas flows, and respiratory rates. Excessive adjustments in these parameters may result in ventilator-induced lung injury (VILI). VILI is manifested clinically as volutrauma (excessive generalized mechanical stress and strain on the lung) and atelectrauma (injury caused by shearing forces as adjacent alveoli collapse and re-expand during mechanical ventilation). VILI tends to be heterogeneous, with injured or atelectatic areas adjacent to relatively normal aerated areas.

Ventilator strategies in the past utilized large tidal volumes (10–15 mg/kg) and high PEEP (12 cm H2O or greater) in an effort to recruit and maintain open small airways. Lung recruitment maneuvers, which entail the application of high airway pressures and or PEEP for variable duration of time, were also used in an attempt to open collapsed lung units. The salutary effects of increased PEEP in improving oxygenation and mitigating atelectrauma are often offset by the attendant damaging consequences of high alveolar pressures and volumes. The adverse effects of these high pressure strategies are further aggravated by the inhomogeneity of lung damage in ARDS, causing some alveolar units to be under more mechanical stress than others. Convincing evidence from aggregate studies has demonstrated increased volutrauma and 28-day mortality among patients with severe ARDS when these strategies were applied [112].

The intent of mechanical ventilation, to rest the respiratory muscles and maintain adequate gas exchange while the underlying cause of lung injury is being treated, must be balanced by efforts to mitigate the deleterious effects of VILI. Efforts to achieve these goals have been the subject of many clinical trials. More recent approaches advocate lowering airway pressures, which offers the dual benefit of minimizing over distension of the aerated areas and mitigating trauma from repeated opening and closing of the alveoli. The American Thoracic Society (ATS), the European Society of Intensive Care Medicine (ESICM), and the Society of Critical Care Medicine (SCCM) met in 2013–2014 to analyze evidence regarding the use of ventilatory strategies established by the ARDSNET trial. Key recommendations that emerged from these meetings included lowering of targets for tidal volumes (4–8 ml/kg predicted body weight) and inspiratory pressures to maintain plateau pressures of <30 mm H20. Low tidal volume strategies have been associated with a 22% relative reduction in mortality when tidal volumes are maintained at 6 mL/kg PBW compared with 12 mL/kg [96]. However, this strategy is limited by subsequent hypercapnia and respiratory acidosis as ARDS progresses. In addition, attendant low lung volumes and atelectasis contribute to increased pulmonary vascular resistance. The utility of an extracorporeal carbon dioxide gas exchanger device or the veno-venous extracorporeal membrane oxygenation (VV ECMO) for removal of carbon dioxide has been studied with promising results, although this strategy remains experimental [113–115]. Investigations probing the utility of ECMO and VV ECMO systematically excluded cancer patients with less than a 5-year life expectancy from many of the larger clinical trials. Thus, even less is known regarding the utility of these invasive mechanical devices in patients with ARDS in the cancer setting.

The ATS, the ESICM, and the SCCM also recommend prone positioning. This approach promotes more uniform distribution of mechanical forces throughout the injured lung, thereby facilitating more homogeneous lung inflation and, as a result, improved oxygenation and reduced VILI. The adoption of prone positioning as adjunctive therapy for ARDS had been stalled for many years, based on early clinical trials that demonstrated improved oxygenation, but no survival gains with this intervention. This observation, coupled with concerns regarding possible adverse events from proning patients, including facial edema, of pressure necrosis with skin break-down, transient desaturation, hemodynamic instability, dislodgement of lines and endotracheal tubes, lead to only sporadic use of this treatment modality over the years. However, findings from a patient meta-analysis of four major clinical studies as well as the PROSEVA trial clearly demonstrate a mortality benefit with prone positioning among a subgroup of patients with severe ARDS [5, 116–123]. Based on these observations, prone positioning for patients with severe ARDS is recommended. This recommendation, which is strongly endorsed by major critical care and thoracic societies, marks a major shift in advised care for ARDS. Prone positioning for a minimum of 12 h per day is recommended for patients with severe ARDS. P/F ratios of 100 are also recommended.

Theoretically, the concept behind high-frequency oscillatory ventilation (HFOV), which uses very small tidal volumes oscillating a very high mean pressure, should improve ARDS-related mortality as a result of its mitigating effects on both volutrauma and atelectrauma. However, two large clinical trials failed to discern any mortality advantage using this ventilator strategy. In fact, the OSCILLATE trial, which compared ARDS outcomes among patients undergoing early application of HFOV to patients undergoing low tidal volume/high PEEP ventilator strategies, was discontinued prematurely due to safety concerns, including hemodynamic issues and higher 28-day mortality. Thus, studies do not support the use of HFOV in patients with ARDS, except perhaps in the patient with very severe ARDS (P/F ratio <64 mmHg), although more research is needed [124–128].

The past three decades has witnessed a proliferation of newer modes of assisted mechanical ventilation, including airway pressure release ventilation (APRV), proportional assist ventilation (PAV), mandatory minute ventilation (MMV), neurally adjusted ventilatory assist (NAVA), adaptive support ventilation (ASV), and SmartCare. In the conventional volume/pressure "open loop" ventilator strategies, delivered parameters are fixed and lack ability to integrate patient feedback into adjusted ventilator settings.

The newer "closed-loop" ventilator strategies are designed to adjust ventilator settings based on patient feedback, thereby optimizing patient-ventilator synchrony, improving patient safety and comfort, and mitigating the work of breathing [129, 130]. Earlier liberation from the ventilator is also facilitated by closed-loop ventilator strategies. However, long-term studies are needed to prove efficacy and to define their true advantages and benefits compared to conventional ventilation strategies, particularly as they relate to mechanically ventilated patients with ARDS.

Sedation and Neuromuscular Blockade

Sedation and neuromuscular blockade are important components of strategies aimed at optimization of patient-ventilator interactions and minimizing patient discomfort and agitation while on the ventilator. Neuromuscular-blocking agents (NBA) are indicated when asynchrony persists despite sedation and ventilator adjustments [131]. When prescribed early in the course of ARDS, these agents may reduce VILI by several pathophysiologic mechanisms. Paralytic agents eliminate patient-initiated double triggering, ensuring delivery of low tidal volumes. In addition, atelectrauma is reduced by eliminating active exhalation and loss of PEEP. Finally, the high ventilator demands and hypercapnia-associated escalations in respiratory drive that are intrinsic to severe lung injury are mitigated. These benefits may translate to favorable survivals. At least one study has demonstrated survival gains among NBA-treated patients with severe ARDS (P/F ratio <150) compared to nonparalyzed controls [132, 133].

Conclusion

Over the past two decades, ALI/ARDS definitions have crystallized. ARDS is increasingly recognized as a heterogeneous condition, fueled by a variety of triggers. Specific triggers are now accepted as important contributors to unique ARDS phenotypes as well as prognosis and response to treatment. Thus, early and aggressive reversal of the inciting event is as pertinent as specialized treatment options, including ventilator strategies and other supportive measures. Furthermore, recognition of different ARDS phenotypes may assist in developing personalized ventilator strategies that consider each patient's unique physiology, thereby mitigating VILI and improving ARDS outcomes. Recent decades have witnessed pivotal advances in evidence-based ARDS treatment strategies. These advances have resulted in significant overall improvements in ARDS mortality in the general population. Survival gains have been largely attributed to optimized approaches to pneumonia and other underlying causes of ARDS, as well as increased utilization of multimodal treatment strategies that include lung-protective ventilation. ARDS prognosis among ventilated patients in the cancer setting have evolved from dismal to encouraging, although mortality rates remain high. The unique vulnerability of cancer patients to respiratory complications caused by the cancer itself, infections, toxic effects of cancer therapies, immune suppression, and cancer- and treatment-related cytopenias frequently contributes to severe lung injury that results in delays and oftentimes discontinuation of cancer therapy. Moreover, long-term morbidity and decreased quality of life among cancer survivors may be substantial. Because of the propensity for severe manifestations of ARDS at presentation, NIV may not be the best option for many cancer patients with acute lung injury. The prognosis following transition to mechanical ventilation following NIV failure remains bleak. These considerations underscore the urgent need for upfront conversations with the patient and family members, together with the oncologist and ICU team in an effort to design a realistic critical care treatment plan that avoids therapeutic intransigence while simultaneously considering the patient's wishes and life expectancy. Treatment strategies for ARDS in the cancer setting have largely been extrapolated from investigations that focus on ARDS in the general population. Studies that focus on the unique challenges of the cancer patient with ARDS are urgently needed.

References

1. Ashbaugh D, Bigelow D, Petty T. Acute respiratory distress in adults. Lancet. 1967;2:319–23.
2. Bernard GR, Artigas A, Brigham KL, Carlet J, Falke K, Hudson L, Lamy M, Legall JR, Morris A, Spragg R. The American-European consensus conference on ARDS. Definitions, mechanisms, relevant outcomes, and clinical trial coordination. Am J Respir Crit Care Med. 1994;149:818–24.
3. Ranieri VM, Rubenfeld GD, Thompson BT, Ferguson ND, Caldwell E, Fan E, Camporota L, Slutsky AS. Acute respiratory distress syndrome: the Berlin definition. JAMA. 2012;307:2526–33.
4. Murray J, Mathay M, Luce J, et al. An expanded definition of the adult respiratory distress syndrome. Am Rev Respir Dis. 1988;138:720–3.
5. Fan E, Brodie D, Slutsky AS. Acute respiratory distress syndrome: advances in diagnosis and treatment. JAMA. 2018;319:698–710.
6. Steinberg K, Ruzinski J, Caldwell E, Radella F 2nd, Davis D, Treece P, Hudson L, Martin T. The heterogeneity of BAL cells and protein in patients at risk for and with ARDS. Chest. 1999;116:98S.
7. Martin TR. Lung cytokines and ARDS*: Roger S. Mitchell Lecture 41st Annual Thomas L. Petty Aspen Lung Conference: acute lung injury. Chest. 1999;116:2S–8S.
8. Katzenstein AL, Bloor CM, Leibow AA. Diffuse alveolar damage – the role of oxygen, shock, and related factors. A review. Am J Pathol. 1976;85:209–28.
9. Hamacher J, Lucas R, Lijnen HR, Buschke S, Dunant Y, Wendel A, Grau GE, Suter PM, Ricou B. Tumor necrosis factor-alpha and angiostatin are mediators of endothelial cytotoxicity in bronchoalveolar lavages of patients with acute respiratory distress syndrome. Am J Respir Crit Care Med. 2002;166:651–6.
10. Pittet JF, Mackersie RC, Martin TR, Matthay MA. Biological markers of acute lung injury: prognostic and pathogenetic significance. Am J Respir Crit Care Med. 1997;155:1187–205.
11. Bellingan GJ. The pulmonary physician in critical care * 6: the pathogenesis of ALI/ARDS. Thorax. 2002;57:540–6.
12. Nelson S, Belknap SM, Carlson RW, Dale D, DeBoisblanc B, Farkas S, Fotheringham N, Ho H, Marrie T, Movahhed H, Root R, Wilson J. A randomized controlled trial of filgrastim as an adjunct to antibiotics for treatment of hospitalized patients with community-acquired pneumonia. CAP study group. J Infect Dis. 1998;178:1075–80.
13. Katz JN, Kolappa KP, Becker RC. Beyond thrombosis: the versatile platelet in critical illness. Chest. 2011;139:658–68.
14. Kor DJ, Carter RE, Park PK, Festic E, Banner-Goodspeed VM, Hinds R, Talmor D, Gajic O, Ware LB, Gong MN. Effect of aspirin on development of

ARDS in at-risk patients presenting to the emergency department: the LIPS-A randomized clinical trial. JAMA. 2016;315:2406–14.

15. Abdulnour RE, Gunderson T, Barkas I, Timmons JY, Barnig C, Gong M, Kor DJ, Gajic O, Talmor D, Carter RE, Levy BD. Early intravascular events are associated with development of acute respiratory distress syndrome. A substudy of the LIPS-A clinical trial. Am J Respir Crit Care Med. 2018;197:1575–85.

16. Abdulnour RE, Howrylak JA, Tavares AH, Douda DN, Henkels KM, Miller TE, Fredenburgh LE, Baron RM, Gomez-Cambronero J, Levy BD. Phospholipase D isoforms differentially regulate leukocyte responses to acute lung injury. J Leukoc Biol. 2018;103:919–32.

17. Reilly JP, Christie JD. Linking genetics to ARDS pathogenesis: the role of the platelet. Chest. 2015;147:585–6.

18. Zhai R, Gong MN, Zhou W, Thompson TB, Kraft P, Su L, Christiani DC. Genotypes and haplotypes of the VEGF gene are associated with higher mortality and lower VEGF plasma levels in patients with ARDS. Thorax. 2007;62:718–22.

19. Bauer T, Ferrer R, Angrill J, Schultze-Werninghaus G, Torres A. Ventilator-associated pneumonia: incidence, risk factors, and microbiology. Semin Respir Infect. 2000;15:272–9.

20. Dolinay T, Kim YS, Howrylak J, Hunninghake GM, An CH, Fredenburgh L, Massaro AF, Rogers A, Gazourian L, Nakahira K, Haspel JA, Landazury R, Eppanapally S, Christie JD, Meyer NJ, Ware LB, Christiani DC, Ryter SW, Baron RM, Choi AM. Inflammasome-regulated cytokines are critical mediators of acute lung injury. Am J Respir Crit Care Med. 2012;185:1225–34.

21. Makabe H, Kojika M, Takahashi G, Matsumoto N, Shibata S, Suzuki Y, Inoue Y, Endo S. Interleukin-18 levels reflect the long-term prognosis of acute lung injury and acute respiratory distress syndrome. J Anesth. 2012;26:658–63.

22. Meduri GU, Headley S, Kohler G, Stentz F, Tolley E, Umberger R, Leeper K. Persistent elevation of inflammatory cytokines predicts a poor outcome in ARDS. Plasma IL-1 beta and IL-6 levels are consistent and efficient predictors of outcome over time. Chest. 1995;107:1062–73.

23. Calfee CS, Delucchi KL, Sinha P, Matthay MA, Hackett J, Shankar-Hari M, McDowell C, Laffey JG, O'Kane CM, McAuley DF. Acute respiratory distress syndrome subphenotypes and differential response to simvastatin: secondary analysis of a randomised controlled trial. Lancet Respir Med. 2018;6:691–8.

24. Pepe PE, Potkin RT, Reus DH, Hudson LD, Carrico CJ. Clinical predictors of the adult respiratory distress syndrome. Am J Surg. 1982;144:124–30.

25. Soubani AO, Shehada E, Chen W, Smith D. The outcome of cancer patients with acute respiratory distress syndrome. J Crit Care. 2014;29:183 e187–12.

26. Garcia CS, Pelosi P, Rocco PR. Pulmonary and extrapulmonary acute respiratory distress syndrome: are they different? Rev Bras Ter Intensiva. 2008;20:178–83.

27. Thille AW, Richard JC, Maggiore SM, Ranieri VM, Brochard L. Alveolar recruitment in pulmonary and extrapulmonary acute respiratory distress syndrome: comparison using pressure-volume curve or static compliance. Anesthesiology. 2007;106:212–7.

28. Shannon VR. Pneumotoxicity associated with immune checkpoint inhibitor therapies. Curr Opin Pulm Med. 2017;23:305–16.

29. Dimopoulou I, Bamias A, Lyberopoulos P, Dimopoulos MA. Pulmonary toxicity from novel antineoplastic agents. Ann Oncol. 2006;17:372–9.

30. Matsuno O. Drug-induced interstitial lung disease: mechanisms and best diagnostic approaches. Respir Res. 2012;13:39.

31. Sakai F, Johkoh T, Kusumoto M, Arakawa H, Takahashi M. Drug-induced interstitial lung disease in molecular targeted therapies: high-resolution CT findings. Int J Clin Oncol. 2012;17:542–50.

32. Azoulay E, Lemiale V, Mokart D, Pene F, Kouatchet A, Perez P, Vincent F, Mayaux J, Benoit D, Bruneel F, Meert AP, Nyunga M, Rabbat A, Darmon M. Acute respiratory distress syndrome in patients with malignancies. Intensive Care Med. 2014;40:1106–14.

33. Wong JL, Evans SE. Bacterial pneumonia in patients with cancer: novel risk factors and management. Clin Chest Med. 2017;38:263–77.

34. Bellani G, Laffey JG, Pham T, Fan E, Brochard L, Esteban A, Gattinoni L, van Haren F, Larsson A, McAuley DF, Ranieri M, Rubenfeld G, Thompson BT, Wrigge H, Slutsky AS, Pesenti A. Epidemiology, patterns of care, and mortality for patients with acute respiratory distress syndrome in intensive care units in 50 countries. JAMA. 2016;315:788–800.

35. Cortegiani A, Russotto V, Raineri SM, Gregoretti C, Giarratano A. Dying with or because of invasive fungal infection? The role of immunity exhaustion on patient outcome. Turk J Anaesthesiol Reanim. 2016;44:285–6.

36. Azoulay E, Darmon M. Acute respiratory distress syndrome during neutropenia recovery. Crit Care. 2010;14:114.

37. Leoni D, Encina B, Rello J. Managing the oncologic patient with suspected pneumonia in the intensive care unit. Expert Rev Anti-Infect Ther. 2016;14:943–60.

38. Young AY, Leiva Juarez MM, Evans SE. Fungal pneumonia in patients with hematologic malignancy and hematopoietic stem cell transplantation. Clin Chest Med. 2017;38:479–91.

39. Pergam SA. Fungal pneumonia in patients with hematologic malignancies and hematopoietic cell transplantation. Clin Chest Med. 2017;38:279–94.

40. Taccone FS, Van den Abeele AM, Bulpa P, Misset B, Meersseman W, Cardoso T, Paiva JA, Blasco-Navalpotro M, De Laere E, Dimopoulos G, Rello J,

Vogelaers D, Blot SI. Epidemiology of invasive aspergillosis in critically ill patients: clinical presentation, underlying conditions, and outcomes. Crit Care. 2015;19:7.

41. Eggimann P, Garbino J, Pittet D. Epidemiology of Candida species infections in critically ill non-immunosuppressed patients. Lancet Infect Dis. 2003;3:685–702.

42. Shah RD, Wunderink RG. Viral pneumonia and acute respiratory distress syndrome. Clin Chest Med. 2017;38:113–25.

43. Vakil E, Evans SE. Viral pneumonia in patients with hematologic malignancy or hematopoietic stem cell transplantation. Clin Chest Med. 2017;38:97–111.

44. Mikkelsen ME, Shah CV, Meyer NJ, Gaieski DF, Lyon S, Miltiades AN, Goyal M, Fuchs BD, Bellamy SL, Christie JD. The epidemiology of acute respiratory distress syndrome in patients presenting to the emergency department with severe sepsis. Shock. 2013;40:375–81.

45. Seethala RR, Blackney K, Hou P, Kaafarani HMA, Yeh DD, Aisiku I, Tainter C, deMoya M, King D, Lee J. The association of age with short-term and long-term mortality in adults admitted to the intensive care unit. J Intensive Care Med. 2017;32:554–8.

46. Dhokarh R, Li G, Schmickl CN, Kashyap R, Assudani J, Limper AH, Gajic O. Drug-associated acute lung injury: a population-based cohort study. Chest. 2012;142:845–50.

47. Shannon V, Price K. Pulmonary complications of cancer therapy. Anesthesiol Clin North Am. 1998;16:563–85.

48. Ryu JH. Chemotherapy-induced pulmonary toxicity in lung cancer patients. J Thorac Oncol. 2010;5:1313–4.

49. Sadowska AM, Specenier P, Germonpre P, Peeters M. Antineoplastic therapy-induced pulmonary toxicity. Expert Rev Anticancer Ther. 2013;13:997–1006.

50. Gibelin A, Parrot A, Maitre B, Brun-Buisson C, Mekontso Dessap A, Fartoukh M, de Prost N. Acute respiratory distress syndrome mimickers lacking common risk factors of the Berlin definition. Intensive Care Med. 2016;42:164–72.

51. Mathes DD. Bleomycin and hyperoxia exposure in the operating room. Anesth Analg. 1995;8:624–9.

52. Couderc LJ, Stelianides S, Frachon I, Stern M, Epardeau B, Baumelou E, Caubarrere I, Hermine O. Pulmonary toxicity of chemotherapy and G/GM-CSF: a report of five cases. Respir Med. 1999;93:65–8.

53. Goldiner PL, Schweizer O. The hazards of anesthesia and surgery in bleomycin-treated patients. Semin Oncol. 1979;6:121–4.

54. Forshag MS, Cooper AD Jr. Postoperative care of the thoracotomy patient. Clin Chest Med. 1992;13:33–45.

55. Reilly JJ Jr. Benefits of aggressive perioperative management in patients undergoing thoracotomy. Chest. 1995;107:312s–5s.

56. Hyde BR, Woodside KJ. Postoperative acute respiratory distress syndrome development in the thoracic surgery patient. Semin Thorac Cardiovasc Surg. 2006;18:28–34.

57. Ahya VN. Noninfectious acute lung injury syndromes early after hematopoietic stem cell transplantation. Clin Chest Med. 2017;38:595–606.

58. Yadav H, Nolan ME, Bohman JK, Cartin-Ceba R, Peters SG, Hogan WJ, Gajic O, Kor DJ. Epidemiology of acute respiratory distress syndrome following hematopoietic stem cell transplantation. Crit Care Med. 2016;44:1082–90.

59. Looney MR, Gilliss BM, Matthay MA. Pathophysiology of transfusion-related acute lung injury. Curr Opin Hematol. 2010;17:418–23.

60. Looney MR, Roubinian N, Gajic O, Gropper MA, Hubmayr RD, Lowell CA, Bacchetti P, Wilson G, Koenigsberg M, Lee DC, Wu P, Grimes B, Norris PJ, Murphy EL, Gandhi MJ, Winters JL, Mair DC, Schuller RM, Hirschler NV, Rosen RS, Matthay MA, Toy P. Prospective study on the clinical course and outcomes in transfusion-related acute lung injury*. Crit Care Med. 2014;42:1676–87.

61. Vlaar AP, Binnekade JM, Prins D, van Stein D, Hofstra JJ, Schultz MJ, Juffermans NP. Risk factors and outcome of transfusion-related acute lung injury in the critically ill: a nested case-control study. Crit Care Med. 2010;38:771–8.

62. Rizk A, Gorson KC, Kenney L, Weinstein R. Transfusion-related acute lung injury after the infusion of IVIG. Transfusion. 2001;41:264–8.

63. Silliman CC, McLaughlin NJ. Transfusion-related acute lung injury. Blood Rev. 2006;20:139–59.

64. Vlaar AP, Juffermans NP. Transfusion-related acute lung injury: a clinical review. Lancet. 2013;382:984–94.

65. van Stein D, Beckers EA, Sintnicolaas K, Porcelijn L, Danovic F, Wollersheim JA, Brand A, van Rhenen DJ. Transfusion-related acute lung injury reports in the Netherlands: an observational study. Transfusion. 2010;50:213–20.

66. Eder AF. Improving safety for young blood donors. Transfus Med Rev. 2012;26:14–26.

67. Juffermans NP, Vlaar AP. Possible TRALI is a real entity. Transfusion. 2017;57:2539–41.

68. Marik PE, Sibbald WJ. Effect of stored-blood transfusion on oxygen delivery in patients with sepsis. JAMA. 1993;269:3024–9.

69. Walsh TS, McArdle F, McLellan SA, Maciver C, Maginnis M, Prescott RJ, McClelland DB. Does the storage time of transfused red blood cells influence regional or global indexes of tissue oxygenation in anemic critically ill patients? Crit Care Med. 2004;32:364–71.

70. Klein H, Natanson C, Flegel W. Transfusion of fresh vs. older red blood cells in the context of infection. ISBT Sci Ser. 2015;10:275–85.

71. Remy KE, Sun J, Wang D, Welsh J, Solomon SB, Klein HG, Natanson C, Cortes-Puch I. Transfusion of recently donated (fresh) red blood cells (RBCs) does not improve survival in comparison with current practice, while safety of the oldest stored units is yet to be

established: a meta-analysis. Vox Sang. 2016;111:43–54.

72. Toy P, Gajic O, Bacchetti P, Looney MR, Gropper MA, Hubmayr R, Lowell CA, Norris PJ, Murphy EL, Weiskopf RB, Wilson G, Koenigsberg M, Lee D, Schuller R, Wu P, Grimes B, Gandhi MJ, Winters JL, Mair D, Hirschler N, Sanchez Rosen R, Matthay MA. Transfusion-related acute lung injury: incidence and risk factors. Blood. 2012;119:1757–67.

73. Wallis JP. Transfusion-related acute lung injury (TRALI) – under-diagnosed and under-reported. Br J Anaesth. 2003;90:573–6.

74. Looney MR, Gropper MA, Matthay MA. Transfusion-related acute lung injury: a review. Chest. 2004;126:249–58.

75. Lucas CE, Ledgerwood AM. Fresh frozen plasma/red blood cell resuscitation regimen that restores pro-coagulants without causing adult respiratory distress syndrome. J Trauma Acute Care Surg. 2012;72:821–7.

76. Lucas G, Win N, Calvert A, Green A, Griffin E, Bendukidze N, Hopkins M, Browne T, Poles A, Chapman C, Massey E. Reducing the incidence of TRALI in the UK: the results of screening for donor leucocyte antibodies and the development of national guidelines. Vox Sang. 2012;103:10–7.

77. Reesink HW, Lee J, Keller A, Dennington P, Pink J, Holdsworth R, Schennach H, Goldman M, Petraszko T, Sun J, Meng Y, Qian K, Rehacek V, Turek P, Krusius T, Juvonen E, Tiberghien P, Legrand D, Semana G, Muller JY, Bux J, Reil A, Lin CK, Daly H, McSweeney E, Porretti L, Greppi N, Rebulla P, Okazaki H, Sanchez-Guerrero SA, Baptista-Gonzalez HA, Martinez-Murillo C, Guerra-Marquez A, Rodriguez-Moyado H, Middelburg RA, Wiersum-Osselton JC, Brand A, van Tilburg C, Dinesh D, Dagger J, Dunn P, Brojer E, Letowska M, Maslanka K, Lachert E, Uhrynowska M, Zhiburt E, Palfi M, Berlin G, Frey BM, Puig Rovira L, Muniz-Diaz E, Castro E, Chapman C, Green A, Massey E, Win N, Williamson L, Silliman CC, Chaffin DJ, Ambruso DR, Blumberg N, Tomasulo P, Land KJ, Norris PJ, Illoh OC, Davey RJ, Benjamin RJ, Eder AF, McLaughlin L, Kleinman S, Panzer S. Measures to prevent transfusion-related acute lung injury (TRALI). Vox Sang. 2012;103:231–59.

78. Tynell E, Andersson TM, Norda R, Edgren G, Nyren O, Shanwell A, Reilly M. Should plasma from female donors be avoided? A population-based cohort study of plasma recipients in Sweden from 1990 through 2002. Transfusion. 2010;50:1249–56.

79. Azoulay E, Fieux F, Moreau D, Thiery G, Rousselot P, Parrot A, Le Gall JR, Dombret H, Schlemmer B. Acute monocytic leukemia presenting as acute respiratory failure. Am J Respir Crit Care Med. 2003;167:1329–33.

80. Stucki A, Rivier AS, Gikic M, Monai N, Schapira M, Spertini O. Endothelial cell activation by myeloblasts:

molecular mechanisms of leukostasis and leukemic cell dissemination. Blood. 2001;97:2121–9.

81. Porcu P, Danielson CF, Orazi A, Heerema NA, Gabig TG, McCarthy LJ. Therapeutic leukapheresis in hyperleucocytic leukaemias: lack of correlation between degree of cytoreduction and early mortality rate. Br J Haematol. 1997;98:433–6.

82. Tryka AF, Godleski JJ, Fanta CH. Leukemic cell lysis pneumonopathy. A complication of treated myeloblastic leukemia. Cancer. 1982;50:2763–70.

83. Fowler A, Hamman R, Good J, Benson K, Baird M, Eberle D, Petty T. Adult respiratory distress syndrome: risk with common predispositions. Ann Intern Med. 1983;98:593–7.

84. Hilbert G, Gruson D, Vargas F, Valentino R, Gbikpi-Benissan G, Dupon M, Reiffers J, Cardinaud JP. Noninvasive ventilation in immunosuppressed patients with pulmonary infiltrates, fever, and acute respiratory failure. N Engl J Med. 2001;344:481–7.

85. Azoulay E, Mokart D, Pene F, Lambert J, Kouatchet A, Mayaux J, Vincent F, Nyunga M, Bruneel F, Laisne LM, Rabbat A, Lebert C, Perez P, Chaize M, Renault A, Meert AP, Benoit D, Hamidfar R, Jourdain M, Darmon M, Schlemmer B, Chevret S, Lemiale V. Outcomes of critically ill patients with hematologic malignancies: prospective multicenter data from France and Belgium – a groupe de recherche respiratoire en reanimation onco-hematologique study. J Clin Oncol. 2013;31:2810–8.

86. Azoulay E, Schlemmer B. Diagnostic strategy in cancer patients with acute respiratory failure. Intensive Care Med. 2006;32:808–22.

87. Azoulay E, Thiery G, Chevret S, Moreau D, Darmon M, Bergeron A, Yang K, Meignin V, Ciroldi M, Le Gall JR, Tazi A, Schlemmer B. The prognosis of acute respiratory failure in critically ill cancer patients. Medicine (Baltimore). 2004;83:360–70.

88. de Montmollin E, Tandjaoui-Lambiotte Y, Legrand M, Lambert J, Mokart D, Kouatchet A, Lemiale V, Pene F, Bruneel F, Vincent F, Mayaux J, Chevret S, Azoulay E. Outcomes in critically ill cancer patients with septic shock of pulmonary origin. Shock. 2013;39:250–4.

89. Mokart D, Azoulay E, Schnell D, Bourmaud A, Kouatchet A, Pene F, Lemiale V, Lambert J, Bruneel F, Vincent F, Legrand M, Rabbat A, Darmon M. Acute respiratory failure in neutropenic patients is associated with a high post-ICU mortality. Minerva Anestesiol. 2013;79:1156–63.

90. Azoulay E, Alberti C, Bornstain C, Leleu G, Moreau D, Recher C, Chevret S, Le Gall JR, Brochard L, Schlemmer B. Improved survival in cancer patients requiring mechanical ventilatory support: impact of noninvasive mechanical ventilatory support. Crit Care Med. 2001;29:519–25.

91. Kraguljac AP, Croucher D, Christian M, Ibrahimova N, Kumar V, Jacob G, Kiss A, Minden MD, Mehta S. Outcomes and predictors of mortality

for patients with acute leukemia admitted to the intensive care unit. Can Respir J. 2016;2016:3027656.

92. Price KJ, Thall PF, Kish SK, Shannon VR, Andersson BS. Prognostic indicators for blood and marrow transplant patients admitted to an intensive care unit. Am J Respir Crit Care Med. 1998;158:876–84.

93. Afessa B, Tefferi A, Hoagland HC, Letendre L, Peters SG. Outcome of recipients of bone marrow transplants who require intensive-care unit support. Mayo Clin Proc. 1992;67:117–22.

94. Suchyta MR, Orme JF Jr, Morris AH. The changing face of organ failure in ARDS. Chest. 2003;124:1871–9.

95. Mokart D, Lambert J, Schnell D, Fouche L, Rabbat A, Kouatchet A, Lemiale V, Vincent F, Lengline E, Bruneel F, Pene F, Chevret S, Azoulay E. Delayed intensive care unit admission is associated with increased mortality in patients with cancer with acute respiratory failure. Leuk Lymphoma. 2013;54:1724–9.

96. Brower RG, Matthay MA, Morris A, Schoenfeld D, Thompson BT, Wheeler A. Ventilation with lower tidal volumes as compared with traditional tidal volumes for acute lung injury and the acute respiratory distress syndrome. N Engl J Med. 2000;342:1301–8.

97. Peter JV, John P, Graham PL, Moran JL, George IA, Bersten A. Corticosteroids in the prevention and treatment of acute respiratory distress syndrome (ARDS) in adults: meta-analysis. BMJ. 2008;336:1006–9.

98. Brun-Buisson C, Brochard L. Corticosteroid therapy in acute respiratory distress syndrome: better late than never? JAMA. 1998;280:182–3.

99. Meduri GU, Headley AS, Golden E, Carson SJ, Umberger RA, Kelso T, Tolley EA. Effect of prolonged methylprednisolone therapy in unresolving acute respiratory distress syndrome: a randomized controlled trial. JAMA. 1998;280:159–65.

100. Tang BM, Craig JC, Eslick GD, Seppelt I, McLean AS. Use of corticosteroids in acute lung injury and acute respiratory distress syndrome: a systematic review and meta-analysis. Crit Care Med. 2009;37:1594–603.

101. Conner BD, Bernard GR. Acute respiratory distress syndrome. Potential pharmacologic interventions. Clin Chest Med. 2000;21:563–87.

102. Schuller D, Mitchell JP, Calandrino FS, Schuster DP. Fluid balance during pulmonary edema. Is fluid gain a marker or a cause of poor outcome? Chest. 1991;100:1068–75.

103. Schuster DP. Fluid management in ARDS: "keep them dry" or does it matter? Intensive Care Med. 1995;21:101–3.

104. Chang DW, Huynh R, Sandoval E, Han N, Coil CJ, Spellberg BJ. Volume of fluids administered during resuscitation for severe sepsis and septic shock and the development of the acute respiratory distress syndrome. J Crit Care. 2014;29:1011–5.

105. Cheng IW, Eisner MD, Thompson BT, Ware LB, Matthay MA. Acute effects of tidal volume strategy on hemodynamics, fluid balance, and sedation in acute lung injury. Crit Care Med. 2005;33:63–70; discussion 239–240

106. Krzak A, Pleva M, Napolitano LM. Nutrition therapy for ALI and ARDS. Crit Care Clin. 2011;27:647–59.

107. Ball J, Venn R. The 21st International Symposium on Intensive Care and Emergency Medicine, Brussels, Belgium, 20–23 March 2001. Crit Care. 2001;5:138–41.

108. Kramer N, Meyer TJ, Meharg J, Cece RD, Hill NS. Randomized, prospective trial of noninvasive positive pressure ventilation in acute respiratory failure. Am J Respir Crit Care Med. 1995;151:1799–806.

109. Bellani G, Laffey JG, Pham T, Madotto F, Fan E, Brochard L, Esteban A, Gattinoni L, Bumbasirevic V, Piquilloud L, van Haren F, Larsson A, McAuley DF, Bauer PR, Arabi YM, Ranieri M, Antonelli M, Rubenfeld GD, Thompson BT, Wrigge H, Slutsky AS, Pesenti A. Noninvasive ventilation of patients with acute respiratory distress syndrome. Insights from the LUNG SAFE study. Am J Respir Crit Care Med. 2017;195:67–77.

110. Depuydt PO, Soares M. Cancer patients with ARDS: survival gains and unanswered questions. Intensive Care Med. 2014;40:1168–70.

111. Tonetti T, Vasques F, Rapetti F, Maiolo G, Collino F, Romitti F, Camporota L, Cressoni M, Cadringher P, Quintel M, Gattinoni L. Driving pressure and mechanical power: new targets for VILI prevention. Ann Transl Med. 2017;5:286.

112. Cavalcanti AB, Suzumura EA, Laranjeira LN, Paisani DM, Damiani LP, Guimaraes HP, Romano ER, Regenga MM, Taniguchi LNT, Teixeira C, Pinheiro de Oliveira R, Machado FR, Diaz-Quijano FA, Filho MSA, Maia IS, Caser EB, Filho WO, Borges MC, Martins PA, Matsui M, Ospina-Tascon GA, Giancursi TS, Giraldo-Ramirez ND, Vieira SRR, Assef M, Hasan MS, Szczeklik W, Rios F, Amato MBP, Berwanger O, Ribeiro de Carvalho CR. Effect of lung recruitment and titrated positive end-expiratory pressure (PEEP) vs low PEEP on mortality in patients with acute respiratory distress syndrome: a randomized clinical trial. JAMA. 2017;318:1335–45.

113. Morelli A, Del Sorbo L, Pesenti A, Ranieri VM, Fan E. Extracorporeal carbon dioxide removal (ECCO2R) in patients with acute respiratory failure. Intensive Care Med. 2017;43:519–30.

114. Combes A, Hajage D, Capellier G, Demoule A, Lavoue S, Guervilly C, Da Silva D, Zafrani L, Tirot P, Veber B, Maury E, Levy B, Cohen Y, Richard C, Kalfon P, Bouadma L, Mehdaoui H, Beduneau G, Lebreton G, Brochard L, Ferguson ND, Fan E, Slutsky AS, Brodie D, Mercat A. Extracorporeal membrane oxygenation for severe acute respiratory distress syndrome. N Engl J Med. 2018;378:1965–75.

115. Raiker NK, Cajigas H. Early initiation of venovenous extracorporeal membrane oxygenation in a mechanically ventilated patient with severe acute respiratory distress syndrome. BMJ Case Rep. 2018; pii: bcr-2018-226223.

116. Gattinoni L, Carlesso E, Taccone P, Polli F, Guerin C, Mancebo J. Prone positioning improves survival in severe ARDS: a pathophysiologic review and individual patient meta-analysis. Minerva Anestesiol. 2010;76:448–54.

117. Sud S, Friedrich JO, Taccone P, Polli F, Adhikari NK, Latini R, Pesenti A, Guerin C, Mancebo J, Curley MA, Fernandez R, Chan MC, Beuret P, Voggenreiter G, Sud M, Tognoni G, Gattinoni L. Prone ventilation reduces mortality in patients with acute respiratory failure and severe hypoxemia: systematic review and meta-analysis. Intensive Care Med. 2010;36:585–99.

118. Gattinoni L, Protti A, Caironi P, Carlesso E. Ventilator-induced lung injury: the anatomical and physiological framework. Crit Care Med. 2010;38:S539–48.

119. Protti A, Andreis DT, Milesi M, Iapichino GE, Monti M, Comini B, Pugni P, Melis V, Santini A, Dondossola D, Gatti S, Lombardi L, Votta E, Carlesso E, Gattinoni L. Lung anatomy, energy load, and ventilator-induced lung injury. Intensive Care Med Exp. 2015;3:34.

120. Kamo T, Aoki Y, Fukuda T, Kurahashi K, Yasuda H, Sanui M, Nango E, Abe T, Lefor AK, Hashimoto S. Optimal duration of prone positioning in patients with acute respiratory distress syndrome: a protocol for a systematic review and meta-regression analysis. BMJ Open. 2018;8:e021408.

121. Kim WY, Kang BJ, Chung CR, Park SH, Oh JY, Park SY, Cho WH, Sim YS, Cho YJ, Park S, Kim JH, Hong SB. Prone positioning before extracorporeal membrane oxygenation for severe acute respiratory distress syndrome: a retrospective multicenter study. Med Intensiva. 2018. pii: S0210–5691(18)30160–8.

122. Lucchini A, De Felippis C, Pelucchi G, Grasselli G, Patroniti N, Castagna L, Foti G, Pesenti A, Fumagalli R. Application of prone position in hypoxaemic patients supported by veno-venous ECMO. Intensive Crit Care Nurs. 2018;48:61–8.

123. Munshi L, Del Sorbo L, Adhikari NKJ, Hodgson CL, Wunsch H, Meade MO, Uleryk E, Mancebo J, Pesenti A, Ranieri VM, Fan E. Prone position for acute respiratory distress syndrome. A systematic review and meta-analysis. Ann Am Thorac Soc. 2017;14:S280–s288.

124. Ferguson ND, Cook DJ, Guyatt GH, Mehta S, Hand L, Austin P, Zhou Q, Matte A, Walter SD, Lamontagne F, Granton JT, Arabi YM, Arroliga AC, Stewart TE, Slutsky AS, Meade MO. High-frequency oscillation in early acute respiratory distress syndrome. N Engl J Med. 2013;368:795–805.

125. Young D, Lamb SE, Shah S, MacKenzie I, Tunnicliffe W, Lall R, Rowan K, Cuthbertson BH, Group OS. High-frequency oscillation for acute respiratory distress syndrome. N Engl J Med. 2013;368:806–13.

126. Ferguson ND. High-frequency oscillatory ventilation in adults: handle with care. Crit Care. 2014;18:464.

127. Goligher EC, Munshi L, Adhikari NKJ, Meade MO, Hodgson CL, Wunsch H, Uleryk E, Gajic O, Amato MPB, Ferguson ND, Rubenfeld GD, Fan E. High-frequency oscillation for adult patients with acute respiratory distress syndrome. A systematic review and meta-analysis. Ann Am Thorac Soc. 2017;14: S289–s296.

128. Meade MO, Young D, Hanna S, Zhou Q, Bachman TE, Bollen C, Slutsky AS, Lamb SE, Adhikari NKJ, Mentzelopoulos SD, Cook DJ, Sud S, Brower RG, Thompson BT, Shah S, Stenzler A, Guyatt G, Ferguson ND. Severity of hypoxemia and effect of high-frequency oscillatory ventilation in acute respiratory distress syndrome. Am J Respir Crit Care Med. 2017;196:727–33.

129. Esnault P, Prunet B, Nguyen C, Forel JM, Guervilly C, Zhou Y, Kang Y. Early application of airway pressure release ventilation in acute respiratory distress syndrome: a therapy for all? Intensive Care Med. 2018;44:135–6.

130. Chatburn RL, Mireles-Cabodevila E. Closed-loop control of mechanical ventilation: description and classification of targeting schemes. Respir Care. 2011;56:85–102.

131. Slutsky AS. Neuromuscular blocking agents in ARDS. N Engl J Med. 2010;363:1176–80.

132. Alhazzani W, Alshahrani M, Jaeschke R, Forel JM, Papazian L, Sevransky J, Meade MO. Neuromuscular blocking agents in acute respiratory distress syndrome: a systematic review and meta-analysis of randomized controlled trials. Crit Care. 2013;17:R43.

133. Papazian L, Forel JM, Gacouin A, Penot-Ragon C, Perrin G, Loundou A, Jaber S, Arnal JM, Perez D, Seghboyan JM, Constantin JM, Courant P, Lefrant JY, Guerin C, Prat G, Morange S, Roch A. Neuromuscular blockers in early acute respiratory distress syndrome. N Engl J Med. 2010;363:1107–16.

134. Türkoğlu M, Erdem GU, Suyanı E, Sancar ME, Yalçın MM, Aygencel G, Akı Z, Sucak G. Acute respiratory distress syndrome in patients with hematological malignancies. Hematology. 2013;18(3):123–30.

Diffuse Alveolar Hemorrhage in Critically Ill Cancer Patients

38

Brian W. Stephenson, Allen H. Roberts II, and Charles A. Read

Contents

Introduction 584

Epidemiology 584

Etiology 584

Pathophysiology 584

Clinical Features 585

Diagnosis 585

Management 586

Prognosis 591

Conclusion 591

References 591

Abstract

Diffuse alveolar hemorrhage (DAH) is a syndrome classically defined by the triad of anemia, hemoptysis, and bilateral infiltrates on chest imaging. DAH can progress rapidly toward respiratory failure and death. It is paramount that critical care practitioners be familiar with the diagnosis and treatments available for this syndrome. This chapter reviews the etiologies of DAH, the pathophysiology, the clinical presentation, and diagnostic evaluation, and concludes with the evidence supporting treatment options with a focus on DAH in the oncologic patient. The reader will be able to distinguish infectious, bland hemorrhage, and connective tissue disease-associated causes of DAH from those caused by cytotoxic drugs and graft versus host disease (GVHD). With appropriate and timely treatment, the prognosis of DAH can be dramatic improved.

Keywords

Diffuse alveolar hemorrhage · alveolar infiltrates · hemoptysis · respiratory failure · vasculitis

B. W. Stephenson · A. H. Roberts II · C. A. Read (✉)
Division of Pulmonary, Critical Care, and Sleep Medicine, Department of Medicine, MedStar Georgetown University Hospital, Washington, DC, USA
e-mail: brian.w.stephenson@gunet.georgetown.edu; ahr8@gunet.georgetown.edu; readc@georgetown.edu

© Springer Nature Switzerland AG 2020
J. L. Nates, K. J. Price (eds.), *Oncologic Critical Care*,
https://doi.org/10.1007/978-3-319-74588-6_49

Introduction

Diffuse alveolar hemorrhage (DAH) is a syndrome in which there is an accumulation of intra-alveolar red blood cells (RBCs) originating from the alveolar capillaries. DAH is distinct from other entities causing hemoptysis, such as bronchiectasis or endobronchial malignancies, where the bleeding source often originates from the bronchial arteries resulting in focal hemorrhage. This chapter focuses solely on DAH. DAH has the clinical constellation of hemoptysis, anemia, and diffuse pulmonary infiltrates leading to often devastating hypoxic respiratory failure [10]. DAH presents diagnostic and management challenges for the intensivist which we address in this chapter. We review the histopathology, clinical features, etiologies, and the management of DAH.

Epidemiology

There is a spectrum of disorders associated with DAH, but there is no estimate on the relative frequency. In a review of 34 cases of biopsy-proven DAH, capillaritis occurred 88% of the time. In one report, the most common cause was granulomatous polyangitits (GPA) (32%) followed by Goodpasture syndrome (13%), idiopathic hemosiderosis (13%), collagen vascular diseases (13%), and microscopic polyangiitis (9%) [25]. DAH has been reported to occur between 5% and 20% of patient undergoing BMT and is associated with a dismal 60–100% mortality rate. Risk factors for this condition include total body radiation and GVHD.

Etiology

There is a spectrum of diseases and mechanisms which lead to capillaritis and ultimately DAH. The most common of these is the direct effect of autoantibodies on the alveolar capillary endothelium as seen in granulomatosis polyangiitis (GPA) or microscopic polyangiitis (MPA). Additionally, autoantibodies may be directed against the alveolar basement membrane as seen in Goodpasture syndrome. There may be immune complex-mediated injury to the capillaries such as that seen in systemic lupus erythematosus. Finally, direct alveolar injury may lead to diffuse alveolar damage as seen with cytotoxic drugs and allogeneic bone marrow transplantation [42]. The systemic vasculitides, however, accounts for approximately half the cases [45].

Pathophysiology

Alveolar hemorrhage can develop by one of the following three pathologic processes: pulmonary capillaritis, bland hemorrhage without capillaritis, and diffuse alveolar damage [36]. Capillaritis refers specifically to the microcirculation containing the arterioles, capillaries, and venules. Capillaritis is the predominant histologic finding in DAH and is identified by neutrophilic infiltration, fibrinoid necrosis of the capillary wall, and leukocytoclasis which leads to destruction of the alveolar-capillary basement membrane and red blood cell infiltration into the alveoli [9, 27]. DAH most commonly refers to pulmonary capillaritis and is a separate entity from bland alveolar hemorrhage and diffuse alveolar damage with hemorrhage. Bland hemorrhage occurs when red blood cells leak into the alveolar space without underlying destruction of the vasculature and can be seen with etiologies such as mitral stenosis or with coagulopathy. In diffuse alveolar damage (DAD), lung injury to the alveolar epithelium and vascular endothelium, likely triggered by various inflammatory mediators, causes fluid to leak into the alveoli. DAD is the histologic pattern of acute respiratory distress syndrome (ARDS). Occasionally, DAD may have hemorrhage and the identification of capillaritis can help differentiate DAH from DAD [21]. Interstitial and alveolar hemosiderin deposition helps to distinguish biopsy-related bleeding from DAH [11]. Other histologic findings of DAH include hyperplasia of the type II alveolar cells, monocyte infiltration, and microthrombi. Immunofluorescence may be applied to distinguish Goodpasture syndrome from SLE and microscopic polyangiitis.

Clinical Features

The classic presentation of DAH consists of hemoptysis, anemia, hypoxic respiratory failure, and bilateral infiltrates on imaging. Hemoptysis may not be present in up to one third of patients [25]. A dropping hemoglobin in the setting of respiratory failure should prompt consideration of DAH. Nonspecific signs and symptoms may be present including fevers, dyspnea, and chest discomfort. The distribution of the alveolar infiltrates is most often bilateral but can be focal in rare cases. The classic chest X-ray will show patchy bilateral alveolar infiltrates. High-resolution CT scan will show scattered ground glass infiltrates and airspace consolidations (Fig. 1). Although not often obtained in the setting of acute respiratory compromise, pulmonary function testing may reveal an elevated diffusion capacity for carbon monoxide (DLCO), due to intra-alveolar hemoglobin binding of CO [18]. Progressive respiratory failure may evolve within hours of presentation.

Diagnosis

Many disease processes can present with hemoptysis and are thus in the differential for DAH. These include bland hemorrhage associated with coagulopathies, diffuse alveolar damage from various drug or toxic insults, endobronchial tumors, bronchiectasis, respiratory infections and necrotizing pneumonias, pulmonary embolism,

arteriovenous malformations, and vasculitides. The patient's history can be crucial to determining the diagnosis and etiology of DAH.

The most common infectious causes of DAH include influenza A and *Staphylococcus aureus.* Worldwide, they include dengue, leptospirosis, and malaria [15]. In those who are immunosuppressed, DAH occurs secondary to hematologic malignancies, organ transplantation, drug reactions, or in association with AIDS.

Drug exposures should be noted with special attention to the most common causes of DAH including anticoagulants, amphotericin B, cytarabine, penicillamine, nitrofurantoin, cocaine, and cyclophosphamide. Immunosuppressive drugs such as azathioprine and cyclophosphamide may lead to thrombocytopenia or incite DAH through other mechanisms. Hematopoietic stem cell transplant and solid organ transplant recipients are at an increased risk of DAH. Immunotherapy with agents such as bevacizumab has also been associated with DAH. Prior radiation can cause capillary leak, leading to DAH.

DAH can be primary or secondary to an underlying systemic disease. If secondary, physical exam features may suggest an associated connective tissue disease or vasculitis. Crackles maybe heard on lung auscultation but are not uniformly present. Clinical signs of volume overload can suggest heart failure or transfusion-associated circulatory overload as possible etiologies. The presence of a systolic heart murmur should raise the possibility of mitral regurgitation (MR), a known cause of DAH.

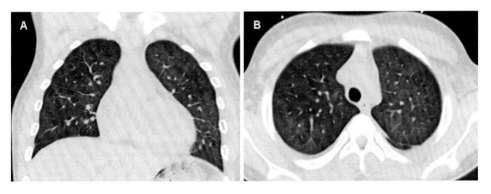

Fig. 1 (**a**) Coronal reconstruction of the lung window of a computed tomographic image and (**b**) axial image showing diffuse bilateral ground glass opacities and linear septal thickening

Chest radiograph typically reveals alveolar infiltrates as the alveoli are filled with red blood cells. Infiltrates may coalesce to form areas of dense consolidation. The distribution is generally bilateral and diffuse but rarely DAH can be focal. Over time, the consolidations start to resolve and give rise to a more reticular pattern. Computed tomography is useful for clarifying the location and extent of airspace disease, seen often as ground-glass opacity, but is unhelpful in terms of establishing an etiologic diagnosis. Pleural effusions are infrequent and should prompt investigation into heart failure and other etiologies of volume overload. Lymphadenopathy is not associated with DAH and may suggest an underlying infectious or malignant condition.

The diagnosis of DAH is confirmed with bronchoscopy and bronchoalveolar lavage (BAL); the typical finding is equal or progressively bloody return on sequential lavage aliquots (Fig. 2). Because of the potential for rapid progression of disease, bronchoscopy with BAL should not be delayed, and may yield an alternate diagnosis such as infection or focal hemorrhage. In time, alveolar macrophages will consume erythrocytes and yield hemosiderin-laden macrophages on lavage. A scoring system has been developed in animal models but is not routinely used in clinical practice. Transbronchial biopsies may exacerbate bleeding and the amount of tissue obtained may

be insufficient to clarify the pathology. For this reason, if BAL is inconclusive and the diagnosis must be confirmed, video-assisted thorascopic biopsy may be required; in this situation, the risk of surgery with general anesthesia must be weighed alongside potential benefit of obtaining this specimen. If features of renal failure are present, suggesting a possible pulmonary-renal syndrome, a renal biopsy may be sufficient for treatment considerations.

Basic laboratory data such as platelet count, prothrombin time, and partial thromboplastin time can identify the underlying coagulopathies found in bland alveolar hemorrhage. If no clear cause is identified by history and physical examination, then serologic testing is performed to rule out a rheumatologic or vasculitic etiology. The workup should include a sedimentation rate and urinalysis to identify red blood cell casts, proteinuria, or sediment. Other laboratory testing to consider includes rheumatoid factor (RF), antibodies against cyclic citrullinated peptides (anti-CCP), anti-DNA antibodies, complement levels, anti-neutrophil cytoplasmic antibodies (ANCA), anti-glomerular basement membrane antibodies (anti-GMB), antinuclear antibody (ANA), and anti-phospholipid antibodies. If GPA is suspected, cytoplasmic proteinase-3 (PR3) for GPA has been reported to have a high sensitivity and specificity, 93% and 97%, respectively, for disease activity and relapse. Culture data should be obtained for bacterial, viral, and fungal causes. The 1-3-β-d-glucan assay should be sent in at risk patients as *Pneumocystis jirovecii* can mimic DAH radiographically. The diagnostic algorithm is summarized in Diagram 1.

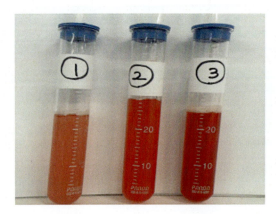

Fig. 2 Three specimens from a bronchoalveolar lavage using serial aliquots of saline. The specimens are labeled sequentially. They reveal a progressively bloodier return. (Image from Moon et al. [30]; Permission from The Korean Society of Critical Care Medicine)

Management

Management of acute respiratory compromise takes precedence over DAH specific treatment and is considered first. Acute or subacute hypoxemia is universally present in diffuse alveolar hemorrhage and is the result of an increased shunt fraction due to alveolar filling by blood, as well as ventilation-perfusion (V/Q) mismatch as blood may occlude the smaller airways.

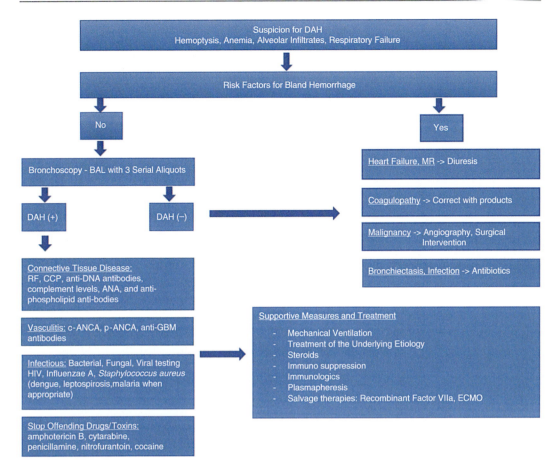

Diagram 1 Diagnostic and management algorithm for diffuse alveolar hemorrhage. *DAH* diffuse alveolar hemorrhage, *BAL* bronchoalveolar lavage, *MR* mitral regurgitation, *RF* Rheumatoid factor, *CCP* anticyclic citrullinated peptides, *anti-DNA* anti-deoxyribonucleic acid, *ANA* antinuclear antibody, *c-ANCA* cytoplasmic antineutrophil cytoplasmic antibodies, *p-ANCA* perinuclear antineutrophil cytoplasmic antibodies, *anti-GBM* antiglomerular basement membrane antibodies

Additionally, there is a concomitant increase in physiologic dead space ventilation (increased dead space to tidal volume ration, V_D/V_T), which may result in an increased work of breathing to maintain $PaCO_2$ homeostasis. Finally, many patients with malignancy have preexisting pulmonary disease and limited respiratory or cardiovascular reserve, and if the patient presents late in the course of evolving respiratory failure, the patient's sensorium may be altered and airway protection lost. Thus, patients with severe DAH may present with combined hypoxemic and hypercapnic respiratory failure; the critical care practitioner will likely encounter the cancer patient with DAH at a moment when acute intervention to provide respiratory support is essential.

Frequently, the precise etiology for respiratory failure in a given patient is not clear, and acute respiratory interventions must precede the establishment of a definitive diagnosis. Indications for and methods of acute airway management are well established [34]. It is recommended to proceed with intubation, and when possible, with a size 8 mm I.D. or larger endotracheal tube (ETT) to facilitate diagnostic bronchoscopy and to minimize the likelihood of ETT occlusion by blood clots. In patients who have suspected intravascular volume depletion related to pulmonary hemorrhage and insensible losses secondary to increased work of breathing, a pre-intubation infusion of isotonic fluid may attenuate the commonly encountered post-intubation hypotension related to the effects of positive pressure in the volume deplete state. In all cases, vasopressors such as phenylephrine or norepinephrine should be readily available for intravenous administration to support the blood pressure, as needed. In the patient who is hemodynamically unstable prior to intubation, the use of etomidate as an anesthesia induction agent for this procedure has been recommended, given its hemodynamic-sparing properties [22]. In the profoundly hypoxemic patient, rapid sequence intubation (RSI) is recommended [43].

In patients with respiratory failure due to other alveolar filling processes, such as pulmonary edema, ARDS, or pneumonia, a trial of noninvasive positive pressure ventilation (NIPPV) may be merited, and in some cases may serve as sufficient a bridge to recovery as to obviate the need for intubation [2]. In patients with DAH, NIPPV may be used as a temporary bridge to improve oxygenation. However, the unpredictability of DAH, with its potential for catastrophic respiratory failure, as well as the need for diagnostic bronchoscopy, renders NIPPV inadvisable as the definitive mode of ventilation. For the same reasons, while the use of high-flow humidified oxygen delivery by nasal cannula may improve oxygenation and, in some cases, reduce the work of breathing [29], it should be used cautiously in DAH.

Ventilator management in the patient with DAH does not differ significantly from that used for any other disease entity [38]. Generally, it is appropriate to initiate mechanical ventilation (MV) in a volume assist-control (V-AC) mode, with initial FiO_2 and PEEP settings of 100% and 5 cm H_2O, respectively. The FiO_2 may be subsequently decreased, based on acceptable oxygenation as determined by pulse oximetry (SaO_2) or arterial blood gas (ABG) analysis. Given the presence of shunt physiology in patients with DAH, as in ARDS, additional PEEP may be required to achieve adequate oxygenation by reducing the shunt fraction. An evolving body of literature endorses the use of the minimum level of FiO_2 needed to support oxygenation, based upon the risk of superoxide radical-mediated lung injury seen at higher levels of inspired oxygen [19]. The titration of FiO_2 and PEEP may be acceptably accomplished by means of the ARDSNET protocol. Use of a tidal volume (VT) = 6–8 cc/kg of ideal body weight (IBW) is now considered to be "lung-protective," and, while this technique was originally described in the treatment of ARDS, it has become the standard of care for virtually all patients [15, 45].

Alternative, nonconventional, or "rescue" modes of ventilation may be employed in circumstances where conventional V-AC with the ARDSNET management protocol has failed satisfactorily to support oxygenation. Whereas to date, no specific ventilator strategy (other than standard low VT lung-protection) has a demonstrated survival benefit; a number of these alternative methods have been described anecdotally in cases of alveolar hemorrhage of various etiologies.

Transitioning a patient with ARDS from the supine to the prone position at intervals is reported to improve alveolar recruitment, oxygenation, and, in certain subgroups, survival [17, 21]. Hayes-Bradley and Choi describe successful management of patients with DAH related to c-ANCA positive vasculitis and organic dust exposure, respectively, with sequential proning during treatment with corticosteroids, cytotoxics, and plasma exchange.

General principles of airway pressure release ventilation (APRV) have been described by Frawley and Habashi [16]. This mode of mechanical ventilation involves sustained extrinsic positive pressure in a de-recruitment prevention strategy which reliably improves oxygenation in patients who fail conventional modes. Ozaki reports the use of APRV in two patients with hypoxemic respiratory failure due to bronchoscopically confirmed DAH complicating systemic lupus erythematosus (SLE), one of whom required sequential courses of mechanical ventilation for recurrent bleeding. Both patients were treated with high-dose corticosteroids; both improved and were extubated [35].

High frequency oscillator ventilation (HFOV) improves oxygenation while minimizing risk of volu- and baro-trauma. This mode of mechanical ventilation has been deployed across adult and pediatric patient populations; however, there is limited experience with and support for HFOV in the latter group; consequently, this modality is not widely available in adult ICUs [33]. Regardless, HFOV has been used successfully in adult and pediatric patients who suffered DAH related to vasculitis [3], leptospirosis [28], and other etiologies [12], as reported anecdotally or in small case series.

Extracorporeal membrane oxygenation (ECMO) has gained traction in recent years as a potentially life-saving intervention for patients in acute respiratory failure whose oxygenation requirements are not met by conventional mechanical ventilation. In cases of pure respiratory failure with preserved hemodynamics, a venovenous (VV) technique is employed [26]. Despite concerns regarding the need for anticoagulation in the ECMO circuit in patients with active alveolar bleeding, ECMO has previously been used successfully as rescue therapy in children with DAH and has more recently been used in adults with DAH related to granulomatous polyangiitis (GPA) [4] and SLE [8]. As of this writing, the technology and requisite expertise is becoming more widespread but is not universally available in all hospital settings. It has been our practice to establish protocols for early identification of patients who may benefit from ECMO, to arrange timely transfer to a center with experience in this method of life support. The superiority of ECMO to more conventional modes of respiratory support is yet to be established in robust, prospective studies [7].

In addition to the life-sustaining measures detailed above, a number of general principles govern the treatment of DAH. If the patient is being medicated with a drug that is suspected as an etiology for DAH, it should be discontinued; anticoagulation should be reversed; and coagulopathy and thrombocytopenia treated with appropriate blood products. Recommendations for specific treatment for DAH fall under several categories, namely, plasma exchange, corticosteroids, cytotoxic agents, and immunotherapy.

While the removal of anti-glomerular basement membrane antibodies in anti-glomerular basement membrane (anti-GBM) disease by plasmapheresis has clear therapeutic benefit, its use in DAH due to GPA or SLE is less well established and is based on small case series [23, 32, 41]. Patient outcomes in these series are mixed; in all cases, plasmapheresis therapy was used concomitantly with aggressive immune suppression.

The administration of high-dose (pulse) corticosteroids for 3–5 days, followed by a tapering dose regimen, is the standard of care for acute reversal of alveolar inflammation-mediated hemorrhage in pulmonary vasculitis. This therapy should be initiated simultaneously with supportive and diagnostic interventions and should be extended to cancer patients with DAH patients in whom the establishment of a definitive underlying etiology is pending [24].

Cytotoxic agents have been used in conjunction with corticosteroids for most forms of vasculitis; while the use of cyclophosphamide is considered standard, dosing regimens are variable, as are outcomes, and the potential for side effects is considerable. Krause and co-workers advise against the use of methotrexate in vasculitis complicated by DAH. All patients who are treated with a combined regimen of corticosteroids and cytotoxic agents should receive pharmaco-prophylaxis for the prevention of *Pneumocystis jirovecii* pneumonia.

Rituximab, a specific anti-CD20-antigen B-cell antibody, has been deployed successfully alongside immunosuppressive therapy in the treatment of recurrent DAH complicating SLE [1], in cases of cytotoxic treatment failure [31], and as a cyclophosphamide alternative [46].

The poor prognosis of DAH following HSCT has prompted the trial of alternative agents. Of these is aminocaproic acid (ACA). Aminocaproic acid blocks the conversion of plasminogen to plasmin and therefore reduces fibrinolysis in bleeding. It is used most frequently in cardiac surgery, intracranial hemorrhage, and procedural related bleeding. ACA is associated with an increase in the incidence of serious complications including venous thromboembolism and stroke.

A retrospective study of 14 patients following HSCT complicated by DAH examined the use of ACA [47]. All patients received steroid therapy. Eight patients were also treated with ACA by physician discretion and were determined to have a survival benefit from the addition of ACA. Infections were more common in those patients treated with steroids alone. Importantly, there were no observed complications from the administration of ACA. This study reported 100-day mortality of 60% overall and median transplantation survival of 99 days. In the patients treated with steroids and aminocaproic acid, the 100-day mortality was 44% and the median transplantation survival was 167 days. In the steroid alone group, the 100 day mortality was notably worse at 83% and median survival was only 96.5 days.

A subsequent retrospective single center study examined 119 patients who underwent HSCT complicated by DAH and examined varying doses of steroids and the addition of ACA to the outcome of hospital and ICU mortality [40]. Steroid treatment was divided into methyprednisolone low dose (250 mg/day), medium dose (250–1000 mg/day), and high dose (≥1000 mg/day). Dosing for the first 5 days of therapy was measured. The dosing/duration of steroids and the addition of ACA were determined by the judgment of the oncologist and/or intensivist. Severity of illness scores was similar between the different dosing groups and the ACA subgroup. A total of 82 patients received ACA in addition to either low-, medium-, or high-dose steroids. The study found no significant differences in 30 day, 60 day, 100 day, ICU, or hospital mortality. There were also no differences detected in ventilator days, ICU length of stay (LOS), and hospital LOS. Interestingly, medium- and high-dose steroids were associated with a higher ICU mortality and medium-dose steroids were associated with a higher hospital mortality in noninfectious cases. Prospective studies are needed to determine if ACA is truly beneficial. The low incidence of adverse reactions may make it a reasonable option in the HSCT patient with DAH who is failing alternative treatments.

Intrapulmonary recombinant factor VIIa (rFVIIa) has been used with some success in DAH. The rFVIIa works by binding tissue factor and activating factor X, leading to initiation of thrombin and ultimately fibrin formation. Data on the use of rFVIIa, thus far, is limited to case reports and cases series and has been used intravenously as well as by endobronchial instillation.

Intravenous rFVIIa was examined in a retrospective single center study of 23 cases of DAH due to a variety of disease including vasculitis, bone marrow transplant, cryoglobulinemia, idiopathic thrombocytopenia, systemic lupus erythematosus, and Goodpasture syndrome [5, 37]. Doses ranged from 35 to 120 mcg/kg rFVIIa every 2 h for total of four doses per day in addition to other standard treatments. The study reports hemostatis in 22 of 23 patients with a mean required dose of 5 mg. No adverse thrombotic events were observed. A multicentre randomized trial of intravenous rFVIIa was performed for the treatment of all bleeding following HSCT. The subset of these patients with DAH was 7%. The study did not demonstrate a benefit in bleeding or the need for transfusions [39].

Bronchoscopically instilled doses of rFVIIa used in the treatment of DAH range from 30mcg/kg to 100 mcg/kg in 50 ml of saline. One small case series of six patients used 30mcg/kg instilled 1–2 times and reported success in 5 of the 6 patients studied [6]. The etiologies included 2 patients with BMT, use of clopidogrel, inhalation injury, SLE, and ARDS. The majority were treated with steroids and additional agents. Another retrospective study compared 23 patients receiving steroids and instilled rFVIIa compared with 14 patients receiving steroids alone. This study found no difference in time to resolution of hemorrhage, duration on mechanical ventilation, or hospital mortality. This study had a significantly higher number of lower respiratory infections. About 4 patients had thrombotic events including endotracheal tube clot, basilic vein thrombosis, and disseminated intravascular coagulation (DIC) [13]. Future studies are needed to determine the appropriate patients for bronchial rFVIIa, the dosing and duration, and the ideal timing of its use.

Prognosis

A retrospective study of 112 immunocompetent patients with DAH in a tertiary hospital in France compared four subgroups of immune, congestive heart failure, miscellaneous, and idiopathic DAH. Collectively the mortality was 35%. The subgroup mortality rates were determined to be 45.4% in those with heart failure, 34.6% in miscellaneous, 30.8% in immune, and 21.4% in idiopathic although there was no statistically significant difference between the groups. The use of corticosteroids and cyclophosphamide for DAH associated with systemic vasculitis has improved the 5-year mortality from 75% to 12% [36]. The mortality from DAH following HSCT is reported between 60% and 100% [13].

Conclusion

The initial management of DAH should include respiratory support with attention to the need for bronchoscopy, hematologic repair with blood products when indicated, bronchoscopic differentiation of DAH from focal pulmonary hemorrhage, and, in the absence of contraindications, prompt administration of pulse-dose steroids. Timely exclusion of infectious and autoimmune disease is necessary before concluding drugs or toxins as the etiology of DAH. The fundamental treatment of DAH is to treat the underlying pathology and provide sufficient respiratory support. The prognosis varies depending upon the underlying etiology. The mortality of DAH has improved with the use of aggressive therapies. Unfortunately, the majority of the existing literature is limited to case series and case reports and therefore patients must be treated on a case-by-case basis.

References

1. Aakjaer S, et al. Continuous rituximab treatment for recurrent diffuse alveolar hemorrhage in a patient with systemic lupus erythematosus and antiphospholipid syndrome. Respirat Med Case Rep. 2017;22:263–5.

2. Abousouan L, Ricauarte B. Noninvasive positive pressure ventilation: increasing use in acute care. Cleve Clin J Med. 2015;77(5):307–16.

3. Afridi F, et al. High-frequency oscillatory ventilation in diffuse alveolar hemorrhage of ANCA-associated vasculitis. Crit Care Med. 2018;46((1) Supplement):512.

4. Ahmed S, et al. Use of extracorporeal membrane oxygenation in a patient with diffuse alveolar hemorrhage. Chest. 2004;126(1):305–9.

5. Alabed A. Treatment of diffuse alveolar hemorrhage in systemic lupus erythematosus with local pulmonary instillation of factor VIIa (rFVIIa). Medicine. 2014;93(14):1–4.

6. Baker M, et al. Intrapulmonary recombinant factor VII as an effective treatment for diffuse alveolar hemorrhage: a case series. J Bronchol Intervent Pulmonol. 2016;23(3):255–8.

7. Brodie D, et al. Research in extracorporeal life support: a call to action. Chest. 2018;153(4):788–91.

8. Claudie C, et al. Extracorporeal membrane oxygenation in diffuse alveolar hemorrhage secondary to systemic lupus erythematosus. J Clin Med Res. 2014;6(2):145–8.

9. Colby T, et al. Pathologic approach to pulmonary hemorrhage. Ann Diagn Pathol. 2001;5(5):309–19.

10. Collard HR, Schwarz MI. Diffuse alveolar hemorrhage. Clin Chest Med. 2004;25:583–92.

11. Collard HR, King TE, Schwarz MI. Alveolar hemorrhage and rare infiltrative diseases. In: Broaddus C, editor. Murray and Nadel's textbook of respiratory medicine. Philadelphia: Saunders, an imprint of Elsevier Inc.; 2016. p. 67.1207–1220.e11.

12. Duval ELIM, Markhorst DG, Ramet J, van Vught AJ. High-frequency oscillatory ventilation in severe lung hemorrhage: a case study of three centres. Respirat Med CME. 2009;2:92–8.

13. Elinoff J, et al. Recombinant human factor viia for alveolar hemorrhage following allogeneic stem cell transplantation. Biol Blood Marrow Transplant. 2014;20:969–78.

14. El-Khatib M, Bou-Khalil P. Clinical review: liberation from mechanical ventilation. Crit Care. 2008;12(221):1–11, Available at http://ccforum.com/content/12/4/221

15. Escuissatoa DL, Warszawiaka D, Marchiorib E. Differential diagnosis of diffuse alveolar haemorrhage in immunocompromised patients. Curr Opin Infect Dis. 2015;28:337–42.

16. Frawley P, Habashi N. Airway pressure release ventilation: theory and practice. AACN Clin Issues. 2001;12(2):234–46.

17. Gattinoni L, et al. Prone position in acute respiratory distress syndrome: rationale, indications and limits. AJRCCM. 2013;188(11):1286–93.

18. Greening A, Hughes J. Serial estimations of carbon monoxide diffusion capacity in intrapulmonary haemorrhage. Clin Sci. 1981;60:507–12.

19. Hafner S, et al. Hyperoxia in intensive care, emergency, and peri-operative medicine: Dr. Jekyll or

Mr. Hyde – a 2015 update. Ann Intensive Care. 2015;5 (42):1–14.

20. Hayes-Bradley C. Hypoxia from vasculitic pulmonary haemorrhage improved by prone position ventilation. Br J Anaesth. 2004;92(5):754–7.

21. Hughes KT, Beasley MB. Pulmonary manifestations of acute lung injury: more than just diffuse alveolar damage. Arch Pathol Lab Med. 2017;141(7):916–22.

22. Jackson W. Should we use etomidate as an induction agent for endotracheal intubation in patients with septic shock? Chest. 2005;127(3):1031–8.

23. Klemmer P, et al. Plasmapheresis therapy for diffuse alveolar hemorrhage in patients with small-vessel vasculitis. Am J Kidney Dis. 2003;42(6):1149–53.

24. Krause M, et al. Update on diffuse alveolar hemorrhage and pulmonary vasculitis. Immunol Allergy Clin N Am. 2012;32(4):587–600.

25. Lara AR, Schwarz MI. Diffuse alveolar hemorrhage. Chest. 2010;137(5):1164–71.

26. Makdisi G, Wang I. Extra corporeal membrane oxygenation (ECMO) review of a lifesaving technology. J Thorac Dis. 2015;7(7):E166–76.

27. Mark E, Ramirez J. Pulmonary capillaritis and hemorrhage in patients with systemic vasculitis. Arch Pathol Lab Med. 1985;109:413–8.

28. Mat Nor MB, Md Ralib A, Ibrahim NA, Abdul-Ghani MR. High frequency oscillatory ventilation in leptospirosis pulmonary hemorrhage syndrome: a case series study. Indian J Crit Care Med. 2016;20(6): 342–8.

29. Mauri T, et al. Physiologic effects of high-flow oxygen by nasal cannula in hypoxemic respiratory failure. AJRCCM. 2016;195(9):1207–15.

30. Moon KM, et al. Diffuse alveolar hemorrhage confirmed by Bronchoalveolar lavage in a patient with hemoptysis after sildenafil use for erectile dysfunction. Korean J Crit Care Med. 2015;30:31–3.

31. Narshi C, et al. Rituximab as early therapy for pulmonary hemorrhage in systemic lupus erythematosus. Rheumatology. 2010;49:394–6.

32. Nguyen T, et al. Plasmapheresis for diffuse alveolare hemorrhage in a patient with Wegener's granulomatosis: case report and review of the literature. J Clin Apher. 2005;20(4):230–4.

33. Nguyen AP, Schmidt UH, MacIntyre NR. Should high-frequency ventilation in the adult be abandoned? Respir Care. 2016;61(6):791–800.

34. O'Connor M, Glick D. Chapter 45: airway management. Principles of critical care. 4th ed. New York: McGraw Hill Education; 2015. p. 384–96.

35. Ozaki Y, Nomura S. Chapter XI: Airway pressure support ventilation (APRV) as supportive management for diffuse alveolar hemorrhage in systemic lupus erythematosus. Lupus: Symptoms, Treatments, and Potential Complications Nova Science Publishers Inc.; 2012. p. 197–203.

36. Park M. Diffuse alveolar hemorrhage. Tuberc Respir Dis. 2013;74:151–62.

37. Pathak V, et al. Use of activated factor VII in patients with diffuse alveolar hemorrhage: a 10 years institutional experience. Lung. 2015;193:375–9.

38. Pham T, et al. Mechanical ventilation: state of the art. Mayo Clin Proc. 2017;92(9):1382–400.

39. Pihusch M, et al. Recombinant activated factor VII in treatment of bleeding complications following hematopoietic stem cell transplantation. J Thromb Haemost. 2005;3:1935–44.

40. Rathi N, et al. Low-, medium- and high-dose steroids with or without aminocaproic acid in adult hematopoietic SCT patients with diffuse alveolar hemorrhage. Bone Marrow Transplant. 2015;50:420–6.

41. Ravindran V, Watts R. Pulmonary haemorrhage in ANCA-associated vasculitis. Rheumatology. 2010;49:1412–4.

42. Shwarz M, Brown K. Small vessel vasculitis of the lung. Thorax. 2000;55:402–510.

43. Sinclair R, Luxton M. Rapid sequence induction. Br J Anaesth. 2005;5(2):65–6.

44. The Acute Respiratory Distress Syndrome Network. Ventilation with lower tidal volumes as compared with traditional tidal volumes for acute lung injury and the acute respiratory distress syndrome. NEJM. 2000;342:1301–8.

45. Travis W, Colby T, Lombard C, Carpenter H. A clincopathologic study of 34 cases of diffuse pulmonary hemorrhage with biopsy confirmation. Am J Surg. 1990;14:1112–25.

46. Tse J, et al. Rituximab: an emerging treatment for recurrent diffuse alveolar hemorrhage in systemic lupus erythematosus. Lupus. 2015;24(7):756–9.

47. Wanko S, et al. Diffuse alveolar hemorrhage: retrospective review of clinical outcome in allogeneic transplant recipients treated with Aminocaproic acid. Biol Blood Marrow Transplant. 2006;12:949–53.

Differentiation (Retinoic Acid) Syndrome in Critically Ill Cancer Patients

39

Cristina Prata Amendola, Ricardo André Sales Pereira Guedes, and Luciana Coelho Sanches

Contents

Introduction 594

Etiology 594

Epidemiology 594

Pathogenesis 594

Physiopathology 595

Clinical Features 597
Symptoms and Signs 598
Laboratory 599
Imaging 600

Diagnosis 600

Differential Diagnosis 601

Management 602
Pharmacologic 602
Non-pharmacologic 602
Management Algorithm 602

Prognosis 602

Summary 602

References 603

Abstract

In patients with acute promyelocytic leukemia, induction therapy, primarily with all-trans retinoic acid (ATRA), or arsenic trioxide (ATO), capable of inducing the differentiation of leukemic cells, may lead to the development of a syndrome of differentiation, formerly known as all-trans-retinoic acid syndrome. In this situation, patients who develop the severe form present a high morbimortality rate. The diagnosis requires a high degree of suspicion, and the criteria used are clinical. Originally, the

C. Prata Amendola (✉) · R. A. S. P. Guedes · L. C. Sanches
Fundação Pio XII – Hospital de Câncer de Barretos, Barretos, São Paulo, Brazil
e-mail: cp.amendola@uol.com.br; sprico@hotmail.com; zucoelho65@yahoo.com.br

© Springer Nature Switzerland AG 2020
J. L. Nates, K. J. Price (eds.), *Oncologic Critical Care*,
https://doi.org/10.1007/978-3-319-74588-6_50

diagnostic criteria were established by Frankel et al. (Ann Intern Med 117(4):292–296, 1992) who were based on seven clinical findings: fever, weight gain (from capillary leak and soft tissue edema, secondary a storm of cytokines), respiratory distress, radiographic opacities, pleural or pericardial effusion, hypotension, and renal failure (usually from hypotension, although disseminated intravascular coagulation may also be present). In this scenario, the use of corticosteroids against suspicion promotes a significant decrease in the mortality rate, changing the prognosis and therefore the course of the disease.

Keywords

Differentiation syndrome · All-trans-retinoic acid syndrome · Acute promyelocytic leukemia · Differentiation therapy · Tretinoin

Introduction

The differentiation syndrome (DS), previously called retinoic acid syndrome, is a complication of induction chemotherapy in patients with acute promyelocytic leukemia (APL). Although its occurrence is related mainly with the all-trans retinoic acid (ATRA, also known as tretinoin) or arsenic trioxide (ATO), agents capable of inducing the differentiation of leukemic cells, it is also seen in untreated patients or after other cytotoxic therapies. The pathogenesis of DS has not been entirely clarified; however, it is known that there is the release of cytokines from malignant promyelocytes, independent of their differentiation to segmented neutrophils [10, 34].

This complication needs a high degree of suspicion to be recognized early, allowing the aggressive institution of therapeutics and increasing the chances of survival.

So, it is important to be aware of the appearance of the clinical picture: unexplained fever, weight gain, peripheral edema, dyspnea with interstitial pulmonary infiltrates, pleuro-pericardial effusion, hypotension, and acute renal failure [12].

Etiology

Currently, the most consistent evidence points to the release of cytokines during the maturation process of promyelocytes, mainly induced by the use of ATRA or ATO. So the presence of malignant promyelocytes cells is fundamental for the onset of the syndrome [1].

Epidemiology

According to statistical data taken from case series studies, most of the registries occurred when using ATRA or ATO, during induction therapy in patients with acute promyelocytic leukemia, something around 25%. It is important to emphasize that only when using these drugs in the induction phase and not in the consolidation or maintenance therapies, besides occurring only in patients with acute promyelocytic leukemia and not in other malignant diseases.

Several studies have tried to point out risk factors involved in the onset of this syndrome, and although some of them reports the elevated white blood cell count as a risk factor, the syndrome may occur in its absence; so far the only one that had recurrent demonstration was the high body mass index [3, 15, 16, 31].

Pathogenesis

For understanding the origin of the problem, it is essential to understand the genetic process involved in acute promyelocytic leukemia, where a blockage in myeloid differentiation occurs in the promyelocytic phase. The genetic hallmark of APL is a balanced reciprocal translocation t(15;17)(q22;q11–12), leading to the fusion of the promyelocytic gene (PML) on chromosome 15 and the retinoic acid receptor alpha gene (RARA) on chromosome 17, and generating the PML/RARA fusion gene and protein [24].

RARA is a member of the RA nuclear receptor family that binds DNA as heterodimers with its cofactor, the retinoid X receptor (RXR) [22]. The PML-RARA/RXR complex binds to specific retinoic acid response elements (RARE) yielding transcriptional repression in the absence of the RA ligand [11] (Fig. 1).

In addition, another stage involved in the onset of differentiation syndrome takes into consideration the participation of the drugs used in induction therapy: ATRA and ATO, as demonstrated above. In view of the different mechanisms of action of these drugs, it is possible to understand more clearly the clinical results achieved. Leukemic initiating cells (LICs) possess high self-renewal capability and give rise to leukemic blasts that form the bulk of the disease. Both ATRA and ATO promote remission of disease by targeting leukemic blasts. Pharmacological doses of ATRA predominantly drive differentiation of leukemic blasts but are unable to efficiently eliminate LICs that can drive disease relapse. In contrast, ATO induces both apoptosis and differentiation of leukemic blasts and can also target LICs and is therefore more effective than ATRA as a monotherapy (left). ATRA acts synergistically with ATO and/or chemotherapy, and these combination therapies definitively cure APL in the vast majority of cases (extracted: Santos et al. [9]) (Fig. 2).

In synthesis what occurs during induction therapy is an increase in the number of differentiated cells that participate in the pathogenesis of the differentiation syndrome. Currently, several theories have been postulated to explain the clinical manifestations, among them are: the storm of cytokines, implicated in the systemic capillary extravasation syndrome; the migration of mature cells with subsequent infiltration of organs, and the increase in the expression of cellular adhesion molecules that would facilitate the adhesion of the leukocytes to the capillary endothelium [13, 14, 18, 20].

Physiopathology

In this scenario, one of the most prominent mechanisms is undoubtedly the hypercytokinemia believed to be the underlying cause of systemic capillary extravasation syndrome, where there is a loss of protein-rich fluid from the intravascular to the interstitial space.

Loss of protein-rich fluid from the intravascular space leads to intravascular volume depletion, resulting in secondary activation of the renin, angiotensin, and aldosterone system; the sympathetic nervous system; and the release of vasopressin. The resulting sodium and water retention results in systemic edema and exudative serous cavity effusions. In the most severe cases, all causes of capillary leak syndrome can result in hypovolemic shock [19].

In relation to pulmonary manifestations, one of the most frequent clinical findings is the appearance of pleural effusions that may be accompanied or not by noncardiogenic pulmonary edema [12]. Differentiation therapy with ATRA and/or ATO alters the expression of integrins and adhesion molecules and chemoattractant factors that mediate transmigration of APL cells across the vascular endothelium into the tissue. Differentiation therapy induces the expression of constitutively active b2-integrins on the surface of APL cells and the expression of ICAM-1 in the lung as well as on the APL cells. Binding of b2-integrins to ICAM-1 mediates adhesion of APL cells to the vascular endothelium in the lung (heterotypic aggregation), and the adhesion of APL cells to each other (homotypic aggregation), which both facilitate transmigration of differentiating APL cells into the underlying pulmonary tissue. Differentiation therapy results in massive production of chemokines by the lung and by APL cells. Due to the upregulation of chemokine receptors on the surface of differentiating APL cells, these cells can easily transmigrate in response to the pulmonary chemokine production (initiation phase of DS). Pulmonary infiltration of differentiating APL cells, which massively produce chemokines, further enhances transmigration of leukemic cells from the bloodstream into the lung, aggravating the hyperinflammatory reaction in the lung (aggravation phase of DS) [19].

AKI is a common manifestation of capillary leak syndrome. The most common causes of AKI are prerenal due to intravascular volume depletion followed by ATN. As such, in addition to hypotension, a role for cytokines in the development of ATN in capillary leak syndrome seems likely.

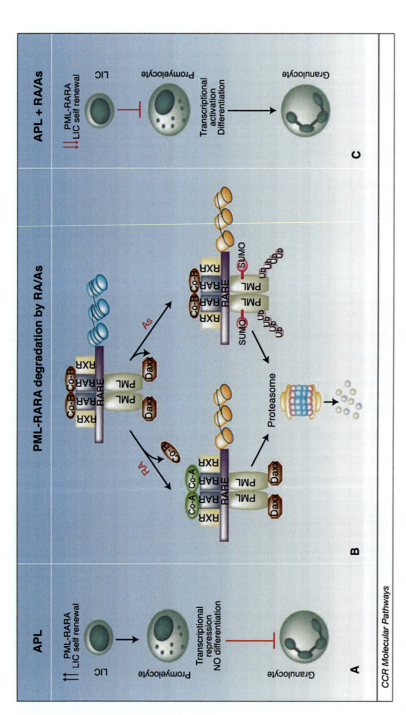

Fig. 1 APL pathogenesis and mechanisms of action of the curable combination RA-As. (**a**) APL is characterized by the expression of PML/RARA that confers self-renewal properties to committed cells and blocks promyelocyte differentiation. (**b**) in APL cells, PML/RARA heterodimerize with RXR and recruit corepressors onto master genes that control promyelocyte differentiation. RA releases corepressors and recruits the coactivators, leading to transcriptional activation of targets and differentiation. RA also induces the recruitment of the proteasome that degrades PML/RARA. Arsenic enhances sumoylation of PML/RARA on Lys 160, which modulates Daxx binding (and thus repression) but also triggers SUMO-dependent polyubiquitination proteasome-dependent degradation of PML and PML/RARA. This will modulate Daxx binding to PML/RARA, leading to the release of transcriptional repression. (**c**) PML/RARA degradation is responsible for the eradication of APL LIC. RA and As also induce PML/RARA transcriptional activation that leads to the differentiation of promyelocytes. However, only loss of LIC self-renewal is correlated to the cure from APL. (Extracted: Nasr et al. [27])

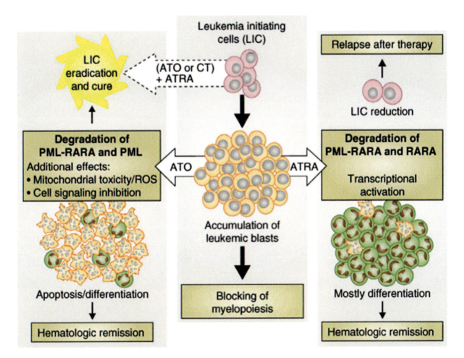

Fig. 2 Elimination of leukemic blasts and LICs is necessary for definitive cure of APL. LICs possess high self-renewal capability and give rise to leukemic blasts that form the bulk of the disease (middle). Both ATRA and ATO promote remission of disease by targeting leukemic blasts. Pharmacological doses of ATRA predominantly drive differentiation of leukemic blasts but are unable to efficiently eliminate LICs that can drive disease relapse (right). In contrast, ATO induces both apoptosis and differentiation of leukemic blasts and can also target LICs and is therefore more effective that ATRA as a monotherapy (left). ATRA acts synergistically with ATO and/or CT, and these combination therapies definitively cure APL in the vast majority of cases (dashed arrow). (Extracted: Santos et al. [9])

In another example of systemic involvement, we have the gastrointestinal tract, with the presentation of abdominal pain, nausea, or vomiting, as a result of edema developed throughout the body. It is likely that many other systems will be affected, justifying a varied clinical picture (Fig. 3).

As already reported, besides the cytokine storm, there are other mechanisms by which the clinical manifestation and the appearance of the complications related to this pathology are damaged. In these processes, we have the involvement of organs and systems by cellular infiltration, promoted by the induction of adhesion of APL cells to the endothelium, through the expression of constitutively active b2-integrins on the surface of APL cells and the expression of ICAM-1 in the organ involvement, both facilitate transmigration of differentiating APL cells into the underlying tissue (Fig. 4).

Clinical Features

There is a divergence in the literature regarding the incidence of the syndrome of differentiation, ranging from 2–27%. This can be explained not only by the different treatment regimens employed and by the methods of prevention but also by the variability in the criteria used in the diagnosis and graduation of this syndrome.

Much of the information related to the clinical picture comes from the Programa Español de Tratamientos en Hematología (PETHEMA) study involving 739 patients diagnosed with acute promyelocytic leukemia and treated with ATRA plus idarubicin. Pau Montesinos et al. through the analysis of this series of cases revealed data on the incidence, characteristics, prognostic factors, and outcome of the

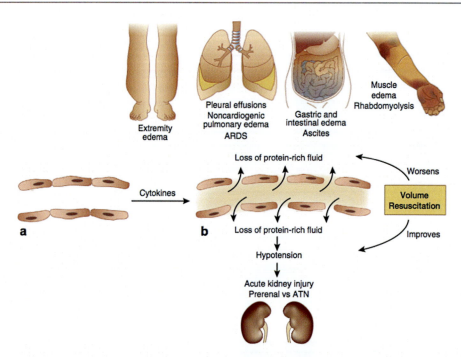

Fig. 3 Clinical manifestations of capillary leak syndrome. (**a**) In the resting state, capillary permeability is normal, and there is limited movement of fluid and proteins from the intravascular to the interstitial space. (**b**) In response to cytokines, vascular permeability increases. The increase in capillary permeability facilitates the movement of protein-rich fluid from the intravascular to the interstitial space. Subsequent intravascular volume depletion causes hypotension of varying severity. Hypotension causes decreased perfusion to the kidneys, resulting in prerenal acute kidney injury or acute tubular necrosis (ATN) in more severe cases. Cytokines themselves may also contribute to renal injury. Accumulation of protein-rich fluid in the interstitial space causes systemic pitting edema, effusions of the thoracic and abdominal cavities, noncardiogenic pulmonary edema, and/or acute respiratory distress syndrome (ARDS) in the lung, gastric, and intestinal edema and muscle edema, which can rarely lead to rhabdomyolysis. Volume resuscitation can increase the intravascular volume and thus improve blood pressure and renal function. Volume resuscitation also expands the interstitial volume and thus potentially worsens systemic edema, increases effusions, and worsens pulmonary, gut, and muscle edema. (Extract: Eric Siddall et al. [35])

differentiation syndrome. Overall, 183 patients (24.8%) experienced DS, 93 with a severe form (12.6%) and 90 with a moderate form (12.2%). Severe but not moderate form was associated with an increase in mortality. A bimodal incidence was observed, with peaks occurring in the first and third weeks after the start of ATRA therapy. The most frequent clinical manifestations of severe DS were dyspnea (95%), pulmonary infiltrates (81%), unexplained fever (74%), weight gain of more than 5 kg (68%), pleural effusion (58%), and renal failure (46%). The frequencies of these symptoms were considerably lower in moderate than in severe form. The frequency of hypotension in late severe DS was significantly higher than in early severe DS, whereas the frequencies of other signs and symptoms did not differ significantly between patients with late and early severe form. A multivariate analysis indicated that a WBC count greater than $5 \times 10\ 9/L$ and an abnormal serum creatinine level correlated with an increased risk of developing severe DS [26].

Symptoms and Signs

Originally, Frankel et al. defined ATRA syndrome in the presence of the following five signs and symptoms: fever, dyspnea, pleural and/or pericardial effusion, pulmonary infiltrates on chest radiograph, and unexplained weight gain greater than 5 kg [12].

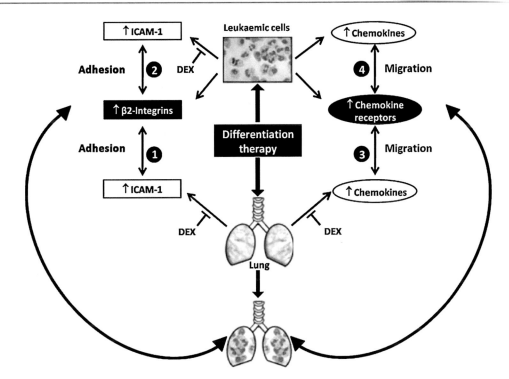

Fig. 4 Mechanisms of pulmonary infiltration of APL cells during differentiation therapy. Differentiation therapy with ATRA and/or ATO alters the expression of integrins and adhesion molecules (left) and chemoattractant factors (right) that mediate transmigration of APL cells across the vascular endothelium into the tissue. Left: Differentiation therapy induces the expression of constitutively active b2-integrins on the surface of APL cells and the expression of ICAM-1 in the lung as well as on the APL cells. Binding of b2-integrins to ICAM-1 mediates adhesion of APL cells to the vascular endothelium in the lung (1: heterotypic aggregation), and the adhesion of APL cells to each other (2: homotypic aggregation), which both facilitate transmigration of differentiating APL cells into the underlying pulmonary tissue. Dexamethasone (DEX) can suppress the expression of ICAM-1 and thereby reduce the adhesion of APL cells to the endothelium (1) and to each other (2). Right: Differentiation therapy results in massive production of chemokines by the lung and by APL cells. Due to the upregulation of chemokine receptors on the surface of differentiating APL cells, these cells can easily transmigrate in response to the pulmonary chemokine production ((3) initiation phase of DS). Pulmonary infiltration of differentiating APL cells, which massively produce chemokines, further enhances transmigration of leukemic cells from the bloodstream into the lung, aggravating the hyperinflammatory reaction in the lung ((4) aggravation phase of DS). Reduction of the pulmonary chemokine secretion by DEX may eliminate the initial trigger for migration of APL cells towards the lung (3). As DEX cannot abrogate the massive chemokine production by differentiating APL cells, pulmonary infiltration of APL cells may induce an uncontrollable hyperinflammatory reaction in the lung (4). (Source extracted: Luesink and Jansen [19])

Over the years, other clinical findings have been described and are listed in the table below (Table 1).

More recently, case reports have been published, associating the appearance of clinical complications with the syndrome of differentiation, among them: ocular manifestations (bilateral reduction in visual acuity) [29], cutaneous lesion (Purulent transformation of granulocytic sarcoma) [6], Sweet syndrome [36], edematous pancreatitis [8], bradycardia [23], cardiac stunning [7], and pulmonary hemorrhage [30].

Laboratory

In laboratory evaluation, there are no specific findings and what is most frequently observed are hematological alterations, which can also be found in patients without the syndrome, attributed to acute promyelocytic leukemia or to the myelosuppressive effect of the chemotherapeutic treatment, such as anemia, thrombocytopenia, and disturbances coagulation. Although some studies attempt to establish a number of leukocytes as

Table 1 Signs and symptoms (Source extracted: Cardinale et al. [4])

Differentiation syndrome: Sign and symptoms	
Elevated white blood cell count	Weight gain >5 kg
Dyspnea	Bone pain
Respiratory distress	Headache
Fever	Hypotension
Pulmonary edema	Congestive heart failure
Pulmonary infiltrates	Acute renal failure
Pleural and pericardial effusion	Hepatotoxicity

a risk factor for development or even as a diagnostic criterion for the differentiation syndrome, there is no cut-off point.

Imaging

Chest radiographs: Radiologic features may be explained by the proposed hypotheses of pathophysiology of the DS. Most of the patients with DS showed cardiomegaly, widening of the vascular pedicle width, increased pulmonary blood volume, peribronchial cuff, ground-glass opacity, septal lines, pleural effusion, parenchymal consolidation, nodular opacities, and air bronchogram (Fig. 5) [17].

It is important to note that these radiographic findings are nonspecific and can be found in other pathologies that make a differential diagnosis with the reported picture. Another observation that is worthy to be mentioned is that a normal X-ray examination not always excludes pulmonary involvement in a considerable number of cases.

Computed tomography: Chest radiographs and CT images obtained in patients with retinoic acid syndrome show nonspecific findings of pulmonary edema and/or hemorrhage. An increased cardiothoracic ratio, increase in vascular pedicle width, increase in pulmonary blood volume, peribronchial cuffing, ground-glass opacities, septal lines, and pleural effusion may be seen, resembling the findings in patients with pulmonary edema due to other causes. Other possible findings, including poorly defined nodules and areas of consolidation, may be due to hemorrhage from damaged endothelial cells (Fig. 6) [5].

Other elements that may constitute the diagnostic armament are bronchoscopy with bronchoalveolar lavage and pulmonary biopsy. They are more used to contribute to make differential diagnosis or to evaluate associated complications than to establish a diagnostic criterion.

Diagnosis

Originally the diagnostic criteria were established by Frankel et al. [12] which were based on seven clinical findings: fever, weight gain (from capillary leak and soft tissue edema), respiratory distress, radiographic opacities, pleural or pericardial effusion, hypotension, and renal failure (usually from hypotension, although disseminated intravascular coagulation may also be present).

However, over time there was no consensus regarding the number of findings necessary to establish the diagnosis. In a report from the Gruppo Italiano Malattie Ematologiche dell'Adulto (GIMEMA group), the diagnosis DS was made by the presence of 5 out of 7 symptoms [21]. In a report by the Program for the Study and Treatment of Malignant Hemopathy (PETHEMA) group, less strict criteria were used (two symptoms) [25]. These variations in the number of criteria, regardless of the therapeutic modalities and the use of preventive measures, contributed to different rates of incidence of the syndrome of differentiation among patients with acute promyelocytic leukemia in treatment with induction therapy ranging from 2% to 25%. The incidence of DS was comparable in the reports from the Breccia et al. [2] (single center study GIMEMA: 14%) and Botton et al. [1] (European APL study group: 15%) who both made the diagnosis of DS in the presence of three or more symptoms. Breccia et al. [2] (Single center study GIMEMA) and Botton et al. [1] (European APL study group) used for the diagnosis of DS in the presence of three or more symptoms and had similar incidences around 15%. Currently it is recommended the utilization of three or more of these findings as a criterion for the diagnosis and early treatment with corticosteroids.

Differential Diagnosis

A confusing point occurs due to the list of differential diagnoses, where pulmonary infections, sepsis, pulmonary thromboembolism, and heart failure appear and there may be coexistence of these with the syndrome of differentiation. Thus, the presence of another diagnosis at the moment of the patient's evaluation does not exclude the possibility of DS.

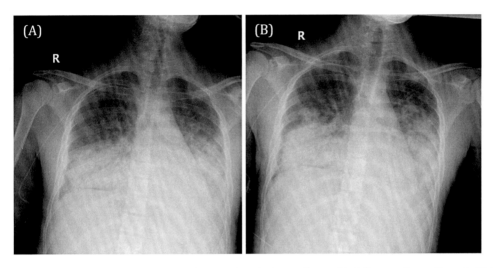

Fig. 5 19-year-old man with all-trans-retinoic acid (ATRA) syndrome, progressing into acute respiratory distress syndrome. (**a**) Chest radiograph 12 days after ATRA treatment shows increased cardiothoracic ratio and increased vascular pedicle width. Poorly defined nodules and ground-glass opacity are noted in entire lung and are considered to be ATRA syndrome. (**b**) Follow-up chest radiograph 42 days after ATRA treatment. Left lung is entirely opacified and coalescent; patchy consolidations are found in right lung, suggesting acute respiratory distress syndrome. (Extracted: ICU from Barretos Cancer Hospital)

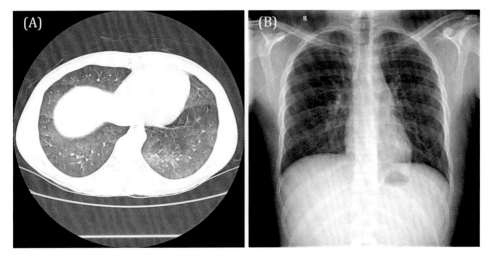

Fig. 6 Retinoic acid syndrome in a patient with acute promyelocytic leukemia (AML subtype M3 in the French-American-British classification system). (**a**) CT image obtained 2 days after treatment with ATRA shows diffuse ground-glass opacities, areas of consolidation, and septal thickening are seen in both lungs. (**b**) Chest radiograph after treatment with corticosteroids. (Extracted: ICU from Barretos Cancer Hospital)

Management

Pharmacologic

Prevention: Despite the lack of scientific evidence for the prophylactic use of corticosteroids in face of the risk of developing the syndrome of differentiation, some authors have followed the recommendation of dexamethasone in the dose of 10 mg intravenously twice daily in patients with compromised renal function (i.e., creatinine >1.4 mg/dL) or total white blood cell count above $5 \times 10^9/L$ (Sanz and Montesinos [32]), while others use a leukocyte count greater than $10 \times 10^9/L$ as a reference [28]. In this scenario of prevention, the criteria regarding the use or not of corticosteroids depend on randomized studies for a better indication.

Treatment: According to the National Comprehensive Cancer Network (NCCN) [28] and European Leukemia Network (ELN) [33] recommendations, all patients with suspected differentiation syndrome should receive intravenous dexamethasone (DEX) 10 mg twice a day and be maintained for at least three consecutive days or until complete remission of signs and symptoms. Dexamethasone can suppress the expression of ICAM-1 and thereby reduce the adhesion of APL cells to the endothelium. Reduction of the pulmonary chemokine secretion by DEX may eliminate the initial trigger for migration of APL cells towards the lung. As DEX cannot abrogate the massive chemokine production by differentiating APL cells, pulmonary infiltration of APL cells may induce an uncontrollable hyperinflammatory reaction in the lung. These patients should continue to receive the differentiation agent involved in the onset of the syndrome (ATRA or ATO), unless there are signs of severity (i.e., presence of progressive worsening of organ dysfunctions such as renal and respiratory insufficiency [19] (Fig. 3).

Non-pharmacologic

Many patients who progress to more severe conditions require intensive care and should receive hemodynamic support (use of vasoactive drugs, for example, for maintenance of pressure levels,

guaranteeing adequate perfusion of the organs), ventilatory (ranging from supplemental oxygen uptake to use of noninvasive ventilatory strategies or even invasive mechanical ventilation), control of the water balance and urinary flow with control of the potential risk factors, and the onset or worsening of renal injury. Moreover, empiric antibiotics should be used when faced with the difficulty of differentiating the syndrome of differentiation and sepsis or even of the overlap of these complications (Table 2).

Management Algorithm

See Fig. 7.

Prognosis

Patients with differentiation syndrome had a high mortality rate in case series studies. This rate fell over the years when the use of corticoids was instituted with the recommended regimen, from 30% to 5%. There is a dramatic improvement of the picture when it was instituted at the time of early diagnosis [26].

Summary

- Differentiation syndrome occurs in patients with acute promyelocytic leukemia after induction chemotherapy with all-trans

Table 2 Measures at suspicion of differentiation syndrome (Source extracted: Cardinale et al. [4])

Measures at suspicion of DS
Chest X-ray, renal function (creatinine and urea), hepatic function (amino transferases and bilirubin), blood cell counts, coagulation test, oxygen saturation
Weight monitoring
Ventilatory support/O_2 supplementation
Blood pressure maintenance measures
Fluid restriction (renal failure)
Steroid administration at first suspicion: dexamethasone 10 mg twice daily until clinical resolution, then tapered dose for a few days
Suspend ATRA or ATO in severe cases, which can be restarted after clinical improvement. If DS recurs after restart, ATRA must be definitively discontinued during induction

Fig. 7 Current algorithm for the management of DS in the PETHEMA trials. (**a**) Prophylaxis. (**b**) Treatment. (Sanz and Montesinos [32])

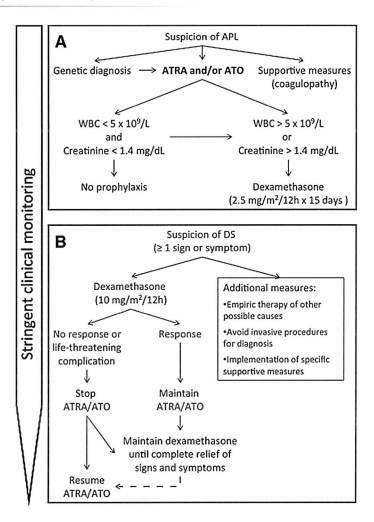

retinoic acid (ATRA) or arsenic trioxide (ATO).

- Its pathophysiological mechanism mainly involves the release of pro-inflammatory cytokines that cause capillary hyper-permeability and lead to the appearance of the most frequent clinical findings: fever, peripheral edema, radiographic pulmonary opacities, hypoxemia, respiratory distress, hypotension, renal and hepatic dysfunction, and serositis resulting in pleural and pericardial effusions.

- As a prophylactic measure to prevent the onset of the syndrome, some authors recommend the administration of 2.5 mg/m² twice daily for 15 days in patients with acute promyelocytic leukemia with WBC >5×109

liter or Cr >1.4 mg/dl and will be dosed with any of the above drugs.

- Other authors advise that dexamethasone is only used for patients presenting with clinical presentation, and the dose of 10 mg twice daily is recommended.

References

1. Botton S, Dombret H, Sanz M, San Miguel J, Caillot D, Zittoun R, Gardembas M, Stamatoulas A, Conde E, Guerci A, Gardin C, Geiser K, Cony Makhoul D, Reman O, de la Serna J, Lefrere F, Chomienne C, Chastang C, Degos L, Fenaux P. Incidence, clinical features, and outcome of all trans-retinoic acid syndrome in 413 cases of newly diagnosed acute promyelocytic leukemia. The European APL Group. Blood. 1998;92:2712–8.

2. Breccia M, Latagliata R, Carmosino I, Cannella L, Diverio D, Guarini A, De Propris MS, Petti MC, Avvisati G, Cimino G, Mandelli F, Lo-Coco F. Clinical and biological features of acute promyelocytic leukemia patients developing retinoic acid syndrome during induction treatment with all-trans retinoic acid and idarubicin. Haematologica. 2008;93:1918–20.

3. Breccia M, Mazzarella L, Bagnardi V, et al. Increased BMI correlates with higher risk of disease relapse and differentiation syndrome in patients with acute promyelocytic leukemia treated with the AIDA protocols. Blood. 2012;119:49.

4. Cardinale L, Asteggiano F, Moretti F, Torre F, Ulisciani S, Fava C, Rege-Cambrin G. Pathophysiology, clinical features and radiological findings of differentiation syndrome/all-trans-retinoic acid syndrome. World J Radiol. 2014;6(8):583–8.

5. Choi MH, Jung JI, Do Chung W, Kim Y-J, Lee S-E, Han DH, Ahn MI, Park SH. Acute pulmonary complications in patients with hematologic malignancies. Radiographics. 2014;34(6):1755–68.

6. Collinge E, Tigaud I, Balme B, Gerland LM, Sujobert P, Carlioz V, Salles G, Thomas X, Paubelle E. Case report: purulent transformation of granulocytic sarcoma: an unusual pattern of differentiation in acute promyelocyticleukemia. Medicine (Baltimore). 2018;97(8):e9657.

7. De Santis GC, Madeira MI, de Oliveira LC, Falcao RP, Rego EM. Cardiac stunning as a manifestation of ATRA differentiation syndrome in acute promyelocytic leukemia. Med Oncol. 2012;29(1):248–50.

8. De D, Nath UK, Chakrabarti P. Pancreatitis in acute promyelocytic leukemia: drug-induced or differentiation syndrome? Indian J Med Paediatr Oncol. 2017;38(3):371–3.

9. Dos Santos GA, Kats L, Pandolfi PP. Synergy against PML-RARa: targeting transcription, proteolysis, differentiation, and self-renewal in acute promyelocytic leukemia. J Exp Med. 2003;210(13):2793–802.

10. Dubois C, Schlageter MH, de Gentile A, et al. Hematopoietic growth factor expression and ATRA sensitivity in acute promyelocytic blast cells. Blood. 1994;83(11):3264–70.

11. Farboud B, Hauksdottir H, Wu Y, Privalsky ML. Isotype-restricted corepressor recruitment: a constitutively closed helix 12 conformation in retinoic acid receptors beta and gamma interferes with corepressor recruitment and prevents transcriptional repression. Mol Cell Biol. 2003;23:2844–58.

12. Frankel SR, Eardley A, Lauwers G, Weiss M, Warrell RP Jr. The "retinoic acid syndrome" in acute promyelocytic leukemia. Ann Intern Med. 1992;117(4):292–6.

13. Gordon M, Jakubowski A, Frankel S, et al. Neutrophil (PMN) function in patients with acute promyelocytic leukemia (APL) treated with all-trans retinoic acid (ATRA) (abstract). Proc Annu Meet Am Soc Clin Oncol. 1991;10:A761.

14. Hickstein DD, Hickey MJ, Collins SJ. Transcriptional regulation of the leukocyte adherence protein beta subunit during human myeloid cell differentiation. J Biol Chem. 1988;263:13863.

15. Jeddi R, Kacem K, Ben Neji H, et al. Predictive factors of all-trans-retinoic acid related complications during induction therapy for acute promyelocyticleukemia. Hematology. 2008;13:142.

16. Jeddi R, Ghédira H, Mnif S, et al. High body mass index is an independent predictor of differentiation syndrome in patients with acute promyelocytic leukemia. Leuk Res. 2010;34:545.

17. Jung JI, Choi JE, Hahn ST, Min CK, Kim CC, Park SH. Radiologic features of all-trans-retinoic acid syndrome. AJR. 2002;178:475–80.

18. Larson RS, Brown DC, Sklar LA. Retinoic acid induces aggregation of the acute promyelocytic leukemia cell line NB-4 by utilization of LFA-1 and ICAM-2. Blood. 1997;90:2747.

19. Luesink M, Jansen JH. Advances in understanding the pulmonary infiltration in acute promyelocyticleukaemia. Br J Haematol. 2010;151:209–20.

20. Luesink M, Pennings JL, Wissink WM, Linssen PC, Muus P, Pfundt R, de Witte TJ, van der Reijden BA, Jansen JH. Chemokine induction by all-trans retinoic acid and arsenic trioxide in acute promyelocytic leukemia: triggering the differentiation syndrome. Blood. 2009;114(27):5512.

21. Mandelli F, Diverio D, Avvisati G, Luciano A, Barbui T, Ber- nasconi C, Broccia G, Cerri R, Falda M, Fioritoni G, Leoni F, Liso V, Petti MC, Rodeghiero F, Saglio G, Vegna ML, Visani G, Jehn U, Willemze R, Muus P, Pelicci PG, Biondi A, Lo-Coco F. Molecular remission in PML/RAR alpha-positive acute promyelocytic leukemia by combined all-trans retinoic acid and idarubicin (AIDA) therapy. Gruppo Italiano-MalattieEmatologiche Maligne dell'AdultoandAssociazione Italiana di E- matologiaed Oncologia Pediatrica Cooperative Groups. Blood. 1997;90:1014–21.

22. Mangelsdorf DJ, Thummel C, Beato M, et al. The nuclear receptor superfamily: the second decade. (Overview). Cell. 1995;83:835–9.

23. McGregor A, Hurst E, Lord S, Jones G. Bradycardiafollowing retinoic acid differentiation syndrome in a patient with acute promyelocyticleukaemia. BMJ Case Rep. 2012;9:2012.

24. Melnick A, Licht JD. Deconstructing a disease: RARalpha, its fusion partners, and their roles in the pathogenesis of acute promyelocytic leukemia. Blood. 1999;93:3167–215.

25. Montesinos P, Bergua JM, Vellenga E, Rayon C, Parody R, de la Serna J, Leon A, Esteve J, Milone G, Deben G, Rivas C, Gonzalez M, Tormo M, Diaz-Mediavilla J, Gonzalez JD, Negri S, Amutio E, Brunet S, Lowenberg B, Sanz MA. Differentiation syndrome in patients with acute promyelocyticleukemia treated with all-transretinoic acid and anthracycline

chemotherapy: characteristics, outcome and prognostic factors. Blood. 2008;113:775–83.

26. Montesinos P, Bergua JM, Vellenga E, CheloRayon RP, de laSerna J, Leon A, Esteve J, Milone G, Deben G, Rivas C, Gonzalez M, Tormo M, Díaz-Mediavilla J, Gonzalez JD, Negri S, Amutio E, Brunet S, Lowenberg B, Sanz MA. Differentiation syndrome in patients with acute promyelocytic leukemia treated with all-trans retinoic acid and anthracycline chemotherapy: characteristics, outcome, and prognostic factors. Blood. 2009; 113(4):775–83.

27. Nasr R, ValérieLallemand-Breitenbach JZ, Guillemin M-C, de Thé H. Therapy-induced PML/RARA proteolysis and acute promyelocytic leukemia cure. Clin Cancer Res. 2009;15(20):6321–6.

28. National Comprehensive Cancer Network (NCCN). NCCN Clinical practice guidelines in oncology. Acute Myeloid Leuk Version 1.2018 – Feb 7

29. Newman AR, Leung B, Richards A, Campbell TG, Wellwood J, Imrie FR. Two cases of differentiation syndrome with ocular manifestations in patients with acute promyelocyticleukaemia treated with all-trans retinoic acid and arsenic trioxide. Am J Ophthalmol Case Rep. 2018;9:106–11.

30. Raanani P, Segal E, Levi I, Bercowicz M, Berkenstat H, Avigdor A, Perel A, Ben-Bassat I. Diffuse alveolar hemorrhage in acute promyelocytic leukemia patients treated with ATRA–a manifestation of the basic disease or the treatment. Leuk Lymphoma. 2000;37(5–6):605.

31. Santos FL, Dore AI, Lima AS, et al. Hematological features and expression profile of myeloid antigens of acute promyelocytic leukemia patients: analysis of prognostic factors for development of the retinoic acid syndrome. Rev Assoc Med Bras (1992). 2004;50:286.

32. Sanz MA, Montesinos P. How we prevent and treat differentiation syndrome in patients with acute promyelocytic leukemia. Blood. 2014;123(18):2777–82.

33. Sanz MA, Grimwade D, Tallman MS, Lowenberg B, Fenaux P, Estey EH, Naoe T, Lengfelder E, Büchner T, Döhner H, Burnett AK, Lo-Coco F. Management of acute promyelocytic leukemia: recommendations from an expert panel on behalf of the European Leukemia Net. Blood. 2009;113(9):1875.

34. Seale J, Delva L, Renesto P, et al. All-trans retinoic acid rapidly decreases cathepsin G synthesis and mRNA expression in acute promyelocytic leukemia. Leukemia. 1996;10(1):95–101.

35. Siddall E, Khatri M, Radhakrishnan J. Capillary leak syndrome: etiologies, pathophysiology, and management. Kidney Int. 2017;92:37–46.

36. Solano-López G, Llamas-Velasco M, Concha-Garzón MJ, Daudén E. Sweet syndrome and differentiation syndrome in a patient with acute promyelocytic leukemia. World J Clin Cases. 2015;3(2):196–8.

Pneumonia in the Cancer Patient

40

Ala Eddin S. Sagar and Scott E. Evans

Contents

Introduction 608

Mechanisms of Susceptibility 608
Anatomical Contributions 608
Innate Immune Dysfunction 609
Neutrophil Defects 609
Lymphocyte Dysfunction 609
Other Mechanisms 610
Critical Illness 610

Notable Pathogens 610
Bacteria 610
Fungi 611
Viruses 612

Epidemiology 613

Clinical Presentation 613

Diagnostic Studies 614
Imaging 614
Respiratory Samples 615
Non-respiratory Samples 616

Management 617
Prevention 617
Pharmacologic Therapies 617
Non-pharmacologic Therapies 618

Prognosis 618

Conclusion 619

References 619

A. E. S. Sagar · S. E. Evans (✉)
Department of Pulmonary Medicine, Division of Internal
Medicine, The University of Texas MD Anderson Cancer
Center, Houston, TX, USA
e-mail: ASagar@mdanderson.org;
seevans@mdanderson.org

© Springer Nature Switzerland AG 2020
J. L. Nates, K. J. Price (eds.), *Oncologic Critical Care*,
https://doi.org/10.1007/978-3-319-74588-6_53

Abstract

Pneumonia is a ubiquitous killer in all patient populations but presents a particular risk for morbidity and mortality among immunosuppressed cancer patients. The enhanced susceptibility of cancer patients to pneumonia arises from the aggregate effects of disease- and treatment-related immune dysfunction, disease- and treatment-related anatomic derangements, and healthcare-associated pathogen exposures, with the exact nature of an individual patient's susceptibility being highly unique. Further, while prompt initiation of adequate antimicrobial therapy is essential to improved pneumonia outcomes, the initial diagnosis of pneumonia is often challenging in this population, as cancer patients with pneumonia frequently present with attenuated clinical signs and symptoms and very often have competing diagnoses that might explain new radiographic infiltrates, fever, or respiratory symptoms. This chapter addresses the mechanisms underlying pneumonia susceptibility in cancer patients, discusses the pathogens most often encountered, and provides an overview of pneumonia preventative, diagnostic, and therapeutic strategies in this vulnerable patient group.

Keywords

Pneumonia · Immunocompromised host · Host-pathogen interactions · Neutropenia · Antibiotic resistance · Bronchoscopy · Hematologic malignancy · Stem cell transplantation · Orogastric aspiration · CT chest · Bacteria · Viruses · Fungi

Introduction

Pneumonia is an important cause of death in all populations worldwide and kills more people than any other nosocomial infections [23]. In cancer patients, pneumonia has a particularly staggering impact, resulting in more deaths than any other infection, despite the widespread use of prophylactic antibiotics [21]. Indeed, the case fatality rates of pneumonia in patients with hematological malignancies have been estimated at 40–80% and may be as high as 90% in some recipients of hematopoietic stem cell transplantation (HSCT) [35]. Despite the extreme acute lethality caused by pneumonia-induced cardiopulmonary instability, these figures fail to adequately capture the additional deaths among cancer patients who are not offered potentially lifesaving cancer treatments due to concerns about therapy-induced immune compromise in the setting of possible lower respiratory tract infections [76]. This chapter addresses etiologies, clinical features, and management of pneumonia in cancer patients.

Mechanisms of Susceptibility

Cancer patients' proclivity for respiratory infections arises from their individual expressions of myriad immune defects, anatomical derangements, and constitutional/nutritional factors related to cancer and/or its treatment [5]. Further, the frequent healthcare encounters that characterize cancer management substantially increase the risk of acquiring nosocomial and drug-resistant pathogens [5]. Moreover, cancer patients may develop new or worsening immunosuppression when critically ill [62], potentially contributing to further pneumonia susceptibility [88].

Anatomical Contributions

Aspiration of orogastric contents is the most common portal of entry for pathogens causing respiratory infections, and disordered laryngoesophageal function is a frequent complication of cancer and its treatment. Swallow function and airway protective responses may be disrupted by central neurological lesions, mucositis of the upper aerodigestive tract, mass lesions in the swallow apparatus, or indwelling devices that bypass protective mechanisms. Alternately, patients with lung cancer or other solid tumors involving the thorax may develop airway obstruction, either by endoluminal airway occlusion or extrinsic compression, leading to atelectasis, impaired mucociliary clearance, and post-obstructive pneumonia [100]. Similarly, airway distortions caused by surgery or radiotherapy may also predispose to infections by impeding pathogen clearance. As in patients without cancer, preexisting anatomic lung diseases such as bronchiectasis and cavitary lung disease predispose to colonization and infection [25]. Relatedly, patients with tumors involving the esophagus are at elevated risk of pneumonia due to contributions of gastric reflux and tracheoesophageal fistulae [70]. Anatomical and immune derangements may coexist in a single patient, increasing their risk of acquiring various forms of infections. Further, non-aspiration routes of pneumonia establishment may also result from cancer-related anatomic issues, such as hematogenous spread or regional progression of infection from infected tumor sites or septic emboli associated with deep venous thrombosis, lines, or grafts.

Innate Immune Dysfunction

The constitutive defenses of the lungs prominently include contributions of airway and alveolar epithelial cells, alveolar macrophages, and the mucociliary escalator system. Epithelial cells confer a barrier preventing pathogen translocation. In addition, the epithelial cell express antimicrobial effectors (e.g., cationic antimicrobial peptides, lactoferrin, lysozyme, cathelicidin, and reactive oxygen species) that activate leukocyte-mediated immunity, enhance pathogen opsonization, and have direct microbiocidal effects, reducing the pathogen burden [104]. Alveolar macrophages phagocytose pathogens and activate the complement system, while the mucociliary escalator entraps and expels inhaled pathogens [32]. The innate defense barriers are often compromised in patients with cancer, either due to the presence of devices that may serve as nidus for pathogen colonization including nasogastric and endotracheal tubes or from chemotherapy- or radiotherapy-induced mucositis that disrupts the epithelial barrier and impairs mucociliary clearance. Mucositis frequently occurs in the gastrointestinal tract due to the rapid turnover rate of the intestinal epithelium and has been classically described with drugs manipulating DNA synthesis such as methotrexate, 5-fluorouracil, and cytarabine, although other antineoplastic drugs including targeted therapy (tyrosine kinase, mammalian target of rapamycin, epidermal growth factor, and vascular growth factor) have also been implicated [57]. Mucositis may also follow head and neck or thoracoabdominal radiation [8], with the severity of mucositis increasing with repetitive cycles of therapy [2].

Neutrophil Defects

Neutropenia is a frequent and important complication of many chemotherapeutic agents, particularly nucleoside analogues and alkylating agent. Severe neutropenia (<500 cells/mL) is clearly associated with both bacterial and fungal pneumonias [43]. While cytotoxic chemotherapy is classically associated with severe neutropenia, both qualitative neutrophil defects and qualitative neutrophil dysfunction may occur as a result of radiation therapy, hypovolemia, acidosis, hyperglycemia, or corticosteroid use [76]. Chemotherapy can also affect multiple neutrophil functions, including chemotaxis and phagocytosis, independent of the quantitative defect [37]. Up to 60% of patients who develop chemotherapy-induced neutropenia will develop pulmonary opacities [97]. Both the degree and duration of neutropenia are associated with increased risk of infection, as is cyclic or recurrent neutropenia.

Lymphocyte Dysfunction

Exposure of cancer patients to agents such as corticosteroids, tacrolimus, calcineurin inhibitors, antithymocyte globulins, and IL-2 inhibitors can contribute to absolute or functional lymphopenia. These defects may persist long after completion of therapy with T cell-depleting chemotherapeutic agents such as alemtuzumab, antithymocyte globulin, and fludarabine, and clinically meaningful lymphocyte dysfunction may continue after lymphocyte counts have recovered to normal levels [79]. Deficiencies of functional leukocytes may result as a consequence of excessive expansion of clonal leukemia population leading to cytopenia and immune dysfunction. Lymphocyte defects notably increase risk for pneumonia caused by organisms such as *Pneumocystis jirovecii*, *Toxoplasma*, *Listeria monocytogenes*, *Salmonella*, *Legionella*, *Cytomegalovirus*, varicella-zoster infection, and human herpesvirus 6, with particular risk in the setting of severe lymphopenia (absolute lymphocyte count <200 cells/mL).

Other Mechanisms

Patients with cancer are prone to specific immunologic derangements depending on the type of malignancy and the antineoplastic therapy they receive [5]. Disproportionate depletion of CD4 T cells relative to CD8 T cells may be caused by alkylating agents causing immune dysfunction. Other chemotherapeutic agents associated with increased risk of pneumonia via non-neutropenic mechanisms including topoisomerase inhibitors, taxanes, anthracyclines, and vinca alkaloids [36]. Waldenstrom's macroglobulinemia and chronic lymphocytic leukemia patients are prone to immunoglobulin dyscrasias and defects in opsonization, just as multiple myeloma may be associated with immune defects due to immunoglobulin deficiency and class switching. Hodgkin's lymphoma, adult T cell leukemia, lymphocytic leukemia, and graft versus host disease (GVHD) are frequently associated with defects of cell-mediated immunity leading to reduced T cell counts and function [24].

Steroid-refractory acute GVHD patients have been shown to have a high 1-year incidence of fatal bacterial, CMV, and invasive fungal infections [24]. Alternately, intensifying immunotherapy to manage GVHD also increases susceptibility to pneumonia.

Ibrutinib, a Bruton tyrosine kinase (BTK), has been described to contribute to immunosuppression by leading to severe hypogammaglobulinemia, mainly affecting immunoglobulin G.

This occurs due to a mutation in the BTK gene, located on the long arm of X chromosome, which has been recognized as the cause of X-linked agammaglobulinemia that puts patients at risk of developing recurrent bacterial infections [75]. Ibrutinib has also been found to inhibit IL2-inducible T cell kinase, an important component of T cell receptor (TCR)-mediated signaling [49]. Ibrutinib has been associated with severe pneumonias occurring as early as 1 week after initiation of treatment and as late as 3 years [45]. Recent studies have suggested that polymorphisms of toll-like receptors are associated with a significant increase in risk of developing pneumonia in AML patients undergoing chemotherapy [80]. Defects in antibody-dependent lymphocyte cytolytic activity increase the risk of severe parasitic infections.

Critical Illness

Critical illness, in the presence or absence of cancer, may contribute to impaired Th1 immune responses, resulting in increased susceptibility to pneumonia [84]. Other immune dysregulations thought to occur secondary to critical illness include lymphocyte anergy, leukocyte apoptosis, and deactivated monocyte functions [62]. Lymphocyte anergy subsequently leads to the loss of delayed-type hypersensitivity reaction to skin tests antigens seen in critically ill patients [96]. The severity of the lymphocyte anergy has been linked with worse outcomes, increased rates of infectious complications, and organ failure [96].

Notable Pathogens

Bacteria

Bacteria frequently cause pneumonia in patients with cancer. Although there is significant overlap with the spectrum of bacterial organisms causing pneumonia in otherwise healthy patients, patients with cancer are at risk of developing pneumonia following a smaller microbial inoculum. As with other populations, microbial epidemiology varies widely with patient age and geography. Cancer-associated immune impairments and the frequent healthcare visits also increase the risk of acquiring pneumonias due to multidrug-resistant (MDR) pathogens.

Although no formal society guidelines address initial antibiotic selection for cancer patients suspected of having pneumonia, making the distinction between community-acquired pneumonia (CAP) and hospital-acquired pneumonia (HAP) remains essential in considering initial management of cancer patients with suspected pneumonia, just as in other populations, due to the differences in bacteria species and susceptibility associated with these distinct processes [94]. The pathogens that cause ventilator-associated pneumonia (VAP) represent a component of the HAP spectrum. Up to 80% of HAPs occurring in the ICU occur among patients receiving ventilatory support, and VAP has been linked to prolonged ventilator days, ICU, and hospital length of stay [72]. The entity of healthcare-associated pneumonia (HCAP) is no longer included in current management guidelines but may still be considered an appropriate descriptor of pneumonias that arise in community-dwelling cancer patients who have frequent exposures to healthcare environments, such as through receipt of parenteral therapies in outpatient settings, putting them at higher than typical risk of nosocomial pathogens [39].

The most common bacterial cause of pneumonia in patients with and without cancer is *Streptococcus pneumoniae*. Frequently encountered Gram-negative pathogens in cancer patients with suspected pneumonia include *Enterobacteriaceae* (*Klebsiella, Escherichia coli, Enterobacter, Citrobacter, Serratia*), *Pseudomonas aeruginosa*, and *Proteus* species. Other bacterial organisms often noted to cause cancer-associated pneumonias include *Stenotrophomonas, Burkholderia, Achromobacter, Chryseobacterium*, and *Alcaligenes* spp., as well as atypical pathogens such as *Mycoplasma pneumoniae, Chlamydia pneumoniae*, and *Legionella* spp. Due to the nosocomial exposures noted above, multidrug-resistant organisms such as methicillin-resistant *Staphylococcus aureus* (MRSA) and extended spectrum beta-lactamase-producing *Enterobacteriaceae* must be considered in initial coverage. Bacterial post-obstructive pneumonias tend to be polymicrobial, often including Gram-negative bacilli, staphylococci, and anaerobes.

Asplenic patients with hypocomplementemia are at increased risk of infections with encapsulated bacterial organisms. Intracellular organisms such as *Listeria monocytogenes, Legionella* spp., and *Salmonella* spp. more commonly cause pneumonia in cancer patients with cellular immune dysfunction.

The incidence of documented *Stenotrophomonas* infection in patients with cancer has substantially increased over the past two decades. Prolonged exposure to carbapenems has been linked to the development of *Stenotrophomonas* infections [77]. Prolonged mechanical ventilation and recent antibiotic administration increase the risk of developing pneumonia due to *P. aeruginosa, Enterobacter* spp., *Acinetobacter, Stenotrophomonas, Alcaligenes*, and *Burkholderia* [72].

Nocardia spp. typically affect patients with impaired cellular immunity, HSCT patients, patients on high-doses of corticosteroids, and patients with GVHD. Indolent cases of *Nocardia* pneumonia may be difficult to distinguish from actinomycetes infections [91].

Although uncommon in many populations in the developed world, *Mycobacterium tuberculosis* remains an important bacterial pathogen to be considered in severely immunosuppressed and/or foreign-born patients with cancer, including those on chronic systemic corticosteroid therapy. The risk seems to be greatest in patients with lung, head and neck, and breast cancers. The disease most often occurs due to reactivation of a latent infection, rather than a primary disease, and may follow a virulent bacterial infection [17].

Fungi

Invasive mold infections are leading causes of morbidity in patients with hematological malignancies, HSCT recipients, and patients on immunosuppressive therapy and frequently present with pneumonias more severe than encountered in non-cancer populations [7]. *Aspergillus* spp. are the most common fungal cause of invasive lung infections. In the United States, *A. fumigatus* is the most common species, followed by *A. flavus*, *A. terreus*, and *A. ustus* [82]. Common non-*Aspergillus* fungal pathogens encountered in lung infections of cancer patients include *Fusarium* spp. (e.g., *F. solani*, *F. oxysporum*, and *F. moniliforme*) and, increasingly, *Mucorales* (e.g., *Mucor*, *Rhizopus*, *Rhizomucor*, and *Lichtheimia* spp.) [89]. Other reported invasive mold infections affecting cancer patients include *Trichosporon*, *Scedosporium*, and *Alternaria* [19]. Rising incidence of non-fumigatus species is suspected to have been driven in part by the frequent use of *Aspergillus*-active prophylaxis in patients at high risk for fungal infections and a pervasive shift of initial empiric antifungal selection away from amphotericin B [44].

Prolonged (>1 week) severe neutropenia, allogenic HSCT, GVHD, refractory leukemia, and corticosteroids are important risk factors for developing invasive pulmonary fungal infections [55]. GVHD has been linked to enhanced fungal susceptibility due to macrophage dysfunction, immunoglobulin subclass deficiencies, and impaired neutrophil chemotaxis [31]. T cell depletion or dysfunction has also been recognized as a risk factor for fungal pneumonia even in the absence of neutropenia [47]. Decreased host defenses to fungal infection may also arise in hematological malignancies complicated by immunoglobulin dyscrasias, which may include impaired production, inappropriate class switching, and increased antibody catabolism [41]. More recently, studies have identified antibodies that promote complement activation and phagocytosis and inhibit adhesion and germination, which may have a protective role against *Aspergillus*, *Histoplasma*, and *Pneumocystis* spp. [9].

The risk *Pneumocystis jirovecii* pneumonia is elevated among patients with lymphopenia, low CD4 counts, preexisting lung disease, ALL, CLL, non-Hodgkin's lymphoma, and multiple myeloma [68], whereas it is relatively less common in patients with AML or myelodysplastic syndrome [68, 73]. In addition to classical association

with corticosteroid exposures, chemotherapeutic agents that have been reported to increase the risk of *Pneumocystis* pneumonia include cyclophosphamide, vincristine, methotrexate, fludarabine, cytarabine, and rituximab [73].

Interestingly, Transplant-Associated Infection Surveillance Network (TRANSNET) data suggest that the rate of pneumonias in HSCT patients caused by the endemic fungi *Histoplasma capsulatum*, *Blastomyces dermatitidis*, and *Coccidioides immitis* is similar to that observed in the non-HSCT population. This is suspected to be due to widespread use of antifungal prophylaxis and systematic avoidance of outdoor activities before engraftment and while on intensive immunosuppression for GVHD [40].

Viruses

HSCT patients with severe lymphopenia have a higher risk of viral pneumonia than patients with absolute lymphocyte counts greater than 200 cells/dL. Susceptibility in the setting of lymphopenia has been demonstrated for CMV, influenza viruses, human rhinovirus and enterovirus, and parainfluenza virus [11]. The risk is particularly the signification among patients receiving intensive myeloablative conditioning regimens prior to HSCT. CMV pneumonia is the most common opportunistic viral complication in cancer patients with defected cellular immunity and typically develops from reactivation of disease rather than de novo virus acquisition. Reactivation risk is significant in HSCT recipients who are seropositive for CMV prior to transplant regardless of donor status [28]. Notably, CMV risk appears to be much greater following HSCT than during acute myeloablative chemotherapy [64]. Additional risk factors for viral pneumonia that have been observed in cancer patients include hypoalbuminemia, chronic or prolonged corticosteroid exposure, and age greater than 65 years [11]. General debility has also been identified as a risk factor for developing pneumonia in patients with cancer. In a retrospective study, hypoxia at diagnosis, elevated creatinine, and respiratory coinfection were associated with a significant increase in 60-day mortality [98]. It is postulated that this effect may arise from a deficiency of essential fatty acids and polyribonucleotides that alter the normal cytotoxic and inflammatory response [34]. GVHD has been associated with a twofold increase in risk of developing viral pneumonia in HSCT patients [56].

Seasonal variations in viral carriage alter the risk of acquiring viral pneumonias. The risk peaks in later autumn and continues through winter for influenza, RSV, and *Human metapneumovirus* (hMPV) infections. A biphasic peak in both autumn and spring is observed with human rhinovirus (HRV), while parainfluenza virus infections typically peak in spring and summer [14].

Epidemiology

Pneumonia is believed to either cause or complicate around 10% of hospital admissions among patients with cancer. A diagnosis of bacterial pneumonia is associated with poorer overall outcomes in cancer patients [103]. The risk of pneumonia during the course of treatment of patients with hematological malignancies exceeds 30% [21]. The risk is even higher in hematopoietic stem cell transplant (HSCT) recipients, among whom as many as 80% of patients will experience at least one episodes of pneumonia throughout the course of their disease. As many as 20% of HSCT patients may ultimately die from pneumonia, making it the leading cause of death among patients with acute leukemia in the transfusion era [21]. The incidence of invasive fungal pneumonias in patients with cancer has been reported to be as high as 48%. The incidence appears to be decreasing due to the implementation of antifungal prophylaxis [107], though improving diagnostic technologies may mask some of this effect.

Epidemiological studies estimated that up to one in five patients admitted to the intensive care unit with sepsis have cancer. Sepsis is the leading cause of ICU admissions in patients with cancer. The most frequent organ infected is the lung [74]. Patients with hematological cancers have more pulmonary dysfunction during their ICU

stay compared to patients without cancer [88]. Furthermore, cancer patients who are critically ill with sepsis in the ICU have longer ICU length of stays compared with those without cancer, putting them at higher risk of developing hospital-acquired infections [74].

Clinical Presentation

The cardinal clinical features of pneumonia, such as fever, cough, purulent secretions, and leukocytosis, may be blunted or absent in cancer patients due to the impairment of the host immune status discussed above. Moreover, the impaired immune status makes these patients more prone to uncommon, atypical, or opportunistic organisms. Therefore, a high index of suspicion is required to avoid missing the diagnosis of pneumonia in cancer patients.

When present, some symptoms may be suggestive of a particular pathogen. For example, RSV pneumonia classically presents with fever, cough, dyspnea, and wheezing and less frequently with sore throat and rhinorrhea [20]. HEV frequently presents with cough, while HRV may worsen preexisting symptoms of chronic lung disease leading to dyspnea and wheezing [99]. CMV pneumonia typically presents with cough, dyspnea, and hypoxia and occasionally fever [93]. Generalized symptoms of malaise, fever, and arthralgia may accompany CMV disease, though these are highly nonspecific. While symptom patterns may be helpful in reminding the clinician to consider specific pathogen when devising an initial treatment regimen, they cannot be used to reliably distinguish between the various forms of pneumonia [15].

The clinical presentation of *Pneumocystis* pneumonia in patients with hematological malignancies differs from the characteristic presentation of that seen in patients with HIV disease. *Pneumocystis* pneumonia presents more acutely and is associated with more inflammation and few organisms than is usually observed in patients with HIV. *Pneumocystis* pneumonia most often affects patients receiving corticosteroids and those not receiving adequate prophylaxis. The mortality rate of PJP pneumonia in patients with hematological malignancies is estimated between 30% and 60% and is likely slightly higher in HSCT patients [58].

The clinician is advised to recall in patients with cancer and HSCT recipients many numerous potential causes for fever, dyspnea, and radiographic infiltrates, such as bronchiolitis obliterans, diffuse alveolar hemorrhage, and cryptogenic organizing pneumonia [13]. Therefore, even when the clinical presentation is strongly suggestive of pneumonia, alternate diagnoses must be considered and addressed.

Diagnostic Studies

The relative paucity and unreliability of symptoms in the presentation of cancer-associated pneumonia has not supported the development of clinically meaningful symptom-based prediction rules for the diagnosis of pneumonia in this population [15]. Thus, the clinician must remain vigilant and systematic in his or her efforts to diagnose pneumonia in the immunosuppressed cancer patient.

Imaging

Radiographic imaging of the chest is a mainstay in the diagnosis of pneumonia, though no modality is without limitations. Much like clinical symptoms, the generation of infiltrates is dependent upon host responses to the presence of a lower respiratory pathogen. Furthermore, the presence of a lung infiltrate on imaging is not specific for a pneumonia diagnosis. In fact, a retrospective study of asymptomatic patients with AML demonstrated that 88% of the patients had radiographic abnormalities at baseline, regardless of respiratory symptoms [95]. Conversely, the absence of radiographic opacities on a chest x-ray does not exclude a pneumonia diagnosis in the proper clinical context, as almost half of patients with febrile neutropenia who had a CT scan of the chest suggestive of pneumonia had a normal chest x-ray and up to 10% or

patients with invasive pulmonary aspergillosis will present with a normal chest x-ray [18].

Although CT scans are considerably more sensitive than conventional chest x-rays for identifying pulmonary opacities and identifying apical disease [87], there is no CT pattern that reliably confirms a pneumonia diagnosis nor differentiates between pathogens. That said, there are certain CT patterns that are characteristically observed with certain pathogens/pathogen classes, such the findings of lobar consolidation or peribronchial nodules that are most typically seen with bacterial pneumonias [65].

Viral pneumonias most often present with CT evidence of ground-glass opacities (GGOs), nodules, interlobular septal thickening, and bronchial wall thickening. The opacities noted on imaging reflect airspace accumulation of fluid, leukocytes, and/or debris [106]. Influenza pneumonia is often associated with mucus plugging of the terminal bronchioles in addition to the more common GGOs, bronchial thickening, and nodules. These opacities may become more diffuse and confluent as the disease progresses [67]. RSV pneumonia in patients with HSCT may demonstrate bronchial wall thickening, airspace consolidation, GGOs, and subcentimeter nodules [26]. And PIV typically manifests with GGOs and peribronchial nodules [22]. A miliary pattern or diffuse interstitial pneumonitis pattern with GGOs and centrilobular nodules has been described in CMV pneumonia [27].

Chest CT findings that raise suspicion for fungal pneumonia include well-circumscribed nodules, cavitary lesions, or the presence of the halo or air-crescent signs [18]. Although not currently the standard of care, CT angiography has been suggested to be more sensitive than conventional CT in diagnosing fungal pneumonia in HSCT patients through demonstration of the occluded vessel sign, an interruption of a vessel at the border of a focal lesion without depiction of the vessel inside the lesion or peripheral to the lesion that suggests pathological angioinvasion [85]. Patients with septic emboli may demonstrate multicentric, pleomorphic lung nodules, with asymmetric, thick-walled cavities.

Chest x-ray may be normal in the early course of *Pneumocystis* pneumonia [1]. CT scans of the chest may demonstrate bilateral patchy ground-glass opacities predominantly in the perihilar regions and sparing the periphery of the lung. Cysts may also be later observed and typically occur in the upper lobes and can potentially lead to pneumothorax. Although pleural effusions are rarely seen in other instances of *Pneumocystis* pneumonia, this finding may be present in HSCT patients [33].

Respiratory Samples

The demonstration of a pathogenic organism from normally sterile respiratory secretions is generally the most convincing means to establish a diagnosis of pneumonia in cancer patients. The role of sputum samples is increasingly debated in both cancer and non-cancer patients that are suspected of having pneumonia. Certainly, identifying a definite pathogen on sputum culture can be helpful in directing appropriate care. However, both negative cultures and the detection of oropharyngeal contaminants or organisms that are occasional or opportunistic pathogens can be challenging to interpret. Although practice patterns vary between centers, bronchoscopy with bronchoalveolar lavage remains the diagnostic tool of choice for immunocompromised host pneumonia. Nonetheless, the yield of traditional BAL cultures is only 25–51% [35], though recent evidence suggests that the yield is enhanced in HSCT patients when the procedure is performed soon after the onset of pneumonia-suggestive symptoms, especially if prior to the initiation of antimicrobial therapy [29].

The current standard clinical practice is to perform serial dilution cultures of BAL fluid for bacterial pathogen detection. This is due to the vast array of organisms that can be identified, quantified, and subcultured for susceptibility using this technique. The role of bronchial washing and protected specimen brush samples remains unclear, as neither have been clearly shown to improve diagnosis. In intubated patients, non-bronchoscopic sample collections (e.g., mini-BAL) offers an opportunity to directly obtain lower respiratory samples, though the current evidence does not allow conclusions regarding overall utility of this approach [86]. Modern molecular techniques, such as polymerase chain reaction (PCR)-based strategies, have recently been used as a supplement to culture-based methods to diagnose bacterial pneumonia and may supplant the conventional approach in the coming years. The rapid results obtained with PCR techniques may aid in improving estimates of pneumonia burden and may facilitate earlier de-escalation from broad-spectrum antibiotics sooner, in hopes of reducing cultivation of antibiotic-resistant organisms. PCR assays can also help in the situations in which sterile cultures are obtained due to delayed sampling, as PCR can detect genomic material even from nonviable bacteria [38].

Molecular techniques have become the principal means in many clinical labs of detecting viral respiratory pathogens. Viral nucleic acid amplification techniques (PCR, microarray, and DNA chip) have been validated in patients with HSCT and are superior to conventional direct fluorescent antibody stains and viral cultures for diagnosing viral pneumonias [63]. It has been suggested that isolating the virus from the lower respiratory tract carries a worse prognosis compared to patients with viruses detected only in the upper respiratory tract (i.e., nasal wash) [81]. Demonstration of intracytoplasmic inclusions on cytologic examination is highly specific for CMV pneumonia, although it lacks sensitivity [69]. PCR carries a high sensitivity and specificity for identifying CMV pneumonia in the right clinical setting. PCR may be falsely positive in asymptomatic patients due to shedding of the virus without tissue invasion [48]. The presence of CMV viremia in a patient with a pulmonary process increases the likelihood of CMV pneumonia.

Demonstration of angioinvasion is formally required to diagnose definite invasive pulmonary infections. Fungal pathogens may be directly visualized via histopathology stains (e.g., Gomori methenamine silver "GMS" staining) or may be grown in cultures. However, isolation of fungi in respiratory samples may not necessarily confirm the etiology of pulmonary opacities, just as isolation of molds from the blood in severely immunosuppressed allogenic HSCT recipients may not prove disseminated mycosis [78]. Therefore, interpretation of fungal organism detection from respiratory samples must take into consideration predisposing risk factors (e.g., neutropenia, immunosuppressive therapy, GVHD), clinical presentation, radiographic features, and competing diagnoses. Molecular detection of antigens such as galactomannan and $(1,3)$-β-D glucan may also aid the diagnosis of fungal pneumonia. Galactomannan is an *Aspergillus* cell wall component that is upregulated during the invasive hyphal phase, suggesting active infection. $(1,3)$-β-D glucan is a cell wall component produced by many fungal species, excluding *Cryptococcus* spp. and *Mucorales*, thereby offering broad specificity. Both antigens are detected via commercial immunoassays. Recent studies suggest that galactomannan detection in the BAL fluid or serum may be informative both as a screening agent for subclinical fungal infections and a means to diagnose fungal pulmonary infections [102]. This test is not necessarily specific for *Aspergillus* infection, as positive results may occur with other fungal infections sharing cross-reacting antigens, including *Fusarium* spp. and *Histoplasma capsulatum* [92]. Galactomannan's diagnostic utility is markedly compromised in the setting of antifungal therapy, but this may offer an opportunity to use galactomannan as a marker of response to antifungal therapy [54]. $(1,3)$-β-D glucan testing may yield false-positive results following patient exposures to hemodialysis with cellulose membranes, use of IV immunoglobulin and albumin, and infections with certain bacteria containing β-glucans (e.g., *Pseudomonas aeruginosa*) [59]. The specificity is slightly higher in allogenic HSCT recipients [71]. Unlike serum galactomannan, $(1,3)$-β-D glucan is not affected by ongoing antifungal treatment [6].

Bronchoscopy with BAL is the gold standard method for diagnosis *Pneumocystis* pneumonia in patients with hematological malignancies. As the number of cysts detected in cancer patients is generally lower than those detected in HIV patients with *Pneumocystis* pneumonia, the chances of obtaining the diagnosis via sputum samples is low [3]. The sensitivity and specificity of LDH is also poorer in cancer patients with *Pneumocystis* pneumonia than in those with HIV [58].

Although transbronchial biopsies may demonstrate definite proof of fungal angioinvasion, this approach is often precluded in cancer patients by thrombocytopenia/bleeding risk and clinical instability. Culture of samples obtained by transbronchial biopsy has not been shown to be superior to BAL-obtained samples, though additional investigations may be warranted [10]. Recognizing the challenges of diagnosing invasive fungal infection, the European Organization for Research and Treatment of Cancer/Invasive Fungal Infections Cooperative Group (*EORTC*) and the National Institute of Allergy and Infectious Diseases Mycoses Study Group (*MSG*) have adopted a clinical classification scheme to define individual cases of suspected fungal infection as none, possible, probable, or proven [18]. This approach allows for pragmatic consideration of cases and homogenizes definitions for clinical research. Current studies suggest that these categorizations offer excellent sensitivity, though they may lack specificity [4].

Non-respiratory Samples

Certainly, failing to culture a pathogen from BAL or sputum does not exclude the existence of a pneumonia. Identifying a respiratory pathogen from an alternate, typically sterile site such as pleural space or blood by conventional culture can provide insight into a potential lower respiratory tract infection. Further, testing for urinary antigens associated with respiratory pathogens (*S. pneumoniae* and *Legionella* spp.) improves the overall sensitivity for diagnosing bacterial pneumonia compared to respiratory sample alone. It is presumed that similar to non-cancer patients, these tests can provide rapid and valuable data to inform initial antibiotic coverage in cancer patients with suspected pneumonia. However, it should be noted that urine antigen testing has not been formally validated in cancer populations. Strong correlations between urine antigen levels and various markers of intact host responses (e.g., procalcitonin, C-reactive protein) have been demonstrated, raising question about their diagnostic accuracy in cancer patients with impaired immune function [60].

Management

Prevention

In pneumonia-susceptible cancer patients, preventative measures can reduce the burden of infections and should be implemented in a manner tailored to each patient's level of immune dysfunction and exposure.

Minimizing pathogen exposure via the use of proper hand hygiene is the most effective intervention to prevent the spread of pneumonia-causing organisms, especially given the frequent healthcare encounters these patients require [21], and should be emphasized for all individuals that come in contact with cancer patients.

Frequent upper airway suctioning and pulmonary toilet may be required in patients at risk of aspiration. In addition, as immunosuppressed patients and those receiving chemotherapy and radiotherapy are at risk of developing periodontal disease, maintaining proper dental hygiene can help minimize the risk of preventable pneumonias.

Patient education and daily patient-performed spirometry have been reported as a potential tool for early detection of pneumonia in patients with acute leukemia. A 15% decline in the patient's expired volumes compared to baseline showed high sensitivity and specificity for predicting pneumonia development [61].

Prophylactic antimicrobial regimens are broadly recommended for neutropenic patients and others with an estimated risk of infection exceeding 20%. This strategy has resulted in a decline in the incidence of many infections. For example, prophylactic trimethoprim-sulfamethoxazole in the early posttransplant period has led to a significant decrease in the incidence of *Pneumocystis* pneumonia, whereas this infection remains problematic in patients allergic to sulfa and those receiving dapsone prophylaxis [83]. The incidence of CMV pneumonia in allogenic HSCT recipients has decreased following the use of posttransplant CMV prophylaxis [51]. Primary antifungal prophylaxis is routinely administered in immunocompromised patients and in patients with AML during remission induction chemotherapy.

Routine vaccination of cancer patients against *S. pneumoniae* with the 23-valent polysaccharide vaccine (PSV23) and the conjugated 13-valent pneumococcal vaccine (PCV13) is recommended, as is annual quadrivalent vaccination against influenza viruses. Patients with asplenia and patients receiving anti-CD20 may have a poor humoral response to vaccination, especially if given during cytoreductive therapy. The current recommendation from the Centers for Disease Control and Prevention is that immunosuppressed patients with cancer receive both PCV13 followed by PSV23 at least 8 weeks apart. The effectiveness of this approach remains unclear [90].

Pharmacologic Therapies

Timely initiation of adequate antimicrobial treatment is crucial to achieve favorable outcomes in the setting of cancer-related immune dysfunction. Aside from instances when bronchoscopically obtained samples can be obtained immediately, initiation of antimicrobial treatment of suspected cancer-related pneumonia should not be delayed to obtain specimens or while awaiting laboratory results. Delays in appropriate antibiotic therapy increase the risk of infection-associated deaths and of secondary complications. As with non-cancer patients, critically ill cancer patients admitted to the ICU with septic shock have better overall survival when antibiotics are administered in the early hours of the ICU admission, with increased mortality and organ failure following delays in antibiotic administration [46].

The initial antimicrobial therapy for cancer patients with febrile neutropenia and pulmonary opacities is recommended to be sufficiently broad to cover the commonly encountered pathogens described above, with prompt de-escalation of therapy based on pathogen identification and evidence of clinical improvement. Antibiotic selection should take into consideration prior antibiotic exposures (including prophylaxis), previously documented pathogens, and their susceptibilities if available, with particular emphasis on consideration of multidrug-resistant staphylococcal and pseudomonal infections [53]. Anaerobic coverage should be considered for patients with periodontal disease or those with a suspected gastrointestinal source of infection.

Initial antimicrobial coverage should also include antifungal coverage in high-risk cancer patients and HSCT recipients. Current recommendations for initial treatment for severe invasive pulmonary aspergillosis endorse liposomal amphotericin B or intravenous voriconazole followed by oral voriconazole after demonstration of clinical improvement [50]. Caspofungin may be considered for salvage therapy of refractory invasive pulmonary aspergillosis [52], as may posaconazole or micafungin. Response to anti-*Aspergillus* therapy may be monitored by serum galactomannan levels, and this approach has been demonstrated to correlate with better survival [66].

Patients with poor clinical response to therapy, those with severe and persistent neutropenia, or those requiring active immunosuppressive therapy often require prolonged durations of antimicrobial therapy.

A critical element of the management of pneumonia in cancer patients is the augmentation of disease- and/or treatment-impaired immune function. Wherever possible, immunosuppressive therapies should be reduced or withdrawn to allow active intrinsic immune defense activity. Colony-stimulating factors are widely used to prevent and treat infections and have clearly demonstrated their ability to improve granulocyte counts, though this alone does not reverse all immune defects, so additional study is warranted to determine the optimal use of this approach [12]. Although not presently the standard of care, observational studies suggest that donor lymphocyte infusion and adjuvant recombinant T_H1 cytokines may improve outcomes in neutropenic cancer patients and in high-risk allogenic HSCT recipients with opportunistic infections [101]. It is worth noting that radiographic findings may paradoxically worsen after initiation of host-augmenting therapies or recovery from neutropenia, due to increases in generation of tissue inflammation [42].

An alternately investigated strategy to protect immunosuppressed cancer patients against pneumonia is therapeutic induction of antimicrobial responses directly from resident lung cells. Targeted inhaled therapies may exert effects on the lung epithelium to stimulate protective innate immune responses, initiating production of microbial effector molecules and modulating local immune responses [16].

Non-pharmacologic Therapies

Many cancer-related pneumonias result in part from anatomical derangements that cause airway obstruction and impaired mucociliary clearance. Where safe and feasible, relief of obstruction can improve rapidity and completeness of pneumonia resolution. This is most often undertaken utilizing advanced bronchoscopic techniques, including tumor destruction and stent placement, depending on the nature of the lesion. Except for lung abscesses that develop in patients who cannot tolerate surgical intervention, transthoracic drainage of the lung parenchyma is rarely undertaken, due to frequent and persistent complications. Surgical resection of non-resolving necrotizing pneumonias is occasionally warranted, particularly for localized lesions that are refractory to conventional antimicrobial therapies [105].

Alternately, pleural disease is commonly investigated and managed via a transthoracic approach. Although thrombocytopenia may increase the challenges of drainage, in most cases it is safe to carefully sample parapneumonic effusions via thoracentesis to exclude the presence or complicated effusion or empyema. Complicated parapneumonic effusions, empyemas, and hemothoraces are best managed with tube drainage whenever possible.

Prognosis

The prognosis of pneumonia in patients with cancer varies widely and depends on many of the host and microbial factors described above. Unfortunately, most available prediction tools were derived for use in community-dwelling non-cancer patients that present with suspected pneumonia; thus common tools such as the CURB65 and the pneumonia severity index (PSI) tend to underestimate the physiologic disturbances, the need for higher levels of care, and the likelihood of death in cancer patients [30]. In particular, features such as having received HSCT or having undergone radiotherapy are not captured in CURB65 or PSI but portend worse outcomes. Whereas the majority of immunocompetent patients suspected of having pneumonia can be safely managed with outpatient antibiotic therapy, most cancer patients with suspected pneumonia must be managed in an inpatient setting. Despite receiving more intensive care, as described above, pneumonia-attributable case fatality rates remain much higher than in the general population.

Conclusion

Pneumonia is a major risk to patients with cancer and a common cause of critical illness and death in this population. Understanding the mechanisms that underlie patient's individual susceptibility and knowledge of prior antibiotic and microbial exposures can inform the clinician about likely pathogens, predict adequate initial antimicrobial therapies, and inform about potential host-directed therapies.

References

1. Ainoda Y, Hirai Y, Fujita T, Isoda N, Totsuka K. Analysis of clinical features of non-HIV *Pneumocystis jirovecii* pneumonia. J Infect Chemother. 2012;18:722–8. https://doi.org/10.1007/s10156-012-0408-5. Epub 2012 Mar 30.
2. Al-Ansari S, Zecha JA, Barasch A, de Lange J, Rozema FR, Raber-Durlacher JE. Oral Mucositis induced by anticancer therapies. Curr Oral Health Rep. 2015;2:202–11. https://doi.org/10.1007/s40496-015-0069-4. Epub 2015 Oct 19.
3. Alanio A, et al. ECIL guidelines for the diagnosis of *Pneumocystis jirovecii* pneumonia in patients with haematological malignancies and stem cell transplant recipients. J Antimicrob Chemother. 2016;71:2386–96. https://doi.org/10.1093/jac/dkw156. Epub 2016 May 12.
4. Anantasit N, Nuntacharruksa N, Incharoen P, Preutthipan A. Clinical and pathological correlation in pediatric invasive pulmonary Aspergillosis. Front Pediatr. 2018;6:31. https://doi.org/10.3389/fped.2018.00031. eCollection 2018.
5. Ashour HM, el-Sharif A. Microbial spectrum and antibiotic susceptibility profile of gram-positive aerobic bacteria isolated from cancer patients. J Clin Oncol. 2007;25:5763–9. https://doi.org/10.1200/JCO.2007.14.0947.
6. Azoulay E, et al. (1, 3)-beta-D-glucan assay for diagnosing invasive fungal infections in critically ill patients with hematological malignancies. Oncotarget. 2016;7:21484–95. https://doi.org/10.18632/oncotarget.7471.
7. Bitar D, et al. Population-based analysis of invasive fungal infections, France, 2001–2010. Emerg Infect Dis. 2014;20:1149–55. https://doi.org/10.3201/eid2007.140087.
8. Bonomi M, Batt K. Supportive management of mucositis and metabolic derangements in head and neck cancer patients. Cancers (Basel). 2015;7:1743–57. https://doi.org/10.3390/cancers7030862.
9. Casadevall A, Pirofski LA. Immunoglobulins in defense, pathogenesis, and therapy of fungal diseases. Cell Host Microbe. 2012;11:447–56. https://doi.org/10.1016/j.chom.2012.04.004.
10. Chellapandian D, et al. Bronchoalveolar lavage and lung biopsy in patients with cancer and hematopoietic stem-cell transplantation recipients: a systematic review and meta-analysis. J Clin Oncol. 2015;33:501–9. https://doi.org/10.1200/JCO.2014.58.0480. Epub 2015 Jan 5.
11. Chemaly RF, et al. The characteristics and outcomes of parainfluenza virus infections in 200 patients with leukemia or recipients of hematopoietic stem cell transplantation. Blood. 2012;119:2738–45; quiz 2969. https://doi.org/10.1182/blood-2011-08-3711 12. Epub 2012 Jan 12.
12. Cherif H, Axdorph U, Kalin M, Bjorkholm M. Clinical experience of granulocyte transfusion in the management of neutropenic patients with haematological malignancies and severe infection. Scand J Infect Dis. 2013;45:112–6. https://doi.org/10.3109/00365548.2012.714906.
13. Chi AK, Soubani AO, White AC, Miller KB. An update on pulmonary complications of hematopoietic stem cell transplantation. Chest. 2013;144:1913–22. https://doi.org/10.1378/chest.12-1708.
14. Chu HY, et al. Nosocomial transmission of respiratory syncytial virus in an outpatient cancer center. Biol Blood Marrow Transplant. 2014;20:844–51. https://doi.org/10.1016/j.bbmt.2014.02.024. Epub 2014 Mar 6.
15. Claus JA, Hodowanec AC, Singh K. Poor positive predictive value of influenza-like illness criteria in adult transplant patients: a case for multiplex respiratory virus PCR testing. Clin Transplant. 2015;29:938–43. https://doi.org/10.1111/ctr.12600. Epub 2015 Sep 3.

16. Cleaver JO, et al. Lung epithelial cells are essential effectors of inducible resistance to pneumonia. Mucosal Immunol. 2014;7:78–88. https://doi.org/10.1038/mi.2013.26.

17. De La Rosa GR, Jacobson KL, Rolston KV, Raad II, Kontoyiannis DP, Safdar A. Mycobacterium tuberculosis at a comprehensive cancer centre: active disease in patients with underlying malignancy during 1990–2000. Clin Microbiol Infect. 2004;10:749–52. https://doi.org/10.1111/j.1469-0691.2004.00954.x.

18. De Pauw B, et al. Revised definitions of invasive fungal disease from the European Organization for Research and Treatment of Cancer/Invasive Fungal Infections Cooperative Group and the National Institute of Allergy and Infectious Diseases Mycoses Study Group (EORTC/MSG) Consensus Group. Clin Infect Dis. 2008;46:1813–21. https://doi.org/10.1086/588660.

19. Delia M, et al. Fusariosis in a patient with acute myeloid leukemia: a case report and review of the literature. Mycopathologia. 2016;181:457–63. https://doi.org/10.1007/s11046-016-9987-5. Epub 2016 Mar 23.

20. Ebbert JO, Limper AH. Respiratory syncytial virus pneumonitis in immunocompromised adults: clinical features and outcome. Respiration. 2005;72:263–9. https://doi.org/10.1159/000085367.

21. Evans SE, Ost DE. Pneumonia in the neutropenic cancer patient. Curr Opin Pulm Med. 2015;21:260–71. https://doi.org/10.1097/MCP.0000000000000156.

22. Ferguson PE, Sorrell TC, Bradstock K, Carr P, Gilroy NM. Parainfluenza virus type 3 pneumonia in bone marrow transplant recipients: multiple small nodules in high- resolution lung computed tomography scans provide a radiological clue to diagnosis. Clin Infect Dis. 2009;48:905–9. https://doi.org/10.1086/597297.

23. Flanders SA, Collard HR, Saint S. Nosocomial pneumonia: state of the science. Am J Infect Control. 2006;34:84–93. https://doi.org/10.1016/j.ajic.2005.07.003.

24. Garcia-Cadenas I, et al. Patterns of infection and infection-related mortality in patients with steroid-refractory acute graft versus host disease. Bone Marrow Transplant. 2017;52:107–13. https://doi.org/10.1038/bmt.2016.225.

25. Garcia-Vidal C, et al. Pneumococcal pneumonia presenting with septic shock: host- and pathogen-related factors and outcomes. Thorax. 2010;65:77–81. https://doi.org/10.1136/thx.2009.123612.

26. Gasparetto EL, Escuissato DL, Marchiori E, Ono S, Fraree Silva RL, Muller NL. High-resolution CT findings of respiratory syncytial virus pneumonia after bone marrow transplantation. AJR Am J Roentgenol. 2004a;182:1133–7. https://doi.org/10.2214/ajr.182.5.1821133.

27. Gasparetto EL, Ono SE, Escuissato D, Marchiori E, Roldan L, Marques HL, Fraree Silva RL.

Cytomegalovirus pneumonia after bone marrow transplantation: high resolution CT findings. Br J Radiol. 2004b;77:724–7. https://doi.org/10.1259/bjr/70800575.

28. George B, et al. Pre-transplant cytomegalovirus (CMV) serostatus remains the most important determinant of CMV reactivation after allogeneic hematopoietic stem cell transplantation in the era of surveillance and preemptive therapy. Transpl Infect Dis. 2010;12:322–9. https://doi.org/10.1111/j.1399-3062.2010.00504.x. Epub 2010 May 11.

29. Gilbert CR, Lerner A, Baram M, Awsare BK. Utility of flexible bronchoscopy in the evaluation of pulmonary infiltrates in the hematopoietic stem cell transplant population – a single center fourteen year experience. Arch Bronconeumol. 2013;49:189–95. https://doi.org/10.1016/j.arbres.2012.11.012. Epub 2013 Feb 27.

30. Gonzalez C, Johnson T, Rolston K, Merriman K, Warneke C, Evans S. Predicting pneumonia mortality using CURB-65, PSI, and patient characteristics in patients presenting to the emergency department of a comprehensive cancer center. Cancer Med. 2014;3:962–70. https://doi.org/10.1002/cam4.240.

31. Centers for Disease Control and Prevention, Infectious Disease Society of America, American Society of Blood and Marrow Transplantation. Guidelines for preventing opportunistic infections among hematopoietic stem cell transplant recipients. Biol Blood Marrow Transplant. 2000;6:7–83.

32. Guzman-Bautista ER, Ramirez-Estudillo MC, Rojas-Gomez OI, Vega-Lopez MA. Tracheal and bronchial polymeric immunoglobulin secretory immune system (PISIS) development in a porcine model. Dev Comp Immunol. 2015;53:271–82. https://doi.org/10.1016/j.dci.2015.07.010. Epub 2015 Jul 15.

33. Hardak E, Brook O, Yigla M. Radiological features of *Pneumocystis jirovecii* pneumonia in immunocompromised patients with and without AIDS. Lung. 2010;188:159–63. https://doi.org/10.1007/s00408-009-9214-y. Epub 2010 Jan 5.

34. Heys SD, Gough DB, Khan L, Eremin O. Nutritional pharmacology and malignant disease: a therapeutic modality in patients with cancer. Br J Surg. 1996;83:608–19.

35. Hohenthal U, et al. Bronchoalveolar lavage in immunocompromised patients with haematological malignancy–value of new microbiological methods. Eur J Haematol. 2005;74:203–11. https://doi.org/10.1111/j.1600-0609.2004.00373.x.

36. Hummel M, Hofheinz R, Buchheidt D. Severe *Chlamydia pneumoniae* infection in a patient with mild neutropenia during treatment of Hodgkin's disease. Ann Hematol. 2004;83:441–3. https://doi.org/10.1007/s00277-003-0799-6.

37. Ibrahim EH, Tracy L, Hill C, Fraser VJ, Kollef MH. The occurrence of ventilator-associated pneumonia in a community hospital: risk factors and clinical outcomes. Chest. 2001;120:555–61.

38. Jiang L, Ren H, Zhou H, Qin T, Chen Y. Simultaneous detection of nine key bacterial respiratory pathogens using Luminex xTAG((R)) technology. Int J Environ Res Public Health. 2017;14. https://doi.org/10.3390/ijerph14030223.

39. Kalil AC, et al. Management of Adults with hospital-acquired and ventilator-associated Pneumonia: 2016 clinical practice guidelines by the Infectious Diseases Society of America and the American Thoracic Society. Clin Infect Dis. 2016;63:e61–e111. https://doi.org/10.1093/cid/ciw353. Epub 2016 Jul 14.

40. Kauffman CA, et al. Endemic fungal infections in solid organ and hematopoietic cell transplant recipients enrolled in the Transplant-Associated Infection Surveillance Network (TRANSNET). Transpl Infect Dis. 2014;16:213–24. https://doi.org/10.1111/tid.12186.

41. Khayr W, Haddad RY, Noor SA. Infections in hematological malignancies. Dis Mon. 2012;58:239–49. https://doi.org/10.1016/j.disamonth.2012.01.001.

42. Kojima R, et al. Chest computed tomography of late invasive aspergillosis after allogeneic hematopoietic stem cell transplantation. Biol Blood Marrow Transplant. 2005;11:506–11. https://doi.org/10.1016/j.bbmt.2005.03.005.

43. Kontoyiannis DP. Antifungal prophylaxis in hematopoietic stem cell transplant recipients: the unfinished tale of imperfect success. Bone Marrow Transplant. 2011;46:165–73. https://doi.org/10.1038/bmt.2010.256.

44. Kontoyiannis DP, et al. Zygomycosis in a tertiary-care cancer center in the era of Aspergillus-active antifungal therapy: a case-control observational study of 27 recent cases. J Infect Dis. 2005;191:1350–60. https://doi.org/10.1086/428780. Epub 2005 Mar 16.

45. Kreiniz N, Bejar J, Polliack A, Tadmor T. Severe pneumonia associated with ibrutinib monotherapy for CLL and lymphoma. Hematol Oncol. 2018;36:349–54. https://doi.org/10.1002/hon.2387.

46. Larche J, et al. Improved survival of critically ill cancer patients with septic shock. Intensive Care Med. 2003;29:1688–95. https://doi.org/10.1007/s00134-003-1957-y. Epub 2003 Sep 12.

47. Lass-Florl C, Roilides E, Loffler J, Wilflingseder D, Romani L. Minireview: host defence in invasive aspergillosis. Mycoses. 2013;56:403–13. https://doi.org/10.1111/myc.12052. Epub 2013 Feb 14.

48. Lee HY, Choi JY, Lee HY, Rhee CK, Lee DG. Clinical utility of quantitative cytomegalovirus detection in bronchial washing fluid in patients with hematologic malignancies. Eur Respir J. 2015;46. https://doi.org/10.1183/13993003.congress-2015.PA572.

49. Li D, Rebecca P, Nurieva R, Molldrem JJ, Champlin RE, Ma Q. Ibrutinib treatment modulates T cell activation and polarization in immune response. Blood. 2015;126:3435.

50. Limper AH, et al. An official American Thoracic Society statement: treatment of fungal infections in adult pulmonary and critical care patients. Am J Respir Crit Care Med. 2011;183:96–128. https://doi.org/10.1164/rccm.2008-740ST.

51. Ljungman P, et al. Risk factors for the development of cytomegalovirus disease after allogeneic stem cell transplantation. Haematologica. 2006;91:78–83.

52. Maertens J, et al. Efficacy and safety of caspofungin for treatment of invasive aspergillosis in patients refractory to or intolerant of conventional antifungal therapy. Clin Infect Dis. 2004;39:1563–71. https://doi.org/10.1086/423381. Epub 2004 Nov 9.

53. Mandell LA, Bartlett JG, Dowell SF, File TM Jr, Musher DM, Whitney C, Infectious Diseases Society of America. Update of practice guidelines for the management of community-acquired pneumonia in immunocompetent adults. Clin Infect Dis. 2003;37:1405–33. https://doi.org/10.1086/380488.

54. Marr KA, Balajee SA, McLaughlin L, Tabouret M, Bentsen C, Walsh TJ. Detection of galactomannan antigenemia by enzyme immunoassay for the diagnosis of invasive aspergillosis: variables that affect performance. J Infect Dis. 2004;190:641–9. https://doi.org/10.1086/422009.

55. Marr KA, Carter RA, Crippa F, Wald A, Corey L. Epidemiology and outcome of mould infections in hematopoietic stem cell transplant recipients. Clin Infect Dis. 2002;34:909–17. https://doi.org/10.1086/339202.

56. Martino R, et al. Prospective study of the incidence, clinical features, and outcome of symptomatic upper and lower respiratory tract infections by respiratory viruses in adult recipients of hematopoietic stem cell transplants for hematologic malignancies. Biol Blood Marrow Transplant. 2005;11:781–96. https://doi.org/10.1016/j.bbmt.2005.07.007.

57. Martins F, de Oliveira MA, Wang Q, Sonis S, Gallottini M, George S, Treister N. A review of oral toxicity associated with mTOR inhibitor therapy in cancer patients. Oral Oncol. 2013;49:293–8. https://doi.org/10.1016/j.oraloncology.2012.11.008. Epub 2013 Jan 9.

58. McKinnell JA, et al. Pneumocystis pneumonia in hospitalized patients: a detailed examination of symptoms, management, and outcomes in human immunodeficiency virus (HIV)-infected and HIV-uninfected persons. Transpl Infect Dis. 2012;14:510–8. https://doi.org/10.1111/j.1399-3062.2012.00739.x. Epub 2012 May 1.

59. Mennink-Kersten MA, Ruegebrink D, Verweij PE. *Pseudomonas aeruginosa* as a cause of 1,3-beta-D-glucan assay reactivity. Clin Infect Dis. 2008;46:1930–1. https://doi.org/10.1086/588563.

60. Molinos L, et al. Sensitivity, specificity, and positivity predictors of the pneumococcal urinary antigen test in community-acquired Pneumonia. Ann Am Thorac Soc. 2015;12:1482–9. https://doi.org/10.1513/AnnalsATS.201505-304OC.

61. Moller T, et al. Early warning and prevention of pneumonia in acute leukemia by patient education, spirometry, and positive expiratory pressure: a

randomized controlled trial. Am J Hematol. 2016;91:271–6. https://doi.org/10.1002/ajh.24262.

62. Monneret G, Venet F, Pachot A, Lepape A. Monitoring immune dysfunctions in the septic patient: a new skin for the old ceremony. Mol Med. 2008;14:64–78. https://doi.org/10.2119/2007-00102.Monneret.

63. Murali S, Langston AA, Nolte FS, Banks G, Martin R, Caliendo AM. Detection of respiratory viruses with a multiplex polymerase chain reaction assay (MultiCode-PLx Respiratory Virus Panel) in patients with hematologic malignancies. Leuk Lymphoma. 2009;50:619–24. https://doi.org/10.1080/10428190902777665.

64. Nakamae H, et al. Effect of conditioning regimen intensity on CMV infection in allogeneic hematopoietic cell transplantation. Biol Blood Marrow Transplant. 2009;15:694–703. https://doi.org/10.1016/j.bbmt.2009.02.009.

65. Nambu A, Ozawa K, Kobayashi N, Tago M. Imaging of community-acquired pneumonia: roles of imaging examinations, imaging diagnosis of specific pathogens and discrimination from noninfectious diseases. World J Radiol. 2014;6:779–93. https://doi.org/10.4329/wjr.v6.i10.779.

66. Neofytos D, et al. Correlation between circulating fungal biomarkers and clinical outcome in invasive aspergillosis. PLoS One. 2015;10:e0129022. https://doi.org/10.1371/journal.pone.0129022. eCollection 2015.

67. Oikonomou A, Muller NL, Nantel S. Radiographic and high-resolution CT findings of influenza virus pneumonia in patients with hematologic malignancies. AJR Am J Roentgenol. 2003;181:507–11. https://doi.org/10.2214/ajr.181.2.1810507.

68. Pagano L, et al. Pneumocystis carinii pneumonia in patients with malignant haematological diseases: 10 years' experience of infection in GIMEMA centres. Br J Haematol. 2002;117:379–86.

69. Paradis IL, Grgurich WF, Dummer JS, Dekker A, Dauber JH. Rapid detection of cytomegalovirus pneumonia from lung lavage cells. Am Rev Respir Dis. 1988;138:697–702. https://doi.org/10.1164/ajrccm/138.3.697.

70. Quint LE. Thoracic complications and emergencies in oncologic patients. Cancer Imaging. 2009;9 Spec No A: S75–82. https://doi.org/10.1102/1470-7330.2009.9031.

71. Reischies FM, Prattes J, Woelfler A, Eigl S, Hoenigl M. Diagnostic performance of 1,3-beta-D-glucan serum screening in patients receiving hematopoietic stem cell transplantation. Transpl Infect Dis. 2016;18:466–70. https://doi.org/10.1111/tid.12527. Epub 2016 May 10.

72. Rello J, Ollendorf DA, Oster G, Vera-Llonch M, Bellm L, Redman R, Kollef MH. Epidemiology and outcomes of ventilator-associated pneumonia in a large US database. Chest. 2002;122:2115–21.

73. Roblot F, et al. Risk factors analysis for pneumocystis jiroveci pneumonia (PCP) in patients with haematological malignancies and pneumonia. Scand J Infect Dis. 2004;36:848–54. https://doi.org/10.1080/00365540410021180.

74. Rosolem MM, et al. Critically ill patients with cancer and sepsis: clinical course and prognostic factors. J Crit Care. 2012;27:301–7. https://doi.org/10.1016/j.jcrc.2011.06.014.

75. Sachanas S, et al. Malakoplakia of the urinary bladder in a patient with chronic lymphocytic leukemia under Ibrutinib therapy: a case report. Anticancer Res. 2016;36:4759–62. https://doi.org/10.21873/anticanres.11032.

76. Safdar A, Armstrong D. Infectious morbidity in critically ill patients with cancer. Crit Care Clin. 2001;17:531–70, vii–viii.

77. Safdar A, Rolston KV. Stenotrophomonas maltophilia: changing spectrum of a serious bacterial pathogen in patients with cancer. Clin Infect Dis. 2007;45:1602–9. https://doi.org/10.1086/522998.

78. Safdar A, Singhal S, Mehta J. Clinical significance of non-Candida fungal blood isolation in patients undergoing high-risk allogeneic hematopoietic stem cell transplantation (1993–2001). Cancer. 2004;100: 2456–61. https://doi.org/10.1002/cncr.20262.

79. Schiffer JT, Kirby K, Sandmaier B, Storb R, Corey L, Boeckh M. Timing and severity of community acquired respiratory virus infections after myeloablative versus non-myeloablative hematopoietic stem cell transplantation. Haematologica. 2009;94:1101–8. https://doi.org/10.3324/haematol.2008.003186.

80. Schnetzke U, et al. Polymorphisms of toll-like receptors (TLR2 and TLR4) are associated with the risk of infectious complications in acute myeloid leukemia. Genes Immun. 2015;16:83–8. https://doi.org/10.1038/gene.2014.67.

81. Seo S, Xie H, Campbell AP, Kuypers JM, Leisenring WM, Englund JA, Boeckh M. Parainfluenza virus lower respiratory tract disease after hematopoietic cell transplant: viral detection in the lung predicts outcome. Clin Infect Dis. 2014;58: 1357–68. https://doi.org/10.1093/cid/ciu134. Epub 2014 Mar 5.

82. Smith JA, Kauffman CA. Pulmonary fungal infections. Respirology. 2012;17:913–26. https://doi.org/10.1111/j.1440-1843.2012.02150.x.

83. Souza JP, Boeckh M, Gooley TA, Flowers ME, Crawford SW. High rates of Pneumocystis carinii pneumonia in allogeneic blood and marrow transplant recipients receiving dapsone prophylaxis. Clin Infect Dis. 1999;29:1467–71. https://doi.org/10.1086/313509.

84. Spolarics Z, Siddiqi M, Siegel JH, Garcia ZC, Stein DS, Denny T, Deitch EA. Depressed interleukin-12-producing activity by monocytes correlates with adverse clinical course and a shift toward Th2-type lymphocyte pattern in severely injured male trauma patients. Crit Care Med. 2003;31:1722–9. https://doi.org/10.1097/01.ccm.00000635 79.43470.aa.

85. Stanzani M, et al. High resolution computed tomography angiography improves the radiographic

diagnosis of invasive mold disease in patients with hematological malignancies. Clin Infect Dis. 2015;60:1603–10. https://doi.org/10.1093/cid/civ154. Epub 2015 Feb 25.

86. Svensson T, Lundstrom KL, Hoglund M, Cherif H. Utility of bronchoalveolar lavage in diagnosing respiratory tract infections in patients with hematological malignancies: are invasive diagnostics still needed? Ups J Med Sci. 2017;122:56–60. https://doi.org/10.1080/03009734.2016.1237595.

87. Syrjala H, Broas M, Suramo I, Ojala A, Lahde S. High-resolution computed tomography for the diagnosis of community-acquired pneumonia. Clin Infect Dis. 1998;27:358–63.

88. Taccone FS, Artigas AA, Sprung CL, Moreno R, Sakr Y, Vincent JL. Characteristics and outcomes of cancer patients in European ICUs. Crit Care. 2009;13: R15. https://doi.org/10.1186/cc7713. Epub 2009 Feb 6.

89. Tacke D, Koehler P, Markiefka B, Cornely OA. Our 2014 approach to mucormycosis. Mycoses. 2014;57:519–24. https://doi.org/10.1111/myc.12203. Epub 2014 May 15.

90. Toleman MS, Herbert K, McCarthy N, Church DN. Vaccination of chemotherapy patients–effect of guideline implementation. Support Care Cancer. 2016;24:2317–21. https://doi.org/10.1007/s00520-015-3037-6.

91. Torres HA, et al. Nocardiosis in cancer patients. Medicine (Baltimore). 2002;81:388–97.

92. Tortorano AM, Esposto MC, Prigitano A, Grancini A, Ossi C, Cavanna C, Cascio GL. Cross-reactivity of *Fusarium* spp. in the Aspergillus Galactomannan enzyme-linked immunosorbent assay. J Clin Microbiol. 2012;50:1051–3. https://doi.org/10.1128/JCM.05946-11.

93. Travi G, Pergam SA. Cytomegalovirus pneumonia in hematopoietic stem cell recipients. J Intensive Care Med. 2014;29:200–12. https://doi.org/10.1177/0885066613476454.

94. Tschernig T. Hospital-acquired pneumonia and community-acquired pneumonia: two guys? Ann Transl Med. 2016;4:S22. https://doi.org/10.21037/atm.2016.10.10.

95. Vallipuram J, et al. Chest CT scans are frequently abnormal in asymptomatic patients with newly diagnosed acute myeloid leukemia. Leuk Lymphoma. 2017;58:834–41. https://doi.org/10.1080/10428194.2016.1213825.

96. Venet F, Chung CS, Monneret G, Huang X, Horner B, Garber M, Ayala A. Regulatory T cell populations in sepsis and trauma. J Leukoc Biol. 2008;83:523–35. https://doi.org/10.1189/jlb.0607371.

97. Vento S, Cainelli F, Temesgen Z. Lung infections after cancer chemotherapy. Lancet Oncol. 2008;9:982–92. https://doi.org/10.1016/S1470-2045(08)70255-9.

98. Vilar-Compte D, Shah DP, Vanichanan J, Cornejo-Juarez P, Garcia-Horton A, Volkow P, Chemaly RF. Influenza in patients with hematological malignancies: experience at two comprehensive cancer centers. J Med Virol. 2018;90:50–60. https://doi.org/10.1002/jmv.24930.

99. Waghmare A, Pergam SA, Jerome KR, Englund JA, Boeckh M, Kuypers J. Clinical disease due to enterovirus D68 in adult hematologic malignancy patients and hematopoietic cell transplant recipients. Blood. 2015;125:1724–9. https://doi.org/10.1182/blood-2014-12-616516. Epub 2015 Jan 15.

100. Waheed Z, Irfan M, Fatimi S, Shahid R. Bronchial carcinoid presenting as multiple lung abscesses. J Coll Physicians Surg Pak. 2013;23:229–30. 03.2013/JCPSP.229230.

101. West KA, Gea-Banacloche J, Stroncek D, Kadri SS. Granulocyte transfusions in the management of invasive fungal infections. Br J Haematol. 2017;177: 357–74. https://doi.org/10.1111/bjh.14597. Epub 2017 Mar 14.

102. Wheat LJ, Walsh TJ. Diagnosis of invasive aspergillosis by galactomannan antigenemia detection using an enzyme immunoassay. Eur J Clin Microbiol Infect Dis. 2008;27:245–51. https://doi.org/10.1007/s10096-007-0437-7. Epub 2008 Jan 9.

103. Whimbey E, Goodrich J, Bodey GP. Pneumonia in cancer patients. Cancer Treat Res. 1995;79:185–210.

104. Whitsett JA, Alenghat T. Respiratory epithelial cells orchestrate pulmonary innate immunity. Nat Immunol. 2015;16:27–35. https://doi.org/10.1038/ni.3045.

105. Wu GX, et al. Survival following lung resection in immunocompromised patients with pulmonary invasive fungal infection. Eur J Cardiothorac Surg. 2016;49:314–20. https://doi.org/10.1093/ejcts/ezv026.

106. Yamamoto K, et al. Roles of lung epithelium in neutrophil recruitment during pneumococcal pneumonia. Am J Respir Cell Mol Biol. 2014;50:253–62. https://doi.org/10.1165/rcmb.2013-0114OC.

107. Young AY, Leiva Juarez MM, Evans SE. Fungal pneumonia in patients with hematologic malignancy and hematopoietic stem cell transplantation. Clin Chest Med. 2017;38:479–91. https://doi.org/10.1016/j.ccm.2017.04.009. Epub 2017 May 31.

Late Noninfectious Pulmonary Complications in Hematopoietic Stem Cell Transplantation

41

Kevin Dsouza, Cameron Pywell, and Victor J. Thannickal

Contents

Introduction 626

Bronchiolitis Obliterans 626
Clinical Features and Diagnosis 627
Risk Factors and Pathogenesis 629
Treatment 629
Clinical Course and Prognosis 630

Idiopathic Pneumonia Syndrome 630
Pathogenesis and Risk Factors 630
Clinical Features and Diagnosis 631
Treatment 631
Clinical Course and Prognosis 632

Organizing Pneumonia 632
Clinical Features and Diagnosis 632
Risk Factors and Pathogenesis 632
Treatment 634
Clinical Course and Prognosis 634

Pulmonary Venocclusive Disease 634
Clinical Features, Pathogenesis, and Diagnosis 634
Treatment and Prognosis 634

Pulmonary Cytolytic Thrombi 634

Pleuroparenchymal Fibroelastosis 635

Thoracic Air Leak Syndrome 635

K. Dsouza · V. J. Thannickal (✉)
Division of Pulmonary, Allergy and Critical Care
Medicine, Department of Medicine, University of
Alabama at Birmingham, Birmingham, AL, USA
e-mail: kdsouza@uabmc.edu; vthannickal@uabmc.edu

C. Pywell
Department of Medicine, University of Alabama at
Birmingham, Birmingham, AL, USA
e-mail: cameronpywell@uabmc.edu

© Springer Nature Switzerland AG 2020
J. L. Nates, K. J. Price (eds.), *Oncologic Critical Care*,
https://doi.org/10.1007/978-3-319-74588-6_51

Post-transplant Lymphoproliferative Disorder 635

Conclusion 636

References 636

Abstract

Hematopoietic stem cell transplantation (HSCT) is an established therapeutic modality for a number of malignant and nonmalignant conditions. Pulmonary complications following HSCT are associated with increased mortality and morbidity. These complications may be classified into infectious *versus* noninfectious, and early *versus* late based on the time of occurrence post-transplant. Thus, exclusion of infectious etiologies is the first step in the diagnoses of pulmonary complications. Late onset noninfectious pulmonary complications typically occur 3 months post-transplant. Bronchiolitis obliterans is the major contributor to late-onset pulmonary complications, and its clinical presentation, pathogenesis, and current therapeutic approaches are discussed. Idiopathic pneumonia syndrome is another important complication which usually occurs early, although its onset may be delayed. Organizing pneumonia is important to recognize due to its responsiveness to corticosteroids. Other late onset noninfectious pulmonary complications discussed here include pulmonary venoocclusive disease, pulmonary cytolytic thrombi, pleuroparenchymal fibroelastosis, thoracic air leak syndrome, and posttransplant lymphoproliferative disorders.

Keywords

Bronchiolitis obliterans · Hematopoietic stem cell transplant · Pulmonary complications · Organizing pneumonia

Introduction

Hematopoietic stem cell transplantation (HSCT) is an established form of therapy for a number of malignant as well as nonmalignant conditions. More than 21,000 HSCTs were conducted in the United States in 2016 (https://www.cibmtr.org). The two main types of HSCTs are autologous and allogenic. Autologous HSCT involves collection of stem cells from the patient that are then infused back after chemotherapy. Allogenic HSCT involves infusion of stem cells from a donor.

The morbidity and mortality from HSCT-related complications have been on the decline over the past several years. These complications are broadly categorized based on etiology, namely, whether they are infectious or noninfectious, and the time of onset of such complications, early vs. late. Pulmonary complications are the most common life-threatening complications post HSCT occurring in 30–60% of patients [1]. We define late onset complications are occurring 3 months after post-HSCT (Fig. 1). In this chapter, we discuss late noninfectious pulmonary complications in HSCT, and current concepts on their pathogenesis, diagnosis, and management. The primary focus will be on bronchiolitis obliterans (BO) which is the most common and carries the highest mortality of the late onset noninfectious complications [81]. The other late onset noninfectious complications that will be discussed include idiopathic pneumonia syndrome, organizing pneumonia, pulmonary venoocclusive disease, pulmonary cytolytic thrombi, pleuroparenchymal fibroelastosis, thoracic air leak syndrome, and posttransplant lymphoproliferative disorders.

Bronchiolitis Obliterans

BO typically occurs between 3 months to several years post HSCT and is inclusive of the spectrum of chronic graft versus host disease (cGVHD) [29, 60]. BO is characterized by progressive, irreversible airway narrowing due to circumferential small airway fibrosis. There is limited understanding of BO pathogenesis. BO

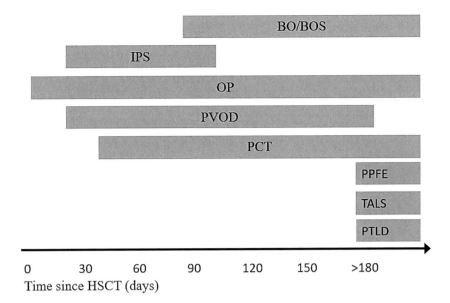

Fig. 1 Timeline of noninfectious HSCT pulmonary complications. *BO/BOS* bronchiolitis obliterans/bronchiolitis obliterans syndrome, *IPS* idiopathic pneumonia syndrome, *OP* organizing pneumonia, *PVOD* pulmonary venoocclusive disease, *PCT* pulmonary cytolytic thrombi, *PPFE* pleuroparenchymal fibroelastosis, *TALS* thoracic air leak syndrome, *PTLD* post-transplant lymphoproliferative disorder

is a pathological diagnosis requiring invasive surgical lung biopsy, which is uncommonly performed in the clinical setting. BO syndrome (BOS) is a more useful clinical diagnosis that is made based on irreversible airflow limitation on pulmonary function testing (PFT) without the need for lung biopsy.

BO is the most common late onset noninfectious complication of HSCT. The reported incidence of BO/BOS after allogeneic HSCT varies based on the diagnostic criteria used, ranging from 2% to 30% in retrospective studies [60]. A recent prospective study to evaluate the epidemiology of late non onset noninfectious complications after allogenic stem cell transplant reported a cumulative incidence of BOS 36 months posttransplant at 10.7% [9]. BO/BOS following autologous HSCT is rare but has been reported [31, 61].

Clinical Features and Diagnosis

Clinical features of BO/BOS are nonspecific. In early stages of the disease, patients are asymptomatic and are identified by airflow limitation on PFTs. Nonproductive cough, dyspnea on exertion, and decreased exercise tolerance are common [14]. Physical examination may be normal or reveal signs of airflow obstruction such as wheezing, hyperinflation, or diffuse crackles. Other causes of such presentations, in particular, respiratory infections, should be ruled out.

The chest radiograph may be normal or reveal hyperinflation. High resolution chest tomography (HRCT) reveals small airway involvement with features of air trapping evidenced by mosaic attenuation on expiratory views (Fig. 2). Histopathology, when available, shows narrowing or complete occlusion of the bronchiolar lumen due to subepithelial inflammatory fibrosis is a hallmark of BO (Fig. 3) [5]. Transbronchial biopsies are insufficient to yield a diagnosis and surgical lung biopsies often prohibitively expose patients to procedural risks. In most cases, BOS can be diagnosed without a histopathological diagnosis using PFTs in the appropriate clinical setting.

The updated National Institutes of Health (NIH) guidelines for diagnosing BOS are based on the following criteria [43]:

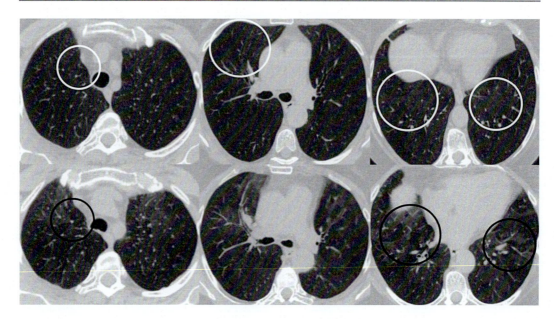

Fig. 2 62-year-old woman with history of allogenic bone marrow transplant for diffuse large B-cell lymphoma 2.5 years back. She presented with progressive shortness of breath. High Resolution Computed Tomography (HRCT) images in inspiration (top row) show subtle mosaic abnormalities (white circles) and the images in expiration (bottom row) show decreased attenuation of these areas (black circles), consistent with air trapping. This appearance is highly concerning for bronchiolitis obliterans syndrome in this setting. (Image courtesy: Dr. Sushilkumar Sonvane, MD – University of Alabama at Birmingham, Department of Radiology)

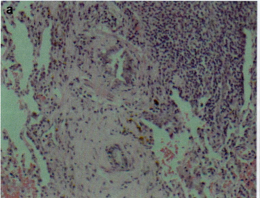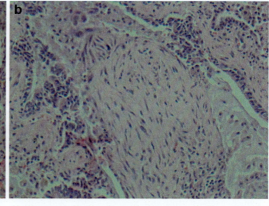

Fig. 3 High power view demonstrating early lesion in bronchiolitis obliterans (**a**) with peribronchial fibrosis and inflammation progressing to frank interalveolar fibroblastic plug formation (**b**). (Image courtesy: Dr. David Ralph Crowe, MD – University of Alabama Birmingham, Department of Pathology)

1. Forced expiratory volume in one second (FEV1)/vital capacity <0.7 or the fifth percentile of predicted.
   (a) Vital capacity includes forced vital capacity or slow vital capacity, whichever is greater.
   (b) The fifth percentile of predicted is the lower limit of the 90% confidence interval.
   (c) For pediatric or elderly patients, use the lower limits of normal, defined according to National Health and Nutrition Examination Survey III calculations [36].

2. FEV1 <75% of predicted with ≥10% decline over less than 2 years. FEV1 should not correct to >75% of predicted with albuterol, and the absolute decline for the corrected values should still remain at ≥10% over 2 years.
3. Absence of infection in the respiratory tract, documented with investigations directed by clinical symptoms, such as chest radiographs, computed tomographic (CT) scans, or microbiologic cultures (sinus aspiration, upper respiratory tract viral screen, sputum culture, bronchoalveolar lavage).
4. One of the two supporting features of BOS:
   (a) Evidence of air trapping by expiratory CT or small airway thickening or bronchiectasis by high-resolution chest CT or
   (b) Evidence of air trapping by PFTs: residual volume >120% of predicted or residual volume/total lung capacity elevated outside the 90% confidence interval

It is important to recognize that a significant number of bronchioles must be involved to manifest airflow limitation on PFTs or to develop clinical symptoms. Hence, early stages of BO may be missed.

Risk Factors and Pathogenesis

Several risk factors for the development of BOS have been identified, and most of these are closely associated with the occurrence of cGVHD [98]. Increasing age of the donor/recipient, development of acute GVHD [26], ABO incompatibility [24], the presence of extra thoracic GVHD, low circulating IgG, and non-Caucasian race [4] have been identified in several retrospective studies. Additional risk factors include the type of transplant procedure such a peripheral blood stem cell transplant [57] and busulfan-based conditioning regimens [69]. Use of antithymocyte globulin (ATG) as part of the pretransplant conditioning regimen is associated with a decreased incidence of BOS [22].

Prior to meeting established criteria for BOS, a decrease in FEV1 from pretransplant levels has also been identified to be a risk factor for the subsequent development of BOS [13]. More recently, a 10% decline in FEV1 from pretransplant to day 100 posttransplant has shown to be predictive for the development of BOS [9].

The precise pathogenetic mechanisms involved in the development of BO are unclear. The pathogenesis appears to be multifactorial and may involve diverse etiologies [5]. Airway epithelial injury is the inciting factor secondary to gastroesophageal reflux disease, respiratory infections, and chemotherapeutic drugs. This is typically followed by a dysregulated immune response that leads to the development of fibrotic changes in small airways. T cells and humoral mechanisms have been implicated [23, 76]. Genetic polymorphisms in NOD2/CARD15 have been linked to susceptibility to BOS [39].

Treatment

There are currently no effective treatments for BOS complicating HSCT. Most treatment protocols are based on combinations of immunosuppressive drugs and, until recently, were largely based on expert opinion. Traditionally, immunosuppression in the form of systemic steroids for extended periods has been used; alternatively, calcineurin inhibitors and azathioprine, agents that impair lymphocyte activation and proliferation, have been employed. Long-term, high-intensity immunosuppression is no longer recommended due to the increased risk of infections [91].

Most clinical studies of treatments for BOS are difficult to interpret due to small sample sizes, their retrospective nature, and confounding effects of treatment for cGVHD. These studies have included systemic corticosteroids [28, 65, 82], rituximab [10, 46], imatinib [59], etanercept [12, 95], as well as extracorporeal photopheresis [52]. A recent retrospective matched cohort study recently showed that extracorporeal photopheresis improves survival in HSCT patients with BOS [37].

Treatment with inhaled budesonide/formoterol led to significant FEV1 improvements in patients with mild/severe BOS after allogeneic HSCT [7]. Another trial showed FEV1 stabilization using a combination of fluticasone, azithromycin, and montelukast along with pulse dosed systemic steroids [92]. A randomized, double-blinded, placebo-controlled trial of azithromycin alone did not reveal any change in FEV1 in late BOS post HSCT [48]. Prophylactic azithromycin has been shown to prevent the onset of lung transplant–related BOS, as well as stabilize FEVI in post-lung transplant BOS [19, 88]. However, prophylactic azithromycin has not shown to be effective in BOS post-HSCT in retrospective studies [44]. A prospective study on the prophylactic use of azithromycin to prevent airflow decline resulted in early termination secondary to hematological relapses [8]; an FDA warning was issued in August 2018 until further review (https://www.fda.gov/Drugs/DrugSafety/ucm614085.htm). Prospective trials of azithromycin, bortezomib, inhaled cyclosporine, and neutrophil elastase inhibitors for prophylaxis and/or treatment of BOS are underway (www.clinicaltrials.gov).

Current treatment strategies include high-dose inhaled glucocorticoid with or without a long acting inhaled beta agonist based on symptoms, with close monitoring of lung function with PFTs. If progressive decline in FEV1 occurs with this regimen, initiation of a combination of fluticasone, azithromycin, and montelukast (FAM) therapy can be considered [91]. Occasionally, patients with chronic GVHD and refractory BOS may respond to increased immunosuppression. In patients who progress despite medical therapies, lung transplantation may be the only option [40, 86].

Novel therapeutic approaches for BO/BOS are currently being investigated. The pleiotropic small molecule p38 MAK inhibitor, pirfenidone, has been shown to ameliorate BO in a murine model of cGVHD [25]. An early phase clinical study evaluating the safety and tolerability of pirfenidone in BOS is currently underway (www.clinicaltrials.gov; NCT03315741).

Clinical Course and Prognosis

The clinical course of BOS is variable, with some patients experiencing rapid declines in lung function, while others stabilize or improve. Mortality from BOS is most commonly due to progressive respiratory failure. BOS confers a 1.6 fold increased risk of death after diagnosis [4]. Early onset of BOS and lower FVC, especially within a year of transplant, is associated with a worse prognosis [13, 26]. Recent estimates indicate a 2–3 year survival of 60–75%, and a 5-year survival of 40–50%; this is an improvement in overall survival from a decade ago, when 2-year survival was 40%, and 5-year survival was 20%. Early recognition, newer treatment strategies, and better supportive care likely account for this improved survival [91].

Idiopathic Pneumonia Syndrome

Idiopathic pneumonia syndrome (IPS) is a severe noninfectious complication of HSCT with an incidence of 12% when it was first described in the 1990s; more recently, incidence is cited at 3–15% [14, 60]. IPS is more common as an early complication of HSCT but can occur after 3 months. Median time of onset is 19 days posttransplant, with a range from 4 to 106 days [60]. IPS is an acute lung injury process characterized by diffuse alveolar damage in the absence of an identifiable lower respiratory tract infection.

Pathogenesis and Risk Factors

Although the exact cause of IPS remains unknown, immune involvement has been invoked; murine models involving immune mismatches between donor and recipient support this concept [15, 73]. Elevated levels of lipopolysaccharide (LPS) and tumor necrosis factor-alpha (TNF-α) have been observed in BAL samples of murine IPS models [16]. TNF-α may contribute to pathogenesis by direct toxicity, upregulation of major histocompatibility complex (MHC), increased leukocyte recruitment, and cell-mediated apoptosis [60]. Donor T lymphocytes secrete chemokines which further amplify the inflammatory cascade [38]. Decreased level of pulmonary surfactant has also been associated with IPS development [27, 56, 94].

Risk factors for IPS include full-intensity conditioning regimens such as total body irradiation and busulfan, acute GVHD, advanced age, and underlying acute leukemia and myelodysplastic syndrome (MDS) [33, 68, 90]. Reduced-intensity conditioning regimens have decreased the incidence of IPS [33]. In children, risk factors for IPS include the underlying disease and busulfan-based conditioning regimens [66]. Interestingly, risk of IPS increases with the number of platelet transfusions received, though the transfusion requirement could be a marker of disease severity [84, 85].

Clinical Features and Diagnosis

The definition of IPS, updated in the 2011 American Thoracic Society guidelines, is based on the following criteria [60]:

1. Evidence of widespread alveolar injury
   (a) Multilobar infiltrates on routine chest radiographs or computed tomography
   (b) Symptoms and signs of pneumonia (cough, dyspnea, tachypnea, rales)
   (c) Evidence of abnormal pulmonary physiology
      (i) Increased alveolar to arterial oxygen difference
      (ii) New or increased restrictive pulmonary function test abnormality
2. Absence of active lower respiratory tract infection based upon:
   (a) Bronchoalveolar lavage negative for significant bacterial pathogens including acid-fast bacilli, *Nocardia,* and *Legionella* species
   (b) Bronchoalveolar lavage negative for pathogenic nonbacterial microorganisms:
      (i) Routine culture for viruses and fungi
      (ii) Shell vial culture for CMV and respiratory RSV
      (iii) Cytology for CMV inclusions, fungi, and *Pneumocystis jirovecii (carinii)*
      (iv) Direct fluorescence staining with antibodies against CMV, RSV, HSV, VZV, influenza virus, parainfluenza virus, adenovirus, and other organisms
   (c) Other organisms/tests to also consider:
      (i) Polymerase chain reaction for human metapneumovirus, rhinovirus, coronavirus, and HHV6
      (ii) Polymerase chain reaction for *Chlamydia, Mycoplasma*, and *Aspergillus* species
      (iii) Serum galactomannan ELISA for *Aspergillus* species
   (d) Transbronchial biopsy if condition of the patient permits
3. Absence of cardiac dysfunction, acute renal failure, or iatrogenic fluid overload as etiology for pulmonary dysfunction

Radiographic findings can be nonspecific, but HRCT findings include ground glass opacities that are bilateral, central, symmetric, with consolidation seen in more severe cases [75]. Recent advances in diagnostic capabilities have increased detection of occult infections which help separate IPS from infectious HSCT complications; the distinction is critical due to their vastly distinct treatment approaches. Many patients diagnosed with IPS were later discovered to have detectable pathogens, most commonly HHV-6, human rhinovirus, and aspergillus, when their BAL samples were re-examined [72].

Treatment

Historically, treatment of IPS has been largely supportive. Once infections have been ruled out, systemic corticosteroids are the mainstay of treatment; IPS in association with diffuse alveolar hemorrhage may require higher doses [60]. The results of other immunotherapeutic agents such as the soluble TNF-α inhibitor, etanercept, has been mixed. A retrospective single-center study over two distinct time-periods comparing steroids alone (earlier time-period) versus combined steroids and etanercept showed significant improvement in survival to hospital discharge [80]. However, the more recent use of reduced-intensity conditioning regimens and improved supportive care may have accounted for this improvement. Patients with late-onset IPS who responded to etanercept have greatly improved short- and long-term mortality [79]. Results in children have been similarly promising, with complete response in 20% of patients [97]. A randomized, double-blind, placebo-controlled trial comparing corticosteroids with placebo to corticosteroids with etanercept was inconclusive due to slow patient accrual and early termination [96]. Other potential therapies are under investigation. Blockade of NF-κB, a transcription factor downstream of the TNF-α receptor, has shown promise in murine models [30]. Pulmonary surfactant replacement is also being studied as an intervention to treat IPS [60].

Clinical Course and Prognosis

Outcomes for IPS remain poor, with mortality rates between 60% and 80%. Rapid clinical deterioration can occur and >95% of patients requiring mechanical ventilation succumb to the disease [20, 33, 45]. Veno-venous extracorporeal membrane oxygenation (ECMO) as a rescue therapy or bridge-to-recovery has met with mixed results [47, 51]. Short-term survival has improved with treatment advances, but 2-year survival remains low. Based on a small study, a more rapid peak and decline in severity of infiltrates on HRCT has been linked to a more favorable prognosis [75]. Biomarkers to predict patients who at risk for IPS and who respond to biologic therapy are being studied [71].

Organizing Pneumonia

Organizing Pneumonia (OP), formerly known as bronchiolitis organizing pneumonia (BOOP), is a complication of HSCT. It can occur as a part of the IPS spectrum or as a stand-alone late onset pulmonary complication of HSCT [6]. OP as a complication of HSCT was first described by Thirman et al. in 1992 [78]. Although it has been described as a complication of both autologous and allogenic HSCT, it is more common following the latter. The incidence of OP post-allogenic HSCT ranges from 0.9% to 10.3% with a median time of onset post-HSCT of 108 days [74]. Among 5340 patients, who underwent allogenic HSCT, 49 cases of histological BOOP/OP was reported, an incidence of 0.9% [32].

Clinical Features and Diagnosis

OP presents with fever, nonproductive cough, and dyspnea and can be precipitated by a recent taper of immunosuppressive regimen. PFTs commonly reveal a restrictive pattern, but could be normal, obstructive, or mixed with a decreased diffusion capacity of carbon monoxide (DLCO) [32, 58]. High resolution chest tomographic scans in patients with OP are notable for airspace consolidations, ground glass opacities, and nodular opacities (Fig. 4) [50]. In a study of 16 patients with biopsy-proven OP post-HSCT, ground glass opacities were noted to be the most common radiological feature [63]. Bronchoalveolar lavage is useful to exclude infections. Surgical lung biopsy is the gold standard for diagnosis of OP, as transbronchial biopsies have lower yield; however, the latter approach may be useful in certain clinical settings [2, 64]. Histopathological features on biopsy include presence of the buds of granulation tissue which contain myofibroblasts and a loose connective tissue (Fig. 5). These buds are intra-alveolar and can extend into the bronchioles causing obstruction with associated mild interstitial inflammation [18].

Risk Factors and Pathogenesis

A prior history of acute or chronic GVHD was found to be a strong risk factor for OP [32] and suggests a common pathogenesis. In a study of 9550 patients of post-allogenic HCST recipients, HLA disparity, female-to-male HSCT, and peripheral blood stem cell transplant (PBSCT) were associated with an increased risk of developing OP. In contrast, busulfan-based or fludarabine-based reduced-intensity conditioning compared to total body irradiation and T cell depletion regimens were associated with a lower risk [58]. The precise

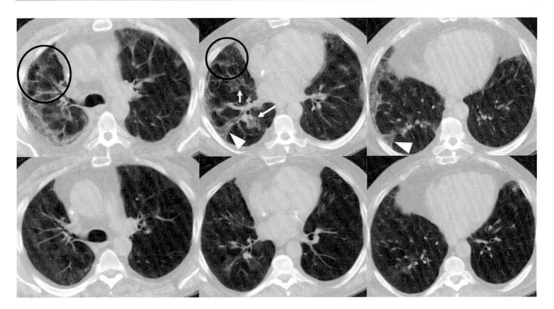

Fig. 4 69-year-old man with history of bone marrow transplant for AML a few years back. He presented with cough and increased shortness of breath. Noncontrast Computed Tomography (CT) of chest (top row) showed patchy consolidations scattered in peribronchiolar (arrow), perilobular distribution (circle), and peripheral, wedge shaped distribution (arrowhead) that were concerning for atypical infection or organizing pneumonia. The patient underwent bronchoscopy with biopsy. No infectious etiology was identified and a provisional diagnosis of cryptogenic organizing pneumonia was made. Patient was started on steroids and showed symptomatic improvement. Follow-up chest CT scan performed after 2 months (bottom row) showed marked improvement in parenchymal consolidations. (Image courtesy: Dr. Sushilkumar Sonvane, MD – University of Alabama at Birmingham, Department of Radiology)

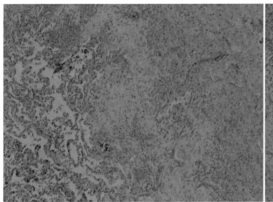
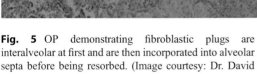
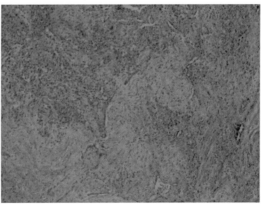

Fig. 5 OP demonstrating fibroblastic plugs are interalveolar at first and are then incorporated into alveolar septa before being resorbed. (Image courtesy: Dr. David Ralph Crowe, MD – University of Alabama at Birmingham, Department of Pathology)

pathogenetic mechanisms of post-HSCT OP are unclear. The association with GVHD and increased incidence post-allogeneic HSCT suggests alloimmune-mediated lung injury. Murine models of OP after respiratory reovirus infections have demonstrated the role of T cells and cytokines such as interferon-α in the development of the process [53].

Treatment

HSCT-associated OP, as in most other cases of OP, is primarily treated with high-dose systemic corticosteroids. There are no specific guidelines on the dose and duration of steroid therapy. Current recommendations are based on expert opinion, and clinical judgment should be exercised. Prednisone in doses ranging from 0.75–1.5 mg/kg/day have been used for 1–3 months with a slow taper over 6–12 months [17]. Further studies are needed to establish ideal doses and duration of corticosteroid therapy. Erythromycin in combination with corticosteroids has been reported with favorable outcomes [42], although the role of macrolides for treatment of OP is unclear.

Clinical Course and Prognosis

About 80% of patients with HSCT-associated OP have a favorable prognosis with resolution or stabilization after corticosteroid therapy [1]. Clinical improvement is seen usually within a week of starting therapy followed by radiological improvement. Failure to respond to treatment may result in progressive respiratory failure and death [32].

Pulmonary Venocclusive Disease

Pulmonary venoocclusive disease (PVOD) resulting in pulmonary hypertension is a rare late onset complication of both autologous and allogeneic HSCT [98]. In reported cases, it was noted in patients less than 25 years old and presented several weeks to months posttransplant [11].

Clinical Features, Pathogenesis, and Diagnosis

Presenting complaints are usually nonspecific, primarily fatigue and exertional dyspnea. Physical examination findings are similar to those of pulmonary hypertension which may be normal in early stages and become more apparent in later stages: Elevated JVD, peripheral edema, and hepatomegaly. Elevated second heart sound, parasternal lift and palpable second heart sounds in the second left intercostal space can be recognized in some patients along with tricuspid regurgitation murmur. Computed tomographic (CT) scans of the chest may show septal thickening, diffuse or mosaic ground glass opacities, small nodules, and areas of consolidation. Right heart catheterization reveals an increased pulmonary artery pressure and normal pulmonary capillary pressure. The triad of severe pulmonary hypertension in the setting of normal pulmonary artery occlusion pressure and radiographic evidence of pulmonary edema could be suggestive of PVOD but is not diagnostic. PVOD can be definitively diagnosed only by surgical biopsy and is characterized by the progressive intimal proliferation, fibrosis, and occlusion of the pulmonary venules as well as small veins [54]. The pathogenesis of PVOD post HSCT is unclear and has been attributed to toxic endothelial injury secondary to chemotherapeutic conditioning regimens and/or viral infections [74] but does not seem to be associated with cGVHD [6].

Treatment and Prognosis

There are no effective treatments for PVOD and prognosis is poor. Conventional arterial vasodilator therapy for pulmonary hypertension could worsen pulmonary edema in PVOD and if initiated should be done with close monitoring [11, 74]. Reported cases of PVOD post HSCT have shown some favorable response to steroid therapy [11, 35, 41].

Pulmonary Cytolytic Thrombi

Pulmonary cytolytic thrombi (PCT) is a complication of allogenic HSCT and primarily occurs in children with GVHD [93]. The incidence is between 1.2% and 4% with a median onset of 3 months post HSCT [83]. Patients typically present with fever, cough, and dyspnea. CT scans of the chest shows peripheral pulmonary and pleural nodules [93]. Bronchoalveolar lavage is indicated to exclude infectious etiology. The diagnosis of PCT is based on surgical biopsy of the lung nodules which are characterized by vascular occlusive and hemorrhagic infarcts secondary to thrombi containing intensely basophilic amorphous material as well as entrapped leucocytes [34]. The prognosis of PCT is favorable as it responds to treatment with systemic corticosteroids. There has not been any mortality attributed to PCT in the reported literature.

Pleuroparenchymal Fibroelastosis

Pleuroparenchymal fibroelastosis (PPFE) is a rare complication of HSCT, grouped under rare interstitial pneumonias with a prevalence of around 0.3% in HSCT recipients [55]. It is characterized by progressive sub pleural fibrosis predominantly in the upper lobes. PPFE has been reported post allogeneic and autologous HSCT. The etiology of PPFE post HSCT is unclear. Chemotherapeutic drugs, radiation therapy and a possible association with cGVHD have been hypothesized [87] to be predisposing factors.

Patients can present with dry cough, exertional dyspnea, and chest pain secondary to spontaneous pneumothorax [89]. PFTs reveal a restrictive or mixed picture of obstruction and restriction. CT scan is characteristic of pleural thickening, fibrosis, subpleural reticulations, and traction bronchiectasis predominantly in the upper lobes [55]. Histopathological exam reveals alveolar collapse, subpleural fibrosis, and extensive elastic deposition [87]. The disease is progressive with worsening symptoms and poor prognosis. Currently no therapeutic options are available except for lung transplantation [6].

Thoracic Air Leak Syndrome

Thoracic air leak syndrome (TALS) consists of a spectrum of conditions that includes spontaneous pneumothorax, subcutaneous emphysema, pneumomediastinum, interstitial emphysema, and pneumopericardium. It occurs as a late onset complication of allogenic HSCT and is associated with cGVHD. According to reported literature, prevalence of TALS post allogenic HSCT is reported to be 0.83–5.7% with a median time range of 202–575 days post HSCT [6]. The mechanism of air leak in BOS is secondary to increased intra-alveolar pressure leading to alveolar rupture into the pulmonary interstitium with subsequent retrograde dissection of air into the mediastinum and subcutaneous tissue causing pneumomediastinum and subcutaneous emphysema. Similarly, rupture into the pleural space causes pneumothorax [62]. CT scan of the chest is the imaging modality of choice and can detect air in the pleural space, mediastinum, and subcutaneous tissue. Infections, cough, emesis, and other causes of a similar presentation should be ruled out. Prognosis is poor with 1-year and 3-year survival of 45% and 15%, respectively [67].

Post-transplant Lymphoproliferative Disorder

Post-transplant lymphoproliferative disorder (PTLD) is a rare complication following allogeneic HSCT and has a cumulative incidence of 1% [21]. In a study of 21,686 HSCT patients' risk factors such as unrelated or HLA mismatched donors, use of ATG or monoclonal antibodies against T cells for GVHD prophylaxis or treatment, T cell depleted donor marrow, age >50 years and second HSCT were identified. The incidence of PTLD ranged from 0.2% in patients with no risk factors to more than 8% with more than 3 risk factors [49]. The pathogenesis of post HSCT PTLD is attributed to proliferation of donor Epstein–Barr Virus (EBV) infected B cells in the setting of weakened T-cell immunity. Though post HSCT is common in the lymph nodes, spleen, and liver, pulmonary involvement occurs in about 20% of the cases. Median onset is around 4–6 months post HSCT [3]. Clinical presentation varies and could range from asymptomatic to fulminant tumor lysis syndrome. CT scans of the chest are notable for multiple pulmonary nodules with basal and peripheral predominance, mediastinal and hilar lymphadenopathy, patchy consolidation, pleural effusion, and chest wall or pleural-based masses [70]. Diagnosis may require a biopsy or could be made via noninvasive methods in the appropriate clinical setting. A probable diagnosis is made by increased EBV DNA levels in the setting of lymphadenopathy or hepatosplenomegaly and when other causes have been ruled out, proven disease requires a biopsy. Treatment strategies include rituximab, reduction of immunosuppression, donor lymphocyte infusion, chemotherapy, and EBV-specific cytotoxic T lymphocyte infusions [77]. The prognosis of PTLD post HSCT is poor compared to that occurring after solid organ transplantation [62].

Conclusion

Late onset pulmonary complications following HSCT are a major cause of mortality and morbidity. Advances in transplant techniques, earlier diagnosis, prevention, and management of infectious complications have led to better outcomes as well as shifted the focus to late noninfectious pulmonary complications in HSCT. These complications are myriad and require further studies to develop more effective screening, preventative, and treatment strategies.

References

1. Afessa B, Peters SG. Major complications following hematopoietic stem cell transplantation. Semin Respir Crit Care Med. 2006;27(3):297–309. https://doi.org/10.1055/s-2006-945530.
2. Alasaly K, Muller N, Ostrow DN, Champion P, FitzGerald JM. Cryptogenic organizing pneumonia. A report of 25 cases and a review of the literature. Medicine (Baltimore). 1995;74(4):201–11.
3. Al-Mansour Z, Nelson BP, Evens AM. Post-transplant lymphoproliferative disease (PTLD): risk factors, diagnosis, and current treatment strategies. Curr Hematol Malig Rep. 2013;8(3):173–83. https://doi.org/10.1007/s11899-013-0162-5.
4. Au BK, Au MA, Chien JW. Bronchiolitis obliterans syndrome epidemiology after allogeneic hematopoietic cell transplantation. Biol Blood Marrow Transplant. 2011;17(7):1072–8. https://doi.org/10.1016/j.bbmt.2010.11.018.
5. Barker AF, Bergeron A, Rom WN, Hertz MI. Obliterative bronchiolitis. N Engl J Med. 2014;370(19):1820–8. https://doi.org/10.1056/NEJMra1204664.
6. Bergeron A. Late-onset noninfectious pulmonary complications after allogeneic hematopoietic stem cell transplantation. Clin Chest Med. 2017;38(2):249–62. https://doi.org/10.1016/j.ccm.2016.12.013.
7. Bergeron A, Chevret S, Chagnon K, Godet C, Bergot E, Peffault de Latour R, Dominique S, de Revel T, Juvin K, Maillard N, Reman O, Contentin N, Robin M, Buzyn A, Socie G, Tazi A. Budesonide/formoterol for bronchiolitis obliterans after hematopoietic stem cell transplantation. Am J Respir Crit Care Med. 2015;191(11):1242–9. https://doi.org/10.1164/rccm.201410-1818OC.
8. Bergeron A, Chevret S, Granata A, Chevallier P, Vincent L, Huynh A, Tabrizi R, Labussiere-Wallet H, Bernard M, Chantepie S, Bay JO, Thiebaut-Bertrand A, Thepot S, Contentin N, Fornecker LM, Maillard N, Risso K, Berceanu A, Blaise D, Peffault de La Tour R, Chien JW, Coiteux V, Socie G, ALLOZITHRO Study Investigators. Effect of azithromycin on airflow decline-free survival after allogeneic hematopoietic stem cell transplant: the ALLOZITHRO randomized clinical trial. JAMA. 2017;318(6):557–66. https://doi.org/10.1001/jama.2017.9938.
9. Bergeron A, Chevret S, Peffault de Latour R, Chagnon K, de Margerie-Mellon C, Riviere F, Robin M, Mani J, Lorillon G, Socie G, Tazi A. Noninfectious lung complications after allogeneic haematopoietic stem cell transplantation. Eur Respir J. 2018;51(5). https://doi.org/10.1183/13993003.02617-2017.
10. Brownback KR, Thomas LA, McGuirk JP, Ganguly S, Streiler C, Abhyankar S. Effect of rituximab on pulmonary function in bronchiolitis obliterans syndrome due to graft-versus-host-disease. Lung. 2017;195(6):781–8. https://doi.org/10.1007/s00408-017-0051-0.
11. Bunte MC, Patnaik MM, Pritzker MR, Burns LJ. Pulmonary veno-occlusive disease following hematopoietic stem cell transplantation: a rare model of endothelial dysfunction. Bone Marrow Transplant. 2008;41(8):677–86. https://doi.org/10.1038/sj.bmt.1705990.
12. Busca A, Locatelli F, Marmont F, Ceretto C, Falda M. Recombinant human soluble tumor necrosis factor receptor fusion protein as treatment for steroid refractory graft-versus-host disease following allogeneic hematopoietic stem cell transplantation. Am J Hematol. 2007;82(1):45–52. https://doi.org/10.1002/ajh.20752.
13. Cheng GS, Storer B, Chien JW, Jagasia M, Hubbard JJ, Burns L, Ho VT, Pidala J, Palmer J, Johnston L, Mayer S, Crothers K, Pusic I, Lee SJ, Williams KM. Lung function trajectory in bronchiolitis obliterans syndrome after allogeneic hematopoietic cell transplant. Ann Am Thorac Soc. 2016;13(11):1932–9. https://doi.org/10.1513/AnnalsATS.201604-262OC.
14. Clark JG, Crawford SW, Madtes DK, Sullivan KM. Obstructive lung disease after allogeneic marrow

transplantation. Clinical presentation and course. Ann Intern Med. 1989;111(5):368–76.

15. Cooke KR, Kobzik L, Martin TR, Brewer J, Delmonte J Jr, Crawford JM, Ferrara JL. An experimental model of idiopathic pneumonia syndrome after bone marrow transplantation: I. The roles of minor H antigens and endotoxin. Blood. 1996;88(8):3230–9.

16. Cooke KR, Hill GR, Gerbitz A, Kobzik L, Martin TR, Crawford JM, Brewer JP, Ferrara JL. Tumor necrosis factor-alpha neutralization reduces lung injury after experimental allogeneic bone marrow transplantation. Transplantation. 2000;70(2):272–9.

17. Cordier JF. Organising pneumonia. Thorax. 2000;55(4):318–28.

18. Cordier JF. Cryptogenic organising pneumonia. Eur Respir J. 2006;28(2):422–46. https://doi.org/10.1183/09031936.06.00013505.

19. Corris PA, Ryan VA, Small T, Lordan J, Fisher AJ, Meachery G, Johnson G, Ward C. A randomised controlled trial of azithromycin therapy in bronchiolitis obliterans syndrome (BOS) post lung transplantation. Thorax. 2015;70(5):442–50. https://doi.org/10.1136/thoraxjnl-2014-205998.

20. Crawford SW, Hackman RC. Clinical course of idiopathic pneumonia after bone marrow transplantation. Am Rev Respir Dis. 1993;147(6 Pt 1):1393–400. https://doi.org/10.1164/ajrccm/147.6_Pt_1.1393.

21. Curtis RE, Travis LB, Rowlings PA, Socie G, Kingma DW, Banks PM, Jaffe ES, Sale GE, Horowitz MM, Witherspoon RP, Shriner DA, Weisdorf DJ, Kolb HJ, Sullivan KM, Sobocinski KA, Gale RP, Hoover RN, Fraumeni JF Jr, Deeg HJ. Risk of lymphoproliferative disorders after bone marrow transplantation: a multi-institutional study. Blood. 1999;94(7):2208–16.

22. Dirou S, Malard F, Chambellan A, Chevallier P, Germaud P, Guillaume T, Delaunay J, Moreau P, Delasalle B, Lemarchand P, Mohty M. Stable long-term pulmonary function after fludarabine, antithymocyte globulin and i.v. BU for reduced-intensity conditioning allogeneic SCT. Bone Marrow Transplant. 2014;49(5):622–7. https://doi.org/10.1038/bmt.2014.15.

23. Ditschkowski M, Elmaagacli AH, Trenschel R, Peceny R, Koldehoff M, Schulte C, Beelen DW. T-cell depletion prevents from bronchiolitis obliterans and bronchiolitis obliterans with organizing pneumonia after allogeneic hematopoietic stem cell transplantation with related donors. Haematologica. 2007;92(4):558–61.

24. Ditschkowski M, Elmaagacli AH, Koldehoff M, Gromke T, Trenschel R, Beelen DW. Bronchiolitis obliterans after allogeneic hematopoietic SCT: further insight–new perspectives? Bone Marrow Transplant. 2013;48(9):1224–9. https://doi.org/10.1038/bmt.2013.17.

25. Du J, Paz K, Flynn R, Vulic A, Robinson TM, Lineburg KE, Alexander KA, Meng J, Roy S, Panoskaltsis-Mortari A, Loschi M, Hill GR, Serody JS, Maillard I, Miklos D, Koreth J, Cutler CS,

Antin JH, Ritz J, MacDonald KP, Schacker TW, Luznik L, Blazar BR. Pirfenidone ameliorates murine chronic GVHD through inhibition of macrophage infiltration and TGF-beta production. Blood. 2017;129(18):2570–80. https://doi.org/10.1182/blood-2017-01-758854.

26. Dudek AZ, Mahaseth H, DeFor TE, Weisdorf DJ. Bronchiolitis obliterans in chronic graft-versus-host disease: analysis of risk factors and treatment outcomes. Biol Blood Marrow Transplant. 2003;9(10):657–66. https://doi.org/10.1016/S1083.

27. Epaud R, Ikegami M, Whitsett JA, Jobe AH, Weaver TE, Akinbi HT. Surfactant protein B inhibits endotoxin-induced lung inflammation. Am J Respir Cell Mol Biol. 2003;28(3):373–8. https://doi.org/10.1165/rcmb.2002-0071OC.

28. Even-Or E, Ghandourah H, Ali M, Krueger J, Sweezey NB, Schechter T. Efficacy of high-dose steroids for bronchiolitis obliterans syndrome post pediatric hematopoietic stem cell transplantation. Pediatr Transplant. 2018;22(2). https://doi.org/10.1111/petr.13155.

29. Filipovich AH, Weisdorf D, Pavletic S, Socie G, Wingard JR, Lee SJ, Martin P, Chien J, Przepiorka D, Couriel D, Cowen EW, Dinndorf P, Farrell A, Hartzman R, Henslee-Downey J, Jacobsohn D, McDonald G, Mittleman B, Rizzo JD, Robinson M, Schubert M, Schultz K, Shulman H, Turner M, Vogelsang G, Flowers ME. National Institutes of Health consensus development project on criteria for clinical trials in chronic graft-versus-host disease: I. Diagnosis and staging working group report. Biol Blood Marrow Transplant. 2005;11(12):945–56. https://doi.org/10.1016/j.bbmt.2005.09.004.

30. Fowler KA, Jania CM, Tilley SL, Panoskaltsis-Mortari A, Baldwin AS, Serody JS, Coghill JM. Targeting the canonical nuclear factor-kappaB pathway with a high-potency IKK2 inhibitor improves outcomes in a mouse model of idiopathic pneumonia syndrome. Biol Blood Marrow Transplant. 2017;23(4):569–80. https://doi.org/10.1016/j.bbmt.2017.01.083.

31. Frankovich J, Donaldson SS, Lee Y, Wong RM, Amylon M, Verneris MR. High-dose therapy and autologous hematopoietic cell transplantation in children with primary refractory and relapsed Hodgkin's disease: atopy predicts idiopathic diffuse lung injury syndromes. Biol Blood Marrow Transplant. 2001;7(1):49–57. https://doi.org/10.1053/bbmt.2001.v7.pm11215699.

32. Freudenberger TD, Madtes DK, Curtis JR, Cummings P, Storer BE, Hackman RC. Association between acute and chronic graft-versus-host disease and bronchiolitis obliterans organizing pneumonia in recipients of hematopoietic stem cell transplants. Blood. 2003;102(10):3822–8. https://doi.org/10.1182/blood-2002-06-1813.

33. Fukuda T, Hackman RC, Guthrie KA, Sandmaier BM, Boeckh M, Maris MB, Maloney DG, Deeg HJ,

Martin PJ, Storb RF, Madtes DK. Risks and outcomes of idiopathic pneumonia syndrome after non-myeloablative and conventional conditioning regimens for allogeneic hematopoietic stem cell transplantation. Blood. 2003;102(8):2777–85. https://doi.org/10.1182/blood-2003-05-1597.

34. Gulbahce HE, Manivel JC, Jessurun J. Pulmonary cytolytic thrombi: a previously unrecognized complication of bone marrow transplantation. Am J Surg Pathol. 2000;24(8):1147–52.

35. Hackman RC, Madtes DK, Petersen FB, Clark JG. Pulmonary venoocclusive disease following bone marrow transplantation. Transplantation. 1989;47(6):989–92.

36. Hankinson JL, Odencrantz JR, Fedan KB. Spirometric reference values from a sample of the general U.S. population. Am J Respir Crit Care Med. 1999;159(1):179–87. https://doi.org/10.1164/ajrccm.159.1.9712108.

37. Hefazi M, Langer KJ, Khera N, Adamski J, Roy V, Winters JL, Gastineau DA, Jacob EK, Kreuter JD, Gandhi MJ, Hogan WJ, Litzow MR, Hashmi SK, Yadav H, Iyer VN, Scott JP, Wylam ME, Cartin-Ceba R, Patnaik MM. Extracorporeal photopheresis improves survival in hematopoietic cell transplant patients with bronchiolitis obliterans syndrome without significantly impacting measured pulmonary functions. Biol Blood Marrow Transplant. 2018. https://doi.org/10.1016/j.bbmt.2018.04.012.

38. Hildebrandt GC, Corrion LA, Olkiewicz KM, Lu B, Lowler K, Duffner UA, Moore BB, Kuziel WA, Liu C, Cooke KR. Blockade of CXCR3 receptor: ligand interactions reduces leukocyte recruitment to the lung and the severity of experimental idiopathic pneumonia syndrome. J Immunol. 2004;173(3):2050–9.

39. Hildebrandt GC, Granell M, Urbano-Ispizua A, Wolff D, Hertenstein B, Greinix HT, Brenmoehl J, Schulz C, Dickinson AM, Hahn J, Rogler G, Andreesen R, Holler E. Recipient NOD2/CARD15 variants: a novel independent risk factor for the development of bronchiolitis obliterans after allogeneic stem cell transplantation. Biol Blood Marrow Transplant. 2008;14(1):67–74. https://doi.org/10.1016/j.bbmt.2007.09.009.

40. Holm AM, Riise GC, Hansson L, Brinch L, Bjortuft O, Iversen M, Simonsen S, Floisand Y. Lung transplantation for bronchiolitis obliterans syndrome after allo-SCT. Bone Marrow Transplant. 2013;48(5):703–7. https://doi.org/10.1038/bmt.2012.197.

41. Hosokawa K, Yamazaki H, Nishitsuji M, Kobayashi S, Takami A, Fujimura M, Nakao S. Pulmonary veno-occlusive disease following reduced-intensity allogeneic bone marrow transplantation for acute myeloid leukemia. Intern Med. 2012;51(2):195–8.

42. Ishii T, Manabe A, Ebihara Y, Ueda T, Yoshino H, Mitsui T, Hisakawa H, Yagasaki H, Kikuchi A, Yoshimasu T, Tanaka R, Takahashi T, Masunaga A, Sugita KI, Nakahata T, Asano S, Tsuji K. Improvement in bronchiolitis obliterans organizing pneumonia in a child after allogeneic bone marrow transplantation by a combination of oral prednisolone and low dose erythromycin. Bone Marrow Transplant. 2000;26(8):907–10. https://doi.org/10.1038/sj.bmt.1702642.

43. Jagasia MH, Greinix HT, Arora M, Williams KM, Wolff D, Cowen EW, Palmer J, Weisdorf D, Treister NS, Cheng GS, Kerr H, Stratton P, Duarte RF, McDonald GB, Inamoto Y, Vigorito A, Arai S, Datiles MB, Jacobsohn D, Heller T, Kitko CL, Mitchell SA, Martin PJ, Shulman H, Wu RS, Cutler CS, Vogelsang GB, Lee SJ, Pavletic SZ, Flowers ME. National Institutes of Health consensus development project on criteria for clinical trials in chronic graft-versus-host disease: I. The 2014 diagnosis and staging working group report. Biol Blood Marrow Transplant. 2015;21(3):389–401. e381. https://doi.org/10.1016/j.bbmt.2014.12.001.

44. Jo KW, Yoon S, Song JW, Shim TS, Lee SW, Lee JS, Kim DY, Lee JH, Lee JH, Choi Y, Lee KH. The efficacy of prophylactic azithromycin on bronchiolitis obliterans syndrome after hematopoietic stem cell transplantation. Int J Hematol. 2015;102(3):357–63. https://doi.org/10.1007/s12185-015-1830-0.

45. Kantrow SP, Hackman RC, Boeckh M, Myerson D, Crawford SW. Idiopathic pneumonia syndrome: changing spectrum of lung injury after marrow transplantation. Transplantation. 1997;63(8):1079–86.

46. Kim SJ, Lee JW, Jung CW, Min CK, Cho B, Shin HJ, Chung JS, Kim H, Lee WS, Joo YD, Yang DH, Kook H, Kang HJ, Ahn HS, Yoon SS, Sohn SK, Min YH, Min WS, Park HS, Won JH. Weekly rituximab followed by monthly rituximab treatment for steroid-refractory chronic graft-versus-host disease: results from a prospective, multicenter, phase II study. Haematologica. 2010;95(11):1935–42. https://doi.org/10.3324/haematol.2010.026104.

47. Koinuma T, Nunomiya S, Wada M, Koyama K, Suzuki T. Concurrent treatment with a tumor necrosis factor-alpha inhibitor and veno-venous extracorporeal membrane oxygenation in a post-hematopoietic stem cell transplant patient with idiopathic pneumonia syndrome: a case report. J Intensive Care. 2014;2(1):48. https://doi.org/10.1186/s40560-014-0048-1.

48. Lam DC, Lam B, Wong MK, Lu C, Au WY, Tse EW, Leung AY, Kwong YL, Liang RH, Lam WK, Ip MS, Lie AK. Effects of azithromycin in bronchiolitis obliterans syndrome after hematopoietic SCT–a randomized double-blinded placebo-controlled study. Bone Marrow Transplant. 2011;46(12):1551–6. https://doi.org/10.1038/bmt.2011.1.

49. Landgren O, Gilbert ES, Rizzo JD, Socie G, Banks PM, Sobocinski KA, Horowitz MM, Jaffe ES, Kingma DW, Travis LB, Flowers ME, Martin PJ, Deeg HJ, Curtis RE. Risk factors for lymphoproliferative disorders after allogeneic hematopoietic cell transplantation. Blood. 2009;113(20):4992–5001. https://doi.org/10.1182/blood-2008-09-178046.

50. Lee KS, Kullnig P, Hartman TE, Muller NL. Cryptogenic organizing pneumonia: CT findings in

43 patients. AJR Am J Roentgenol. 1994;162(3): 543–6. https://doi.org/10.2214/ajr.162.3.8109493.

51. Liao WI, Tsai SH, Chiu SK. Successful use of extracorporeal membrane oxygenation in a hematopoietic stem cell transplant patient with idiopathic pneumonia syndrome. Respir Care. 2013;58(2):e6–10. https://doi.org/10.4187/respcare.01716.

52. Lucid CE, Savani BN, Engelhardt BG, Shah P, Clifton C, Greenhut SL, Vaughan LA, Kassim A, Schuening F, Jagasia M. Extracorporeal photopheresis in patients with refractory bronchiolitis obliterans developing after allo-SCT. Bone Marrow Transplant. 2011;46 (3):426–9. https://doi.org/10.1038/bmt.2010.152.

53. Majeski EI, Paintlia MK, Lopez AD, Harley RA, London SD, London L. Respiratory reovirus 1/L induction of intraluminal fibrosis, a model of bronchiolitis obliterans organizing pneumonia, is dependent on T lymphocytes. Am J Pathol. 2003;163(4): 1467–79. https://doi.org/10.1016/S0002-9440(10) 63504-3.

54. Mandel J, Mark EJ, Hales CA. Pulmonary veno-occlusive disease. Am J Respir Crit Care Med. 2000;162(5):1964–73. https://doi.org/10.1164/ajrccm.162.5.9912045.

55. Mariani F, Gatti B, Rocca A, Bonifazi F, Cavazza A, Fanti S, Tomassetti S, Piciucchi S, Poletti V, Zompatori M. Pleuroparenchymal fibroelastosis: the prevalence of secondary forms in hematopoietic stem cell and lung transplantation recipients. Diagn Interv Radiol. 2016;22(5):400–6. https://doi.org/10.5152/dir.2016.15516.

56. McCormack FX, Whitsett JA. The pulmonary collectins, SP-A and SP-D, orchestrate innate immunity in the lung. J Clin Invest. 2002;109(6):707–12. https://doi.org/10.1172/JCI15293.

57. Nakaseko C, Ozawa S, Sakaida E, Sakai M, Kanda Y, Oshima K, Kurokawa M, Takahashi S, Ooi J, Shimizu T, Yokota A, Yoshiba F, Fujimaki K, Kanamori H, Sakai R, Saitoh T, Sakura T, Maruta A, Sakamaki H, Okamoto S. Incidence, risk factors and outcomes of bronchiolitis obliterans after allogeneic stem cell transplantation. Int J Hematol. 2011;93(3): 375–82. https://doi.org/10.1007/s12185-011-0809-8.

58. Nakasone H, Onizuka M, Suzuki N, Fujii N, Taniguchi S, Kakihana K, Ogawa H, Miyamura K, Eto T, Sakamaki H, Yabe H, Morishima Y, Kato K, Suzuki R, Fukuda T. Pre-transplant risk factors for cryptogenic organizing pneumonia/bronchiolitis obliterans organizing pneumonia after hematopoietic cell transplantation. Bone Marrow Transplant. 2013;48 (10):1317–23. https://doi.org/10.1038/bmt.2013.116.

59. Olivieri A, Locatelli F, Zecca M, Sanna A, Cimminiello M, Raimondi R, Gini G, Mordini N, Balduzzi A, Leoni P, Gabrielli A, Bacigalupo A. Imatinib for refractory chronic graft-versus-host disease with fibrotic features. Blood. 2009;114(3):709–18. https://doi.org/10.1182/blood-2009-02-204 156.

60. Panoskaltsis-Mortari A, Griese M, Madtes DK, Belperio JA, Haddad IY, Folz RJ, Cooke KR,

American Thoracic Society Committee on Idiopathic Pneumonia Syndrome. An official American Thoracic Society research statement: noninfectious lung injury after hematopoietic stem cell transplantation: idiopathic pneumonia syndrome. Am J Respir Crit Care Med. 2011;183(9):1262–79. https://doi.org/10.1164/rccm.2007-413ST.

61. Paz HL, Crilley P, Patchefsky A, Schiffman RL, Brodsky I. Bronchiolitis obliterans after autologous bone marrow transplantation. Chest. 1992;101(3): 775–8.

62. Pena E, Souza CA, Escuissato DL, Gomes MM, Allan D, Tay J, Dennie CJ. Noninfectious pulmonary complications after hematopoietic stem cell transplantation: practical approach to imaging diagnosis. Radiographics. 2014;34(3):663–83. https://doi.org/10.1148/rg.343135080.

63. Pipavath SN, Chung JH, Chien JW, Godwin JD. Organizing pneumonia in recipients of hematopoietic stem cell transplantation: CT features in 16 patients. J Comput Assist Tomogr. 2012;36(4):431–6. https://doi.org/10.1097/RCT.0b013e31825ba274.

64. Poletti V, Cazzato S, Minicuci N, Zompatori M, Burzi M, Schiattone ML. The diagnostic value of bronchoalveolar lavage and transbronchial lung biopsy in cryptogenic organizing pneumonia. Eur Respir J. 1996;9(12):2513–6.

65. Ratjen F, Rjabko O, Kremens B. High-dose corticosteroid therapy for bronchiolitis obliterans after bone marrow transplantation in children. Bone Marrow Transplant. 2005;36(2):135–8. https://doi.org/10.1038/sj.bmt.1705026.

66. Sakaguchi H, Takahashi Y, Watanabe N, Doisaki S, Muramatsu H, Hama A, Shimada A, Yagasaki H, Kudo K, Kojima S. Incidence, clinical features, and risk factors of idiopathic pneumonia syndrome following hematopoietic stem cell transplantation in children. Pediatr Blood Cancer. 2012;58(5):780–4. https://doi.org/10.1002/pbc.23298.

67. Sakai R, Kanamori H, Nakaseko C, Yoshiba F, Fujimaki K, Sakura T, Fujisawa S, Kawai N, Onoda M, Matsushima T, Maruta A, Sakamaki H, Okamoto S. Air-leak syndrome following allo-SCT in adult patients: report from the Kanto Study Group for Cell Therapy in Japan. Bone Marrow Transplant. 2011;46 (3):379–84. https://doi.org/10.1038/bmt.2010. 129.

68. Sampath S, Schultheiss TE, Wong J. Dose response and factors related to interstitial pneumonitis after bone marrow transplant. Int J Radiat Oncol Biol Phys. 2005;63(3):876–84. https://doi.org/10.1016/j.ijrobp.2005.02.032.

69. Santo Tomas LH, Loberiza FR Jr, Klein JP, Layde PM, Lipchik RJ, Rizzo JD, Bredeson CN, Horowitz MM. Risk factors for bronchiolitis obliterans in allogeneic hematopoietic stem-cell transplantation for leukemia. Chest. 2005;128(1):153–61. https://doi.org/10.1378/chest.128.1.153.

70. Scarsbrook AF, Warakaulle DR, Dattani M, Traill Z. Post-transplantation lymphoproliferative disorder: the

spectrum of imaging appearances. Clin Radiol. 2005;60(1):47–55. https://doi.org/10.1016/j.crad. 2004. 08.016.

71. Schlatzer DM, Dazard JE, Ewing RM, Ilchenko S, Tomcheko SE, Eid S, Ho V, Yanik G, Chance MR, Cooke KR. Human biomarker discovery and predictive models for disease progression for idiopathic pneumonia syndrome following allogeneic stem cell transplantation. Mol Cell Proteomics. 2012;11(6):M111 015479. https://doi.org/10.1074/mcp.M111.015479.

72. Seo S, Renaud C, Kuypers JM, Chiu CY, Huang ML, Samayoa E, Xie H, Yu G, Fisher CE, Gooley TA, Miller S, Hackman RC, Myerson D, Sedlak RH, Kim YJ, Fukuda T, Fredricks DN, Madtes DK, Jerome KR, Boeckh M. Idiopathic pneumonia syndrome after hematopoietic cell transplantation: evidence of occult infectious etiologies. Blood. 2015;125(24):3789–97. https://doi.org/10.1182/blood-2014-12-617035.

73. Shankar G, Scott Bryson J, Darrell Jennings C, Kaplan AM, Cohen DA. Idiopathic pneumonia syndrome after allogeneic bone marrow transplantation in mice. Role of pretransplant radiation conditioning. Am J Respir Cell Mol Biol. 1999;20(6):1116–24. https:// doi.org/10.1165/ajrcmb.20.6.3455.

74. Soubani AO, Pandya CM. The spectrum of non-infectious pulmonary complications following hematopoietic stem cell transplantation. Hematol Oncol Stem Cell Ther. 2010;3(3):143–57.

75. Spira D, Faul C, Schaup V, Wirths S, Schulze M, Sauter A, Horger M. HRCT findings in idiopathic pneumonia syndrome with documentation of the disease course. Eur J Radiol. 2012;81(2):e147–52. https:// doi.org/10.1016/j.ejrad.2011.01.055.

76. Srinivasan M, Flynn R, Price A, Ranger A, Browning JL, Taylor PA, Ritz J, Antin JH, Murphy WJ, Luznik L, Shlomchik MJ, Panoskaltsis-Mortari A, Blazar BR. Donor B-cell alloantibody deposition and germinal center formation are required for the development of murine chronic GVHD and bronchiolitis obliterans. Blood. 2012;119(6):1570–80. https://doi.org/10.1182/blood-2011-07-364414.

77. Styczynski J, van der Velden W, Fox CP, Engelhard D, de la Camara R, Cordonnier C, Ljungman P, Sixth European Conference on Infections in Leukemia, a joint venture of the Infectious Diseases Working Party of the European Society of Blood and Marrow Transplantation, the Infectious Diseases Group of the European Organization for Research and Treatment of Cancer, the International Immunocompromised Host Society and the European Leukemia Net. Management of Epstein-Barr Virus infections and post-transplant lymphoproliferative disorders in patients after allogeneic hematopoietic stem cell transplantation: Sixth European Conference on Infections in Leukemia (ECIL-6) guidelines. Haematologica. 2016;101(7):803–11. https://doi.org/10.3324/haematol. 2016.144428.

78. Thirman MJ, Devine SM, O'Toole K, Cizek G, Jessurun J, Hertz M, Geller RB. Bronchiolitis

obliterans organizing pneumonia as a complication of allogeneic bone marrow transplantation. Bone Marrow Transplant. 1992;10(3):307–11.

79. Thompson J, Yin Z, D'Souza A, Fenske T, Hamadani M, Hari P, Rizzo JD, Pasquini M, Saber W, Shah N, Shaw BE, Shahir K, Banerjee A, Drobyski WR. Etanercept and corticosteroid therapy for the treatment of late-onset idiopathic pneumonia syndrome. Biol Blood Marrow Transplant. 2017;23(11):1955–60. https://doi.org/10.1016/j.bbmt. 2017.07.019.

80. Tizon R, Frey N, Heitjan DF, Tan KS, Goldstein SC, Hexner EO, Loren A, Luger SM, Reshef R, Tsai D, Vogl D, Davis J, Vozniak M, Fuchs B, Stadtmauer EA, Porter DL. High-dose corticosteroids with or without etanercept for the treatment of idiopathic pneumonia syndrome after allo-SCT. Bone Marrow Transplant. 2012;47(10):1332–7. https://doi.org/10.1038/bmt. 2011.260.

81. Ueda K, Watadani T, Maeda E, Ota S, Kataoka K, Seo S, Kumano K, Hangaishi A, Takahashi T, Imai Y, Ohtomo K, Fukayama M, Nannya Y, Kurokawa M. Outcome and treatment of late-onset noninfectious pulmonary complications after allogeneic haematopoietic SCT. Bone Marrow Transplant. 2010;45(12):1719–27. https://doi.org/10.1038/bmt. 2010.48.

82. Uhlving HH, Buchvald F, Heilmann CJ, Nielsen KG, Gormsen M, Muller KG. Bronchiolitis obliterans after allo-SCT: clinical criteria and treatment options. Bone Marrow Transplant. 2012;47(8):1020–9. https://doi. org/10.1038/bmt.2011.161.

83. Vande Vusse LK, Madtes DK. Early onset non-infectious pulmonary syndromes after hematopoietic cell transplantation. Clin Chest Med. 2017;38(2): 233–48. https://doi.org/10.1016/j.ccm.2016.12.007.

84. Vande Vusse LK, Madtes DK, Guthrie KA, Gernsheimer TB, Curtis JR, Watkins TR. The association between red blood cell and platelet transfusion and subsequently developing idiopathic pneumonia syndrome after hematopoietic stem cell transplantation. Transfusion. 2014;54(4):1071–80. https://doi.org/ 10.1111/trf.12396.

85. Vande Vusse LK, Madtes DK, Bolgiano D, Watkins TR. The association between platelet transfusion and idiopathic pneumonia syndrome is unaffected by platelet product type. Transfusion. 2016;56(2): 489–96. https://doi.org/10.1111/trf.13361.

86. Vogl UM, Nagayama K, Bojic M, Hoda MA, Klepetko W, Jaksch P, Dekan S, Siersch V, Mitterbauer M, Schellongowski P, Greinix HT, Petkov V, Schulenburg A, Kalhs P, Rabitsch W. Lung transplantation for bronchiolitis obliterans after allogeneic hematopoietic stem cell transplantation: a single-center experience. Transplantation. 2013;95(4):623–8. https://doi.org/10.1097/TP.0b013e318277e29e.

87. von der Thusen JH, Hansell DM, Tominaga M, Veys PA, Ashworth MT, Owens CM, Nicholson AG. Pleuroparenchymal fibroelastosis in patients with

pulmonary disease secondary to bone marrow transplantation. Mod Pathol. 2011;24(12):1633–9. https://doi.org/10.1038/modpathol.2011.114.

88. Vos R, Vanaudenaerde BM, Verleden SE, De Vleeschauwer SI, Willems-Widyastuti A, Van Raemdonck DE, Schoonis A, Nawrot TS, Dupont LJ, Verleden GM. A randomised controlled trial of azithromycin to prevent chronic rejection after lung transplantation. Eur Respir J. 2011;37(1):164–72. https://doi.org/10.1183/09031936.00068310.

89. Watanabe K. Pleuroparenchymal fibroelastosis: its clinical characteristics. Curr Respir Med Rev. 2013;9:299–37. https://doi.org/10.2174/1573398X09 04140129125307.

90. Weiner RS, Bortin MM, Gale RP, Gluckman E, Kay HE, Kolb HJ, Hartz AJ, Rimm AA. Interstitial pneumonitis after bone marrow transplantation. Assessment of risk factors. Ann Intern Med. 1986;104(2):168–75.

91. Williams KM. How I treat bronchiolitis obliterans syndrome after hematopoietic stem cell transplantation. Blood. 2017;129(4):448–55. https://doi.org/10.1182/blood-2016-08-693507.

92. Williams KM, Cheng GS, Pusic I, Jagasia M, Burns L, Ho VT, Pidala J, Palmer J, Johnston L, Mayer S, Chien JW, Jacobsohn DA, Pavletic SZ, Martin PJ, Storer BE, Inamoto Y, Chai X, Flowers MED, Lee SJ. Fluticasone, azithromycin, and montelukast treatment for new-onset bronchiolitis obliterans syndrome after hematopoietic cell transplantation. Biol Blood Marrow Transplant. 2016;22(4):710–6. https://doi.org/10.1016/j.bbmt.2015.10.009.

93. Woodard JP, Gulbahce E, Shreve M, Steiner M, Peters C, Hite S, Ramsay NK, DeFor T, Baker KS. Pulmonary cytolytic thrombi: a newly recognized complication of stem cell transplantation. Bone Marrow Transplant. 2000;25(3):293–300. https://doi.org/10.1038/sj.bmt.1702137.

94. Yang S, Milla C, Panoskaltsis-Mortari A, Ingbar DH, Blazar BR, Haddad IY. Human surfactant protein a suppresses T cell-dependent inflammation and attenuates the manifestations of idiopathic pneumonia syndrome in mice. Am J Respir Cell Mol Biol. 2001;24(5):527–36. https://doi.org/10.1165/ajrcmb.24.5.4400.

95. Yanik GA, Mineishi S, Levine JE, Kitko CL, White ES, Vander Lugt MT, Harris AC, Braun T, Cooke KR. Soluble tumor necrosis factor receptor: enbrel (etanercept) for subacute pulmonary dysfunction following allogeneic stem cell transplantation. Biol Blood Marrow Transplant. 2012;18(7):1044–54. https://doi.org/10.1016/j.bbmt.2011.11.031.

96. Yanik GA, Horowitz MM, Weisdorf DJ, Logan BR, Ho VT, Soiffer RJ, Carter SL, Wu J, Wingard JR, Difronzo NL, Ferrara JL, Giralt S, Madtes DK, Drexler R, White ES, Cooke KR. Randomized, double-blind, placebo-controlled trial of soluble tumor necrosis factor receptor: enbrel (etanercept) for the treatment of idiopathic pneumonia syndrome after allogeneic stem cell transplantation: blood and marrow transplant clinical trials network protocol. Biol Blood Marrow Transplant. 2014;20(6):858–64. https://doi.org/10.1016/j.bbmt.2014.02.026.

97. Yanik GA, Grupp SA, Pulsipher MA, Levine JE, Schultz KR, Wall DA, Langholz B, Dvorak CC, Alangaden K, Goyal RK, White ES, Collura JM, Skeens MA, Eid S, Pierce EM, Cooke KR. TNF-receptor inhibitor therapy for the treatment of children with idiopathic pneumonia syndrome. A joint Pediatric Blood and Marrow Transplant Consortium and Children's Oncology Group Study (ASCT0521). Biol Blood Marrow Transplant. 2015;21(1):67–73. https://doi.org/10.1016/j.bbmt.2014.09.019.

98. Yoshihara S, Yanik G, Cooke KR, Mineishi S. Bronchiolitis obliterans syndrome (BOS), bronchiolitis obliterans organizing pneumonia (BOOP), and other late-onset noninfectious pulmonary complications following allogeneic hematopoietic stem cell transplantation. Biol Blood Marrow Transplant. 2007;13(7):749–59. https://doi.org/10.1016/j.bbmt.2007.05.001.

Pleural Disease: Malignant and Benign Pleural Effusions

42

María F. Landaeta and Macarena R. Vial

Contents

Introduction 644

Epidemiology 644

Pathophysiology 644

Etiology 645

Diagnosis 645
Confirmation of the Effusion: Imaging Studies 646
Classification as Transudates or Exudates 646
Identifying the Underlying Cause 647

Clinical Relevance 647

Pleural Effusion Drainage 648
Continuous or Repetitive Drainage 648
Permanent Catheters 649

Pleural Effusion in Malignant Neoplasms 649

Conclusion 649

References 649

M. F. Landaeta
Lincoln Medical and Mental Health Center, New York, NY, USA
e-mail: mafelandaeta@gmail.com

M. R. Vial (✉)
Interventional Pulmonology Unit, Clínica Alemana de Santiago-Universidad del Desarrollo, Santiago, Chile

Servicio de Enfermedades Respiratorias, Unidad de Neumologia Intervencional, Clinica Alemana de Santiago, Vitacura, Santiago, Chile
e-mail: mrodriguezvi@alemana.cl

Abstract

Pleural effusion is a common problem in intensive care unit (ICU) patients. Proper diagnosis involves three steps: confirmation of the effusion with imaging studies, classification as transudates or exudates and identifying the underlying cause. Imaging studies such as chest X-ray, ultrasound, and CT scan are useful to confirm the diagnosis and may also suggest the underlying cause. Ultrasound is particularly helpful in the ICU setting due to its portability and ability to characterize the effusion and guide pleural procedures. If an effusion is clinically significant or

© Springer Nature Switzerland AG 2020
J. L. Nates, K. J. Price (eds.), *Oncologic Critical Care*,
https://doi.org/10.1007/978-3-319-74588-6_62

the diagnosis is unknown, then drainage and fluid analysis are essential. Mechanical ventilation is not associated with increased complications of pleural drainage and can be safely performed if indicated. Drainage also has a therapeutic objective, and it is mandatory and urgent if an infection is suspected but also indicated in patients with large effusions, a noncompliant chest wall, or severe respiratory failure requiring higher positive end-expiratory pressures (PEEP). In patients with a suspected malignant effusion, effusion will recur, and a definitive treatment may be considered if the patient survives the ICU.

Keywords

Pleural effusion · Malignancy · Exudate · Transudate · Empyema · Chest tube · Ultrasound · Thoracentesis · Pleurodesis · Mesothelioma · Indwelling pleural catheter

Introduction

Pleural effusion is a frequent problem in patients admitted to intensive care units (ICUs). While some effusions are small or have no clinical significance, others may have a negative impact on the patients' health condition or represent the primary cause of admission. Identifying the presence of pleural effusion and the underlying cause is critical to establish an appropriate treatment plan. Pleural effusions can worsen gas exchange, respiratory mechanics, and cause hemodynamic instability. Drainage can improve oxygenation, and fluid analysis provides essential information to establish the underlying cause of the effusion [13]. This chapter reviews the leading causes, diagnostic tools, and management of patients with pleural effusion, with a particular focus on the critically ill patient.

Epidemiology

An estimated 1.5 million people per year develop pleural effusions in the United States, and approximately 178,000 undergo thoracentesis [8]. Prevalence of pleural effusions is unusually high in

patients admitted to ICU, with studies showing effusions in up to 62% of patients when assessed by ultrasound [23]. The majority of these effusions, however, is not significant and may have small or no clinical impact.

Several reasons explain the high prevalence of pleural effusions in the ICU setting. First, pneumonia is a common cause of admission and also a complication of hospitalization and mechanical ventilation. Second, patients undergoing heart, pulmonary, or abdominal surgeries often develop pleural effusions in the postoperative period. Third, patients usually have volume overload due to large amounts of fluids administered during resuscitation.

Oncologic patients may develop pleural effusions due to all the above reasons; they frequently receive immunosuppressive treatments increasing the risk of pleural, pulmonary, or other infections, they may undergo surgeries with either curative or palliative intent, and often receive drugs that can cause heart failure or pleural effusion directly. Additionally, oncologic patients can present with malignant pleural effusions (MPE), a condition that affects approximately 15% of patients with cancer [6] and is likely to rise due to increased life expectancy, increased cancer incidence, and increased cancer survival [1].

Pathophysiology

The pleural cavity is the space between the visceral and the parietal pleura. Under physiological conditions, only a thin layer of fluid separates the pleural membranes. This cavity has negative pressure due to the opposing forces between the elasticity of the lung and the chest wall. The role of the pleural fluid is not completely understood. Some studies claim the pleural cavity has an important role in respiratory physiology, facilitating the lung expansion, and reducing friction with respiratory movements [42]. However, patients who undergo pleurodesis, even at young ages, don't appear to have any clinical deterioration, supporting the idea that the role is limited, if any.

Pleural fluid is produced at a constant rate of approximate 0.01 mL/Kg/h and depends on the combination of hydrostatic and oncotic pressures between the blood vessels and the pleural space [20]. Fluid is also continuously absorbed by the lymphatics at the parietal pleura at a rate that equals production and can dramatically increase in the presence of increased fluid production [25]. In normal conditions, the volume of fluid in each pleural cavity is 0.26 ml/kg of body mass and undergoes continuous turnover [27]. Accumulation of fluid in the pleural cavity occurs due to an imbalance between the mechanisms of production and reabsorption of pleural fluid. Considering the large reserve capacity of the absorption mechanism and the fast rates at which fluid can accumulate, most times both processes need to be affected for fluid to collect in the pleural cavity. Accumulation of fluid can occur due to diseases involving thoracic structures such as pleura, lungs, mediastinum, or diaphragm, or conditions that involve primarily extrathoracic organs. Whatever the underlying disease, the general approach and management of these patients requires a diagnosis of the primary mechanism, if the primary cause of the effusion is an imbalance between the hydrostatic and the oncotic pressure, it is called a transudate, while exudates are effusions in which the primary mechanism is an increased permeability of the pleural membrane.

Etiology

Differential diagnosis of pleural effusion in critically ill patients is broad and not different from non-ICU patients. Some causes, however, are more common in the ICU setting and often the etiology is multifactorial. In a study of pleural effusions in 3 medical ICUs, 85 patients underwent thoracentesis, and the etiologies were as follows: 35 infectious exudates, 25 non-infectious exudates, and 20 transudates [9]. Other study found transudates to be the most common cause of effusion in the ICU, with 61% of transudative effusions in a group of 229 mechanically ventilated patients [24].

Heart failure is one of the most common causes of pleural effusions accounting for 35% of all effusions in a study of medical ICU patients [23]. An increase of left side filling pressure causes a rise in capillary hydrostatic pressures and therefore extravasation of fluid to the alveoli with subsequent pulmonary edema. Aggressive fluid resuscitation is usual in ICU patients and may contribute to the development of pleural effusions in the setting of heart failure, but fluids can also cause effusions in the absence of heart failure [4]. Pleural effusions are also commonly seen in infections, with 42% of effusions in medical ICUs resulting from a parapneumonic effusion or empyema [9]. Iatrogenic pleural effusions should also be considered among the differential diagnosis; parenteral formulas, for example, have been introduced in the pleural space due to catheter migration or malpositioning [28]. Hemothorax may present as a complication of central venous catheterization or a pleural procedure such as thoracentesis, pleural biopsy, or chest tube placement [38].

Oncologic patients may present pleural effusions due to all the above reasons, but some causes are exclusive of these patients. In particular, oncologic patients may present MPE, a condition defined by the presence of an exudate with malignant cells or tumor tissue in the pleural cavity. The most common tumors that cause MPE are lung, breast, and lymphoma. It represents an advanced stage of disease with an average survival of 4–6 months after diagnosis, and treatment is oriented to palliate the symptoms [31]. Oncologic patients can also present effusions as a consequence of treatment such as lung resections, chest radiation, or associated with drugs like dasatinib.

Diagnosis

Diagnosis of pleural effusions in critically ill patients requires a different approach due to limitations for mobilization and communication. They may present nonspecific signs such as fever, agitation, or increase in the oxygen and ventilator requirements. When suspected on a routine X-ray, a comprehensive diagnosis should follow, including three components: confirmation of the effusion, classification as transudates or exudates, and identification of the underlying cause.

Confirmation of the Effusion: Imaging Studies

Considering the limitations of the physical exam to identify pleural effusions in ICU patients, images are essential and necessary for verification. The initial test is generally a chest X-ray with the advantages of being cheap, safe, and widely available. The sensitivity of chest X-ray in the diagnosis of pleural effusion is around 51%, and specificity is 91% with slight variations according to the amount of fluid and the patient's position [44].

Ultrasound is significantly superior to chest X-ray with a sensitivity of 93% in effusions as small as 20 ml [36]. It is particularly useful in mechanically ventilated patients since it can be performed at the bedside. Additionally, it allows for the identification of loculations, assessment of the fluid density, pleural thickness, and pleural masses [21, 39]. In good hands, ultrasound has a sensitivity of 79% and a specificity of 100% to identify MPE [32]. Thickening of the pleura greater than 1 cm, thickening of the diaphragm greater than 7 mm, and pleural nodularity are all characteristics suggestive of malignancy. Ultrasound is also helpful to guide thoracentesis or chest tube insertion resulting in increased success rate and safety [15]. (Fig. 1).

Contrast-enhanced CT scans, ideally performed after drainage of the effusion, can provide additional information of pleural anatomy. Pleural thickening, nodularity, pleural-based masses, loculations can be all identified on CT scan. Some studies have reported good discrimination of benign and malignant effusions by using a combination of pleural characteristics [39]. At the same time, it allows for the assessment of airways, lung parenchyma, and mediastinum. The main disadvantages are the risks and complexities of transferring a critically ill patient to the radiology unit.

A PET-CT scan is not accurate to discriminate benign from malignant effusions, but in cases where malignant effusion is suspected due to metastasis from an unknown primary, it can help identify the primary lesion.

Classification as Transudates or Exudates

Determining the fluid characteristics is an essential part of the approach to a patient with pleural effusion just as in other non-ICU settings. Fluid characteristics allow classification in two broad groups: transudates and exudates. The most common and sensitive criteria to distinguish exudates

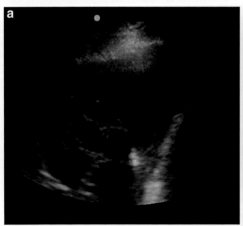
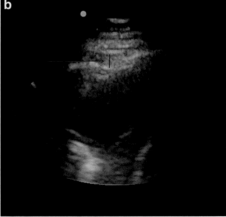

Fig. 1 (**a**) Ultrasound image showing a complex pleural effusion with multiple loculations, in a patient with empyema. (**b**) Ultrasound image showing an anechoic pleural effusion and pleural thickening seen as a hypoechoic band (red arrow) in a patient with malignant pleural effusion

from transudates are Light's criteria and include two indicators, LDH and proteins [22]. Pleural fluid cholesterol, triglycerides, albumin, amylase, bilirubin, and pH have also been studied, but none of these parameters have shown improved diagnostic performance compared to Light's criteria [43].

Transudates are noninflammatory effusions caused by imbalances in hydrostatic and oncotic pressures, and the clinical scenario generally allows the clinician to recognize the underlying cause. The most common causes are congestive heart failure, cirrhosis, and nephrotic syndrome. In oncologic patients, superior vena cava obstruction, constrictive pericarditis, and drugs should be considered.

Exudates are due to pleural inflammation with a consequent increase in pleural permeability. Exudates are classified as such if they present any of the following criteria: protein pleural fluid/blood ratio greater than 0.5, LDH pleural fluid/blood ratio greater than 0.6, or an LDH value in pleural fluid greater than 200 U/L. If the fluid is an exudate, other fluid characteristics are essential to identify the underlying disease process. The causes of exudative effusions include an extensive list of diagnosis, the most common being malignant or paramalignant effusions, parapneumonic effusions, and pulmonary embolism. In approximately 30% of cases, a transudate may be mislabeled as an exudate, due to an increase in the protein gradient; this is seen in patients with acute diuresis and increased protein concentration in serum. In these cases, a plasma/pleural albumin gradient greater than 1.2 g/L or a plasma/pleural protein concentration > 3.1 g/dL suggests a transudate [35].

Identifying the Underlying Cause

Exudative pleural effusions generally need further study to determine and confirm the underlying cause. Even after imaging studies with a high suspicion of malignancy, fluid analysis and sometimes a biopsy are needed. A neutrophilic predominant fluid suggests an acute process such as a parapneumonic effusion, while a lymphocyte-predominant fluid indicates a more chronic disease such as cancer or tuberculosis. Adenosine deaminase level (ADA), an enzyme important in lymphocyte differentiation, rises in the setting of tuberculosis and has a sensitivity of 90–100% when a cutoff of 40 U/L is used. A pleural fluid pH < 7.2 or glucose <60 mg/dL suggest a complicated parapneumonic effusion. Cultures for both aerobic and anaerobic bacteria may help identify the responsible organism in approximately 40% of cases. Cytology is positive in only 60% of malignant pleural effusions. Other markers such as procalcitonin or brain natriuretic peptide (BNP) have limited utility. If a complete study of the pleural fluid is not enough to obtain a confident diagnosis of the underlying etiology, a pleural biopsy may be indicated. The benefits of these procedures should be weight against the risks, particularly in patients requiring mechanical ventilation, and may be postponed if the patient's general health is expected to improve and the diagnosis is not urgent. If an MPE is suspected and tissue diagnosis is considered crucial, a good option in ICU patients may be an ultrasound-guided biopsy, a procedure with low risks and a reasonable sensitivity in selected cases [16].

Clinical Relevance

The clinical significance of pleural effusion in respiratory mechanics is not fully understood. Animal studies have shown lung volume decreases by only one-third of the volume added to the pleural space at functional residual capacity and even less at total lung capacity [19]. These findings mean that in patients with pleural effusions, chest wall compliance increases to accommodate the excess fluid, while lung compliance decreases. The reduction in lung compliance is mostly due to a collapse of the dependent areas of the lung, areas where pleural pressures are significantly increased [26]. These areas of airspace collapse generate ventilation-perfusion mismatch or shunt, leading to oxygenation abnormalities. Therefore, recruitment maneuvers such as increased PEEP may improve lung compliance and increase lung volumes, displacing the pleural fluid in a compliant chest wall.

In mechanically ventilated patients, thoracentesis has demonstrated variable effects on oxygenation. A meta-analysis of five studies including 118 patients reported a mean improvement in the PaO_2FiO_2 ratio of 18% (95% CI: 9–33%) [14]. Later studies have reported even better results after pleural fluid drainage with increases of the partial pressure of oxygen of 40% after the procedure [40, 41]. Despite the described benefits, there is no evidence that this procedure reduces the duration of mechanical ventilation or hospital stay. Of note, the magnitude of the effect on oxygenation is not related to the volume removed, and although poorly understood, it seems that patients with a noncompliant chest wall or a high PEEP will benefit the most.

Pleural Effusion Drainage

Indications for drainage of the pleural cavity will depend on the nature of the pleural effusion and the clinical setting. Drainage has a diagnostic and often therapeutic purpose and is recommended in any new or unexplained pleural effusion. In mechanically ventilated patients, routine thoracentesis has proven to change management in 33% of patients [9].

Pleural drainage can be safely performed in mechanically ventilated ICU patients. Main complications include pneumothorax, hemothorax, and re-expansion pulmonary edema. Pneumothorax is relatively common with an estimated rate of 6% in a recent meta-analysis [15]. The common belief that patients receiving positive pressure ventilation have an increased risk of pneumothorax is not supported by current evidence with rates of pneumothorax that range from 0% to 9%, similar to patients without MV [11, 12]. The procedure is safer if performed with ultrasound guidance [24, 34].

The incidence of hemothorax related to thoracentesis in this population has been reported between %0 and 5% [14]. Hematological malignancies, anticoagulant treatment, and renal failure are often seen in these patients, and all coagulation abnormalities should be corrected when possible. In general, patients with platelets <50,000 and INR > 1.5 are considered at high risk of bleeding. [18].

Re-expansion pulmonary edema is a feared but infrequent complication of this procedure. In ICU patients who often have pulmonary opacities and already have respiratory failure, the frequency of this complication is difficult to determine. Unfortunately, there are no apparent risk factors, and the pathophysiology is poorly understood. It may be due to excessive negative of fast drop in pleural pressure and an increase in alveolo-capillary permeability [29]. Given the fact that drops of intrapleural pressure are associated with symptoms, some authors recommend symptom-limited drainage while others recommend volume limited drainage [2]. Advocating a maximum amount to drain is not supported by evidence, but drainage should be performed cautiously in these patients, considering the already-compromised respiratory function and the little value of symptoms in sedated patients.

Pleural fluid drainage can be performed as a single procedure; thoracentesis or a more continuous fashion by the use of a pleural catheter. Catheters and tubes of different caliber and materials are inserted in the pleural cavity for more continuous drainage of the effusion.

Continuous or Repetitive Drainage

Pleural effusions that require continuous drainage, such as those associated with pleural infections, can be drained by using a catheter connected to a closed system, and then removed as needed. This objective can be achieved by using a traditional chest tube, meaning a large bore catheter (usually with a diameter above 14 Fr) or smaller and softer catheters, such as pigtails. Using a small bore catheter to drain an infected viscous fluid is not associated with a higher risk of tube obstruction and seems to be as useful as a large bore chest tube, but with significantly less pain [33]. Small-bore catheters have also been used successfully in the management of pneumothorax [10]. Pleurodesis may be performed through a catheter by instillation of a sclerosant agent such as talc. Rahman N et al.

studied the use of smaller diameter tubes (<12 Fr) in talc pleurodesis, and the success rate was not different from that obtained with the 24 Fr tubes, traditionally used to perform this procedure [33]. A more recent study, however, found that small-bore catheters suffer from blockage or unintentional removal more commonly and catheters equal to or smaller than 12 Fr are not the best option for pleurodesis. [17].

Permanent Catheters

Indwelling pleural catheters (IPCs) are composed of a soft and flexible material that allows subcutaneous insertion and tunneling, and ambulatory drainage pleural fluid even by nonexpert hands. The primary indication is malignant pleural effusion although it is increasingly being used for recurrent benign effusions. In MPE, it can successfully alleviate symptoms in up to 90% of patients and lead to spontaneous pleurodesis in approximately 45% of cases [30, 37]. Complications such as infection of the chest wall or the pleural cavity are less than 5%, with low mortality [7].

Pleural Effusion in Malignant Neoplasms

If a patient is confirmed to have MPE, the effusion will reproduce after drainage and a more definitive therapeutic procedure may be needed. The short life expectancy of patients with MPE, probably even shorter for the patient in intensive care, must be considered when deciding if a definitive treatment is necessary. A predictive model of mortality has been developed for MPE, known as the LENT score for its acronym L: LDH, E: ECOG score or performance status, N: neutrophils lymphocytes ratio in serum, and T: tumor pathology [5]. Although it is worth mentioning, this predictive model was not explicitly developed in ICU patients and therefore should be used carefully.

Options for definitive management include indwelling pleural catheters and chemical pleurodesis. More recently, combined alternatives such as chemical pleurodesis through an IPC have been used. If the lung re-expands after draining the pleural fluid, then pleurodesis may be performed by the installation of a chemical agent in the pleural cavity through a pleural tube, a catheter, or in the course of a video-assisted thoracoscopy. Complications of this procedure include pneumonitis and acute respiratory distress syndrome [3] and therefore it seems reasonable to avoid performing pleurodesis until the patient no longer needs mechanical ventilation. In the setting of a nonexpandable lung, however, an IPC may be the only option for definitive management and can be placed at the bedside with local anesthesia.

Conclusion

Pleural effusion is a common problem in ICU patients. Imaging studies, including chest X-ray, ultrasound, and CT scan, can confirm the presence of an effusion and suggest the cause. Ultrasound is particularly helpful in the ICU setting due to its portability and ability to guide pleural procedures. Thoracentesis is a relatively safe procedure with no evidence of increased complications in patients with mechanical ventilation.

Thoracentesis should be considered in the setting of an effusion of unknown cause, particularly if a pleural infection is suspected. In patients with large effusions, decreased chest wall compliance, or high PEEP requirements, thoracentesis may have therapeutic effects, but there is no evidence to support the fact that the procedure reduces the length of mechanical ventilation or hospital stay.

References

1. American Thoracic Society. Management of malignant pleural effusions. Am J Respir Crit Care. 2000;162:1987–2001.
2. Ault MJ, Rosen BT, Scher J, Feinglass J, Barsuk JH. Thoracentesis outcomes: a 12-year experience. Thorax. 2015;70(2):127–32.
3. Bintcliffe OJ, Lee GY, Rahman NM, Maskell NA. The management of benign non-infective pleural effusions. European respiratory review: an official journal of the European respiratory. Society. 2016;25(141):303–16.

4. Broaddus VC, Wiener-Kronish JP, Staub NC. Clearance of lung edema into the pleural space of volume loaded anesthetized sheep. J Appl Physiol. 1990;68(6): 2623–30.

5. Clive AO, Kahan BC, Hooper CE, Bhatnagar R, Morley AJ, Zahan-Evans N, et al. Predicting survival in malignant pleural effusion: development and validation of the LENT prognostic score. Thorax. 2014;69 (12):1098–104.

6. Clive A, Jones H, Bhatnagar R, Preston N, Maskell N. Interventions for the management of malignant pleural effusions: a network meta-analysis. Cochrane Database Syst Rev. 2016;8:CD010529.

7. Corcoran JP, Psallidas I, Wrightson JM, Hallifax RJ, Rahman NM. Pleural procedural complications: prevention and management. J Thorac Dis. 2015;7 (6):1058–67.

8. DeBiasi EM, Pisani MA, Murphy TE, Araujo K, Kookoolis A, Argento AC, et al. Mortality among patients with pleural effusion undergoing thoracentesis. Eur Respir J. 2015;46(2):495–502.

9. Fartoukh M, Azoulay E, Galliot R, Le Gall JR, Baud F, Chevret S, et al. Clinically documented pleural effusions in medical ICU patients: how useful is routine thoracentesis? Chest. 2002;121(1):178–84.

10. Gammie JS, Banks MC, Fuhrman CR, Pham SM, Griffith B, Keenan RJ, et al. The pigtail catheter for pleural drainage: a less invasive alternative to tube Thoracostomy. J Soc Laparoendosc Surg. 1999;3(1):57–61.

11. Gervais DA, Petersein A, Lee MJ, Hahn PF, Saini S, Mueller PR. US-guided thoracentesis: requirement for postprocedure chest radiography in patients who receive mechanical ventilation versus patients who breathe spontaneously. Radiology. 1997;204(2):503–6.

12. Godwin JE, Sahn SA. Thoracentesis: a safe procedure in mechanically ventilated patients. Ann Intern Med. 1990;113(10):800–2.

13. Goligher EC, Leis JA, Fowler RA, Pinto R, Adhikari NK, Ferguson ND. Utility and safety of draining pleural effusions in mechanically ventilated patients: a systematic review and meta-analysis. Crit Care (London). 2011;15(1):1.

14. Goligher EC, Ferguson ND. Utility of draining pleural effusions in mechanically ventilated patients. Curr Opin Pulm Med. 2012;18(4):359–65.

15. Gordon CE, Feller-Kopman D, Balk EM, et al. Pneumothorax following thoracentesis: a systematic review and meta-analysis. Arch Intern Med. 2010;170:332–9.

16. Hallifax RJ, Corcoran JP, Ahmed A, et al. Physician-based ultrasound-guided biopsy for diagnosing pleural disease. Chest. 2014;146:1001–6.

17. Hallifax RJ, Psallidas I, Rahman NM. Chest drain size: the debate continues. Curr Pulmonol Rep. 2017;6(1):26–9.

18. Hooper C, Lee YC, Maskell N, BTS Pleural Guideline Group. Investigation of a unilateral pleural effusion in adults: British Thoracic Society pleural disease guideline 2010. Thorax. 2010;65(Suppl 2):ii4–17.

19. Krell WS, Rodarte JR. Effects of acute pleural effusion on respiratory system mechanics in dogs. J Appl Physiol. 1985;59:1458–63.

20. Lai-Fook SJ. Pleural mechanics and fluid exchange. Physiol Rev. 2004;84(2):385–410.

21. Lichtenstein D, Goldstein I, Mourgeon E, Cluzel P, Grenier P, Rouby J-J. Comparative diagnostic performances of auscultation, chest radiography, and lung ultrasonography in acute respiratory distress syndrome. Anesthesiology. 2004;100(1):9–15.

22. Light RW. Pleural effusion. N Engl J Med. 2002;346(25):1971–7.

23. Mattison LE, Coppage L, Alderman DF, Herlong JO, Sahn SA. Pleural effusions in the medical ICU: prevalence, causes, and clinical implications. Chest. 1997;111(4):1018–23.

24. Mayo PH, Goltz HR, Tafreshi M, Doelken P. Safety of ultrasound-guided thoracentesis in patients receiving mechanical ventilation. Chest. 2004;125 (3):1059–62.

25. Miserocchi G. Physiology and pathophysiology of pleural fluid turnover. Eur Respir J. 1997;10:219–25.

26. Miserocchi G, D'Angelo E, Agostoni E. Topography of pleural surface pressure after pneumo- or hydrothorax. J Appl Physiol. 1972;32:296–303.

27. Noppen M, De Waele M, Li R, Gucht KV, D'Haese J, Gerlo E, Vincken W. Volume and cellular content of normal pleural fluid in humans examined by pleural lavage. Am J Respir Crit Care Med. 2000;162(3 Pt 1):1023–6.

28. Oakes DD, Wilson RE, Malposition of a subclavian line. Resultant pleural effusions, interstitial pulmonary edema, and chest wall abscess during total parenteral nutrition. JAMA. 1975;233(6):532–3.

29. Pannu J, DePew ZS, Mullon JJ, Daniels CE, Hagen CE, Maldonado F. Impact of pleural manometry on the development of chest discomfort during thoracentesis: a symptom-based study. J Bronchol Interv Pulmonol. 2014;21(4):306–13.

30. Patil M, Dhillon SS, Attwood K, Saoud M, Alraiyes AH, Harris K. The management of benign pleural effusions using indwelling pleural catheters – a systematic review and meta-analysis. Chest. 2016;150:582A.

31. Porcel JM, Azzopardi M, Koegelenberg CF, Maldonado F, Rahman NM, Lee YC. The diagnosis of pleural effusions. Expert Rev Respir Med. 2015;9(6):801–15.

32. Qureshi NR, Rahman NM, Gleeson FV. Thoracic ultrasound in the diagnosis of malignant pleural effusion. Thorax. 2009;64(2):139–43.

33. Rahman NM, Maskell NA, Davies CW, Hedley EL, Nunn AJ, Gleeson FV, et al. The relationship between chest tube size and clinical outcome in pleural infection. Chest. 2010;137(3):536–43.

34. Raptopoulos V, Davis LM, Lee G, Umali C, Lew R, Irwin RS. Factors affecting the development of pneumothorax associated with thoracentesis. AJR Am J Roentgenol. 1991;156(5):917–20.

35. Romero-Candeira S, Fernández C, Martín C, Sánchez-Paya J, Hernández L. Influence of diuretics on the concentration of proteins and other components of pleural transudates in patients with heart failure. Am J Med. 2001;110(9):681–6.

36. Soni NJ, Franco R, Velez MI, Schnobrich D, Dancel R, Restrepo MI, et al. Ultrasound in the diagnosis and

management of pleural effusions. J Hosp Med. 2015;10(12):811–6.

37. Stokes LS. Percutaneous Management of Malignant Fluid Collections. Semin Interv Radiol. 2007;24(4):398–408.

38. Strange C. Pleural complications in the intensive care unit. Clin Chest Med. 1999;20:317–27.

39. Traill ZC, Davies RJ, Gleeson FV. Thoracic computed tomography in patients with suspected malignant pleural effusions. Clin Radiol. 2001;56(3):193–6.

40. Walden AP, Garrard CS, Salmon J. Sustained effects of thoracocentesis on oxygenation in mechanically ventilated patients. Respirology. 2010;15(6):986–92.

41. Walden AP, Jones QC, Matsa R, Wise MP. Pleural effusions on the intensive care unit; hidden morbidity with therapeutic potential. Respirology. 2013;18(2):246–54.

42. Wang NS. Anatomy of the pleura. Clin Chest Med. 1998;19:229–40.

43. Wilcox ME, Chong CA, Stanbrook MB, Tricco AC, Wong C, Straus SE. Does this patient have an exudative pleural effusion? The rational clinical examination systematic review. JAMA. 2014;311(23):2422–31.

44. Yousefifard M, Baikpour M, Ghelichkhani P, Asady H, Shahsavari Nia K, Moghadas Jafari A, et al. Screening performance characteristic of ultrasonography and radiography in detection of pleural effusion; a meta-analysis. Emergency. 2016;4(1):1–10.

Management of Tracheobronchial Diseases in Critically Ill Cancer Patients

43

Donald R. Lazarus and George A. Eapen

Contents

Introduction 654

Hemoptysis 654
Etiology, Severity, and Prognosis of Hemoptysis 654
Initial Evaluation of Hemoptysis 655
Management of Hemoptysis 657

Central Airway Obstruction 660
Clinical Presentation and Evaluation of Central Airway Obstruction 660
Management of Central Airway Obstruction 660

Conclusion 663

References 663

Abstract

Tracheobronchial diseases are uncommon in critically ill oncologic patients but are responsible for significant morbidity and risk of mortality in this population. The most significant tracheobronchial diseases of relevance in oncologic critical care are hemoptysis and central airway obstruction. In the inpatient setting, hemoptysis is most often related to lung cancer or bronchiectasis. After initial stabilization of the airway, localizing the source of bleeding and resuscitation are paramount. Then intervention to control bleeding and prevent recurrence with bronchial artery embolization or therapeutic bronchoscopy is indicated, with surgery most appropriately used for those patients refractory to less invasive management. Central airway obstruction refers to narrowing of the trachea or mainstem bronchi and can result from the direct effect of malignant tumors or complications of treatment. Patients often have severe obstruction before becoming symptomatic. If surgical resection is not possible, therapeutic bronchoscopy is the mainstay of treatment. Effective techniques used in central airway obstruction include laser photoresection, electrocautery, argon plasma coagulation, microdebrider bronchoscopy, bronchoplasty, and stenting. Complex stenoses often require

D. R. Lazarus
Baylor College of Medicine, Houston, TX, USA

G. A. Eapen (✉)
Department of Pulmonary Medicine, Division of Internal Medicine, The University of Texas MD Anderson Cancer Center, Houston, TX, USA
e-mail: geapen@mdanderson.org

© Springer Nature Switzerland AG 2020
J. L. Nates, K. J. Price (eds.), *Oncologic Critical Care*,
https://doi.org/10.1007/978-3-319-74588-6_46

multimodality therapy. A multidisciplinary approach is recommended.

Keywords
Hemoptysis · Airway obstruction · Tracheobronchial

Introduction

Although not common, tracheobronchial diseases in oncologic patients convey significant morbidity and risk of mortality. The most significant of these to the critical care practitioner are hemoptysis and central airway obstruction. This chapter will define and describe them and review their management.

Hemoptysis

Hemoptysis is defined as the expectoration of blood arising from a source within the lower respiratory tract – the bronchial tree or lungs [3]. Hemoptysis may be related to a wide variety of conditions seen in oncologic patients. Most cases of hemoptysis are self-limited and of mild or moderate severity, but massive hemoptysis is a life-threatening emergency necessitating urgent and aggressive management by a multidisciplinary team [28, 71]. Because massive hemoptysis is more relevant to the critical care of the oncologic patient, it will be the focus of the majority of our discussion.

Etiology, Severity, and Prognosis of Hemoptysis

Causes of hemoptysis are listed in Table 1 [39, 50, 51, 71, 79, 85]. The clinical setting determines the relative frequency of the various causes of hemoptysis. While tuberculosis remains the most common cause of hemoptysis worldwide, other etiologies are more frequent in the developed world [43, 71]. In an outpatient primary care setting in the United Kingdom, acute respiratory tract infections were found to be the most

Table 1 Causes of hemoptysis [2, 4–8]

Bronchiectasis	Vascular
Bronchitis	Arteriovenous malformations
Neoplasm	Bronchial telangiectasias
Lung cancer	Heart failure
Pulmonary metastases	Mitral stenosis
Bronchial adenomas	Arteriobronchial fistula
Endobronchial tumors (carcinoid, adenoid cystic carcinoma, etc.)	Pulmonary embolism
	Bronchial artery aneurysm
Infections	Pulmonary artery aneurysm
Tuberculosis	Iatrogenic
Fungal infection/mycetoma	Pulmonary artery catheterization
Lung abscess	Bronchoscopy
Necrotizing bacterial pneumonia	Trauma
Parasitic	Foreign body aspiration
Coagulopathy	Idiopathic/ cryptogenic
Vasculitis	Silicosis

common cause of hemoptysis [25, 44]. Bronchiectasis and lung cancer are found more commonly in the inpatient setting [39, 85]. The etiology of hemoptysis also differs among patients who are smokers and nonsmokers, with malignancy and chronic bronchitis being much more frequent among smokers [85]. Despite aggressive diagnostic evaluation, the etiology of hemoptysis remains unknown in 8–33% of patients [36, 39, 46, 53, 55, 73, 88]. Approximately 90% of cases of hemoptysis originate from the bronchial arteries, which carry only around 2% of cardiac output but at systemic blood pressures. They typically arise from the thoracic aorta but in some cases branch from the intercostal arteries [51, 93]. The pulmonary arterial circulation is a lower pressure system, but hemoptysis from a pulmonary arterial source can be particularly severe since it carries almost the entire cardiac output. It is responsible for only around 5% of episodes of hemoptysis [51, 93].

It is important to distinguish true hemoptysis from pseudohemoptysis and hematemesis, which have a different source of the expectorated blood and also different management. In pseudohemoptysis the source of expectorated blood is the upper respiratory tract – the nose or larynx – and for hematemesis the source of bleeding is the gastrointestinal tract [3]. Pseudohemoptysis from a nasopharyngeal source may often be confirmed by careful history and examination of the nasopharynx. Expectorated blood arising from the respiratory tract is often bright red, alkaline, and foamy and may be associated with dyspnea. Blood arising from the gastrointestinal tract is more often associated with nausea and abdominal pain and may appear dark red or brown with an acidic pH [25, 43].

Hemoptysis is usually mild or moderate in severity, but massive hemoptysis, which accounts for 5–15% of episodes, may be acutely life threatening and requires urgent management to stabilize the patient and then localize and control the source of bleeding [51, 71]. There is no current consensus regarding the definition of massive hemoptysis [51, 71]. Some authors use an estimation of the volume of blood expectorated over time to define massive hemoptysis. Such volumetric definitions range from 100 to 1000 mL in 24 h, with typical definitions ranging from 200 to 600 mL/24 h [1, 16, 42, 93]. Others argue that a strictly volumetric definition is problematic. It is frequently difficult to quantify accurately the amount of blood expectorated, and given that the anatomic dead space of the airways is between 100 and 200 mL, volumes in the low end of that range are more than sufficient to obstruct the airway and cause death by asphyxiation if not cleared [42, 51]. A more practical definition of massive hemoptysis might then be any volume of hemoptysis that has a life-threatening magnitude of effect by causing airway obstruction, impaired gas exchange, or hemodynamic instability [42, 51, 71].

The prognosis of hemoptysis is also variable. The mortality rate for submassive hemoptysis is relatively low, between 2% and 6%, while massive hemoptysis results in a mortality ranging from 8% to 38% even with aggressive treatment

[39, 48, 53, 60, 69, 77]. Perhaps the most important factor affecting prognosis is the rate of bleeding [16, 18]. The mortality rate of massive hemoptysis with less than 1000 mL blood loss in 24 h is 9%, whereas the rate of death when blood loss exceeds that amount was 58% [16]. The underlying etiology of hemoptysis also influences the prognosis, with higher mortality for patients with a malignant cause than for those with infectious or inflammatory causes [16]. Another important factor influencing the prognosis of massive hemoptysis is the management strategy undertaken. Increasing use of bronchial artery embolization with a concomitant reduction in emergent surgery for hemoptysis has also been shown to have reduced mortality in some centers [77]. A prediction score has been developed and validated to estimate in-hospital mortality using 1087 patients admitted for hemoptysis to the ICU of a single French tertiary hospital. Independent predictors of death included cancer, aspergillosis, need for mechanical ventilation, chronic alcoholism, pulmonary artery involvement, and presence of abnormalities on two or more quadrants of the admission chest x-ray [28]. While not yet validated in other settings, such models may prove useful in estimating prognosis on admission and helping treating clinicians appropriately triage patients with hemoptysis.

Initial Evaluation of Hemoptysis

The initial evaluation of hemoptysis should be carried out in tandem with its initial management. The most important initial step is to determine the risk of hemoptysis to the patient's airway, gas exchange, and hemodynamic stability and intervene to address those issues immediately [43, 51, 71]. Localizing the site or at least the side of the source of bleeding is of critical importance. If the source of bleeding can be lateralized, then the bleeding side should be placed in the dependent position to avoid flooding the good lung with blood and further impairing gas exchange [43]. Lateralizing the source of bleeding may also facilitate early bronchial artery embolization (BAE) in patients who are too

Fig. 1 Right upper lobe cavitary lesion seen on chest x-ray of a patient with hemoptysis

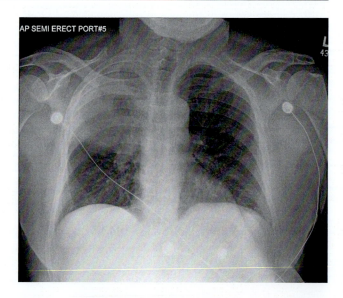

unstable for additional testing. Once the patient has been stabilized, a careful history and physical exam should be rapidly undertaken to rule out non-pulmonary causes of bleeding and search for likely possible causes.

This evaluation should also include routine laboratory testing with coagulation studies, a complete blood count, basic chemistry, and a blood type and antibody screen. Serologic tests for vasculitis and sputum samples for microbiologic testing should also be considered [43]. A chest x-ray should also be obtained rapidly. Plain chest films are able to localize the site of bleeding in 19–80% of cases and determine the underlying cause as often as 35% of the time [35, 39, 47, 55, 60, 69, 71] (Fig. 1). If the location and cause of bleeding are not evident after chest x-ray (CXR), then evaluation should continue with bronchoscopy and computed tomography (CT).

Bronchoscopy is an important tool for localizing the source of bleeding as well as for early intervention to control it. It is most useful for localizing bleeding in massive hemoptysis and when the source of bleeding is a central endobronchial lesion visible within the airway. In cases of massive hemoptysis, bronchoscopy is able to identify the site of bleeding 73–93% of the time [35, 41, 47, 69] (Fig. 2). In submassive hemoptysis, bronchoscopy is less useful for

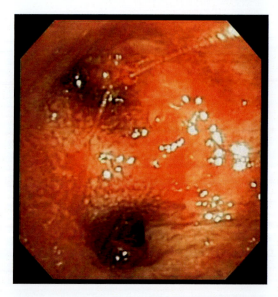

Fig. 2 Hemoptysis arising from an endobronchial tumor in the left upper lobe

localizing the site of bleeding, with rates of success between 31% and 40% [55, 59]. In either case early bronchoscopy (within 24–48 h of presentation) seems to be more effective at localizing the site of bleeding than bronchoscopy performed later [31, 72]. Bronchoscopy is less useful for identifying the cause of bleeding than it is for identifying the site. The cause of bleeding is identified by bronchoscopy in only about 3–43% of patients with hemoptysis [39, 47, 64, 69, 75].

CT is slightly more accurate than bronchoscopy for localizing the site of bleeding, particularly when the source is in the peripheral lung beyond the reach of bronchoscopy. The rate of localization using CT is 70–88% including both massive and submassive hemoptysis [47, 55, 69]. CT is also significantly more accurate than bronchoscopy at identifying the cause of hemoptysis, with the etiology identified by CT in 60–77% of cases [39, 47, 55, 59, 69, 75]. CT does have limitations, most notably the inability to obtain samples for tissue diagnosis or culture and difficulty distinguishing endobronchial tumor from endobronchial blood clots [47, 50].

It should be emphasized that chest x-ray, bronchoscopy, and CT are not mutually exclusive diagnostic techniques but rather complementary in scope. Bronchoscopy is better than CT for identifying small endobronchial lesions of the central airways. Conversely CT is clearly superior for identifying peripheral sources of bleeding, especially when the rate of bleeding is submassive. The use of CT and bronchoscopy together has a higher rate of localization of the site of bleeding than either modality alone and ranges from 81% to 96% [39, 47, 55, 85].

Management of Hemoptysis

The management of massive hemoptysis requires the initial stabilization of the patient, rapid localization of the bleeding site, and then definitive treatment of the cause of bleeding. Involvement of a multidisciplinary team including intensivists, pulmonologists, thoracic surgeons, and interventional radiologists is recommended [77]. Temporizing measures to control bleeding until more definitive management can be pursued are often necessary [43, 71]. Patients with massive hemoptysis should be admitted to an intensive care unit for close monitoring [51]. As discussed in the previous section, initial efforts should be targeted at assessing the status of the patient's airway, gas exchange, and hemodynamic stability [43, 51, 71]. If the side from which the patient is bleeding can be determined, the patient should be positioned with the bleeding side dependent so as to prevent aspiration of blood into the non-bleeding lung [51, 71]. Volume resuscitation and transfusion to correct coagulopathies that may be present are also indicated [51, 71].

Stabilizing the airway is of paramount importance and may also allow the treating team to tamponade the area of bleeding as well as ensuring adequate oxygenation and ventilation of the good lung [51, 71]. If rigid bronchoscopy by an experienced operator is immediately available, it is perhaps the most efficient way to clear the airway of blood and clots, tamponade the bleeding area, and intervene on visible sources of bleeding in the central airways [71]. However, because most pulmonologists and intensivists are not as facile with the rigid bronchoscope as with the flexible bronchoscope, other methods are generally preferred for initial airway management in massive hemoptysis [51]. In general, intubation with a large caliber endotracheal tube (ETT) should be performed with immediate flexible bronchoscopy. In addition to securing the airway, this allows immediate clearance of blood and clots from the bronchial tree in order to improve ventilation. This also may allow for rapid determination of the location of bleeding, facilitating further interventions to tamponade the bleeding area and protect the non-bleeding lung [71]. Several techniques are available to accomplish this. Perhaps the most common method to position a single-lumen ETT can be in the mainstem bronchus of the non-bleeding lung with the cuff inflated, allowing ventilation of the good lung while protecting it from aspiration of blood from the bad lung. This works best for right-sided bleeding. In patients with left-sided bleeding, intubating the right mainstem bronchus often occludes the right upper lobe bronchus as well [51, 71]. In the case of left-sided bleeding, intubating the trachea and then positioning a blocking balloon to occlude the left mainstem bronchus is also effective without compromising ventilation to the right upper lobe [51, 71]. A number of balloon catheters have been used for this purpose. They include catheters contained within and secured to the ETT, catheters advanced beside the ETT and positioned with the help of the bronchoscope, and a few specialized catheters designed to be placed through the working channel of the flexible bron-choscope [51, 71]. Double-lumen endotracheal tubes can also be used to isolate the bleeding lung, but their smaller inner diameter limits the ability to use bronchoscopy to clear the airways, and they are also more difficult to place and maintain [51]. Once the airway has been secured, the bleeding lung isolated, and the patient stabilized, additional interventions to more definitively control bleeding should be undertaken (Fig. 3).

The mainstay of treatment for massive hemoptysis is arterial embolization. Bronchial artery embolization (BAE), first reported in 1973, is most often used since the bronchial circulation is the source of 90% of hemoptysis episodes, though embolization of branches of the pulmonary arterial system is also sometimes required [67, 68, 71]. In BAE the interventional radiologist performs an aortogram to identify the location of any dilated or ectatic bronchial arteries that are likely to be the source of bleeding. Extravasation of contrast is not usually seen but when present is helpful in localizing the bleeding vessel [93]. Once the abnormal vessel is identified, embolization is performed using one of a number of materials, including Gelfoam, absorbable sponges, cyanoacrylates, coils, gelatin microspheres, and polyvinyl alcohol [7, 53, 56, 92, 93] (Fig. 4). Although rare, the most feared complication of BAE is spinal cord ischemia resulting

from inadvertent embolization of spinal arteries. Superselective embolization using microcatheters allows the abnormal vessels to be embolized distal to the origin of the spinal arteries, greatly reducing the chance of spinal ischemia [71, 84, 93]. BAE has a high rate of immediate success, with control of bleeding achieved in 73–98% of patients [7, 53, 56, 83, 84, 93]. Recurrence rates range from 10% to 50%, with increased risk of recurrence seen in patients with hemoptysis due to aspergillomas, tuberculosis, and cancer [7, 53, 83, 93]. BAE may be safely repeated for recurrent episodes in most patients [93].

Bronchoscopy in the treatment of hemoptysis is most appropriately used to intervene on visible lesions located in the central airways and to deliver topical therapies in order to slow bleeding from more distal lesions. The majority of bronchoscopic techniques used to intervene upon visible lesions within the central airways are thermal therapies. Photocoagulation using laser, most commonly the neodymium-doped yttrium-aluminum garnet (Nd:YAG) laser, has been used successfully to treat hemoptysis [26, 34, 37]. Most patients with sources of bleeding amenable to photocoagulation also have some degree of airway obstruction, and so laser can be used to palliate both conditions [37]. Argon plasma coagulation (APC) is a noncontact form of electrocautery which uses ionized argon gas to

Fig. 3 Chest x-ray of a patient after massive hemoptysis. Endotracheal tube and right mainstem endobronchial blocking balloon (white arrow) are seen. A bullet fragment is seen in the lower right chest, and endovascular coils within a pulmonary artery pseudoaneurysm are seen in the middle right chest

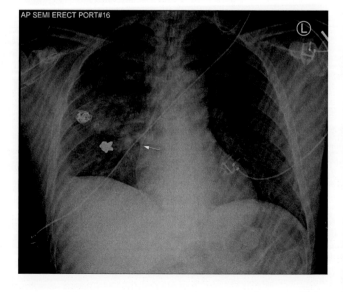

Fig. 4 Pulmonary artery angiogram reveals the source of massive hemoptysis in a pulmonary arterial pseudoaneurysm

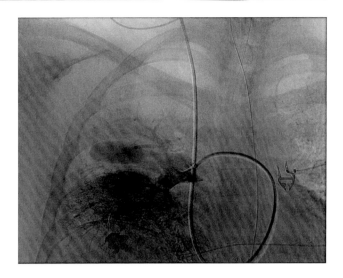

conduct electricity to the target tissue, producing coagulation and devitalization of the target tissue [58]. One advantage of APC over laser photocoagulation is the ability of the plasma beam to travel in a direction other than the axial plane to the nearest point of contact, including "side-firing" or even retrograde coagulation [66]. A number of small studies have shown APC to be effective for achieving hemostasis in bleeding lesions within reach of the bronchoscope [45, 58, 66]. Contact electrocautery has also been reported to be effective for control of hemoptysis of central origin in small series but is less widely used for this indication than laser or APC [71, 81]. Endobronchial cryotherapy has been used successfully to treat submassive hemoptysis in patients with endoluminal tumors [54, 91]. However, cryotherapy is less useful for hemorrhage control in massive hemoptysis because its effects are delayed. It is, however, very useful for clearing the airway of organized clots that are difficult to remove by simple suction [71]. Other bronchoscopic techniques that can be utilized to control hemoptysis include the application of vasoconstrictors and topical procoagulants. These may be effective even in hemoptysis originating beyond the view of the bronchoscope. Vasoconstrictors include iced saline, epinephrine, and derivatives of vasopressin [71]. Lavage with iced saline was able to achieve control of hemoptysis in all 12 patients evaluated by Conlan and

colleagues, with a recurrence rate of 17% [15]. Topical application of epinephrine (diluted to concentrations between 1:10,000 and 1:100,000), glypressin, ornipressin, and terlipressin has shown some efficacy mainly in case series. Hemodynamic effects of these medications on heart rate and blood pressure have also been demonstrated, and their real effectiveness for massive hemoptysis remains unknown [6, 23, 87]. Topical procoagulants including thrombin, thrombin combined with fibrinogen, and oxidized regenerated cellulose mesh have also been used successfully in case series but may be most useful as a temporizing measure while awaiting embolization [19, 86, 88].

Surgical treatment of hemoptysis carries a high morbidity, and the mortality for emergent surgery for hemoptysis ranges from 15% to 25% [18, 29, 32, 77]. The adoption of new protocols with BAE used as the initial treatment rather than emergent surgery has improved outcomes in some centers, and delaying surgery by at least 48 h in patients who are able to be sufficiently stabilized is associated with reduced mortality [77]. Surgery for hemoptysis is now reserved primarily for hemoptysis that is refractory to embolization, due to complex vascular malformations, due to mycetomas unresponsive to other treatment, and due to aortic aneurysm or ruptured pulmonary arteries and for patients too unstable to be transported to the angiography suite [51, 71].

Central Airway Obstruction

Central airway obstruction (CAO) refers to obstruction of the trachea and mainstem bronchi [2, 27]. While benign causes such as post-intubation tracheal stenosis, postradiation stenosis, and strictures related to connective tissue diseases are also described, malignancy is likely to be the most commonly encountered etiology of CAO in the oncologic critical care setting. Malignant CAO most often arises from lung cancer with direct invasion or compression of the airway, but less common primary tracheal tumors as well as other cancers that have metastasized to the airways or mediastinum can also cause life-threatening obstruction of the central airways [2, 27]. Among patients with lung cancer, between 20% and 30% may develop complications associated with CAO during the course of their illness, and symptoms may be severe [27]. The degree of airway stenosis determines the severity of symptoms. Most patients with CAO are not symptomatic until the airway is narrowed by more than 50% [8]. Tracheal stenosis therefore typically produces dyspnea with exertion at a diameter of 8 mm and resting symptoms at a diameter of 5 mm [27, 30, 40].

Clinical Presentation and Evaluation of Central Airway Obstruction

The symptoms of central airway obstruction may develop suddenly or more gradually over time depending on the severity, location, and rate of progression of the stenosis [27]. The hallmark symptom is dyspnea with exertion, although cough, hemoptysis, and symptoms related to the compression of adjacent vascular structures may also be prominent [2, 27]. By the time dyspnea is present at rest, tracheal stenosis is frequently critical in severity, and urgent intervention may be required [4]. In addition to a history of progressive dyspnea and prior malignant involvement of the thorax, other symptoms and signs suggesting CAO include stridor, wheezing, hoarseness, orthopnea, facial plethora, and engorgement of upper extremity veins [2, 4, 27]. If spirometry is

obtained, a flow-volume loop with blunting or squaring suggesting a fixed or variable obstruction may be seen [57, 80]. In addition to clinical assessment, CT of the chest and neck is helpful for excluding suspected CAO as well as defining the nature of the obstruction [27]. A normal CT does not conclusively exclude CAO, since volume averaging may cause thin, weblike strictures to go unnoticed on CT. Direct visualization with bronchoscopy is sometimes required to confirm the diagnosis. Bronchoscopy is also useful for defining more precisely the extent and nature of the obstruction, information which is useful when planning therapeutic intervention [27]. Bronchoscopy is also required to obtain tissue diagnosis [27].

In addition to their underlying etiology, airway stenosis is classified by the nature of the obstruction. Some obstructing lesions are caused primarily by endoluminal growth of tumor and others predominantly by extrinsic compression of the airway with intact mucosa. The third type of obstruction, which is the most common in malignant CAO, is caused by a combination of endoluminal tumor growth and extrinsic compression [2, 4]. It is important to distinguish these three types of obstruction when evaluating a patient with CAO since the optimal treatment differs among them.

Management of Central Airway Obstruction

The primary goal of the management of central airway obstruction is to alleviate dyspnea by restoring the patency of the airway. If the area of obstruction or stenosis is short and amenable to surgical resection, this is the preferred treatment, but in many cases surgical treatment is not possible, so other methods are required [4, 13, 33, 62]. The mainstay of nonsurgical treatment of CAO is therapeutic bronchoscopy, and the involvement of a multidisciplinary team including interventional pulmonologists, thoracic surgeons, or otolaryngologists is crucial. Unstable patients should have the airway secured with an ETT, rigid bronchoscope, or via tracheostomy with the method chosen determined by the location and severity of the obstruction and availability of local expertise [27]. Once the airway is secured, then the remainder of the therapeutic intervention can be planned and executed. While bronchoscopic therapeutic modalities for CAO which have a delayed effect such as photodynamic therapy, endobronchial brachytherapy, and topical endobronchial cryotherapy exist, they are only appropriately used in stable patients and therefore have at most a very limited role in oncologic critical care [90].

For lesions primarily causing obstruction by the presence of tumor within the lumen, ablative therapy with thermal or mechanical means is recommended [2, 4]. Such ablative therapies include laser photocoagulation, argon plasma coagulation, electrocautery, microdebrider bronchoscopy, and mechanical debulking. The thermal ablative techniques used for CAO are the same ones described above for hemoptysis (Figs. 5 and 6).

Laser photocoagulation, most often using the Nd:YAG laser, has shown effectiveness in multiple case series and cohort studies of patients with malignant CAO [4, 27]. The overall rate of success for bronchoscopic laser photocoagulation used to treat CAO is 76–94% [10, 12, 22, 49, 70]. Locations of obstruction which are most amenable to a successful result with laser are the trachea, right mainstem bronchus, and bronchus intermedius [10]. Additional lesional characteristics that predict success with laser are primarily endobronchial nature, length less than 4 cm, and the presence of a visible distal lumen beyond the area of obstruction [10, 27]. Complications of laser in bronchoscopy are rare, occurring in 2–8% of cases [11, 63]. The most commonly seen complications are bleeding, hypoxemia, and pneumothorax [11, 63]. Risk factors for early complications include age older than 60 years and the presence of hypertension or chronic obstructive pulmonary disease [63].

Bronchoscopic electrocautery is another thermal ablative method used to treat CAO. In electrocautery a high-frequency electrical current is transformed into heat at the point of contact with tissue, thereby desiccating and destroying the targeted lesion. The tissue effect is determined

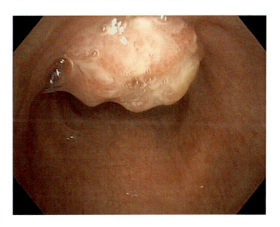

Fig. 5 Endoluminal squamous cell carcinoma obstructing the mid-trachea

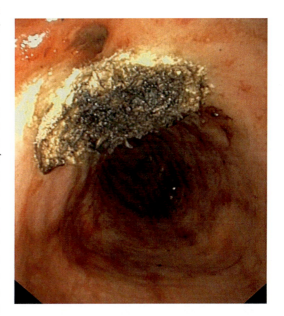

Fig. 6 Mid-trachea after cautery snare resection and argon plasma coagulation treatment of endoluminal squamous cell carcinoma

by the voltage, duration and area of contact, and the density and water content of the tissue [27, 76, 89]. The effect progresses from coagulation starting at around 70° centigrade through vaporization at temperatures above 200° centigrade [76]. A variety of electrocautery instruments are available, including blunt probes, forceps, blades, and loop snares [17]. A number of small studies have shown electrocautery to be as effective as laser photocoagulation for endoluminal tumors causing CAO, with rates of success between 70% and 90% [5, 17, 82]. Complications of electrocautery include bleeding, respiratory failure, airway fire, shock to the patient or operator, and malfunction of implanted cardiac devices.

Argon plasma coagulation (APC) is a non-contact form of electrocautery in which a monopolar current travels between the probe and the tissue at the point of nearest contact. It is there transformed into heat for coagulation and destruction of the targeted tissue [58, 76]. Because the tissue develops increased resistance as it is coagulated, the depth of penetration of APC is limited, reducing the risk of perforation relative to laser or contact electrocautery [27, 66]. Although most useful for control of bleeding, APC is also very effective for palliation of central airway obstruction, especially when combined with mechanical debridement [58, 66]. Complications of APC are rare and seen in less than 4% of patients treated. They include bleeding, perforation, airway fire, and gas embolism [58, 65, 66].

Mechanical ablative techniques for treatment of CAO from endoluminal tumor include forceps debulking, coring out of lesions using the rigid bronchoscope, microdebrider bronchoscopy, and more recently cryorecanalization. Rigid or flexible forceps can be used to remove portions of the obstructing lesion piecemeal until the airway is recanalized. Forceps debulking is often combined with laser or APC to improve hemostatic control during debulking [4]. The contact cryotherapy probe can also be used for mechanical debulking. The probe is extended from the working channel of the bronchoscope until it is in contact with the endoluminal tumor. After freezing for a few seconds, the surrounding tissue adheres to the freezing tip of the cryotherapy probe. The bronchoscope, cryotherapy probe, and adherent tissue are then removed en bloc to rapidly recanalize the airway [38]. Significant bleeding is possible after cryorecanalization, so this technique is also often combined with ablative thermal methods to improve hemostasis before the tumor is removed. The rigid bronchoscope itself can be used to core out endobronchial tumors, resulting in rapid recanalization of the obstructed airway. The beveled edge of the rigid scope is placed against the airway wall involved with tumor while keeping its orientation parallel to the airway to avoid perforation. The bronchoscope is then rotated in a corkscrew motion to shave off parts of the tumor which can then be easily removed. This technique is also frequently combined with thermal therapy to enhance hemostasis during debulking [4]. The microdebrider is a device consisting of a rotary blade enclosed within a hollow metal tube having integrated suction. The blade cuts tissue between 1000 and 5000 revolutions per minute, and the debrided tissue is then suctioned clear of the airway through the hollow shaft of the microdebrider [52]. It has shown excellent results for both benign and malignant CAO and offers the advantages of precise tissue debridement with integrated suction [9, 52, 78]. The potential disadvantages of the microdebrider are the requirement for rigid bronchoscopy, its inability to reach distal lesions, and the risk of accidental resection of normal tissue.

For lesions primarily causing obstruction by extrinsic compression of the airway, mechanical dilation and stenting if needed are appropriate. Mechanical dilation (bronchoplasty) can be accomplished using the barrel of the rigid bronchoscope, serial metal dilators advanced through the rigid bronchoscope, or sequential dilating balloons [27]. While all three methods are effective, the dilating balloons may produce less mucosal trauma than use of the rigid bronchoscope for dilation [27].

If an extrinsically compressed airway does not respond durably to balloon bronchoplasty, an airway stent may need to be placed in order to maintain luminal patency. Airway stents keep obstructed airways open via two distinct functions. First they offer a splinting effect – the radial force of the expanded stent opposes extrinsic pressure from the compressive lesion to keep the airway open. Secondly, stents provide a barrier to ingrowth of mucosal tumor into the lumen. This combination of effects is very effective at maintaining airway patency [8, 27]. The first dedicated airway stents were made of silicone and pioneered by Dumon in the late 1980s [21]. They are customizable and easy to remove but also prone to migrate and require rigid bronchoscopy for placement [8, 61]. Y-shaped silicone stents have also been developed and are often ideal for lesions involving or near the main carina [8, 24] (Figs. 7 and 8). Self-expandable metal stents (SEMS) were later developed in the 1990s [20]. SEMS are able to be placed using rigid or flexible bronchoscopes and are less prone to migration but cannot be customized and are more difficult to remove than silicone stents [8]. Hybrid stents have a nitinol metal frame covered with a silicone or polyurethane coating. They are designed to combine the ease of deployment of SEMS with the relative ease of removal of silicone stents but are associated with increased infectious risk and are also prone to migration

[8, 61]. All types of airway stents are effective at palliating dyspnea from CAO [8]. The differences among the types of stents in size, shape, and flexibility affect their type and rate of complications, difficulty of placement and removal, and suitability for different lesion types and location [8, 14, 61, 74].

For complex lesions involving both endoluminal tumor and extrinsic compression, multimodality treatments including both ablative therapy and dilation with possible stenting are most effective [4, 27]. The general approach for the mixed-type obstructions is to use ablative techniques to clear endoluminal tumor and then consider dilation or stenting if the caliber is still narrowed by more than 50% after ablation.

Brachytherapy and photodynamic therapy are not commonly used for severe CAO because they work more slowly and have less predictable results than the aforementioned treatments which produce an immediate effect. For patients who have been successfully temporarily recanalized with rapid-acting treatments, these modalities may be useful for longer-term treatment of obstruction [90].

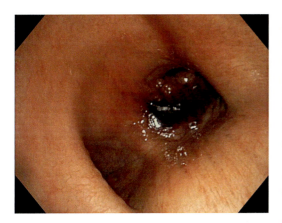

Fig. 7 Obstructing tumor at main carina and proximal right mainstem bronchus

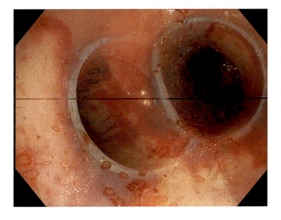

Fig. 8 Main carina and patent bilateral mainstem bronchi after debulking of tumor at main carina and right mainstem bronchus with placement of a Y-stent

Conclusion

The most serious tracheobronchial disorders affecting the oncologic critical care patient are hemoptysis and central airway obstruction. Both cause serious morbidity and may be acutely lifethreatening. Aggressive management by a multidisciplinary team is crucial for their successful management.

References

1. Amirana M, Frater R, Tirschwell P, Janis M, Bloomberg A, State D. An aggressive surgical approach to significant hemoptysis in patients with pulmonary tuberculosis. Am Rev Respir Dis. 1968;97:187–92. https://doi.org/10.1164/arrd.1968.97.2.187.
2. Beamis JF Jr. Interventional pulmonology techniques for treating malignant large airway obstruction: an update. Curr Opin Pulm Med. 2005;11:292–5.
3. Bidwell JL, Pachner RW. Hemoptysis: diagnosis and management. Am Fam Physician. 2005;72:1253–60.

4. Bolliger CT, Sutedja TG, Strausz J, Freitag L. Therapeutic bronchoscopy with immediate effect: laser, electrocautery, argon plasma coagulation and stents. Eur Respir J. 2006;27:1258–71. https://doi.org/10.1183/09031936.06.00013906.

5. Boxem T, Muller M, Venmans B, Postmus P, Sutedja T. Nd-YAG laser vs bronchoscopic electrocautery for palliation of symptomatic airway obstruction: a cost-effectiveness study. Chest. 1999;116:1108–12.

6. Breuer HW, Charchut S, Worth H, Trampisch HJ, Glanzer K. Endobronchial versus intravenous application of the vasopressin derivative glypressin during diagnostic bronchoscopy. Eur Respir J. 1989;2:225–8.

7. Brinson GM, Noone PG, Mauro MA, Knowles MR, Yankaskas JR, Sandhu JS, Jaques PF. Bronchial artery embolization for the treatment of hemoptysis in patients with cystic fibrosis. Am J Respir Crit Care Med. 1998;157:1951–8. https://doi.org/10.1164/ajrccm.157.6.9708067.

8. Casal RF. Update in airway stents. Curr Opin Pulm Med. 2010;16:321–8. https://doi.org/10.1097/MCP.0b013e32833a260.

9. Casal RF, et al. Safety and effectiveness of micro-debrider bronchoscopy for the management of central airway obstruction. Respirology. 2013;18:1011–5. https://doi.org/10.1111/resp.12087.

10. Cavaliere S, Foccoli P, Farina PL. Nd:YAG laser bronchoscopy. A five-year experience with 1,396 applications in 1,000 patients. Chest. 1988;94:15–21.

11. Cavaliere S, Foccoli P, Toninelli C, Feijo S. Nd:YAG laser therapy in lung cancer: an 11-year experience with 2253 applications in 1585 patients. J Bronchol. 1994;1:105–11.

12. Cavaliere S, Venuta F, Foccoli P, Toninelli C, La Face B. Endoscopic treatment of malignant airway obstructions in 2,008 patients. Chest. 1996;110:1536–42.

13. Charokopos N, Foroulis CN, Rouska E, Sileli MN, Papadopoulos N, Papakonstantinou C. The management of post-intubation tracheal stenoses with self-expandable stents: early and long-term results in 11 cases. Eur J Cardiothorac Surg. 2011;40:919–24. https://doi.org/10.1016/j.ejcts.2010.12.042.

14. Chhajed PN, et al. Therapeutic bronchoscopy for malignant airway stenoses: choice of modality and survival. J Cancer Res Ther. 2010;6:204–9. https://doi.org/10.4103/0973-1482.65250.

15. Conlan AA, Hurwitz SS. Management of massive haemoptysis with the rigid bronchoscope and cold saline lavage. Thorax. 1980;35:901–4.

16. Corey R, Hla KM. Major and massive hemoptysis: reassessment of conservative management. Am J Med Sci. 1987;294:301–9.

17. Coulter TD, Mehta AC. The heat is on: impact of endobronchial electrosurgery on the need for Nd-YAG laser photoresection. Chest. 2000;118:516–21.

18. Crocco JA, Rooney JJ, Fankushen DS, DiBenedetto RJ, Lyons HA. Massive hemoptysis. Arch Intern Med. 1968;121:495–8.

19. de Gracia J, de la Rosa D, Catalan E, Alvarez A, Bravo C, Morell F. Use of endoscopic fibrinogen-thrombin in the treatment of severe hemoptysis. Respir Med. 2003;97:790–5.

20. Ducic Y, Khalafi RS. Use of endoscopically placed expandable nitinol tracheal stents in the treatment of tracheal stenosis. Laryngoscope. 1999;109:1130–3.

21. Dumon JF. A dedicated tracheobronchial stent. Chest. 1990;97:328–32.

22. Dumon JF, Reboud E, Garbe L, Aucomte F, Meric B. Treatment of tracheobronchial lesions by laser photoresection. Chest. 1982;81:278–84.

23. Dupree HJ, Lewejohann JC, Gleiss J, Muhl E, Bruch HP. Fiberoptic bronchoscopy of intubated patients with life-threatening hemoptysis. World J Surg. 2001;25:104–7.

24. Dutau H, Toutblanc B, Lamb C, Seijo L. Use of the Dumon Y-stent in the management of malignant disease involving the carina: a retrospective review of 86 patients. Chest. 2004;126:951–8. https://doi.org/10.1378/chest.126.3.951.

25. Earwood JS, Thompson TD. Hemoptysis: evaluation and management. Am Fam Physician. 2015;91:243–9.

26. Edmondstone WM, Nanson EM, Woodcock AA, Millard FJ, Hetzel MR. Life threatening haemoptysis controlled by laser photocoagulation. Thorax. 1983;38:788–9.

27. Ernst A, Feller-Kopman D, Becker HD, Mehta AC. Central airway obstruction. Am J Respir Crit Care Med. 2004;169:1278–97. https://doi.org/10.1164/rccm.200210-1181SO.

28. Fartoukh M, et al. Early prediction of in-hospital mortality of patients with hemoptysis: an approach to defining severe hemoptysis. Respiration. 2012;83:106–14. https://doi.org/10.1159/000331501.

29. Garzon AA, Gourin A. Surgical management of massive hemoptysis. A ten-year experience. Ann Surg. 1978;187:267–71.

30. Geffin B, Grillo HC, Cooper JD, Pontoppidan H. Stenosis following tracheostomy for respiratory care. JAMA. 1971;216:1984–8.

31. Gong H Jr, Salvatierra C. Clinical efficacy of early and delayed fiberoptic bronchoscopy in patients with hemoptysis. Am Rev Respir Dis. 1981;124:221–5. https://doi.org/10.1164/arrd.1981.124.3.221.

32. Gourin A, Garzon AA. Operative treatment of massive hemoptysis. Ann Thorac Surg. 1974;18:52–60.

33. Grillo HC. Reconstruction of the trachea. Experience in 100 consecutive cases. Thorax. 1973;28:667–79.

34. Han CC, Prasetyo D, Wright GM. Endobronchial palliation using Nd:YAG laser is associated with improved survival when combined with multimodal adjuvant treatments. J Thorac Oncol. 2007;2:59–64. https://doi.org/10.1097/JTO.0b013e31802bff2d.

35. Haponik EF, Britt EJ, Smith PL, Bleecker ER. Computed chest tomography in the evaluation of hemoptysis. Impact on diagnosis and treatment. Chest. 1987;91:80–5.

36. Herth F, Ernst A, Becker HD. Long-term outcome and lung cancer incidence in patients with hemoptysis of unknown origin. Chest. 2001;120:1592–4.

37. Hetzel MR, Smith SG. Endoscopic palliation of tracheobronchial malignancies. Thorax. 1991;46:325–33.

38. Hetzel M, Hetzel J, Schumann C, Marx N, Babiak A. Cryorecanalization: a new approach for the immediate management of acute airway obstruction. J Thorac Cardiovasc Surg. 2004;127:1427–31. https://doi.org/10.1016/j.jtcvs.2003.12.032.

39. Hirshberg B, Biran I, Glazer M, Kramer MR. Hemoptysis: etiology, evaluation, and outcome in a tertiary referral hospital. Chest. 1997;112:440–4.

40. Hollingsworth HM. Wheezing and stridor. Clin Chest Med. 1987;8:231–40.

41. Hsiao EI, Kirsch CM, Kagawa FT, Wehner JH, Jensen WA, Baxter RB. Utility of fiberoptic bronchoscopy before bronchial artery embolization for massive hemoptysis. AJR Am J Roentgenol. 2001;177:861–7. https://doi.org/10.2214/ajr.177.4.1770861.

42. Ibrahim WH. Massive haemoptysis: the definition should be revised. Eur Respir J. 2008;32:1131–2. https://doi.org/10.1183/09031936.00080108.

43. Ittrich H, Bockhorn M, Klose H, Simon M. The diagnosis and treatment of hemoptysis. Dtsch Arztebl Int. 2017;114:371–81. https://doi.org/10.3238/arztebl.2017.0371.

44. Jones R, Charlton J, Latinovic R, Gulliford MC. Alarm symptoms and identification of non-cancer diagnoses in primary care: cohort study. BMJ. 2009;339:b3094. https://doi.org/10.1136/bmj.b3094.

45. Keller CA, Hinerman R, Singh A, Alvarez F. The use of endoscopic argon plasma coagulation in airway complications after solid organ transplantation. Chest. 2001;119:1968–75.

46. Khalil A, Fartoukh M, Tassart M, Parrot A, Marsault C, Carette MF. Role of MDCT in identification of the bleeding site and the vessels causing hemoptysis. AJR Am J Roentgenol. 2007;188:W117–25. https://doi.org/10.2214/AJR.05.1578.

47. Khalil A, Soussan M, Mangiapan G, Fartoukh M, Parrot A, Carette MF. Utility of high-resolution chest CT scan in the emergency management of haemoptysis in the intensive care unit: severity, localization and aetiology. Br J Radiol. 2007;80:21–5. https://doi.org/10.1259/bjr/59233312.

48. Knott-Craig CJ, Oostuizen JG, Rossouw G, Joubert JR, Barnard PM. Management and prognosis of massive hemoptysis. Recent experience with 120 patients. J Thorac Cardiovasc Surg. 1993;105:394–7.

49. Kvale PA, Eichenhorn MS, Radke JR, Miks V. YAG laser photoresection of lesions obstructing the central airways. Chest. 1985;87:283–8.

50. Larici AR, et al. Diagnosis and management of hemoptysis. Diagn Interv Radiol. 2014;20:299–309. https://doi.org/10.5152/dir.2014.13426.

51. Lordan JL, Gascoigne A, Corris PA. The pulmonary physician in critical care * Illustrative case 7: assessment and management of massive haemoptysis. Thorax. 2003;58:814–9.

52. Lunn W, Garland R, Ashiku S, Thurer RL, Feller-Kopman D, Ernst A. Microdebrider bronchoscopy: a new tool for the interventional bronchoscopist. Ann Thorac Surg. 2005;80:1485–8. https://doi.org/10.1016/j.athoracsur.2004.12.023.

53. Mal H, Rullon I, Mellot F, Brugiere O, Sleiman C, Menu Y, Fournier M. Immediate and long-term results of bronchial artery embolization for life-threatening hemoptysis. Chest. 1999;115:996–1001.

54. Mathur PN, Wolf KM, Busk MF, Briete WM, Datzman M. Fiberoptic bronchoscopic cryotherapy in the management of tracheobronchial obstruction. Chest. 1996;110:718–23.

55. McGuinness G, Beacher JR, Harkin TJ, Garay SM, Rom WN, Naidich DP. Hemoptysis: prospective high-resolution CT/bronchoscopic correlation. Chest. 1994;105:1155–62.

56. Mehta AS, et al. Bronchial artery embolization for malignant hemoptysis: a single institutional experience. J Thorac Dis. 2015;7:1406–13. https://doi.org/10.3978/j.issn.2072-1439.2015.07.39.

57. Miller RD, Hyatt RE. Evaluation of obstructing lesions of the trachea and larynx by flow-volume loops. Am Rev Respir Dis. 1973;108:475–81. https://doi.org/10.1164/arrd.1973.108.3.475.

58. Morice RC, Ece T, Ece F, Keus L. Endobronchial argon plasma coagulation for treatment of hemoptysis and neoplastic airway obstruction. Chest. 2001;119:781–7.

59. Naidich DP, Funt S, Ettenger NA, Arranda C. Hemoptysis: CT-bronchoscopic correlations in 58 cases. Radiology. 1990;177:357–62. https://doi.org/10.1148/radiology.177.2.2217769.

60. Ong TH, Eng P. Massive hemoptysis requiring intensive care. Intensive Care Med. 2003;29:317–20. https://doi.org/10.1007/s00134-002-1553-6.

61. Ost DE, et al. Respiratory infections increase the risk of granulation tissue formation following airway stenting in patients with malignant airway obstruction. Chest. 2012;141:1473–81. https://doi.org/10.1378/chest.11-2005.

62. Pearson FG, Todd TR, Cooper JD. Experience with primary neoplasms of the trachea and carina. J Thorac Cardiovasc Surg. 1984;88:511–8.

63. Perin B, et al. Patient-related independent clinical risk factors for early complications following Nd: YAG laser resection of lung cancer. Ann Thorac Med. 2012;7:233–7. https://doi.org/10.4103/1817-1737.10 2184.

64. Poe RH, et al. Utility of fiberoptic bronchoscopy in patients with hemoptysis and a nonlocalizing chest roentgenogram. Chest. 1988;93:70–5.

65. Reddy C, Majid A, Michaud G, Feller-Kopman D, Eberhardt R, Herth F, Ernst A. Gas embolism following bronchoscopic argon plasma coagulation: a case series. Chest. 2008;134:1066–9. https://doi.org/10.1378/chest.08-0474.

66. Reichle G, Freitag L, Kullmann HJ, Prenzel R, Macha HN, Farin G. Argon plasma coagulation in

bronchology: a new method – alternative or complementary? Pneumologie. 2000;54:508–16. https://doi.org/10.1055/s-2000-8254.

67. Remy J, et al. Treatment, by embolization, of severe or repeated hemoptysis associated with systemic hypervascularization. Nouv Presse Med. 1973;2:2060.

68. Remy J, Lemaitre L, Lafitte JJ, Vilain MO, Saint Michel J, Steenhouwer F. Massive hemoptysis of pulmonary arterial origin: diagnosis and treatment. AJR Am J Roentgenol. 1984;143:963–9. https://doi.org/10.2214/ajr.143.5.963.

69. Revel MP, Fournier LS, Hennebicque AS, Cuenod CA, Meyer G, Reynaud P, Frija G. Can CT replace bronchoscopy in the detection of the site and cause of bleeding in patients with large or massive hemoptysis? AJR Am J Roentgenol. 2002;179:1217–24. https://doi.org/10.2214/ajr.179.5.1791217.

70. Ross DJ, Mohsenifar Z, Koerner SK. Survival characteristics after neodymium: YAG laser photoresection in advanced stage lung cancer. Chest. 1990;98:581–5.

71. Sakr L, Dutau H. Massive hemoptysis: an update on the role of bronchoscopy in diagnosis and management. Respiration. 2010;80:38–58. https://doi.org/10.1159/000274492.

72. Saumench J, Escarrabill J, Padro L, Montana J, Clariana A, Canto A. Value of fiberoptic bronchoscopy and angiography for diagnosis of the bleeding site in hemoptysis. Ann Thorac Surg. 1989;48:272–4.

73. Savale L, et al. Cryptogenic hemoptysis: from a benign to a life-threatening pathologic vascular condition. Am J Respir Crit Care Med. 2007;175:1181–5. https://doi.org/10.1164/rccm.200609-1362OC.

74. Seijo LM, Ancochea J. In search of the ideal tracheobronchial stent: metal or silicone? Arch Bronconeumol. 2004;40:293–4.

75. Set PA, Flower CD, Smith IE, Chan AP, Twentyman OP, Shneerson JM. Hemoptysis: comparative study of the role of CT and fiberoptic bronchoscopy. Radiology. 1993;189:677–80. https://doi.org/10.1148/radiology.189.3.8234690.

76. Sheski FD, Mathur PN. Endobronchial electrosurgery: argon plasma coagulation and electrocautery. Semin Respir Crit Care Med. 2004;25:367–74. https://doi.org/10.1055/s-2004-832709.

77. Shigemura N, et al. Multidisciplinary management of life-threatening massive hemoptysis: a 10-year experience. Ann Thorac Surg. 2009;87:849–53. https://doi.org/10.1016/j.athoracsur.2008.11.010.

78. Simoni P, Peters GE, Magnuson JS, Carroll WR. Use of the endoscopic microdebrider in the management of airway obstruction from laryngotracheal carcinoma. Ann Otol Rhinol Laryngol. 2003;112:11–3. https://doi.org/10.1177/000348940311200103.

79. Soares Pires F, Teixeira N, Coelho F, Damas C. Hemoptysis – etiology, evaluation and treatment in a university hospital. Rev Port Pneumol. 2011;17:7–14.

80. Stoller JK. Spirometry: a key diagnostic test in pulmonary medicine. Cleve Clin J Med. 1992;59:75–8.

81. Sutedja G, van Kralingen K, Schramel FM, Postmus PE. Fibreoptic bronchoscopic electrosurgery under local anaesthesia for rapid palliation in patients with central airway malignancies: a preliminary report. Thorax. 1994;49:1243–6.

82. Sutedja T, Van Boxem TJ, Schramel FM, Van Felius C, Postmus P. Endobronchial electrocautery is an excellent alternative to Nd:YAG laser to treat airway tumors. J Bronchol. 1997;4:101–5.

83. Swanson KL, Johnson CM, Prakash UB, McKusick MA, Andrews JC, Stanson AW. Bronchial artery embolization: experience with 54 patients. Chest. 2002;121:789–95.

84. Tanaka N, et al. Superselective bronchial artery embolization for hemoptysis with a coaxial microcatheter system. J Vasc Interv Radiol. 1997;8:65–70.

85. Tsoumakidou M, Chrysofakis G, Tsiligianni I, Maltezakis G, Siafakas NM, Tzanakis N. A prospective analysis of 184 hemoptysis cases: diagnostic impact of chest x-ray, computed tomography, bronchoscopy. Respiration. 2006;73:808–14. https://doi.org/10.1159/000091189.

86. Tsukamoto T, Sasaki H, Nakamura H. Treatment of hemoptysis patients by thrombin and fibrinogen-thrombin infusion therapy using a fiberoptic bronchoscope. Chest. 1989;96:473–6.

87. Tuller C, Tuller D, Tamm M, Brutsche MH. Hemodynamic effects of endobronchial application of ornipressin versus terlipressin. Respiration. 2004;71:397–401. https://doi.org/10.1159/000079646.

88. Valipour A, Kreuzer A, Koller H, Koessler W, Burghuber OC. Bronchoscopy-guided topical hemostatic tamponade therapy for the management of life-threatening hemoptysis. Chest. 2005;127:2113–8. https://doi.org/10.1378/chest.127.6.2113.

89. van Boxem TJ, Venmans BJ, Schramel FM, van Mourik JC, Golding RP, Postmus PE, Sutedja TG. Radiographically occult lung cancer treated with fibreoptic bronchoscopic electrocautery: a pilot study of a simple and inexpensive technique. Eur Respir J. 1998;11:169–72.

90. Vergnon JM, Huber RM, Moghissi K. Place of cryotherapy, brachytherapy and photodynamic therapy in therapeutic bronchoscopy of lung cancers. Eur Respir J. 2006;28:200–18. https://doi.org/10.1183/09031936.06.00014006.

91. Walsh DA, Maiwand MO, Nath AR, Lockwood P, Lloyd MH, Saab M. Bronchoscopic cryotherapy for advanced bronchial carcinoma. Thorax. 1990;45:509–13.

92. Wong ML, Szkup P, Hopley MJ. Percutaneous embolotherapy for life-threatening hemoptysis. Chest. 2002;121:95–102.

93. Yoon W, Kim JK, Kim YH, Chung TW, Kang HK. Bronchial and nonbronchial systemic artery embolization for life-threatening hemoptysis: a comprehensive review. Radiographics. 2002;22:1395–409. https://doi.org/10.1148/rg.226015180.

Tracheostomy

44

Appropriateness and Indications in Cancer Patients

Macarena R. Vial and Joseph L. Nates

Contents

Introduction 668

Epidemiology 668

Indications 669
Upper Airway Obstruction 669
Respiratory Failure and Prolonged Mechanical Ventilation 669

Expected Benefits 669
Mortality 669
Patient Comfort and Sedation Requirements 670
Long-Term Airway Complications 670
Reduce the Length of Mechanical Ventilation or ICU Stay 670
Reduce the Risk of Ventilator-Associated Pneumonia 671

Contraindications 671

Appropriate Timing 671

Appropriate Technique 672

Conclusion 672

References 672

M. R. Vial (✉)
Interventional Pulmonology Unit, Clínica Alemana de
Santiago-Universidad del Desarrollo, Santiago, Chile

Servicio de Enfermedades Respiratorias, Unidad de
Neumologia Intervencional, Clínica Alemana de Santiago,
Vitacura, Santiago, Chile
e-mail: macarena.r@gmail.com;
mrodriguezvi@alemana.cl

J. L. Nates
Department of Critical Care and Respiratory Care,
The University of Texas MD Anderson Cancer Center,
Houston, TX, USA
e-mail: jlnates@mdanderson.org

Abstract

Increased survival in cancer patients and increased use of immunosuppressive treatments has resulted in a higher number of cancer patients admitted to intensive care units (ICUs). Tracheostomy is the most commonly performed procedure in ICUs, so the question of the appropriateness of tracheostomy is one clinicians will face even more in the coming years. The main benefits of tracheostomy in critically ill cancer patients are often clear in cases with upper airway obstruction, but

© Springer Nature Switzerland AG 2020
J. L. Nates, K. J. Price (eds.), *Oncologic Critical Care*,
https://doi.org/10.1007/978-3-319-74588-6_61

this is not the case in prolonged mechanical ventilation. The main benefit appears to be an overall reduction in the duration of mechanical ventilation. In order to maximize this benefit, tracheostomy should be performed as early as possible, but unfortunately, clinicians are not good at predicting who will require prolonged mechanical ventilation. Therefore, the benefit has to be weighed against the risk of performing unnecessary procedures, and ideally, it should not be performed before 7 days of endotracheal intubation. Finally and more importantly, appropriateness will depend on the overall plan of care and prognosis of the underlying malignancy.

Keywords

Tracheostomy · Acute respiratory failure · Mechanical ventilation · Percutaneous tracheostomy · Airway obstruction

Introduction

Increasing life expectancy, increasing incidence of cancer, and improved survival of several malignancies have increased the total number of cancer patients that seek medical care in general. This goes along with an increasing use of immunosuppressive drugs as part of cancer treatments and an associated increase in patients with severe infections and respiratory failure requiring mechanical ventilation. Given that tracheostomy is one of the most common procedures in intensive care units (ICUs) [6, 9] and the major indication is prolonged mechanical ventilation [3], the question of appropriateness of tracheostomy in this setting will become increasingly more relevant.

Appropriateness of performing a tracheostomy in cancer patients depends on the benefits and risks of tracheostomy in general, just like in non-cancer patients, but it also depends on the overall plan of care of the underlying malignancy. Will the patient return to his prior level of care after discharge from the ICU? Will he attain a reasonable quality of life afterwards? What is a reasonable quality of life for this particular patient? Will this procedure act as a bridge so the patient can pursue further cancer treatment?

What is the prognosis? All these questions should be considered in the decision-making process and discussed with the treating physician, usually the medical oncologist. Also, and very importantly, they need to be discussed in advance with patients and their families, clarifying expectations and understanding their desires and beliefs. This will allow establishing a consented plan of care that will facilitate further decisions and communication among the ICU team, family members, and treating physician.

Of note, while reviewing the evidence, it is important to keep in mind some of the problems in tracheostomy research: (i) there is minimal data comparing tracheostomy versus prolonged mechanical intubation in order to assess the benefits of tracheostomy independent of timing; (ii) most prospective studies comparing early versus late tracheostomy include patients that never undergo a tracheostomy in the "late" group; (iii) consequently, retrospective studies comparing "early" versus "late" tracheostomy suffer from significant selection bias; (iv) significant heterogeneity in study design regarding definitions and procedure techniques makes it difficult to compare different studies and obtain pooled estimates (particularly for definitions of early or late and multiple percutaneous techniques); and finally (v) blinding the ICU team to treatment assignment is not possible. In this chapter, we will review the evidence regarding the major benefits and risks of performing a tracheostomy in adult cancer patients admitted to the ICU and also briefly address the appropriate timing and techniques.

Epidemiology

Tracheostomy is one of the oldest and most frequently performed procedures in patients admitted to the ICU with an average number of tracheostomies performed annually in the United States of 100,000 [24]. A few epidemiologic studies have evaluated the main indications for tracheostomy. In a large study, surveying 152 ICUs in France, prolonged mechanical ventilation and failed extubation were the most commonly stated reasons when performing a tracheostomy [3]. Similarly, among intensive care physicians in Switzerland, the most common indication was the need for prolonged mechanical ventilation followed by persistent coma, airway toilet, and airway protection [9].

Only a few studies have assessed the indications of tracheostomy in critically ill cancer patients. Indications are similar than those in the general ICU population, but upper airway obstruction appears to be more common. According to a prospective study on 463 critically ill cancer patients with respiratory failure, the leading cause was sepsis; however, in up to 11% of them, the cause was airway or lung involvement by tumor [19]. A study that looked specifically into the indications of tracheostomy in 130 oncologic patients found that head and neck cancers together constituted the most common indication for this procedure with 47% of cases [2].

Indications

There are several indications for tracheostomy, but in the critically ill patient, it is mainly performed in two circumstances: (i) patients with upper airway obstruction in order to ensure an appropriate safe airway and (ii) patients with prolonged mechanical ventilation as an alternative to endotracheal intubation, generally believed to carry more complications and higher patient discomfort compared to tracheostomy. In any of these conditions, the decision-making process should always consider the overall patient's prognosis and the treatment plan for the underlying malignancy. Other indications specific to patients with head and neck cancers, such as elective postoperative tracheostomy, will not be reviewed here.

Upper Airway Obstruction

Upper airway obstruction can be caused by a mechanical effect of the tumor itself or by a laryngeal dysfunction, such as bilateral recurrent laryngeal nerve palsy. In cases where the level of the obstruction is close to or above the vocal cords, the obstruction needs to be bypassed. In these cases, tracheostomy will be the treatment of choice providing a long-term solution to assure the airway. If the airway obstruction is below the level of the vocal cords, the possibility of removing the obstruction and recovering airway function should always be assessed.

Respiratory Failure and Prolonged Mechanical Ventilation

In patients with respiratory failure and prolonged mechanical ventilation, tracheostomy is indicated based on several potential benefits of tracheostomy. Many of these potential benefits are not supported by the evidence with studies showing negative or contradicting results. Of note, the vast majority of studies have not compared tracheostomy to prolonged endotracheal intubation, but have evaluated whether performing an early tracheostomy results in improved outcomes compared to waiting and determining the need for a tracheostomy later on during the disease. We will briefly review some of them here.

Expected Benefits

Mortality

Several studies have assessed the effect of tracheostomy on survival in patients with prolonged mechanical ventilation. Tracheostomy compared to prolonged endotracheal intubation appears to have no benefit on mortality [4]. Also, there is no clear benefit on mortality when comparing early versus late tracheostomy, despite several randomized controlled trials (RCT). The largest RCT comparing early versus late tracheostomy in mechanically ventilated subjects is the TracMan trial (Young et al. 2013), a multicenter trial performed in the United Kingdom in 72 ICUs. A total of 909 mechanically ventilated subjects were enrolled at day 4 after endotracheal intubation. Patients were randomized only if the estimated length of mechanical ventilation was at least 7 more days, according to the treating physician. Subjects were randomized to early tracheostomy (day 4) or late tracheostomy (after day 10 if it was still indicated). They found no difference in 30-day mortality (30.8% early vs. 31.5% late) or 2-year mortality (51.0% early vs. 53.7% late). Interestingly, in the late tracheostomy group, only 45.5% of subjects were still requiring mechanical ventilation at day 10 and thus underwent a tracheostomy, despite the treating physician's predictions.

Additionally, several meta-analyses have compared mortality in early versus late tracheostomy. Only one of them reported a mortality benefit for the early tracheostomy group [1], but the remaining ones have only confirmed the results of the TracMan trial, with no mortality benefit [10–12, 17].

Patient Comfort and Sedation Requirements

Tracheostomy as opposed to endotracheal intubation allows the patient to eat and communicate. It is generally believed to increase patient comfort while on mechanical ventilation which may translate into decreased sedation requirements. This was evaluated in a retrospective study including all 72 patients who underwent a tracheostomy in a French ICU during a 14-month period. To achieve a predetermined level of Sedation-Agitation Scale score (SAS), sedation dose requirements were significantly different after tracheostomy, compared to doses before tracheostomy [13]. These findings are consistent with those reported in the TracMan trial randomizing early to late tracheostomy, which reported significantly decreased days on sedation in the early tracheostomy compared to the late tracheostomy group [23]. However, this benefit comes at a cost, and as the lead author stated, "If you had 100 patients requiring tracheostomy, doing it early results in 2.4 days less sedation overall, but you would perform 48 more, with 3 more procedural complications and no effect on mortality or ICU stay."

Unfortunately, due to the lack of blinding in this studies and variability in weaning protocols, it is unclear if the reduction in sedative and analgesic medication doses after tracheostomy is due to increased patient comfort, or they are just a result of changes in clinician's perception of patient's discomfort, thus changing sedation prescription.

Long-Term Airway Complications

Prolonged airway intubation may induce airway injury, generally at the cuff site due to pressure in the mucosal wall with subsequent scarring and airway stenosis. Only a few studies have compared tracheostomy to prolonged endotracheal intubation. The largest one included 123 ICU patients and assessed airway injury with both laryngeal symptoms and fiber-optic airway examination [4]. This study failed to demonstrate any difference regarding laryngotracheal complications although it was not designed with airway injury as the primary outcome. These findings are consistent with another prospective study of 120 critically ill patients who underwent bronchoscopy and computed tomography, during the in-hospital stay and 10 weeks post-intubation. Results were not different among patients with early tracheostomy, late tracheostomy, or prolonged intubation. In summary, the belief that tracheostomy may reduce airway injury is not supported by evidence and both devices; tracheostomy and endotracheal tubes can induce airway damage.

Reduce the Length of Mechanical Ventilation or ICU Stay

Tracheostomy reduces dead space and airway resistance, decreasing the work of breathing. These physiologic advantages could theoretically facilitate weaning, decreasing the length of mechanical ventilation. Also, the easy fashion in which a tracheostomy tube can be connected and reconnected to the ventilator may induce the clinician to a more aggressive attitude toward weaning. Many studies have shown that early tracheostomy results in increased ventilator-free days, regardless of the definition of early tracheostomy and the method used to measure the length of mechanical ventilation [5, 15, 20, 21]. One of the largest RCTs [20] reported a significant difference favoring early tracheostomy with a median of ventilator days of 6 in the early group compared to 11 in the late tracheostomy group.

However, unless studies use a predetermined weaning protocol, we cannot conclude the improved outcome is related to the tracheostomy and its physiologic benefits, as much as from changes in clinician's behavior.

Reduce the Risk of Ventilator-Associated Pneumonia

Ventilator-associated pneumonia (VAP) is defined as pneumonia that occurs 48–72 h or after that following endotracheal intubation. If tracheostomy reduces the length of mechanical ventilation, then almost by definition, performing a tracheostomy early on after intubation would decrease the risk of pneumonia. Also, endotracheal intubation is associated with micro-aspiration, and microaspiration is believed to be part of the physiopathology of VAP; thus by early removal of the endotracheal tube, one would expect a reduction in VAP.

However, the evidence supporting a decreased risk of VAP after tracheostomy is contradictory; while some studies have shown early tracheostomy decreased the risk of VAP [15, 20, 25], some found no difference [8, 21]. Several meta-analyses have also informed on the effects of early tracheostomy on the risk of VAP [1, 11, 17]. Unfortunately, they found significant variability on methodologies and statistical heterogeneity, so two of these studies did not present pooled estimates on this outcome.

Contraindications

Tracheostomy has been reported to result in serious and potentially life-threatening complications. Some of these complications are related to the inexperience of the operator, while others are related to the patient's characteristics. Immediate complications include hemorrhage, hypoxemia, accidental extubation, pneumothorax, pneumomediastinum,

and tracheal injury [16, 22]. Patients who are at high risk for any of these complications have a relative contraindication, and the risk factor should be corrected when possible, or the procedure should be deferred until the risk is lower. High risk for these complications generally includes severe hypoxemia (defined as $PaO2/FiO2$ <100 mmHg or positive expiratory pressure >10 cmH_2O) and bleeding disorders (platelets <50,000/mm^3, international normalized ratio >1.5 and partial thromboplastin time >2 normal). Intracranial hypertension is often mentioned as a contraindication because minimally invasive procedures such as percutaneous tracheostomy may significantly increase intracranial pressure. If the benefits of tracheostomy are felt to be higher than the risk of neurological deterioration, then it should be performed with continuous ICP monitoring.

Appropriate Timing

In patients with upper airway obstruction, tracheostomy should ideally be performed before symptoms or stridor appears, because intubation or mask ventilation may be difficult or even impossible. Emergent airway interventions are associated with a significantly higher risk of complications compared to elective procedures. Unfortunately, in a study including only oncologic patients, 55% of tracheostomies were considered emergent, defined as a patient presenting with stridor [2].

Although not specifically in cancer patients, the issue of the most appropriate timing of tracheostomy in patients with prolonged mechanical ventilation (mostly due to acute respiratory failure) has been widely examined. The answer, however, is not clear due in part to the challenges expressed in the introduction section. We referred to some of these studies when discussing the potential benefits of tracheostomy, but one of the most important lessons in terms of timing came from the TracMan trial. Clinician's predictions on patients who would require prolonged mechanical ventilation, defined as 10 or more days, failed in 54.5% of cases when the prediction was performed at day 4 of endotracheal intubation. This suggests that tracheostomy in patients with mechanical ventilation should be deferred at least after day 4 of intubation, to avoid performing unnecessary procedures.

Appropriate Technique

There are two main techniques to perform a tracheostomy: surgical and percutaneous, with a wide range of devices used to perform a percutaneous tracheostomy. Some cancer patients are not adequate candidates to undergo a percutaneous tracheostomy, particularly patients with large head and neck tumors or abnormal neck anatomy, for example, secondary to radiation treatment. Due to a higher risk of complications, a surgical procedure is generally more appropriate in this case. Obesity and short neck are other commonly stated contraindications of a percutaneous technique, but these are relative, and an experienced operator may be able to overcome them.

If an ICU patient is a good candidate for both, percutaneous or surgical procedure, then a percutaneous tracheostomy is generally preferred. This is based on shorter operative time, decreased incidence of stoma infection and inflammation, and possibly a reduced time from indication to the execution of the procedure. There is no evidence of a difference in significant complications or death.

In a meta-analysis of 17 RCTs, PT was associated with significantly fewer stoma infections, odds ratio (OR) of 0.28 (95%CI 0.16 to 0.49), compared with ST [7]. Similar findings were reported in a more recent meta-analysis with lower risks of minor inflammation of the stoma (OR, 0.38; 95% CI, 0.19 to 0.76) and infectious complications (OR, 0.22; 95% CI 0.11 to 0.41) in patients undergoing PT compared to ST [14]. The reduced risk of infections may be particularly significant in cancer patients who are often immunosuppressed and should be considered when determining the best technique.

PT also offers a logistical advantage over ST when performed by the intensivists, with a shorter time between the indication and the actual execution of the procedure [18].

Conclusion

Tracheostomy is a useful and safe method to ensure the airway in patients with malignant diseases. In patients with upper airway involvement and impending airway obstruction, the decision is more straightforward considering that tracheostomy will provide an effective long-term solution. In patients with mechanical ventilation, the benefits of tracheostomy are less evident and appear to be mainly a decreased length of mechanical ventilation and easier airway management compared to endotracheal tubes. Tracheostomy should be performed soon after intubation to maximize the benefits, but not before the fourth day of mechanical ventilation since this will result in many unnecessary procedures.

In any of the situations described above, the appropriateness of a tracheostomy in cancer patients depends highly on the prognosis and overall plan of care as well as on patient's expectations. Hence, the decision should be a team decision that considers the views of all the physicians involved (critical care, oncologist, surgeon, radiation oncologist as appropriate) and the patient or family members.

References

1. Andriolo BN, Andriolo RB, Saconato H, Atallah AN, Valente O. Early versus late tracheostomy for critically ill patients. Cochrane Database Syst Rev. 2015;1: CD007271.
2. Bhatti AB, Iqbal H, Hussain R, Syed AA, Jamshed A. Tracheotomy in cancer patients: experience from a Cancer Hospital in Pakistan. Indian J Surg. 2015;77 (Suppl 3):906–9.
3. Blot F, Melot C, Commission d'Epidémiologie et de Recherche Clinique. Indications, timing, and techniques of tracheostomy in 152 French ICUs. Chest. 2005;127(4):1347–52.
4. Blot F, Similowski T, Trouillet JL, Chardon P, Korach JM, Costa MA, Journois D, Thiéry G, Fartoukh M, Pipien I, Bruder N, Orlikowski D, Tankere F, Durand-Zaleski I, Auboyer C, Nitenberg G, Holzapfel L, Tenaillon A, Chastre J, Laplanche A. Early tracheotomy versus prolonged endotracheal intubation in unselected severely ill ICU patients. Intensive Care Med. 2008;34(10):1779–87.
5. Bösel J, Schiller P, Hook Y, Andes M, Neumann JO, Poli S, Amiri H, Schönenberger S, Peng Z,

Unterberg A, Hacke W, Steiner T. Stroke-related early tracheostomy versus prolonged orotracheal intubation in neurocritical care trial (SETPOINT): a randomized pilot trial. Stroke. 2013;44(1):21–8.

6. Cox CE, Carson SS, Holmes GM, Howard A, Carey TS. Increase in tracheostomy for prolonged mechanical ventilation in North Carolina, 1993–2002. Crit Care Med. 2004;32:2219–26.

7. Delaney A, Bagshaw SM, Nalos M. Percutaneous dilatational tracheostomy versus surgical tracheostomy in critically ill patients: a systematic review and meta-analysis. Crit Care. 2006;10(2):R55

8. Diaz-Prieto A, Mateu A, Gorriz M, et al. A randomized clinical trial for the timing of tracheotomy in critically ill patients: factors precluding inclusion in a single center study. Crit Care. 2014;18:585.

9. Fischler L, Erhart S, Kleger GR, Frutiger A. Prevalence of tracheostomy in ICU patients. A nation-wide survey in Switzerland. Intensive Care Med. 2000;26:1428–33.

10. Griffiths J, Barber VS, Morgan L, et al. Systematic review and meta-analysis of studies of the timing of tracheostomy in adult patients undergoing artificial ventilation. BMJ. 2005;330(7502):1243.

11. Liu CC, Livingstone D, Dixon E, Dort JC. Early versus late tracheostomy: a systematic review and meta-analysis. Otolaryngol Head Neck Surg. 2015;152:219–27.

12. Meng L, Wang C, Li J, et al. Early vs late tracheostomy in critically ill patients: a systematic review and meta-analysis. Clin Respir J. 2016;10(6):684–92.

13. Nieszkowska A, Combes A, Luyt CE, Ksibi H, Trouillet JL, Gibert C, Chastre J. Impact of tracheotomy on sedative administration, sedation level, and comfort of mechanically ventilated intensive care unit patients. Crit Care Med. 2005;33(11):2527–33.

14. Putensen C, Theuerkauf N, Guenther U, Vargas M, Pelosi P. Percutaneous and surgical tracheostomy in critically ill adult patients: a meta-analysis. Crit Care. 2014;18(6):544.

15. Rumbak MJ, Newton M, Truncale T, Schwartz SW, Adams JW, Hazard PB. A prospective, randomized, study comparing early percutaneous dilational tracheotomy to prolonged translaryngeal intubation (delayed tracheotomy) in critically ill medical patients. Crit Care Med. 2004;32:1689–94.

16. Raimondi N, et al. Evidence-based guidelines for the use of tracheostomy in critically ill patients. J Crit Care. 2017;38:304–18.

17. Siempos II, Ntaidou TK, Filippidis FT, Choi AM. Effect of early versus late or no tracheostomy on mortality and pneumonia of critically ill patients receiving mechanical ventilation: a systematic review and meta-analysis. Lancet Respir Med. 2015;3:150–8.

18. Silvester W, Goldsmith D, Uchino S, Bellomo R, Knight S, Seevanayagam S, Brazzale D, McMahon M, Buckmaster J, Hart GK, Opdam H, Pierce RJ, Gutteridge GA. Percutaneous versus surgical tracheostomy: a randomized controlled study with long-term follow-up. Crit Care Med. 2006;34(8):2145–52.

19. Soares M, Salluh JI, Spector N, Rocco JR. Characteristics and outcomes of cancer patients requiring mechanical ventilatory support for >24 hrs. Crit Care Med. 2005;33(3):520–6.

20. Terragni PP, Antonelli M, Fumagalli R, et al. Early vs late tracheotomy for prevention of pneumonia in mechanically ventilated adult ICU patients: a randomized controlled trial. JAMA. 2010;303:1483–9.

21. Trouillet JL, Luyt CE, Guiguet M, et al. Early percutaneous tracheotomy versus prolonged intubation of mechanically ventilated patients after cardiac surgery: a randomized trial. Ann Intern Med. 2011;154:373–83.

22. Trouillet JL, Collange O, Belafia F, Blot F, Capellier G, Cesareo E, Constantin JM, Demoule A, Diehl JL, Guinot PG, Jegoux F, L'Her E, Luyt CE, Mahjoub Y, Mayaux J, Quintard H, Ravat F, Vergez S, Amour J, Guillot M, French Intensive Care Society, French Society of Anaesthesia and Intensive Care. Tracheotomy in the intensive care unit: guidelines from a French expert panel: the French Intensive Care Society and the French Society of Anaesthesia and Intensive Care Medicine. Anaesth Crit Care Pain Med. 2018;37(3):281–94.

23. Young D, Harrison DA, Cuthbertson BH, Rowan K, TracMan Collaborators. Effect of early vs late tracheostomy placement on survival in patients receiving mechanical ventilation: the TracMan randomized trial. JAMA. 2013;309(20):2121–9.

24. Yu M. Tracheostomy patients on the ward: multiple benefits from a multidisciplinary team? Crit Care. 2010;14(1):109.

25. Zheng Y, Sui F, Chen XK, et al. Early versus late percutaneous dilational tracheostomy in critically ill patients anticipated requiring prolonged mechanical ventilation. Chin Med J. 2012;125:1925–30.

Pulmonary Hypertension in an Oncologic Intensive Care Unit

45

Lilit A. Sargsyan and Saadia A. Faiz

Contents

Introduction 676

Etiology 677
Pulmonary Arterial Hypertension (PAH) 679

Epidemiology 682
PAH 682

Pathophysiology 682
Preload 683
Afterload 684
Contractility and Perfusion 684
Chronic PH 684

Clinical Features 685

Diagnosis 685
Echocardiography 685
Right Heart Catheterization (RHC) 688

Management 688
Stabilize and Identify Triggers 688
Optimize Preload 689
Oxygenation and Ventilation 690
Reduce Right Ventricular (RV) Afterload 690

L. A. Sargsyan
Divisions of Critical Care, Pulmonary, and Sleep
Medicine, Department of Internal Medicine, McGovern
Medical School at The University of Texas Health Science
Center at Houston, Houston, TX, USA
e-mail: lilit.a.sargsyan@uth.tmc.edu

S. A. Faiz (✉)
Department of Pulmonary Medicine, Division of Internal
Medicine, The University of Texas MD Anderson Cancer
Center, Houston, TX, USA
e-mail: safaiz@mdanderson.org

© Springer Nature Switzerland AG 2020
J. L. Nates, K. J. Price (eds.), *Oncologic Critical Care*,
https://doi.org/10.1007/978-3-319-74588-6_47

Optimize RV Contractility and Perfusion 691
Pharmacologic Treatment Modalities 692
Nonpharmacologic Treatment Modalities 692
End-of-Life Care 694

Prognosis 694

Conclusion 694

References 695

Abstract

Pulmonary hypertension (PH) is the condition of elevated pressures in the pulmonary circulation. PH can develop acutely in patients with critical illness such as acute respiratory distress syndrome, sepsis, massive pulmonary embolism, left ventricular dysfunction, or after surgery. In a cancer patient, unique etiologies such as myeloproliferative disorders, tyrosine kinase inhibitors, or tumor emboli may result in PH. Early recognition and treatment of the causative condition may reverse acute PH or return chronic PH to its baseline status. Progression of the disease or its decompensation due to infection, a thromboembolic event, or other triggers can lead to admission to an intensive care unit. Regardless of etiology, the development or worsening of PH may precipitate hypoxemia, hemodynamic instability, or right ventricular failure, which can be challenging to manage or even fatal. In select cases, rapid institution of advanced treatment modalities may be warranted. This chapter reviews the etiology, epidemiology, pathophysiology, clinical features, diagnosis, and prognosis of PH and presents a comprehensive analysis of PH and right heart failure management strategies in the critical care setting. In particular, a unique perspective on oncologically relevant PH is provided.

Keywords

Pulmonary hypertension · Intensive care · Critical care · Cancer · Myeloproliferative disorders · Pulmonary embolism · Cor pulmonale · PAH · TKI · RV failure

Introduction

Pulmonary hypertension (PH) represents a complex and challenging dimension in the management of critically ill patients. Historically, the left heart was considered to be the only pump and the dominant force in the cardiovascular system, while the right heart was seen as a passive conduit through which blood flowed for reoxygenation. The function and importance of the right ventricle (RV) is now much better understood, largely due to the growing experience with right ventricular failure (RVF). Moreover, recent studies have identified RV function as a major determinant of outcomes including mortality, especially after myocardial infarction, in acute pulmonary embolism, and in moderate left heart failure [26]. In the intensive care unit (ICU), acute RV dysfunction has been well described with septic shock and acute respiratory distress syndrome (ARDS), and a decompensated RV, especially in those with chronic PH, portends limited survival [13]. Thus, early detection and treatment of PH and impending RVF can significantly improve outcomes. The RV differs from the left ventricle in both structure and function, and management of a failing RV is fundamentally different. Distinct etiologies for PH exist in the oncologic patient. The purpose of this chapter is to review the etiologies, epidemiology, and clinical features of PH in the oncologic patient, followed by a broad discussion of the pathophysiology, diagnosis, management strategies, and prognosis for subsequent RVF in the critical care setting.

Etiology

PH in the ICU may be associated with a number of causative factors (Table 1), with the most common being left heart failure, sepsis, acute respiratory insufficiency with hypoxia, pulmonary embolism, ARDS, or decompensation of chronic PH. PH is defined as mean pulmonary artery pressure greater than or equal to 25 mm Hg. The World Health Organization (WHO) classifies PH into groups based on etiology, hemodynamics, and treatment options. This classification has evolved from two to five categories as follows: group 1, pulmonary arterial hypertension (PAH); group 2, PH due to left heart disease; group 3, PH due to hypoxia or lung disease; group 4, chronic thromboembolic pulmonary hypertension (CTEPH); and group 5, PH caused by multifactorial mechanisms [80].

The most common cause of right heart failure is left heart failure. In fact, PH secondary to left heart disease (WHO group 2) was recently shown to comprise 69% of all PH, of which 49% was due to valvular disease, 31% to left ventricular systolic dysfunction, and 21% to left ventricular diastolic dysfunction [90]. In addition, PH was found in up to 60% of patients with severe systolic heart failure, up to 70% in those with heart failure with preserved ejection fraction, up to 65% in those with symptomatic aortic stenosis, and in practically everyone with severe symptomatic mitral valve disease [47, 65]. WHO group 2 PH is associated with mean left atrial pressures of >14 mmHg which can result in pulmonary venous hypertension, also known as post-capillary PH. Conditions in this category include left ventricular systolic and diastolic dysfunction, constrictive pericarditis, left atrial myxoma, valvular disease, congenital or acquired left heart inflow/outflow tract obstruction, and congenital cardiomyopathies. Chemotherapy-induced cardiotoxicity may occur in patients having received anthracycline-based regimens, tyrosine kinase inhibitors, alkylating agents, or taxanes [79]. Radiation fields that involve the heart may also accelerate coronary atherosclerosis and induce acute or chronic pericardial disease, valvular heart disease, conduction system disease,

and cardiomyopathy [92]. Young age and left anterior thoracic radiation place patients at higher risk for cardiac damage [31]. Infiltrative diseases such as amyloidosis may also manifest with restrictive cardiomyopathy or PH.

Patients in WHO group 3 have PH due to lung disease and/or hypoxia, including chronic obstructive pulmonary disease (COPD), interstitial lung disease (ILD), other lung diseases with mixed restrictive and obstructive patterns, sleep-disordered breathing such as obstructive sleep apnea, alveolar hypoventilation disorders such as obesity hypoventilation syndrome, and neuromuscular weakness. ARDS promotes hypoxic vasoconstriction, increases alveolar dead space, and releases pro-inflammatory cytokines and pulmonary microthrombi, all of which may result in RVF in up to 30–56% of cases [28]. Predictors of RVF in ARDS include pneumonia-induced ARDS, partial pressure of arterial oxygen/fraction of inspired oxygen ratio <150, partial pressure of carbon dioxide >47 mmHg, and a driving pressure (end-inspiratory plateau pressure minus the positive end-expiratory pressure, PEEP) >18 cm H_2O [61]. Pneumonitis from infections, aspiration, radiation therapy, or drugs can also cause hypoxic pulmonary vasoconstriction resulting in PH. A myriad of chemotherapeutic agents including anti-epidermal growth factor receptor, small-molecule tyrosine kinase inhibitors, mTOR inhibitors, anti-lymphocyte monoclonal antibodies, and even immunotherapy may result in lung injury [3, 71]. Degree of hypoxemic respiratory insufficiency may be compounded if new infiltrates are superimposed on underlying COPD, ILD, or metastatic or primary lung cancer.

Cancer is a well-known cause of venous thromboembolism, and pulmonary embolism may certainly present with PH and, potentially, hemodynamic instability. In a large population-based, case-controlled study to identify risk factors for venous thrombosis, a sevenfold increase in patients with malignancy compared to patients without malignancy was found [7]. Interestingly, there was a 28-fold increase in those with hematologic malignancies, followed by lung cancer and gastrointestinal cancer. Certain anti-

Table 1 Etiologies of pulmonary hypertension (PH) and precipitants of acute right heart failure

	General PH	Oncologic-related PH
Cardiac	• Acute LV failure (systolic, diastolic) • LV ischemia or infarction • RV ischemia or infarction • Arrhythmias (SVT or VT) • Congenital heart disease (e.g., ASD, VSD, Ebstein's anomaly) • Valvulopathies (TR, pulmonary valve stenosis) • Cardiomyopathies including infiltrative disorders • Myocarditis or other inflammatory disorders • Pericardial disease (tamponade, constrictive pericarditis)	• Amyloidosis • Carcinoid heart disease • Cardiac tumors • Radiation therapy • SVC syndrome • Anthracyclines (doxorubicin, epirubicin, idarubicin) • Anthraquinone (mitoxantrone) • Alkylating agents (cyclophosphamide, ifosfamide) • Taxanes (docetaxel) • Tyrosine kinase inhibitors (monoclonal antibody, trastuzumab, bevacizumab; small molecules, sunitinib, dasatinib, imatinib, lapatinib; antimetabolites, clofarabine; proteasome inhibitor, bortezomib)
Endocrine	• Thyrotoxicosis • Pregnancy	• Thyroid cancer • Immunotherapy
Hematologic	• Acute chest syndrome in sickle cell disease • Beriberi syndrome • Anemia	• Chronic myeloproliferative disorders (PAH, CTEPH) • Multiple myeloma
Infection	• Systemic inflammatory states and sepsis	• Cancer patients susceptible due to immunosuppression
Surgery	• Cardiac surgery (e.g., cardiac transplant or LVAD implantation, CAB, valvular) • Noncardiac surgery (e.g., abdominal, vascular)	• Surgery involving tumors around and in the pulmonary circulation and lung resection

Pulmonary	• ARDS
	• Acute pulmonary embolism
	• Hypoxic pulmonary vasoconstriction related to parenchymal lung injury (pneumonia)
	• Mechanical ventilation
	• Exacerbation of lung disease (COPD, ILD, bronchiectasis)
	• Withdrawal of chronic PH therapy
	  • PH (WHO groups 1–5)
	  • Group 1, pulmonary arterial hypertension (PAH)
	    – Group 1, PVOD and/or PCH
	  • Group 2, PH due to left heart disease
	  • Group 3, PH due to lung disease and/or hypoxia including OSA/OHS
	  • Group 4, chronic thromboembolic pulmonary hypertension (CTEPH)
	  • Group 5, pulmonary hypertension with unclear multifactorial mechanisms
		• Pneumonitis from drugs
		• Radiation injury (acute and chronic)
		• Pulmonary emboli
		• PAH (tyrosine kinase inhibitors, chronic myeloproliferative disease)
		• CTEPH
		• Pulmonary circulation tumors (pulmonary artery sarcoma, pulmonary vein sarcoma)
		• Fibrosing mediastinitis (radiation, fungal infection)
		• Tumor emboli (adenocarcinoma)
		• PVOD

Definition of abbreviations: LV, left ventricular; RV, right ventricular; SVT, supraventricular tachycardia; VT, ventricular tachycardia; ASD, atrial septal defect; VSD, ventricular septal defect; TR, tricuspid regurgitation; SVC, superior vena cava; LVAD, left ventricular assist device; CAB, coronary artery bypass; ARDS, acute respiratory distress syndrome; COPD, chronic obstructive pulmonary disease; ILD, interstitial lung disease; WHO, World Health Organization; PAH, pulmonary arterial hypertension; PVOD, pulmonary veno-occlusive disease; PCH, pulmonary capillary hemangiomatosis; OSA, obstructive sleep apnea; OHS, obesity hypoventilation syndrome; CTEPH, chronic thrombo-embolic pulmonary hypertension

angiogenic agents such as thalidomide and vascular endothelial growth factor inhibitors such as bevacizumab may increase the incidence of pulmonary emboli during therapy. Cancer patients often have incidental pulmonary emboli on routine imaging. CTEPH has been described in patients with chronic myeloproliferative disease, subsequently treated with pulmonary vasodilator therapy or thromboendarterectomy [30]. The incidence of CTEPH in cancer populations has not been established, likely due to limitation in long-term follow-up.

PH due to mixed or unclear mechanisms in miscellaneous malignant and nonmalignant conditions is classified under WHO group 5. Such conditions include hematologic disorders (chronic hemolytic anemia, myeloproliferative disorders, splenectomy), systemic disorders (sarcoidosis, pulmonary histiocytosis, lymphangioleiomyomatosis), metabolic disorders (glycogen storage diseases, Gaucher disease, thyroid disorders), as well as tumoral obstruction, fibrosing mediastinitis, chronic renal failure, and segmental PH. Chronic myeloproliferative disorders comprise a rare cause of PH. The potential mechanisms include splenectomy, direct obstruction of pulmonary arteries, chronic thromboembolism, portal hypertension, high cardiac output, and left heart failure [80]. Attributing PH solely to chronic myeloproliferative disease is difficult, as many of the reported cases did not have a right heart catheterization (RHC) needed to definitively diagnose PAH and rule out other causes such as left heart disease [54]. Multiple myeloma has also been associated with PH with potential etiologies that include concomitant amyloidosis, left heart dysfunction, chronic kidney failure, and treatment-related toxicities [50]. Other etiologies of PH in group 5 may be from obstruction of pulmonary vasculature from metastatic disease or primary tumors of the pulmonary vasculature (e.g., pulmonary artery sarcoma), or fibrosing mediastinitis due to previous radiation therapy or fungal infection such as histoplasmosis. Finally, an autopsy series has estimated that 6 to 26% of patients with solid tumors, primarily adenocarcinoma, have pulmonary tumor emboli [74], and these patients may sometimes present antemortem with acute or subacute cor pulmonale [23].

Pulmonary Arterial Hypertension (PAH)

PAH is a disease state that directly affects the pulmonary vasculature and includes idiopathic and heritable PAH, PAH caused by drugs or toxins, PAH associated with connective tissue disease, human immunodeficiency virus (HIV) infection, portal hypertension, congenital heart disease, schistosomiasis, pulmonary veno-occlusive disease (PVOD), and pulmonary capillary hemangiomatosis (PCH). In order to be recognized as WHO group 1, specific criteria for PAH based on RHC must be met (Table 2). PAH has a progressive clinical course studded with episodes of acute decompensation, eventually leading to severe symptoms and heart failure. Death from PAH may occur suddenly in an out-of-hospital setting or slowly from inexorable right heart failure, often necessitating a hospitalization and, frequently, an ICU admission. Even mild, typically reversible events (e.g., infection, new anemia, a small pulmonary embolism) can trigger clinical deterioration.

Sepsis is the most common reason for a patient with PAH to be admitted to the ICU [83], and it should be diagnosed and treated according to the Surviving Sepsis Campaign International guidelines [72]. Special care should be taken to closely monitor hemodynamic status and administer crystalloids cautiously as part of the initial resuscitation in order to prevent volume overload. Pericardial effusion in PAH typically occurs in 13 to 44% of cases, but this number rises with conditions that independently carry a higher incidence of pericardial effusion, such as cancer or collagen vascular disease. Given the chronically elevated right-sided pressures, cardiac tamponade manifests atypically with left atrial and ventricular diastolic collapse [75]. Pulsus paradoxus is also often absent due to the inability of the stiff and dilated RV to pull in more volume during inspiration [19].

There are a few cancer-related etiologies for PAH. Dasatinib, a tyrosine kinase inhibitor used to treat acute and chronic leukemia, has been reported to cause PAH, and in most cases cessation of the drug resolves the PAH [62]. The new generation of tyrosine kinase inhibitors

Table 2 Diagnostic testing for pulmonary hypertension and right ventricular failure

Cardiac	
Electrocardiographic signs	• Right axis deviation, right bundle branch block, anteroseptal ST and T wave changes, P pulmonale (right atrial enlargement), RV hypertrophy, QTc prolongation, and RV strain • Signs of possible PE: sinus tachycardia, "S1Q3T3"

Echocardiographic signs	• Pulmonary artery systolic pressure >40 mmHg is suggestive of PH
	  - Depends on peak TR jet + estimated right atrial pressure [45]
	  - Underestimated when TR jet is minimal
	  - Overestimated in significant anemia
	• RV size and function
	  - RVEF <45%, RV enlargement and hypertrophy
	  - TAPSE <18 mm (normal 2.4–2.7 cm)
	  - RV/LV basal diameter ratio >1.0
	  - IVS flat ("D sign") or bowed into LV (in systole → RV pressure overload, in diastole → RV volume overload)
	  - McConnell sign: early and specific sign of an acute PE
	    • Regional pattern of RV dysfunction with akinesia of the mid-free wall and a normal RV apex [57]
	• Severity of TR: peak TR velocity ≥3 m/s is suggestive of PH
	• Pericardial fluid: poor prognostic sign in PAH
	• Clues for causes of PH
	  - Left heart disease: depressed LVEF, diastolic dysfunction, valvular disease, infiltrative cardiomyopathies
	  - Interatrial shunts seen with an agitated saline bubble study
	• Signs of volume overload
	  - Inferior vena cava diameter >21 mm with decreased respiratory collapse
	  - Right end-systolic atrial area >18 cm^2 [23]
	  - Systolic flow reversal in hepatic veins from severe TR, RV overload, RV stiffness

Right heart catheterization	• Normal: mean pulmonary artery pressures are considered to be around 14 ± 3 mmHg with upper limit of normal of 20 mmHg [37]
	• At risk for PH: mean PAPs of 21–24 mmHg
	• PAH: mean pulmonary artery pressure ≥25 mmHg, pulmonary capillary wedge pressure (PCWP) ≤15 mmHg, pulmonary vascular resistance (PVR) >3 wood units [23]
	• Markers of poor survival: CI <2.2 L/min/m^2, elevated RAP [4]
	  - Pre-capillary PH: PAH, PH due to lung disease, chronic thromboembolic PH (CTEPH), PH with unclear etiology or with multifactorial etiologies, end-expiratory PCWP of ≤15 mmHg [37]
	  - Post-capillary PH: PH from left heart disease, PH of unclear etiology and/or multifactorial mechanisms, PCWP >15 mmHg
	  - DPG (diastolic PAP minus mean PCWP) and the pulmonary vascular resistance (PVR) can help distinguish between isolated post-capillary and combined pre- and post-capillary PH [23]
	    • DPG <7 mmHg and PVR <3 WU = isolated post-capillary PH
	    • DPG of ≥7 mmHg or PVR ≥3 WU = both pre- and post-capillary PH

Imaging	
Chest radiography	• Enlarged cardiac silhouette, decreased retrosternal air space on lateral film (RV enlargement), enlarged central pulmonary arteries
Computed tomography	• Enlarged RV, increased PA diameter of >28 mm, PA: ascending aorta >1 - 73% sensitive and 84% specific for the presence of PH at rest [44] • Reflux of contrast into IVC and hepatic veins • Chronic thromboembolic disease • Signs of PVOD: interstitial edema with diffuse central ground-glass opacification and thickening of interlobular septa • Signs of PCH: diffuse bilateral thickening of the interlobular septa and presence of small, centrilobular poorly circumscribed nodular opacities

(continued)

Table 2 (continued)

Ventilation/perfusion (V/Q) scan	• More sensitive for CTEPH than computed tomography showing one or more segmental or larger mismatched perfusion defects • Tumor emboli: perfusion defects are numerous, symmetric, and more peripheral • Less radiation, most cost-effective, and contrast-free than a CT chest
Cardiac magnetic resonance imaging (MRI)	• Cardiac MRI: Better in delineating RV anatomy, estimating RV end-diastolic volume, RV mass, RV/LV interactions, and RV ejection fraction than echocardiography [4] • Limited use in intensive care unit
Laboratory	
Biomarkers	• BNP >100 pg/mL, NT-proBNP >900 pg/mL: correlate with the degree of RV dysfunction • Good markers for monitoring response to treatment • Increased troponins indicate acute myocardial injury (acute coronary syndrome, myocarditis, acute PE, arrhythmias) and possibly predict poor outcomes in PAH
Pulmonary	
Pulmonary function testing	• Normal spirometry (may have obstruction with COPD or restriction with ILD) • Decreased DLCO
CPET	• Increased VE/VCO$_2$: more dead space and less ventilatory efficiency • Steeper VE to VCO$_2$ slope • Lack of expected decrease in Vd/Vt • Reduced peak VO$_2$ as reduced O$_2$ pulse • VO$_2$ at anaerobic threshold is decreased, earlier lactic acidosis [39]

Definition of abbreviations: RV, right ventricular; PE, pulmonary embolism; P2, pulmonary valve closure sound; PH, pulmonary hypertension; TR, tricuspid regurgitation; RVEF, right ventricular ejection fraction; TAPSE, tricuspid annular plane systolic excursion; LV, left ventricular; IVS, interventricular septum; PAH, pulmonary arterial hypertension; LVEF, left ventricular ejection fraction; PAP, pulmonary artery pressure; PA, pulmonary artery; PCWP, pulmonary capillary wedge pressure; PVR, pulmonary vascular resistance; RAP, right atrial pressure; DPG, diastolic pressure gradient; WU, Wood units; IVC, inferior vena cava; PVOD, pulmonary veno-occlusive disease; PCH, pulmonary capillary hemangiomatosis; CTEPH, chronic thromboembolic pulmonary hypertension; CT, computed tomography; MRI, magnetic resonance imaging; BNP, brain natriuretic peptide; NT-proBNP, N-terminal-proBNP; COPD, chronic obstructive pulmonary disease; ILD, interstitial lung disease; DLCO, diffusing capacity for carbon monoxide; VE/VCO$_2$, minute ventilation relative to CO$_2$ exhalation; Vd/Vt, dead space to tidal volume ratio; VO$_2$, oxygen consumption

(bosutinib, ponatinib, lapatinib) has also been implicated as causing PAH [36, 73, 78]. PAH has also been described in patients with chronic myeloproliferative disorders [5, 30], and, along with pulmonary vasodilator therapy, treatment of the cancer and hematopoietic stem cell transplantation have been described to stabilize, improve, and even resolve the PAH [21, 54, 85].

PVOD is rare and characterized by obliteration of small pulmonary veins by fibrous intimal thickening and patchy capillary proliferation [63]. It may occur after hematopoietic stem cell transplantation [15] or in association with several chemotherapeutic classes, including alkylating agents (most notoriously with cyclophosphamide), antimetabolites, plant alkaloids and naturally occurring molecules, cytotoxic antibiotic and related molecules, cyclosporine, asparaginase, mycophenolate mofetil, anagrelide, interferon, antithymocyte globulin, and monoclonal antibodies [70]. PVOD portends a poor prognosis, and rapid referral should be made to a specialized PAH center for management and possible transplantation.

Surgery in Patients with Preexisting PAH

Patients with chronic PAH, who present for unrelated outpatient surgery, should receive careful perioperative care, preferably in an expert care facility familiar with and equipped for handling RV failure and cardiogenic shock [81]. A consideration should be made to switching oral PAH therapy to parenteral (inhaled or intravenous) ahead of time, as swallowing function and gut absorption may not be predictable perioperatively [23]. PAH patients carry a very large risk of mortality when surgery becomes emergent; and preoperative RV dysfunction, a higher NYHA functional class with worse exercise tolerance, and longer and more intricate surgery are associated with worse outcomes [68]. Induction of general anesthesia poses significant risks due to vasodilation and systemic hypotension, as well as adverse effects of positive pressure ventilation. Additively, surgery itself poses the usual risks, which patients with PAH are hemodynamically less equipped to tolerate. These surgical risks include fluid shifts, the need for continuous anesthetic use and neuromuscular blockade, and unfavorable positioning affecting lung volumes, all with resultant hypoventilation and hypoxemia that raise RV afterload [68]. In contrast, regional anesthetic techniques including nerve blocks and epidural anesthesia are better tolerated and preferentially recommended when possible [23].

Epidemiology

The prevalence of PH in the ICU is difficult to estimate, but the most common causes include left heart failure, pulmonary emboli, sepsis, and ARDS. In acute left heart failure, 3–9% of admissions will have PH and subsequent RVF [35]. In severe COPD, approximately 3–5% have PH at baseline, and exacerbation or pneumonia may result in an ICU admission [13]. CTEPH occurs in 3.8% of patients suffering from an acute pulmonary embolism [67]. In general, WHO groups 2 to 5 are more common and thus more likely to require admission to higher-level care, primarily due to the risk of RVF [13].

PAH

Various national and international registries of patients with PAH (such as the REVEAL registry in the United States) have provided a framework for describing patient characteristics, natural history, and prognostication with data on treatment outcomes of PAH [59]. An important lesson from the current registries is the realization that subpopulations of PAH have significantly different outcomes and that overall survival has improved in the current era of new emerging treatments [58]. The prevalence of idiopathic (IPAH) and heritable PAH (HPAH) is estimated at 5–15 per one million in the general population [43, 52, 58], while European registries estimate prevalence of PAH at 5–52 per one million [2, 47, 66]. The mean age of patients with idiopathic PAH has risen from 36 years to a mean age at diagnosis between 50 and 65 years in the current registries. In addition, the usual female predominance is less certain among older patients. Presentation to the ICU with RVF due to undiagnosed PAH has become increasingly rare and can be explained by improved awareness and earlier recognition of PAH. Furthermore, the newer PAH therapies have stabilized outpatient PAH and may have improved survival; thus ICU admissions are now more frequently due to triggering factors than decompensated PAH itself.

Pathophysiology

In order to treat PH with consequent RVF, it is important to understand the normal physiology of the RV. The thin-walled crescent-shaped RV differs substantially from the muscular and ellipsoidal left ventricle (LV). The RV performs six times less work than the LV while moving the same volume of blood [27, 41]. The RV pumps the entire systemic venous return into the highly compliant, low-resistance pulmonary circulation for gas exchange. In addition, the RV is easily distensible and can accommodate various changes in venous return due to posture, volume status, and respiration while maintaining adequate cardiac output [27].

The interaction of the forces transmitted from one ventricle to the other through the myocardium and pericardium is referred to as ventricular interdependence, and it is vital for ventricular synchrony [29, 41]. The pressure difference between the two ventricles is referred to as the transseptal gradient and is typically around 100 mmHg [82]. The pressure in the LV is normally much higher than in the RV, and the interventricular septum (IVS) in its normal state

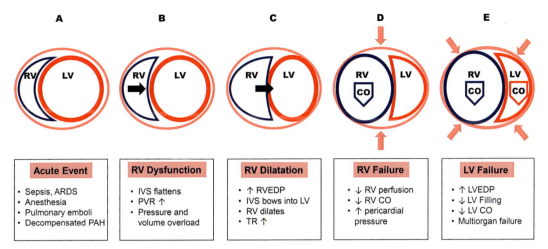

Fig. 1 Pathophysiology of right ventricular (RV) failure. An acute event (**A**) triggers right ventricular pressure and volume overload and dysfunction (**B**), causing flattening of the interventricular septum (black arrow). Subsequently, the right ventricular end-diastolic pressure begins to rise, the right ventricle begins to dilate (**C**), and tricuspid regurgitation worsens. As the interventricular septum further bows into the left ventricle with concomitant pericardial constriction (pink arrows), the right ventricle becomes ischemic from decreased perfusion and begins to fail (**D**), dropping its cardiac output (blue arrow). The failing right ventricle then compromises left ventricular filling (**E**), causing rising left ventricular end-diastolic pressures and left ventricular failure. As systemic cardiac output drops (red arrow), ensuing hypotension results in multi-organ failure and possibly death. Definition of abbreviations: RV, right ventricular; LV, left ventricle; CO, cardiac output; ARDS, adult respiratory distress syndrome; PAH, pulmonary arterial hypertension; IVS, interventricular septum; PVR, pulmonary vascular resistance; RVEDP, right ventricular end-diastolic pressure; TR, tricuspid regurgitation; LVEDP, left ventricular end-diastolic pressure

bulges into the RV, acting as a splint against which the RV contracts.

Cardiac output for both the RV and LV is governed by the same three factors: preload, afterload, and myocardial contractility. Coronary perfusion to the RV occurs during both systole and diastole, while LV perfusion occurs during diastole, thus making the RV dependent on systolic blood pressure. Perturbations in the normal physiology lead to RV dysfunction and eventually RVF (Fig. 1).

Preload

Both underfilling and overfilling of the RV can be detrimental. Decreased preload, as seen with an underfilled RV, leads to reduced stroke volume and cardiac output. Sepsis can exacerbate the underfilled RV with a low effective intravascular volume. Subsequent initiation of mechanical ventilation further increases intrathoracic pressures and negatively affects venous return, and the effect may be augmented with high levels of PEEP. Conversely, factors that excessively increase venous return result in volume overload for the RV, leading to tension and possible ischemia of its free wall, stretching of the tricuspid valve annulus, and flattening and bowing of the IVS into the LV. Thus, the RV cardiac output decreases and negatively affects LV filling and cardiac output as well. Conditions that manifest with an increased RV preload include tricuspid or pulmonic regurgitation, atrial septal defect, anomalous pulmonary venous return, and states of overall volume overload such as renal failure or after resuscitation for shock. Myocardial depression and decreased LV contractility often occur with sepsis in part due to oxygen supply and demand mismatch [40] and in part because of the effects of circulating cytokines such as tumor necrosis factor-alpha [8, 25]. As a result, the RV develops diastolic dysfunction as well as decreased contractility by the same mechanisms of myocyte hypoxia and circulating pro-inflammatory mediators. As sepsis resolves, both LV and RV function may normalize.

Afterload

The pulmonary vascular bed represents the afterload for the RV. In normal circumstances of increased oxygen demand, such as during exercise, the pulmonary circulation is able to both recruit and distend more vessels, thus realizing its great capacitance. Pulmonary blood flow and the ability to oxygenate are enhanced to match oxygen demand and rising systemic cardiac output. Conditions that affect the pulmonary circulation by increasing the pulmonary vascular resistance (PVR) include acute pulmonary embolism, RV outflow tract obstruction, hypoxic pulmonary vasoconstriction, pulmonary stenosis, and all chronic forms of PH. Sepsis causes vasoactive, microthrombotic, and inflammatory damage to the pulmonary circulation, raising the PVR [68]. In the ICU, volume loss (atelectasis, consolidation, pleural effusions, mainstem intubation) and overdistension (dynamic hyperinflation, high tidal volumes or PEEP) as well as acidemia, hypercarbia, hypoxemia, and hypothermia may also raise the PVR [82]. Alveolar hypoxia leads to hypoxic pulmonary vasoconstriction, decreased nitric oxide (NO), and increased endothelin production in the pulmonary circulation, causing further local vasoconstriction [25] Lastly, disseminated intravascular coagulation, commonly part of sepsis, may cause microthrombi to form in the pulmonary arterial tree [9].

Contractility and Perfusion

Conditions that manifest with decreased RV contractility include RV infarction, arrhythmias, cardiomyopathy, and sepsis. In conditions of acute RV failure, such as during a massive PE, pressure in the pulmonary vascular bed rapidly increases, thus causing RV pressure to increase. Although the RV can dilate to accommodate the increased preload, its thin free wall precludes adequate acute adaptation to increased afterload. Once myocyte recruitment per the Frank-Starling mechanism has been maximized, any further increase in afterload will trigger a precipitous decrease in RV contractile function [27]. The dilated RV free wall experiences increased tension and ischemia, which further reduces free wall contractility. RV dilatation also results in stretching of the tricuspid annulus with subsequent tricuspid regurgitation (TR). The pericardial pressure also rises concurrently with the rising RV pressures and can constrain the cardiac chambers, further reducing their compliance, filling, and output [32].

Under excessive volume and pressure, the globular RV eventually pushes the IVS toward and into the LV cavity, compromising LV filling, stroke volume, and cardiac output. The resulting systemic hypotension further reduces coronary flow, RV perfusion, and RV cardiac output [51]. Thus, the cycle propagates, with a failing RV compromising LV function, and a struggling LV increasing the demand on the RV thus leading to worsened RV function followed closely by multi-organ hypoperfusion and failure.

Chronic PH

In cases of chronic PH (of either pre- or post-capillary etiology), the RV responds to increased pressures in the pulmonary vascular bed with progressive hypertrophy, thus maintaining cardiac output at rest over long periods of time [35]. In the end stage, the RV dilates, which leads to worsened TR and ultimately decreased cardiac output. Acute decompensation of chronic pulmonary hypertension may be clinically indistinguishable from acute RVF.

PAH in particular is a progressive vasculopathy, in which the pulmonary vascular bed undergoes intimal and smooth muscle hypertrophy, adventitial remodeling complicated with fibrosis, in situ vasoconstriction, and microthrombosis [42]. The histopathologic hallmark of PAH is the plexiform lesion, which consists of obliterative endothelial cell proliferation and vascular smooth muscle cell hypertrophy in small pre-capillary pulmonary arterioles. These changes over time cause an increase in pulmonary artery pressures and subsequently PVR. With a gradual rise in PVR, the RV can adapt by means of hypertrophy in order to preserve its cardiac output and ventriculoarterial coupling [64].

Clinical Features

PH may be suspected due to presenting signs and symptoms or, not infrequently, due to incidentally noted features on a diagnostic test (Table 2) such as electrocardiogram, echocardiography (Fig. 2), or other imaging (Fig. 3). Cardinal symptoms of volume overload such as jugular venous distention, peripheral edema, and ascites indicate RVF, also referred to as cor pulmonale. In the absence of an established diagnosis, presenting clinical features may point in the direction of an underlying cause of PH. For example, obesity and awake alveolar hypoventilation may indicate obesity hypoventilation syndrome, inspiratory crackles and clubbing may point toward interstitial lung disease, while sclerodactyly and digital ulcers may suggest systemic sclerosis.

As the pulmonary artery enlarges further, it may exert mass effect on adjacent structures to cause wheezing from compression of airways, hoarseness from compression of the recurrent laryngeal nerve, or cardiac ischemia from compression of the left main coronary artery [23, 68]. A massively enlarged pulmonary artery is also at risk for dissection or spontaneous rupture, potentially causing cardiac tamponade or dramatic hemodynamic collapse and death [23].

On cardiac examination, presence of a right parasternal lift, an accentuated pulmonary component of a second heart sound (loud P2), a right-sided third heart sound (S3), pansystolic murmur of TR, or a diastolic murmur of pulmonary regurgitation may all raise suspicion for PH, while jugular venous distention, hepatic enlargement and tenderness, and hepatojugular reflux may indicate right heart failure. Signs of left-sided heart failure may include a left-sided third heart sound (S3), crackles on lung examination, displaced apical impulse, or cool cyanotic extremities.

Diagnosis

Certain conditions may initially present as PH in the ICU but then return to normal pulmonary pressures days to weeks after treatment. Airway exacerbation caused by underlying COPD or ILD, acute decompensated left heart failure, pulmonary embolism, and sepsis are prime examples. A subset of these patients already has or will develop PH as a sequela of their disease. Chronic PH is often a comorbidity that becomes destabilized by an acute insult or critical illness. If chronic PH is suspected during an ICU admission, an attempt should be made to confirm the diagnosis adequately and classify it appropriately, for pulmonary vasodilator therapy could be part of the treatment.

Detection of PH in the ICU centers around two main tools: echocardiography and pulmonary artery catheterization. A thorough history may provide information regarding risk factors for heart disease, pulmonary emboli or chronic PH, as well as symptoms that preceded ICU admission. Other studies (Table 2) may also be suggestive of PH.

Echocardiography

Echocardiography is a dependable tool for screening and serial follow-up of pulmonary pressures and both left and right heart function in outpatient PH. Its role in the ICU is indispensable in quick and noninvasive measurement of the pulmonary artery systolic pressure (PASP), assessment of RV structure and function, estimation of volume status, evaluation of TR severity, evaluation of the pericardium, and search for causes of PH such as intracardiac shunts and left heart disease [60] (Table 2). Measuring the PASP depends on the peak TR jet Doppler velocity plus an estimate of the right atrial pressure [45]. An estimated PASP greater than 40 mmHg or a peak TR jet velocity ≥ 3 m/s is predictive of PH [45]. The tricuspid

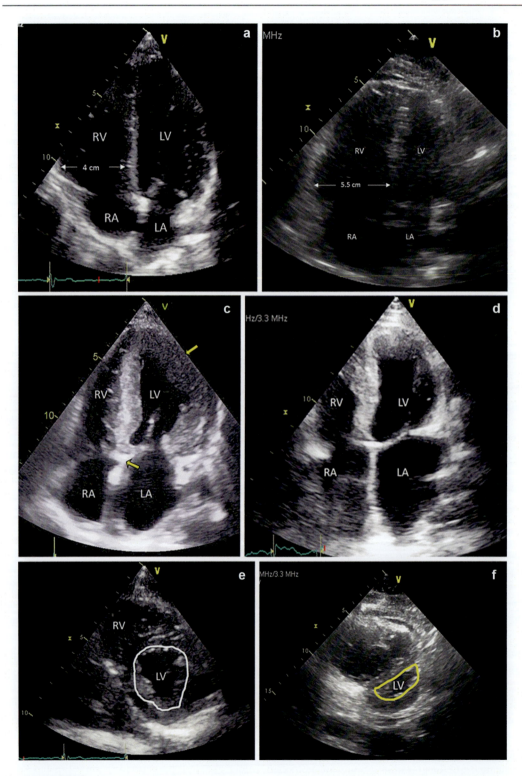

Fig. 2 (continued)

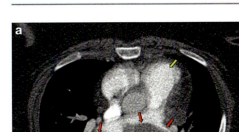
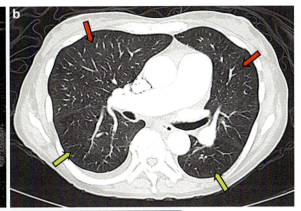
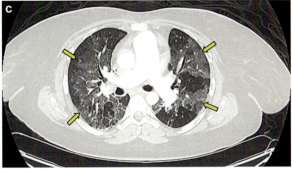

Fig. 3 CT imaging of pulmonary hypertension. (**a**) Saddle embolus (red arrows) that bridges across the pulmonary artery from the heart as it divides into right and left main pulmonary arteries with enlarged pulmonary artery (yellow arrow). (**b**) Myelofibrosis with severe pulmonary arterial hypertension (a mean pulmonary artery pressure of 49, pulmonary capillary wedge pressure of 9, pulmonary vascular resistance of 9.4) with CT angiogram revealing no pulmonary embolism but prominent enlarged main pulmonary artery with mosaic attenuation (yellow arrows, decreased lung perfusion; red arrow, increased lung perfusion) within lung parenchyma. (**c**) Ovarian cancer (status post five cycles of vinblastine, cisplatin, cyclophosphamide, bleomycin, doxorubicin, and etoposide) with hypoxic respiratory insufficiency, new bilateral infiltrates, and pulmonary hypertension on echocardiogram thought to be related to bleomycin toxicity. Oxygen was limited due to concern for bleomycin toxicity, and she was treated with high-dose steroids and empiric antimicrobial therapy. Definition of abbreviations: CT, computed tomography

annular plane systolic excursion (TAPSE) should be about 2.4–2.7 cm, while values below 1.8 cm have been shown to correlate well with a decreased stroke volume index and RV ejection fraction, as well as increased hospitalizations for RHF and decreased survival in those with PAH [86]. Higher PASPs often imply that the PH is chronic, and the RV may have had time to hypertrophy, or there is acute-on-chronic PH. Dilation or hypokinesis of the RV or a flattened (or bowing) IVS suggests RV pressure and volume overload. Echocardiography also rules out or confirms pericardial effusion, measures cardiac chamber sizes,

Fig. 2 Transthoracic echocardiogram. Four-chamber view in diastole of a normal right ventricle base (**a**) measuring 4 cm (should be less than 4.2 cm), dilated right ventricle (**b**) in pulmonary hypertension, restrictive cardiomyopathy (**c**) in an amyloid in patient with thickened septum (yellow arrow between RA and LA) and left ventricular cavity wall (yellow arrow next to LV), and diastolic heart failure (**d**) with enlarged left atrium and ventricle. Parasternal view with normal right and left ventricle (**e**) and dilated right ventricle (**f**) with D-shaped left ventricular (yellow outline) suggestive of volume and pressure overload (Echocardiographic images courtesy of Juan Lopez-Mattei, MD, MD Anderson Cancer Center, Houston, Texas). Definition of abbreviations: LA, left atrium; LV, left ventricle; RA, right atrium; RV right ventricle

and may reveal constrictive physiology and/or the presence of infiltrative cardiomyopathy.

Right Heart Catheterization (RHC)

A RHC procedure is done to confirm elevated pulmonary artery pressures and aids in classifying PH, grading its severity, and assessing for vasoreactivity. Pressures in right-sided heart chambers and the pulmonary artery can be directly measured, while the left atrial pressure can be estimated by measuring the pulmonary capillary wedge pressure (PCWP). In addition, cardiac output, cardiac index, as well as systemic vascular resistance (SVR) and PVR can be calculated. Vasoreactivity studies with NO, adenosine, or prostacyclins may be performed at baseline to evaluate the responsiveness of the pulmonary circulation and also provide prognostic information, but they should be avoided in patients with significant evidence of post-capillary PH [60]. In those who respond, calcium channel blockers could be a potential treatment option.

Management

Regardless of the etiology, the natural progression of PH inevitably leads to RVF. Treatment directed toward the underlying cause is important; however, the exact trigger may not always be obvious. Strategies are crucial to optimize preload and cardiac contractility, enhance systemic arterial perfusion, and reduce right ventricular afterload. In cases of new or decompensated PAH, coordination of care and potential transfer to a specialized PH center should be arranged early, if possible.

In order to maximize hemodynamic recovery in RVF, a few overarching principles need to be considered and optimized concurrently (Fig. 4). It is useful to have an arterial catheter and a central venous catheter in the internal jugular or subclavian position for close hemodynamic monitoring. These allow for serial measurements of central venous pressure (CVP), arterial blood gases, central venous oxygen saturation (ScvO2), and lactic

acid levels. A rising lactic acid and a dropping or low ScvO2 level can be used as surrogates for end-organ hypoperfusion from a decreasing cardiac output. Other signs of acute end-organ injury may include elevated serum creatinine or decreasing urine output indicating renal insufficiency, while elevated liver enzymes or new coagulopathy may suggest liver injury. It is important to note that venous congestion seen with an overdistended RV and that from reduced cardiac output from RV underfilling may have similar presentations, which necessitates accurate measurement of CVP. In certain complex cases, such as a mixed shock state, a case where trending PVR and PCWP are important, or post cardiac surgery, a pulmonary artery catheter may be necessary to optimize management of RVF.

Stabilize and Identify Triggers

Among the first priorities of treating RVF is proper identification and control of exacerbating factors. Sepsis, pulmonary embolism, and acute coronary syndrome are notorious culprits of PH in the ICU. In patients with septic shock, empiric antimicrobial therapy and identification of infectious etiology are vital. Institution of high-flow oxygen or noninvasive positive pressure ventilation may help stabilize patients with hypoxic or hypercapnic respiratory insufficiency. Patients with pulmonary embolism and hemodynamic compromise should be evaluated for systemic thrombolytics, and in nonresponders or those who cannot receive them, surgical embolectomy, catheter-directed thrombolysis, as well as mechanical circulatory support devices such as extracorporeal membrane oxygenation (ECMO) and right ventricular assist devices (RVAD) can be considered when appropriate [48, 56, 76, 88]. Ensuring that RV ischemia is not a result of an acute coronary syndrome is important since rapid revascularization by percutaneous coronary intervention could be necessary to restore RV perfusion. Prompt cessation of any pharmacologic agents that may have precipitated PH, such as tyrosine kinase inhibitors, chemotherapy,

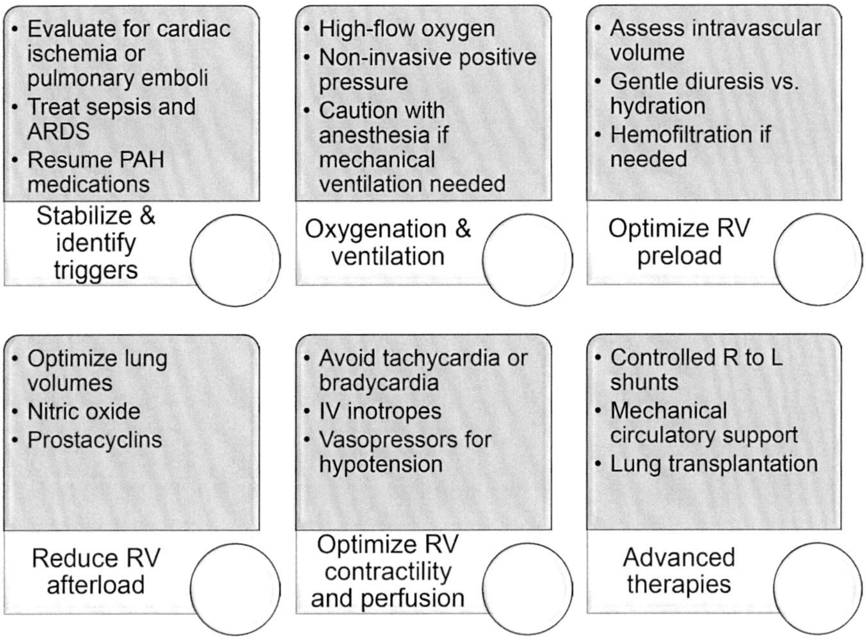

• Evaluate for cardiac ischemia or pulmonary emboli • Treat sepsis and ARDS • Resume PAH medications	• High-flow oxygen • Non-invasive positive pressure • Caution with anesthesia if mechanical ventilation needed	• Assess intravascular volume • Gentle diuresis vs. hydration • Hemofiltration if needed
Stabilize & identify triggers	Oxygenation & ventilation	Optimize RV preload
• Optimize lung volumes • Nitric oxide • Prostacyclins	• Avoid tachycardia or bradycardia • IV inotropes • Vasopressors for hypotension	• Controlled R to L shunts • Mechanical circulatory support • Lung transplantation
Reduce RV afterload	Optimize RV contractility and perfusion	Advanced therapies

Fig. 4 Management of right ventricular failure. Strategies to stabilize should be taken swiftly and concomitantly rather than sequentially. Consultation and transfer of patients with pulmonary arterial hypertension (PAH) to a specialized pulmonary hypertension center should be considered. Definition of abbreviations: ARDS, adult respiratory distress syndrome; PAH, pulmonary arterial hypertension; RV, right ventricular; IV, intravenous; R, right heart; L, left heart

anorexigens, or illicit drugs, is imperative. The use of steroids and/or nebulized therapy could be a part of the treatment for exacerbations of COPD or ILD. In cases of PAH therapy withdrawal, restarting pulmonary vasodilators is crucial. In those with suspected CTEPH, review with and/or referral to a specialized surgical center for consideration of pulmonary endarterectomy is imperative. Finally, continuous vigilance to correct metabolic abnormalities including acidosis, hypoxemia, hypercapnia, hypothermia, and hypocalcemia is vital to sustain RV contractility negatively affected by these factors.

Optimize Preload

Patients with RV failure, especially those with chronic PH, may be preload-dependent, so ensuring adequate RV filling without allowing overload is crucial to maintain RV function. Using invasive or noninvasive measurements of CVP and cardiac output is necessary to determine optimal RV filling. Aggressive volume resuscitation or vigorous diuresis should be discouraged, and cautious fluid replacement or gradual diuresis with monitoring should be considered especially since concomitant hypotension may be present. Aiming for a CVP of around 10–14 mmHg is usually recommended.

Often a dysfunctional RV may be distended and overloaded, requiring volume removal in addition to providing inotropic support. If the kidneys are functioning, diuresis with intravenous loop diuretic agents can be tried initially, using careful continuous infusion in case of hypotension. As heart failure induces a hyperaldosterone state, addition of spironolactone, barring any contraindications, such as hyperkalemia, may be helpful [68]. Furthermore, dopamine has been used in low doses to improve renal perfusion, thus aiding in natriuresis [20, 24]. Lastly, tolvaptan, an oral selective vasopressin antagonist, has been studied with promising results [84], but needs further validation. The goal is to attain 1–1.5 L of net negative fluid balance per day to avoid large hemodynamic swings and any acute drastic decrease in RV preload. In cases of profound RVF leading to dense renal injury (or acute or chronic renal insufficiency of other etiologies), ultrafiltration through continuous renal replacement therapy may be required.

Oxygenation and Ventilation

Oxygen is the most important physiologic vasodilator of the pulmonary system, and it may ameliorate hypoxic pulmonary vasoconstriction and reduce PVR. High-flow oxygen may be especially useful in avoiding or preventing intubation. In those with underlying lung disease or concomitant left heart dysfunction, noninvasive positive pressure therapy may help reduce the labor of breathing and improve ventilation. Positive airway pressure, however, can negatively affect RV function. In those with hemodynamic instability, altered mentation, or persistent hypoxemia, intubation with mechanical ventilation may be unavoidable despite its risks of significant metabolic and hemodynamic adverse effects. Hypotension with induction is common from sedating agents and neuromuscular blockade, and it may also occur from withdrawal of the potent sympathetic drive when work of breathing is relieved. Lastly, placing the patient in the supine position worsens hypoxemia through physiologic shunting. Therefore, in cases of decompensated PH and RVF, intubation should be avoided if at all possible. When intubation is necessary, precautions must be taken to prevent hypotension, acidosis, hypercarbia, and hypoxemia. Typically, medications that are considered relatively safe to use include opiates, benzodiazepines, etomidate, and ketamine at the lowest effective doses. If possible, propofol and paralysis should be avoided to prevent hypotension or, if needed, should be co-administered with a vasopressor empirically to prevent hypotension. It is also wise to have a vasopressor infusion

prepared and ready to administer if sudden hypotension occurs.

Reduce Right Ventricular (RV) Afterload

Reduction of RV afterload essentially implies reduction of PVR, and when possible, non-pharmacologic strategies to reduce RV afterload should be instituted rapidly. In those who are mechanically ventilated, a high PEEP may increase PVR and decrease venous return thereby affecting preload, so limiting plateau and PEEP pressures is important. Attaining and maintaining optimal lung volumes is crucial as both over-distension and atelectasis of lung units increase the PVR. Atelectatic alveoli compress extra-alveolar vessels, resulting in an increase in PVR. Overdistension of alveoli compresses intra-alveolar vessels, still causing an increase in PVR [11]. Other helpful strategies include drainage of significant pleural effusions, sedation to prevent ventilator dyssynchrony, and appropriate positioning of the patient (including proning).

Pharmacologic therapy will almost invariably be required. Significant improvement in RV function can be achieved only with significant decrease in PVR [91]. Inhaled pulmonary artery vasodilators are effective by directly lowering the PVR, and the improved perfusion then optimizes ventilation/perfusion matching in well-ventilated parts of lung [17]. As hypoxemia improves, PVR is reduced further. Inhaled NO can easily be administered in either ventilated or non-ventilated patients in doses of 10–40 ppm. NO is often used in severe ARDS and also perioperatively for cardiac surgery in heart failure. Prolonged use at high doses, though, can cause accumulation of methemoglobin as well as other oxidants such as NO_2 [89]. In addition, abrupt withdrawal of NO may cause devastating rebound of PH [12]; therefore it needs to be weaned slowly.

Much of the evidence for use of medications in PAH pertains to chronic outpatient management rather than critical care in an ICU setting. Because of the lack of robust evidence, most current practices are specific to individual preferences, facility culture, and expert opinion. Moreover, a large majority of targeted PAH medications that are revolutionizing outpatient PAH treatment are not indicated in the majority of patients with RVF without PAH. For those patients with chronic PAH, all chronic pulmonary vasodilator therapy should be resumed. In patients with decompensated PAH and RVF, intravenous or inhaled prostanoids should be emergently initiated, and ideally invasive monitoring should be started to guide titration based on hemodynamic measures. Concurrent inotropic support with dobutamine or dopamine, as well as vasopressor support with norepinephrine or vasopressin, may be necessary during this process to maintain hemodynamic stability. Targets of end-organ perfusion such as lactic acid, ScvO2, urine output, and liver function tests should also be serially monitored. Abrupt discontinuation of IV prostacyclin can lead to rapid deterioration from rebound PH; therefore interruptions should be carefully anticipated and avoided. Longer-acting analogues of prostacyclin (iloprost and treprostinil) can be administered through nebulization [10]. Inhaled milrinone has also been studied alone as well as in combination with inhaled prostacyclin in the context of cardiovascular surgery, but it is not widely used at this time [6, 16, 34]. Sildenafil, a phosphodiesterase-5 inhibitor, can be used in treating acute cardiogenic RV shock from PH [22]. Percutaneous balloon pulmonary angioplasty (BPA) is an alternative option to pulmonary endarterectomy in CTEPH and carries a significant risk of reperfusion injury, embolism, and pulmonary artery perforation [1]. Therefore, these procedures are best performed at specialized centers.

Optimize RV Contractility and Perfusion

Treating systemic hypotension should be one of the earliest steps in management of RV failure. Vasopressors must be initiated rapidly in order to restore adequate mean arterial pressure, but those that raise SVR and not PVR should be preferentially selected. Norepinephrine is used as the first-line agent and does not significantly raise PVR [46]. Vasopressin acts through non-adrenergic V1 receptors and is either PVR neutral or potentially may even lower it slightly [68].

Milrinone, a phosphodiesterase-3 inhibitor, and to a lesser extent dobutamine, a beta agonist, decrease the PVR while increasing contractility. Both agents, but especially milrinone, cause systemic vasodilation that can result in or exacerbate hypotension. Therefore, while necessary to improve forward flow through the pulmonary vasculature with inotropic agents, norepinephrine or vasopressin may be concurrently necessary to maintain an adequate SVR. Dobutamine is typically the first choice for inotropic support, but dopamine and milrinone are also options. All catecholamines carry a risk of causing or worsening tachycardia, and milrinone may also cause atrial arrhythmias. Aside from cases of concomitant left heart failure, digoxin does not have much of a role in the treatment of RVF. Levosimendan, a calcium sensitizer and phosphodiesterase-3 inhibitor, enhances cardiac contractility without increasing myocardial oxygen demand, but it may result in systemic and pulmonary vasodilation [68] and atrial arrhythmias. In a recent meta-analysis, levosimendan showed significant increase in TAPSE and ejection fraction, with decrease in PASP and PVR [69].

The preservation and restoration of sinus rhythm are also a high priority with an optimal heart rate range of 80–100 beats per minute. Bradycardia seen with conduction abnormalities can reduce RV stroke volume by allowing more time for TR, while supraventricular tachycardias (SVT) can reduce RV stroke volume by decreasing the time for RV filling; neither are well tolerated and should be treated expeditiously if they occur [33]. Direct current cardioversion should be done early to restore normal sinus rhythm, ventricular filling, and cardiac output. Although amiodarone has a slower onset of action, it does not have negative inotropic effects, and is beneficial for maintaining sinus rhythm after cardioversion. When an SVT involves the atrioventricular node, adenosine may be considered prior to cardioversion [68]. The use of beta-blockers and calcium channel blockers is controversial and, if pursued, should be done cautiously, since both may have a detrimental effect on the RV.

Malignant arrhythmias such as ventricular tachycardia, torsades de pointes, and ventricular fibrillation can occur for variety of reasons. Triggering factors for arrhythmias, including electrolyte abnormalities, metabolic disturbances (thyroid disease), myocardial ischemia, and medication interactions (QTC prolongation), should be uncovered and treated.

Pharmacologic Treatment Modalities

Pharmacologic therapies and their properties are detailed in Table 3. The vasopressors recommended for use are typically norepinephrine and vasopressin, but phenylephrine may be considered. The inotropes include dobutamine, dopamine, and epinephrine, while the inodilators include milrinone and levosimendan. In addition, in order to decrease RV afterload, pulmonary vasodilators, most commonly NO, are a crucial part of acute RVF treatment.

Nitric oxide

Inhaled NO is very short acting and is quickly inactivated in the pulmonary capillaries, causing little to no systemic effects [93]. Thus, NO or its donors (inhaled nitroglycerin or sodium nitroprusside) rapidly and effectively lower the PVR and can be easily administered as an inhaled gas. Several targeted PAH agents exploit the NO pathway for treatment of PAH.

Prostacyclins

Inhaled prostacyclins, iloprost and treprostinil, are both options for PH. Prostacyclin was the first agent used and was shown to improve outcomes in PH, RV dysfunction, and refractory hypoxemia after cardiovascular surgery [18], and it may be more economical and more available than inhaled NO in many ICUs.

Other pulmonary vasodilators

In the outpatient setting, endothelin receptor agonists (bosentan, ambrisentan, macitentan), phosphodiesterase-5 inhibitors (sildenafil and tadalafil), the soluble guanylate cyclase agonist (riociguat), as well as oral prostanoids (selexipag, Orenitram) are all widely used for PAH. Combination therapy is now the standard for a significantly lower risk of clinical failure events. However, these oral agents do not have a role in acute management of RVF in the ICU.

Nonpharmacologic Treatment Modalities

Balloon Atrial Septostomy (BAS)

An artificial surgical atrial septal right-to-left shunt can be created in order to decompress the right heart chambers, thus decreasing RV wall stress, volume, and pressure overload and increasing LV preload and cardiac output. BAS is indicated in patients with functional class IV symptoms with RHF from PH who are optimized and refractory to all other medical therapy. In these cases, BAS can serve either as a bridge to lung transplantation or as a palliative care measure [77]. Since BAS carries a risk of further oxygen desaturation and a higher risk of complications in patients with baseline mean RAP >20 mmHg or oxygen saturation at rest of <85% on room air [23], it should be avoided in these cases.

Mechanical Circulatory Support

Mechanical circulatory support should be considered in those with persistent RVF who are optimized on medical therapy. Transfer to a specialized center is essential, and device selection is based on etiology of RVF and expected duration of mechanical support. The timing of placement ideally occurs prior to end-organ damage, for multi-organ failure is the leading cause of death in unsuccessful cases [35]. RVF due to RV myocardial infarction, acute pulmonary embolism, following left ventricular assist device (LVAD) implantation, or primary graft failure after heart transplantation are clinical scenarios in which acute mechanical circulatory support may be required.

In cases of primary pulmonary etiology, ECMO is the most appropriate therapy, as an

Table 3 Pharmacotherapy available to treat pulmonary hypertension or decompensation of right ventricular failure

Agent (receptor & MOA)	Primary goal Secondary effect	Usual dosing	Adverse effects other notes
Increased inotropy			
Dopamine Low to medium dose (D, β1 > α1) High dose (α1 = β1, D)	↑ Inotropy ↑ Renal perfusion ↑ CI ↑ SVR at higher doses	2–10 μg/kg/min 10–50 μg/kg/min	Tachycardia Arrhythmias ↑ PVR at higher doses
Dobutamine (β1 > β2)	↑ Inotropy ↑ CI, ↓ PVR	2.5–15 μg/kg/min	Tachycardia, arrhythmias Hypotension (↓ SVR)
Epinephrine (α1 = β1 > β2)	↑ CI ↓ PVR, ↑ SVR	0.1–0.5 μg/kg/min	Tachycardia, arrhythmias
Milrinone (PDE$_3$I)	↑ Inotropy ↑ CI, ↓ PVR	Load: 50 μg/kg 0.25–0.75 μg/kg/min	Tachycardia, arrhythmias Hypotension (↓ SVR)
Levosimendan (Ca^{2+} sensitizer and PDE$_3$I)	↑ Inotropy ↑ CI, ↓ PVR	Load: 6–12 μg/kg 0.05–0.2 μg/kg/min	Tachycardia, arrhythmias Hypotension (↓ SVR)
Digitalis	↑ Inotropy ↓ HR	Rhythm control in atrial fibrillation	AV blocks Use when ↓ LVEF
Decreased pulmonary vascular resistance			
Inhaled NO	↓ PVR	10–40 ppm	Methemoglobinemia Hypotension
Inhaled prostanoids Iloprost Treprostinil	↓ PVR	2.5–5 μg 6–9/day 6–54 μg QID	Hypotension, headache Flushing Jaw pain
IV/SC prostanoids Epoprostenol (IV) Treprostinil (IV/SC)	↓PVR	1–40 ng/kg/min	Hypotension, headache Flushing, jaw pain
Sildenafil IV/SL (PDE$_5$I)	↓ PVR	5–20 mg TID	Hypotension
Increased mean arterial pressure			
Norepinephrine (α1 > β1)	↑ SVR ↑ CI	0.01–3 μ/kg/min	Tachycardia, arrhythmias PVR neutral at low doses ↑ PVR at higher doses
Vasopressin (V1, D)	↑ SVR	0.01–0.03 IU/min	PVR, CI neutral Heart rate neutral
Phenylephrine (α1)	↑ SVR	0.5–5 μg/kg/min	↓ CI, ↑ PVR Reflex bradycardia

Medications are grouped by their primary goal effect. Pink, increased inotropy; blue, decreased pulmonary vascular resistance; yellow, increased mean arterial pressure.

Definition of abbreviations: PH, pulmonary hypertension; RVF, right ventricular failure; MOA, mechanism of action; D, dopamine receptor; β1, beta-1 adrenergic receptor; β2, beta-2 adrenergic receptor; α1, alpha-1 adrenergic receptor; PDE$_3$I, phosphodiesterase-3 inhibitor; NO, nitric oxide; IV, intravenous; SC, subcutaneous; SL, sublingual; PDE$_5$I, phosphodiesterase-5 inhibitor; V1, vasopressin-1 receptor; PVR, peripheral vascular resistance; CI, cardiac index; SVR, systemic vascular resistance; HR, heart rate; QID, four times a day; TID, three times a day; IU, international units; ppm, parts per million; AV, atrioventricular; LVEF, left ventricular ejection fraction

right ventricular assist device (RVAD) may further increase PASP and potentially precipitate pulmonary hemorrhage [49, 55]. An RVAD is more appropriate when RHF is from an isolated RV etiology. Advanced heart failure from an LV etiology usually requires an LVAD, while biventricular failure or RHF following LVAD implantation or heart transplantation may necessitate placement of a biventricular assist device or a total artificial heart device [49, 55]. The use of permanent mechanical support devices in RHF caused by chronic PH is contentious, off-label and needs further study [49, 55].

Transplantation

Cardiac transplant is the ultimate treatment for refractory RVF [35]. Of note, presence of an RVAD support before heart transplantation is associated with a higher mortality [53].

In those with PAH, referral should be made before severe RHF develops. Patients with PVOD and PCH have the worst prognosis and should be listed for transplantation at diagnosis, given the lack of treatment options [23]. Patients with PAH associated with connective tissue disease also have a relatively poor prognosis compared with idiopathic PAH patients, while those with congenital heart disease PAH have a better survival. The overall survival following transplantation for PAH has increased to 52–75% at 5 years and 45–66% at 10 years [23]. Double-lung, isolated heart, and heart-lung transplantation have been done for PAH, but a double-lung transplant is the most commonly performed modality. Typically, the right heart has a good ability to recover its function after elimination of PAH, but in certain situations, a heart transplant is also necessary [23].

End-of-Life Care

Prognosis of RVF in the ICU is guarded, and in cases of RVF refractory to aggressive medical management, focus on symptom control and supportive care may be prudent. Ideally, in an oncologic setting the conversation regarding end-of-life care has already been initiated, but often the intensivist may have to focus on the goals of care early during the admission. Frank discussions regarding potential treatment options and prognosis are recommended. Assistance from a dedicated palliative care team may be helpful.

Due to the natural course of PAH and unpredictability of deterioration and adverse outcomes, discussions of prognosis, prospects for transplantation, and the patient's wishes regarding end-of-life care should be held early and readdressed with changes in condition. The multidisciplinary PAH care team most familiar with each patient and family should carry this responsibility in a stable, calm environment. If transplant is not a possibility, then the patient may elect to decline any advanced therapies, including admission to an ICU or resuscitation in case of cardiac arrest.

Prognosis

Estimates of in-hospital mortality of patients with RVF range from 5% to 17% [35]. Evidence for all patients with PH and RVF is scarce, but there is more data available in the cohort with PAH. The most common cause of death in patients with PAH is RVF, which is also the major determinant of outcomes [14, 87]. In fact, patients with PAH or CTEPH and a pulmonary artery diameter of >48 mm have a 7.5-fold increased risk of death [94]. Cardiopulmonary resuscitation for cardiac arrest in PAH was shown in a large retrospective review to be unsuccessful in 79% of cases, despite 96% of the arrests taking place in hospitalized patients (74% in ICU setting), with only 6% surviving more than 90 days neurologically intact. In those who survived, almost all had a rapidly reversible cause for their circulatory arrest [38].

Conclusion

PH in the ICU continues to be a challenging and complex clinical issue. Multiple potential etiologies of PH exist in a cancer center. A keen understanding of the pathophysiology for PH and consequent RVF is imperative. A high clinical index of suspicion and systematic testing can help identify PH rapidly. Prompt management with continued escalation as needed, along with referral to a specialized center, is helpful. With the advent of new pulmonary vasodilator therapy and increased survival for those with PAH, familiarity with etiology, natural history, and available therapies for PAH is needed. As technologies and targeted therapies emerge, new etiologies and effects on the RV will continue to evolve.

References

1. Andreassen AK, Ragnarsson A, Gude E, et al. Balloon pulmonary angioplasty in patients with inoperable chronic thromboembolic pulmonary hypertension. Heart. 2013;99:1415–20.
2. Badesch DB, Raskob GE, Elliott CG, et al. Pulmonary arterial hypertension: baseline characteristics from the REVEAL registry. Chest. 2010;137:376–87.
3. Barber NA, Ganti AK. Pulmonary toxicities from targeted therapies: a review. Target Oncol. 2011;6:235–43.
4. Bartolome SD, Torres F. Severe pulmonary arterial hypertension: stratification of medical therapies, mechanical support, and lung transplantation. Heart Fail Rev. 2016;21:347–56.
5. Bashoura L, Eapen GA, Faiz SA. Pulmonary manifestations of lymphoma and Leukemia. Clin Chest Med. 2017;38:187–200.
6. Bednarczyk J, Strumpher J, Jacobsohn E. Inhaled milrinone for pulmonary hypertension in high-risk cardiac surgery: silver bullet or just part of a broader management strategy? Can J Anaesth. 2016; 63:1122–7.
7. Blom JW, Doggen CJ, Osanto S, et al. Malignancies, prothrombotic mutations, and the risk of venous thrombosis. JAMA. 2005;293(6):715–22.
8. Carlson DL, Willis MS, White DJ, et al. Tumor necrosis factor-α-induced caspase activation mediates endotoxin-related cardiac dysfunction. Crit Care Med. 2005;33:1021–8.
9. Chan CM, Klilnger JR. The right ventricle in sepsis. Clin Chest Med. 2008;29(4):661–76. https://doi.org/10.1016/j.ccm.2008.07.002.
10. Channick RN, Voswinckel R, Rubin LJ. Inhaled treprostinil: a therapeutic review. Drug Des Devel Ther. 2012;6:19–28. https://doi.org/10.2147/DDDT.S19281.
11. Cherpanath TGV, Lagrand WK, Schultz MJ, Groeneveld ABJ. Cardiopulmonary interactions during mechanical ventilation in critically ill patients. Neth Heart J. 2013;21:166–72.
12. Christenson J, Lavoie A, O'connor M, et al. The incidence and pathogenesis of cardiopulmonary deterioration after abrupt withdrawal of inhaled nitric oxide. Am J Respir Crit Care Med. 2000;161:1443–9.
13. Coz Yataco A, Aguinaga MM, Buck KP, et al. Hospital and intensive care unit management of decompensated pulmonary hypertension and right ventricular failure. Heart Fail Rev. 2016;21(3):323–46.
14. D'Alonzo GE, Barst RJ, Ayres SM, et al. Survival in patients with primary pulmonary hypertension. Results from a national prospective registry. Ann Intern Med. 1991;115:343–9.
15. Dandoy CE, Hirsch R, Chima R, et al. Pulmonary hypertension after hematopoietic stem cell transplantation. Biol Blood Marrow Transplant. 2013; 19:1546–56.
16. Denault AY, Bussières JS, Arellano R, et al. A multicentre randomized-controlled trial of inhaled milrinone in high-risk cardiac surgical patients. Can J Anaesth. 2016;63(10):1140–53. https://doi.org/10.1007/s12630-016-0709-8.
17. Denault AY, Haddad F, Jacobsohn E, et al. Perioperative right ventricular dysfunction. Curr Opin Anaesthesiol. 2013;26:71–81.
18. De Wet CJ, Affleck DG, Jacobsohn E, et al. Inhaled prostacyclin is safe, effective, and affordable in patients with pulmonary hypertension, right heart dysfunction, and refractory hypoxemia after cardiothoracic surgery. J Thorac Cardiovasc Surg. 2004;127:1058–67.
19. Dudzinski DM, Mak GS, Hung JW. Pericardial diseases. Curr Probl Cardiol. 2012;37(3):75–118.
20. Elkayam U, Ng TMH, Hatamizadeh P, et al. Renal vasodilatory action of dopamine in patients with heart failure: magnitude of effect and site of action. Circulation. 2008;117:200–5.
21. Faiz SA, Iliescu C, Lopez-Mattei J, et al. Resolution of myelofibrosis-associated pulmonary arterial hypertension following allogeneic hematopoietic stem cell transplantation. Pulm Circ. 2016;6:611–3.
22. Freitas AF Jr, Bacal F, Oliveira Jde L Jr, et al. Impact of sublingual sildenafil on pulmonary hypertension in patients with heart failure. Arq Bras Cardiol. 2009;92:116–26.
23. Galiè N, Humbert M, Vachiery J-L, et al. 2015 ESC/ERS guidelines for the diagnosis and treatment of pulmonary hypertension: the joint task force for the diagnosis and treatment of pulmonary hypertension of the European Society of Cardiology (ESC) and the European Respiratory Society (ERS): endorsed by: Association for European Paediatric and Congenital Cardiology (AEPC), International Society for Heart and Lung Transplantation (ISHLT). Eur Heart J. 2016;37:67–119.
24. Gildea JJ. Dopamine and angiotensin as renal counterregulatory systems controlling sodium balance. Curr Opin Nephrol Hypertens. 2009;18:28–32.
25. Greer JR. Pathophysiology of cardiovascular dysfunction in sepsis. BJA Edu. 2015;15:316–21.
26. Greyson CR. Evaluation of right ventricular function. Curr Cardiol Rep. 2011;13:194–202.
27. Greyson CR. Pathophysiology of right ventricular failure. Crit Care Med. 2008;36:S57–65.
28. Grignola JC, Domingo E. Acute right ventricular dysfunction in intensive care unit. Biomed Res Int. 2017; https://doi.org/10.1155/2017/8217105.
29. Grinstein J, Gomberg-Maitland M. Management of pulmonary hypertension and right heart failure in the intensive care unit. Curr Hypertens Rep. 2015;17(5):32. https://doi.org/10.1007/s11906-015-0547-z.
30. Guilpain P, Montani D, Damaj G, et al. Pulmonary hypertension associated with myeloproliferative disorders: a retrospective study of ten cases. Respiration. 2008;76:295–302.

31. Gurghean AL, Savulescu-Fiedler I, Mihailescu A. Multiple cardiac complications after adjuvant therapy for breast cancer: the importance of echocardiography. A case report and review of the literature. Med Ultrason. 2017;19:117–20.

32. Haddad F, Doyle R, Murphy DJ, et al. Right ventricular function in cardiovascular disease, part II: pathophysiology, clinical importance, and Management of Right Ventricular Failure. Circulation. 2008a;117:1717–31.

33. Haddad F, Hunt SA, Rosenthal DN, et al. Right ventricular function in cardiovascular disease, part I: anatomy, physiology, aging, and functional assessment of the right ventricle. Circulation. 2008b;117:1436–48.

34. Haraldsson s A, Kieler-Jensen N, Ricksten SE. The additive pulmonary vasodilatory effects of inhaled prostacyclin and inhaled milrinone in postcardiac surgical patients with pulmonary hypertension. Anesth Analg. 2001;93(6):1439–45.

35. Harjola V-P, Mebazaa A, Čelutkienė J, et al. Contemporary management of acute right ventricular failure: a statement from the heart failure association and the working group on pulmonary circulation and right ventricular function of the European Society of Cardiology. Eur J Heart Fail. 2016;18:226–41.

36. Hickey PM, Thompson AAR, Charalampopoulos A, et al. Bosutinib therapy resulting in severe deterioration of pre-existing pulmonary arterial hypertension. Eur Respir J. 2016;48:1514–6.

37. Hoeper MM, Bogaard HJ, Condliffe R, et al. Definitions and diagnosis of pulmonary hypertension. J Am Coll Cardiol. 2013;62:D42–50.

38. Hoeper MM, Galiè N, Murali S, et al. Outcome after cardiopulmonary resuscitation in patients with pulmonary arterial hypertension. Am J Respir Crit Care Med. 2002;165:341–4.

39. Hossri CAC, Almeida RL, da C, Teixeira FR, et al. Cardiopulmonary exercise testing in pulmonary hypertension. Int J Cardiovas Sci. 2016; https://doi.org/10.5935/2359-4802.20160062.

40. Hotchkiss RS, Karl IE. Reevaluation of the role of cellular hypoxia and bioenergetic failure in sepsis. JAMA. 1992;267:1503–10.

41. Hrymak C, Strumpher J, Jacobsohn E. Acute right ventricle failure in the intensive care unit: assessment and management. Can J Cardiol. 2017;33:61–71.

42. Humbert M, Morrell NW, Archer SL, et al. Cellular and molecular pathobiology of pulmonary arterial hypertension. J Am Coll Cardiol. 2004;43:13S–24S.

43. Humbert M, Sitbon O, Chaouat A, et al. Pulmonary arterial hypertension in France. Am J Respir Crit Care Med. 2006;173:1023–30.

44. Iyer AS, Wells JM, Vishin S, et al. CT scan-measured pulmonary artery to aorta ratio and echocardiography for detecting pulmonary hypertension in severe COPD. Chest. 2014;145:824–32.

45. Jentzer JC, Mathier MA. Pulmonary hypertension in the intensive care unit. J Intensive Care Med. 2016;31:369–85.

46. Kerbaul F, Rondelet B, Motte S, et al. Effects of norepinephrine and dobutamine on pressure load-induced right ventricular failure*. Crit Care Med. 2004;32:1035–40.

47. Kiely DG, Elliot CA, Sabroe I, et al. Pulmonary hypertension: diagnosis and management. BMJ. 2013; https://doi.org/10.1136/bmj.f2028.

48. Kolkailah AA, Hirji S, Piazza G, et al. Surgical pulmonary embolectomy and catheter-directed thrombolysis for treatment of submassive pulmonary embolism. J Card Surg. 2018;33:252–9.

49. Konstam MA, Kiernan MS, Bernstein D, et al. Evaluation and Management of Right-Sided Heart Failure: a scientific statement from the American Heart Association. Circulation. 2018;137:e578–622.

50. Krishnan U, Mark TM, Niesvizky R, et al. Pulmonary hypertension complicating multiple myeloma. Pulm Circ. 2015;5:590–7.

51. Lang IM. Management of acute and chronic RV dysfunction. Eur Heart J Suppl. 2007;9:H61–7.

52. Ling Y, Johnson MK, Kiely DG, et al. Changing demographics, epidemiology, and survival of incident pulmonary arterial hypertension: results from the pulmonary hypertension registry of the United Kingdom and Ireland. Am J Respir Crit Care Med. 2012;186:790–6.

53. Lund LH, Edwards LB, Kucheryavaya AY, et al. The registry of the International Society for Heart and Lung Transplantation: thirty-second official adult heart transplantation report–2015; focus theme: early graft failure. J Heart Lung Transplant. 2015;34:1244–54.

54. Machado RF, Farber HW. Pulmonary hypertension associated with chronic Hemolytic Anemia and other blood disorders. Clin Chest Med. 2013;34:739–52.

55. Machuca TN, de Perrot M. Mechanical support for the failing right ventricle in patients with precapillary pulmonary hypertension. Circulation. 2015;132:526–36.

56. Mangi MA, Rehman H, Bansal V, et al. Ultrasound assisted catheter-directed thrombolysis of acute pulmonary embolism: a review of current literature. Cureus. 2017; https://doi.org/10.7759/cureus.

57. McConnell MV, Solomon SD, Rayan ME, et al. Regional right ventricular dysfunction detected by echocardiography in acute pulmonary embolism. Am J Cardiol. 1996;78:469–73.

58. McGoon MD, Benza RL, Escribano-Subias P, et al. Pulmonary arterial hypertension: epidemiology and registries. J Am Coll Cardiol. 2013;62:D51–9.

59. McGoon MD, Krichman A, Farber HW, et al. Design of the REVEAL registry for US patients with pulmonary arterial hypertension. Mayo Clin Proc. 2008;83:923–31.

60. McLaughlin VV, Shah SJ, Souza R, et al. Management of pulmonary arterial hypertension. J Am Coll Cardiol. 2015;65:1976–97.

61. Mekontso Dessap A, Boissier F, Charron C, et al. Acute cor pulmonale during protective ventilation for acute respiratory distress syndrome: prevalence,

predictors, and clinical impact. Intensive Care Med. 2016;42:862–70.

62. Montani D, Bergot E, Günther S, et al. Pulmonary arterial hypertension in patients treated by dasatinib. Circulation. 2012;125:2128–37.

63. Montani D, Lau EM, Dorfmüller P, et al. Pulmonary veno-occlusive disease. Eur Respir J. 2016; 47:1518–34.

64. Naeije R, Manes A. The right ventricle in pulmonary arterial hypertension. Eur Respir Rev. 2014;23:476–87.

65. Oudiz RJ. Pulmonary hypertension associated with left-sided heart disease. Clin Chest Med. 2007;28:233–41.

66. Peacock AJ, Murphy NF, McMurray JJV, et al. An epidemiological study of pulmonary arterial hypertension. Eur Respir J. 2007;30:104–9.

67. Pengo V, Lensing AWA, Prins MH, et al. Incidence of chronic thromboembolic pulmonary hypertension after pulmonary embolism. N Engl J Med. 2004; 350:2257–64.

68. Price LC, Dimopoulos K, Marino P, et al. The CRASH report: emergency management dilemmas facing acute physicians in patients with pulmonary arterial hypertension. Thorax. 2017;72:1035–45.

69. Qiu J, Jia L, Hao Y, et al. Efficacy and safety of levosimendan in patients with acute right heart failure: a meta-analysis. Life Sci. 2017;184:30–6.

70. Ranchoux B, Günther S, Quarck R, et al. Chemotherapy-induced pulmonary hypertension: role of alkylating agents. Am J Pathol. 2015;185:356–71.

71. Rashdan S, Minna JD, Gerber DE. Diagnosis and management of pulmonary toxicity associated with cancer immunotherapy. Lancet Respir Med. 2018;6:472–8.

72. Rhodes A, Evans LE, Alhazzani W, et al. Surviving sepsis campaign: international guidelines for Management of Sepsis and Septic Shock: 2016. Crit Care Med. 2017;45:486–552.

73. Riou M, Seferian A, Savale L, et al. Deterioration of pulmonary hypertension and pleural effusion with bosutinib following dasatinib lung toxicity. Eur Respir J. 2016;48:1517–9.

74. Roberts KE, Hamele-Bena D, Saqi A, et al. Pulmonary tumor embolism: a review of the literature. Am J Med. 2003;115:228–32.

75. Sahay S, Tonelli AR. Pericardial effusion in pulmonary arterial hypertension. Pulm Circ. 2013;3:467–77.

76. Salsano A, Sportelli E, Olivieri GM, et al. RVAD support in the setting of submassive pulmonary embolism. J Extra Corpor Technol. 2017;49:304–6.

77. Sandoval J, Gaspar J, Pulido T, et al. Graded balloon dilation atrial septostomy in severe primary pulmonary hypertension. J Am Coll Cardiol. 1998;32:297–304.

78. Seegobin K, Babbar A, Ferreira J, et al. A case of worsening pulmonary arterial hypertension and pleural effusions by bosutinib after prior treatment with dasatinib. Pulm Circ. 2017;7:808–12.

79. Shaikh AY, Shih JA. Chemotherapy-induced cardiotoxicity. Curr Heart Fail Rep. 2012;9:117–27.

80. Simonneau G, Gatzoulis MA, Adatia I, et al. Updated clinical classification of pulmonary hypertension. J Am Coll Cardiol. 2013;62:D34–41.

81. Steppan J, Diaz-Rodriguez N, Barodka VM, et al. Focused review of perioperative Care of Patients with pulmonary hypertension and proposal of a perioperative pathway. Cureus. 2018; https://doi.org/10.7759/cureus.2072.

82. Strumpher J, Jacobsohn E. Pulmonary hypertension and right ventricular dysfunction: physiology and perioperative management. J Cardiothorac Vasc Anesth. 2011;25:687–704.

83. Sztrymf B, Souza R, Bertoletti L, et al. Prognostic factors of acute heart failure in patients with pulmonary arterial hypertension. Eur Respir J. 2010;35:1286–93.

84. Tamura Y, Kimura M, Takei M, et al. Oral vasopressin receptor antagonist tolvaptan in right heart failure due to pulmonary hypertension. Eur Respir J. 2015; 46:283–6.

85. Trow TK, Christina Argento A, Rubinowitz AN, et al. A 71-year-old woman with myelofibrosis, hypoxemia, and pulmonary hypertension. Chest. 2010;138:1506–10.

86. Ventetuolo CE, Klinger JR. Management of acute right ventricular failure in the intensive care unit. Ann Am Thorac Soc. 2014;11:811–22.

87. Vonk Noordegraaf A, Galie N. The role of the right ventricle in pulmonary arterial hypertension. Eur Respir Rev. 2011;20:243–53.

88. Weinberg A, Tapson VF, Ramzy D. Massive pulmonary embolism: extracorporeal membrane oxygenation and surgical pulmonary embolectomy. Semin Respir Crit Care Med. 2017;38:66–72.

89. Weinberger B, Laskin DL, Heck DE, et al. The toxicology of inhaled nitric oxide. Toxicol Sci. 2001;59:5–16.

90. Weitsman T, Weisz G, Farkash R, et al. Pulmonary hypertension with left heart disease: prevalence, temporal shifts in Etiologies and outcome. Am J Med. 2017;130:1272–9.

91. Westerhof BE, Saouti N, van der Laarse WJ, et al. Treatment strategies for the right heart in pulmonary hypertension. Cardiovasc Res. 2017;113:1465–73.

92. Yusuf SW, Venkatesulu BP, Mahadevan LS, et al. Radiation-induced cardiovascular disease: a clinical perspective. Front Cardiovasc Med. 2017;4:66. https://doi.org/10.3389/fcvm.2017.00066.

93. Zamanian RT, Haddad F, Doyle RL, et al. Management strategies for patients with pulmonary hypertension in the intensive care unit. Crit Care Med. 2007;35: 2037–50.

94. Żyłkowska J, Kurzyna M, Florczyk M, et al. Pulmonary artery dilatation correlates with the risk of unexpected death in chronic arterial or thromboembolic pulmonary hypertension. Chest. 2012;142:1406–16.

Sleep Disorders in Critically Ill Cancer Patients

46

Matthew Scharf, Niki Kasinathan, and Jag Sunderram

Contents

Introduction 699

Sleep Disturbances in the Cancer Patient 701

Sleep in the ICU 702
Sleep in the Critically Ill Cancer Patient 704

Conclusion 705

References 705

Abstract

Sleep disorders are common in society and are common in patients with cancer. Patients with cancer frequently complain of sleep problems and daytime sleepiness. The diagnosis of cancer, cancer treatments, and psychological issues in dealing with a cancer diagnosis and treatment may cause sleep disruption. Furthermore, in the course of cancer treatment, many patients with cancer require intensive care unit (ICU) care which can cause additional sleep disruption. This sleep disruption in an ICU can be due to environmental factors, frequent interventions, and use of various sedative medications. Therefore, patients with cancer, particularly those requiring ICU care, commonly develop sleep problems. Treatment of sleep problems in these patients may improve the morbidity and possibly mortality associated with cancer.

M. Scharf (✉)
Department of Medicine, Division of Pulmonary and Critical Care, Rutgers-Robert Wood Johnson Medical School, New Brunswick, NJ, USA

Department of Neurology, Rutgers-Robert Wood Johnson Medical School, New Brunswick, NJ, USA
e-mail: Matthew.scharf@rwjms.rutgers.edu

N. Kasinathan · J. Sunderram
Department of Medicine, Division of Pulmonary and Critical Care, Rutgers-Robert Wood Johnson Medical School, New Brunswick, NJ, USA
e-mail: nkasinathan4@gmail.com; sunderja@rwjms.rutgers.edu

Keywords

Sleep · Cancer · Oncology · ICU

Introduction

Sleep is a fundamental biological need and is necessary for optimal functioning. Sleep disruption has been associated with diseases, including dementia [1, 2], cancer [3–5], heart disease [6], stroke [7], and early mortality [8]. Sleep disruption is also associated with functional impairments, including worsened mood [9], impaired cognition [2], and an increased risk of motor vehicle accidents [10]. Therefore, ensuring adequate sleep is important and remains a major public health issue.

Adequate sleep consists of both an appropriate amount of sleep and sleeping at a biologically appropriate time of day. In one popular formulation of this concept, sleep is divided into two components. The first component is a homeostatic one – the longer a person is awake, the sleepier that person becomes. The second component is a circadian one – sleepiness increases at certain times of day independent of how long a person has been awake. This is commonly referred to as the two process model of sleep and highlights the importance of length of sleep in addition to the timing of sleep [11]. Therefore, sleep disorders can be caused by disruption of either the homeostatic or circadian components of sleep.

Disorders which affect the timing of sleep are broadly classified as circadian rhythm disorders. These disorders include conditions where the biological circadian clock is misaligned with the light/dark cycle. For example, patients with a delayed sleep phase will sleep well when allowed a late bedtime and late wake time, but when forced to follow a "normal" schedule will often report poor sleep and significant daytime sleepiness. Also included in this category are conditions where the patient has a biological circadian clock which is appropriately entrained to the light/dark cycle, but has sleep disruption due to extrinsic factors which interrupt the ability to sleep at biologically appropriate times. These problems are often encountered when a patient has a job which requires evening or overnight shifts. Misalignment between the biological circadian clock and the sleep schedule is a common cause of sleep problems [12, 13].

Sleep disorders which predominantly affect the amount of sleep include the sleep-related breathing disorders, such as obstructive sleep apnea (OSA), sleep-related movement disorders, hypersomnias such as narcolepsy, and insomnia. The amount of sleep can also be adversely affected by inadequate sleep opportunity where patients simply do not allow enough time to sleep. OSA and insomnia are common sleep disorders [14–16].

Insomnia is the inability to fall asleep, stay asleep, or both. Insomnia is often a transient and self-limited problem which requires no specific intervention. However, in some patients, insomnia persists for longer periods of time and is both distressing to the patient and associated with significant morbidity and mortality.

The process by which short-term insomnia becomes chronic insomnia has been extensively studied and remains an active area of investigation. Spielman and colleagues proposed the "3P" model of insomnia which posits that there are predisposing, precipitating, and perpetuating factors that regulate the transformation of acute to chronic insomnia [17]. According to this model, chronic insomnia ensues when a susceptible individual (predisposing) experiences a stressor (precipitating) and adopts behaviors and beliefs that continue to interfere with sleep once the stressor has resolved (perpetuating). There are many types of precipitating and perpetuating factors which helps explain how ubiquitous insomnia is in modern society.

Patients with insomnia often complain of being sleepy despite the difficulty they have with actually sleeping. For this reason, when evaluating patients with sleep complaints, it is important to understand what constitutes sleepiness. Sleepiness is often defined as an abnormal propensity to sleep, not necessarily a complaint of being "sleepy." Patients may complain of being tired, sleepy, or fatigued, but when questioned explicitly, may in fact have a low likelihood of abnormally falling asleep.

One commonly used tool to assess sleepiness according to this understanding is the Epworth Sleepiness Scale. This scale asks patients to rate their likelihood of falling asleep in different situations rather than how tired or sleepy they feel. A higher score indicates a higher propensity to fall asleep. Interestingly, comparison between the two common disorders of OSA and insomnia reveals a sharp divergence in scores: patients with OSA have high scores and patients with insomnia have low scores [18] even though patients with either problem may complain of being sleepy. The decreased propensity of patients with insomnia to fall asleep has been borne out by objective testing [19]. These observations highlight the fact that a complaint of being sleepy does not necessarily mean an abnormal propensity to fall asleep and often requires further elucidation.

One term often used to encompass a feeling of being tired, run down, and not able to function normally is fatigue. Although there is no broad consensus of what actually constitutes fatigue [20], there are a number of scales used to quantify it. Although fatigue and sleepiness may be related, it is important to not equate fatigue and sleepiness as patients with fatigue do not necessarily have an increased propensity to sleep, and fatigue may not necessarily imply an underlying sleep disorder. Whether patients with fatigue have an underlying sleep disorder often requires investigation.

Sleep Disturbances in the Cancer Patient

Patients with cancer may be predisposed to have sleep disturbances. The stress of dealing with a cancer diagnosis, the various treatments these patients undergo, and the sequelae of these factors can increase the likelihood of developing a sleep disturbance. Sleep disturbances can be distressing to the patient and can be associated with significant morbidity.

Determining the prevalence of sleep disturbances in patients with cancer is complicated not only by the varied nature of different types of cancer and their associated treatments, but also by a lack of objective data [21]. Most of the data are comprised of questionnaires rather than objective sleep testing. Furthermore, many of these surveys assess for fatigue rather than sleepiness per se. These factors make it difficult to establish accurate prevalence estimates of specific sleep disorders in patients with cancer but may suggest that sleep problems are present and likely to be common.

Sleep disturbances appear to be present through all phases of cancer care, including before treatment has occurred, and are often related to the diagnosis [22]. On the basis of questionnaire data,

the prevalence of sleep disturbances has been described to be twice as high in patients with cancer compared to the general population with a prevalence in the range of 30–50% [23]. One study involving a sleep survey questionnaire demonstrated decreased number of hours of sleep (sleep duration), increased number of minutes to fall asleep (sleep latency), more nighttime awakenings (sleep disruption), as well as overall decreased sleep quality [24]. However, formal evaluation for sleep disorders such as OSA and sleep-related movement disorders such as periodic limb movement disorder has seldom been performed [21]. These studies suggest that sleep disruption is common in patients with cancer but do not elucidate the specific types of sleep disturbance.

A number of studies have shown that patients with cancer have fatigue. For example, the Brief Fatigue Inventory, a validated questionnaire to assess fatigue, is elevated in patients with cancer [24, 25]. Although fatigue and sleepiness are not identical, sleep disturbance (as assessed by validated and unvalidated questionnaires) is more common in those with fatigue (assessed by the Brief Fatigue Inventory and other questionnaires, such as the RAND-36 item Health Survey) than in those without fatigue. Furthermore, sleep disturbance is a significant predictor of fatigue [25–27]. This correlation between fatigue and sleep disturbance has also been found specifically in cancer patients [24]. In fact, in a study of patients with multiple types of cancer, 35% of variation in fatigue was attributable to sleep disturbance [28]. These observations suggest that while sleepiness and fatigue are not identical, there is a direct relationship between sleep disturbance and fatigue in patients with cancer.

Whether fatigue can cause sleep disturbance or sleep disturbance can cause fatigue is unclear. Some authors have suggested that fatigue from chemotherapy can lead to more inactivity and longer time in bed during the day. These behaviors may precipitate insomnia and, in turn, exacerbate daytime fatigue [22]. These data suggest that fatigue can lead to maladaptive behaviors (spending more time in bed) which can cause or worsen sleep disturbance. It may be that cancer causes both sleep disturbance and fatigue, but it may also be the case that fatigue and sleep disturbance may exacerbate one another.

The presence of fatigue or sleepiness in patients with cancer has functional consequences. Longitudinal data suggests that the presence of either sleep disturbance or fatigue adversely affect functional status as assessed by the Karnofsky Performance Scale [29] and are each independent predictors of functional status 8 weeks after the cancer diagnosis compared with 3 months prior to diagnosis [30]. Correlation between sleep problems and fatigue persists even a year after completion of treatment [26, 31] suggesting that fatigue in cancer patients is likely mediated, at least in part, by sleep disturbance and may have deleterious consequences. The importance of an appropriate amount of sleep in patients with cancer was highlighted by a recent study which showed that too little or too much sleep time in patients with advanced cancer is associated with mortality [32]. Therefore, sleep in patients with cancer is important and sleep problems are associated with worse functioning and may even reduce survival.

There are a number of factors that can increase the risk of sleep disturbance in patients with cancer compared to the general population:

1. Disease-related factors: Altered physiology directly related to the presence of cancer may play a role in dampening the circadian regulatory processes [23]. The secretion of melatonin, which is important for sleep onset, is blunted in colorectal, lung, breast, and ovarian cancers [33–36]. Tumor-induced release of cytokines such as TNF-α and IL6 could result in excessive daytime sleepiness [37]. Pain, which is present in 80% of patients with cancer, can lead to disrupted sleep, and poor sleep enhances pain sensitivity leading to a vicious cycle of pain and sleep disruption [23].
2. Psychological factors: Anxiety and depression related to cancer diagnosis can lead to sleep-onset and sleep-maintenance insomnia [38, 39].
3. Demographic factors: Since cancers commonly affect the elderly, and sleep disturbance is common with aging, patients with cancer may be at an increased risk of having a baseline sleep disturbance.
4. Treatment-related factors: Side effects of chemotherapy and radiation therapy, particularly in combination with agents such as antihistamines and steroids, may lead to either excessive sleepiness or insomnia [23, 40].
5. Coexisting sleep disorders: Anemia precipitated by the cancer or treatments can lead to iron deficiency and restless leg syndrome and periodic limb movement disorder [41, 42]. Additionally, weight gain from corticosteroid use and cancers of the head and neck are associated with a high prevalence of obstructive sleep apnea [43, 44], while tumors of the central nervous system involving the brainstem could lead to central sleep apnea [45].

Sleep in the ICU

Patients with cancer may require admission to the ICU during the course of the disease. Cancer and its associated treatments put patients at increased risk for a litany of problems including infections, metabolic derangements, and respiratory and cardiac issues which often necessitate admission to the ICU. These patients may experience complications, such as graft versus host disease, sepsis, and acute renal and respiratory failure eventually requiring mechanical ventilation, dialysis, vasopressor support, and continuous medications for sedation. Therefore, the ICU is often an important component of treatment for patients with cancer.

Sleep in the ICU is an often overlooked component of ICU care. During acute illness, sleep is important since disrupted sleep has been linked to slow recovery, decreased immune function, impaired cognition, and increased mortality [46]. Furthermore, recognition of sleep disturbances in the ICU is essential as lack of identification and treatment can lead to chronic fatigue, delirium, increased length of ICU stay, and diminished capacity for patients to participate in their own care [47]. Despite the importance of sleep in the ICU, recognition and treatment of sleep disturbances are often suboptimal in the critical care setting [48]. Identifying characteristics of cancer-related sleep disturbances may facilitate diagnosis and treatment.

While sleep is an important component of ICU care, there is a dearth of objective sleep data on patients in the ICU. This is especially important since comparison of objective sleep data by polysomnography correlates poorly with data from actigraphy or nurse assessment of sleep characteristics [49]. Patient-reported sleep characteristics do accurately represent sleep [49]; however, given the fact that patients in the ICU are often cognitively impaired due to sedation or delirium, the ability of patients to report on their sleep is somewhat limited.

The limited amount of data we have on sleep in the ICU suggests that sleep is often fragmented in patients in the ICU. In patients in the ICU, there is a relatively high percentage of the lighter stages of sleep at the expense of deeper stages of sleep such as slow wave sleep and rapid eye movement (REM) sleep [46, 50]. Interestingly, a similar pattern of an increased amount of light sleep and a decreased amount of deep sleep is seen in intrinsic sleep disorders, such as OSA [51], suggesting that sleep in the ICU may share some of the characteristics of an organic sleep disorder. The lack of consolidated sleep in the ICU at night can lead to daytime sleepiness and more sleep occurring during the day [52]. This may have the unintended consequence of both causing sleep disruption and altering the normal circadian rhythm [52].

There are a number of factors that can lead to sleep disturbances in the ICU setting:

1. **Altered light/dark and feeding schedules**: The circadian clock has an endogenous, approximately 24 h rhythm, but is altered by environmental cues such as light and feeding. In an ICU, exposure to natural light is often limited, daytime lighting may be low, and there may be extensive light exposure at night. Additionally, in patients requiring enteral nutrition, feeding may be provided continuously throughout the day and night rather than intermittently throughout the day. These changes in the normal light/dark and feeding patterns may cause circadian rhythm disruption [53]. Interestingly, in a small study where healthy subjects were subjected to ICU light and noise conditions and then given the simple intervention of eye masks and ear plugs at night, there was an improvement in sleep quality as reflected by a decrease in the number of electrophysiologic awakenings and an increase in REM sleep [54]. There was also an increase in nocturnal urinary secretion of 6-sulphatoxymelatonin (a metabolite of melatonin), suggesting that the endogenous circadian rhythm was being restored in these subjects [54]. Furthermore, in another small study utilizing actigraphy, patients in the ICU had very fragmented sleep and had a blunted nocturnal peak in melatonin, suggesting a breakdown of the normal circadian rhythm in these ICU patients [55]. Interestingly, exogenous administration of melatonin to ICU patients improved actigraphically determined sleep [56]. These studies are consistent with the notion that circadian realignment can improve sleep in ICU patients.

2. **Environmental noise**: Loud noise is common in hospitals and ICUs. Given the recognized role of loud noise causing sleep disruption, the World Health Organization recommends that background noise levels in hospital wards should not exceed 35 decibels (dB) [57]. However, average noise levels in ICUs often exceed 50 dB and peaks of above 85 dB are common [58]. Potential sources of noise include common ICU equipment, frequent alarms on ICU equipment, and communication among care providers. Surveys of nursing staff have noted a false conception that in patients who are intubated and sedated there is no need for noise reduction [59]. This is important because a small study demonstrated that the number of noise peaks above 80 dB was strongly correlated with electrophysiologic arousals [60]. Although, it should be noted that in a larger study of ICU patients, environmental noise was only responsible for approximately 10% of the electrophysiologic arousals observed and only responsible for about two arousals per hour [61]. Nonetheless, noise may be a factor in causing sleep disruption in ICU patients.

3. **Clinical interactions**: Monitoring and intervention often increase substantially as patients

become critically ill. Frequent interactions with patients at night for fluid balance assessments, medication administration, blood draws, and hourly vital sign checks are standard in ICUs. One study recorded an average of 51 interactions by nursing staff per night in patients in the ICU. Certain types of nursing activity such as decubitus ulcer care were done more frequently between midnight and 5 AM, suggesting that many of these interactions could have been safely deferred to normal waking hours [62].

4. **Sedation**: Sedative medications are commonly used in the ICU, often in mechanically-ventilated patients. Although sleep and sedation share some similarities as both states are associated with decreased interaction with the environment, sleep and pharmacologic-induced sedation are distinct in a number of ways, including in cortical electrophysiology. The extent to which sedative medications mimic natural sleep is dependent on the particular agent and the dosing regimen [63]. Sedation can be achieved by a number of different agents which exert different pharmacologic effects. Interestingly, use of the α2 agonist dexmedetomidine for sedation in the ICU compared to the benzodiazepine GABA-A agonist lorazepam was associated with less delirium,

fewer days of mechanical ventilation, and a decrease in 28-day mortality in patients with sepsis [64]. Since endogenous sleep structures are causally involved in dexmedetomidine-induced sedation [65], it is possible that part of the beneficial effect of dexmedetomidine may have been due to its effects on sleep. Although the data is not clear on which sedation regimens are ideal in ICU patients, it seems likely that different regimens and their different effects on sleep may be an important factor in the success of ICU care.

Sleep in the Critically Ill Cancer Patient

There is a paucity of data on sleep disturbances that occur specifically in the critically ill cancer patient. However, as previously discussed, cancer patients have a high propensity to develop sleep disturbances, and sleep in patients in the ICU is often disrupted. It is very likely that among patients with cancer that are cared for in an ICU there is a high prevalence of sleep disruption. There may be baseline sleep disorders, worsening of sleep during the diagnosis and treatment of cancer, and a further exacerbation of sleep problems by ICU care. Fig. 1 provides a schematic of the interaction between baseline conditions, cancer, and the ICU which can

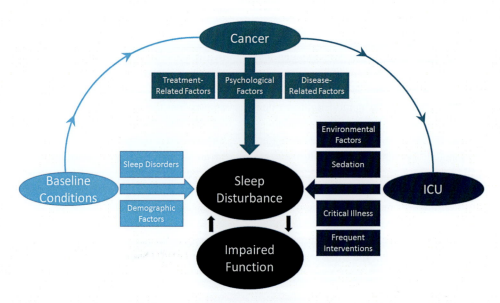

Fig. 1 Schematic of factors associated with sleep disturbance in critically ill cancer patients

lead to sleep disturbance and impaired function. Thus, addressing and improving sleep in the ICU in patients with cancer, who often have a long-term treatment course and a higher propensity to develop sleep disorders, may be of particular importance.

Conclusion

Sleep complaints are common in patients with cancer. Preexisting conditions, cancer-related factors, various cancer treatments, and psychological issues pertaining to a cancer diagnosis and treatment can all lead to sleep disruptions. In the course of cancer care, patients may require ICU care. While often necessary in the course of ICU care, patients are often exposed to disruptions of the normal light/dark cycle, altered feeding schedules, frequent clinical interactions during the night, sedation, and often critical illness itself which can cause further sleep disruptions. Sleep disruption is associated with significant morbidity and may even be associated with mortality. Therefore, optimization of sleep and treatment of sleep disorders is a critical component of care in the cancer patients. A low threshold should be set for further evaluation of sleep disturbances in patients with cancer.

References

1. Porter VR, Buxton WG, Avidan AY. Sleep, cognition and dementia. Curr Psychiatry Rep. 2015;17:97. https://doi.org/10.1007/s11920-015-0631-8.
2. Yaffe K, Falvey CM, Hoang T. Connections between sleep and cognition in older adults. Lancet Neurol. 2014;13:1017–28. https://doi.org/10.1016/S1474-4422(14)70172-3.
3. Davis S, Mirick DK, Stevens RG. Night shift work, light at night, and risk of breast cancer. J Natl Cancer Inst. 2001;93:1557–62.
4. Hansen J. Night shift work and risk of breast cancer. Curr Environ Health Rep. 2017;4:325–39. https://doi.org/10.1007/s40572-017-0155-y.
5. Kubo T, et al. Prospective cohort study of the risk of prostate cancer among rotating-shift workers: findings from the Japan collaborative cohort study. Am J Epidemiol. 2006;164:549–55. https://doi.org/10.1093/aje/kwj232.
6. Nagai M, Hoshide S, Kario K. Sleep duration as a risk factor for cardiovascular disease- a review of the recent literature. Curr Cardiol Rev. 2010;6:54–61. https://doi.org/10.2174/157340310790231635.
7. Patyar S, Patyar RR. Correlation between sleep duration and risk of stroke. J Stroke Cerebrovasc Dis. 2015;24:905–11. https://doi.org/10.1016/j.jstrokecerebrovasdis.2014.12.038.
8. Yin J, et al. Relationship of sleep duration with all-cause mortality and cardiovascular events: a systematic review and dose-response meta-analysis of prospective cohort studies. J Am Heart Assoc. 2017;6. https://doi.org/10.1161/JAHA.117.005947.
9. Zhai L, Zhang H, Zhang D. Sleep duration and depression among adults: a meta-analysis of prospective studies. Depress Anxiety. 2015;32:664–70. https://doi.org/10.1002/da.22386.
10. Gottlieb DJ, Ellenbogen JM, Bianchi MT, Czeisler CA. Sleep deficiency and motor vehicle crash risk in the general population: a prospective cohort study. BMC Med. 2018;16:44. https://doi.org/10.1186/s12916-018-1025-7.
11. Borbely AA, Daan S, Wirz-Justice A, Deboer T. The two-process model of sleep regulation: a reappraisal. J Sleep Res. 2016;25:131–43. https://doi.org/10.1111/jsr.12371.
12. Sack RL, et al. Circadian rhythm sleep disorders: part I, basic principles, shift work and jet lag disorders. An American Academy of Sleep Medicine review. Sleep. 2007a;30:1460–83.
13. Sack RL, et al. Circadian rhythm sleep disorders: part II, advanced sleep phase disorder, delayed sleep phase disorder, free-running disorder, and irregular sleep-wake rhythm. An American Academy of Sleep Medicine review. Sleep. 2007b;30:1484–501.
14. Peppard PE, Young T, Barnet JH, Palta M, Hagen EW, Hla KM. Increased prevalence of sleep-disordered breathing in adults. Am J Epidemiol. 2013;177:1006–14. https://doi.org/10.1093/aje/kws342.
15. Punjabi NM. The epidemiology of adult obstructive sleep apnea. Proc Am Thorac Soc. 2008;5:136–43. https://doi.org/10.1513/pats.200709-155MG.
16. Roth T. Insomnia: definition, prevalence, etiology, and consequences. J Clin Sleep Med. 2007;3:S7–10.
17. Spielman AJ, Caruso LS, Glovinsky PB. A behavioral perspective on insomnia treatment. Psychiatr Clin North Am. 1987;10:541–53.
18. Johns MW. A new method for measuring daytime sleepiness: the Epworth sleepiness scale. Sleep. 1991;14:540–5.
19. Roehrs TA, Randall S, Harris E, Maan R, Roth T. MSLT in primary insomnia: stability and relation to nocturnal sleep. Sleep. 2011;34:1647–52. https://doi.org/10.5665/sleep.1426.
20. Ream E, Richardson A. Fatigue: a concept analysis. Int J Nurs Stud. 1996;33:519–29.
21. Otte JL, et al. Systematic review of sleep disorders in cancer patients: can the prevalence of sleep disorders be ascertained? Cancer Med. 2015;4:183–200. https://doi.org/10.1002/cam4.356.
22. Roscoe JA, et al. Cancer-related fatigue and sleep disorders. Oncologist. 2007;12(Suppl 1):35–42. https://doi.org/10.1634/theoncologist.12-S1-35.

23. Berger AM, et al. Sleep wake disturbances in people with cancer and their caregivers: state of the science. Oncol Nurs Forum. 2005;32:E98–126. https://doi.org/10.1188/05.ONF.E98-E126.

24. Davidson JR, MacLean AW, Brundage MD, Schulze K. Sleep disturbance in cancer patients. Soc Sci Med. 2002;54:1309–21.

25. Anderson KO, Getto CJ, Mendoza TR, Palmer SN, Wang XS, Reyes-Gibby CC, Cleeland CS. Fatigue and sleep disturbance in patients with cancer, patients with clinical depression, and community-dwelling adults. J Pain Symptom Manag. 2003;25:307–18.

26. Bower JE, Ganz PA, Desmond KA, Rowland JH, Meyerowitz BE, Belin TR. Fatigue in breast cancer survivors: occurrence, correlates, and impact on quality of life. J Clin Oncol. 2000;18:743–53. https://doi.org/10.1200/JCO.2000.18.4.743.

27. Redeker NS, Lev EL, Ruggiero J. Insomnia, fatigue, anxiety, depression, and quality of life of cancer patients undergoing chemotherapy. Sch Inq Nurs Pract. 2000;14:275–90; discussion 291–278

28. Beck SL, Dudley WN, Barsevick A. Pain, sleep disturbance, and fatigue in patients with cancer: using a mediation model to test a symptom cluster. Oncol Nurs Forum. 2005;32:542. https://doi.org/10.1188/04.ONF.E48-E55.

29. Dodd MJ, Miaskowski C, Paul SM. Symptom clusters and their effect on the functional status of patients with cancer. Oncol Nurs Forum. 2001;28:465–70.

30. Given B, Given C, Azzouz F, Stommel M. Physical functioning of elderly cancer patients prior to diagnosis and following initial treatment. Nurs Res. 2001;50:222–32.

31. Broeckel JA, Jacobsen PB, Horton J, Balducci L, Lyman GH. Characteristics and correlates of fatigue after adjuvant chemotherapy for breast cancer. J Clin Oncol. 1998;16:1689–96. https://doi.org/10.1200/JCO.1998.16.5.1689.

32. Collins KP, et al. Sleep duration is associated with survival in advanced cancer patients. Sleep Med. 2017;32:208–12. https://doi.org/10.1016/j.sleep.2016.06.041.

33. Bartsch C, Bartsch H. Melatonin in cancer patients and in tumor-bearing animals. Adv Exp Med Biol. 1999;467:247–64.

34. Khoory R, Stemme D. Plasma melatonin levels in patients suffering from colorectal carcinoma. J Pineal Res. 1988;5:251–8.

35. Payne JK. The trajectory of fatigue in adult patients with breast and ovarian cancer receiving chemotherapy. Oncol Nurs Forum. 2002;29:1334–40. https://doi.org/10.1188/02.ONF.1334-1340.

36. Viviani S, Bidoli P, Spinazze S, Rovelli F, Lissoni P. Normalization of the light/dark rhythm of melatonin after prolonged subcutaneous administration of interleukin-2 in advanced small cell lung cancer patients. J Pineal Res. 1992;12:114–7.

37. Ardestani SK, Inserra P, Solkoff D, Watson RR. The role of cytokines and chemokines on tumor progression: a review. Cancer Detect Prev. 1999;23:215–25.

38. Ancoli-Israel S, et al. Sleep, fatigue, depression, and circadian activity rhythms in women with breast cancer before and after treatment: a 1-year longitudinal study. Support Care Cancer. 2014;22:2535–45. https://doi.org/10.1007/s00520-014-2204-5.

39. Cimprich B. Pretreatment symptom distress in women newly diagnosed with breast cancer. Cancer Nurs. 1999;22:185–94; quiz 195

40. Savard J, Ivers H, Savard MH, Morin CM. Cancer treatments and their side effects are associated with aggravation of insomnia: Results of a longitudinal study. Cancer. 2015;121:1703–11. https://doi.org/10.1002/cncr.29244.

41. Enderlin CA, et al. Sleep measured by polysomnography in patients receiving high-dose chemotherapy for multiple myeloma prior to stem cell transplantation. Oncol Nurs Forum. 2013;40:73–81. https://doi.org/10.1188/13.Onf.73-81.

42. Savard J, Simard S, Blanchet J, Ivers H, Morin CM. Prevalence, clinical characteristics, and risk factors for insomnia in the context of breast cancer. Sleep. 2001;24:583–90.

43. Nesse W, Hoekema A, Stegenga B, van der Hoeven JH, de Bont LG, Roodenburg JL. Prevalence of obstructive sleep apnoea following head and neck cancer treatment: a cross-sectional study. Oral Oncol. 2006;42:108–14. https://doi.org/10.1016/j.oraloncology.2005.06.022.

44. Payne RJ, et al. High prevalence of obstructive sleep apnea among patients with head and neck cancer. J Otolaryngol. 2005;34:304–11.

45. Rosen GM, Bendel AE, Neglia JP, Moertel CL, Mahowald M. Sleep in children with neoplasms of the central nervous system: case review of 14 children. Pediatrics. 2003;112:e46–54.

46. Kamdar BB, Needham DM, Collop NA. Sleep deprivation in critical illness: its role in physical and psychological recovery. J Intensive Care Med. 2012;27:97–111. https://doi.org/10.1177/0885066610394322.

47. Matthews EE. Sleep disturbances and fatigue in critically ill patients. AACN Adv Crit Care. 2011;22:204–24. https://doi.org/10.1097/NCI.0b013e31822052cb.

48. Friese RS. Sleep and recovery from critical illness and injury: a review of theory, current practice, and future directions. Crit Care Med. 2008;36:697–705. https://doi.org/10.1097/CCM.0B013E3181643F29.

49. Beecroft JM, Ward M, Younes M, Crombach S, Smith O, Hanly PJ. Sleep monitoring in the intensive care unit: comparison of nurse assessment, actigraphy and polysomnography. Intensive Care Med. 2008;34:2076–83. https://doi.org/10.1007/s00134-008-1180-y.

50. Elliott R, McKinley S, Cistulli P, Fien M. Characterisation of sleep in intensive care using 24-hour polysomnography: an observational study. Crit Care. 2013;17:R46. https://doi.org/10.1186/cc12565.

51. Sforza E, Haba-Rubio J, De Bilbao F, Rochat T, Ibanez V. Performance vigilance task and sleepiness in patients with sleep-disordered breathing. Eur Respir J. 2004;24:279–85.

52. Pulak LM, Jensen L. Sleep in the intensive care unit: a review. J Intensive Care Med. 2016;31:14–23. https://doi.org/10.1177/0885066614538749.

53. Sunderram J, Sofou S, Kamisoglu K, Karantza V, Androulakis IP. Time-restricted feeding and the realignment of biological rhythms: translational opportunities and challenges. J Transl Med. 2014;12:79. https://doi.org/10.1186/1479-5876-12-79.

54. Hu RF, Jiang XY, Zeng YM, Chen XY, Zhang YH. Effects of earplugs and eye masks on nocturnal sleep, melatonin and cortisol in a simulated intensive care unit environment. Crit Care. 2010;14:R66. https://doi.org/10.1186/cc8965.

55. Shilo L, et al. Patients in the intensive care unit suffer from severe lack of sleep associated with loss of normal melatonin secretion pattern. Am J Med Sci. 1999;317:278–81.

56. Shilo L, Dagan Y, Smorjik Y, Weinberg U, Dolev S, Komptel B, Shenkman L. Effect of melatonin on sleep quality of COPD intensive care patients: a pilot study. Chronobiol Int. 2000;17:71–6.

57. Berglund B, Lindvall T, Schwela DH (1999) Guidelines for Community Noise. World Health Organization: Protection of the Human Environment. http://apps.who.int/iris/handle/10665/66217. Accessed 08 July 2018.

58. Darbyshire JL, Young JD. An investigation of sound levels on intensive care units with reference to the WHO guidelines. Crit Care. 2013;17:R187. https://doi.org/10.1186/cc12870.

59. Christensen M. Noise levels in a general intensive care unit: a descriptive study. Nurs Crit Care. 2007;12:188–97. https://doi.org/10.1111/j.1478-5153.2007.00229.x.

60. Aaron JN, Carlisle CC, Carskadon MA, Meyer TJ, Hill NS, Millman RP. Environmental noise as a cause of sleep disruption in an intermediate respiratory care unit. Sleep. 1996;19:707–10.

61. Freedman NS, Gazendam J, Levan L, Pack AI, Schwab RJ. Abnormal sleep/wake cycles and the effect of environmental noise on sleep disruption in the intensive care unit. Am J Respir Crit Care Med. 2001;163:451–7. https://doi.org/10.1164/ajrccm.163.2.9912128.

62. Celik S, Oztekin D, Akyolcu N, Issever H. Sleep - disturbance: the patient care activities applied at the night shift in the intensive care unit. J Clin Nurs. 2005;14:102–6. https://doi.org/10.1111/j.1365-2702.2004.01010.x.

63. Scharf MT, Kelz MB. Sleep and anesthesia interactions: a pharmacological appraisal. Curr Anesthesiol Rep. 2013;3:1–9. https://doi.org/10.1007/s40140-012-0007-0.

64. Pandharipande PP, et al. Effect of dexmedetomidine versus lorazepam on outcome in patients with sepsis: an a priori-designed analysis of the MENDS randomized controlled trial. Crit Care. 2010;14:R38. https://doi.org/10.1186/cc8916.

65. Nelson LE, Lu J, Guo T, Saper CB, Franks NP, Maze M. The alpha2-adrenoceptor agonist dexmedetomidine converges on an endogenous sleep-promoting pathway to exert its sedative effects. Anesthesiology. 2003;98:428–36.